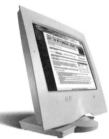
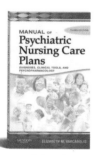
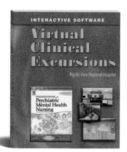

Comprehensive Nursing Assessment Tool

Client History

I. GENERAL HISTORY OF CLIENT

Name _____ Age _____ Sex _____

Racial and ethnic data _____

Marital status _____

Number and ages of children/siblings _____

Living arrangements _____

Occupation _____

Education _____

Religious affiliation _____

II. PRESENTING PROBLEM

A. Statement in the client's own words of why he or she is hospitalized or seeking help

_____

_____

B. Recent difficulties/alterations in _____

    1. Relationships

    2. Usual level of functioning

    3. Behavior

    4. Perceptions or cognitive abilities

C. Increased feelings of _____

    1. Depression

    2. Anxiety

    3. Hopelessness

    4. Being overwhelmed

    5. Suspiciousness

    6. Confusion

D. Somatic changes, such as _____

    1. Constipation

    2. Insomnia

    3. Lethargy

    4. Weight loss or gain

    5. Palpitations

III. RELEVANT HISTORY—PERSONAL

A. Previous hospitalizations and illnesses _____

B. Educational background _____

C. Occupational background _____

    1. If employed, where? _____

    2. How long at that job? _____

    3. Previous positions and reasons for leaving _____

    4. Special skills _____

D. Social patterns

    1. Describe friends. _____

    2. Describe a usual day. _____

E. Sexual patterns

    1. Sexually active? _____

    2. Sexual orientation _____

    3. Sexual difficulties _____

    4. Practice safe sex or birth control? _____

F. Interests and abilities

    1. What does the client do in his or her spare time? _____

    2. What is the client good at? _____

    3. What gives the client pleasure? _____

G. Substance use and abuse

    1. What medication does the client take? _____

      How often? _____ How much? _____

    2. What herbal or over-the-counter medications does the client take? _____

      How often? _____ How much? _____

    3. What psychotropic drugs does the client take? _____

      How often? _____ How much? _____

    4. How many drinks of alcohol does the client take per day? _____

      Per week? _____

    5. Does the client identify use of drugs as a problem? _____

H. How does the client cope with stress? _____

    1. What does the client do when he or she gets upset? _____

    2. Whom can the client talk to? _____

    3. What usually helps to relieve stress? _____

    4. What did the client try this time? _____

IV. RELEVANT HISTORY—FAMILY

A. Childhood

    1. Who was important to the client growing up? _____

    2. Was there physical or sexual abuse? _____

    3. Did the parents drink or use drugs? _____

4. Who was in the home when the client was growing up? _____

B. Adolescence

1. How would the client describe his or her feelings in adolescence? _____

2. Describe the client's peer group at that time. _____

C. Use of drugs

1. Was there use or abuse of drugs by any family member? _____

Prescription _____ Street _____ By whom? _____

2. What was the effect on the family? _____

D. Family physical or mental problems

1. Is there any family history of violence or physical or sexual abuse? _____

2. Who in the family had physical or mental problems? _____

3. Describe the problems. _____

4. How did they affect the family? _____

E. Was there an **unusual** or **outstanding event** the client would like to mention? _____

_____

Mental and Emotional Status

A. Appearance

Physical handicaps _____

Dress: Appropriate _____ Sloppy _____

Grooming: Neat _____ Poor _____

Eye contact held _____ Posture _____

B. Behavior

Restless _____ Agitated _____ Lethargic _____

Mannerisms _____ Facial expressions _____ Other _____

C. Speech

Clear _____ Mumbled _____ Rapid _____ Slurred _____

Constant _____ Mute or silent _____ Barriers to communications _____

Specify (e.g., client has delusions or is confused, withdrawn, or verbose) _____

_____

D. Mood

What mood does the client convey? _____

_____

E. Affect

Is the client's affect bland, apathetic, dramatic, bizarre, or appropriate? Describe.

_____

F. Thought process

1. Characteristics

Flights of ideas _____ Looseness of association _____ Blocking _____
Concrete thinking _____ Confabulation _____

Describe the characteristics of the client's responses. _____

_____

2. Cognitive ability

Proverbs: Concrete _____ Abstract _____

Serial sevens: How far does the client go? _____ Can the client do simple math? _____

What seems to be the reason for poor concentration? _____

Orientation to time? _____ Place? _____ Person? _____

G. Thought content

1. Central theme: What is important to the client? _____

   Describe. _____

2. Self-concept: How does the client view himself or herself? _____

   _____

   What does the client want to change about himself or herself? _____

   _____

3. Insight: Does the client realistically assess his or her symptoms? _____

   Realistically appraise his or her situation? _____

   Describe. _____

4. Suicidal or homicidal ideation? _____ What is suicide potential? _____
   Family history of suicide or homicide attempt or successful completion? _____

   Explain. _____

5. Preoccupations: Does the client have hallucinations? _____ Delusions? _____

   Obsessions? _____ Rituals? _____ Phobias? _____ Grandiosity? _____

   Religiosity? _____ Worthlessness? _____

   Describe. _____

H. Spiritual assessment

1. What importance does religion or spirituality have in the client's life? _____

   _____

2. Do the client's religious or spiritual beliefs influence the way the client takes care of himself or herself or his or her illness? _____ How? _____

3. Who or what supplies the client with hope? _____

I. Cultural influences

1. With what cultural group does the client identify? _____

2. Has the client tried any cultural remedies or practices for his or her condition? If so, what?

   _____

3. Does the client use any alternative or complementary medicines/herbs/practices?

   _____

FOUNDATIONS OF
Psychiatric Mental Health Nursing

FOUNDATIONS OF Psychiatric Mental Health Nursing

A CLINICAL APPROACH

FIFTH EDITION

ELIZABETH M. VARCAROLIS, RN, MA
Professor Emeritus
Formerly Deputy Chairperson, Department of Nursing
Borough of Manhattan Community College
New York, New York;
Associate Fellow
Albert Ellis Institute for Rational Emotional Behavioral Therapy (REBT)
New York, New York

VERNA BENNER CARSON, PhD, APRN/PMH
National Director of Restore Behavioral Home Health Care
Tender Loving Care Home Health Care
Lake Success, New York;
Formerly Associate Professor of Psychiatric Nursing
School of Nursing
University of Maryland
Baltimore, Maryland

NANCY CHRISTINE SHOEMAKER, APRN/PMH, BC
Nurse Psychotherapist
University of Maryland Medical System
Baltimore, Maryland;
Faculty Associate
School of Nursing
University of Maryland
Baltimore, Maryland

SAUNDERS

ELSEVIER

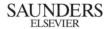

11830 Westline Industrial Drive
St. Louis, Missouri 63146

FOUNDATIONS OF PSYCHIATRIC MENTAL HEALTH NURSING:	ISBN-13 978-1-4160-0088-4
A CLINICAL APPROACH, FIFTH EDITION	ISBN-10 1-4160-0088-7

Notice

Knowledge and best practice in this field are constantly changing. As new research and experience broaden our knowledge, changes in practice, treatment and drug therapy may become necessary or appropriate. Readers are advised to check the most current information provided (i) on procedures featured or (ii) by the manufacturer of each product to be administered, to verify the recommended dose or formula, the method and duration of administration, and contraindications. It is the responsibility of the practitioner, relying on their own experience and knowledge of the patient, to make diagnoses, to determine dosages and the best treatment for each individual patient, and to take all appropriate safety precautions. To the fullest extent of the law, neither the Publisher nor the Authors assume any liability for any injury and/or damage to persons or property arising out or related to any use of the material contained in this book.

The Publisher

ISBN-13 978-1-4160-0088-4
ISBN-10 1-4160-0088-7

Executive Editor: Tom Wilhelm
Developmental Editor: Jill Ferguson
Publishing Services Manager: Deborah L. Vogel
Senior Project Manager: Deon Lee
Design Manager: Teresa McBryan

Printed in China

Last digit is the print number: 9 8 7 6 5 4 3 2 1

To the memory of Josiah and Ruth Merrill, to whom I owe so much and think of everyday.

And to my husband, Paul, whose love and devotion mean everything to me.

Betsy Varcarolis

To my husband of 35 years, John, who provided me with unwavering support throughout this project. He never complained and kept me company during many late nights as I toiled over the computer. I especially appreciated the jokes he emailed me while I wrote. Laughter is certainly good for my soul!

I also thank my personal cheering squad—my three sons, Adam, Johnny, and Rob; my lovely daughter-in-law, Michelle; and Adele and Kathy, who are my best friends.

Verna Benner Carson

To my grandchildren, Mackenzie and Nathan, you are the light of my life.

Nancy Shoemaker

Acknowledgments

I owe a great deal to many for their support and contributions to this text.

First, the fifth edition is richer and broader with the hard work and dedication of Verna Benner Carson and Nancy Shoemaker. I thank them for sharing a burden that is now too heavy for one person and for making this edition stronger and better than ever.

My coauthors and I express our gratitude to the authors who either have written new chapters for this edition or have updated previous chapters, keeping the material current and relevant. We are fortunate to work with professionals who brought their clinical expertise, knowledge, and clarity of thought to the readers of this text.

My thanks to contributors of past editions, whose influence on the content and completeness of this text is still apparent: Denise Saint Arnault, Jeannemarie Baker, Barbara B. Bauer, Beth Bonham, Helene S. (Kay) Charron, Brenda Lewis Cleary, Mattie Collins, Michelle Conant Dan-El, Jeffery S. Grunberg, Mary Ursula Guthomsen, Mary Jane Herron, William G. Herron, Anne Cowley Herzog, Signe S. Hill, Suzanne Lego, Kem B. Louie, Margie Lovett-Scott, Mary McAndrew, Susan Mejo, Peggy Miller, Jane Bryant Neese, Hildegard E. Peplau, Margaret H. Pipchick, Francesca Profiri, Carla E. Randall, Marcia A. Ullman, Lorenza M. Valvo, Judith Sutherland, Ardis R. Swanson, Juliet L. Tien-Hyatt, and Thomas Wenzka.

Special thanks to Kay Charron, Lee Murray, and Jane Young for their creative work on the instructor ancillaries to accompany this edition.

To Steven Leopold, who supplied unit opening photographs. He worked hard to find creative and poignant photos to add a compassionate dimension. Thanks, Steve—again—an artful job.

Pivotal in the production of a successful text are the people who balance, advise, supply, figure out, support, suggest, and solve the thousands of details, questions, and dilemmas that are inherent in any undertaking of this kind.

Tom Wilhelm, Executive Editor, worked hard to keep the many threads and tone of this edition consistent. He supported and guided us all when support and guidance were needed. His planning and input were crucial.

Jill Ferguson, our Developmental Editor, worked tirelessly with an eagle's eye on reams of manuscripts with grace and efficiency. The balancing act here was incredible.

Deon Lee, Senior Project Manager, managed consistency to the minutest detail.

Janet Lincoln, whose copyediting skills are a bit amazing, made this edition as error free as possible.

Teresa McBryan, Design Manager, created an appealing and inviting design.

Always, a huge debt of gratitude to the educators and clinicians who reviewed the manuscript pages and offered valuable suggestions, ideas, opinions, criticisms, and contributions. All were welcomed and greatly helped refine and strengthen the individual chapters. These contributions were invaluable. We thank you all.

Betsy Varcarolis

Contributors

Penny Simpson Brooke, APRN, MS, JD
Professor and Director of Outreach
College of Nursing
University of Utah
Salt Lake City, Utah
Chapter 8: Legal and Ethical Guidelines for Safe Practice

Cherrill W. Colson, MA, CS, EdD
Assistant Professor
Department of Nursing
Hostos Community College
City University of New York, Bronx;
Clinical Specialist
Leake and Watts Children's Services
Yonkers, New York
Chapter 32: Disorders of Children and Adolescents

Judith W. Coram, RN, MN, CNS, BCFE, FACFE
Clinical Faculty
University of Washington
Seattle, Washington;
Adjunct Faculty
University of Colorado
Colorado Springs, Colorado;
Special Deputy
Spokane County Sheriff's Department
Spokane, Washington
Chapter 31: Psychiatric Forensic Nursing

Charlotte Eliopoulos, RN, MPH, ND, PhD
President
Health Education Network
Glen Arm, Maryland
Chapter 21: Cognitive Disorders
Chapter 37: Integrative Care

Kathleen Ibrahim, MA, APRN, BC
Assistant Director of Nursing for Staff Development
New York State Psychiatric Institute
New York, New York
Chapter 17: Eating Disorders

Miriam Jacik, MSN, MSPsy
Coordinator, Grief Support Group
Lanham, Maryland
Unit Three A Nurse Speaks

Kathy A. Kramer-Howe, MA, MSW, CMSW
Member NASW
Member National Council of Hospice Professionals
Paradise Valley, Arizona
Chapter 30: Care for the Dying and for Those Who Grieve

Mary Curry Narayan, MSN, APRN, CTN
Transcultural Nurse Specialist
Visiting Nurse Service Network
Chantilly, Virginia
Chapter 7: Culturally Relevant Mental Health Nursing: A Global Perspective

John A. Payne, MA, BS (Deceased)
Formerly Assistant Professor of Nursing
Borough of Manhattan Community College;
Formerly Director of Nursing/Senior Management Consultant for Long Term Care and Psychiatry
NYC Department of Hospitals;
Formerly Director of Nursing Services
Harlem Hospital Center
New York, New York
Unit One A Nurse Speaks

John Raynor, PhD
Professor
Borough of Manhattan Community College
City University of New York
New York, New York
Chapter 3: Biological Basis for Understanding Psychotropic Drugs

Carolyn M. Scott, MS, RN
Team Leader, Wellness Center
Home Health of Illinois
Breakers Senior Living at Edgewater Beach
Chicago, Illinois
Chapter 22: Crisis

Sharon Shisler, RN, CS
Clinical Nurse Specialist—Mental Health;
Psychiatric Liaison
Greenwich Hospital;
Group Therapist
Greenwich AIDS Alliance
White Plains Day Care Center
Greenwich, Connecticut
Unit Nine A Nurse Speaks

Kathleen Smith-DiJulio, MA, RN
Research Scientist
Seattle Midlife Women's Health Study
Department of Family and Child Nursing
University of Washington
Seattle, Washington;
Doctoral Student
School of Nursing
University of Washington
Seattle, Washington
Chapter 27: Care of the Chemically Impaired

Margaret Swisher, MSN, RN
Assistant Professor of Nursing
Montgomery County Community College
Blue Bell, Pennsylvania
Chapter 5: Mental Health Nursing in Acute Care Settings

Evelyn L. Yap, MS, APRN-PMH
Nurse Psychotherapist—Adult (Board Certified)
Carruthers Clinic
University of Maryland Medical System
Baltimore, Maryland
Chapter 34: Psychosocial Needs of the Older Adult

Reviewers

Carla Abel-Zieg, RN, MS, CNS, APRN
Assistant Professor
School of Nursing
Creighton University
Omaha, Nebraska

Angela Frederick Amar, PhD, APRN, BC
Assistant Professor
School of Nursing and Health Sciences
Georgetown University
Washington, District of Columbia

Lois Angelo, RN, MSN, CS
Psychiatric Clinical Nurse Specialist
Massachusetts General Hospital
Boston, Massachusetts

Dorit Golan Breiter, MSN, ARNP
Instructor
College of Nursing
University of South Florida
Tampa, Florida

Carolyn Pierce Buckelew, RN, MA, APNC, CHYC, NBCC
Senior Instructor
C.E. Gregory School of Nursing
Raritan Bay Medical Center
Perth Amboy, New Jersey

Sue S. Butell, RN, MS
Associate Professor
School of Nursing
Linfield College
Portland, Oregon

Carissa Enright, MSN, RN
Clinical Assistant Professor
College of Nursing
Texas Woman's University
Dallas, Texas

Patricia A. Graham, APRN, BC
RN Manager, Staff Development
Western State Hospital
Staunton, Virginia

Patricia A. Griffin, MSN
Associate Professor of Nursing
University Assessment Coordinator
Anderson University
Anderson, Indiana

Margaret J. Halter, PhD, APRN
Professor
School of Nursing
Malone College
Canton, Ohio

Connie S. Heflin, MSN, RN
Professor of Nursing
West Kentucky Community and Technical College
Paducah, Kentucky

Melinda Stanley Hermanns, MSN, RN, BC
Senior Lecturer and Course Coordinator
College of Nursing and Health Sciences
The University of Texas at Tyler
Tyler, Texas

Cheryl Hilgenberg, BSN, MS, EdD, RN, CTN
Associate Professor
School of Nursing
Millikin University
Decatur, Illinois

Theresa Inott, MSN
Instructor
School of Nursing
Vanderbilt University
Nashville, Tennessee

Deborah Kindy, PhD, RN
Associate Professor of Nursing
Sonoma State University
Rohnert Park, California

Nancy Kostin, RN, MSN
Assistant Professor of Nursing
Madonna University
Livonia, Michigan

Charlotte Lorentson, MSN, RN, CS, BC
Clinical Nurse Specialist
Hancock Geriatric Treatment Center
Eastern State Hospital
Williamsburg, Virginia

Christine W. Massey, MSN, RN, BC, CSE
Associate Professor of Nursing
Barton College
Wilson, North Carolina

Marilyn K. Miller, RN, BSN, MSN
Associate Professor of Nursing
St. Charles Community College
St. Charles, Missouri

R. Lea Montgomery, RN, MSN
Instructor
Harris School of Nursing
Texas Christian University
Fort Worth, Texas

Agnes A. Natale, RN, MS, MSN
Assistant Professor
College of Nursing
University of Nebraska Medical Center
Lincoln, Nebraska

Paul Philippe, RN
Nurse Manager
St. Luke's-Roosevelt Hospital Center
New York, New York

Robin L. Pigg, MSN
Department Chair, Nursing
Edgecombe Community College
Tarboro, North Carolina

Anne W. Ryan, MPH, MSN, RN, C
Associate Professor
MGW Nursing Program
Chesapeake College
Wye Mills, Maryland

Patricia Ann Saylor, MSN
Assistant Professor
College of Nursing—Kearney Division
University of Nebraska Medical Center
Kearney, Nebraska

Janet Stuckman, MSN
Nursing Instructor
John Wood Community College
Quincy, Illinois

Joan D. Thomas, RN, PhD, CS
Assistant Professor
Loewenberg School of Nursing
University of Memphis
Memphis, Tennessee

Dorothy A. Varchol, MSN, MA, RN, C
Nursing Instructor
Cincinnati State Technical and Community College
Cincinnati, Ohio

Judith A. Wilson, APRN, BC
Clinical Nurse Specialist
Geriatric Psychiatry
University Hospital
Birmingham, Alabama

Jane Ellen Young, MSN, FNP, RN, MPH
Nursing Instructor
Wake Technical Community College
Raleigh, North Carolina

Psychiatric nursing challenges us to understand human behavior. In the chapters that follow, you will learn about people with psychiatric disorders and how to provide them with quality nursing care. As you read, keep in mind these special features.

KEY TERMS AND CONCEPTS and OBJECTIVES introduce the topics of each chapter and provide a concise overview of the material discussed.

KEY POINTS TO REMEMBER appear at the end of each chapter to reinforce essential information.

CRITICAL THINKING AND CHAPTER REVIEW at the end of each chapter provide scenario-based critical thinking problems and multiple-choice questions for study and review. Answers to the multiple-choice questions are provided in Appendix D, and rationales and text page references can be found on the Evolve website.

CHAPTER 15

Somatoform and Dissociative Disorders

NANCY CHRISTINE SHOEMAKER ■ ELIZABETH M. VARCAROLIS

KEY TERMS and CONCEPTS

The key terms and concepts listed here appear in color where they are defined or first discussed in this chapter.

alternate personality (alter) or subpersonality, 267
body dysmorphic disorder, 259
conversion disorder, 259
depersonalization disorder, 265
dissociative amnesia, 265
dissociative disorders, 264
dissociative fugue, 266
dissociative identity disorder (DID), 266
factitious disorder, 253
hypochondriasis, 258
la belle indifférence, 259
malingering, 253
pain disorder, 259
psychosomatic illness, 253
secondary gains, 260
somatization, 253
somatization disorder, 258
somatoform disorders, 252

OBJECTIVES

After studying this chapter, the reader will be able to

1. Compare and contrast essential characteristics of the somatoform and the dissociative disorders.
2. Differentiate symptoms of somatoform disorders from (a) malingering, (b) factitious disorder, and (c) psychosomatic illness.
3. Give a clinical example of what would be found in each of the somatoform disorders.
4. Describe five psychosocial interventions that would be appropriate for a client with somatic complaints.
5. Plan interventions for a client with conversion disorder who is receiving a great deal of secondary gain from his or her "blindness." Include self-care and family teaching.
6. Explain the key symptoms of the four dissociative disorders.
7. Compare and contrast dissociative amnesia and dissociative fugue.
8. Identify three specialized elements in the assessment of a client with a dissociative disorder.

evolve Visit the Evolve website at http://evolve.elsevier.com/Varcarolis for a pretest on the content in this chapter.

As noted in the previous chapter, anxiety exerts a powerful influence on the mind and may lead to clinical conditions known as anxiety disorders. Although clients with anxiety disorders often have some somatic symptoms, the predominant complaint is mental or emotional distress. This chapter introduces the somatoform and dissociative disorders, in which anxiety has a major impact on the body with secondary but significant effects on the mind. These disorders are relatively rare in the psychiatric setting, but the nurse may encounter clients with these disorders in the general medical setting or in specialized units. The placement of these disorders on the mental health continuum can be seen in Figure 15-1.

Somatoform Disorders

Somatoform disorders are defined in the *Diagnostic and Statistical Manual of Mental Disorders*, fourth edi-

252

Somatoform and Dissociative Disorders **CHAPTER 15** 273

■■■ KEY POINTS to REMEMBER

- Somatoform disorders are characterized by the presence of multiple real physical symptoms for which there is no evidence of medical illness.
- Dissociative disorders involve a disruption in consciousness with a significant impairment in memory, identity, or perceptions of self.
- Somatoform and dissociative disorders are believed to be responses to psychological stress, although the client shows no insight into the potential stressors.
- Clients with somatoform and dissociative disorders often have comorbid psychiatric illness, primarily depression, anxiety, or substance abuse.
- The course of these disorders may be brief, with acute onset and spontaneous remission, or chronic, with a gradual onset and prolonged impairment.

- Because these clients may not seek psychiatric treatment, the nurse does not usually see them in the acute psychiatric setting, except during a period of crisis such as suicidal risk.
- The nursing assessment is especially important to clarify the history and course of past symptoms, as well as to obtain a complete picture of the current physical and mental status.
- Although these clients do respond to crisis intervention, they usually require referral for psychotherapy to attain sustained improvement in level of functioning.

Visit the Evolve website at http://evolve.elsevier.com/Varcarolis for a posttest on the content in this chapter.

Critical Thinking and Chapter Review

Visit the Evolve website at http://evolve.elsevier.com/Varcarolis for additional self-study exercises.

■■■ CRITICAL THINKING

1. A client with suspected somatization disorder has been admitted to the medical-surgical unit after an episode of chest pain with possible electrocardiographic changes. While on the unit, she frequently complains of palpitations, asks the nurse to check her vital signs, and begs staff to stay with her. Some nurses take her pulse and blood pressure when she asks. Others evade her requests. Most staff try to avoid spending time with her. Consider why staff wish to avoid her. Design interventions to cope with the client's behaviors. Give rationales for your interventions.

2. A client with body dysmorphic disorder talks incessantly about how big her nose is, how those around her are offended by her appearance, and how her appearance has negatively affected her employment and her social life. What interventions could you make to reduce her anxiety?

3. A client with DID has been admitted to the crisis unit for a short-term stay after a suicide threat. On the unit, the client has repeated the statement that she will kill herself to get rid of "all the others," meaning her subpersonalities. The client refuses to sign a "no harm" contract. Design a care plan to meet her safety and security needs.

■■■ CHAPTER REVIEW

Choose the most appropriate answer.

1. Nurses working with clients with somatization and dissociative disorders can expect that these clients will fit on the continuum of psychobiological disorders at the
   1. mild level.
   2. moderate to severe level.
   3. severe to psychotic level.
   4. They do not belong on the continuum, because anxiety has been reduced by ego defense mechanisms.

2. Mr. R. presents with a history of having assumed a new identity in a distant locale and of having no recollection of his former identity. Which *DSM-IV-TR* diagnosis can the nurse expect the psychiatrist to make?
   1. Hypochondriasis
   2. Conversion disorder
   3. Dissociative fugue
   4. Depersonalization disorder

3. The information that is least relevant when assessing a client with a suspected somatoform disorder is
   1. determination of whether the symptom is under voluntary control.
   2. results of diagnostic workups.
   3. limitations in activities of daily living.
   4. potential for violence.

4. A suitable outcome criterion for the nursing diagnosis *ineffective coping* related to dependence on pain relievers to treat chronic pain of psychological origin is which of the following?
   1. Client will resume preillness roles.
   2. Client will cope adaptively as evidenced by use of alternative coping strategies.
   3. Client will demonstrate improved self-esteem as evidenced by focusing less on weaknesses.
   4. Client will replace demanding, manipulative behaviors with more socially acceptable behavior.

5. Which nursing diagnosis would be least likely to be used for a client with hypochondriasis?
   1. Disturbed personal identity
   2. Ineffective denial
   3. Disturbed body image
   4. Interrupted family processes

396 UNIT FIVE Psychobiological Disorders: Severe to Psychotic

during assessment is crucial for the following reasons (Tandon et al., 2003):

- Depression affects a majority of people with schizophrenia.
- Depression may herald a psychotic relapse and rehospitalization.
- Depression increases the likelihood of substance abuse.
- Depression increases the likelihood of suicide.
- Depression is associated with impaired functioning.

Self-Assessment

Working with individuals diagnosed with schizophrenia produces strong emotional reactions in most health care workers, including nurses. The psychotic client is intensely anxious, lonely, dependent, and distrustful. The intensity of these emotions evokes similarly intense, uncomfortable, and frightening emotions in others. It is important for the nurse to identify personal feelings and responses to clients with schizophrenia; otherwise, the nurse may experience helplessness and increased anxiety. Without support and the opportunity and willingness to explore these reactions with more experienced nursing staff, the nurse may adopt defensive behaviors such as denial, withdrawal, and avoidance. These behaviors not only thwart the client's progress but also undermine the nurse's self-esteem. Statements such as "These clients are hopeless," "You can't understand these people," and "You waste your time with them" are examples of unexamined or unrecognized emotional reactions to clients' behaviors or feelings.

For nurses new to the psychiatric setting, especially for student nurses, supportive supervision must be available if learning is to take place. The student's part in the supervisory process is a willingness to discuss and identify personal feelings and problem behaviors. This can be, and often is, accomplished in group supervision. Experienced psychiatric nurses call this process **peer group supervision.**

Years ago Menninger (1984) noted that staff experience extreme frustration because of the slow progress of clients with schizophrenia. This sense of frustration and accompanying feelings of helplessness are precursors to burnout. The antidote to this downward spiral is a team approach involving periodic reassessment of treatment outcomes with a willingness to scale down unrealistic expectations as well as periodic reassessment of clients who cause frustration to better understand each client's strengths and weaknesses. A team approach to reevaluating and establishing realistic, obtainable outcomes can increase nurses' skills and confidence and improve the quality of interpersonal relationships with clients, as well as relationships with others.

Assessment Guidelines Schizophrenia and Other Psychotic Disorders

1. Assess whether the client has had a medical workup; if so, was medical or substance-induced psychosis ruled out?
2. Assess whether the client is dependent on alcohol or drugs.
3. Assess for command hallucinations (e.g., voices telling the person to harm self or another). If present, ask the client:
   - Do you plan to follow the command?
   - Do you believe the voices are real?
   - Do you recognize the voices?
4. Assess the client's belief system. Is it fragmented, poorly or well organized? Is it systematized? Is the system of beliefs unsupported by reality (delusion)? If yes, then
   - Assess whether delusions focus on someone trying to harm the client; assess whether the client is planning to retaliate against a person or organization.
   - Assess whether precautions need to be taken.
5. Assess for co-occurring disorders:
   - Depression (suicidality)
   - Anxiety
   - Substance dependency
   - History of violence
6. Assess which medications the client is taking. Assess whether the client is adhering to the medication regimen.
7. Assess the family's response to increased symptoms. Are they overprotective? Hostile? Suspicious?
8. Assess the manner in which family members and the client relate.
9. Assess the support system. Is the family well informed about the disease? Does the family understand the need for medication adherence? Is the family familiar with what family support groups are available in the community or where to go for respite and family support? Have family members received or been referred for psychoeducation?
10. Assess the client's global functioning (using the Global Assessment of Functioning [GAF] Scale in Box 1-2).

NURSING DIAGNOSIS

People with schizophrenia have multiple disturbing and disabling symptoms that invite a multifaceted approach to care and treatment of the client as well as the client's family. See Table 20-4 for potential nursing diagnoses for a person with schizophrenia.

ASSESSMENT GUIDELINES at the end of each Assessment section in the nursing process part of the clinical chapters provide summary points for client assessment.

VIGNETTES describe and individualize clients with specific psychiatric disorders.

282 UNIT FOUR Psychobiological Disorders: Moderate to Severe

DSM-IV-TR AND THE CLINICAL PICTURE OF CLUSTER B DISORDERS (DRAMATIC, EMOTIONAL, ERRATIC)

Individuals with cluster B PDs are described as dramatic, emotional, or erratic. Refer to Figure 16-3 for the diagnostic criteria for each disorder in this group. In general, individuals with these disorders seek out interpersonal relationships but cannot maintain them because of excessive demands and emotional instability. They are manipulative in their interactions; that is, although they demonstrate charm and superficial warmth for others, their main goal is to use others to meet their own needs. They often display a sense of entitlement: they unconsciously feel that their needs are more important than the needs of others, and they deny the negative effects of hurting others (Kerr, 2002). Many individuals with cluster B disorders receive psychiatric care, either voluntarily because of affective distress, or involuntarily because of illegal behavior. Key attributes for each disorder are described in the following sections (Kay et al., 2000) and are illustrated in the vignettes.

Antisocial Personality Disorder

Antisocial personality disorder has the main features of consistent disregard for others with exploitation and repeated unlawful actions. Persons with antisocial PD were previously called psychopaths or sociopaths. There is a clear history of conduct disorder in childhood (see Chapter 32), and the individuals show no remorse for hurting others. They repeatedly neglect responsibilities, tell lies, and perform destructive or illegal acts, without developing any insight into predictable consequences. This disorder may be underdiagnosed in women and overdiagnosed in clients of lower socioeconomic status. These individuals do not voluntarily seek psychiatric care, but they are often seen for court-referred evaluation or treatment.

VIGNETTE

Mr. Rouse is a 25-year-old divorced cab driver who is referred to the hospital by the court for competency evaluation after an assault charge. He told the arresting officer that he has bipolar disorder. He has a history of substance abuse and multiple arrests for disorderly conduct or assault. During his intake interview he is polite and even flirtatious with the female RN. He insists that he is not responsible for his behavior because he is manic. The only symptom that he describes is irritability. He points out that he cannot tolerate any psychotropic medications because of the side effects. He also notes that he has dropped out of three clinics after several visits because "the staff don't understand me."

Borderline Personality Disorder

Borderline personality disorder has the central characteristic of instability in affect, identity, and relationships. Individuals with borderline PD desperately seek relationships to avoid feeling abandoned. But they often drive others away because of their excessive demands, impulsive behavior, or uncontrolled anger. Their frequent use of the defense of splitting strains personal relationships and creates turmoil in health care settings. Borderline PD is one of the most common PDs seen in psychiatric treatment settings. Under stress, these clients may show psychosis-like symptoms, and they may demonstrate chronic depression or self-destructive behavior. Clients with borderline PD may have a history of multiple or dramatic suicidal gestures, and there is a significant risk of suicide: one in ten clients can be expected to complete suicide (Paris, 2002).

VIGNETTE

Ms. Bracey is a 28-year-old divorced female who attends the dual diagnosis group at a mental health clinic. She has a history of five hospitalizations for suicidal ideation and self-mutilation. Her main theme in the group involves repeated failures in intimate relationships. In each case, she initially describes a warm, supportive person who will be her "soul mate." But within several months, she reports episodes of disappointment seemingly related to minor events. She then breaks off the relationship, concluding that the boy friend is "just another loser." When a peer in the group suggests that there is a pattern to her behavior, she bursts into tears and runs out of the meeting.

Histrionic Personality Disorder

Histrionic personality disorder has the key ingredient of emotional attention-seeking behavior, in which the person needs to be the center of attention. The histrionic person is impulsive and melodramatic, and may act flirtatious or provocative to get the spotlight. Relationships do not last because the partner often feels smothered or reacts to the insensitivity of the histrionic person. The individual with histrionic PD does not have insight into his or her role in breaking up relationships and may seek treatment for depression or another comorbid condition. In the treatment setting, the person demands "the best of everything" and can be very critical.

VIGNETTE

Ms. Lombard is a 35-year-old twice-divorced female admitted to an inpatient unit after an overdose of asthma medications and antibiotics. She took all of her pills after her primary care doctor refused to order a sleeping pill for her. On the first night, she is withdrawn and tearful in her room. But

A NURSE SPEAKS

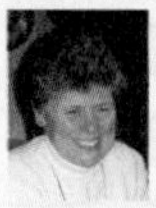

Communication with a psychiatric client that can convey knowledge, caring, encouragement, and support can lead that client along a path that endorses wellness and well-being. This is termed *therapeutic communicating* or *therapeutic relating*. Let me share a story from my own experience that illustrates the power of such communication.

I was working in a psychiatric day treatment program when I met Sue. Sue was brand new to the program. I could see the same confusion and denial in Sue that I so often see in persons newly diagnosed with mental health problems. Sue truly did not believe that she was facing a diagnosis of schizophrenia. She believed she was overly stressed but certainly not mentally ill. If the health care team would just listen to her, believe her, and help her, she could get over this. She described the attacks "they" were making upon her person and her life. "They" followed her, repeated to her segments of conversations she had with her family, invaded the privacy of her home, and harassed her at her job.

As Sue's psychiatric nurse, I perceived that she was experiencing fear, panic, and feelings that her life was totally out of control. I acknowledged the feelings that this frightened woman expressed. I offered Sue support and help as treatment with medications and therapy began. Adjusting to an antipsychotic medication was difficult, especially because Sue really did not think she needed it. After all, she believed that she was just very stressed and talking to someone about it was bound to help.

I provided Sue with some simple explanations about how the antipsychotic medication would work to correct the chemical imbalance that existed in her brain. I was fully aware that these explanations and ongoing teaching would mean nothing if Sue did not feel that I cared and was sincerely interested in her. Sue needed to feel safe, cared about, and protected at a time when her world was so foreboding.

As medication dulled the delusional thoughts that raced through Sue's mind, I could see her transform into a calmer, more trusting person. Sue's gifts became apparent—she was smart and very creative. I acknowledged these gifts and called them into play. This bolstered Sue's self-confidence, which had been badly battered by the symptomatology of the illness.

I was determined to focus on Sue's personal gifts and talents, as well as the evident manifestations of the disease, addressing both as I could. Sue's response to this approach was positive. She began to feel less like a "sick, overwhelmed person." She was encouraged to grasp and hold on to that which had been good and positive in her life before the onset of her illness. I truly believe that reaching out to the well person that Sue could and would become was helpful.

The progress was slow and painstaking. I believed it was worth all of the effort involved. My hope was that Sue would leave treatment stabilized, less stressed, and aware that a nurse she met at the day program believed in her, reached out to her, and walked the road to wellness with her.

Miriam Jacik

A NURSE SPEAKS provides personal stories of individual nurses in various practice settings. *A Client Speaks* and *A Family Speaks* also introduce select units and bring to life disorders and their effects on clients, their families, and those who care for them.

CULTURALLY SPEAKING boxes reinforce the importance of culturally competent care.

FORENSIC HIGHLIGHTS boxes focus on the nurse's role in this expanding area of practice, which deals with sexual assault, family violence, and incarcerated persons.

Sigmund Freud taught that anxiety resulted from the threatened breakthrough of repressed ideas or emotions from the unconscious into consciousness. Freud also suggested that ego defense mechanisms are used by the individual to keep anxiety at manageable levels. Later in this chapter, Table 14-7 defines and gives examples of defense mechanisms commonly used by individuals with anxiety disorders. The use of defense mechanisms results in behavior that is not wholly adaptive because of its rigidity and repetitive nature. Chapters 2 and 13 provide the reader with more details on the dynamics of defense mechanisms.

Harry Stack Sullivan placed anxiety in an interpersonal context. He believed that all anxiety is linked either to the emotional distress caused when early needs go unmet or to the anxiety transmitted to the infant from the caregiver through the process of empathy. Thus, the anxiety experienced early in life becomes the prototype for that experienced when unpleasant events occur later in life.

Learning theories provide another view. Behavioral psychologists conceptualize anxiety as a learned response that can be unlearned. Some individuals may learn to be anxious from the modeling provided by parents or peers. For example, a mother who is fearful of thunder and lightning and who hides in closets during storms may transmit her anxiety to her children, who continue to adopt her behavior even into adult life. Such individuals can unlearn this behavior by observing others who react normally to a storm.

Cognitive theorists take the position that anxiety disorders are caused by distortions in an individual's thinking and perceiving. Because individuals with such distortions believe that any mistake they make will have catastrophic results, they experience acute anxiety.

Cultural Considerations

Reliable data on the incidence of anxiety disorders in this and other cultures are sparse, but sociocultural variation in symptoms of anxiety disorders has been noted. In some cultures, individuals express anxiety through somatic symptoms, whereas in other cultures, cognitive symptoms predominate. Panic attacks in Latin Americans and Northern Europeans often involve sensations of choking, smothering, numbness, or tingling, as well as fear of dying. In other cultural groups, panic attacks involve fear of magic or witchcraft. Social phobias in Japanese and Korean cultures may relate to a belief that the individual's blushing, eye contact, or body odor is offensive to others (APA, 2000).

The *Diagnostic and Statistical Manual of Mental Disorders*, fourth edition, text revision *(DSM-IV-TR)* (APA, 2000) notes cultural aspects of each psychiatric disorder to alert the clinician to consider cultural context before making a psychiatric diagnosis. The Culturally Speaking box discusses factors relevant to one anxiety disorder. Also review Chapter 7 for more discussion of cultural issues.

CLINICAL PICTURE

The term *anxiety disorders* refers to a number of disorders, including the following:

- Panic disorders
- Phobias
- OCD
- GAD
- PTSD
- Acute stress disorder
- Anxiety due to substance use
- Anxiety due to medical conditions
- Anxiety not otherwise specified

CULTURALLY SPEAKING

Posttraumatic Stress Disorder

Cultural and social factors play a major role in posttraumatic stress disorder (PTSD). Minority groups in the United States have much higher rates of PTSD than do non-Hispanic white persons. African Americans of all ages have a high risk of exposure to violent crime. One study found PTSD in 25% of African American youth who were victims of violence. Likewise, American Indians and Alaska Natives have an increased risk of victimization. This higher rate of trauma results in a 22% prevalence rate of PTSD in these groups compared to 8% in the general population.

Refugees are another group at higher risk of PTSD. Central American Hispanics often fled their homelands during civil wars, and rates of PTSD range from 33% to 60% in this refugee group. Similarly, many Asian Americans from Laos, Vietnam, and Cambodia were severely traumatized before they left their native lands. One study of Southeast Asia refugees seeking mental health care showed that 70% met the criteria for PTSD.

U.S. Department of Health and Human Services. (2001). *Mental Health: Culture, race and ethnicity: A supplement to mental health: A report of the surgeon general.* Rockville, MD: U.S. Department of Health and Human Services, Substance Abuse and Mental Health Services Administration, Center for Mental Health Services.

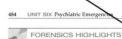

FORENSICS HIGHLIGHTS

Rates of suicide are higher among those in jails and prisons than in the general population. The U.S. Department of Justice Bureau of Justice Statistics estimated that, in 1999, the suicide rate among prison inmates was 14 per 100,000 and the rate among jail inmates was 55 per 100,000 (jails are short-term local facilities, whereas prisons are facilities where longer-term sentences are carried out). Most suicides occur in the first 24 hours of incarceration in a jail. Other risk factors include learning of new legal complications, receiving bad news from home, and experiencing sexual assault. The typical person who commits suicide is young, white, male, single, intoxicated, and has a history of substance abuse. The most common method is hanging. Suicide prevention programs have been shown to be effective in reducing suicide rates. The National Commission on Correctional Health Care had adopted standards for assessment and intervention. Nurses in the forensic setting may play a key role in admission screening and ongoing monitoring of suicidal inmates.

Data from American Psychiatric Association. (2003). Practice guidelines for the assessment and treatment of patients with suicidal behaviors. *American Journal of Psychiatry, 160*(11 Suppl.) 1-60.

Survivors of Completed Suicide: Postvention

A discussion of suicidal clients is incomplete without noting the issues surrounding a completed suicide. Surviving family and friends experience overwhelming guilt and shame, compounded by the difficulty of discussing the taboo subject of suicide (Fine & Myers, 2003). The usual social supports of neighbors and church are sometimes lacking for these mourners. Within 6 months of a suicide, 45% of bereaved adults report mental deterioration, with symptoms of depression or posttraumatic stress disorder. Adolescent siblings of youth suicide victims have a seven times higher risk of developing major depressive disorder over the 6-month period. Adolescent friends who suffer traumatic grief are more likely to report suicidal ideation within 6 years of the suicide (APA, 2003). Family members of a suicide victim develop a higher risk of suicide, 4.5 times greater than the risk in families in which no suicide occurred.

One survivor wrote a personal account 25 years after the suicide of her brother:

> The first year after was a blur. . . . I became so severely depressed that I had to withdraw from school. . . . I am still plagued by what I call the 'if onlys'—if only I could have switched places with him, if only he had been in restraints. . . . despite the progress I have made, the death of anyone close to me rips open the wound. Even fictional suicides on television lead to uncontrollable crying. (Simon, 2003, p. 1597)

Despite their suffering, only approximately 25% of survivors seek treatment (APA, 2003).

Survivors give the following suggestions to health care professionals:

- If being a survivor is the main reason treatment has been sought, remember that the survivor is the client and not the deceased. Focus on the client's thoughts and feelings and do a thorough assessment as you usually would.
- If the deceased was your client, clarify why the relative is coming to you—for more information, for consolation, or for treatment.
- If being a survivor comes out as an incidental finding during an assessment, ask open-ended questions and evaluate how much the loss has been resolved.
- Do not say "successful suicide." More acceptable phrases are "died by suicide" or "killed himself or herself."
- Do recommend community resources and survivor support groups and show empathy about the loss of someone to suicide.
- Do examine you own feelings and countertransference if you treat a suicide survivor. Use clinical supervision or a mentor or therapy to help yourself.

Staff members who have cared for a suicide victim are similarly traumatized by suicide. Staff may also experience symptoms of posttraumatic stress disorder with guilt, shock, anger, shame, and decreased self-esteem (APA, 2003). Group support is essential as the treatment team conducts a thorough psychological postmortem assessment. The event is carefully reviewed to identify the potential overlooked clues, faulty judgments, or changes that are needed in agency protocols. Most facilities have a clear policy about communication with families after suicide. Although some lawyers advise having no contact except through them, others recommend designating a spokesperson who can address the feelings of the family without discussing the details of the client's care. In fact, referrals should be given to family members to try to assist them in dealing with their grief and to address any emotional problems that develop, especially in adolescents. The team needs to discuss any clinician's plan to attend the funeral. As for documentation, all staff need to ensure that the record is complete and that any late entries are identified as such. Legal cases have shown that the courts require that the client be periodically evalu-

EVIDENCE-BASED PRACTICE

Treatment of Generalized Anxiety Disorder

Background

Generalized anxiety disorder (GAD) has a high prevalence rate, results in many visits to primary care providers for somatic complaints, and has an impact on workplace absenteeism. Studies over the past 20 years provide evidence of the benefits of cognitive-behavioral therapy (CBT) in the treatment of GAD.

Studies

Sixteen experimental studies have been reported and were analyzed as a group. The client population was two-thirds women, with an average age of 40 years, average GAD duration of 7 years, and average length of treatment of 11 sessions. CBT included teaching clients to engage in self-monitoring and observe their anxiety triggers, relaxation training, cognitive therapy to reduce expectation of negative events, and rehearsal of coping responses to graduated exposure to stressful situations. CBT was compared to low-dose diazepam therapy, placebo, supportive listening, and no treatment.

Results of Studies

CBT showed superior results compared with control treatments in the majority of studies, as measured by improved scores on standardized anxiety questionnaires. Clients receiving CBT also maintained or increased their degree of improvement at 6-month and 12-month follow-up.

Implications for Nursing Practice

Nurses need to teach clients with GAD that there are effective psychotherapy treatments for this disorder. Nurses may refer clients to appropriate resources in the community. Also, it is beneficial to teach anxious clients about the benefits of relaxation exercises whenever possible.

Borkovec, T. D., Newman, M. G., & Castonguay, L. G. (2003). Cognitive-behavioral therapy for generalized anxiety disorder with integrations from interpersonal and experiential therapies. *CNS Spectrums, 8*(5), 382-389.

Posttraumatic Stress Disorder

Posttraumatic stress disorder (PTSD) is characterized by repeated reexperiencing of a highly traumatic event that involved actual or threatened death or serious injury to self or others, to which the individual responded with intense fear, helplessness, or horror (APA, 2000). PTSD may occur after any traumatic event that is outside the range of usual experience. Examples are military combat; detention as a prisoner of war; natural disasters such as floods, tornadoes, and earthquakes; human disasters such as plane and train accidents; crime-related events such as bombing, assault, mugging, rape, and being taken hostage; or diagnosis of a life-threatening illness. PTSD symptoms often begin within 3 months after the trauma, but a delay of months or years is not uncommon (Figure 14-3). The major features of PTSD are the following:

- Persistent reexperiencing of the trauma through recurrent intrusive recollections of the event, through dreams, and through flashbacks. (Flashbacks are dissociative experiences during which the event is relived and the person behaves as though he or she is experiencing the event at that time.)
- Persistent avoidance of stimuli associated with the trauma, which results in the individual's avoiding talking about the event or avoiding activities, people, or places that arouse memories of the trauma.
- After the trauma, experience of persistent numbing of general responsiveness, as evidenced by the individual's feeling detached or estranged from others, feeling empty inside, or feeling turned off to others.
- After the trauma, experiencing of persistent symptoms of increased arousal, as evidenced by irritability, difficulty sleeping, difficulty concentrating, hypervigilance, or exaggerated startle response.

Difficulty with interpersonal, social, or occupational relationships nearly always accompanies PTSD, and trust is a common issue of concern. Child and spousal abuse may be associated with hypervigilance and irritability. Chemical abuse may begin as an attempt to self-medicate to relieve anxiety.

It is important for health care workers to realize that exposure to stimuli reminiscent of those associated with the original trauma may cause an exacerbation of the trauma. For example, one nurse therapist observed that the attack on the World Trade Center on September 11, 2001, caused an exacerbation of PTSD symptoms in veterans of World War II (Kaiman, 2003). See Case Study and Nursing Care Plan 14-1 at the end of the chapter, which describes a client with PTSD.

Acute Stress Disorder

Acute stress disorder occurs within 1 month after exposure to a highly traumatic event, such as those listed in the section on PTSD. To be diagnosed with acute stress disorder, the individual must display at least three dissociative symptoms either during or after the traumatic event: a subjective sense of numbing, detachment, or absence of emotional responsiveness; a reduction in awareness of surroundings; derealization (a sense of unreality related to the environment); depersonalization (experience of a sense of unreality or self-estrangement); or dissociative amnesia (loss of memory) (APA, 2000). By definition, acute stress disorder resolves within 4 weeks.

EVIDENCE-BASED PRACTICE boxes demonstrate how research findings affect psychiatric nursing practice and standards of care.

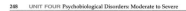

INTEGRATIVE THERAPY

Kava kava

Kava kava is prepared from a South Pacific plant *(Piper methysticum)* and is used as an herbal sedative with antianxiety effects. Before seeking psychiatric treatment, clients with anxiety disorders may try kava kava in the belief that herbs are safer than medications. But kava kava may interact with any drugs metabolized by the liver, especially central nervous system depressants such as the benzodiazepines. There are reports of elevated liver enzyme levels in clients taking kava kava and one documented case of liver failure in a client who took this herb for 2 months.

Before administering medications to clients with anxiety disorders, the nurse must assess for the use of kava kava or other herbal supplements to avoid toxic effects.

Dasgupta, A. (2003). Review of abnormal laboratory test results and toxic effects due to herbal medicines. *American Journal of Clinical Pathology, 120*(1), 127-137.

- Is the client experiencing a reduced level of anxiety?
- Does the client recognize symptoms as anxiety related?
- Does the client continue to display obsessions, compulsions, phobias, worrying, or other symptoms of anxiety disorders? If still present, are they more or less frequent? more or less intense?
- Is the client able to use newly learned behaviors to manage anxiety?
- Can the client adequately perform self-care activities?
- Can the client maintain satisfying interpersonal relations?
- Can the client assume usual roles?

INTEGRATIVE THERAPY boxes discuss the increasing popularity and significance of complementary and alternative therapies.

CASE STUDY and NURSING CARE PLAN 14-1 Posttraumatic Stress Disorder

Mr. Blake is brought to the emergency department by his wife after she finds him writing a suicide note and planning to take a bottle of prescription sleeping pills. Mr. Blake is subdued, shows minimal affect, and has the odor of alcohol on his breath. When asked about his suicidal thoughts, he states that he is worthless and that his wife and family would be better off if he were dead. He refuses to contract for safety. The decision is made to hospitalize him to protect him from danger to self.

Mr. Blake's wife gives further history. Her husband is a 50-year-old retired firefighter who was part of the emergency team that responded to the World Trade Center terrorist attack on September 11, 2001. He lost half of his crew members in the fire. A few months later, he decided to take an early retirement so that he and his wife could move south to be near their daughter's family. Initially, he showed no signs of anxiety and refused offers of crisis treatment: "I was in Vietnam, I can handle stress." But 6 months later, Ms. Blake noticed that he had trouble sleeping, his mood was irritable or withdrawn, he avoided news reports on television, and he started drinking daily. He complained of nightmares but would not talk to her about his fears. He only agreed to go to the primary care physician to request sleeping medication.

Mr. Blake is admitted to the psychiatric unit and is assigned to a nurse, Ms. Dawson. He is passive as she orients him to the unit, but she observes that he looks all around carefully and is easily startled by sounds on the unit.

Self-Assessment

Ms. Dawson is a registered nurse with an AA degree and 3 years of experience on this unit. Initially, she feels sympathy for Mr. Blake, and he reminds her of her Uncle James, who also served in Vietnam. She is concerned because his suicide plan was lethal and he is guarded in his speech, not revealing his thoughts or feelings. She realizes that as she implements suicide precautions, she must demonstrate an attitude of hope and acceptance to encourage him to develop trust. Also, she must stay neutral and not convey any pity or sympathy. As a firefighter, Mr. Blake was once a care provider, and he already feels like a failure because he could not save his friends or prevent his own symptoms.

ASSESSMENT

Objective Data
- Sleep difficulty, nightmares
- Hypervigilance
- Alcohol use
- Withdrawn mood
- Guarded affect
- Avoidance of news coverage with potential for emergency reports
- Refusal of treatment and safety contract
- Plan for suicide

Subjective Data
- "I don't deserve to live, I should have died with the others."
- "You can't stop me."

CASE STUDIES AND NURSING CARE PLANS present individualized histories of clients with specific psychiatric disorders and follow the steps of the nursing process. Interventions with rationales and evaluation statements are presented for each client goal.

NURSING DIAGNOSIS (NANDA)

Risk for suicide related to anger and hopelessness due to severe trauma, as evidenced by suicidal plan and verbalization of intent
- Lethal plan with saved prescription medication and alcohol
- Refusal to contract for safety
- Emotional withdrawal from wife

OUTCOME CRITERIA (NOC)

Client will consistently refrain from attempting suicide.

PLANNING

The initial plan is to maintain safety for Mr. Blake while encouraging him to express feelings and recognize that his situation is not hopeless.

INTERVENTION (NIC)

Mr. Blake's plan of care is personalized as follows:

Short-Term Goal	Intervention	Rationale	Evaluation
1. Client will speak to staff whenever experiencing self-destructive thoughts.	1a. Administer medications with mouth checks.	1a. Addresses risk of hiding medications.	GOAL MET After 8 hours, client contracts for safety every shift and starts to discuss feelings of self-harm.
	1b. Provide ongoing surveillance of client and environment.	1b. Provides one-to-one monitoring for safety.	
	1c. Contract for "no self-harm" for specified periods.	1c. Encourages increased self-control.	
	1d. Use direct, nonjudgmental approach in discussing suicide.	1d. Shows acceptance of client's situation with respect.	
	1e. Provide illness teaching regarding PTSD.	1e. Offers reality of treatment.	
2. Client will express feelings by the third day of hospitalization.	2a. Interact with client at regular intervals to convey caring and openness and to provide an opportunity to talk.	2a. Encourages development of trust.	GOAL MET By second day, client occasionally answers questions about feelings and admits to anger and grief.
	2b. Use silence and listening to encourage expression of feelings.	2b. Shows positive expectation that client will respond.	
	2c. Be open to expressions of loneliness and powerlessness.	2c. Allows client to voice these uncomfortable feelings.	
	2d. Share observations or thoughts about client's behavior or response.	2d. Directs attention to here-and-now treatment situation.	
3. Client will express will to live by discharge from unit.	3a. Listen to expressions of grief.	3a. Supports client that such feelings are natural.	GOAL MET By third day, client becomes tearful and states that he does not want to hurt his wife and daughter.
	3b. Encourage client to identify own strengths and abilities.	3b. Affirms client's worth and potential to survive.	
	3c. Explore with client previous methods of dealing with life problems.	3c. Reinforces client's past coping skills and ability to problem-solve now.	
	3d. Assist in identifying available support systems.	3d. Addresses fact that anxiety has narrowed client's perspective, distorting reality about loved ones.	
	3e. Refer to spiritual advisor of individual's choice.	3e. Allows opportunity to explore spiritual values and self-worth.	

EVALUATION

See individual outcomes and evaluation within the care plan.

evolve Visit the Evolve website at **http://evolve.elsevier.com/Varcarolis** for a full case study of this client and more case studies and nursing care plans.

To the Instructor

The role of the health care provider continues to become more challenging as our health care system is compromised by increasing federal cuts, lack of trained personnel, and the dictates of Health Maintenance Organizations (HMOs) and Behavioral Health Maintenance Organizations (BHMOs). Our clients are from increasingly diverse cultural and religious backgrounds, bringing with them a wide spectrum of cultural and religious practices. To compound these complexities, we are living in an age of fast-paced research in neurobiology, genetics, and psychopharmacology, as well as research to find the most effective evidence-based approaches for clients and their families. Needless to add, the legal issues and ethical dilemmas faced by the health care system are magnified accordingly. Given these challenges, knowing how best to teach our students and/or serve our clients can seem overwhelming.

It is therefore with gratitude that I welcome the contributions of Verna Benner Carson and Nancy Shoemaker to bring to you, the reader, the most recent and comprehensive trends and evidence-based practices in psychiatric mental health nursing. Great effort has been made to keep the material comprehensible and reader friendly in the style of previous editions. It should also be evident throughout the text that an assessment and understanding of cultural, religious/spiritual, and social practices can be a cornerstone in the administration of appropriate and effective nursing care. Verna and Nancy bring a great deal of background and expertise, and I think the reader will find this fifth edition stronger and more comprehensive than ever.

Content New to This Edition

New content for the fifth edition includes the following:

- **Culturally relevant mental health nursing** (Chapter 7)
- **Psychiatric forensic nursing** (Chapter 31)

- Adult issues including **sleep disorders, attention deficit hyperactivity disorder**, and **sexual disorders** (Chapter 33)

The most current information in the field provides the foundation for the text:

- *DSM-IV-TR* (2000) taxonomy and criteria are used throughout.
- **Psychotropic drug information,** both new and updated, is found in all clinical chapters and on the Evolve website.
- **NANDA-approved nursing diagnoses** are used in all nursing process sections.
- **NIC/NOC classifications for interventions and for outcomes** are introduced in Chapter 9 and used throughout when appropriate.
- **Standards of Care** from *Scope and Standards of Psychiatric–Mental Health Nursing Practice* (2000) of the American Nurses Association, American Psychiatric Nurses Association, and International Society of Psychiatric–Mental Health Nurses are incorporated throughout and included opposite the inside back cover for easy reference.

New Features

While many familiar features are retained and updated, we have added the following to inform, heighten understanding, and engage the reader:

- **A Client Speaks** and **A Family Speaks** join *A Nurse Speaks* at the beginning of units to bring to life disorders and their effects on clients, families, and those who care for them. Clients describe their experiences living with a dual diagnosis (**obsessive compulsive disorder and cocaine dependence** in Unit Four and **bipolar disorder and alcohol dependence** in Unit Six), **major depressive disorder** (Unit Five), and **schizophrenia** (Unit Seven), and the daughter of a woman with **Alzheimer's disease** shares her story (Unit Eight).

- **Evidence-Based Practice** boxes demonstrate how research findings affect psychiatric nursing practice and standards of care.
- **Integrative Therapy** boxes discuss the increasing popularity and significance of complementary and alternative therapies.
- **Culturally Speaking** boxes reinforce the importance of culturally competent care.
- **Forensic Highlights** boxes help focus students on the nurse's role in dealing with sexual assault, family violence, and incarcerated persons and further develop student awareness in this expanding area.
- **Key Points to Remember** reinforce essential information in bulleted summaries at the end of each chapter.

Familiar Features with a New Perspective

The following features have been updated to reflect new knowledge and to introduce students to the clients they may encounter in psychiatric nursing and the nurses who care for them:

- **Mental health continuum** is a visual representation of the way in which psychobiological mental disorders are placed on a range from moderate to severe (anxiety, somatoform/dissociative, personality, and eating disorders) and from severe to psychotic (mood-depression and mania, schizophrenia, and other psychotic disorders and cognitive disorders).
- **Assessment Guidelines** are summary points for client assessment and are found at the end of each assessment step in the nursing process section of all clinical chapters.
- **Case Studies and Nursing Care Plans** in clinical chapters present individualized histories of clients with specific psychiatric disorders and corresponding care plans, helping the reader translate theory into practice. Additional nursing diagnoses for care plans in the book as well as additional case studies and nursing care plans are found on the Evolve website.
- **Vignettes** with a personal touch are brief, descriptive characterizations of clients with specific psychiatric disorders, to enhance the text discussion.
- **A Nurse Speaks** showcases nurses who speak from personal experience in their own practice to a variety of real issues that psychiatric nurses face in clinical practice. For example, a **psychiatric homecare nurse** describes a psychiatric emergency involving a client with dementia and a learning opportunity for the nursing staff of an assisted living facility (Unit Two). A nurse working in a psychiatric day treatment program discusses the importance and power of **therapeutic communication** (Unit Three). Another nurse dis-

cusses her experience as the leader in **group therapy** (Unit Nine). One of my favorites is a personal account of the **growth of psychiatry and the role of the psychiatric nurse** since the Korean War (Unit One).

- **Vibrant, full-color design** gives the book an open, spacious feeling, while incorporating a wealth of information.

Organization of the Text

Organized by units, chapters have been grouped to emphasize the clinical perspective and to facilitate locating information. All clinical chapters are organized in a clear, logical, and consistent format with nursing process as the strong, visible framework. Prevalence of disorders and comorbidity are included, because knowing that comorbid disorders are often part of the clinical picture of specific disorders helps students as well as clinicians understand how to better assess and treat their clients. The basic outline for clinical chapters is:

- Prevalence
- Comorbidity
- Theory
- Assessment
  Overall Assessment—Appropriate assessment for a specific disorder, including assessment tools and rating scales. The rating scales included help to highlight important areas in the assessment of a variety of behaviors or mental conditions. Because many of the answers are subjective in nature, experienced clinicians use these tools as a guide when planning care, in addition to their knowledge of their clients.
  Self-Assessment—Discusses the nurse's own thoughts and feelings that may need to be addressed to give maximum care to the client and enhance self-growth in the nurse.
  Assessment Guidelines—Summary of specific areas to assess by disorder.
- Nursing Diagnosis
- Outcome Criteria
- Planning
- Interventions
  Interventions follow the categories set by the *Scope and Standards of Psychiatric-Mental Health Care* (2000). Various interventions for each of the clinical disorders are chosen based on which of them most fit specific client needs. There are **Basic Interventions** (counseling, self-care, milieu therapy, health teaching, case management, psychobiological interventions, health promotion, and health maintenance) and **Advanced Practice Interventions** (psychotherapy, prescriptive authority, and treatment and consultation). **Alternative and Complementary Therapies** are included for specific disorders.
- Evaluation

Exciting Teaching Aids

Resources for instructors include a print **Instructor's Resource Manual**, an **Instructor's Electronic Resource** on CD-ROM, and **Evolve Resources** for faculty.

The **Instructor's Manual** includes an expansive Introduction with course preparation guidelines and teaching tips, and then by chapter, Objectives and Key Terms lists from the book, annotated Chapter Outlines, Thoughts About Teaching the Topic, and Concept Maps. **Lecture Slides** offer approximately 750 text and graphic slides including cartoons that characterize client behaviors. The **Test Bank** has over 1200 test items, complete with the correct answer, rationale, cognitive level of each question, corresponding stage of the nursing process, appropriate NCLEX label, and corresponding text page reference.

I am always grateful to the educators who send suggestions and provide feedback. I hope this fifth edition continues to help students learn and appreciate the wide range and scope of the practice of psychiatric mental health nursing.

Betsy Varcarolis

Contents

UNIT FIVE

PSYCHOBIOLOGICAL DISORDERS: SEVERE TO PSYCHOTIC, 324

A NURSE SPEAKS

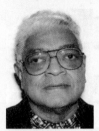

Fifty years ago psychiatry was practiced in an environment vastly different from the one in which it is practiced today. Most clients were treated in large state hospitals, which were like small towns with their own stores, restaurants, churches, farms, power plants, carpentry shops, and buildings housing thousands of clients and staff. There were buildings for admission and for treatment, infirmaries, chronic quiet units, and chronic disturbed units.

As nursing students, we were taught to care for clients who were receiving sedation, insulin shock, electric shock, malaria therapy, continuous hydrotherapy, wet packs, supraorbital lobotomies, physical restraints, and seclusion. All of these treatments were designed to make the clients more amenable to psychotherapy, to calm them, or for the safety of themselves or others. The disturbed wards were usually noisy and very active places in which clients acted out their psychoses both physically and vocally. Care for these clients was mostly custodial and involved keeping them clean, fed, safe, and calm.

I distinctly remember one client who was almost continuously kept in seclusion because of his bizarre and aggressive behavior. He would not keep his clothes on, could not safely use eating utensils, and roared like a lion. Because of his behavior, he was frequently referred to as the Lion Man.

Keeping him clean and fed was a major project for the staff and always required several people. It was a frustrating experience because we all wanted to help him and see him behave in a more acceptable manner.

During the Korean War, I was away in the Air Force for four years. For three years I was a part of a system that treated young men for psychiatric problems by using many of the same modalities that were used in the state hospitals. The treatment there was somewhat more successful than that provided in the state hospitals because most of the men's visible signs of psychoses were of recent origin, having been caused by the stress of basic training or the stress of being in battle.

During my fourth year in the Air Force, psychotropic drugs were introduced. We began to use them cautiously on our clients, with very limited success. As the doctors became more familiar with the drugs and increased the dosages, we saw much improved behavior in most clients. Gradually no clients were being put into packs, and the hydrotherapy room was seldom used.

After being discharged from the Air Force, I returned to the hospital in which I had trained. As I went to the different buildings, I was surprised to see that here too there had been a decrease in the use of the old treatment modalities. Clients for the most part appeared much calmer; no clients were in seclusion all of the time, not even the Lion Man.

One day, while I was walking on the grounds with one of the charge attendants, he asked me if I knew who a client sitting on a bench talking with another client was. I said, "No. Who is he?" "That is the guy we used to call the Lion Man." What a change! The attendant told me that they had given him Thorazine and that within one week he was out of seclusion and keeping his clothes on. Gradually he began to socialize with staff and other clients. Within one month he was playing checkers, and within one year he was granted ground privileges.

John A. Payne

John Payne died in April 2001 after a long illness.

FOUNDATIONS IN THEORY

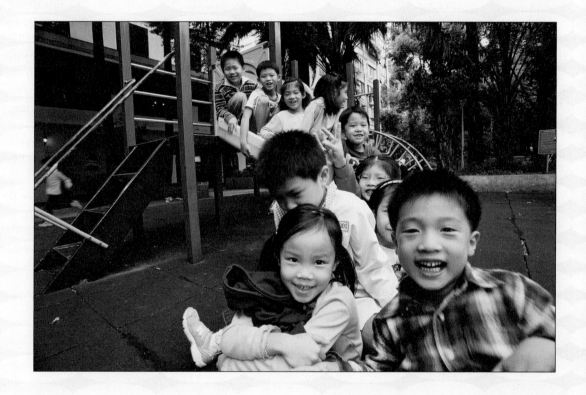

NOTHING GREAT WAS EVER ACHIEVED WITHOUT ENTHUSIASM.

Ralph Waldo Emerson

CHAPTER 1

Mental Health and Mental Illness

ELIZABETH M. VARCAROLIS ▪ JULIUS TRUBOWITZ

■ KEY TERMS and CONCEPTS

The key terms and concepts listed here appear in color where they are defined or first discussed in this chapter.

biologically based mental illnesses, 6

clinical epidemiology, 5

Diagnostic and Statistical Manual of Mental Disorders (DSM-IV-TR), 3

epidemiology, 4

mental disorders, 3

mental health, 2

mental illness, 2

myths and misconceptions (regarding mental illness), 3

prevalence rate, 6

psychiatry's definition of normal (mental health), 3

psychobiological disorder, 6

■ OBJECTIVES

After studying this chapter, the reader will be able to

1. Assess his or her own mental health using the seven signs of mental health identified in this chapter (Table 1-1 and Figure 1-1).
2. Summarize factors that can affect the mental health of an individual and the ways that these factors influence conducting a holistic nursing assessment.
3. Discuss some dynamic factors (including social climate, politics, myths, and biases) that contribute to making a clear-cut definition of mental health elusive.
4. Explain how epidemiological studies can improve medical and nursing care.
5. Demonstrate how the *DSM-IV-TR* multiaxial system can influence a clinician to consider a broad range of information before making a *DSM-IV-TR* diagnosis.
6. Compare and contrast a *DSM-IV-TR* diagnosis with a nursing diagnosis.
7. Give examples from his or her own culture of how consideration of norms and other cultural influences can affect making an accurate *DSM-IV-TR* diagnosis.

evolve Visit the Evolve website at **http://evolve.elsevier.com/Varcarolis** for a pretest on the content in this chapter.

Mental health is defined as successful performance of mental functions, resulting in the ability to engage in productive activities, enjoy fulfilling relationships, and change or cope with adversity. Mental health provides people with the capacity for rational thinking, communication skills, learning, emotional growth, resilience, and self-esteem (U.S. Department of Health and Human Services, 1999). Mental illness is considered a clinically significant behavioral or psychological syndrome experienced by a person and marked by distress, disability, or the risk of suffering disability or loss of freedom (American Psychiatric Association [APA], 2000). In the past, the term *mental illness* was applied to behaviors described as "strange" and "dif-

ferent" that occurred infrequently and deviated from an established norm. Such criteria are inadequate because they suggest that mental health is based on conformity. If such definitions were used, nonconformists and independent thinkers such as Abraham Lincoln, Mahatma Gandhi, and Socrates would be judged mentally ill. In addition, there is a further problem in viewing people whose behavior is "strange" or "different" as mentally ill. For example, the sacrifices of a Mother Teresa and the dedication of Martin Luther King, Jr., are uncommon, but none of us would consider these much-admired behaviors to be signs of mental illness.

This chapter discusses concepts of mental health and mental illness. You are introduced to the concept of mental disorders as medical diseases that can be identified along a mental health continuum. You will come to understand how mental disorders are categorized using the *Diagnostic and Statistical Manual of Mental Disorders (DSM-IV-TR)* (APA, 2000). The *DSM* is a manual that classifies mental disorders. The *DSM-IV-TR* (fourth edition, text revision) focuses on research and clinical observation when constructing diagnostic categories for a discrete mental disorder. The chapter describes how nursing diagnoses can be used to ensure appropriate care. Mental health and managed care are addressed, and the need to assess a person's ethnic background and culture before a valid diagnosis can be made is emphasized.

CONCEPTS OF MENTAL HEALTH AND ILLNESS

One approach to differentiating mental health from mental illness is based on what a particular culture regards as acceptable or unacceptable. In this view the mentally ill are those who violate social norms and thus threaten (or make anxious) those observing them. This definition seems partly true. For example, the callous psychopathic person fits the definition, as does the sometimes wild manic person and the schizophrenic person who is displaying strange behaviors. However, this definition explicitly makes mental illness a relative concept. Many forms of unusual behavior can be tolerated, depending on the prevailing cultural norms. The difficulty with defining mental illness through a particular behavior that is unacceptable to society is that it does not tell us what behavior a society should accept. Some totalitarian governments, to serve their own repressive goals, have classed all political dissidents as "mentally ill."

The field of mental illness is plagued by a host of myths and misconceptions. One myth is that to be mentally ill is to be different and odd. Another misconception is that to be healthy, a person must be logical and rational. All of us dream "irrational" dreams every night, and "irrational" emotions are not only universal human experiences but also essential to a fulfilling life. There are people who show extremely abnormal behavior and are characterized as mentally ill who are far more like the rest of us than different from us. There is no obvious and consistent line between mental illness and mental health. In fact, all human behavior lies somewhere along a continuum of mental health and mental illness.

Many psychiatrists still consider mental health, or normalcy, as the absence of psychopathology, but to many, mental health is far more than the absence of disease. Normal people may have medical deviation or disease, but as long as this does not impair their reasoning, judgment, intellectual capacity, and the ability to make harmonious personal and social adaptation, they may be regarded as psychically sound or normal (Sadock & Sadock, 2003).

Psychiatry's definition of normal (mental health) changes over time and reflects changes in cultural norms, society's expectations and values, professional biases, individual differences, and the political climate of the time (Sadock & Sadock, 2003). For example, criticisms have come from various groups who believe that they were or are stereotyped (and unfairly) in the psychiatric community. Their concerns include the way in which the psychiatric community places an emphasis on the group's psychopathology rather than on health attributes. The psychology of women and the issues surrounding homosexuality are two very important examples but are by no means the only ones. This topic is discussed in more detail in the section on the *DSM-IV-TR* axis system later in this chapter.

We are taught to evaluate our clients with mental health issues to identify their strengths and their areas of high functioning. You will find many attributes of mental health in some of your clients with mental health issues. It is these strengths that we build upon and encourage. By the same token, those who are "normal" or "mentally healthy" may have several areas of dysfunction at different times in their lives. We are all different, have different backgrounds (even siblings), and reflect different cultural influences even within the same subculture. We grow at different rates intellectually and emotionally, make different decisions at different times in our lives, choose or choose not to evaluate our behaviors and grow within ourselves, have deep-seated spiritual beliefs or not, and so on. Understandably, then, there can be no one definition of mental health that fits all. However, there are some traits that mentally healthy people share and that contribute to a better quality of life. Some of these traits of mentally healthy people are depicted in Figure 1-1.

The following comments of a 40-year-old woman illustrate the continuum between illness and health as her condition changes from (1) deep depression to (2) mania to (3) health:

1. It was horror and hell. I was at the bottom of the deepest and darkest pit there ever was. I was worthless and unforgivable. I was as good as—no, worse than—dead.
2. I was incredibly alive. I could sense and feel everything. I was sure I could do anything, accomplish any task, create whatever I wanted, if only other people wouldn't get in my way.
3. Yes, I am sometimes sad and sometimes happy and excited, but nothing as extreme as before. I am much more calm. I realize now that, when I was manic, it was a pressure-cooker feeling. When I am happy now, or loving, it is more peaceful and real. I have to admit that I some-

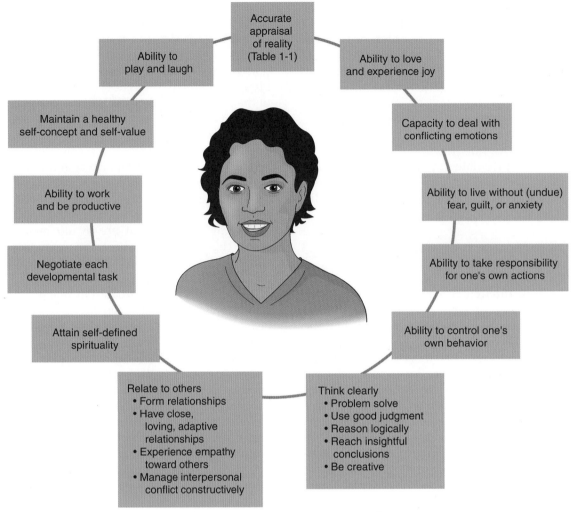

FIGURE 1-1 Some attributes of mental health.

times miss the intensity—the sense of power and creativity—of those manic times. I never miss anything about the depressed times, but of course the power and the creativity never bore fruit. Now I do get things done, some of the time, like most people. And people treat me much better now. I guess I must seem more real to them. I certainly seem more real to me. (Altrocchi, 1980)

Finally, many people think that mental illness is incurable or that mental health treatment is not successful. However, the success rates for the treatment of many common mental disorders equal or exceed the success rates for treatment of many other medical disorders (Goldberg, 1998). For example, people with panic disorder or bipolar disorder may have an 80% treatment success rate; those with major depression, a 60% to 80% rate; and those with schizophrenia, 60%. Contrast that with the success rates of various treatments for people who have cardiovascular disease (Goldberg, 1998):

- Arthrectomy—52%
- Angioplasty—41%

Table 1-1 compares some important aspects of mental health with those of specific mental disorders. These aspects include degree of (1) happiness, (2) control over behavior, (3) appraisal of reality, (4) effectiveness in work, (5) healthy self-concept, (6) satisfying relationships, and (7) effective coping strategies.

EPIDEMIOLOGY OF MENTAL DISORDERS

Applications of Epidemiology

Epidemiology is the quantitative study of the distribution of mental disorders in human populations. Once the distribution of mental disorders has been determined quantitatively, then epidemiologists can identify high-risk groups and high-risk factors. Study of these high-risk factors may lead to important clues about the etiology of various mental disorders.

The various applications of epidemiology are dependent on three levels of investigation (Sadock & Sadock, 2003):

TABLE 1-1

Mental Health Versus Mental Illness

Signs of Mental Health	Signs of Mental Illness
Happiness	**Major Depressive Episode**
A. Finds life enjoyable B. Can see in objects, people, and activities their possibilities for meeting his or her needs	A. Loses interest or pleasure in all or almost all usual activities and pastimes B. Describes mood as depressed, sad, hopeless, discouraged, "down in the dumps"
Control over Behavior	**Control Disorder, Undersocialized, Aggressive**
A. Can recognize and act on cues to existing limits B. Can respond to the rules, routines, and customs of any group to which he or she belongs	A. Shows repetitive and persistent pattern of aggressive conduct in which the basic rights of others are violated
Appraisal of Reality	**Schizophrenic Disorder**
A. Accurate picture of what is happening around the individual B. Good sense of the consequences, both good and bad, that will follow his or her acts C. Can see the difference between the "as if" and "for real" in situations	A. Shows bizarre delusions, such as delusions of being controlled B. Has auditory hallucinations C. Manifests delusions with persecutory or jealous content
Effectiveness in Work	**Adjustment Disorder with Work (or Academic) Inhibition**
A. Within limits set by abilities, can do well in tasks attempted B. When meeting mild failure, persists until determines whether or not he or she can do the job	A. Shows inhibition in work or academic functioning whereas previously there was adequate performance
A Healthy Self-Concept	**Dependent Personality Disorder**
A. Sees self as approaching individual ideals, as capable of meeting demands B. Has reasonable degree of self-confidence that helps in being resourceful under stress	A. Passively allows others to assume responsibility for major areas of life because of inability to function independently B. Lacks self-confidence (e.g., sees self as helpless, stupid)
Satisfying Relationships	**Borderline Personality Disorder**
A. Experiences satisfaction and stability in relationships B. Socially integrated and can rely on social supports	A. Shows pattern of unstable and intense interpersonal relationships B. Has chronic feelings of emptiness
Effective Coping Strategies	**Substance Dependencies**
A. Uses stress reduction strategies that address the problem, issue, threat (e.g., problem solving, cognitive restructuring) B. Uses coping strategies in a healthy way that does not cause harm to self or others	A. Repeatedly self-administers substances despite significant substance-related problems (e.g., threat to job, family, social relationships)

Modified from Redl F., & Wattenberg, W. (1959). *Mental hygiene in teaching* (pp. 198-201). New York: Harcourt, Brace & World; American Psychiatric Association. (2000). *Diagnostic and statistical manual of mental disorders* (4th ed., text rev.). Washington, DC: Author; and Farber, E. W., & Kaslow, F. W. (2003). Social psychology: Theory, research, and mental health implications. In A. Tasman, J. Kay, & J. A. Lieberman (Eds.). *Psychiatry* (2nd ed.). West Sussex, England: Wiley.

1. **Descriptive**—studies that produce basic estimates of the rates of disorder in a general population and its subgroups
2. **Analytic**—studies that explore the rates of variation in illness among different groups, to identify risk factors that may contribute to development of a disorder
3. **Experimental**—studies that test the presumed assumption between a risk factor and a disorder and seek to reduce the occurrence of the illness by controlling risk factors

Each level of investigation supplies information that can be used to improve clinical practice and plan public health policies.

Clinical epidemiology is a broad field that addresses what happens to people with illnesses who are seen by providers of clinical care. Studies use traditional epidemiological methods and are conducted in groups that are usually defined by illness or symptoms, or by diagnostic procedures or treatments given for the illness or symptoms. Clinical epidemiology includes the following:

- Studies of the natural history of an illness
- Studies of diagnostic screening tests
- Observational and experimental studies of interventions used to treat people with the illness or symptoms

Results of epidemiological studies are now routinely included in the *DSM-IV-TR* to describe the frequency of mental disorders. Analysis of epidemiological studies can assess the frequency with which symptoms appear together. For example, epidemiological studies demonstrated the significance of depression as a risk factor for death in people with cardiovascular disease and for premature death in people with breast cancer.

Prevalence

The prevalence rate is the proportion of a population with a mental disorder at a given time. The National Institute of Mental Health (NIMH) provides a summary of statistics describing the prevalence of mental disorders in the United States (NIMH, 2001). According to this summary an estimated 21.1% of Americans aged 18 and older—about one in five adults—suffer from a diagnosable mental disorder annually. When this percentage is applied to the 1998 U.S. Census residential population estimate, the figure translates into 44.3 million people. In addition, mental disorders—specifically major depression, schizophrenia, bipolar disorder, and obsessive-compulsive disorder—comprise 4 of the 10 leading causes of disability in the United States as well as in other developed countries. Many individuals have more than one mental disorder at a time.

Table 1-2 shows the prevalence of some psychiatric disorders in the United States.

MENTAL ILLNESS AND THE MENTAL HEALTH CONTINUUM

In 1996, the Mental Health Parity Act was passed by Congress. This legislation required insurers that provide mental health coverage to offer benefits at the same level provided for medical and surgical coverage. In 2000, the Government Accounting Office found that, although 86% of health plans complied with the 1996 law, 87% of health plans that complied with the law imposed new limits on mental health coverage. On April 29, 2002, President George W. Bush endorsed parity and established a new mental health commission. In February 2003, the Senator Paul Wellstone Mental Health Equitable Treatment Act was introduced into the Senate and the House of Representatives. In July 2003, the President's New Freedom Commission on Mental Health also endorsed parity. The legislation became stalled in Congress in 2003 and 2004 (National Mental Health Association, 2004). Passage of this legislation would require full insurance parity for the most severe, biologically based mental illnesses, that is, mental disorders caused by neurotransmitter dysfunction, abnormal brain structure, inherited genetic factors, or other biological causes. Another term for such an illness is psychobiological disorder. These biologically influenced illnesses include:

- Schizophrenia
- Bipolar disorder
- Major depression
- Obsessive-compulsive and panic disorders

- Posttraumatic stress disorder
- Autism

Other severe and disabling mental disorders include the following:

- Anorexia nervosa
- Attention deficit hyperactivity disorder

Thus, many (not necessarily all) of the most prevalent and disabling mental disorders have been found to have strong biological influences. Therefore, we can look at these disorders as "diseases." It is helpful to visualize these disorders along the mental health continuum. This continuum is used in each of the clinical chapters to identify the severity of the biologically influenced disorders. See Figure 1-2 for a conceptualization of biologically based disorders on the mental health continuum.

The *DSM-IV-TR* cautions that the emphasis on the term *mental disorder* implies a distinction between "mental" disease and "physical" disorder, which is an outdated concept, and stresses mind-body dualism: "there is much 'physical' in 'mental' disorders and much 'mental' in 'physical' disorders" (APA, 2000, p. xxx).

As nurses, we do not treat diseases; we care for people by providing effective nursing care using the nursing process as a guide. If we believe that human beings have biological, psychological, social, and spiritual components and needs, then we believe in holistic nursing. Our task as nurses is to assess and plan care for the whole individual under our care. Nurses and physicians are two parts of a multidisciplinary team that, when well coordinated, can provide optimal care for the biological, psychological, social, and spiritual needs of clients.

There are many factors that can affect the severity and progress of a mental health illness, biologically based or otherwise, and these same factors can affect a "normal" person's mental health as well. Some of these factors include available support systems, family influences, developmental events, cultural or subcultural beliefs and values, health practices, and negative influences impinging on an individual's life. If possible, these influences need to be evaluated and factored into an individual's plan of care. Figure 1-3 identifies some influences that can have an impact on a person's mental health. In fact, the *DSM-IV-TR* states that there is evidence suggesting that the symptoms and causes of a number of disorders listed in the *DSM-IV-TR* are influenced by cultural and ethnic factors (APA, 2000).

MEDICAL DIAGNOSIS AND NURSING DIAGNOSIS OF MENTAL ILLNESS

To carry out their professional responsibilities, clinicians and researchers need clear and accurate guidelines for identifying and categorizing mental illness.

TABLE 1-2

Prevalence of Psychiatric Disorders in the United States

Disorder	Prevalence over 12 Months (%)	Estimated No. of People Affected by Disorder in U.S.	
Schizophrenia	1.1	2.2 million	▪ Affects men and women equally ▪ May appear earlier in men than in women
Any affective (mood) disorder (includes major depression, dysthymic disorder, and bipolar disorder)	9.5	18.8 million	▪ Women affected 2 times more than men (12.4 million women, 6.4 million men) ▪ Depressive disorders may be appearing earlier in life in those born in recent decades compared to past ▪ Often co-occurs with anxiety and substance abuse
Major depressive disorder	5	9.9 million	▪ Leading cause of disability in U.S. and established economies worldwide ▪ Nearly twice as many women (6.5%) as men (3.3%) suffer from major depressive disorder every year
Bipolar affective disorder	1.2	2.3 million	▪ Affects men and women equally
Anxiety disorders (includes panic disorder, obsessive-compulsive disorder, posttraumatic stress disorder, generalized anxiety disorder, and phobias)	13.3	19.1 million	▪ Anxiety disorders frequently co-occur with depressive disorders, eating disorders, and/or substance abuse
Panic disorder	1.7	2.4 million	▪ Typically develops in adolescence or early adulthood ▪ About 1 in 3 people with panic disorder develops agoraphobia
Obsessive-compulsive disorder	2.3	3.3 million	▪ First symptoms begin in childhood or adolescence
Posttraumatic stress disorder (PTSD)	3.6	5.2 million	▪ Can develop at any time ▪ About 30% of Vietnam veterans experienced PTSD after the war; percentage high among first responders to 9/11/01 terrorist attacks on the U.S.
Generalized anxiety disorder	2.8	4.0 million	▪ Can begin across life cycle; risk is highest between childhood and middle age
Social phobia	3.7	5.3 million	▪ Typically begins in childhood or adolescence
Agoraphobia	2.2	3.2 million	
Specific phobia	4.4	6.3 million	
Any substance abuse	11.3		
Alcohol dependence	7.2		

Data from National Institute of Mental Health. (2001; updated April 2004). *The numbers count: Mental disorders in America* (NIH Publication No. 01-4584). Retrieved August 1, 2004, from http://www.nimh.nih.gov/publicat/numbers.cfm.

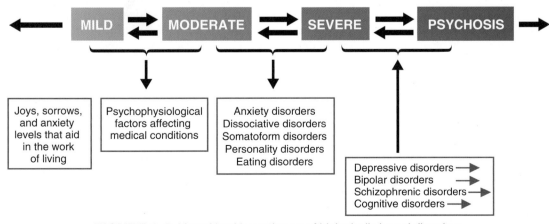

FIGURE 1-2 Mental health continuum of biologically based disorders.

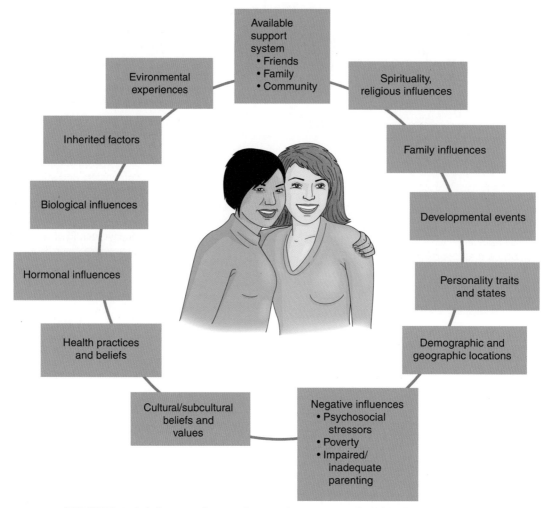

FIGURE 1-3 Influences that can have an impact on an individual's mental health.

Such guidelines help clinicians plan and evaluate treatment for their clients. A necessary element for categorization includes agreement regarding which behaviors constitute a mental illness.

Medical Diagnoses and the *DSM-IV-TR*

In the *DSM-IV-TR*, each of the mental disorders is conceptualized as a clinically significant behavioral or psychological syndrome or pattern that occurs in an individual and is associated with present **distress** (e.g., a painful symptom) or **disability** (i.e., impairment in one or more important areas of functioning) or with a significantly increased risk of suffering death, pain, disability, or an important loss of freedom (APA, 2000). This syndrome or pattern must not be merely an expected and culturally sanctioned response to a particular event, such as the death of a loved one. Whatever its original cause, it must currently be considered a manifestation of a behavioral, psychological, or biological dysfunction in the individual. Deviant behavior (e.g., political, religious, or sexual) and conflicts between the individual and society are not considered

mental disorders unless the deviance or conflict is a symptom of a dysfunction in the individual.

A common misconception is that a classification of mental disorders classifies *people* when actually the *DSM-IV-TR* classifies disorders that people have. For this reason, the text of the *DSM-IV-TR* avoids the use of expressions such as "a schizophrenic" or "an alcoholic" and instead uses the more accurate terms "an individual with schizophrenia" or "an individual with alcohol dependence."

Since the third edition of the *DSM* appeared in 1980, the criteria for classification of mental disorders have been sufficiently detailed for clinical, teaching, and research purposes. As an example, Box 1-1 shows the specific criteria provided by the *DSM-IV-TR* for the diagnosis of generalized anxiety disorder.

The *DSM-IV-TR* in Culturally Diverse Populations

Special efforts have been made in the *DSM-IV-TR* to incorporate an awareness that the manual is used in culturally diverse populations in the United States and internationally. Clinicians evaluate individuals from

DSM-IV-TR Criteria for Generalized Anxiety Disorder

A. Excessive anxiety and worry (apprehensive expectation), occurring more days than not for at least 6 months, about a number of events or activities (such as work or school performance).

B. The person finds it difficult to control the worry.

C. The anxiety and worry are associated with three (or more) of the following six symptoms (with at least some symptoms present for more days than not for the past 6 months). *Note:* Only one item is required in children.
   (1) Restlessness or feeling keyed up or on edge
   (2) Being easily fatigued
   (3) Difficulty concentrating or mind going blank
   (4) Irritability
   (5) Muscle tension
   (6) Sleep disturbance (difficulty falling or staying asleep; or restless, unsatisfying sleep)

D. The focus of the anxiety and worry is not confined to features of an Axis I disorder, for example, the anxiety or worry is not about having a panic attack (as in panic disorder), being embarrassed in public (as in social phobia), being contaminated (as in obsessive-compulsive disorder), being away from home or close relatives (as in separation anxiety disorder), gaining weight (as in anorexia nervosa), having multiple physical complaints (as in somatization disorder), or having a serious illness (as in hypochondriasis), and the anxiety and worry do not occur exclusively during posttraumatic stress disorder.

E. The anxiety, worry, or physical symptoms cause significant distress or impairment in social, occupational, or other important areas of functioning.

F. The disturbance is not due to the direct physiologic effects of a substance (e.g., a drug of abuse, a medication) or a general medical condition (e.g., hyperthyroidism) and does not occur exclusively during a mood disorder, a psychotic disorder, or a pervasive developmental disorder.

From American Psychiatric Association. (2000). *Diagnostic and statistical manual of disorders* (4th ed., text rev.). Washington, DC: Author.

numerous ethnic groups and cultural backgrounds (including many who are recent immigrants). Diagnostic assessment can be especially challenging when a clinician from one ethnic or cultural group uses the *DSM-IV-TR* classification to evaluate an individual from a different ethnic or cultural group. For example, among certain cultural groups, particular religious practices or beliefs (e.g., hearing or seeing a deceased relative during bereavement) may be misdiagnosed as manifestations of a psychotic disorder; furthermore, a syndrome often takes different superficial forms in different cultures. Also, people from minority or migrant populations may have good reason to be distrustful, and it should not be assumed that

these clients are suffering from paranoia or paranoid schizophrenia. Refer to Chapter 7 for more on culturally based syndromes.

The *DSM-IV-TR* Multiaxial System

The *DSM-IV-TR* axis system, by requiring judgments to be made on each of five axes, forces the diagnostician to consider a broad range of information (Table 1-3).

Axis I refers to the collection of signs and symptoms that together constitute a particular disorder, for example, schizophrenia, or a condition that may be a focus of treatment (refer to Appendix A for a list of all the mental disorders catalogued in the *DSM-IV-TR*). Axis II refers to personality disorders and mental retardation (refer to Chapters 16 and 32). Thus, axes I and II constitute the classification of abnormal behavior. Axes I and II were separated to ensure that the possible presence of long-term disturbance is considered when attention is directed to the current one. For example, a heroin addict would be diagnosed on axis I as having a substance-related disorder; this client might also have a long-standing antisocial personality disorder, which would be noted on axis II.

Although the remaining three axes are not needed to make the actual diagnosis, their inclusion in the *DSM-IV-TR* indicates the recognition that factors other than a person's symptoms should be considered in an assessment. On axis III the clinician indicates any general medical conditions believed to be relevant to the mental disorder in question. In some individuals, a physical disorder (e.g., a neurological dysfunction) may be the cause of the abnormal behavior, whereas in others, it may be an important factor in the individual's overall condition (e.g., diabetes in a child with a conduct disorder). Axis IV is for reporting psychosocial and environmental problems that may affect the diagnosis, treatment, and prognosis of a mental disorder. These may include occupational problems, educational problems, economic problems, interpersonal difficulties with family members, and a variety of problems in other life areas. Often a psychosocial assessment will uncover these (see Chapter 9). Finally, axis V, called Global Assessment of Functioning (GAF), gives an indication of the person's best level of psychological, social, and occupational functioning during the preceding year, rated on a scale of 1 to 100 (where 1 indicates persistent danger of severely hurting oneself or others, and 100 indicates superior functioning in a variety of activities at the time of the evaluation, as well as the highest level of functioning for at least a few months during the past year). Box 1-2 presents the GAF Scale. Table 1-4 illustrates how the multiaxial system of classification might be applied to a hypothetical case.

Caution must be exercised to avoid labeling or stereotyping when a medical diagnosis or a nursing diagnosis is being formulated. That every society has

TABLE 1-3

DSM-IV-TR Multiaxial System of Evaluation

Axis	Example
Axis I	
Clinical disorders	Major depressive disorder
Other conditions that may be a focus of clinical attention	
Axis II	
Personality disorders	Dependent personality disorder
Mental retardation	
Axis III	
General medical conditions	Diabetes
Axis IV	
Psychosocial and environmental problems	Divorce 3 months previously
Axis V	
Global Assessment of Functioning	31 years old and unable to work or respond to family and friends

From American Psychiatric Association. (2000). *Diagnostic and statistical manual of mental disorders* (4th ed., text rev.). Washington, DC: Author.

BOX 1-2

Global Assessment of Functioning (GAF) Scale

Consider psychological, social, and occupational functioning on a hypothetical continuum of mental health–mental illness. Do not include impairment in functioning due to physical (or environmental) limitations. *Note:* Use intermediate codes when appropriate (e.g., 45, 68, 72).

Code

100 | 91	**Superior functioning in a wide range of activities, life's problems never seem to get out of hand, is sought out by others because of his or her many positive qualities. No symptoms.**
90 | 81	**Absent or minimal symptoms** (e.g., mild anxiety before an exam), **good functioning in all areas, interested and involved in a wide range of activities, socially effective, generally satisfied with life, no more than everyday problems or concerns** (e.g., an occasional argument with family members).
80 | 71	**If symptoms are present, they are transient and expected reactions to psychosocial stressors** (e.g., difficulty concentrating after family argument); **no more than slight impairment in social, occupational, or school functioning** (e.g., temporarily falling behind in schoolwork).
70 | 61	**Some mild symptoms** (e.g., depressed mood and mild insomnia) **OR some difficulty in social, occupational, or school functioning** (e.g., occasional truancy, or theft within the household), **but generally functioning pretty well, has some meaningful interpersonal relationships.**
60 | 51	**Moderate symptoms** (e.g., flat affect and circumstantial speech, occasional panic attacks) **OR moderate difficulty in social, occupational, or school functioning** (e.g., few friends, conflicts with peers or co-workers).
50 | 41	**Serious symptoms** (e.g., suicidal ideation, severe obsessional rituals, frequent shoplifting) **OR any serious impairment in social, occupational, or school functioning** (e.g., no friends, unable to keep a job).
40 | 31	**Some impairment in reality testing or communication** (e.g., speech is at times illogical, obscure, or irrelevant) **OR major impairment in several areas, such as work or school, family relations, judgment, thinking, or mood** (e.g., depressed man avoids friends, neglects family, and is unable to work; child frequently beats up younger children, is defiant at home, and is failing at school).
30 | 21	**Behavior is considerably influenced by delusions or hallucinations OR serious impairment in communication or judgment** (e.g., sometimes incoherent, acts grossly inappropriately, suicidal preoccupation) **OR inability to function in almost all areas** (e.g., stays in bed all day; no job, home, or friends).
20 | 11	**Some danger of hurting self or others** (e.g., suicide attempts without clear expectation of death; frequently violent; manic excitement) **OR occasionally fails to maintain minimal personal hygiene** (e.g., smears feces) **OR gross impairment in communication** (e.g., largely incoherent or mute).
10 | 1	**Persistent danger of severely hurting self or others** (e.g., recurrent violence) **OR persistent inability to maintain minimal personal hygiene OR serious suicidal act with clear expectation of death.**
0	Inadequate information.

From American Psychiatric Association. (2000). *Diagnostic and statistical manual of mental disorders* (4th ed., text rev.). Washington, DC: Author.
The rating of overall psychological functioning on a scale of 0 to 100 was operationalized by Luborsky (1962) in the Health-Sickness Rating Scale. Spitzer and colleagues developed a revision of the Health-Sickness Rating Scale called the Global Assessment Scale (GAS) (Endicott et al., 1976). A modified version of the GAS was included in the *Diagnostic and statistical manual of mental disorders,* third edition, revised (American Psychiatric Association, 1987) as the Global Assessment of Functioning Scale.
This rating scale highlights important areas in the assessment of functioning. Because many of the judgments are subjective, experienced clinicians use this tool as a guide when planning care, and also draw on their knowledge of their clients.

TABLE 1-4

Clinical Example Demonstrating *DSM-IV-TR* Axes

DSM-IV-TR Axis	Clinical Example
Axis I	
Schizophrenic disorder, paranoid	For the past 9 months, Michael, a 33-year-old sales representative, has suffered delusions of grandeur and persecution. Believing himself to be a genius, he became convinced that another salesman in his firm was trying to kill him because the other man could not tolerate Michael's superiority. In the past 2 weeks, Michael has become certain that this other man has had a pale green gas pumped into his office through the air-conditioning ducts, but there is no objective evidence of such gas or any other malfunctioning of the air-conditioning system.
Axis II	
Paranoid traits, no personality disorder	Michael has always tended to be suspicious and distrustful of people. He looks constantly for evidence that others are trying to get the better of him or to harm him, and his manner is guarded. He has trouble relaxing, and others see him as cold and unemotional. He has no close friends and is considered a loner. He was extremely jealous of his wife, from whom he is now separated, and often accused her, falsely, of having affairs with other men.
Axis III	
Colitis	Michael sees a flare-up of his colitis (inflammation of the colon) as evidence that the salesman is poisoning him, even though Michael has had the same symptoms many times before.
Axis IV	
Psychosocial and environmental problems a. Marital separation b. Loss of work responsibility Rated severe	Michael left his wife 10 months ago. Two months ago, the president of Michael's firm reassigned one of Michael's important accounts to the salesman Michael now suspects of hostile intent. Michael thinks this was maneuvered by the other salesman, but in fact, the president acted because the quality of Michael's work was deteriorating. His work had slowed visibly, and coworkers complained that they could not perform their work properly when he was present.
Axis V	
Highest level of adaptive functioning in last year (GAF) Serious symptoms 45-50 Rated moderate to serious	Michael's functioning was adequate until he separated from his wife. At that point, he began to withdraw further from friends and acquaintances. He appeared to concentrate more on his job but actually spent his time checking and rechecking his work. When the firm's president reassigned his major account, Michael's work deteriorated further, and Michael began to air some of his suspicions about the partner who took over the account. When his colitis flared up 2 weeks ago, he requested an appointment with the president and accused the partner openly. Michael was fired.

GAF, Global Assessment of Functioning.
Adapted from Altrocchi, J. (1980). *Abnormal behavior.* New York: Harcourt Brace Jovanovich; American Psychiatric Association. (2000). *Diagnostic and statistical manual of mental disorders* (4th ed., text rev.). Washington, DC: Author.

its own view of health and illness and its own classification of diseases has long been observed by anthropologists, historians, and students of cross-cultural society (Klerman, 1986). The process of psychiatric labeling or stereotyping can have harmful effects on an individual and family, especially if the diagnosis was made on insufficient evidence and proves faulty.

An example of the influence of cultural and social bias on psychiatric diagnosis is the inclusion of homosexuality as a psychiatric disease in both the first and second editions of the *DSM.* All research consistently failed to demonstrate that people with a homosexual orientation were any more maladjusted than heterosexuals, but despite the research data, change occurred in the medical community only when gay rights activists advocated an end to discrimination against lesbians and gay men. No longer is homosexuality classified as a mental disorder. Instances of bias may involve

many other minority groups, including African Americans, elderly persons, children, and women. These biases are often reflected in our power structures and political systems. Awareness of the cultural bias and dangers in labeling and stereotyping has enormous implications for nursing practice, especially in the field of mental health, because nurses often take their cues from the medical structure.

Nursing Diagnoses and the *DSM-IV-TR*

Psychiatric mental health nursing includes the diagnosis and treatment of human responses to actual or potential mental health problems. The North American Nursing Diagnosis Association (NANDA) describes a nursing diagnosis as a clinical judgment about individual, family, or community responses to actual or potential health problems and life processes. Therefore, the *DSM-IV-TR* is used to diagnose a psychiatric disorder, whereas a well-defined nursing diagnosis provides the framework for identifying appropriate nursing interventions for dealing with the phenomena a client with a mental health disorder is experiencing, for example, hallucinations, low self-esteem issues, impaired ability to function (in job and family), and so on. Appendix C lists NANDA-approved nursing diagnoses. The individual clinical chapters offer suggestions for potential nursing diagnoses for the behaviors and phenomena often encountered in association with specific disorders. A more thorough discussion of nursing diagnoses in psychosocial nursing is found in Chapter 9.

INTRODUCTION TO CULTURE AND MENTAL ILLNESS

What should society do with George? Over the past 4 months, George has struck and injured several dozen people, most of whom he hardly knew. Two of them had to be sent to the hospital. George expresses no guilt, no regrets. He says he would attack every one of them again if he got the chance.

- Send him to jail?
- Commit him to a mental hospital?
- Give him an award for being the best defensive lineman in the league?

Before you can answer, you must know the context of George's behavior. Behavior that seems normal at a party might seem bizarre at a business meeting. Behavior that earns millions for a rock singer might earn a trip to the mental hospital for a college professor. Behavior that is perfectly routine in one culture might be considered criminal in another.

Even when we know the context of someone's behavior, we may wonder whether it is normal. Suppose your Aunt Tillie starts to pass out $5 bills to strangers on the street corner and vows that she will keep on doing so until she has exhausted her entire fortune. Is she mentally ill? Should the court commit her to a mental hospital and turn her fortune over to you as her trustee?

A man claims to be Jesus Christ and asks permission to appear before the United Nations to announce God's message to the world. A psychiatrist is sure that he can relieve this man of his disordered thinking by giving him antipsychotic drugs, but the man refuses to take them and insists that his thinking is normal. Should we force him to take the drugs, just ignore him, or put his address on the agenda of the United Nations?

In determining the mental health or mental illness of the individual, we must consider the norms and influence of culture. Throughout history, people (including us) have interpreted health or sickness according to their own current views. People in the Middle Ages, for example, regarded bizarre behavior as a sign that the disturbed person was possessed by a demon. To exorcise the demon, priests resorted to prescribed religious rituals. During the 1880s, when the "germ theory" of illness was popular, physicians interpreted bizarre behavior as stemming from biological causes. A striking example of how cultural change influences the interpretation of mental illness is the diagnosis of hysteria, which is much less common today than it was in the nineteenth century; according to some authors, this is because of a less restrictive family atmosphere, more permissive child rearing, and greater societal tolerance of sexual practices.

Cultures differ not only in their views regarding mental illness but also in the types of behavior categorized as mental illness. For example, one form of mental illness recognized in parts of Southeast Asia is **running amok,** in which someone (usually a male) runs around engaging in furious, almost indiscriminate violent behavior. **Pibloktoq** is an uncontrollable desire to tear off one's clothing and expose oneself to severe winter weather; it is a recognized form of psychological disorder in parts of Greenland, Alaska, and the Arctic regions of Canada. In our own society, we recognize **anorexia nervosa** as a psychobiological disorder that entails voluntary starvation. That disorder is well known in Europe, North America, and Australia, but unheard of in many other parts of the world.

What is to be made of the fact that certain disorders occur in some cultures but are absent in others? One interpretation is that the conditions necessary for causing a particular disorder occur in some places but are absent in other places. Another interpretation is that people learn certain kinds of abnormal behavior by imitation. However, the fact that some disorders may be culturally determined does not prove that all mental illnesses are so determined. The best evidence suggests that schizophrenia and bipolar affective disorders are found throughout the world. The symptom patterns of schizophrenia have been observed among indigenous Greenlanders and West African villagers, as well as in our own Western culture.

The *DSM-IV-TR* includes information specifically related to culture in three areas:

1. A discussion of cultural variations for each of the clinical disorders
2. A description of culture-bound syndromes
3. An outline designed to assist the clinician in evaluating and reporting the impact of the individual's cultural context

Refer to Chapter 7 for a discussion of the differing ways people view the world and a review of discrete cultural syndromes, and to Chapter 9 for a discussion of psychosocial assessment.

■■■ KEY POINTS to REMEMBER

- Mental illness is difficult to define, and people hold many myths regarding mental illness. There are many important aspects of mental health (e.g., happiness, control over behavior, appraisal of reality, effectiveness in work, a healthy self concept, presence of satisfying relationships, and effective coping strategies). Some components of mental health are identified in Figure 1-1.

- The study of epidemiology can help identify high-risk groups and behaviors. In turn, this can lead to a better understanding of the causes of some disorders. Prevalence rates help us identify the proportion of a population who have a mental disorder at a given time.

- With the current recognition that many common mental disorders are biologically based, it is easier to see how these biologically based disorders can be classified as medical disorders as well. Many of the more prevalent mental disorders are placed on a mental health continuum, which is used throughout the clinical chapters (see Figure 1-2).

- The reader is introduced to the *DSM-IV-TR,* the *DSM-IV-TR* multiaxial system, and the GAF Scale. The five axes of the *DSM-IV-TR* make it possible for clinicians to make a more holistic and realistic assessment of their clients, and thus allow for more comprehensive and appropriate interventions.

- Factors that may influence the intensity or cause of a mental illness, as well as affect normal individuals, are illustrated in Figure 1-3. The use of well-thought-out nursing diagnoses helps to target the symptoms and needs of clients so that clients may achieve a higher level of functioning and a better quality of life.

- Lastly, the influence of culture on behavior and the way in which symptoms may reflect a person's cultural patterns are discussed. At times, symptoms need to be understood in terms of a person's cultural background. Caution is recommended for all health care professionals concerning the damage and disservice that stereotyping can cause in the lives of clients in need of medical and mental health services. Lack of knowledge on the part of health care professionals about people from backgrounds and cultures other than our own can result in lack of services or delivery of inappropriate services to those under our care.

Critical Thinking and Chapter Review

Visit the Evolve website at **http://evolve.elsevier.com/Varcarolis** for additional self-study exercises.

■■■ CRITICAL THINKING

1. Timothy Harris is a college sophomore with a grade point average of 3.4. He is brought to the emergency department after a suicide attempt. He has been extremely depressed since the death of his girlfriend 5 months previously when the car he was driving careened out of control and crashed. Timothy's parents have been very distraught since the accident. To compound things, the parent's religious beliefs include the conviction that taking one's own life will prevent a person from going to heaven. Timothy has epilepsy and has had increased seizures since the accident; he refuses help because he says he should be punished for his carelessness and doesn't care what happens to him. He has not been to school and has not showed up for his part-time job of tutoring younger children in reading.

   A. Questions regarding Timothy and the use of the *DSM-IV-TR* multiaxial system

   (1) What might be a possible *DSM-IV-TR* diagnosis for axis I?

   (2) What information should be included on axis III?

   (3) What should be included on axis IV?

   (4) What score (range) might you give to Timothy on the GAF Scale?

   B. Mental health and mental illness

   (1) What are some factors that you would like to assess regarding aspects of Timothy's overall mental health and other influences that can affect mental health before you plan your care?

   (2) If an antidepressant medication could help him with his depression, explain why this alone would not meet his multiple needs. What issues do you think have to be addressed if Timothy is to receive a holistic approach to care?

   (3) Formulate at least two potential nursing diagnoses for Timothy.

   (4) Would Timothy's parents' religious beliefs factor into your plan of care? If so, how?

2. Using Table 1-1, evaluate yourself and one of your clients in terms of mental health.

3. In a small study group, share experiences you have had with others from unfamiliar cultural, ethnic, or racial backgrounds and identify two positive learning experiences from these encounters.

■■■ CHAPTER REVIEW

Choose the most appropriate answer.

1. Which statement about mental illness is true?

   1. Mental illness is a matter of individual nonconformity with societal norms.

   2. Mental illness is present when individual irrational and illogical behavior occurs.

   3. Mental illness changes with culture, time in history, political system, and group defining it.

   4. Mental illness is evaluated solely by considering individual control over behavior and appraisal of reality.

Continued

Critical Thinking and Chapter Review—cont'd

Visit the Evolve website at **http://evolve.elsevier.com/Varcarolis** for additional self-study exercises.

2. A nursing student new to psychiatric nursing asks a peer what resource he or she can use to figure out which symptoms are part of the picture of a specific psychiatric disorder. The best answer would be
   1. Nursing Interventions Classification (NIC).
   2. Nursing Outcomes Classification (NOC).
   3. NANDA nursing diagnoses.
   4. *DSM-IV-TR.*

3. Why is it important for the nurse to be aware of the multiple factors that can influence an individual's mental health?
   1. Rates of illness differ among various groups.
   2. The *DSM-IV-TR* cannot be used without this information.
   3. A holistic nursing assessment requires this awareness.
   4. The nurse must contribute this data for epidemiological research.

4. Epidemiological studies contribute to improvements in care for individuals with mental disorders by
   1. providing information about effective nursing techniques.
   2. identifying risk factors that contribute to the development of a disorder.
   3. identifying who in the general population will develop a specific disorder.
   4. identifying which individuals will respond favorably to a specific treatment.

5. Which statement best describes a major difference between a *DSM-IV-TR* diagnosis and a nursing diagnosis?
   1. There is no functional difference between the two. Both serve to identify a human deviance.
   2. The *DSM-IV-TR* diagnosis disregards culture, whereas the nursing diagnosis takes culture into account.
   3. The *DSM-IV-TR* is associated with present distress or disability, whereas a nursing diagnosis considers past and present responses to actual mental health problems.
   4. The *DSM-IV-TR* diagnosis impacts the choice of medical treatment, whereas the nursing diagnosis offers a framework for identifying interventions for phenomena a client is experiencing.

Visit the Evolve website at **http://evolve.elsevier.com/Varcarolis** for a posttest on the content in this chapter.

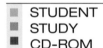

- STUDENT
- STUDY
- CD-ROM

Access the accompanying CD-ROM for animations, interactive exercises, review questions for the NCLEX® examination, and an audio glossary.

REFERENCES

Altrocchi, J. (1980). *Abnormal behavior.* New York: Harcourt Brace Jovanovich.

American Psychiatric Association. (2000). *Diagnostic and statistical manual of mental disorders (DSM-IV-TR)* (4th ed., text rev.). Washington, DC: Author.

Endicott J, et al. (1976). The global assessment scale: A procedure for measuring overall severity of psychiatric disturbance. *Archives of General Psychiatry, 33,* 766-771.

Goldberg, R. J. (1998). *Practical guide to the care of the psychiatric patient* (2nd ed.). St. Louis, MO: Mosby.

Klerman, G. L. (1986). *Contemporary directions in psychopathology: Toward the DSM-IV.* New York: Guilford Press.

Luborsky, L. (1962). Clinicians' judgments of mental health. *Archives of General Psychiatry, 7,* 407-417.

National Institute of Mental Health. (2001; updated April 2004). *The numbers count: Mental disorders in America* (NIH Publication No. 01-4584). Retrieved August 1, 2004, from http://www.nimh.nih.gov/publicat/numbers.cfm.

National Mental Health Association. (2004). *Congress must pass mental health parity now.* Retrieved July 31, 2004, from http://www.nmha.org/federal/parity/parityfactsheet.cfm.

Sadock, B. J., & Sadock, V. A. (2003). *Kaplan and Sadock's synopsis of psychiatry* (9th ed.). Philadelphia: Lippincott Williams & Wilkins.

U.S. Department of Health and Human Services. (1999). *Mental health: A report of the Surgeon General.* Rockville, MD: U.S. Department of Health and Human Services, Center for Mental Health Services, National Institutes of Health.

CHAPTER 2

Relevant Theories and Therapies for Nursing Practice

VERNA BENNER CARSON ■ JULIUS TRUBOWITZ

■ KEY TERMS and CONCEPTS

The key terms and concepts listed here appear in color where they are defined or first discussed in this chapter.

aversion therapy, 29

behavioral therapy, 27

cognitive therapy, 26

conditioning, 21

conscious, 16

countertransference, 25

defense mechanisms, 17

ego, 17

id, 16

interpersonal psychotherapy (IPT), 26

milieu therapy, 30

modeling, 27

operant conditioning, 22

positive reinforcement, 22

preconscious, 16

psychodynamic psychotherapy, 25

reinforcer, 22

security operations, 18

short-term dynamic psychotherapy, 26

superego, 17

systematic desensitization, 29

transference, 25

unconscious, 16

■ OBJECTIVES

After studying this chapter, the reader will be able to

1. Compare and contrast the developmental stages defined by Freud and Erikson.
2. Evaluate the premises behind the various therapeutic models discussed in this chapter.
3. Identify ways that each theorist contributes to the nurse's ability to assess a client's behaviors.
4. Drawing on clinical experience, provide the following:
   a. An example of how a client's irrational beliefs influenced behavior.
   b. An example of countertransference in your relationship with a client.
   c. An example of the use of behavior modification with a client.
5. Identify Peplau's expectation of the nurse-patient relationship.
6. Clarify the difference between the art and the science of nursing.
7. Choose the one therapeutic model that would be most useful, if there were an issue that needed to be resolved.

---

evolve Visit the Evolve website at **http://evolve.elsevier.com/Varcarolis** for a pretest on the content in this chapter.

As important as it is to approach clients with kindness, compassion, and concern, it is just as important to have a structured approach to care. Theory provides us with that structure. Psychiatric mental health nursing uses many theories drawn from a variety of disciplines. We take relevant ideas and concepts from psychology, psychiatry, medicine, sociology, neurology,

philosophy, and of course our own theoretical base of nursing. No one theory offers us everything that we need to understand the lives of our clients.

Our clients challenge us to understand stories that are complex and always unique. We do well to have a broad base of knowledge about personality development, human needs, the ingredients of mental health, the contributing factors to mental illness, and the importance of relationships.

This chapter provides snapshot views of some of the most influential theorists and the contributions they have made to our current state of understanding as well as our practice of psychiatric mental health nursing. We begin our theoretical journey with a look at Sigmund Freud, often referred to as the "father of psychoanalysis." We travel on with a look at Harry Stack Sullivan and Erik Erickson, who initially were devotees of Freud but found Freudian theory lacking and so took divergent paths. Next on our theoretical exploration is Abraham Maslow, who is our representative theorist from the humanistic approach to psychiatry. We continue on with a look at Ivan Pavlov, John B. Watson, and B. F Skinner as representatives of a behaviorist approach. Before we consider nursing theories, we take a brief detour to look at the medical-biological theories. Each of these theoretical approaches is evaluated for its relevance to psychiatric mental health nursing. We end our theoretical journey with an examination of nursing theorists, with a focus on Hildegard Peplau. Next we examine a variety of therapeutic approaches and again look at the value of these approaches to nursing. Let's begin the journey!

MAJOR THEORIES OF PERSONALITY

Psychodynamic Theories

Freud's Psychoanalytic Theory

Sigmund Freud (1856-1939) revolutionized thinking about mental health disorders with his groundbreaking theory of personality structure, levels of awareness, anxiety, the role of defense mechanisms, and the stages of psychosexual development, as well as his insistence on psychological treatment of behavioral symptoms. He believed that the vast majority of mental disorders were due to unresolved issues that originated in childhood. He arrived at this conclusion from his experiences in treating people with hysteria—individuals who were suffering physical symptoms despite the absence of a physiological cause.

As part of treatment, Freud initially used hypnosis, but this provided mixed therapeutic results. He then changed his approach to talk therapy, known as the cathartic method. Today we refer to catharsis as "getting things off of our chests." Talk therapy evolved to include "free association," which requires full and honest disclosure of thoughts and feelings as they come to mind. Freud (1961, 1969) concluded that talking about difficult emotional issues had the potential to heal the wounds of mental illness. Viewing the success of these therapeutic approaches led Freud to construct his theory.

Levels of Awareness. Through the use of talk therapy and free association, Freud (1969) came to believe that there were different levels of psychological awareness in operation. He offered a topographic theory of how the mind functions—a description, if you will, of the landscape of the mind. He used the image of an iceberg to describe three levels of awareness (Figure 2-1).

Conscious. Freud described the conscious part of the mind as the tip of the iceberg. It contains all of the material that the person is aware of at any one time.

Preconscious. Just below the surface of awareness is the preconscious, which contains material that can be retrieved rather easily through conscious effort.

Unconscious. The unconscious includes all repressed memories, passions, and unacceptable urges lying deep below the surface. The unconscious exerts a powerful yet unseen effect on the conscious thoughts and feelings of the individual. The individual is usually unable to retrieve unconscious material without the assistance of a trained therapist; however, with this assistance, unconscious material can be brought into conscious awareness.

Personality Structure. Freud (1960) delineated three major and distinct but interactive systems of the personality: the id, the ego, and the superego.

Id. At birth we are all id. The id is the source of all drives, instincts, reflexes, needs, genetic inheritance, and capacity to respond, as well as all the wishes that motivate us. The id cannot tolerate frustration and seeks to discharge tension and return to a more comfortable level of energy. The id lacks the ability to problem solve; it is not logical and operates according to the pleasure principle. The pleasure principle works to discharge tension through one of two mechanisms: reflex action and primary process. Reflex action is inherent and automatic. We are equipped with many reflexes, including gagging, crying, and laughing. Each of these successfully alleviates certain forms of tension.

Not all tension can be relieved through reflex action. This is especially true of psychic or emotional tension, usually called *anxiety*. In these cases the id employs the primary processes to diminish tension by creating an image of the object that would rectify the

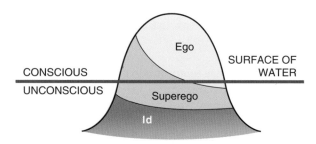

FIGURE 2-1 The mind as an iceberg.

uncomfortable situation. For example, the mirages of water that people see in the desert enable them to experience in their minds the reality of plentiful water. Freud referred to this process as wish fulfillment. It is obvious that primary processes and wish fulfillment offer only temporary relief from tension. In the example given here, the thirsty individual cannot drink imaginary water. The outside environment must be considered, and the id is not able to do so. This is where the ego enters the picture.

Ego. The ego develops because the needs, wishes, and demands of the id cannot be satisfactorily met through primary processes and reflex action. The ego, which emerges sometime in the fourth or fifth month of life, is the problem solver and reality tester. The ego is able to differentiate subjective experiences, memory images, and objective reality, and attempts to negotiate a solution with the outside world. The ego follows the reality principle, which says to the id, "You have to delay gratification for right now." The ego uses secondary processes to plan a course of action and to test this action in an effort to validate the plan. For example, the hungry man feels tension arising from the id. His ego allows him not only to think about his hunger but to plan where he can eat and allows him to seek that destination. This process is known as reality testing because the individual is factoring in reality to implement a plan to decrease tension. It is the ego that coordinates expression of self and is the mediator of various demands from the id, superego, and reality.

Superego. The superego, the last portion of the personality to develop, represents the moral component of personality. The superego consists of the conscience, which is all the "should nots" internalized from parents, and the ego ideal, which is all the "shoulds" internalized from parents. The superego represents the ideal rather than the real; it seeks perfection as opposed to seeking pleasure or engaging reason.

In a mature and well-adjusted individual, the three systems of the personality—the id, the ego, and the superego—work together as a team under the administrative leadership of the ego. If the id is too powerful, the person will lack control over impulses; if the superego is too powerful, the person may be self-critical and suffer from feelings of inferiority.

Defense Mechanisms and Anxiety. Freud (1969) believed that anxiety is an inevitable part of living. The environment we live in presents dangers and insecurities, threats and satisfactions. It can produce pain and increase tension or produce pleasure and decrease tension. The ego develops defenses, or defense mechanisms, to ward off anxiety by preventing conscious awareness of threatening feelings.

Defense mechanisms share two common features: (1) they all (except suppression) operate on an unconscious level, so that we are not aware of their operation; and (2) they deny, falsify, or distort reality to make it less threatening. Although we cannot survive without defense mechanisms, it is possible for our defense mechanisms to distort reality to such a degree that we experience difficulty with healthy adjustment and personal growth (see Chapters 13 and 14 for further discussions of defense mechanisms).

Psychosexual Stages of Development. Freud believed that human development proceeds through five stages from infancy to adulthood. His main focus, however, was on what happens during the first 5 years of life. From Freud's perspective experiences during the early stages determine an individual's lifetime adjustment patterns and personality traits. In fact, Freud thought that personality was formed by the time the child entered school and that subsequent growth consisted of elaborating on this basic structure. Freud's psychosexual stages of development are presented in Table 2-1.

Implications for Psychiatric Mental Health Nursing. Freud's theory has relevance to psychiatric nursing practice at many junctures. First, the theory offers a comprehensive explanation of complex human processes and suggests that the formation of a client's personality is influenced by many diverse sources rooted in past events. Freud's theory of the unconscious is particularly valuable as a baseline for considering the complexity of human behavior. By considering conscious and unconscious influences, a nurse can identify and begin to think about the root causes of client suffering. Freud emphasized the importance of individual talk sessions characterized by attentive listening with a focus on underlying themes as an important tool of healing in psychiatric care.

Sullivan's Interpersonal Theory

Harry Stack Sullivan (1892-1949), an American-born psychiatrist, initially approached patients from a Freudian framework, but he became frustrated by dealing with what he considered unseen and private mental processes within the individual. He turned his attention to interpersonal processes that could be observed in a social framework. Sullivan (1953) defined personality as behavior that can be observed within interpersonal relationships. This premise lead to the development of his interpersonal theory.

According to Sullivan the purpose of all behavior is to get needs met through interpersonal interactions and decrease or avoid anxiety. He viewed anxiety as a key concept and defined it as any painful feeling or emotion arising from social insecurity or blocks to getting biological needs satisfied. Sullivan coined the term *security operations* to describe those measures that

TABLE 2-1

Freud's Psychosexual Stages of Development

Stage (Age)	Source of Satisfaction	Primary Conflict	Tasks	Desired Outcomes	Other Possible Personality Traits
Oral (0-1 yr)	Mouth (sucking, biting, chewing)	Weaning	Mastery of gratification of oral needs; **beginning of ego development** (4-5 mo)	Development of trust in the environment with the realization that needs can be met	Fixation at the oral stage is associated with passivity, gullibility, and dependence; the use of sarcasm; and the development of orally focused habits (e.g., smoking, nail-biting).
Anal (1-3 yr)	Anal region (expulsion and retention of feces)	Toilet training	Beginning of development of a sense of control over instinctual drives; **ability to delay immediate gratification** to gain a future goal	Control over impulses	Fixation at the anal stage is associated with anal retentiveness (stinginess, rigid thought patterns, obsessive-compulsive disorder) or anal expulsive character (messiness, destructiveness, cruelty).
Phallic (oedipal) (3-6 yr)	Genitals (masturbation)	Oedipus and Electra	Sexual identity with parent of same sex; **beginning of superego development**	Identification with parent of the same sex	Lack of successful resolution may result in difficulties with sexual identity and difficulties with authority figures.
Latency (6-12 yr)	—	—	**Growth of ego functions** (social, intellectual, mechanical) and the ability to care about and relate to others outside the home (peers of the same sex)	The development of skills needed to cope with the environment	Fixations can result in difficulty in identifying with others and in developing social skills, leading to a sense of inadequacy and inferiority.
Genital (12 yr and beyond)	Genitals (sexual intercourse)	—	**Development of satisfying** sexual and emotional **relationships** with members of the opposite sex; **emancipation from parents—planning of life goals** and development of a strong **sense of personal identity**	The ability to be creative and find pleasure in love and work	Inability to negotiate this stage could result in difficulties in becoming emotionally and financially independent, lack of strong personal identity and future goals, and inability to form satisfying intimate relationships.

Data from Gleitman, H. (1981). *Psychology.* New York: W. W. Norton.

the individual employs to reduce anxiety and enhance security. Collectively, all of the security operations an individual uses to defend himself or herself against anxiety and ensure self-esteem make up the self-system.

There are many parallels between Sullivan's notion of security operations and Freud's concept of defense mechanisms. Both are processes of which we are unaware, and both are ways in which we reduce anxiety. However, Freud's defense mechanism of repression is an intrapsychic activity, whereas Sullivan's security operations are interpersonal relationship activities that can be observed.

Implications for Psychiatric Mental Health Nursing. Sullivan's theory is the foundation for Hildegard Peplau's nursing theory of interpersonal relationships that we examine later in this chapter. Sullivan believed that therapy should educate patients and assist them in gaining personal insight. Sullivan first used the term *participant observer,* which indicates that professional helpers cannot be isolated from the therapeutic situation if they are to be effective. Sullivan would insist that the nurse interact with the patient as an authentic human being. Mutuality, respect for the patient, unconditional acceptance, and empathy, which are considered essential aspects of modern therapeutic relationships, were important aspects of Sullivan's theory of interpersonal therapy.

Sullivan also demonstrated that a psychotherapeutic environment, characterized by an accepting atmosphere that provided numerous opportunities for practicing interpersonal skills and developing relationships, is an invaluable treatment tool. Group psychotherapy, family therapy, and educational and skill training programs as well as unstructured periods can be incorporated into the design of a psychotherapeutic environment to facilitate healthy interactions. This method is used today in virtually all residential and day hospital settings.

Erikson's Ego Theory

Erik Erikson (1902-1994), an American psychoanalyst, was also a follower of Freud. However, Erikson (1950) believed that Freudian theory was restrictive and negative. Erikson placed greater emphasis on the role of the ego. He also stressed that an individual's development is influenced by more than the limited mother-child-father triangle and that culture and society exert significant influence on personality. Erikson created a developmental model that (1) spans the full life cycle, and (2) allows for corrective emotional experiences beyond the first 5 years. He did not believe that personality was set in stone by 5 years of age but rather felt that personality continued to develop through old age. Erikson studied healthy personalities, emphasizing strengths as well as weaknesses and pointing out that failures at one stage could be rectified by successes at later stages. Table 2-2 lists the major stages in the life cycle as described by Erikson.

Implications for Psychiatric Mental Health Nursing. Nurses use Erikson's developmental model as an important part of patient assessment. Analysis of behavior patterns using Erikson's framework can identify age-appropriate or arrested development of normal interpersonal skills. A developmental framework helps the nurse know what types of interventions are most likely to be effective. For exam-

TABLE 2-2

Erikson's Eight Stages of Development

Approximate Age	Developmental Task	Psychosocial Crisis	Successful Resolution of Crisis	Unsuccessful Resolution of Crisis
Infancy (0-1½ yr)	Forming attachment to mother, which lays foundations for later trust in others	Trust vs. mistrust	Sound basis for relating to other people; trust in people; faith and hope about environment and future	General difficulties relating to people effectively; suspicion; trust-fear conflict; fear of future
Early childhood (1½-3 yr)	Gaining some basic control of self and environment (e.g., toilet training, exploration)	Autonomy vs. shame and doubt	Sense of self-control and adequacy; will power	Independence-fear conflict; severe feelings of self-doubt
Late childhood (3-6 yr)	Becoming purposeful and directive	Initiative vs. guilt	Ability to initiate one's own activities; sense of purpose	Aggression-fear conflict; sense of inadequacy or guilt
School age (6-12 yr)	Developing social, physical, and school skills	Industry vs. inferiority	Competence; ability to work	Sense of inferiority; difficulty learning and working
Adolescence (12-20 yr)	Making transition from childhood to adulthood; developing sense of identity	Identity vs. role confusion	Sense of personal identity; fidelity	Confusion about who one is; submersion of identity in relationships or group memberships
Early adulthood (20-35 yr)	Establishing intimate bonds of love and friendship	Intimacy vs. isolation	Ability to love deeply and commit oneself	Emotional isolation; egocentricity
Middle adulthood (35-65 yr)	Fulfilling life goals that involve family, career, and society; developing concerns that embrace future generations	Generativity vs. self-absorption	Ability to give and to care for others	Self-absorption; inability to grow as a person
Later years (65 yr to death)	Looking back over one's life and accepting its meaning	Integrity vs. despair	Sense of integrity and fulfillment; willingness to face death; wisdom	Dissatisfaction with life; denial of or despair over prospect of death

Data from Erikson, E. H. (1963). *Childhood and society.* New York: W. W. Norton; and Altrocchi, J. (1980). *Abnormal psychology* (p. 196). New York: Harcourt Brace Jovanovich.

ple, children in Erikson's initiative-versus-guilt stage of development respond best if they actively participate and ask questions. Elderly patients respond to a life review strategy that focuses on the integrity of their life as a tapestry of experience. In the therapeutic encounter, individual responsibility and the capacity for improving one's functioning are addressed. Treatment approaches and interventions can be tailored to the patient's developmental level.

Humanistic Theories

Humanistic theories developed as a negative reaction to the psychoanalytic school of thought. These theories focus on human potential and the possibility of choosing life patterns supportive of personal growth. Humanistic frameworks emphasize a person's capacity for self-actualization. This approach focuses on understanding the client's perspective as she or he subjectively experiences it. There are a number of humanistic theorists. Our journey will stop to explore Abraham Maslow and his theory of self-actualization.

Maslow's Humanistic Psychology Theory

Abraham Maslow (1908-1970), considered the father of humanistic psychology, introduced the concept of a "self-actualized personality," associated with high productivity and enjoyment of life (Maslow, 1963, 1968). He criticized psychology for focusing too intently on humanity's frailties and not enough on its strengths. Maslow contended that the focus of psychology must go beyond experiences of hate, pain, misery, guilt, and conflict to include love, compassion, happiness, exhilaration, and well-being.

Hierarchy of Needs. Maslow conceptualized human motivation as a hierarchy of dynamic processes or needs that are critical for the development of all humans. Central to his theory is the assumption that humans are active rather than passive participants in life, striving for self-actualization. Maslow (1968) focused on human need fulfillment, which he categorized into six incremental stages, beginning with physiological survival needs and ending with self-transcendent needs (Figure 2-2). Although these needs are present in all humans, the behaviors that emanate from them differ according to a person's individual biological makeup and environmental factors. Maslow described basic needs as "D-motives" or "deficiency needs," meaning that they are so basic to existence that they must be resolved to reduce the tension associated with them. These needs have the greatest strength and must be satisfied before a person turns attention to higher-level needs. For example, a homeless person is not going to be interested in a support group to get in touch

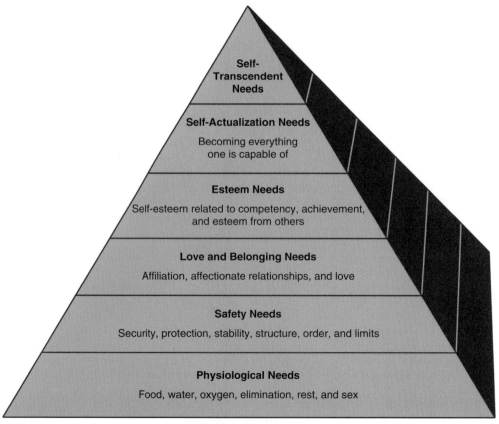

FIGURE 2-2 Maslow's hierarchy of needs. (Adapted from Maslow, A. H. [1972]. *The farther reaches of human nature*. New York: Viking.)

with his or her feelings if issues of basic survival remain unresolved. Maslow described self-esteem and self-actualization as "B-motives" or "being needs," reflective of growth motivation.

Maslow based his theory on the results of clinical investigations of people who represented self-actualized individuals; they moved in the direction of achieving and reaching their highest potentials. Some of those Maslow chose to investigate were historical figures such as Abraham Lincoln, Thomas Jefferson, Harriet Tubman, Walt Whitman, Beethoven, William James, and Franklin D. Roosevelt, whereas others like Albert Einstein, Eleanor Roosevelt, and Albert Schweitzer were living at the time they were studied. This investigation led Maslow (1963, 1970) to identify some basic personality characteristics that distinguished self-actualizing people from what might be called ordinary people (Box 2-1).

Implications for Psychiatric Mental Health Nursing. The value of Maslow's model in nursing practice is twofold. First, an emphasis on human potential and the client's strengths is key to successful nurse-client relationships. The second value of the model is that it helps to establish what is most impor-

tant in the sequencing of nursing actions in the nurse-client relationship. For example, to collect any but the most essential information when a client is struggling with drug withdrawal is inappropriate. Following Maslow's model as a way of prioritizing actions, the nurse meets the client's physiological need for stabilizing vital signs and pain relief before collecting general information for a nursing database.

Behavioral Theories

Behavioral theories also developed as a protest response to Freud's assumption that a person's destiny was carved in stone at a very early age. Behavioral models posit that personality consists of learned behaviors. Consequently, personality becomes synonymous with behavior—if behavior changes, so does the personality.

The development of behavioral models began in the nineteenth century as a result of Ivan Pavlov's laboratory work with dogs and continued into the twentieth century with John B. Watson's application of these models to shape behavior and B. F. Skinner's research on rat behavior. These behavioral theorists developed systematic learning principles that could be applied to humans. Behavioral models emphasize the ways in which observable behavioral responses are learned and can be modified in a particular environment. Pavlov's, Watson's, and Skinner's models focus on the belief that behavior can be influenced through a process referred to as conditioning. Conditioning involves pairing a behavior with a condition that reinforces or diminishes the behavior's occurrence.

Pavlov's Classic Conditioning Theory

Ivan Pavlov (1849-1936) was a Russian physiologist. He won the Nobel Prize for his outstanding contributions to the physiology of digestion, which he studied through his well-known experiments with dogs. In incidental observation of the dogs, Pavlov noticed that the dogs were able to anticipate when food would be forthcoming and would begin to salivate even before actually tasting the meat. Pavlov labeled this process *psychic secretion*. He hypothesized that the psychic component was a learned association between two events: the presence of the experimental apparatus and the serving of meat.

Pavlov formalized his observations of behaviors in dogs in a theory of **classical conditioning.** Pavlov (1928) found that when a neutral stimulus (a bell) was repeatedly paired with another stimulus (food that triggered salivation), eventually the sound of the bell alone could elicit salivation in dogs. From this he developed the concept of stimulus-response or respondent conditioning. Classical conditioning is sometimes referred to as respondent conditioning because the subject responds and is basically a passive agent. Although Pavlov (1928) considered his scientific ob-

---

BOX 2-1

Some Characteristics of Self-Actualized Persons

- Accurate perception of reality. Not defensive in their perceptions of the world.
- Acceptance of themselves, others, and nature.
- Spontaneity, simplicity, and naturalness. Self-actualized individuals (SAs) do not live programmed lives.
- Problem-centered rather than self-centered orientation. Possibly the most important characteristic. SAs have a sense of a mission to which they dedicate their lives.
- Enjoyment of privacy and detachment. Pleasure in being alone; ability to reflect on events.
- Freshness of appreciation. SAs don't take life for granted.
- Mystical or peak experiences. A peak experience is a moment of intense ecstasy, similar to a religious or mystical experience, during which the self is transcended. More recently, Mihaly Csikzentmihalyi developed the term *flow experience* to describe times when people become so totally involved in what they are doing that they lose all sense of time and awareness of self.
- Active social interest.
- An unhostile sense of humor.
- Democratic character structure. SAs display little racial, religious, or social prejudice.
- Creativity, especially in managing their lives.
- Resistance to conformity (enculturation). SAs are autonomous, independent, and self-sufficient.

From Maslow, A. H. (1954). *Motivation and personality.* New York: Harper & Row.

servations to represent physiological responses, rather than psychological ones, his ideas formed the foundation for the evolution of behavioral therapies.

Watson's Behaviorism Theory

John B. Watson (1878-1958) was an American psychologist who developed the school of thought referred to as behaviorism. He was strongly influenced by Pavlov's conditioning principles and began to apply these principles to human beings. Watson (1919) placed a strong emphasis on the role of the social environment in shaping behavior. He is best known for his experiments with a child named Albert. In one experiment, Watson stood behind Albert, who liked animals, and made a loud noise with a hammer every time Albert reached for a large white rat. After a number of repetitions of this noise, Albert became afraid of the white rat and later of all furry animals and objects, even in the absence of the loud noise. One might question the ethics of Watson's experiment, but the results were clear: behavior could be changed or shaped by controlling the stimulus.

Skinner's Operant Conditioning Theory

B. F. Skinner (1904-1990) represented the second wave of behavioral theorists and is recognized as one of the prime movers behind the behavioral movement. Skinner (1987) labeled the most important aspect of his theory **operant conditioning**, which refers to the manipulation of selected reinforcers to elicit and strengthen desired behavioral responses. **Reinforcer** refers to the consequence of behavior and is defined as anything that increases the occurrence of a behavior. The value of a reinforcer lies in its meaning to a particular individual. For example, a dollar bill could be a valuable reinforcer to a poor person, whereas a millionaire might scoff at the power of a dollar to influence behavior.

Skinner (1987) believed that a person performs a behavior (emits an operant) and experiences a consequence (reinforcement) as a result of performing the behavior. The consequence makes it more or less probable that the person will repeat the behavior. **Positive reinforcement** increases the likelihood that the behavior will be repeated. A negative consequence produces a deterrent effect on behavior. Absence of a reinforcer decreases behavior. For instance, if a person tells a joke and no one laughs, the person is less apt to tell jokes because his joke-telling behavior is not being reinforced. The crux of Skinner's theory is that reinforcement ultimately determines the occurrence of behavior.

Figure 2-3 illustrates the differences between respondent and operant conditioning.

Implications for Psychiatric Mental Health Nursing. Skinner's behavioral model provides a concrete method for modifying or replacing behaviors.

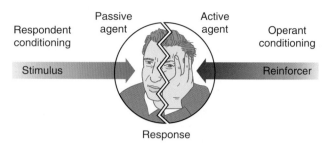

FIGURE 2-3 Respondent versus operant conditioning. (From Carson, V. B. [2000]. *Mental health nursing: The nurse-patient journey* [2nd ed., p. 121]. Philadelphia: Saunders.)

Behavior management and modification programs based on his principles have proven to be successful in altering targeted behaviors. Programmed learning and token economies represent extensions of Skinner's thoughts on learning. Behavioral methods are particularly effective with children, adolescents, and individuals with many forms of chronic mental illness.

Refer to Table 2-3 for information on additional theorists whose contributions influence psychiatric mental health nursing.

Biological Theories

In 1950 a French drug firm synthesized chlorpromazine, a powerful antipsychotic medication, and with this development, psychiatry experienced a revolution. The advent of psychopharmacology presented a direct challenge to psychodynamic approaches to mental illness. The dramatic experience of witnessing clients freed from the bondage of psychosis and mania because of powerful drugs such as chlorpromazine and lithium left those who were witnesses convinced of the critical role of the brain in psychiatric illness. In fact, President George H. Bush declared the 1990s to be the Decade of the Brain, and vast amounts of research monies and effort were directed at study of the structure and functions of the brain.

Since the discovery of chlorpromazine, many other medications have proven effective in controlling psychosis, mania, depression, and anxiety. These medications greatly reduce the need for hospitalization and dramatically improve the lives of people suffering with serious psychiatric difficulties. Today we know that psychoactive medications exert differential effects on different neurotransmitters and help restore brain function, allowing patients with mental illness to continue living productive lives, with greater satisfaction and with far less emotional pain.

A biological model of mental illness focuses on neurological, chemical, biological, and genetic issues and seeks to understand how the body and brain interact to create emotions, memories, and perceptual experiences. A biological perspective views abnormal behavior as part of a disease process or a defect and seeks to

TABLE 2-3

Additional Theorists Whose Contributions Influence Psychiatric Mental Health Nursing

Theorist	School of Thought	Major Contributions	Relevance to Psychiatric Mental Health Nursing
Carl Rogers	Humanism	Developed a person-centered model of psychotherapy. Emphasized the concepts of ■ Congruence—authenticity of the therapist in dealings with the client ■ Unconditional acceptance and positive regard—climate in the therapeutic relationship that facilitates change ■ Empathetic understanding—therapist's ability to apprehend the feelings and experiences of the client as if these things were happening to the therapist	Encourages nurses to view each client as unique. Emphasizes attitudes of unconditional positive regard, empathetic understanding, and genuineness that are essential to the nurse-client relationship.
Jean Piaget	Cognitive development	Identified stages of cognitive development including sensorimotor (0-2 yr); preoperational (2-7 yr); concrete operational (7-11 yr); and formal operational (11 yr–adulthood). These describe how cognitive development proceeds from reflex activity to application of logical solutions to all types of problems.	Provides a broad base for cognitive interventions, especially with clients with negative self-views.
Lawrence Kohlberg	Moral development	Posited a six-stage theory of moral development.	Provides nurses with a framework for evaluating moral decisions.
Albert Ellis	Existentialism	Developed approach of rational emotive behavioral therapy that is active and cognitively oriented; confrontation used to force clients to assume responsibility for behavior; clients are encouraged to accept themselves as they are and are taught to take risks and try out new behaviors.	Encourages nurses to focus on "here and now" issues and to help the client live fully in the present and look forward to the future.
Albert Bandura	Social learning theory	Responsible for concepts of modeling and self-efficacy: person's belief or expectation that he or she has the capacity to affect a desired outcome through his or her own efforts.	Includes cognitive functioning with environmental factors, which provides nurses with a comprehensive view of how people learn.
Viktor Frankl	Existentialism	Developed "logotherapy," a form of support offered to help people find their sense of self-respect. Logotherapy is a future-oriented therapy, focused on one's need to find meaning and value in living as one's most important life task.	Focuses nurse beyond mere behaviors to understanding the meaning of these behaviors to the client's sense of life meaning.

Data from Bandura, A. (1977). *Social learning theory*. Englewood Cliffs, NJ: Prentice-Hall; Bernard, M. E., & Wolfe, J. L. (Eds.). (1993). *The RET resource book for practitioners*. New York: Institute for Rational-Emotive Therapy; Ellis, A. (1989). *Inside rational emotive therapy*. San Diego, CA: Academic Press; Frankl, V. (1969). *The will to meaning*. Cleveland, OH: New American Library; Kohlberg, L. (1986). A current statement on some theoretical issues. In S. Modgil & C. Modgil (Ed.), *Lawrence Kohlberg*. Philadelphia: Palmer; and Rogers, C. R. (1961). *On becoming a person*. Boston: Houghton Mifflin.

stop or alter that disease process or defect; it locates the illness or disease in the body—usually in the limbic system of the brain and the synapse receptor sites of the central nervous system—and targets the site of the illness using physical interventions such as drugs, diet, or surgery.

The recognition that psychiatric illnesses are as much physical in origin as diabetes and coronary heart disease serves to decrease the stigma surrounding psychiatric illnesses. After all, we do not stigmatize a client with diabetes or heart disease and we do not hold them responsible for their illness. In the same way, clients with schizophrenia or bipolar affective disorder are no more responsible for causing their illnesses. Sometimes one of the kindest things we can tell clients and their families is that they are not responsible or to blame for the illness.

Implications for Psychiatric Mental Health Nursing. Historically, psychiatric nurses always attended to the physical needs of psychiatric clients. Nurses administer medications; monitor sleep, activity, nutrition and hydration, elimination, and other functions; and prepare clients for somatic therapies such as electroconvulsive therapy. They will continue to do so with the advancement of the biological model. In addition, the biological model does not eliminate the need for nurses to focus on the qualities of a therapeutic relationship, understand the patient's perspective, and communicate in such a way as to facilitate the client's recovery. One of the risks in adopting a biological model to the exclusion of all other theoretical perspectives is that, when carried to an extreme, a biological perspective suggests social control of behavior through modification of the brain's biochemistry and refutes the idea of personal responsibility. A biological model defines mental illness as an individual disorder. Such a theory ignores the myriad other influences of social, environmental, cultural, economic, spiritual, and educational factors that play a role in the development and treatment of mental illness.

It is imperative for psychiatric mental health nurses to stay abreast of changes in the biological model so that we are able to apply the newest findings in our own care practices.

Nursing Theories

The current practice of psychiatric mental health nursing draws from the contributions of many nursing theorists. Our focus, however, is on Hildegard Peplau, considered the mother of psychiatric nursing.

Peplau and the Therapeutic Relationship

Hildegard Peplau (1909-1999), influenced by the work of Sullivan and learning theory, developed the first systematic theoretical framework for psychiatric nursing in her groundbreaking book *Interpersonal Relations in Nursing* (1952). Not only did Peplau establish the foundation for the professional practice of psychiatric nursing, but she continued to enrich psychiatric nursing theory and worked for the advancement of nursing practice throughout her career.

Peplau (1952) was the first nurse to identify psychiatric nursing both as an essential element of general nursing and as a specialty area that embraces specific governing principles. She was also the first nurse theorist to describe the nurse-patient relationship as the foundation of nursing practice (Forchuk, 1991). In shifting the focus from what nurses do *to* patients to what nurses do *with* patients, Peplau (1989) engineered a major paradigm shift from a model focused on medical treatments to an interpersonal relational model of nursing practice.

Peplau (1987) viewed nursing as an educative instrument designed to help individuals and communities use their capacities in living more productively. Her theory is mainly concerned with the processes by which the nurse helps patients make positive changes in their health care status and well-being. She believed that illness offered a unique opportunity for experiential learning, personal growth, and improved coping strategies and that psychiatric nurses play a unique role in facilitating this growth (Peplau, 1982a, 1982b).

Peplau identified stages of the nurse-patient relationship, which are discussed in Chapter 10; she also used the technique of process recording to help her students hone their communication and relationship skills (see Table 11-1). The skills of the psychiatric nurse include observation, interpretation, and intervention. As the nurse observes and listens to the patient and develops impressions about the meaning of the patient's situation, the nurse's view of the patient is transformed and the patient is seen as a unique individual. The nurse's inferences are then validated with the patient for accuracy.

Peplau proposed an approach in which nurses are both participants and observers in therapeutic conversations. She believed it was essential for nurses to observe not only the behavior of the client, but also their own behavior. This self-awareness of the nurse is essential to keep the focus on the client as well as to keep the social and personal needs of the nurse out of the nurse-patient conversation.

Peplau spent a lifetime illuminating the science and art of professional nursing practice, and her work has had a profound effect on the nursing profession, nursing science, and the clinical practice of psychiatric nursing (Haber, 2000). The art of nursing is the care, compassion, and advocacy that nurses provide to enhance comfort and well-being. The science component of nursing involves the application of knowledge to understand a broad range of human problems and psychosocial phenomena as well as to intervene in relieving clients' suffering and promoting growth (Haber, 2000). In her works Peplau (1995) constantly reminds nurses to look beyond the illness and to "care for the person as well as the illness" and "think exclusively of patients as persons."

Perhaps Peplau's most universal contribution to the everyday practice of psychiatric nursing is her application of Sullivan's theory of anxiety to nursing practice. She described the effects of different levels of anxiety (mild, moderate, severe, and panic levels) on perception and learning. She promoted interventions to lower people's anxiety with the aim of improving clients' ability to think and to function at more satisfactory levels. More on the application of Peplau's theory of anxiety and interventions is presented in Chapter 13.

Table 2-4 lists additional nursing theorists and summarizes their major contributions and the impact of these contributions on psychiatric mental health nursing.

TABLE 2-4

Selected Nursing Theorists, Their Major Contributions, and Their Impact on Psychiatric Mental Health Nursing

Nursing Theorist	Focus of Theory	Contribution to Psychiatric Mental Health Nursing
Patricia Benner	"Caring" as foundation for nursing	Benner encourages nurses to provide caring and comforting interventions; she emphasizes the importance of the nurse-client relationship and the importance of teaching and coaching the client and bearing witness to suffering as the client deals with his or her illness.
Dorothea Orem	Goal of self-care as integral to the practice of nursing	Orem emphasizes the role of the nurse in promoting self-care activities of the client; this has relevance to the seriously and persistently mentally ill client.
Sister Callista Roy	Continual need for people to adapt physically, psychologically, and socially	Roy emphasizes the role of nursing in assisting clients to adapt in order to cope more effectively with changes.
Betty Neuman	Impact of internal and external stressors on the equilibrium of the system	Neuman emphasizes the role of nursing in assisting clients in discovering and using stress-reducing strategies.
Joyce Travelbee	Meaning in the nurse-client relationship and the importance of communication	Travelbee emphasizes the role of nursing in affirming the suffering of the client and being able to alleviate that suffering through communication skills used appropriately through the stages of the nurse-client relationship.

Data from Benner, P., & Wrubel, J. (1989). *The primacy of caring: Stress and coping in health and illness.* Menlo Park, CA: Addison-Wesley; Leddy, S., & Pepper, J. M. (1993). *Conceptual bases of professional nursing* (3rd ed., pp. 174-175). Philadelphia: Lippincott; Neuman, B., & Young, R. (1972). A model for teaching total person approach to patient problems. *Nursing Research, 21,* 264-269; Orem, D. E. (1995). *Nursing: Concepts of practice* (5th ed.). New York: McGraw-Hill; Roy, C., & Andrews, H. A. (1991). *The Roy adaptation model: The definitive statement.* Norwalk, CT: Appleton & Lange; and Travelbee, J. (1961). *Intervention in psychiatric nursing.* Philadelphia: F. A. Davis.

TRADITIONAL THERAPEUTIC APPROACHES

Our journey continues with an overview of traditional therapeutic approaches. Although most of these therapies are beyond the scope of your practice, it is important that you be aware of the range of treatment modalities. However, as you review these therapies, ask yourself, "How does this approach affect my nursing practice?" Those therapies that have proven effective for the treatment of specific mental disorders are addressed at length in the appropriate clinical chapters.

Classical Psychoanalysis

Classical psychoanalysis, developed by Sigmund Freud, is seldom used today because it is too expensive and takes too long, and Freud's premise that all mental illness is caused by early intrapsychic conflict is no longer thought to be valid. However, there are two concepts from classic psychoanalysis that are important for all psychiatric nurses to know: transference and countertransference (Freud, 1969).

A positive transference is developed when the client experiences feelings toward the nurse or therapist that were originally held toward significant others in his or her life. When this occurs, these feelings need to be explored with the client. Such exploration helps the client to better understand his or her own feelings and behaviors. Countertransference is the health care worker's unconscious and personal response to the client. For instance, if the client reminds you of someone that you do not like, you may unconsciously react to the client "as if" the client were the other individual. Countertransference underscores the importance of maintaining self-awareness and seeking supervision regarding the progress of therapeutic relationships. Refer to Chapter 10 for more on countertransference and the nurse-client relationship.

Psychodynamic and Psychoanalytic Psychotherapy

Psychotherapy that follows the psychoanalytic model uses many of the tools of psychoanalysis, such as free association, dream analysis, transference, and countertransference, but the therapist is much more involved and interacts with the client more freely than in traditional psychoanalysis. Psychodynamic psychotherapy is oriented more to the here and now, and less of an attempt is made to reconstruct the developmental origins of conflicts (Ursano & Norwood, 1999).

Advance practice psychiatric mental health nurses, psychiatric social workers, and psychologists with special training at the master's level or above may undertake psychodynamic psychotherapy with clients. The focus of this type of therapy is to uncover unconscious material that appears in the form of symptoms or unsatisfactory life patterns. This is done through an intimate professional relationship between the therapist and the client over a period of months to years.

Short-Term Dynamic Psychotherapy

Today one of the most common approaches to psychotherapy is short-term dynamic psychotherapy in which the duration of therapy is ten sessions or fewer. One of many reasons for the short duration of therapy is the growing reluctance of insurance companies to cover more than perhaps 25 psychotherapy sessions in a given calendar year. The emergence of cognitive and behavioral therapies over the past 20 to 30 years has also played a role; these approaches focus on discrete problems and avoid long-term therapy.

The best candidates for brief psychotherapy are relatively healthy and well-functioning individuals, sometimes referred to as the "worried well," who have a clearly circumscribed area of difficulty and who are intelligent, psychologically minded, and well motivated for change. Clients with psychosis, severe depression, and borderline personality disorders, as well as individuals with severe character disorders, often are not appropriate candidates for this type of treatment. Supportive therapies, which are within the purview of the basic level psychiatric nurse, are useful for these clients. A variety of supportive therapies are described in chapters concerning specific disorders (Chapters 14 to 21).

At the start of treatment, client and therapist agree on what the focus will be and concentrate their work on that focus. Sessions are held weekly, and the total number of sessions to be held is determined at the outset of therapy. There is a rapid, back-and-forth pattern between client and therapist with both participating actively. The therapist intervenes constantly to keep the therapy on track, either by redirecting the client's attention or by interpreting deviations from the focus to the client.

Brief therapies share the following common elements:

- Assessment tends to be rapid and early.
- Clear expectations are established for time-limited therapy with improvement demonstrated within a small number of sessions.
- Goals are concrete and focus on improving the client's worst symptoms, improving coping skills, and helping the client understand what is going on in his or her life.

- Interpretations are directed toward present life circumstances and client behavior rather than toward the historical significance of feelings.
- There is a general understanding that psychotherapy does not cure but that it can help troubled individuals learn to deal better with life's inevitable stressors.

Interpersonal Psychotherapy

Interpersonal psychotherapy (IPT) is an effective psychotherapeutic modality that derives more from the school of psychiatry which originated with Adolph Meyer and Harry Stack Sullivan. The focus is on reassurance, clarification of feeling states, improvement of interpersonal communication, and improvement of interpersonal skills, rather than on personality reconstruction (Ursano & Norwood, 1999). IPT has been found to be successful in the treatment of depression, and it is predicated on the notion that disturbances in important interpersonal relationships (or a deficit in the capacity to form those relationships) can play a role in initiating or maintaining clinical depression. In IPT the therapist identifies the nature of the problem to be resolved and then selects strategies that are consistent with that problem area. Four types of problem areas have been identified (Hollon & Engelhardt, 1997):

1. **Grief**—complicated bereavement following the death or loss of a loved one
2. **Role disputes**—conflicts with a significant other
3. **Role transition**—problematic change in life status or social or vocational role
4. **Interpersonal deficit**—an inability to initiate or sustain close relationships

Cognitive Therapy

Aaron Beck's approach (Beck et al., 1979) to therapy for people suffering from depression illustrates the major components of cognitive therapy. This is an active, directive, time-limited, structured approach used to treat a variety of psychiatric disorders (e.g., depression, anxiety, phobias, and pain problems). It is based on the underlying theoretical principle that how people feel and behave is largely determined by the way in which they think about the world and their place in the world (Beck, 1967, 1976). Their cognitions (verbal or pictorial events in their stream of consciousness) are based on schemata (attitudes or assumptions) developed from previous experiences. For example, if a person interprets all experiences in terms of whether he or she is competent and adequate, thinking may be dominated by the schema "Unless I do everything perfectly, I'm a failure." Consequently, the person reacts to situations in terms of adequacy even when these situations are unrelated to whether he or she is personally competent. Albert Ellis (b. 1913), founder of rational

Relevant Theories and Therapies for Nursing Practice **CHAPTER 2** 27

emotive behavioral therapy, calls these dysfunctional thoughts irrational beliefs. Table 2-5 describes common dysfunctional or irrational thoughts or beliefs that influence many people.

The therapeutic techniques of the cognitive therapist are designed to identify, reality test, and correct distorted conceptualizations and the dysfunctional beliefs (schemata) underlying these cognitions. In other words, the cognitive therapist helps clients to change the way they think and therefore to reduce symptoms. Clients are taught to challenge their own negative thinking and to substitute positive thoughts. They are taught to recognize when their thinking is based on distortions and misconceptions. Homework assignments play an important role in cognitive therapy.

The following is an example of the type of analysis done by a client receiving cognitive therapy.

A 24-year-old nurse recently discharged from the hospital for severe depression presented this record (Beck et al., 1979):

EVENT	FEELING	COGNITIONS	OTHER POSSIBLE INTERPRETATIONS
While at a party, Jim asked me, "How are you feeling?" shortly after I was discharged from the hospital.	Anxious	Jim thinks I am a basket case. I must really look bad for him to be concerned.	He really cares about me. He noticed that I look better than before I went into the hospital and wants to know if I feel better too.

Box 2-2 presents an example of cognitive therapy. Table 2-6 compares and contrasts psychodynamic psy-chotherapy, interpersonal psychotherapy, and cognitive psychotherapy.

Behavioral Therapy

Behavioral therapy is based on the assumption that changes in maladaptive behavior can occur without insight into the underlying cause. This approach works best when it is directed at specific problems and the goals are well defined. Behavioral therapy is effective in treating people with phobias, alcoholism, schizophrenia, and many other conditions. Four types of behavioral therapy are discussed here: modeling, operant conditioning, systematic desensitization, and aversion therapy. Box 2-3 provides a clinical example illustrating several behavioral approaches.

Modeling

In **modeling**, the therapist provides a role model for specific identified behaviors, and the client learns through imitation. The therapist may do the modeling, provide another person to model the behaviors, or present a video for the purpose. Bandura, Blahard, and Ritter (1969) were able to help people reduce their phobias about nonpoisonous snakes by having them first view close-ups of filmed encounters between people and snakes that resulted in successful outcomes and then to view live encounters between people and snakes that also had successful outcomes. In a similar fashion, some behavioral therapists use role playing in the consulting room. They demonstrate to clients patterns of behaving that might prove more effective than those the clients usually engage in and then have the

---

TABLE 2-5

Dysfunctional Versus Functional Thinking

Irrational Thoughts That Cause Disturbance	Rational Thoughts That Promote Emotional Self-Control
How *awful*.	This is disappointing.
I can't stand it.	I can put up with what I don't like.
I'm stupid.	What I *did* was stupid.
He stinks!	He's not perfect either.
This *shouldn't* have happened.	This should have happened because it did!
I am to be blamed.	I am at fault but am not to be blamed.
He has no right.	He has every right to follow his own mind though I wish he hadn't exercised that right!
I *need* him to do that.	I want/desire/prefer him to do that, but I don't have to have what I want.
Things *always* go wrong.	Sometimes—if not frequently—things will go wrong.
Every time I try I fail.	Sometimes—even often—I may fail.
Things *never* work out.	More often than I would like, things don't work out.
This is bigger than life.	This is an important part of my life.
This *should* be easier.	I wish this were easier, but often things that are good for me aren't—no gain without pain. Tough, too bad!
I *should* have done better.	I would have *preferred* to do better, but I did what I could at the time.
I am a failure.	I'm a person who sometimes fails.

From Bernard, M. E., & Wolfe, J. L. (Eds.). (1993). *The RET resource book for practitioners.* New York: Institute for Rational-Emotive Therapy.

BOX 2-2

Example of Cognitive Therapy

The client was an attractive woman in her early twenties. Her depression of 18 months' duration was precipitated by her boyfriend's leaving her. She had numerous automatic thoughts that she was ugly and undesirable. These automatic thoughts were handled in the following manner.

Therapist: Other than your subjective opinion, what evidence do you have that you are ugly?

Client: Well, my sister always said I was ugly.

Therapist: Was she always right in these matters?

Client: No. Actually, she had her own reasons for telling me this. But the real reason I know I'm ugly is that men don't ask me out. If I weren't ugly, I'd be dating now.

Therapist: That is a possible reason why you're not dating. But there's an alternative explanation. You told me that you work in an office by yourself all day and spend your nights alone at home. It doesn't seem like you're giving yourself opportunities to meet men.

Client: I can see what you're saying, but still, if I weren't ugly, men would ask me out.

Therapist: I suggest we run an experiment: that is, for you to become more socially active, stop turning down invitations to parties and social events, and see what happens.

After the client became more active and had more opportunities to meet men, she started to date. At this point, she no longer believed she was ugly.

Therapy then focused on her basic assumption that one's worth is determined by one's appearance. She readily agreed this didn't make sense. She also saw the falseness of the assumption that one must be beautiful to attract men or be loved. This discussion led to her basic assumption that she could not be happy without love (or attention from men). The latter part of treatment focused on helping her to change this belief.

Therapist: On what do you base this belief that you can't be happy without a man?

Client: I was really depressed for a year and a half when I didn't have a man in my life.

Therapist: Is there another reason why you were depressed?

Client: As we discussed, I was looking at everything in a distorted way. But I still don't know if I could be happy if no one was interested in me.

Therapist: I don't know either. Is there a way we could find out?

Client: Well, as an experiment I could not go out on dates for a while and see how I feel.

Therapist: I think that's a good idea. Although it has its flaws, the experimental method is still the best way currently available to discover the facts. You're fortunate in being able to run this type of experiment. Now, for the first time in your adult life you aren't attached to a man. If you find you can be happy without a man, this will greatly strengthen you and also make your future relationships all the better.

In this case, the client was able to stick to a "cold turkey" regimen. After a brief period of dysphoria, she was delighted to find that her well-being was not dependent on another person.

There were similarities between these two interventions. In both, the distorted conclusion or assumption was delineated and the client was asked for evidence to support it. An experiment to gather data was also suggested in both instances. However, to achieve the results, a contrasting version of the same experimental situation was required.

From Beck, A., et al. (1979). *Cognitive theory of depression.* New York: Guilford Press.

clients practice these new behaviors. For example, a student who does not know how to ask a professor for an extension on a term paper would watch the therapist portray a potentially effective way of making the request. The clinician would then help the student practice the new skill in a similar role-playing situation.

Operant Conditioning

Operant conditioning is the basis for behavior modification and uses positive reinforcement to increase desired behaviors. For example, when desired goals are achieved or behaviors are performed, clients might be rewarded with tokens. These tokens can be exchanged for food, small luxuries, or privileges. This reward system is known as a token economy.

Operant conditioning has been useful in improving the verbal behaviors of mute, autistic, and developmentally disabled children. In clients with severe and persistent mental illness, behavior modification has helped to increase levels of self-care, social behavior,

group participation, and more. You may find this a useful technique as you proceed through your clinical rotations.

Each of us uses positive reinforcement in our everyday lives, whether we are aware of it or not. Here is an example of three ways in which behavior can be reinforced. A mother takes her son to the grocery store. The child starts acting out, demanding candy, nagging, crying, and yelling:

ACTION	RESULT
1. The mother gives the child the candy.	The child continues to use this behavior. This is positive reinforcement of negative behavior.
2. The mother scolds the child.	Acting out may continue because the child gets what he or she really wants—attention. This positively rewards negative behavior.
3. The mother ignores the acting out but gives attention to the child when he is acting appropriately.	The child gets a positive reward for appropriate behavior.

TABLE 2-6

Comparison of Psychoanalytic, Interpersonal, and Cognitive Psychotherapies

	Psychodynamic/ Psychoanalytic Psychotherapy	Interpersonal Psychotherapy	Cognitive Psychotherapy
Treatment focus	Internal experience	Interpersonal relationships and social supports	Thoughts and cognitions
Primary disorders treated	Anxiety Depression Personality disorders	Depression Anxiety	Depression Anxiety
Skills needed by therapist	++++	++++	++++
Therapeutic alliance	++++	++++	++++
Nonjudgmental stance	++++	++++	++++
Focus			
Cognitive	+++ (defense mechanisms)	+	++++ (Cognitive distortions)
Interpersonal	++++ (Transference and past relationships)	++++ (Interpersonal withdrawal, attachments, and models)	+
Technique			
Nondirective	++++	+	+
Directive (interventions)	+	++++	++++

From Ursano, R. J., & Norwood, A. E. (1999). Brief psychotherapy. In B. J. Sadock & V. A. Sadock (Eds.), *Kaplan and Sadock's comprehensive textbook of psychiatry* (7th ed., p. 168). Philadelphia: Williams & Wilkins.
Note: Plus signs indicate degree, from low (+) to high (++++).

Systematic Desensitization

Systematic desensitization is another form of behavior modification therapy that involves the development of behavioral tasks customized to the client's specific fears; these tasks are presented to the client while he or she is using learned relaxation techniques. The process involves four steps. First, the client's fear is broken down into its components by exploring the particular stimulus cues to which the client reacts. For example, certain situations may precipitate a phobic reaction, whereas others do not. Crowds at parties may be problematic, whereas similar numbers of people in other settings do not cause the same distress. Second, the client is incrementally exposed to the fear. For example, a client who has a fear of flying is introduced to short periods of visual presentations of flying—first with still pictures, then with videos, and finally in a busy airport. The situations are confronted while the client is in a relaxed state. Gradually, over a period of time, exposure is increased until the anxiety about or fear of the object or situation has ceased. Third, clients are instructed in how to design their own hierarchies of fear. For fear of flying, a client might develop a set of statements representing the stages of a flight, order the statements from the most fearful to the least fearful, and use relaxation techniques to reach a state of relaxation as they progress through the list. Fourth, clients practice these techniques every day.

Aversion Therapy

Today, aversion therapy, which is akin to punishment, is used widely to treat behaviors such as alcoholism, sexual deviation, shoplifting, hallucinations, violent and aggressive behavior, and self-mutilation. Punishment is sometimes the treatment of choice when other less drastic measures have failed to produce the desired effects. Three paradigms for using aversive techniques are the following:
- Pairing of a maladaptive behavior with a noxious stimulus (e.g., pair the sight and smell of alcohol with electric shock), so that anxiety or fear becomes associated with the once-pleasurable stimulus
- Punishment (e.g., applied after the patient has had an alcoholic drink)
- Avoidance training (e.g., the patient avoids punishment by pushing a glass of alcohol away within a certain time limit)

Some other examples of aversive stimuli are electric shock, chemicals inducing nausea and vomiting, noxious odors, unpleasant verbal stimuli such as descriptions of disturbing scenes, costs or fines in a token economy, and denial of positive reinforcement (isolation).

Before initiating any aversive protocol, the therapist, treatment team, or society *must* answer the following questions: Is this therapy in the best interest of the patient? Does its use violate the patient's rights? Is

BOX 2-3

Example of Behavioral Therapy

A 30-year-old married woman, mother of three boys, came to the therapist with a complaint of anxiety and depression as a chronic state for several years. She had become disheveled, with hair and clothes in disarray, and her walk was a shuffling pace—all overt signs of psychomotor retardation.

An attempt was made to get details about the things that were disturbing her. She felt inadequate as a mother, and situations that involved making decisions concerning her three boys, aged 6, 5, and 2½, were distressing to her. In addition, she felt that her husband, to whom she had been married for 9 years, gave her no emotional support, constantly criticized her, and never gave her any positive advice, although he was quick to tell her about the things she did wrong.

The first interview was productive, primarily as an opportunity for her to unburden herself about the things she had not been able to talk about with anyone before, and the therapist felt that an excellent working relationship had been established. It was possible to get some idea about the things that were distressing her, but more details were needed, because she reported being distressed all the time. So far, it was impossible to tell which situations made her feel either worse or better, so she was asked to do some homework: to keep records of any upsetting events that occurred during the ensuing week. In addition, she was asked to fill out and bring in a Fear Survey Schedule.

When she came back the next time, she brought in her homework assignment. She said, "I went to a movie and I became very upset." Only upon closer questioning about what specifically was happening at the time she became distressed did it become apparent that the disturbing scene was one in which people were drinking. The second thing she noted was that her husband would withdraw when they were talking about emotionally laden things, when what she really needed was for him to put his arms around her and give her some comfort. The third event she noted was that she was very sensitive to the fact that her husband had asked her to make an appointment with the dentist that he had not kept. She felt that the dentist wouldn't think her trustworthy. In some way, she felt she would be seen by the dentist as being less of a person; he would be critical of her. The fourth area that she brought up was that any time her children were engaged in fighting or disagreement, she became upset. The fifth observation was that sudden noises distressed her.

In subsequent sessions the therapist went over each of these situations with the client to further clarify them. *Assertiveness training* was begun using a hierarchical approach, by giving her the instruction that between that session and the next session she was to go up and greet anyone that she knew even slightly. A list of people from whom she feared criticism was obtained; these were graded in terms of how distressing criticism from each might be to her.

Relaxation training was begun at this point to prepare for *systematic desensitization* in the areas of criticism and rejection. In subsequent sessions the assignments in assertiveness training were continued, because she was carrying them out effectively.

At termination, the client no longer looked depressed. A 1-year follow-up indicated that she was continuing to function fully, was no longer experiencing depression, and on the whole was enjoying life.

From Goldstein, A. (1978). Behavior therapy. In R. Corsini (Ed.), *Current psychotherapies* (2nd ed., pp. 239-245). Itasca, IL: F. E. Peacock. Reproduced by permission of the publisher, F. E. Peacock Publishers, Inc.

it in the best interest of society? Ongoing supervision, support, and evaluation of those administering the aversion therapy must occur.

For example, mild electric shock and shock in combination with positive reinforcement have been demonstrated to eliminate self-injurious behavior, and application of a bitter-tasting substance to the fingers of nail biters, a mild aversive treatment, has been found effective (Silber & Haynes, 1992). Behaviors such as thumb sucking, hair pulling, and nose picking have responded to mild aversive therapy, which was found to be most effective when the patients cooperated with the treatment program.

Biofeedback, which is also a form of behavioral therapy and is successfully used today, especially for controlling the body's physiological response to stress and anxiety. Biofeedback is discussed in detail in Chapter 12.

Milieu Therapy

In 1948, Bruno Bettelheim coined the term milieu therapy to describe his use of the total environment to treat disturbed children. Bettelheim created a comfortable, secure environment (or milieu) in which psychotic children were helped to form a new world. Staff members were trained to provide 24-hour support and understanding for each child on an individual basis. In 1953, Maxwell Jones in Great Britain wrote the book *The Therapeutic Community*. This book both laid the groundwork for the milieu therapy movement in the United States and defined the nurse's role in this therapy.

Milieu is sometimes a difficult concept to grasp. It is an all-inclusive term that recognizes the people, setting, structure, and emotional climate as all important to healing. Milieu therapy takes naturally occurring events in the environment and uses them as rich learning opportunities for clients. There are certain basic characteristics of milieu therapy, regardless of whether the setting involves treatment of psychotic children, clients in a psychiatric hospital, drug abusers in a residential treatment center, or psychiatric clients in a day hospital. Milieu therapy, or a therapeutic community, has as its locus a living, learning, or working environment. Such therapy may be based on any number of therapeutic modalities, from structured behavioral therapy to spontaneous, humanistically oriented approaches.

Milieu therapy is a basic intervention in nursing practice. Nurses are constantly involved in the assessment and provision of safe and effective milieus for their clients. Common examples include providing a safe environment for the suicidal client or a client with a cognitive disorder (e.g., Alzheimer's disease), referring abused women to safe houses, and advocating for children suspected of being abused in their home environments.

Additional Therapies

You will be introduced to other therapeutic approaches later in the book. Crisis intervention is an approach that you will find useful not only in psychiatric mental health nursing but in other nursing specialties as well; this subject is presented in Chapter 22. There are forms of group therapy that are appropriate for the basic level practitioner, and you will explore these in Chapter 35. Finally, family therapy is discussed in Chapter 36.

■ ■ ■ KEY POINTS to REMEMBER

- Sigmund Freud advanced the first theory of personality development.
- Freud articulated levels of awareness (unconscious, preconscious, conscious) and demonstrated the influence of our unconscious behavior on everyday life, as evidenced by the use of defense mechanisms.
- Freud identified three psychological processes of personality (id, ego, superego) and described how they operate and develop.
- Freud articulated one of the first modern developmental theories of personality based on five psychosexual stages.
- Erik Erikson expanded on Freud's developmental stages to include middle age through old age. Erikson called his stages psychosocial stages and emphasized the social aspect of personality development.
- Harry Stack Sullivan proposed the interpersonal theory of personality development, which focuses on interpersonal processes that can be observed in a social framework.
- Abraham Maslow, the founder of humanistic psychology, offered the theory of self-actualization and human motivation that is basic to all nursing education today.
- Hildegard Peplau's theoretical framework in psychiatric nursing has become the foundation of psychiatric nursing practice.
- A variety of psychotherapeutic interventions are used, including psychodynamic psychotherapy, short-term dynamic therapy, IPT, cognitive-behavioral therapy, and behavior modification.

■ ■ ■

Visit the Evolve website at **http://evolve.elsevier.com/Varcarolis** for a posttest on the content in this chapter.   **evolve**

Critical Thinking and Chapter Review

Visit the Evolve website at **http://evolve.elsevier.com/Varcarolis** for additional self-study exercises.
evolve

■ ■ ■ CRITICAL THINKING

1. What influences can or do the theorists discussed in this chapter have on your practice of nursing?
    A. How does Freud's concepts of the conscious, preconscious, and unconscious affect your understanding of clients' behaviors?
    B. Are Erikson's psychosocial stages a sound basis for identifying disruptions in stages of development in some of your clients? Can you give a clinical example?
    C. What are the implications of Sullivan's focus on the importance of interpersonal relationships for your interactions with clients?
    D. Peplau believed that nurses must exercise self-awareness within the nurse-patient relationship. Describe situations in your student experience in which this self-awareness played a vital role in your relationship(s) with client(s).
    E. Can you think of anyone who seems to be self-actualized? What is your reason for this conclusion? What characteristics does this person have that make you think he or she is a self-actualized individual? How do you make use of Maslow's hierarchy of needs in your nursing practice?
    F. What do you think about the behaviorist point of view that to change behaviors is to change personality?
2. Which of the therapies described here do you think can be the most helpful to you in your nursing practice? What are your reasons for this choice?

Continued

Critical Thinking and Chapter Review—cont'd

Visit the Evolve website at **http://evolve.elsevier.com/Varcarolis** for additional self-study exercises.

■ ■ ■ CHAPTER REVIEW

Choose the most appropriate answer.

1. Which of the following contributions to modern psychiatric nursing practice was made by Freud?
   1. The theory of personality structure and levels of awareness
   2. The concept of a "self-actualized personality"
   3. The thesis that culture and society exert significant influence on personality
   4. Provision of a developmental model that includes the entire life span

2. The theory of interpersonal relationships developed by Hildegard Peplau is based on the foundation provided by which of the following early theorists?
   1. Freud
   2. Piaget
   3. Sullivan
   4. Maslow

3. The concepts at the heart of Sullivan's theory of personality are
   1. needs and anxiety.
   2. basic needs and meta-needs.
   3. schemata, assimilation, and accommodation.
   4. developmental tasks and psychosocial crises.

4. The premise that an individual's behavior and affect are largely determined by the attitudes and assumptions the person has developed about the world underlies
   1. modeling.
   2. milieu therapy.
   3. cognitive therapy.
   4. psychoanalytic psychotherapy.

5. Providing a safe environment for clients with impaired cognition, referring an abused spouse to a "safe house," and conducting a community meeting are nursing interventions that address aspects of
   1. milieu therapy.
   2. cognitive therapy.
   3. behavioral therapy.
   4. interpersonal psychotherapy.

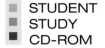

■ STUDENT
■ STUDY
■ CD-ROM

Access the accompanying CD-ROM for animations, interactive exercises, review questions for the NCLEX examination, and an audio glossary.

REFERENCES

Bandura, A., Blahard, E. B., & Ritter, B. (1969). Relative efficacy of desensitization and modeling approaches for inducing behavioral, affective, and attitudinal changes. *Journal of Personality and Social Psychology, 13,* 173-199.

Beck, A. T. (1967). *Depression: Clinical, experimental and theoretical aspects.* New York: Harper & Row.

Beck, A. T. (1976). *Cognitive therapy and the emotional disorders.* New York: New American Library.

Beck, A. T., et al. (1979). *Cognitive theory of depression.* New York: Guilford Press.

Erikson, E. H. (1950). *Childhood and society.* New York: W. W. Norton.

Forchuk, C. (1991). A comparison of the works of Peplau and Orlando. *Archives of Psychiatric Nursing, 5*(1), 38-45.

Freud, S. (1960). *The ego and the id* (J. Strachey, Trans.). New York: W. W. Norton.

Freud, S. (1961). *The interpretation of dreams* (J. Strachey, Ed. & Trans.). New York: Scientific Editions.

Freud, S. (1969). *An outline of psychoanalysis* (J. Strachey, Trans.). New York: W. W. Norton.

Haber, J. (2000). Hildegard E. Peplau: The psychiatric nursing legacy of a legend. *Journal of the American Psychiatric Nurses Association, 6*(2), 56-62.

Hollon, S. D., & Engelhardt, N. (1997). Review of psychosocial treatment of mood disorders. In D. L. Dunner (Ed.), *Current psychiatric therapy II.* Philadelphia: Saunders.

Jones, M. (1953). *The therapeutic community.* New York: Basic Books.

Maslow, A. H. (1963). Self actualizing people. In G. B. Levitas (Ed.), *The world of psychology* (Vol. 2). New York: Braziller.

Maslow, A. H. (1968). *Toward a psychology of being.* Princeton, NJ: Van Nostrand.

Maslow, A. H. (1970). *Motivation and personality* (2nd ed.). New York: Harper & Row.

Pavlov, I. (1928). *Lectures on conditioned reflexes* (W. H. Grant, Ed. & Trans.). New York: International Publishers.

Peplau, H. E. (1952). *Interpersonal relations in nursing: A conceptual frame of reference for psychodynamic nursing.* New York: Putnam.

Peplau, H. E. (1982a). Therapeutic concepts. In S. A. Smoyak & S. Rouslin (Eds.), *A collection of classics in psychiatric nursing literature* (pp. 91-108). Thorofare, NJ: Slack.

Peplau, H. E. (1982b). Interpersonal techniques: The crux of psychiatric nursing. In S. A. Smoyak & S. Rouslin (Eds.), *A collection of classics in psychiatric nursing literature* (pp. 276-281). Thorofare, NJ: Slack.

Peplau, H. E. (1987). Interpersonal constructs for nursing practice. *Nursing Education Today, 7,* 201-208.

Peplau, H. E. (1989). Future directions in psychiatric nursing from the perspective of history. *Journal of Psychosocial Nursing, 27*(2), 18-28.

Peplau, H. E. (1995). Another look at schizophrenia from a nursing standpoint. In C. A. Anderson (Ed.), *Psychiatric nursing 1946-94: The state of the art.* St. Louis, MO: Mosby.

Silber, K. P., & Haynes, C. E. (1992). Treating nailbiting: A comparative analysis of mild aversion and competing response therapies. *Behavioral Research Therapy, 31,* 155-170.

Skinner, B. F. (1987). Whatever happened to psychology as the science of behavior? *American Psychologist, 42,* 780-786.

Sullivan, H. S. (1953). *The interpersonal theory of psychiatry.* New York: W. W. Norton.

Ursano, R. J., & Norwood, A. E. (1999). Brief psychotherapy. In B. J. Sadock & V. A. Sadock (Eds.), *Kaplan & Sadock's comprehensive textbook of psychiatry* (7th ed.). Philadelphia: Williams & Wilkins.

Watson, J. B. (1919). *Psychology from the standpoint of a behaviorist.* Philadelphia: Lippincott.

CHAPTER 3

Biological Basis for Understanding Psychotropic Drugs

JOHN RAYNOR

KEY TERMS and CONCEPTS

The key terms and concepts listed here appear in color where they are defined or first discussed in this chapter.

acetylcholine, 51

antagonists, 50

antianxiety or anxiolytic drugs, 57

anticholinesterase drugs, 59

atypical antipsychotic drugs, 51

atypical or novel antidepressants, 57

basal ganglia, 44

circadian rhythms, 37

γ-aminobutyric acid (GABA), 47

hypnotic, 57

limbic system, 42

lithium, 53

monoamine oxidase (MAO), 56

monoamine oxidase inhibitors (MAOIs), 56

mood-stabilizing drug, 53

neurons, 38

neurotransmitter, 38

pharmacodynamics, 48

pharmacokinetics, 48

receptors, 39

reticular activating system (RAS), 42

reuptake, 39

selective serotonin reuptake inhibitors (SSRIs), 55

standard (first-generation) antipsychotic drugs, 50

synapse, 38

therapeutic index, 53

typical or standard antidepressants, 54

OBJECTIVES

After studying this chapter, the reader will be able to

1. Discuss at least eight functions of the brain and the way these functions can be altered by psychotropic drugs.
2. Describe how a neurotransmitter functions as a neuromessenger.
3. Draw the three major areas of the brain and identify at least three functions of each.
4. Identify how specific brain functions are altered in certain mental disorders (e.g., depression, anxiety, schizophrenia).
5. Describe how the use of imaging techniques can be helpful for understanding mental illness.
6. Apply to a medication teaching plan how the blockage of dopamine at the receptor site can result in motor abnormalities and hyperprolactinemia.
7. Describe the result of blockage of the muscarinic receptors and the α_1 receptors by the standard neuroleptic drugs.
8. Contrast and compare the side-effect profiles of the standard antipsychotics with those of (a) clozapine and (b) risperidone.
9. Briefly identify the main neurotransmitters that are affected by the following psychotropic drugs:
   a. Standard (first-generation) antipsychotics
   b. Tricyclic antidepressants
   c. Selective serotonin reuptake inhibitors
   d. Monoamine oxidase inhibitors
   e. Antianxiety agents (benzodiazepines, buspirone)
   f. Anticholinesterase drugs
10. Apply to a medication teaching plan the knowledge of why a person taking a monoamine oxidase inhibitor would have special dietary and drug restrictions.
11. Identify specific cautions you might incorporate into your medication teaching plan with regard to the following:
   a. Herbal medicine
   b. Genetic pharmacology (variations in effects and therapeutic actions of medications among different ethnic groups)

evolve Visit the Evolve website at **http://evolve.elsevier.com/Varcarolis** for a pretest on the content in this chapter.

Whether conscious or unconscious, focused on the logical or filled with fantasy, all mental activity has its locus in the brain. This implies that a primary goal of psychiatry is to understand both normal and abnormal mental processes in terms of brain function. Ultimately, we would like to be able to apply this understanding to the treatment of mental disease and the alleviation of mental suffering. Approached in terms of brain function, psychiatric problems are explained and treated in the same way as any other biological problems.

Implied in the biological approach to psychiatric illness is the idea that, although the origin of a psychiatric illness may be related to any number of factors (genetics, neurodevelopmental factors, drugs, infection, psychosocial experience), there will eventually be an alteration in cerebral function that accounts for the disturbances in the client's behavior and mental experiences. These physiological alterations are the targets of the psychotropic drugs used to treat mental disease. From a holistic point of view, mental disorders then have neurobiopsychological components that support the efficacy of treating these disorders both pharmacologically and with appropriate psychotherapy.

Reversal of these alterations is the goal of the use of psychotropic drugs in the treatment of these illnesses. During recent years there has been an explosion of information in this area. Earlier theories, such as the dopamine theory of schizophrenia and the monoamine theory of depression, are currently seen as overly simplistic because a large number of other neurotransmitters, hormones, and coregulators are now thought to play important and complex roles. The importance of receptor subtypes and the role of these receptors in normal physiology, pathology, and pharmacology are also receiving increasing attention.

The goal of this chapter is to relate psychiatric disturbances and the psychotropic drugs used to treat these disturbances to normal brain structure and function. We first look at the normal functions of the brain and how these functions are carried out from an anatomical and physiological perspective. We then review current theories of the neuropsychological basis of various types of emotional and physiological dysfunctions. As will be seen, these theories focus primarily on neurotransmitters and their receptors. Finally, we attempt to relate both the beneficial and the untoward effects of psychiatric drugs to their interaction with various transmitter-receptor systems.

Although the modern era of the treatment of mental illness with psychotropic drugs extends back almost half a century, a full understanding of how these drugs improve the symptoms of these illnesses continues to elude investigators. The focus of research is on neurotransmitters—their release from presynaptic cells and their actions on postsynaptic cells—and how psychotropic drugs interact with the physiology of these substances. In recent years many subtypes of receptors for the various neurotransmitters have been discovered, and long-term changes induced in postsynaptic cells have taken on increased significance. This information is becoming increasingly important for nurses to understand. Such an understanding is particularly crucial for advanced practice psychiatric nurses, who in many states have the authority to write prescriptions.

Included in this chapter is an overview of the major drugs used to treat mental disorders and an explanation of how they work. Additional and detailed information regarding adverse and toxic effects, dosage, nursing implications, and teaching tools is presented in the appropriate clinical chapters.

In many ways all of this new information has clouded rather than cleared the water, leaving much to be clarified in understanding the complex ways in which the brain carries out its normal functions, is altered during disease, and is improved by pharmacological intervention. On completing this chapter, students should have a neurobiological framework into which they can fit existing, as well as future, information about mental illness and its treatment.

Structure and Function of the Brain

FUNCTIONS OF THE BRAIN

The regulation of behavior and the carrying out of mental processes are important, but far from the only, responsibilities of the brain. Box 3-1 summarizes some of the major activities for which the brain is responsible. Because all of these brain functions are carried out by similar mechanisms (interactions of neurons), and often in similar locations, it is not surprising that men-

---

BOX 3-1

Functions of the Brain

- Monitor changes in the external world
- Monitor the composition of body fluids
- Regulate the contractions of the skeletal muscles
- Regulate the internal organs
- Initiate and regulate the basic drives: hunger, thirst, sex, aggressive self-protection
- Mediate conscious sensation
- Store and retrieve memories
- Regulate mood (affect) and emotions
- Think and perform intellectual functions
- Regulate the sleep cycle
- Produce and interpret language
- Process visual and auditory data

tal disturbances are often associated with alterations in other brain functions and that the drugs used to treat mental disturbances can also interfere with other activities of the brain.

The brain serves as the coordinator and director of the body's response to both internal and external changes. Appropriate responses require a constant monitoring of the environment, interpretation and integration of the incoming information, and control over the appropriate organs of response. The goal of these responses is to maintain homeostasis and thus to maintain life. Information about the external world is relayed from various sense organs to the brain by the peripheral nerves. This information, which is at first received as gross sensation (light, sound, touch), must ultimately be interpreted (a key, a train whistle, a hand on the back). Interestingly, a component of major psychiatric disturbance (e.g., schizophrenia) is an alteration of sensory experience. Thus, the client may experience a sensation that does not originate in the external world. People with schizophrenia may hear voices talking to them (auditory hallucination), or they may misinterpret incoming information that does originate in the external world—for instance, thinking that a broom is a rifle (illusion). To some extent these types of phenomena are experienced by all of us, such as during dreaming.

The brain not only monitors the external world but also keeps a close watch on the internal one. Thus, information about blood pressure, body temperature, blood gases, and the chemical composition of the body fluids is continuously received by the brain so that it can direct the appropriate responses required to maintain homeostasis.

To respond to external changes, the brain must and does have control over the skeletal muscles. This control involves not only the ability to initiate contraction (e.g., to contract the biceps and flex the arm) but also the ability to fine-tune and coordinate contraction so that a person can, for example, guide the fingers to the correct keys on a piano. Unfortunately, both psychiatric disease and the treatment of psychiatric disease with psychotropic drugs are often associated with disturbance of movement.

It is important to remember that the skeletal muscles controlled by the brain include the diaphragm, which is essential for breathing, and the muscles of the throat, tongue, and mouth, which are essential for speech. Thus, drugs that affect brain function can stimulate or depress respiration or lead to slurred speech.

Adjustments to changes within the body require that the brain exert control over the various internal organs. For example, if blood pressure drops, the brain must direct the heart to pump more blood and the smooth muscles of the arterioles to constrict. This increase in cardiac output and vasoconstriction allows the body to return blood pressure to its normal level.

The autonomic nervous system and the endocrine system serve as the communication links between the brain and the cardiac muscle, smooth muscle, and glands of which the internal organs are composed (Figure 3-1). Thus, if the brain needs to stimulate the heart, it must activate the sympathetic nerves to the sinoatrial node and the ventricular myocardium, and if it needs to bring about vasoconstriction, it must activate the sympathetic nerves to the smooth muscles of the arterioles.

The linkage between the brain and the internal organs that allows for the maintenance of homeostasis may also serve to translate mental disturbances, such as anxiety, into alterations of internal function. For example, anxiety in some people can cause activation of parasympathetic nerves to the digestive tract, leading to hypermotility and diarrhea. Likewise, anxiety can activate the sympathetic nerves to the arterioles, leading to vasoconstriction and hypertension.

The brain exerts its influence over the internal organs not only via the connections of the autonomic nervous system, but also by its regulation of the hormonal secretions of the pituitary gland, which in turn regulate those of a number of other glands. A specific area of the brain, the hypothalamus, secretes hormones called releasing factors that are carried directly to the pituitary gland, where they stimulate or inhibit the synthesis and release of pituitary hormones. These pituitary hormones, in turn, are carried in the general circulation, where they can influence various internal activities. A classic example of this linkage is the release of gonadotropin-releasing hormone by the hypothalamus at the time of puberty. This hormone stimulates the release of two gonadotropins, follicle-stimulating hormone and luteinizing hormone, by the pituitary and consequent activation of the ovaries or testes. Not surprisingly, this linkage may explain why anxiety or depression in some women may lead to disturbances of the menstrual cycle.

The relationship among the brain, the pituitary gland, and the adrenal glands seems to play a particularly important role in normal and abnormal mental function. Specifically, the hypothalamic secretion **corticotropin-releasing hormone (CRH)** stimulates the pituitary to release corticotropin, which in turn stimulates the cortex of each adrenal gland to secrete the hormone cortisol. This system is activated as a normal component of the body's general response to a variety of mental and physical stresses. Among many other actions, all three hormones—CRH, corticotropin, and cortisol—influence the functions of the nerve cells of the brain. There is considerable evidence that in both anxiety and depression this system is overactive and does not respond to the normal limitations of negative feedback.

To understand the neurobiological basis of mental disease and its treatment, it is helpful to distinguish

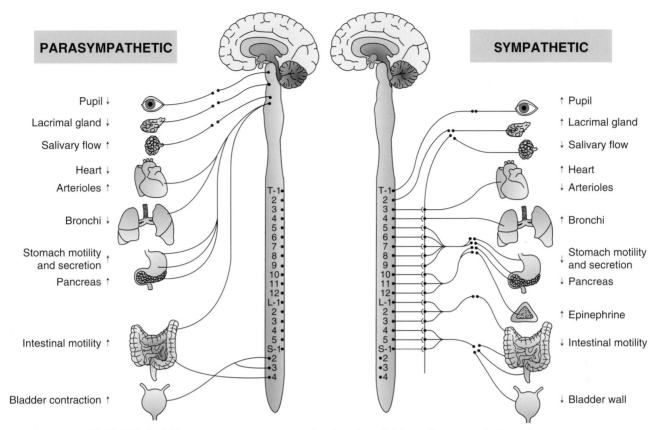

FIGURE 3-1 The autonomic nervous system has two divisions: the sympathetic and parasympathetic. The sympathetic division is dominant in stress situations, such as fear and anger—known as the fight-or-flight response.

between the various types of brain activity that serve as the basis of mental experience and of behavior. An understanding of these activities shows where to look for disturbed function and what to hope for in treatment.

The brain, for example, is responsible for the basic drives such as sex and hunger that play a strong role in molding behavior. Disturbances of these drives (e.g., overeating or undereating, loss of sexual interest) can be an indication of an underlying psychological disease such as depression.

The entire cycle of sleep and wakefulness, as well as the intensity of alertness while the person is awake, are regulated and coordinated by various regions of the brain. Although we are far from a full understanding of the true homeostatic function of sleep, there is no question that it is essential for both physiological and psychological well-being. Sleep disturbances are often a symptom of psychological distress, and an assessment of sleep patterns is part of what is required to determine a psychiatric diagnosis.

When a person is awake, the degree of alertness and the ability to focus attention are regulated in complex ways by the brain. Disturbances in alertness and focus—hypervigilance in a person with paranoid schizophrenia or inability to concentrate in a person with depression—can be indications of mental disturbance.

Unfortunately, many of the drugs used to treat psychiatric problems interfere with the normal regulation of sleep and alertness. Drugs with a sedative-hypnotic effect can blunt the degree to which a person feels alert and is able to focus attention and can make the client feel drowsy and fall asleep. The sedative-hypnotic effect demands caution in using these drugs while engaging in activities that require a great deal of attention, such as driving a car or operating farm machinery. One way of minimizing the danger is to give such drugs at night just before the client goes to sleep. Alteration in this area may also form a component of attention deficit hyperactivity disorder (ADHD) in which a child or adult has difficulty maintaining the focus of attention on one source and is continuously in search of novel and intense stimuli.

The cycle of sleep and wakefulness is only one aspect of what we call circadian rhythms, the fluctuation of various physiological and behavioral parameters over a 24-hour cycle. Other variations include changes in body temperature, the secretion of hormones such as corticotropin and cortisol, and the secretion of neurotransmitters such as norepinephrine and serotonin. Both norepinephrine and serotonin are thought to be involved in mood (affect), whether normal or abnormal; thus, daily fluctuations of mood may be related in part to circadian variations in these transmitters. There is some evidence that the circadian rhythm of neurotransmitter secretion is altered in psychological disease, particularly in disorders that involve alteration of mood.

All aspects of conscious mental experience and sense of self must ultimately result from the neurophysiological activity of the brain. The most basic type of conscious mental activity is probably the loose, meandering stream of consciousness that can jump back and forth between thoughts of future responsibilities, past experience, fantasized activities, interpersonal grievances, and so on. Conscious mental activity must, of course, become much more organized when it is applied to problem solving and the interpretation of the external world. Both the random stream of consciousness and the ability to interpret the environment can become extremely distorted in psychiatric illness. Thus, a person with schizophrenia can show chaotic and seemingly incoherent speech and thought patterns (a jumble of unrelated words known as **word salad,** and unconnected phrases and topics known as **looseness of association**) and delusional interpretations of personal interactions, such as beliefs about people or events that are not supported by data or reality.

An extremely important component of mental activity is memory, the ability to retain and recall past experience. From both an anatomical and a physiological perspective, there is thought to be a major difference in the processing of short- and long-term memory. Clinically, this can be seen dramatically in some forms of cognitive mental disorders such as dementia, in which a person has no recall of the events of the previous 8 minutes but may have vivid recall of events that occurred 80 years earlier.

Conscious mental activity and memory become integrated in complex and still unknown ways in the process of learning. In some cases, such as learning the names of the states in the United States, learning primarily involves memory storage and retrieval. In others, in-depth thought processes (abstract, organizing, categorizing) must be applied along with the retrieval of facts; examples include the analysis of a poem, the solution of a complex mathematical problem, and application of the nursing process for that matter.

A very important, and often neglected, aspect of learning involves the social skills that cement interpersonal relationships. In almost all types of mental illness, from mild anxiety to severe schizophrenia, difficulties in interpersonal relationships are important parts of the disorder and improvements in these relationships are an important part of the cure. The relationship between brain activity and social behavior is an area of intense research. It involves basic genetic drives modified by individual experience. There is evidence that positive reward-based experiential learning and negative avoidance learning may involve different areas of the brain.

CELLULAR COMPOSITION OF THE BRAIN

The brain is composed of nerve cells, or neurons, that conduct electrical impulses and the various types of cells that surround these neurons. Traditionally it has been thought that the types of activity we have discussed thus far, the various functions carried out by the brain, result from the interactions of neurons. The surrounding cells have been thought to provide for the physical, metabolic, and immunological support of the neurons. However, it may well be that the interactions of the various types of cells are more complex than was originally assumed.

Most functions of the brain, from regulation of blood pressure to the conscious sense of self, are thought to result from the actions of individual neurons and the interconnections between these neurons. Although neurons come in a great variety of shapes and sizes, all carry out the same three types of physiological action: (1) they respond to stimuli, (2) they conduct electrical impulses, and (3) they release chemicals called neurotransmitters.

An essential feature of neurons is their ability to conduct an electrical impulse from one end of the cell to the other. This electrical impulse consists of a self-propagating change in membrane permeability that first allows the inward flow of sodium ions and then the outward flow of potassium ions. The inward flow of sodium ions changes the polarity of the membrane from positive on the outside to positive on the inside. Movement of potassium ions out of the cell returns the positive charge to the outside of the cell. Because these electrical charges are self-propagating, a change at one end of the cell is conducted along the membrane until it reaches the other end of the cell (Figure 3-2). The functional significance of this propagation is that the electrical impulse serves as a means of communication between one part of the body and another.

Once an electrical impulse reaches the end of a neuron, a chemical called a neurotransmitter is released. A neurotransmitter is a chemical substance that functions as a neuromessenger. Neurotransmitters are released from the axon terminal at the **presynaptic** neuron on excitation. This transmitter then diffuses across a narrow space, or synapse, to an adjacent **postsynaptic** neuron, where it attaches to specialized receptors on the cell surface and either inhibits or excites the postsynaptic neuron. It is the interaction between transmitter and receptor that allows the activity of one neuron to influence the activity of other neurons. Depending on the chemical structure of the transmitter and the specific type of receptor to which it attaches, the postsynaptic cell will be rendered either more or less likely to initiate an electrical impulse. As we shall see, it is the interaction between transmitter and receptor that is a major target of

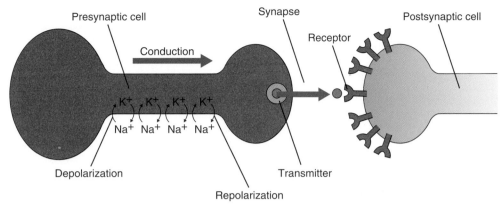

FIGURE 3-2 Activities of neurons. Conduction along a neuron involves the inward movement of sodium ions (Na⁺) followed by the outward movement of potassium ions (K⁺). When the current reaches the end of the cell, a neurotransmitter is released. The transmitter crosses the synapse and attaches to a receptor on the postsynaptic cell. The attachment of transmitter to receptor either stimulates or inhibits the postsynaptic cell.

the drugs used to treat psychiatric disease. Table 3-1 lists some of the most important neurotransmitters and the types of receptors to which they attach. Also listed are the mental disorders that are associated with an increase or decrease in these neurotransmitters.

After attaching to a receptor and exerting its influence on the postsynaptic cell, the transmitter separates from the receptor and is destroyed. The process of transmitter destruction is described in Box 3-2. As can be seen, there are two basic mechanisms by which transmitters are destroyed. Some transmitters (e.g., acetylcholine) are destroyed by specific enzymes at the postsynaptic cell. The enzyme that destroys acetylcholine is called **acetylcholinesterase.** Other transmitters (e.g., norepinephrine) are taken back into the presynaptic cell from which they were originally released by a process called cellular reuptake. Upon their return to these cells, the transmitters are either reused or destroyed by intracellular enzymes. In the case of the monoamine transmitters (e.g., norepinephrine, dopamine, serotonin), the destructive enzyme is called **monoamine oxidase (MAO).**

As a means of regulating the concentration of transmitters at the postsynaptic receptors, many of the transmitters exert a feedback inhibition of their own release. This inhibition is accomplished by the attachment of transmitters to what are called presynaptic receptors at the synapse, which acts to inhibit the further release of transmitters.

In recent years it has become clear that the concept of a neuron releasing a specific transmitter that stimulates or inhibits a postsynaptic membrane receptor and acts via negative feedback on a presynaptic receptor is an accurate but far from complete picture of the interaction between nerve cells. It is now known that in many cases neurons release more than one chemical at the same time. Transmitters such as norepinephrine or acetylcholine, which have immediate effects on postsynaptic membranes, are often joined by larger molecules, neuropeptides, that may initiate long-term changes in the postsynaptic cells. The changes may involve basic cell functions such as genetic expression and lead to modifications of cell shape and responsiveness to stimuli. Ultimately this means that the action of one neuron on another affects not only the immediate response of that neuron but also its sensitivity to future influence. The long-term implications of this for neural development, normal and abnormal mental health, and the treatment of psychiatric disease are being intensively investigated.

It is also becoming increasingly clear that the communication between neurons at a synapse is not unidirectional. *Neurotrophic factors* are proteins and even simple gases such as carbon monoxide and nitrous oxide that are released by postsynaptic cells and influence the growth, shape, and activity of presynaptic cells. These factors are thought to be particularly important during the development of the brain in utero, guiding the growing brain to form the proper neuronal connections. However, it is now apparent that the brain retains anatomical plasticity throughout life and that internal and external influences can alter the synaptic network of the brain. There is much current investigation of the role that altered genetic expression or environmental trauma can play in the action of these factors and the negative and positive consequences of these changes on mental function and psychiatric disease.

The development and responsiveness of neurons is dependent not only on chemicals released by other neurons but also on chemicals brought to the neurons by the blood, particularly the **steroid hormones.** Estrogen, testosterone, and cortisol can bind to neurons, where they can cause short- and long-term changes in neuronal activity. A clear and tragic example of this is seen in the psychosis that can sometimes result from the hypersecretion of cortisol in Cushing's disease or from the use of prednisone in high doses to treat chronic inflammatory disease.

TABLE 3-1

Transmitters and Receptors

Transmitters	Receptors	Effects/Comments	Association with Mental Health
Monoamines			
Dopamine (DA)	D_1, D_2, D_3, D_4, D_5	■ Involved in fine muscle movement ■ Involved in integration of emotions and thoughts ■ Involved in decision making ■ Stimulates hypothalamus to release hormones (sex, thyroid, adrenal)	*Decrease:* ■ Parkinson's disease ■ Depression *Increase:* ■ Schizophrenia ■ Mania
Norepinephrine (NE) (noradrenaline)	α_1, α_2, β_1, β_2	■ Level in brain affects mood ■ Stimulates sympathetic branch of autonomic nervous system for "fight or flight" in response to stress	*Decrease:* ■ Depression *Increase:* ■ Mania ■ Anxiety states ■ Schizophrenia
Serotonin (5-HT)	5-HT, 5-HT_2, 5-HT_3, 5-HT_4	■ Plays a role in sleep regulation, hunger, mood states, and pain perception ■ Plays a role in aggression and sexual behavior	*Decrease:* ■ Depression *Increase:* ■ Anxiety states
Histamine	H_1, H_2	■ Involved in alertness ■ Involved in inflammatory response ■ Stimulates gastric secretion	*Decrease:* ■ Depression ■ Sedation ■ Weight gain
Amino Acids			
γ-aminobutyric acid (GABA)	GABA_A, GABA_B	■ Plays a role in inhibition; reduces aggression, excitation, and anxiety ■ May play a role in pain perception ■ Has anticonvulsant and muscle-relaxing properties	*Decrease:* ■ Anxiety disorders ■ Schizophrenia ■ Huntington's chorea *Increase:* ■ Reduction of anxiety
Glutamate	NMDA, AMPA	■ Is excitatory ■ Plays a role in learning and memory	*Decrease (NMDA):* ■ Psychomimetic state that resembles schizophrenia *Increase (AMPA):* ■ Improvement of cognitive performance in behavioral tasks
Cholinergics			
Acetylcholine (ACh)	Nicotinic, muscarinic (M_1, M_2, M_3)	■ Plays a role in learning, memory ■ Regulates mood: mania, sexual aggression ■ Affects sexual and aggressive behavior ■ Stimulates parasympathetic nervous system	*Decrease:* ■ Alzheimer's disease ■ Huntington's chorea ■ Parkinson's disease *Increase:* ■ Depression
Peptides (Neuromodulators)			
Substance P (SP)	SP	■ Centrally active SP antagonist has antidepressant and antianxiety effects in depression ■ Promotes and reinforces memory ■ Enhances sensitivity to pain receptors to activate	■ Involved in regulation of mood and anxiety ■ Role in pain management
Somatostatin (SRIF)	SRIF	■ Altered levels associated with cognitive disease	*Decrease:* ■ Alzheimer's disease ■ Decreased levels of SRIF found in spinal fluid of some depressed clients *Increase:* ■ Huntington's chorea
Neurotensin (NT)	NT	■ Endogenous antipsychotic-like properties	Decreased levels found in spinal fluid of schizophrenic clients

AMPA, α-Amino-3-hydroxy-5-methyl-4-isoxazolepropionic acid; *NMDA,* N-methyl-D-aspartate.

Destruction of Neurotransmitters

A full explanation of the various ways in which psychotropic drugs alter neuronal activity requires a brief review of the manner in which neurotransmitters are destroyed after attaching to the receptors. To avoid continuous and prolonged action on the postsynaptic cell, the neurotransmitter is released shortly after attaching to the postsynaptic receptor. Once released, the transmitter is destroyed in one of two ways.

One way is the immediate inactivation of the transmitter at the postsynaptic membrane. An example of this method of destruction is the action of the enzyme acetylcholinesterase on the neurotransmitter acetylcholine. Acetylcholinesterase is present at the postsynaptic membrane and destroys acetylcholine shortly after it attaches to nicotinic or muscarinic receptors on the postsynaptic cell.

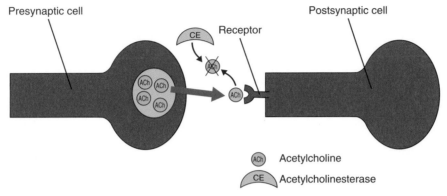

A *second* method of neurotransmitter inactivation is a little more complex. After interacting with the postsynaptic receptor, the transmitter is released and taken back into the presynaptic cell, the cell from which it was released. This process, referred to as the reuptake of neurotransmitter, is a common target for drug action. Once inside the presynaptic cell, the transmitter is either recycled or inactivated by an enzyme within the cell. The monoamine transmitters norepinephrine, dopamine, and serotonin are all inactivated in this manner by the enzyme monoamine oxidase.

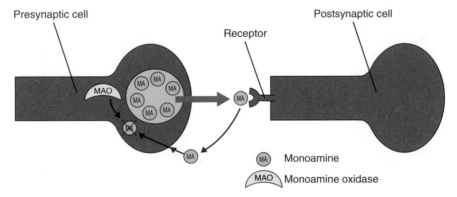

Looking at this second method, you might naturally ask what prevents the enzyme from destroying the transmitter before its release. The answer is that before release the transmitter is stored within a membrane and is thus protected from the degradative enzyme. After release and reuptake, the transmitter is either destroyed by the enzyme or reenters the membrane to be used again.

ORGANIZATION OF THE NERVOUS SYSTEM

Brainstem

The central core of the brainstem regulates the internal organs and is responsible for such vital functions as the regulation of blood gases and the maintenance of blood pressure.

The hypothalamus, a small area in the ventral superior portion of the brainstem, plays a vital role in such basic drives as hunger, thirst, and sex. It also serves as a crucial link between higher brain activities such as thought and emotion and the functioning of the internal organs. It is a crucial psychosomatic link. The brainstem also serves as an initial processing center for sensory information that is then sent on to the cerebral cortex. Through projections of what is called the reticular activating system (RAS), the brainstem regulates the entire cycle of sleep and wakefulness and the ability of the cerebrum to carry out conscious mental activity.

A variety of other ascending pathways, referred to as *mesolimbic* and *mesocortical pathways,* seem to play a strong role in modulating the emotional value of sensory material. These pathways project to those areas of the cerebrum collectively known as the limbic system that play a crucial role in emotional status and psychological function. They use norepinephrine, serotonin, and dopamine as their neurotransmitters. Much attention has been paid to the role of these pathways in normal and abnormal mental activity. For example, it is thought that the release of dopamine from what is called the *ventral tegmental pathway* plays a role in psychological reward and drug addiction. As we shall see, the neurotransmitters released by these neurons are major targets of the drugs used to treat psychiatric disease.

Cerebellum

Located posteriorly to the brainstem, the cerebellum (Figure 3-3) is primarily involved in the regulation of skeletal muscle coordination and contraction and the maintenance of equilibrium. It plays a crucial role in coordinating contractions so that movement is accomplished in a smooth and directed manner.

Cerebrum

The brainstem and cerebellum of the human brain are similar in both structure and function to these same structures in the brains of other mammals. The development of a much larger and more elaborate cerebrum is what distinguishes human beings from the rest of the animal kingdom.

The cerebrum, situated on top of and surrounding the brainstem, is responsible for mental activities and a conscious sense of being. Thus, the cerebrum is respon-

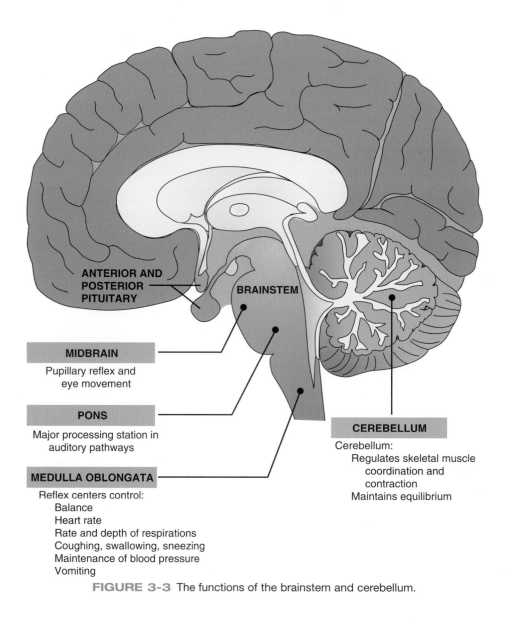

ANTERIOR AND POSTERIOR PITUITARY

BRAINSTEM

MIDBRAIN
Pupillary reflex and eye movement

PONS
Major processing station in auditory pathways

MEDULLA OBLONGATA
Reflex centers control:
Balance
Heart rate
Rate and depth of respirations
Coughing, swallowing, sneezing
Maintenance of blood pressure
Vomiting

CEREBELLUM
Cerebellum:
Regulates skeletal muscle coordination and contraction
Maintains equilibrium

FIGURE 3-3 The functions of the brainstem and cerebellum.

sible for our conscious perception of the external world and our own body, for emotional status, for memory, and for the control of the skeletal muscles that allow the willful direction of movement. The cerebrum is also responsible for language and the ability to communicate.

Anatomically, the cerebrum consists of surface and deep areas of integrating gray matter (the cerebral cortex and basal ganglia) and the connecting tracts of white matter that link these areas with each other and with the rest of the nervous system. The cerebral cortex, which forms the outer layer of the brain, is responsible for conscious sensation and the initiation of movement. It is organized in such a way that specific areas of the cortex are responsible for specific sensations: the parietal cortex is responsible for touch, the temporal cortex for sound, the occipital cortex for vision, and so on. Likewise, the initiation of skeletal muscle contraction is controlled by a specific area of the frontal cortex. Of course, all the areas of the cortex are interconnected so that an integral picture of the world can be formed and, if necessary, linked to an appropriate response (Figure 3-4).

Specialized areas of the cerebral cortex are responsible for language in both its sensory and motor aspects. Sensory language functions include the ability to read, to understand spoken language, and to know the names of

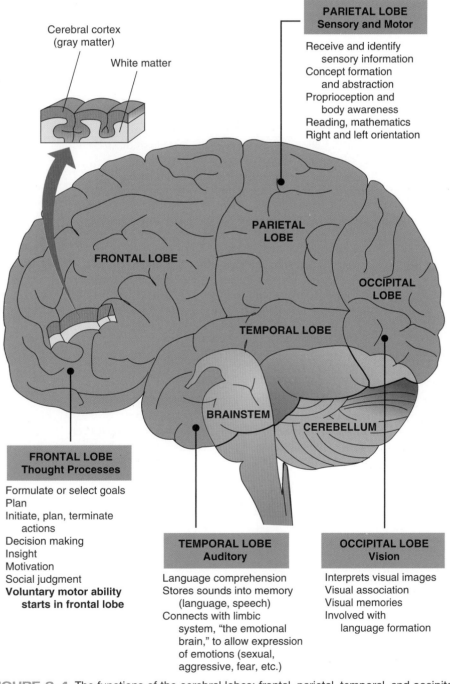

**PARIETAL LOBE
Sensory and Motor**

Receive and identify
    sensory information
Concept formation
    and abstraction
Proprioception and
    body awareness
Reading, mathematics
Right and left orientation

Cerebral cortex
(gray matter)

White matter

PARIETAL
LOBE

FRONTAL LOBE

OCCIPITAL
LOBE

TEMPORAL LOBE

BRAINSTEM

CEREBELLUM

**FRONTAL LOBE
Thought Processes**

Formulate or select goals
Plan
Initiate, plan, terminate
    actions
Decision making
Insight
Motivation
Social judgment
**Voluntary motor ability
    starts in frontal lobe**

**TEMPORAL LOBE
Auditory**

Language comprehension
Stores sounds into memory
    (language, speech)
Connects with limbic
    system, "the emotional
    brain," to allow expression
    of emotions (sexual,
    aggressive, fear, etc.)

**OCCIPITAL LOBE
Vision**

Interprets visual images
Visual association
Visual memories
Involved with
    language formation

FIGURE 3-4 The functions of the cerebral lobes: frontal, parietal, temporal, and occipital.

objects that are perceived by the senses, whereas motor functions involve the ability to use muscles properly for speech and writing. In both neurological and psychological dysfunction, the use of language may become compromised or distorted. The change in linguistic ability may be a factor in determining a diagnosis.

In addition to the gray matter forming the surface of the cerebrum, there are pockets of integrating gray matter deep within the cerebrum. Some of these, the basal ganglia, are involved in the regulation of movement. Others, the amygdala and hippocampus, are involved in emotions, learning, memory, and basic drives. Significantly, there is an overlap of these various areas both anatomically and in the types of neurotransmitters employed. One consequence is that drugs used to treat emotional disturbances may cause move-

ment disorders, and drugs used to treat movement disorders may cause emotional changes.

A variety of noninvasive imaging techniques is used to visualize brain structure, functions, and metabolic activity in clients experiencing various mental disorders. Table 3-2 identifies some common brain imaging techniques and some preliminary findings as they relate to psychiatry. There are basically two types of neuroimaging technique: structural and functional. **Structural imaging techniques** (e.g., computed tomography [CT] and magnetic resonance imaging [MRI]) identify gross anatomical changes in the brain. **Functional imaging techniques** (e.g., positron emission tomography [PET] and single photon emission computed tomography [SPECT]) reveal physiological activity in the brain, as described in Table 3-2.

TABLE 3-2

Common Brain Imaging Techniques

Technique	Description	Uses	Psychiatric Relevance and Preliminary Findings
STRUCTURAL: Show Gross Anatomical Details of Brain Structures			
Computed tomography (CT)	A series of x-ray images are taken of the brain and a computer analysis produces "slices" providing a precise 3D-like reconstruction of each segment.	Can detect: ▪ Lesions ▪ Abrasions ▪ Areas of infarct ▪ Aneurysm	Schizophrenia ▪ Cortical atrophy ▪ Third ventricle enlargement Cognitive disorders ▪ Abnormalities
Magnetic resonance imaging (MRI)	A magnetic field is applied to the brain. The nuclei of hydrogen atoms absorb and emit radio waves that are analyzed by computer, which provides 3D visualization of the brain's structure in sectional images.	Can detect: ▪ Brain edema ▪ Ischemia ▪ Infection ▪ Neoplasm ▪ Trauma	Schizophrenia ▪ Enlarged ventricles ▪ Reduction in temporal lobe and prefrontal lobe
Functional magnetic resonance imaging (fMRI)	A functional imaging approach that avoids exposure to ionizing radiation.		
FUNCTIONAL: Show Some Activity of the Brain			
Position-emission tomography (PET) (uses radioactive tracer)	Radioactive substance is injected, travels to the brain, and shows up as bright spots on the scan. Data collected by the detectors are relayed to a computer, which produces images of the activity and 3D visualization of the CNS.	Can detect: ▪ Oxygen utilization ▪ Glucose metabolism ▪ Blood flow ▪ Neurotransmitter-receptor interaction	Schizophrenia ▪ Increased D_2, D_3 receptors in caudate nucleus ▪ Abnormalities in limbic system Mood disorder ▪ Abnormalities in temporal lobes Adult ADHD ▪ Decreased utilization of glucose
Single photon emission computed tomography (SPECT) (uses radioactive tracer)	Similar to PET but uses radionuclides that emit γ-radiation (photons). Measures various aspects of brain functioning and provides images of multiple layers of the CNS (as does PET).	Can detect: ▪ Circulation of cerebrospinal fluid ▪ Similar functions to PET	

ADHD, Attention deficit hyperactivity disorder; *CNS*, central nervous system; *3D*, three-dimensional.

PET scans are particularly useful in identifying physiological and biochemical changes as they occur in living tissue. Usually, a radioactive "tag" is used to trace compounds such as glucose in the brain. Glucose use is related to functional activity in certain areas of the brain. For example, in clients with schizophrenia, PET scans may show a decreased use of glucose in the frontal lobes of unmedicated individuals. Figure 3-5 shows lower brain activity in the frontal lobe of a twin diagnosed with schizophrenia than in the twin who does not have schizophrenia. The area affected in the frontal cortex of the schizophrenic twin is an area associated with reasoning skills, which are greatly impaired in people with schizophrenia. Scans such as these suggest a location in the frontal cortex as the site of functional impairment in people with schizophrenia.

In people with obsessive-compulsive disorder, brain metabolism is seen to be increased in certain areas of the frontal cortex on PET scans. Figure 3-6 shows increased brain metabolism in such an individual compared with that in a normal control, which suggests altered brain function in people with obsessive-compulsive disorder.

Decreased brain activity may be seen on PET scans in the prefrontal cortex of many depressed individuals. Figure 3-7 shows the results of a PET scan taken af-

ter a form of radioactively tagged glucose was used as a tracer to visualize brain activity. The depressed client shows reduced brain activity compared with a nondepressed control. Finally, Figure 3-8 shows three views of a PET scan of the brain of a client with Alzheimer's disease.

Modern imaging techniques have also become important tools in assessing molecular changes in mental disease and marking the receptor sites of drug action.

From a psychiatric perspective, we would like to be able to understand where in the brain the various components of psychological activity take place and what types of neurotransmitters and receptors underlie this activity physiologically. Currently, our understanding of both of these questions is far from complete. However, it is thought that the limbic system—a group of structures that includes parts of the frontal cortex, the basal ganglia, and the brainstem—is a major locus of psychological activity.

Within these areas the monoamine transmitters (norepinephrine, dopamine, and serotonin), the amino acid transmitters glutamate and γ-aminobutyric acid (GABA), and the neuropeptides CRH and endorphin, as well as acetylcholine, play a major role. Alterations in these areas are thought to form the basis of psychiatric disease and are the target for pharmacological treatment.

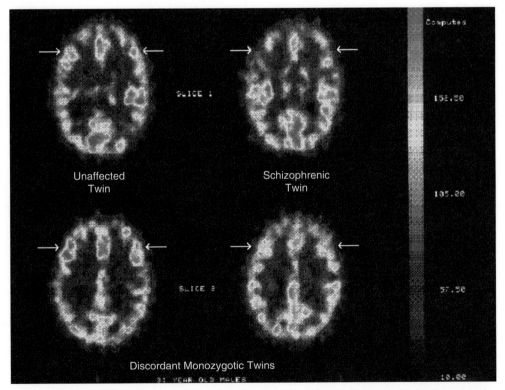

FIGURE 3-5 Positron emission tomographic scans of blood flow in identical twins, one of whom has schizophrenia, illustrate that individuals with this illness have reduced brain activity in the frontal lobes when asked to perform a reasoning task that requires activation of this area. Schizophrenic clients also perform poorly on the task. This suggests a site of functional impairments in schizophrenia (From Karen Berman, MD, courtesy of National Institute of Mental Health, Clinical Brain Disorders Branch.)

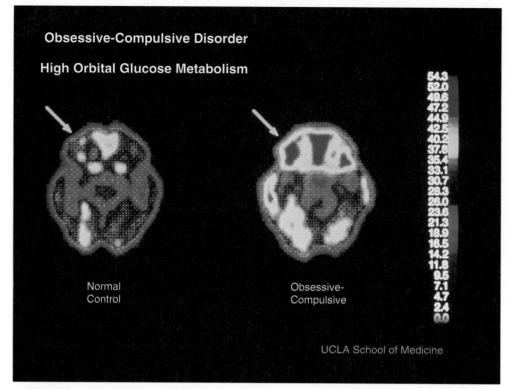

FIGURE 3-6 Positron emission tomographic scans show increased brain metabolism *(brighter colors),* particularly in the frontal cortex, in a client with obsessive-compulsive disorder (OCD), compared with a normal control. This suggests altered brain function in OCD. (From Lewis Baxter, MD, University of Alabama, courtesy National Institute of Mental Health.)

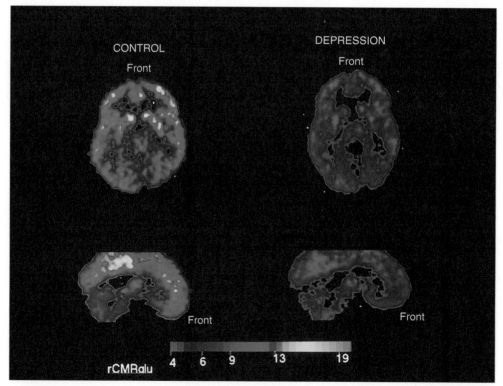

FIGURE 3-7 Positron emission tomographic scans of a normal subject *(left)* and a depressed client *(right)* reveal reduced brain activity *(darker colors)* in depression, especially in the prefrontal cortex. A form of radioactively tagged glucose was used as a tracer to visualize levels of brain activity. (From Mark George, MD, courtesy National Institute of Mental Health, Biological Psychiatry Branch.)

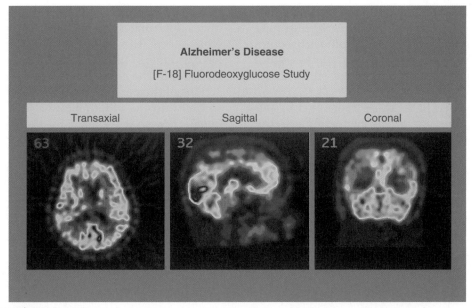

FIGURE 3-8 Positron emission tomographic (PET) scan of a client with Alzheimer's disease demonstrates a classic pattern for areas of hypometabolism in the temporal and parietal regions of the brain. Areas of reduced metabolism *(dark blue and black regions)* are very noticeable in the sagittal and coronal views. (Courtesy PET Imaging Center, Department of Radiology, University of Iowa Hospitals and Clinics, Iowa City.)

DISTURBANCES OF MENTAL FUNCTION

Although in a limited number of clients the cause of mental dysfunction is known, most occurrences are of unknown origin. Among known causes are drugs (e.g., lysergic acid diethylamide [LSD]), long-term use of prednisone, excess levels of hormones (e.g., thyroxine, cortisol), infection (e.g., encephalitis, acquired immunodeficiency syndrome [AIDS]), and physical trauma. Even when the cause is known, however, the link between the causative factor and the mental dysfunction is far from understood.

Results from numerous studies indicate that there is at least in part a genetic component to psychological dysfunction. The incidence of both thought and mood disorders is higher in relatives of people with these diseases than in the general population. There is also a strong concordance, although certainly not 100%, among identical twins even when they are raised apart. Psychosocial stress, either in the family of origin or in contacts with society at large, increases the likelihood of mental problems, as does physical disease. Genetics and environment interact in complex ways so that some people are better able to cope with stress than others.

Researchers ultimately want to be able to understand mental dysfunction in terms of altered activity of neurons in specific areas of the brain; the hope is that such an understanding will lead to better treatments and possible prevention of mental disorders. Current interest is focused on certain neurotransmitters and their receptors, particularly in the limbic system, which links the frontal cortex, basal ganglia, and upper brainstem. **As mentioned earlier, the transmitters that have been most consistently linked to mental activity are norepinephrine, dopamine, serotonin, GABA, glutamate, and CRH.**

Although the underlying physiology is complex, it is thought that a deficiency of norepinephrine or serotonin, or both, may serve as the biological basis of depression. Figure 3-9 shows that an insufficient degree of transmission may be due to a deficient release of transmitters by the presynaptic cell or to a loss of the ability of postsynaptic receptors to respond to the transmitters. Changes in transmitter release and receptor response can be both a cause and a consequence of intracellular changes in the neurons involved. Thought disorders such as schizophrenia are associated physiologically with excess transmission of the neurotransmitter dopamine, among other changes. As illustrated in Figure 3-10, this may be due to either an excess release of transmitter or an increase in receptor responsiveness.

The neurotransmitter γ-aminobutyric acid (GABA) seems to play a role in modulating neuronal excitability and anxiety. Not surprisingly, most antianxiety (anxiolytic) drugs act by increasing the effectiveness of this transmitter. This is accomplished primarily by increasing receptor responsiveness.

It is important to keep in mind that the various areas of the brain are interconnected structurally and functionally by a vast network of neurons. This network serves to integrate the many and varied activities of the brain. A limited number of neurotransmitters are used in the brain, and thus a particular transmitter is often used by different neurons to carry out quite different activities. For example, dopamine is used not only by neurons involved in thought processes but also by neurons involved in the regulation of movement.

As a result of the use of the same transmitter by different types of neurons, alterations in transmitter activity, due to a mental disturbance or to the drugs used to treat the disturbance, can affect more than one area of brain activity. In other words, alterations in mental status, whether arising from disease or from medication, are often accompanied by changes in basic drives, sleep patterns, body movement, and autonomic functions.

Mechanisms of Action of Psychotropic Drugs

Whenever one studies drugs, the important concepts of pharmacodynamics and pharmacokinetics must be kept in mind. Pharmacodynamics refers to the actions of the drug on the person, the types of changes it produces. Pharmacodynamic changes include both large-scale effects (the client feels less depressed) and molecular effects (the enzyme monoamine oxidase is inhibited). The term pharmacokinetics refers to the actions of the person on the drug. How is the drug absorbed into the blood? How is it transformed in the liver? How is it excreted by the kidney? Pharmacokinetics determines the blood level of a drug and is used to guide the dosage schedule. It is also used to determine the type and amount of drug used in cases of liver and kidney disease.

The processes of pharmacokinetics and pharmacodynamics play an extensive role in how genetic factors give rise to interindividual and cross-ethnic variations in drug response (Lin, Smith, & Lin, 2003). The Culturally Speaking box discusses how this new area of pharmacogenetics may influence the way health care providers tailor their prescriptions for clients.

Many drugs are transformed by the liver into active metabolites—chemicals that themselves have pharmacological actions. This knowledge is used by researchers in designing new drugs that make use of the

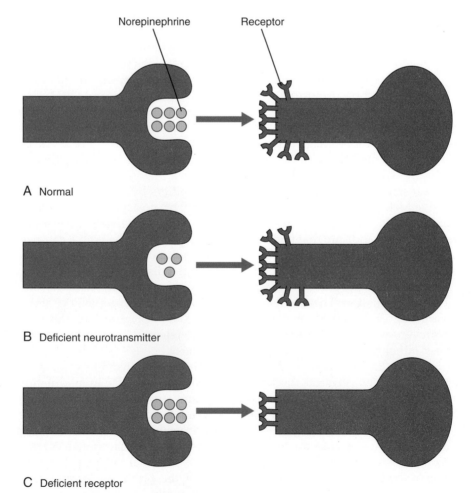

FIGURE 3-9 Normal transmission of neurotransmitters **(A).** Deficiency in transmission may be due to deficient release of transmitter, as shown in **B,** or to a reduction in receptors, as shown in **C.**

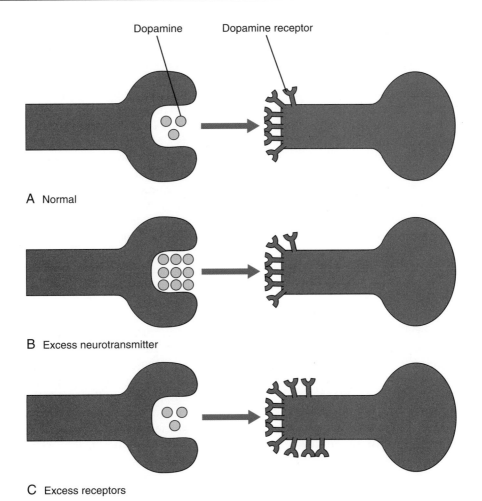

A Normal

B Excess neurotransmitter

C Excess receptors

FIGURE 3-10 Causes of excess transmission of neurotransmitters. Excess transmission may be due to excess release of transmitter, as shown in **B**, or to excess responsiveness of receptors, as shown in **C**.

■ ■ ■ **CULTURALLY SPEAKING**

Pharmacogenetics

Pharmacogenetics is a relatively new area; however, it is able to point out dramatic differences in drug response among various ethnic groups. Olajide and Bhui (1999) provide examples showing how a drug can have different effects in different cultural and ethnic groups. These differences are important for health care providers to take into consideration when prescribing psychopharmacological agents.

- **Lithium** causes greater neuron system toxicity in African Americans than it does in whites.
- **Haloperidol** plasma concentrations are 50% higher in Asian clients with schizophrenia than in white clients taking the same dosage.
- **Clozapine**-induced agranulocytosis has been found to be more prevalent in Ashkenazi Jews than in other ethnic groups.

- **β-blockers such as propranolol** have been found to be relatively ineffective in reducing hypertension in African Americans. However, relatively small dosages are effective in Asians compared with whites. Propranolol is at times used to treat anxiety disorders; it appears that it would not be a very effective anxiolytic for African Americans, whereas Asians would respond to relatively low dosages.

There are many factors that influence compliance with the medical regimen in all groups of people. Individuals from some ethnic and cultural groups have even greater compliance issues for a variety of reasons. For example, cultural and ethnic beliefs surrounding mental illness, attitudes toward the mental health system, and the cultural practices of an ethnic group all impact greatly on a client's degree of engagement and adherence with the medical regimen. This topic is discussed more fully in Chapter 7.

Olajide, D., & Bhui, K. (1999). Psychiatry and cultural relativity. In K. Bhui & D. Olajide (Eds.), *Mental health services provisions for a multi-cultural society.* London: Saunders.

body's own mechanisms to activate a chemical for pharmacological use.

An ideal psychiatric drug would relieve the mental disturbance of the client without inducing untoward cerebral (mental) or somatic (physical) effects. Unfortunately, in psychiatry, as in most areas of pharmacology, there are no drugs that are both fully effective and at the same time free of undesired side effects. Researchers work toward developing medications that target the symptoms while producing no or minimal side effects.

Because all the activities of the brain involve the actions of neurons, neurotransmitters, and receptors, these are the targets of pharmacological intervention. Most psychotropic drugs act by either increasing or decreasing the activity of certain transmitter-receptor systems. It is generally agreed that different transmitter-receptor systems are dysfunctional in persons with different psychiatric conditions. These differences offer more specific targets for drug action. In fact, much of what is known about the relationship between specific transmitters and specific disturbances has been derived from a knowledge of the pharmacology of the drugs used to treat these conditions. For example, it was found that most agents that were effective in reducing the delusions and hallucinations of schizophrenia block the D_2 receptors for dopamine. From this information, it was concluded that delusions and hallucinations result from overactivity of dopamine at these receptors.

ANTIPSYCHOTIC DRUGS

Standard First-Generation Antipsychotics

Figure 3-11 illustrates the proposed mechanism of action of the standard (first-generation) antipsychotic drugs: the phenothiazines, thioxanthenes, butyrophenones, and pharmacologically related agents. These drugs are strong antagonists (blocking the action) of the D_2 receptors for dopamine. By binding to these receptors and blocking the attachment of dopamine, they reduce dopaminergic transmission. It has been postulated that an overactivity of the dopamine system in certain areas of the limbic system may be responsible for at least some of the symptoms of schizophrenia; thus, blockage of dopamine may reduce these symptoms. This is thought to be particularly true of the "positive" symptoms of schizophrenia, such as delusions (e.g., paranoid and grandiose ideas) and hallucinations (e.g., hearing or seeing things not present in reality).

These drugs, however, are also antagonists, to varying degrees, of the muscarinic receptors for acetylcholine, α_1 receptors for norepinephrine, and histamine$_1$ (H_1) receptors for histamine. Although it is unclear if this antagonism plays a role in the beneficial effects of the drugs, it is certain that antagonism is responsible for some of their major side effects (see Chapter 20). For a more detailed description of how these drugs not only block dopamine but also can block muscarinic receptors for acetylcholine and α_1 receptors for norepinephrine, go to the Evolve website.

As summarized in Figure 3-12, many of the untoward side effects of these drugs can be understood as a logical extension of their receptor-blocking activity. Thus, because in the basal ganglia dopamine (D_2) plays a major role in the regulation of movement, it is not surprising that dopamine blockage can lead to motor abnormalities (extrapyramidal side effects) such as parkinsonism, akinesia, akathisia, dyskinesia, and tardive dyskinesia. Nurses and physicians often monitor clients for evidence of involuntary movements after administration of the standard first-generation antipsychotic agents. One popular scale is called the Abnormal Involuntary Movement Scale (AIMS), which is included in Chapter 20. You can practice with a classmate the use of this scale. These disturbances and others are discussed in Chapter 20, which details the clinical use of the antipsychotic drugs along with specific nursing interventions and client teaching strategies.

An important physiological function of dopamine is that it acts as the hypothalamic factor which inhibits the release of prolactin from the anterior pituitary gland; thus, blockage of dopamine transmission can lead to increased pituitary secretion of prolactin. In

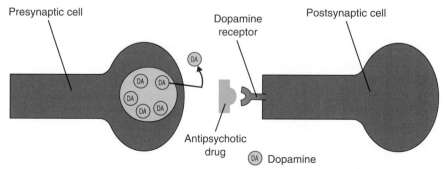

FIGURE 3-11 How the standard (first-generation) antipsychotics block dopamine receptors. *DA,* Dopamine.

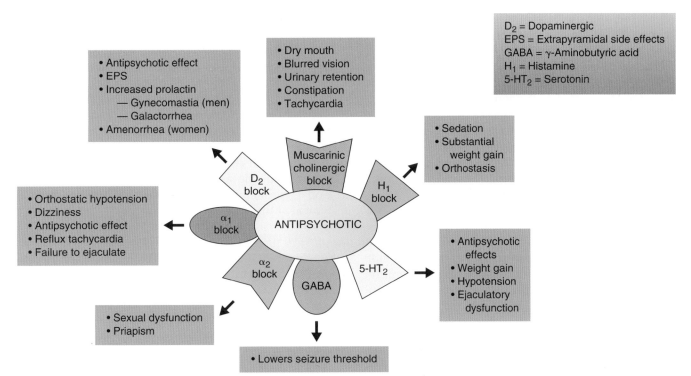

FIGURE 3-12 Adverse effects of receptor blockage of antipsychotic agents. (From Varcarolis, E. [2004]. *Manual of psychiatric nursing care plans* [2nd ed.]. St. Louis: Elsevier.)

women this hyperprolactinemia can result in amenorrhea (absence of the menses) or galactorrhea (milk flow), and in men it can lead to gynecomastia (development of the male mammary glands).

Acetylcholine is the neurotransmitter released by the postganglionic neurons of the parasympathetic nervous system. Through its attachment to muscarinic receptors on internal organs, it serves to help regulate internal function. Blockage of the muscarinic receptors by phenothiazines and a wide variety of other psychiatric drugs can lead to a constellation of untoward effects predictable from knowledge of the normal physiology of the parasympathetic nervous system. These side effects typically involve blurred vision, dry mouth, constipation, and urinary hesitancy.

In addition to blocking dopamine and muscarinic receptors, many of the standards first-generation antipsychotic drugs act as antagonists at the α_1 receptors for norepinephrine. These receptors are found on smooth muscle cells that contract in response to norepinephrine from sympathetic nerves. For example, the ability of sympathetic nerves to constrict blood vessels is dependent on the attachment of norepinephrine to α_1 receptors; thus, blockage of these receptors can bring about vasodilation and a consequent drop in blood pressure. Sympathetic nervous system–mediated vasoconstriction is particularly essential for maintaining normal blood pressure in the upright position; blockage of the α_1 receptors can lead to orthostatic hypotension.

The α_1 receptors are also found on the vas deferens and are responsible for the propulsive contractions leading to ejaculation. Blockage of these receptors can lead to a failure to ejaculate.

Finally, many of these conventional first-generation antipsychotic agents, as well as a variety of other psychiatric drugs, block the H_1 receptors for histamine. The two most significant side effects of blocking these receptors are sedation and substantial weight gain. The sedation may be beneficial in severely agitated clients. It is because of all of these troublesome side effects that nonadherence to the medication regimen is a significant issue, and the atypical antipsychotic agents have now become the drugs of choice.

Atypical Antipsychotics

The newer atypical antipsychotic drugs produce few or no extrapyramidal symptoms and also target the negative as well as the positive symptoms of schizophrenia, as discussed more fully in Chapter 20. These newer agents are often chosen as first-line treatment over the standard and less frequently used antipsychotics described earlier because of their more favorable side effect profile.

These newer drugs seem to show a difference in receptor binding profile from the older agents. They bind to dopamine receptors in the limbic system preferentially over those in the neostriatal areas of the basal ganglia and thus are able to exert psychiatric actions without motor side effects. They are also antagonists at the 5-HT$_2$ receptors for serotonin. This action may explain their efficacy in treating negative as well as positive symptoms in schizophrenia.

Significant disturbances in cognitive function are seen in as many as 85% of people with schizophrenia, and these disturbances progress in most clients. However, there is some evidence that the atypical antipsychotic agents may improve some of the domains of cognition (McGurk et al., 2004). Olanzapine seems to be the most effective for improvement in cognition at the time of this writing (McGurk et al., 2004).

Clozapine

Clozapine (Clozaril), the first of the atypicals, is an antipsychotic drug that is relatively free of the motor side effects of the phenothiazines and other first-generation antipsychotics. It is thought that clozapine preferentially blocks the dopamine receptors in the limbic system rather than those in the neostriatal area of the basal ganglia. This allows this agent to exert an antipsychotic action without leading to difficulties with movement.

Clozapine can produce a possibly fatal side effect in 1% to 2% of clients. This is due to its potential to suppress bone marrow and induce agranulocytosis. Any deficiency in white blood cells renders a person prone to serious infection. For this reason, regular measurement of white blood cell count is mandatory for any client taking clozapine; the count should be measured weekly for the first 6 months, then every other week.

Clozapine also has the potential for inducing convulsions in a small percentage (3%) of clients, and a warning has been issued about its association with myocarditis. This means that all clients taking the drug must be monitored closely.

The most common side effects of clozapine are drowsiness and sedation (40%), hypersalivation (30%), tachycardia (25%), and dizziness (20%). Because of these side effects, **this drug is not a first choice.** The other atypical agents are all good first-line drugs for schizophrenia.

Risperidone

Risperidone (Risperdal) is an antipsychotic drug that shares with clozapine the ability to treat psychotic symptoms of delusions and hallucinations without frequently inducing motor abnormalities. Unlike clozapine, it does not seem to have the potential for inducing agranulocytosis or convulsions. These advantages are offset, however, by the fact that at dosages of risperidone only slightly higher than those that are effective, clients taking this drug may begin to experience motor difficulties. Because risperidone blocks α_1 and H$_1$ receptors, it can cause orthostatic hypotension

and sedation. Keep in mind that orthostatic hypotension can lead to falls, which are a serious problem among the elderly. Weight gain, sedation, and sexual dysfunction are also adverse effects that may affect compliance with the medication regimen and need to be taken into consideration and discussed with clients.

A rare but serious side effect is an increased risk of cerebrovascular accidents in the elderly with dementia who are being treated for agitation (Lee et al., 2004). It is notable that risperidone is the first atypical antipsychotic available as a long-acting injection. Risperdal Consta provides an alternative to the depot form of typical antipsychotics.

Quetiapine

Quetiapine (Seroquel) has a broad receptor-binding profile. This drug binds to and antagonizes D$_1$, D$_2$, 5-HT$_1$, 5-HT$_2$, α_1, α_2, and H$_1$ receptors. Its strong blockage of H$_1$ receptors accounts for the sedation and weight gain associated with use of this drug. It causes moderate blockage of muscarinic and α_1 receptors and associated side effects. At normal dosages it has not been associated with extrapyramidal symptoms.

Other Atypical Antipsychotics

Other atypical antipsychotics include olanzapine (Zyprexa), ziprasidone (Geodon), and the most recent aripiprazole (Abilify). *Olanzapine* is a derivative of clozapine and it is an antagonist of 5-HT$_2$, D$_2$, H$_1$, α, and muscarinic receptors. Side effects include sedation, weight gain, hyperglycemia, and new-onset type 2 diabetes. *Ziprasidone* is a serotonin-norepinephrine reuptake inhibitor and also binds to multiple receptors: 5-HT$_2$, D$_2$, α, and H$_1$. The main side effects are hypotension and sedation. One major safety concern is prolongation of the QT$_c$ interval, which can be fatal if the client has a history of cardiac arrhythmia. A baseline electrocardiogram and blood chemistry testing for magnesium and potassium are recommended prior to treatment. Finally, *aripiprazole* is a unique atypical known as a dopamine system stabilizer. It functions as a partial agonist at the D$_2$ receptor. In areas of the brain with excess dopamine, it lowers the dopamine level by acting as a receptor antagonist; however, in regions with low dopamine, it stimulates receptors to raise the dopamine level (Bristol-Myers Squibb, 2005). Side effects include sedation, hypotension, and anticholinergic effects.

Chapter 20 discusses these agents more fully, and individual drug monographs can be found on the Evolve website. Also included in Chapter 20 is a detailed discussion of the positive, negative, and cognitive symptoms in schizophrenia, and the indications for use of the standard and atypical antipsychotic agents, as well as adverse reactions, dosage, nursing implications, and client and family teaching.

MOOD STABILIZERS

Lithium

Although the efficacy of lithium (Eskalith, Lithobid) as a mood-stabilizing drug in clients with bipolar (manic-depressive) disorder has been established for many years, its mechanism of action is still far from understood. As a positively charged ion, similar in structure to sodium and potassium, lithium may well act by affecting electrical conductivity in neurons.

As discussed earlier, an electrical impulse consists of the inward, depolarizing flow of sodium followed by an outward, repolarizing flow of potassium. These electrical charges are propagated along the neuron so that, if they are initiated at one end of the neuron, they will pass to the other end. Once they reach the end of a neuron, a transmitter is released.

It may be that an overexcitement of neurons in some parts of the brain underlies bipolar disorders and that lithium interacts in some complex way with sodium and potassium at the cell membrane to stabilize electrical activity. Even if such an alteration in electrical conductivity is not responsible for the beneficial effects of lithium, it certainly explains some of the adverse effects and toxicity of the drug.

By altering electrical conductivity, lithium represents a potential threat to all body functions that are regulated by electrical currents. Foremost among these functions, of course, is cardiac contraction, so lithium can induce cardiac dysrhythmias. Extreme alteration of cerebral conductivity can lead to convulsions. Alteration in nerve and muscle conduction can lead to tremor or more extreme motor dysfunction.

The fact that sodium and potassium play a strong role in regulating fluid balance and the distribution of fluid in various body compartments explains the disturbances in fluid balance that can be caused by lithium. These include polyuria (the output of large volumes of urine) and edema (the accumulation of fluid in the interstitial space). There is evidence that long-term use of lithium increases the risk of kidney and thyroid disease.

Primarily because of its effects on electrical conductivity, lithium has the lowest therapeutic index of all psychiatric drugs. The therapeutic index represents the ratio of the lethal dose to the effective dose, and thus indicates the safety of a drug. A low therapeutic index means that the blood level of a drug that can cause death is not far above the blood level required for drug effectiveness. This means that the blood level of lithium needs to be monitored on a regular basis to be sure that the drug is not accumulating and rising to dangerous levels. Table 3-3 lists some of the adverse effects of lithium. Chapter 19 considers lithium treatment in more depth and discusses specific dosage-

TABLE 3-3

Adverse Effects of Lithium

System	Adverse Effects
Nervous and muscular	Tremor, ataxia, confusion, convulsions
Digestive	Nausea, vomiting, diarrhea
Cardiac	Arrhythmias
Fluid and electrolyte	Polyuria, polydipsia, edema
Endocrine	Goiter and hyperthyroidism

related adverse and toxic effects, nursing implications, and the client teaching plan.

Antiepileptic Drugs

Carbamazepine (Tegretol), divalproex (Depakote), and lamotrigine (Lamictal) have demonstrated efficacy in the treatment of bipolar disorders (Preston, O'Neal, & Talaga, 2005). Their anticonvulsant properties derive from the fact that they alter electrical conductivity in membranes; in particular, they reduce the firing rate of very-high-frequency neurons in the brain. It is possible that this membrane-stabilizing effect accounts for the ability of these drugs to reduce the mood swings that occur in clients with bipolar disorders. The drugs are particularly effective in reducing the excitement of the manic phase of this disease; thus, they are sometimes used to calm a manic client before long-term stabilization with lithium. When the client cannot tolerate lithium, valproic acid or carbamazepine may be used for long-term maintenance therapy.

Carbamazepine

Carbamazepine (Tegretol) is structurally similar to the tricyclic antidepressants (TCAs), although it is not clear if it shares the ability of these drugs to treat unipolar depression. Carbamazepine does, however, share the ability of TCAs to serve as a neurological analgesic. It is particularly effective in conditions such as trigeminal neuralgia that involve paroxysms (bursts) of severe pain. The efficacy of carbamazepine as an analgesic may be related to its ability to reduce the firing rate of overexcited neurons as well as to its ability to calm the accompanying psychological agitation associated with the pain. Common side effects include nausea, sedation, and ataxia. Rash may occur in 10% of clients (Sadock & Sadock, 2003). Recommended baseline laboratory work includes liver function tests, complete blood count (CBC), electrocardiogram, and electrolyte levels. The therapeutic blood level is monitored regularly.

Divalproex

Divalproex (Depakote) is structurally different from other anticonvulsant and psychiatric drugs that show efficacy in the treatment of manic depression. Divalproex may be used as a first-line treatment for bipolar disorder, and many clients tolerate it better than lithium or carbamazepine (Sadock & Sadock, 2003). Divalproex is recommended for mixed episodes and has been found useful for rapid cycling. Common side effects include hair loss, tremor, weight gain, and sedation. Occasional serious side effects are thrombocytopenia, pancreatitis, hepatic failure, and birth defects. Baseline levels are measured for liver function indicators and CBC before an individual is started on this medication and measurements are repeated periodically; in addition, the therapeutic blood level of the drug is monitored.

Lamotrigine

Lamotrigine (Lamictal) is a newer agent that is approved by the Food and Drug Administration (FDA) for acute and maintenance therapy (Preston et al., 2005). It is generally well tolerated; however, rare and potentially life-threatening dermatological symptoms are associated with lamotrigine.

Other Agents

Other anticonvulsants used as mood stabilizers are gabapentin (Neurontin) and topiramate (Topamax). Although gabapentin was initially widely used, there is currently no evidence to support first- or second-line use (Preston et al., 2005). There seems to be some promise, however, for people with co-morbid bipolar disorders and chronic pain. Similarly, topiramate is not classified as a mood stabilizer but may be appropriate for some clients when weight loss is desirable (Preston et al., 2005).

Clonazepam (Klonopin) is structurally a benzodiazepine, a type of antianxiety drug discussed later in this chapter. Benzodiazepines have strong sedating properties, which may in part account for the ability of clonazepam to calm a client rapidly in the manic phase of a bipolar disorder. Clonazepam is often used as an adjunct to lithium to increase the time between mood cycles (Sadock & Sadock, 2003). It may be used as part of a multiple-drug regimen to treat clients who show a mixture of anxious and depressive symptoms concomitantly; these individuals are sometimes given both antidepressants and antianxiety agents. The serious drawback of this agent is that clients develop tolerance and dependence. Baseline laboratory studies include CBC, liver function tests, and renal function tests.

Other agents including calcium channel blockers and thyroid hormones are being used with some effectiveness in the treatment of bipolar disorder. Refer to Chapter 19 for a detailed discussion of these drugs and the adverse reactions, dosage, indications for use, nursing implications, and client and family teaching.

Antidepressant Drugs

Our understanding of the neurophysiological basis of mood disorders is far from complete. However, a great deal of evidence seems to indicate that the neurotransmitters norepinephrine and serotonin play a major role in regulating mood. It is thought that a transmission deficiency of one or both of these monoamines within the limbic system underlies depression. One of the lines of evidence pointing in this direction is that all the drugs that show efficacy in the treatment of depression increase the synaptic level of one or both of these transmitters. Figure 3-13 identifies the types of side effects that a person may experience when specific neurotransmitters are blocked or bound. Figure 3-14 illustrates the normal release, reuptake, and destruction of the monoamine transmitters. A grasp of this underlying physiology is essential for understanding the mechanisms by which the antidepressant drugs are thought to act.

Typical or Standard Antidepressants

Typical or standard antidepressants such as the TCAs (e.g., amitriptyline [Elavil], imipramine [Tofranil], and nortriptyline [Pamelor]) are thought to act primarily by blocking the reuptake of norepinephrine and, to a lesser degree, of serotonin. As shown in Figure 3-15, this blocking prevents norepinephrine from coming into contact with its degrading enzyme, MAO, and thus increases the level of norepinephrine at the synapse. Similarly, the TCAs block the reuptake and destruction of serotonin and also increase the synaptic level of this transmitter. Exactly how the increased level of these transmitters alleviates depression is far from clear; however, many controlled scientific studies attest to the efficacy of these drugs. For a more thorough discussion of how tricyclic antidepressants work, refer to the Evolve website.

To varying degrees, many of the tricyclic drugs also block the muscarinic receptors that normally bind acetylcholine. As discussed in the previous section, this blockage leads to typical anticholinergic effects such as blurred vision, dry mouth, tachycardia, and constipation. These adverse effects can be troubling to clients and can limit their compliance with the regimen.

Again to varying degrees, depending on the individual drug, these agents can block H_1 receptors in the brain. Blockage of these receptors by any drug causes sedation and drowsiness, an unwelcome symptom in daily use (see Figure 3-13). People taking the TCAs often have compliance issues with these drugs as well because of their adverse reactions.

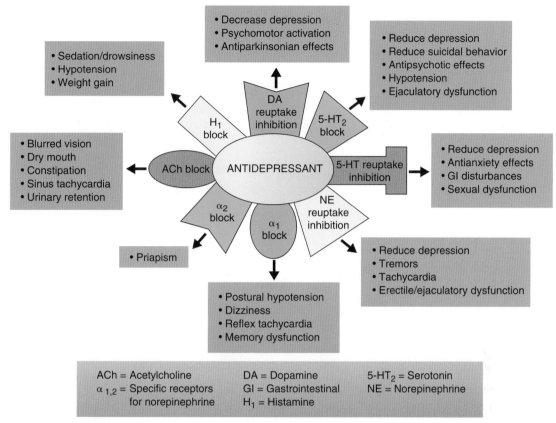

- Decrease depression
- Psychomotor activation
- Antiparkinsonian effects

- Reduce depression
- Reduce suicidal behavior
- Antipsychotic effects
- Hypotension
- Ejaculatory dysfunction

- Sedation/drowsiness
- Hypotension
- Weight gain

- Blurred vision
- Dry mouth
- Constipation
- Sinus tachycardia
- Urinary retention

- Reduce depression
- Antianxiety effects
- GI disturbances
- Sexual dysfunction

- Priapism

- Reduce depression
- Tremors
- Tachycardia
- Erectile/ejaculatory dysfunction

- Postural hypotension
- Dizziness
- Reflex tachycardia
- Memory dysfunction

ACh = Acetylcholine   DA = Dopamine   5-HT$_2$ = Serotonin
$\alpha_{1,2}$ = Specific receptors   GI = Gastrointestinal   NE = Norepinephrine
for norepinephrine   H$_1$ = Histamine

FIGURE 3-13 Possible effects of receptor binding of the antidepressant medications.

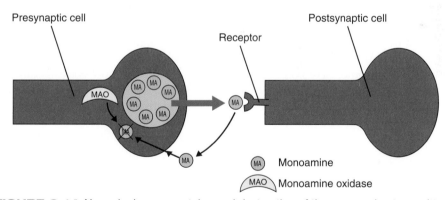

Presynaptic cell   Postsynaptic cell

Receptor

MA   Monoamine

MAO   Monoamine oxidase

FIGURE 3-14 Normal release, reuptake, and destruction of the monoamine transmitters.

Selective Serotonin Reuptake Inhibitors

As the name implies, the selective serotonin reuptake inhibitors (SSRIs), such as fluoxetine (Prozac), sertraline (Zoloft), paroxetine (Paxil), citalopram (Celexa), and escitalopram (Lexapro), preferentially block the reuptake and thus the destruction of serotonin, with little or no effect on the other monoamine transmitters. These drugs, as a group, also have less ability to block the muscarinic and H$_1$ receptors than do the TCAs. As a result of their more selective action, they seem to

show comparable efficacy while not eliciting the anticholinergic and sedating side effects that limit client compliance. Refer to Figure 3-16. For a more detailed explanation of how the SSRIs work, go to the Evolve website.

Monoamine Oxidase Inhibitors

The MAO inhibitors are a group of antidepressant drugs which illustrate the principle that drugs can have a desired and beneficial effect in the brain, while at the same time having possibly dangerous effects

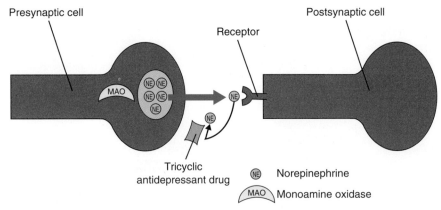

FIGURE 3-15 How the tricyclic antidepressant drugs block the reuptake of norepinephrine.

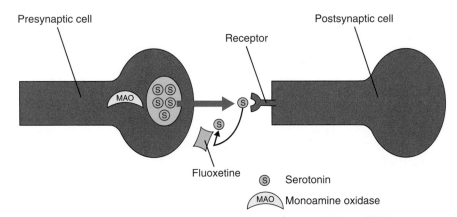

FIGURE 3-16 How the selective serotonin reuptake inhibitors (SSRIs) work.

elsewhere in the body. To understand the action of these drugs, keep in mind the following definitions:

> **Monoamines:** a type of organic compound; include the neurotransmitters norepinephrine, epinephrine, dopamine, and serotonin, as well as many different food substances and drugs
>
> Monoamine oxidase (MAO): an enzyme that destroys monoamines
>
> Monoamine oxidase inhibitors (MAOIs): drugs that prevent the destruction of monoamines by inhibiting the action of MAO

The monoamine neurotransmitters, as well as any monoamine food substance or drugs, are degraded (destroyed) by the enzyme MAO, which is located in neurons and in the liver. Antidepressant drugs such as isocarboxazid (Marplan), phenelzine (Nardil), and tranylcypromine (Parnate) are MAOIs; that is, they act by inhibiting the enzyme and interfering with the destruction of the monoamine neurotransmitters. This in turn increases the synaptic level of the transmitters and makes possible the antidepressant effects of these drugs (Figure 3-17). For a more comprehensive explanation of how MAOIs work, go to the Evolve website.

The use of MAO-inhibiting drugs is complicated by the fact that the enzyme is also present in the liver and is responsible for degrading monoamine substances that enter the body via food or drugs. Of particular importance is the monoamine tyramine, which is present in many food substances such as aged cheeses, pickled or smoked fish, and wine. Tyramine poses a threat of hypertensive crises because it can produce intense vasoconstriction, and thus an elevation in blood pressure, if allowed to circulate freely in the blood. Normally, this does not happen, because tyramine is destroyed by MAO as it passes through the liver before entering the general blood circulation. However, in the presence of MAOIs, tyramine is not destroyed by the liver and can cause serious, even life-threatening, hypertension.

A substantial number of drugs are chemically monoamines. The dosage of these drugs is determined by the rate at which they are destroyed by MAO in the liver. In a client taking MAOIs, the blood level of monoamine drugs can reach high levels and cause serious toxicity.

Because of the dangers that result from inhibition of hepatic MAO, clients taking MAOIs must be given a list of foods and drugs high in tyramine that need to be avoided. Chapter 18 discusses the treatment of depression and contains a list of forbidden foods and foods to be taken in moderation, along with nursing measures and instructions for client teaching.

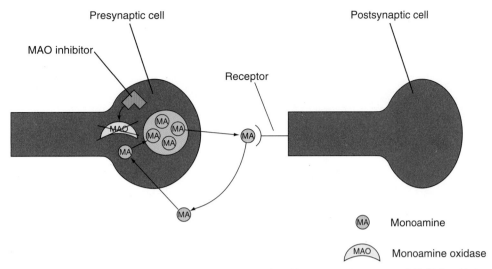

FIGURE 3-17 Blocking of monoamine oxidase (MAO) by inhibiting agents (MAOIs), which prevents the breakdown of monoamine by MAO.

Atypical or Novel Antidepressants

A number of drugs seem to work by mechanisms less clearly defined than those of the TCAs, SSRIs, and MAOIs. These atypical or novel antidepressants differ structurally or in their pharmacological actions from the TCAs, SSRIs, and MAOIs. Included in this group are venlafaxine (Effexor), duloxetine (Cymbalta), bupropion (Wellbutrin), mirtazapine (Remeron), and trazodone (Desyrel).

Venlafaxine, duloxetine, and mirtazapine are dual-action *serotonin-norepinephrine* reuptake inhibitors (SNRIs). Bupropion is an effective antidepressant and first-line agent for smoking cessation. It seems to act as a *dopamine-norepinephrine* reuptake inhibitor and also inhibits nicotinic acetylcholine receptors to reduce the addictive action of nicotine. Trazodone is **not a first choice** for antidepressant treatment, but it is often given along with another agent because somnolence, one of the side effects, helps with sleep disturbance.

On March 22, 2004, the FDA asked that drug companies put out a warning statement that all individuals, especially children and adolescents, should be monitored closely when they start taking antidepressants (especially SSRIs and atypical agents).

Refer to Chapter 18 for a detailed discussion of all classes of antidepressants, their adverse effects, dosages, nursing implications, and client and family teaching. These drugs are included in the drug monographs found on the Evolve website.

ANTIANXIETY OR ANXIOLYTIC DRUGS

The neurotransmitter GABA seems to have an inhibitory effect on neurons in many parts of the brain. Drugs that can enhance this effect exert a sedative-hypnotic action on brain function. Many drugs with this type of effect, called antianxiety or anxiolytic drugs, tend to reduce anxiety and are used as antianxiety agents. The most commonly used anxiolytic agents are the benzodiazepines.

Benzodiazepines

Figure 3-18 shows that benzodiazepines, such as diazepam (Valium), clonazepam (Klonopin), and alprazolam (Xanax), bind to specific receptors adjacent to the GABA receptors. Because of their ability to bind benzodiazepines, these receptors are called benzodiazepine receptors. Binding of benzodiazepines to these receptors at the same time that GABA binds to its receptors allows GABA to inhibit more forcefully than it would if binding alone. The fact that benzodiazepines do not inhibit neurons in the absence of GABA limits the potential toxicity of these drugs.

Of the various benzodiazepines, some, such as flurazepam (Dalmane) and triazolam (Halcion), have a predominantly hypnotic (sleep-inducing) effect, whereas others, such as lorazepam (Ativan) and alprazolam, reduce anxiety without being as **soporific** (sleep producing). Currently, there is no clear explanation for the differential effects of the various benzodiazepines. There seems to be some evidence that there are subtypes of the benzodiazepine receptors in different areas of the brain, and these subtypes differ in their ability to bind the different drugs.

The fact that the benzodiazepines potentiate the ability of GABA to inhibit neurons probably accounts for their efficacy as anticonvulsants and for their ability to reduce the neuronal overexcitement of alcohol withdrawal. When used alone, even at high dosages, these drugs rarely inhibit the brain to the degree that respiratory depression, coma, and death result.

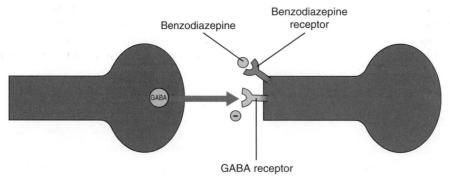

FIGURE 3-18 Action of the benzodiazepines. Drugs in this group attach to receptors adjacent to the receptors for the neurotransmitter γ-aminobutyric acid (GABA). Drug attachment to these receptors results in a strengthening of the inhibitory effects of GABA. In the absence of GABA there is no inhibitory effect of benzodiazepines.

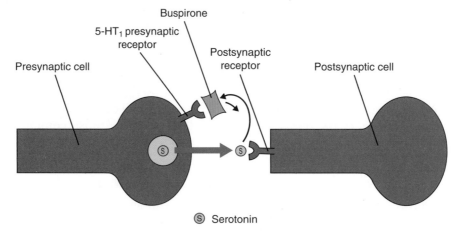

FIGURE 3-19 Action of buspirone. A proposed mechanism of action of buspirone is that it blocks feedback inhibition by serotonin. This leads to increased release of serotonin by the presynaptic cell. *5-HT₁*, Serotonin.

However, when combined with other central nervous system (CNS) depressants, such as alcohol, opiates, or TCAs, the inhibitory actions of the benzodiazepines can lead to life-threatening respiratory depression.

Any drug that inhibits electrical activity in the brain can interfere with motor ability, attention, and judgment. A client taking benzodiazepines must be cautioned about engaging in activities that could be dangerous if reflexes and attention are impaired. These include specialized activities such as working in construction on a tall building and more common activities such as driving a car. In the elderly, the use of benzodiazepines may contribute to falls and broken bones.

Buspirone

Buspirone (BuSpar) is a drug that reduces anxiety without having strong sedative-hypnotic properties. Because this agent does not leave the client sleepy or sluggish, it is often much better tolerated than the benzodiazepines. It is not a CNS depressant and thus does not have as great a danger of interaction with other CNS depressants such as alcohol. Also there is not the potential for addiction that exists with benzodiazepines.

Although at present the mechanism of action of buspirone is not clearly understood, one possibility is illustrated in Figure 3-19. Buspirone seems to act as an antagonist at presynaptic 5-HT₁ receptors. The normal function of these receptors is to monitor the synaptic level of serotonin; that is, serotonin released by the neurons binds not only to postsynaptic receptors to exert its effects on adjacent neurons but also to presynaptic receptors on the neuron from which it is released. Once bound to the presynaptic receptor, serotonin inhibits the further release of this transmitter; this release serves as negative feedback. Buspirone, by blocking these presynaptic receptors, prevents the negative feedback and allows more transmitter to be released. The end result is an increased synaptic level of serotonin that presumably accounts for the beneficial action of this drug.

Refer to Chapter 14 on anxiety disorders for the adverse reactions, dosages, nursing implications, and client and family teaching for the anxiolytic drugs.

ANTIDEPRESSION TREATMENT OF CONDITIONS ASSOCIATED WITH ANXIETY

A variety of psychiatric conditions involve symptom formation in which anxiety is thought to play a major role. Included among these are panic attacks, generalized anxiety disorder, phobias, obsessive-compulsive disorder, social anxiety, and possibly eating disorders. Although the etiologies of these conditions are far from understood, it has been found clinically that antidepressants often show efficacy in their treatment. Antidepressants from all the various classes are being investigated in the treatment of these conditions. There is some indication that specific drugs or drug classes show special efficacy in specific conditions. Thus, imipramine is often used to treat panic attacks, SSRIs to treat obsessive-compulsive disorders, and sertraline to treat social phobias. The relationship between depression and the anxiety disorders is an area of active research.

TREATMENT OF ATTENTION DEFICIT HYPERACTIVITY DISORDER

Children and adults with ADHD show symptoms of short attention span, impulsivity, and overactivity. Paradoxically, the mainstay of treatment for this condition in children, and increasingly in adults, is the administration of psychostimulant drugs. Both methylphenidate (Ritalin) and dextroamphetamines such as Adderall seem to show efficacy in these conditions. These drugs seem to work by increasing the release and blocking the reuptake of monoamines. How this translates into clinical efficacy is far from understood, but it is thought that the monoamines may inhibit an overactive part of the limbic system. Among many concerns with the use of these drugs are the side effects of agitation, exacerbation of psychotic thought processes, hypertension, and long-term growth suppression, as well as their potential for abuse. One nonstimulant medication is available for the treatment of ADHD. Atomoxetine hydrochloride (Strattera) is a norepinephrine reuptake inhibitor that is approved for use in children 6 years and older. Common side effects include decreased appetite and weight loss, fatigue, and dizziness. Refer to Chapters 32 and 33 for more on these agents.

DRUG TREATMENT FOR ALZHEIMER'S DISEASE

The insidious and progressive loss of memory and other higher brain functions brought about by Alzheimer's disease is a great individual family and social tragedy. Because the disease seems to involve progressive structural degeneration of the brain, there are two major pharmacological directions in its treatment. The first is to attempt to prevent or slow the structural degeneration. Although actively pursued, this approach has so far not been successful. The second is to attempt to maintain normal brain function for as long as possible. Much of the memory loss in this disease has been attributed to dysfunction of neurons that secrete acetylcholine. Tacrine and donepezil are anticholinesterase drugs (also called *cholinesterase inhibitors*) that show some efficacy in slowing the rate of memory loss and, in some clients, may even improve memory. The drugs work by interfering with the action of acetylcholinesterase. Inactivation of this enzyme leads to less destruction of the neurotransmitter acetylcholine and, therefore, a higher concentration at the synapse.

Tacrine

Tacrine (Cognex) was the first anticholinesterase approved by the FDA for the treatment of Alzheimer's disease. It has been shown to have moderate efficacy in some clients. Untoward effects include nausea, abdominal distress, tachycardia, and hepatic toxicity in some individuals. Liver enzyme levels should be monitored on a regular basis.

Donepezil

Donepezil (Aricept) shows clinical efficacy in some clients with Alzheimer's disease without the liver toxicity associated with tacrine. Untoward effects include nausea, diarrhea, and sedation. Rivastigmine (Exelon) and galantamine (Reminyl) are two other similar drugs in use today and are further discussed in Chapter 21.

Memantine

Memantine (Namenda, Ebixa) is a new class of drug that has demonstrated effectiveness in clients with moderate to severe Alzheimer's disease. It is an N-methyl-D-aspartate receptor antagonist. Refer to Chapter 21 for a more thorough discussion of these drugs and nursing considerations and teaching.

HERBAL MEDICINE

The growing interest in medicinal herbs is driven by a variety of factors. Many people believe that herbal medications are safer because they are "natural" or that they may have fewer side effects. They are often less costly than traditional medications.

Use of many of the herbal "medicines" taken today by people has been supported by scientific evidence regarding mechanism of action and clinical trials demonstrating safety and efficacy (Brown, Gerberg, & Muskin, 2003). By the same token, many medicinal herbs have been found to be nontherapeutic and some even deadly if taken over long periods of time and in combination with other chemical substances and prescription drugs (Preston et al., 2005).

Among the major concerns of health care professionals regarding herbal medications are the potential long-term effects of some herbal agents (nerve damage, kidney damage, liver damage) and the possibility of adverse chemical reactions when herbal agents are taken in conjunction with other substances, including conventional medications.

As examples, kava can induce hepatitis and can be toxic at doses over 240 mg/day; St. John's wort (SJW), on the other hand, can have serious interactions with a number of conventional medications. Preclinical studies suggest that taking SJW with other serotonin-related psychotropic agents can raise the possibility of mild serotonin syndrome, especially in the elderly (Gelenberg, 2000). SJW also has serious interactions with other drugs. Among healthy volunteers given digoxin, digoxin levels decreased by 28% in those taking SJW but dropped only 9% in a placebo group (Jonte et al., 1999). Breakthrough bleeding has been reported in women taking birth control pills who also take SJW (Brown et al., 2003). Anesthesiologists anecdotally report changes in heart rate and blood pressure in individuals taking herbal medications, particularly in those taking SJW, ginkgo biloba, and ginseng; therefore, it is advisable to discontinue these herbal medications 2 to 3 weeks before undergoing surgery (Voelker, 1999).

A number of other herbal products (ginkgo biloba, feverfew, and garlic) suppress platelet aggregation and therefore increase the risk of bleeding in people taking anticoagulants (heparin, warfarin) or aspirin (Brown et al., 2003).

Another key concern regarding the use of alternative herbs and nutrients is the quality of herbal supplements on the market. Many brands are of poor quality, have dosing inconsistencies, or are of questionable purity or stability. This is partly because herbal preparations are sold as dietary supplements rather than drugs; thus they avoid regulation under the FDA's Federal Food, Drug, and Cosmetic Act. Health care professionals and especially nurses need to stay current using unbiased sources of product information to pass this information on to those clients taking alternative agents (Brown et al., 2003). Independent evaluation of many brands with updates can be found at http://www.consumerlab.com or http://www.supplementwatch.com. Recalls and warnings to stop use of certain brands are available at http://www.fda.gov/medwatch (Brown et al., 2003).

It is most important, therefore, that nurses and other health care professionals explore the client's use of herbal supplements in a nonjudgmental manner, for example, by asking, "What over-the-counter medications or herbs do you take to help your symptoms? Do they help? How much are you taking and how long have you been taking them?" Individuals taking medications or other supplements need to be aware of drug-substance interactions and product safety.

Such discussion should be part of the initial and ongoing interviews with clients. Chapter 37 covers complementary and integrative therapies in more detail.

■ ■ ■ KEY POINTS to REMEMBER

- All actions of the brain—sensory, motor, intellectual—are carried out physiologically through the interactions of nerve cells. These interactions involve impulse conduction, transmitter release, and receptor response. Alterations in these basic processes can lead to mental disturbances and physical manifestations.

- In particular, it seems that excess activity of dopamine, among other factors, is involved in the thought disturbances of schizophrenia and that deficiencies of norepinephrine or serotonin or both underlie the mood disturbances of depression. Insufficient activity of GABA seems to play a role in anxiety.

- Pharmacological treatment of mental disturbances is directed at the suspected transmitter receptor problem. Thus, antipsychotic drugs block dopamine receptors, antidepressant drugs increase synaptic levels of norepinephrine and/or serotonin, and antianxiety drugs increase the effectiveness of GABA.

- Because the immediate target activity of a drug can result in many downstream alterations in neuronal activity, it has been found that drugs with a variety of chemical actions may show efficacy in treating the same clinical condition. Thus, in the treatment of schizophrenia, depression, and anxiety, newer drugs with novel mechanisms of action are being brought into use. This often makes understanding the pharmacology of mental disease more, rather than less, difficult.

- Unfortunately, as is the case for almost all pharmacological agents, the agents used to treat mental disease can cause various undesired effects. Prominent among these can be sedation or excitement, motor disturbances, muscarinic blockage, α antagonism, sexual dysfunction, and weight gain. There is a continuing effort on the part of pharmacologists to develop new drugs that are effective as well as safe and comfortable for people suffering from emotional disorders.

■ ■ ■

Visit the Evolve website at **http://evolve.elsevier.com/Varcarolis** for a posttest on the content in this chapter. **evolve**

Critical Thinking and Chapter Review

Visit the Evolve website at **http://evolve.elsevier.com/Varcarolis** for additional self-study exercises.

evolve

■■■ CRITICAL THINKING

1. With an understanding that, no matter where you practice nursing, many individuals under your care will be taking one psychotropic drug or another (especially an antidepressant, antianxiety medication, or even an antimanic agent), how important is it for you in your nursing practice to understand normal brain structure and function as they relate to mental disturbances and psychotropic drugs? Include the following in your answer:

   ■ Ways nurses can use the knowledge about how normal brain function (control of peripheral nerves, skeletal muscles, the autonomic nervous system, hormones, and circadian rhythms) can be affected by either psychotropic drugs or psychiatric illness

   ■ Ways brain imaging can help in understanding and treating people with mental disorders

   ■ Ways your understanding of how neurotransmitters work may affect your ability to assess your clients' responses to specific medications

2. What specific information could you include in your medication teaching for your client based on your understanding of what symptoms may occur with alterations of the following neurotransmitters?

   ■ Dopamine D_2 (as with use of phenothiazines and other drugs)

   ■ Blockage of muscarinic receptors (as with use of phenothiazines and other drugs)

   ■ α_1 receptors (as with use of phenothiazines and other drugs)

   ■ Histamine (as with use of phenothiazines and other drugs)

   ■ MAO (as with use of an MAOI)

   ■ GABA (as with use of antianxiety drugs)

■■■ CHAPTER REVIEW

Choose the most appropriate answer.

1. A nurse administering a benzodiazepine should understand that the therapeutic effect of benzodiazepines results from potentiating the neurotransmitter
   1. GABA.
   2. dopamine.
   3. serotonin.
   4. acetylcholine.

2. Fluoxetine (an SSRI) exerts its antidepressant effect by blocking the reuptake of
   1. GABA.
   2. dopamine.
   3. serotonin.
   4. norepinephrine.

3. The nurse administers each of the following drugs to various clients. The client who should be most carefully assessed for fluid and electrolyte imbalance is the one receiving
   1. lithium.
   2. clozapine.
   3. diazepam.
   4. amitriptyline.

4. Which drug group calls for nursing assessment for development of parkinsonian movement disorders among individuals who take therapeutic dosages?
   1. SSRIs
   2. Phenothiazines
   3. Benzodiazepines
   4. Tricyclic antidepressants

5. Blockage of dopamine transmission can lead to increased pituitary secretions of prolactin. In women this hyperprolactinemia can result in
   1. dry mouth.
   2. amenorrhea.
   3. increased production of testosterone.
   4. blurred vision.

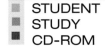

■ STUDENT
■ STUDY
■ CD-ROM

Access the accompanying CD-ROM for animations, interactive exercises, review questions for the NCLEX examination, and an audio glossary.

REFERENCES

Abelson, J. L., & Curtis, G. C. (1996). Hypothalamic-pituitary-adrenal axis activity in panic disorder. *Archives of General Psychiatry, 53,* 323-331.

American College of Neuropsychopharmacology. (1992). Suicidal behavior and psychotropic medication (consensus statement). *Neuropsychopharmacology, 8,* 177.

Andersen, P. H., et al. (1990). Dopamine receptor subtypes. *Trends in Pharmacological Science, 11,* 231.

Baldessarini, R. J., et al. (1990). Clozapine—a novel antipsychotic agent. *New England Journal of Medicine, 324,* 746.

Ballenger, J. C. (1995). Benzodiazepines. In A. F. Schatzberg & C. B. Nemeroff (Eds.), *The American Psychiatric Press textbook of psychopharmacology.* Washington, DC: American Psychiatric Press.

Beare, R. G., & Myers, J. L. (1994). *Principles and practices of adult health nursing* (2nd ed., p. 1167). St. Louis: Mosby.

Boyer, W. E., & Feighner, J. P. (1991). The efficacy of selective serotonin uptake inhibitors in depression. In J. P. Feighner & W. E. Boyer (Eds.), *Selective serotonin re-uptake inhibitors.* Chichester, England: Wiley.

Brown, R., Gerbarg, P. L., & Muskin, P. R. (2003). Complementary and alternative treatment in psychiatry. In A. Tashman, J. Kay, & J. A. Lieberman (Eds.), *Psychiatry* (2nd ed.). London: Wiley.

Burman, R. M., et al. (1999). Principles of the pharmacotherapy of depression. In D. S. Charney, E. J. Nestler, & B. S. Bunney (Eds.), *Neurobiology of mental illness*. New York: Oxford University Press.

Byne, W., et al. (1999). The neurochemistry of schizophrenia. In D. S. Charney, E. J. Nestler, & B. S. Bunney (Eds.), *Neurobiology of mental illness*. New York: Oxford University Press.

Charney, D. S., et al. (1991). Current hypotheses of the mechanism of antidepressant treatment: Implications for the treatment of refractory depression. In J. S. Amsterdam (Ed.), *Advances in neuropsychiatry and psychopharmacology* (Vol. 2). New York: Raven Press.

Charney, D. S., & Bremmer J. D. (1999). The neurobiology of anxiety disorder. In D. S. Charney, E. J. Nestler, & B. S. Bunney (Eds.), *Neurobiology of mental illness*. New York: Oxford University Press.

Cole, J. O., & Yonkers, K. A. (1995). Nonbenzodiazepine anxiolytics. In A. F. Schatzberg & C. B. Nemeroff (Eds.), *The American Psychiatric Press textbook of psychopharmacology*. Washington, DC: American Psychiatric Press.

Cooper, J. R., Bloom, F. E., & Roth, R. H. (1992). *The biochemical basis of neuropharmacology* (6th ed.). New York: Oxford University Press.

Dechant, K. L., & Cissold, S. P. (1991). Paroxetine. *Drugs, 41*, 225.

Dentch, A. Y., & Roth, R. H. (1999). Neurochemical systems in the central nervous systems. In D. S. Charney, E. J. Nestler, & B. S. Bunney (Eds.), *Neurobiology of mental illness*. New York: Oxford University Press.

Duman, R. S. (1999). The neurochemistry of mood disorders: Preclinical studies. In D. S. Charney, E. J. Nestler, & B. S. Bunney (Eds.), *Neurobiology of mental illness*. New York: Oxford University Press.

Faraona, S. V., & Biederman, J. (1999). The neurobiology of attention deficit hyperactivity disorder. In D. S. Charney, E. J. Nestler, & B. S. Bunney (Eds.), *Neurobiology of mental illness*. New York: Oxford University Press.

Fitton, A., & Heel, R. C. (1990). Clozapine—a review of pharmacological properties and therapeutic use in schizophrenia. *Drugs, 40*, 722.

Gelenberg, A. J. (2000). St. John's wort update. *Biological Therapeutic Psychiatry, 23*, 22-24.

Gerlach, J. (1991). New antipsychotics: Classification, efficacy and adverse effects. *Schizophrenia Bulletin, 17*(2), 289.

Goddard, A. W., et al. (1999). Principles of the pharmacotherapy of the anxiety disorders. In D. S. Charney, E. J. Nestler, & B. S. Bunney (Eds.), *Neurobiology of mental illness*. New York: Oxford University Press.

Goodwin, F. K., & Jamison, K. R. (1990). *Manic-depressive illness*. New York: Oxford University Press.

Heninger, G. R. (1999). Special challenges in the investigation of the neurobiology of mental illness. In D. S. Charney, E. J. Nestler, & B. S. Bunney (Eds.), *Neurobiology of mental illness*. New York: Oxford University Press.

Hodgson, B. B., & Kizior, R. J. (2003). *Saunders nursing drug handbook 2003*. Philadelphia: Saunders.

Hollister, L. E. (1995). Antipsychotic agents and lithium. In G. G. Katzung (Ed.), *Basic and clinical pharmacology*. Norwalk, CT: Appleton & Lange.

Hyman, S. E., & Nestler, E. (1996). Initiation and adaptation: A paradigm for understanding psychotropic drugs' action. *American Journal of Psychiatry, 153*, 151-162.

Jonte, A., et al. (1999). Pharmacokinetic interaction of digoxin with an herbal extract from St. John's wort. *Clinical Pharmacology Therapy, 66*, 338-345.

Krishnan, K. R. (1995). Monoamine oxidase inhibitors. In A. F. Schatzberg & C. B. Nemeroff (Eds.), *The American Psychiatric Press textbook of psychopharmacology*. Washington, DC: American Psychiatric Press.

Lavin, M. R., & Rifkin, A. (1992). Neuroleptic induced parkinsonism. In J. M. Kane & J. A. Lieberman (Eds.), *Adverse effects of psychotropic drugs*. New York: Guilford Press.

Lee, P. E., et al. (2004). Atypical antipsychotic drugs in the treatment of behavioural and psychological symptoms of dementia: Systematic review. *British Medical Journal, 329*, 75. Retrieved from: http://bmj.bmjjournals.com/cgi/content/full/329/7457/75.

Lin, K. M., Smith, M. W., & Lin, M. T. (2003). Psychopharmacology. In A. Tashman, J. Kay, & J. A. Lieberman (Eds.), *Psychiatry* (2nd ed.). London: Wiley.

Manji, H. K., et al. (1991). Mechanisms of action of lithium. *Archives of General Psychiatry, 48*, 505.

Mansour, A., et al. (1995). Biochemical anatomy: Insights into the cell biology and pharmacology of neurotransmitter systems in the brain. In A. F. Schatzberg & C. B. Nemeroff (Eds.), *The American Psychiatric Press textbook of psychopharmacology*. Washington, DC: American Psychiatric Press.

Marin, D. B. (1999). Principles of the pharmacotherapy of dementia. In D. S. Charney, E. J. Nestler, & B. S. Bunney (Eds.), *Neurobiology of mental illness*. New York: Oxford University Press.

Maxman, J. S., & Ward, N. G. (2002). *Psychotropic drugs fast facts* (3rd ed.). New York: W. W. Norton.

McGurk, S. R., et al. (2004). Cognitive effects of olanzapine treatment in schizophrenia. *Medscape General Medicine, 6*(2). Retrieved from: http://www.medscape.com/viewarticle/474626.

Modell, S., et al. (1997). Corticosteroid receptor function is decreased in depressed patients. *Neuroendocrinology, 65*, 216-222.

Netsler, E. J., & Hyman, S. E. (1999). Mechanisms of neural plasticity. In D. S. Charney, E. J. Nestler, & B. S. Bunney (Eds.), *Neurobiology of mental illness*. New York: Oxford University Press.

Olajide, D., & Bhui, K. (1999). Psychiatry and cultural relativity. In K. Bhui & D. Olajide (Eds.), *Mental health services provisions for a multi-cultural society*. London: Saunders.

Owens, M. J., & Rich, S. L. (1995). Atypical antipsychotics. In A. F. Schatzberg & C. B. Nemeroff (Eds.), *The American Psychiatric Press textbook of psychopharmacology*. Washington, DC: American Psychiatric Press.

Perl, D. P. (1999). Abnormalities in brain structures on postmortem analysis of dementias. In D. S. Charney, E. J. Nestler, & B. S. Bunney (Eds.), *Neurobiology of mental illness*. New York: Oxford University Press.

Preston, J. D., O'Neal, J. H., & Talaga, M. C. (2005). *Handbook of clinical psychopharmacology for therapists* (3rd ed.). Oakland, CA: New Harbinger.

Ray, W. A. (1992). Psychotropic drugs and injuries among the elderly: A review. *Journal of Clinical Psychopharmacology, 12*, 386.

Risby, E. D., et al. (1991). The mechanisms of action of lithium. *Archives of General Psychiatry, 48*, 513.

Risch, N., & Merileangas, K. (1996). The future of genetic studies of complex human disease. *Science, 273*, 1516-1517.

Rudorfer, M. S. (1994). Comparative tolerability profiles of the newer versus the older antidepressants. *Drug Safety, 10*, 18.

Sadock, B. J., & Sadock, V. A. (2003). *Synopsis of psychiatry behavioral sciences/clinical psychiatry* (9th ed.). Philadelphia: Lippincott Williams & Wilkins.

Seibyl, J. P., et al. (1999). Neuroimaging methodologies. In D. S. Charney, E. J. Nestler, & B. S. Bunney (Eds.), *Neurobiology of mental illness*. New York: Oxford University Press.

Siever, L. J., et al. (1991). Critical issues in defining the role of serotonin in psychiatric disorders. *Pharmacological Reviews, 43*, 509.

Snyder, S. H. (1990). The dopamine connection. *Nature, 247*, 121.

Spencer, T. J., et al. (1996). Pharmacotherapy of ADHA across the life cycle: A literature review. *Journal of the American Academy of Child and Adolescent Psychiatry, 32*, 1031-1037.

Stober, G., et al. (1996). Serotonin transporter gene polymorphism and affective disorder. *Lancet, 347*, 1340-1341.

Tammings, C. A. (1999). Principles of the pharmacology of schizophrenia. In D. S. Charney, E. J. Nestler, & B. S. Bunney (Eds.), *Neurobiology of mental illness*. New York: Oxford University Press.

Theonen, H. (1995). Neurotrophins and neuronal plasticity. *Science, 270*, 593-598.

Tollefson, G. D. (1995). Selective serotonin reuptake inhibitors. In A. F. Schatzberg & C. B. Nemeroff (Eds.), *The American Psychiatric Press textbook of psychopharmacology*. Washington, DC: American Psychiatric Press.

Trevor, A. J., & Way, W. L. (1995). Sedative-hypnotics. In G. G. Katzung (Ed.), *Basic and clinical pharmacology*. Norwalk, CT: Appleton & Lange.

Voelker, R. (1999). Herbs and anesthesia. *JAMA, 281*, 1882.

Wilcox, R. F., & Gonzales, R. A. (1995). Introduction to neurotransmitters, receptors, signal transaction, and second messengers. In A. F. Schatzberg & C. B. Nemeroff (Eds.), *The American Psychiatric Press textbook of psychopharmacology*. Washington, DC: American Psychiatric Press.

Wileng, T., et al. (1995). Pharmacotherapy of adult attention deficit/hyperactivity disorders: A review. *Journal of Clinical Psychopharmacology, 15*, 270-279.

Wyatt, R. J. (1991). Neuroleptics and the natural cause of schizophrenia. *Schizophrenia Bulletin, 17*, 325.

CHAPTER 4

Psychiatric Mental Health Nursing and Managed Care Issues

NANCY CHRISTINE SHOEMAKER ▪ ELIZABETH M. VARCAROLIS

▪ KEY TERMS and CONCEPTS

The key terms and concepts listed here appear in color where they are defined or first discussed in this chapter.

advanced practice registered nurse—psychiatric mental health (APRN-PMH), 65

basic level registered nurse, 65

case management, 67

client advocate, 69

community nursing centers, 66

evidence-based practice, 65

health maintenance organizations, 66

managed behavioral health care organizations (MBHOs), 66

managed care, 66

Nursing Interventions Classification (NIC), 64

Nursing Outcomes Classification (NOC), 64

phenomena of concern, 64

preferred provider organizations, 66

psychiatric nursing, 64

telehealth, 68

▪ OBJECTIVES

After studying this chapter, the reader will be able to

1. Define psychiatric mental health nursing and discuss the client population served by the psychiatric nurse.
2. Explain the reasons for using standardized classification systems (North American Nursing Diagnosis Association, Nursing Interventions Classification, Nursing Outcomes Classification) in psychiatric nursing practice.
3. Compare and contrast the nursing actions of the basic level psychiatric nurse with those of the advanced level psychiatric nurse.
4. Describe recent developments that have increased the biological emphasis in psychiatric mental health nursing.
5. Discuss the impact of managed care on psychiatric nursing roles.
6. Explore emerging roles for the future of psychiatric nursing related to scientific and social trends.
7. Explain how Forchuk's case management model incorporates elements of Peplau's theory.

evolve Visit the Evolve website at **http://evolve.elsevier.com/Varcarolis** for a pretest on the content in this chapter.

In all clinical settings, nurses work with people who are going through crises, including physical, psychological, mental, and spiritual distress. You will encounter clients who are experiencing feelings of hopelessness, helplessness, anxiety, anger, low self-esteem, or confusion. You will meet people who are withdrawn, suspicious, elated, depressed, hostile, manipulative, suicidal, intoxicated, or withdrawing from a substance. Many of you have already come across people who are going through difficult times in their lives. At times you may have handled these situations skillfully, and at other times you may have wished you had additional skills and knowledge. Basic concepts of psychosocial nursing will become central to your practice of nursing and increase your competency as a practitioner in all clinical settings. Your experience in the psychiatric nursing rotation can help you gain insight into yourself and greatly increase your insight into the experiences of others. This part of your nursing education can also give you guidelines and the opportunity to learn new skills for dealing with a variety of challenging behaviors. This chapter presents a brief overview of what professional psychiatric nurses do, the scope of practice, their role in managed care, and the challenges and evolving roles for the future health care environment.

WHAT IS PSYCHIATRIC MENTAL HEALTH NURSING?

Psychiatric mental health nurses work with children, adolescents, adults, and the elderly. Psychiatric mental health nurses work with healthy people who are in crisis or who are experiencing life problems, as well as those with long-term mental illness. Their clients may include people with dual diagnoses (a mental disorder and a coexisting substance disorder), homeless persons and families, people in jail (forensic nursing), people who have survived abusive situations, people with acquired immunodeficiency syndrome, and people in crisis. Psychiatric nurses work with individuals, couples, families, and groups. They work with clients in hospitals, in their homes, in halfway houses, in shelters, in clinics, in storefronts, on the street—virtually everywhere. Because of the diversity of clients and settings, the scope of psychiatric mental health nursing is referred to as phenomena of concern. Refer to Box 4-1 for examples of client problems addressed by the psychiatric nurse.

The specific activities of the psychiatric nurse are defined by the *Scope and Standards of Psychiatric-Mental Health Nursing Practice*. (See the inside back cover of the book for Standards of Care.) This publication, written by the American Nurses Association (ANA), the American Psychiatric Nurses Association, and the International Society of Psychiatric-Mental Health Nurses, defines psychiatric nursing as "the diagnosis and treatment of human responses to actual or potential mental health problems" (2000, p. 10). The psychiatric nurse uses the same nursing process that you have already learned to assess and diagnose clients' illnesses, to identify outcomes, and to plan, implement, and evaluate nursing care.

To provide the most appropriate and scientifically sound care, the psychiatric nurse uses standardized classification systems developed by professional nursing groups. The *Nursing Diagnoses: Definitions and Classification 2005-2006* of the North American Nursing Diagnosis Association (NANDA) provides 172 standardized diagnoses, with more than 40% related to psychosocial care. These diagnoses provide a common language "for selection of nursing interventions to achieve outcomes for which the nurse is accountable" (NANDA, 2003, p. 263).

The Nursing Outcomes Classification (NOC) is one reference that provides "a comprehensive list of standardized outcomes, definitions, and measures to describe client outcomes influenced by nursing practice" (Moorhead, Johnson, & Maas, 2004, p. 11). Outcomes are organized into seven domains: Functional Health, Physiologic Health, Psychosocial Health, Health Knowledge and Behavior, Perceived

---

BOX 4-1

Psychiatric Mental Health Nursing's Phenomena of Concern

Actual or potential mental health problems of clients pertaining to the following:

- Maintenance of optimal health and well-being and prevention of psychobiological illness
- Self-care limitations or impaired functioning related to mental and emotional distress
- Deficits in the functioning of significant biological, emotional, and cognitive systems
- Emotional stress or crisis components of illness, pain, and disability
- Self-concept changes, developmental issues, and life process changes
- Problems related to emotions such as anxiety, anger, sadness, loneliness, and grief
- Physical symptoms that occur along with altered psychological functioning
- Alterations in thinking, perceiving, symbolizing, communicating, and decision making
- Difficulties relating to others
- Behaviors and mental states that indicate the client is a danger to self or others or has a severe disability
- Interpersonal, systematic, sociocultural, spiritual, or environmental circumstances or events that affect the mental and emotional well-being of the individual, family, or community
- Symptom management, side effects and toxicities associated with psychopharmacological intervention and other aspects of the treatment regimen

From American Nurses Association, American Psychiatric Nurses Association, & International Society of Psychiatric-Mental Health Nurses. (2000). *Scope and standards of psychiatric-mental health nursing practice*. Washington, DC: American Nurses Publishing.

Health, Family Health, and Community Health. The Psychosocial Health domain includes four classes: Psychological Well-Being, Psychosocial Adaptation, Self-Control, and Social Interaction.

The Nursing Interventions Classification (NIC) is another tool to define and measure nursing care. A nursing intervention is "any treatment, based upon clinical judgment and knowledge, that a nurse performs to enhance client outcomes," including direct and indirect care through a series of nursing activities (Dochterman & Bulechek, 2004, p. xxiii). There are seven domains: Physiological: Basic; Physiological: Complex; Behavioral; Safety; Family; Health System; and Community. Two domains relate specifically to psychiatric nursing: Behavioral, including communication, coping, and education; and Safety, covering crisis and risk management.

These three classification systems have been extensively researched by nurses across a variety of treatment settings. Thus, they form a foundation for the novice or experienced nurse to provide evidence-based practice; that is, care based on the "collection, interpretation and integration of valid, important, and applicable client-reported, clinician-observed, and research-derived evidence" (ANA et al., 2000, p. 52). In the chapters that follow, you will see examples of application of these classifications to specific clients in vignettes and case studies, along with brief descriptions of other relevant research in the boxes titled Evidence-Based Practice.

Psychiatric nurses must also be familiar with two other classification systems for client diagnosis: the *Diagnostic and Statistical Manual of Mental Disorders* produced by the American Psychiatric Association (2000) and the *International Statistical Classification of Diseases and Related Health Problems* issued by the World Health Organization (1993). Psychiatric nurses often function as members of a multidisciplinary treatment team, and professional language must be consistent.

LEVELS OF PSYCHIATRIC MENTAL HEALTH CLINICAL NURSING PRACTICE

Psychiatric mental health nurses are registered nurses who are educated in nursing and are licensed to practice in their individual states. Psychiatric nurses are qualified to practice at two levels depending on educational preparation: basic and advanced (ANA et al., 2000).

Basic Level

The nurse at the basic level has completed a nursing program and passed the state licensure examination. The basic level registered nurse (RN) is a graduate of a diploma school, a 2-year college, or a 4-year college. The baccalaureate RN may take a basic certification examination sponsored by the ANA through its credentialing center to demonstrate clinical competence. Certification is required by employers in some states for reimbursement purposes. At the basic level, nurses work in various supervised settings and perform multiple roles, for example, staff nurse, case manager, home care nurse, and so on.

Advanced Level

The advanced practice registered nurse—psychiatric mental health (APRN-PMH) is a licensed RN with a master's degree in psychiatric nursing.

The term *APRN-PMH* applies to either a clinical specialist or a nurse practitioner. This clinician is eligible to take an advanced certification examination, which adds another credential to the nurse's title. This certification demonstrates a certain level of clinical expertise and is required in certain positions for third-party reimbursement. The APRN-PMH may function autonomously and is eligible for specialty privileges as described later. Some advanced practice nurses continue their education to the doctoral level.

WHAT DO PSYCHIATRIC NURSES DO?

The main focus of the psychiatric mental health nurse is to promote and maintain optimal mental functioning, to prevent mental illness (or further dysfunction), and to help clients regain or improve their coping abilities. These goals are realized through a variety of nursing activities in diverse hospital and community settings. The *Scope and Standards of Psychiatric-Mental Health Nursing Practice* (ANA et al., 2000) clearly defines nursing actions for the professional nurse, distinguishing between those nursing activities appropriate for the basic level and for the advanced level. Refer to Table 4-1 for a description of basic and advanced psychiatric nursing interventions. Note that not all interventions are used by every nurse or in every client situation. In the following chapters you will find illustrations of basic and advanced nursing activities.

RECENT ISSUES AFFECTING PSYCHIATRIC MENTAL HEALTH NURSING

The 1990s were called the Decade of the Brain by the National Institute of Mental Health due to the multitude of scientific advances growing out of brain research. Numerous imaging techniques expanded our understanding of the neurophysiology and neuroanatomy of the brain. Neurobiological changes were observed in people with mental disorders, which led to a stronger emphasis on psychopharmacological treatment. Many of the most serious psychiatric disorders are now categorized as diseases of the brain.

In 1994, the ANA published the *Psychiatric Mental Health Nursing Psychopharmacology Project*, which recommended that nursing programs prepare nurses with a solid foundation in neuroscience and psychopharmacology as these relate to mental illness (ANA, 1994).

Furthermore, results of the Human Genome Project started to support biological and genetic explanations for psychiatric conditions (Cohen, 2000). Research has begun to validate the effectiveness of some complementary therapies, leading nurses to include these in comprehensive care (Ahmed & Maurana, 1999). The information explosion from daily access to the Internet has provided nurses with a constant stream of new

TABLE 4-1

Psychiatric Mental Health Nursing Interventions: Basic and Advanced Levels

Intervention	Description
Basic Level	
Counseling	Communication techniques including interviewing, problem solving, crisis intervention, conflict resolution, support groups
Milieu therapy	Use of the physical and social environment to influence behavior, such as orienting to the facility and setting verbal and physical limits to maintain safety
Promotion of self-care activities	Assistance with activities of daily living as needed to promote independence (e.g., grooming, eating, and sleeping patterns)
Psychobiological interventions	Administration of medication with evaluation of effects, care during recovery from electroconvulsive therapy, use of relaxation techniques
Health teaching	Formal or informal teaching about medication, illness, physical health, coping skills, relapse prevention
Case management	Coordination of care to promote optimal outcomes with available resources, e.g., communication with family, community resources, third-party payers
Health promotion and health maintenance	Activities to prevent mental illness or enhance mental health (e.g., community screenings, parenting classes, stress management)
Advanced Level	
All of the above plus	
Psychotherapy	Individual, group, or family therapy
Medication prescription and treatment	Prescription of psychotropic medications with appropriate use of diagnostic tests; hospital admitting privileges
Consultation	Clinical feedback to nurses or those in other disciplines to enhance their treatment of clients or address systems issues (e.g., supervision of basic registered nurses)

Data from American Nurses Association, American Psychiatric Nurses Association, & International Society of Psychiatric-Mental Health Nurses. (2000). *Scope and standards of psychiatric-mental health nursing practice.* Washington, DC: American Nurses Publishing.

findings relevant to nursing care. The challenge for the psychiatric mental health nurse is how to absorb all of this new knowledge and skills and yet not lose sight of the core values of psychiatric nursing, for example, the meaning of the nurse-client relationship (Forchuk et al., 2000). NIC still lists establishing trust or rapport as the first activity in treating clients with many identified problems, such as hallucinations, delusions, and difficulty in anger control. To be more than educated technicians, nurses still need to pay attention to the art of nursing, as defined by Hildegard Peplau. Peplau emphasized that nursing combines caring and scientific knowledge to achieve improved quality of life for clients (Peplau, 1952).

MENTAL HEALTH AND MANAGED CARE

Although managed care is now the dominant form of health care, and most consumers report satisfaction with this system, it has caused a revolution for clients and providers over the past 25 years (Britt et al., 1998). Prior to 1980, payment for health care was largely based on fee for service, and the client could choose any provider. Providers or facilities set their own fees, and insurers paid negotiated rates without question. For mental health care, clients had basically two choices: inpatient treatment or office or clinic outpatient treatment (Book, 2000). As health care costs continued to grow, however, insurers, employers, and the government sought to control costs through managed care organizations.

The goal of managed care is to provide coordination of all health services at the appropriate level of care, with an emphasis on preventive care, to control costs. Managed care organizations offer two basic types of health plan. Health maintenance organizations provide comprehensive services to members only within a defined provider network for a fixed yearly rate, using a primary care physician as the gatekeeper for specialty care. Preferred provider organizations give members a choice of using providers in a defined network for a fixed copayment or using providers outside the network for a higher copayment. To provide mental health and substance abuse treatment, managed behavioral health care organizations (MBHOs) were developed separately, or "carved out," from medical services. Both private and public (Medicaid) MBHOs monitor psychiatric care through preadmission reviews, continuing treatment authorizations, or retroactive chart review. MBHOs use written criteria to approve or deny requests for treatment, based on "the most up-to-date research on psychotherapeutic effectiveness" (Keefe & Hall, 1999, p. 151). Initially, there was a paucity of research data on psychiatric outcomes, and few objective clinical guidelines existed.

This lack was a source of severe disagreement between managed care payers and psychiatric providers as they discussed length of stay and level of care. For example, a hospital would request more days to teach coping skills to a suicidal client, but the MBHO would prefer discharge after the suicidal crisis resolved, with teaching provided in a partial hospitalization program.

This external oversight had a dramatic impact on mental health services and providers. To decrease the high cost of inpatient treatment, hospital stays were shortened or admission denied, and outpatient options were enhanced. New levels of outpatient care were developed: partial hospitalization programs, intensive outpatient treatment, assertive community treatment, psychiatric home care, and school-based services. Medicaid, as a major payer for mental health services, supported new approaches to community-based care, including assertive community treatment and alternatives for residential treatment for children (Rowland et al., 2003).

The influence of MBHOs on providers had special significance for the psychiatric nurse. After the initial resistance and negative feelings about external review, hospitals and other agencies realized that they had to document clinical care in measurable, behavioral terms to justify treatment. Research on treatment outcomes proliferated as various disciplines of the psychiatric team clarified their standards of care. This increased emphasis on documentation affected nurses in two major ways. First, psychiatric nurses are significant members of the psychiatric team in most settings and perform much of the direct care with subsequent documentation. The quality of nursing documentation plays a direct role in ensuring that clients receive necessary care. For example, when a suicidal client is admitted to a hospital, the treatment team must assess and document risk behavior, behavioral outcomes that indicate when the risk is resolved, and daily interventions intended to accomplish the specified goals. Daily nursing notes, whenever possible using standardized language from NANDA, NOC, and NIC sources, record the behavioral details that are used to justify payment for the client's stay.

The second impact on the psychiatric nurse related to managed care is the need to assume the role of evaluator, either in the internal utilization review processes of the agency or in the external review process for the MBHO. To effectively communicate with MBHOs, most agencies strengthened their internal quality review departments. Support staff—known as utilization reviewers, case managers, or clinical care managers—are often nurses, who are skilled in the interpretation of significant biopsychosocial data from the chart. Likewise, because of that same nurse expertise, MBHOs employ psychiatric nurses to conduct admission and continued stay reviews.

FUTURE CHALLENGES AND ROLES FOR NURSES

Expected future trends in psychiatric nursing indicate the need to strengthen current roles and to develop novel approaches. Psychiatric illnesses are expected to contribute 11% to 15% of the world's diseases in the next century, and there will be increasing need for psychiatric clinicians (ANA et al., 2000, p. 8). Violence and self-inflicted injuries are considered serious global threats, and in the United States, the 1999 Surgeon General's report focused on suicide as a public health problem (U.S. Department of Health and Human Services, 1999). Violence in the home, school, and workplace, as well as the threat of terrorism, are reported in the news daily. Psychiatric nurses will continue to work with survivors of violence but will also have increased opportunity for preventive counseling and teaching in the community, often through collaboration with other service providers. For example, one innovative role is to provide "postvention" to suicide survivors through collaboration with police officers who report suicides. Clinical teams including nurses can provide immediate counseling to family members after the death to reduce trauma and prevent future risk (Moon, 2003).

As community-based care continues to dominate, psychiatric nurses will need to enhance their **case management** skills. Case management is an integral part of psychiatric home care for the elderly, in-home services for children and adolescents, and long-term treatment of the chronically mentally ill. Refer to Figure 4-1 for a classic model of case management that links to concepts from Peplau's theory of psychiatric nursing. Also, **community nursing centers** will hopefully survive to serve low-income and uninsured people as long as they can secure funding. In this model, psychiatric nurses work with primary care nurses to provide comprehensive care, usually funded by scarce grants from academic centers. As one example of increased nursing skills in fiscal management, some clinics in 2003 decided to break ties with schools of nursing to become federally qualified health centers, eligible for federal reimbursement (Goldsmith, 2003).

Three more significant trends will affect the future of psychiatric nursing: the aging of the population, increasing cultural diversity, and ever-expanding technology. As the number of elderly Americans grows, there will be increased prevalence of Alzheimer's disease and other dementias requiring skilled nursing care in institutions. The healthier aged will also need more services at home, in retirement communities, or in assisted living facilities. By 2003, as many as half a million people resided in assisted living environments, defined by various state laws and regulations as environments providing nursing care (Mitty, 2003,

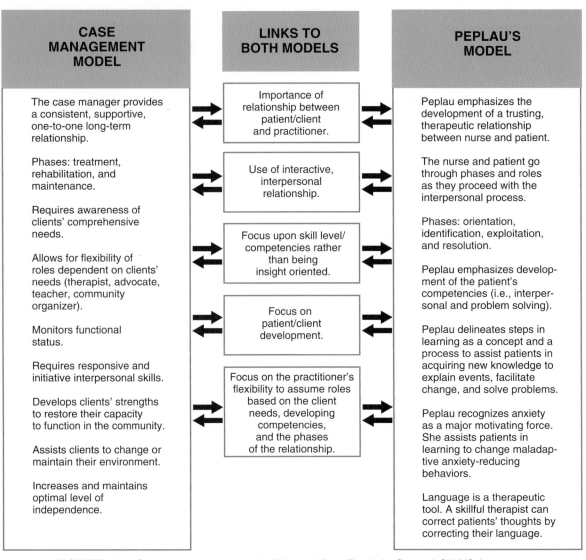

FIGURE 4-1 Case management model. (Adapted from Forchuk, C., et al. [1989]. Incorporating Peplau's theory and case management. *Journal of Psychosocial Nursing*, 27[2], 36.)

p. 32). For more information on the needs of the elderly, refer to Chapters 21 and 34.

Cultural diversity is steadily increasing in the United States; the projection is that by 2050 the majority of the population will be people of color (ANA et al., 2000, p. 8). Psychiatric nurses will need to increase their cultural competence, that is, their sensitivity to different cultural views regarding health, illness, and response to treatment.

Scientific advances through research and technology are certain to shape psychiatric nursing practice. Magnetic resonance imaging research, in addition to comparing healthy people and people diagnosed with mental illness, is now focusing on development of preclinical profiles of children and adolescents. One study in 2003 noted differences in brain organization between healthy adolescents and adolescent children of parents with schizophrenia or bipolar disorder (Goldman, 2003). The hope of this type of research is to identify people at risk for developing mental illness, which allows earlier interventions to try to decrease impairment. Likewise, findings from the Human Genome Project may one day permit genetic testing and counseling for people vulnerable to mental disorders (Merikangas & Risch, 2003). Nurses need to maintain an active role in clinical research, whether it is at the basic level of participating in nursing studies or proposing topics for study, or at the advanced level of conducting formal investigations.

Communication technology is constantly expanding through the Internet and other telehealth services. Telehealth services—that is, health care services provided from a distance—include telephone consultation and triage, Internet communication, and services delivered using other computer-based interactive media. Many health agencies already use nurses to staff help lines or hotlines, and provision of these cost-effective services will likely increase, with more need for bilingual resources. For example, in 2003, the U.S. Department of Health and Human Services funded Su

Familia: The National Hispanic Family Health Helpline, a free health hotline for Hispanic families in the United States (Coleman, 2003).

More than 33 million Americans report using the Internet for health information or peer support (Houston et al., 2002, p. 2062). One study noted significant improvement over a 1-year period in depressed clients who participated in a support group; most clients also continued face-to-face counseling. Psychiatric nurses may become more active in developing websites for mental health education, screening, or support, especially to reach geographically isolated areas.

Finally, the role of the psychiatric nurse as client advocate must continue to evolve. The nurse advocates for the psychiatric client through direct care and indirect community action. In all treatment settings, the nurse has the responsibility to communicate to the client and to uphold the client's rights. Incidents of abuse or neglect are reported to the appropriate officials for immediate action. Computerization of client records poses new challenges regarding confidentiality. Refer to Chapter 8 for more detail on ethics and client rights. With managed care, situations continue to arise in which the client disagrees with the treatment approved. The nurse can teach the client about the appeal process, including internal appeal procedures for the MBHO as well as procedures for appeal to the external review bodies available in most states (Sabin et al., 2003).

At the indirect level, the nurse may participate in consumer mental health groups, such as the National Alliance for the Mentally Ill and state and local mental health associations, to help destigmatize mental illness. The nurse can also be vigilant about reviewing local and national legislation affecting health care to identify potential detrimental effects on the mentally ill. Most professional nursing organizations have a "legislative watchdog" service or even a political action committee to influence laws related to health care or health care providers. Especially during times of fiscal crisis, lawmakers are inclined to decrease or elimi-

nate funding for vulnerable populations who do not have a strong political voice. Current political issues that need monitoring are the Medicare drug benefit and efforts to pass a national mental health parity law.

In closing, one presenter at the 2003 national convention of the National Alliance for the Mentally Ill thoughtfully summarized his knowledge gained from a 45-year career in mental health care as follows: "Mental health services look very different now than they did a half century ago. The good news is that we know more, have better treatment tools, and provide useful services to more people. The bad news is that many signs of neglect remain, particularly for the most poor and most disenfranchised individuals. As the history of mental illness attests, a decent mental health system depends as much on the interest and compassion of the larger public as it does on the concerned professionals who make mental health their work, and this area requires improvement" (Mechanic, 2003, p. 1232).

■ ■ ■ KEY POINTS to REMEMBER

- Psychiatric mental health nurses work with a broad population of clients in diverse settings to promote optimal mental health.
- Nursing standardized classification systems (NANDA, NIC, NOC) are used to communicate about client problems, interventions, and outcomes specific to nursing care.
- Psychiatric mental health nurses function at a basic or advanced level of practice with clearly defined roles.
- Psychiatric mental health nurses need a firm understanding of neuroscience and the role of psychopharmacology.
- Managed care has had a significant impact on mental health services and on the role of the nurse.
- The future holds many challenges for the psychiatric mental health nurse because of social, scientific, and political factors.

Visit the Evolve website at **http://evolve.elsevier.com/Varcarolis** for a posttest on the content in this chapter.

Critical Thinking and Chapter Review

Visit the Evolve website at **http://evolve.elsevier.com/Varcarolis** for additional self-study exercises.

■ ■ ■ CRITICAL THINKING

1. Consider the difference between working with a group of healthy women preparing for parenthood versus a group of depressed women in a mental health clinic. What are the advantages and disadvantages of working with each group?

2. Would you feel comfortable referring a family member to a mental health clinician? What factors make you feel that way?

3. How do basic level and advanced practice psychiatric nurses work together to provide the highest quality of care?

4. Would you consider joining a professional group or advocacy group that promotes mental health? Why or why not?

Continued

Critical Thinking and Chapter Review—cont'd

Visit the Evolve website at **http://evolve.elsevier.com/Varcarolis** for additional self-study exercises.

evolve

■ ■ ■ CHAPTER REVIEW

Choose the most appropriate answer.

1. A nursing student asks the psychiatric nursing instructor, "What's the difference in preparation between a basic level psychiatric nurse and an advanced practice psychiatric nurse?" The instructor should reply,
    1. "The basic level psychiatric nurse needs to have only RN licensure, whereas the advanced practice psychiatric nurse holds a baccalaureate degree in nursing."
    2. "The basic level psychiatric nurse has a baccalaureate degree in nursing, and the advanced practice psychiatric nurse has a baccalaureate degree in nursing and holds certification in the specialty."
    3. "The basic level psychiatric nurse has a baccalaureate degree in nursing, and the advanced practice psychiatric nurse has a master's degree in psychiatric nursing."
    4. "The basic level psychiatric nurse has a master's degree in psychiatric nursing, and the advanced practice psychiatric nurse has a master's degree and certification in psychiatric nursing."

2. The intervention that can be practiced by an advanced practice registered nurse in psychiatric mental health that cannot be practiced by a basic level registered nurse is
    1. advocacy.
    2. psychotherapy.
    3. case management.
    4. community-based care.

3. Only advanced practice psychiatric mental health nurses provide interventions pertaining to
    1. self-care limitations.
    2. self-concept changes.
    3. alterations in thinking and perceiving.
    4. prescription of psychopharmacological treatment.

4. A trend in psychiatric mental health nursing related to cost control imposed in the managed care environment is
    1. approval of longer treatment periods.
    2. decreased use of case management.
    3. increased ease of access to treatment.
    4. shift from inpatient care to community care.

5. An emerging role for psychiatric mental health nurses is
    1. working with the National Alliance for the Mentally Ill.
    2. serving as telehealth service provider.
    3. managing care.
    4. counseling.

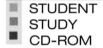 **STUDENT STUDY CD-ROM**

Access the accompanying CD-ROM for animations, interactive exercises, review questions for the NCLEX examination, and an audio glossary.

REFERENCES

Ahmed, S. M., & Maurana, C. A. (1999). Reaching out to the underserved: A collaborative partnership to provide health care. *Journal of Health Care for the Poor and Underserved, 10,* 157-168.

American Nurses Association. (1994). *Psychiatric-mental health nursing psychopharmacology project.* Washington, DC: Author.

American Nurses Association, American Psychiatric Nurses Association, & International Society of Psychiatric-Mental Health Nurses. (2000). *Scope and standards of psychiatric-mental health nursing practice.* Washington, DC: American Nurses Publishing.

American Psychiatric Association. (2000). *Diagnostic and statistical manual of mental disorders (DSM-IV-TR)* (4th ed., rev.). Washington, DC: Author.

Book, J. (2000). Behavioral health care then and now: Significant progress, but more work to do. *Psychiatric Services, 53*(10), 1249-1251.

Britt, R., Schraeder, C., & Shelton, P. (1998). Managed care and capitation: Issues in nursing. Washington, DC: American Nurses Publishing.

Cohen, J. I. (2000). Stress and mental health: A biobehavioral perspective. *Issues in Mental Health Nursing, 21,* 185-202.

Coleman, S. (2003, May 26). A phone call away. *Advance for Nurses,* p. 13.

Dochterman, J. M., & Bulechek, G. M. (2004). *Nursing interventions classification (NIC)* (4th ed.). St. Louis, MO: Mosby.

Forchuk, C., et al. (2000). The developing nurse-client relationship: Nurses' perspectives. *Journal of the American Psychiatric Nurses Association, 6,* 3-10.

Goldman, E. L. (2003). MRI can presage schizophrenia, bipolar disorder. *Clinical Psychiatry News, 31*(12), 22.

Goldsmith, J. (2003). How healthy are nursing clinics? *American Journal of Nursing, 103*(11), 22-23.

Houston, R. K., Cooper, L. A., & Ford, D. E. (2002). Internet support groups for depression: A 1-year prospective cohort study. *American Journal of Psychiatry, 159*(12), 2062-2068.

Keefe, R., & Hall, M. (1999). Private practitioners' documentation of outclient psychiatric treatment: Questioning managed care. *Journal of Behavioral Health Services and Research, 26*(2), 151-164.

Mechanic, D. (2003). Improving mental health services: Some lessons from the past. *Psychiatric Services, 54*(9), 1227-1232.

Merikangas, K. R., & Risch, N. (2003). Will the genome's revolution revolutionize psychiatry? *American Journal of Psychiatry, 160*(4), 625-635.

Mitty, E. L. (2003). Assisted living and the role of nursing. *American Journal of Nursing, 103*(8), 32-43.

Moon, M. A. (2003). "Postvention" imperative for suicide survivors. *Clinical Psychiatry News, 31*(12), 36.

Moorhead, S., Johnson, M., & Maas, M. (2004). *Nursing outcomes classification (NOC)* (3rd ed.). St. Louis, MO: Mosby.

North American Nursing Diagnosis Association. (2005). *NANDA nursing diagnoses: Definitions and classification 2005-2006.* Philadelphia: Author.

Peplau, H. E. (1952). *Interpersonal relations in nursing: A conceptual frame of reference for psychodynamic nursing.* New York: Putnam.

Rowland, D., Garfield, R., & Elias, R. (2003). Accomplishments and challenges in Medicaid mental health. *Health Affairs (Millwood), 22*(5), 73-83.

Sabin, J., Granoff, K., & Daniels, N. (2003). Strengthening the consumer voice in managed care: VI. Initial lessons from independent external review. *Psychiatric Services, 54*(1), 24-25.

U.S. Department of Health and Human Services, U.S. Public Health Service. (1999). *Mental health: A report of the Surgeon General.* Washington, DC: U.S. Government Printing Office.

World Health Organization. (1993). *International statistical classification of diseases and related health problems* (10th rev.) (ICD-10). Geneva: Author.

A NURSE SPEAKS

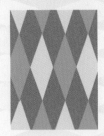

As a psychiatric home care nurse, I took care of an elderly patient named Lucy who was diagnosed with major depression. Lucy resided in an assisted living facility (ALF). Initially, I administered the Geriatric Depression Scale and the Mini-Mental State Exam. These assessments demonstrated that Lucy was seriously depressed and appeared to be suffering with dementia as well. I focused my interventions on depression as well as dementia.

Lucy seemed to be responding to my nursing care until one night at about 10 PM, when one of the staff members called me to report that Lucy was crying and screaming. I provided suggestions to calm Lucy. This same scenario repeated itself the next two nights. On the third night I decided to visit the ALF. I arrived to find Lucy cowering in a corner, crying, wringing her hands, and incredibly distraught. I saw a nursing assistant pointing her finger and yelling at Lucy to stop crying. This made Lucy more upset. I asked the nursing assistant to tell me what had happened, and she explained that for the last few nights Lucy had come out of her room at about 10 PM asking to see Lou. The nursing assistant said, "Every night I tell her the same thing: Lou is dead. He has been dead for ten years. Stop asking to see him when you know he is dead!"

With that explanation of what had occurred, I asked if I could intervene. I walked over to Lucy, placed my arm around her shoulder, and asked her what was wrong. Through her tears Lucy said to me, "They tell me that Lou is dead. How can that be? He is my husband—wouldn't I know if he were dead? Why would they say something so cruel to me?" I said, "Lucy, Lou is not here. He went out. Let's go back to your room and spend a little time together." Lucy immediately calmed. We walked to Lucy's room, where we each had a cup of tea and played cards until Lucy said, "I'm tired now. I think I'll go to sleep."

I left Lucy's room and gathered the nursing staff together to teach them about memory loss and dementia. I instructed them on the value of the "therapeutic fib"—an intervention that recognizes that when a patient has lost certain memories, the patient can no longer handle reality as we know it—and how much kinder it is for us to enter into the patient's reality, even if it means that we have to fib. The staff actually enjoyed this and provided examples of other resident situations in which telling the truth made things worse.

This incident took place years ago, but I remember it as if it happened yesterday. It confirmed that as a psychiatric home care nurse my focus is certainly the patient but it is also everyone else who is involved in the care of that patient. It also reminded me that sometimes the most effective interventions are also the simplest.

Katherine Vanderhorst

FOUNDATIONS FOR PRACTICE

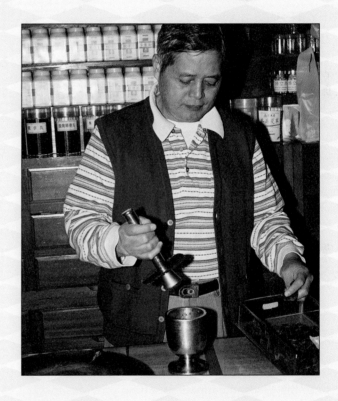

IT'S SO CLEAR THAT YOU HAVE TO CHERISH
EVERYONE . . . EVERY SOUL IS TO BE
CHERISHED . . . EVERY FLOWER IS
TO BLOOM.

Alice Walker

CHAPTER 5
Mental Health Nursing in Acute Care Settings

MARGARET SWISHER

KEY TERMS and CONCEPTS

The key terms and concepts listed here appear in color where they are defined or first discussed in this chapter.

clinical pathway, 77
codes, 81
elopement, 80
intensive case management, 82
managed behavioral health care organizations (MBHOs), 74
multidisciplinary treatment plan, 77
psychiatric case management, 77
psychiatric crisis center, 74
psychosocial rehabilitation, 82

OBJECTIVES

After studying this chapter, the reader will be able to

1. Analyze the psychiatric hospital experience from the client's perspective.
2. Explain how the mental health team collaborates to plan and implement care for the hospitalized client.
3. Describe the role of the nurse as advocate and provider of care for the client.
4. Explain the interrelationships among the managed care system, treatment planning, and the role of the case manager.
5. Discuss the managerial and coordinating roles of nursing on an inpatient acute care unit.
6. Discuss the process for preparing clients to return to the community for ongoing care.

evolve Visit the Evolve website at **http://evolve.elsevier.com/Varcarolis** for a pretest on the content in this chapter.

Hospitalization remains one option for the treatment of clients with mental disorders and emotional crises. Although lengths of stay have decreased from weeks to days since the 1980s, the inpatient setting provides intensive and effective treatment for the acutely ill client. Admission therefore is commonly reserved for those conditions that require immediate assessment, stabilization, and symptom management (Rossi, 2003). Most inpatient treatment today takes place in private general hospitals or psychiatric hospitals as described later. There are also state psychiatric hospitals that exist as a resource for the uninsured and for specialty populations, such as forensic clients referred for evaluation or treatment by the court system. State hospitals also serve as aftercare providers for clients who are not ready for discharge to the community after a brief hospitalization. For example, a client's behavior may continue to pose a danger to self or others, or severe symptoms may persist despite multiple medication trials.

ADMISSION AND GOALS

Inpatient psychiatric care is available in specialty units of general hospitals as well as in psychiatric hospitals that provide only mental health services. Although admission to either may be planned, it is common for a client to enter treatment through a **psychiatric crisis center** that is located in the admissions area or is part of emergency department services. Most **managed behavioral health care organizations (MBHOs)** and other third-party payers require that at least one of the following criteria be met to justify admission:

- Clear risk of the client's danger to self or others
- Dangerous decompensation of a client under long-term treatment
- Failure of community-based treatment with a clearly demonstrable need for more intensive and structured treatment to avoid harmful consequences

- Medical need, either unassociated with psychiatric treatment (such as intractable pain experienced by a depressed person) or associated with treatment (such as serious adverse reactions to a psychotropic medication)

Currently, therefore, goals for acute psychiatric hospitalization tend to include the following:

- Prevention of self-harm to the client
- Prevention of harm to others by the client
- Stabilization of crisis with a return to community-based services
- Initiation or modification of a psychotropic medication regimen for clients requiring careful titration or observation
- Brief, specific problem solving that is designed to enable the client to gain or regain a state of compensation
- Rapid establishment of a plan for outpatient therapy, especially referral to a partial hospitalization program that provides intensive daily services

Table 5-1 illustrates common nursing diagnoses, sample nursing interventions, and sample nursing outcomes to guide the nurse in evidence-based practice for the client during an acute admission for psychiatric care.

The following two vignettes demonstrate the application of the admission criteria.

■ ■ ■ VIGNETTE

Allen G., a 49-year-old computer programmer, has arrived at the emergency department in tears, stating that he has had suicidal thoughts after losing his job during corporate restructuring. He has been divorced for the past 6 months. The psychiatric crisis center located in the emergency department is notified and Allen is brought there for evaluation. The psychiatric nurse practitioner who interviews him determines that his risk of suicide is not high at this time: he has no history of suicidal behavior, his religious beliefs forbid suicide, and he currently resides with a supportive sister. (Refer to Chapter 23 for assessment of suicide risk.) Allen responds to crisis counseling and agrees to make an appointment to come to the partial hospitalization program the next morning. The nurse helps Allen to identify supports and to begin to recognize coping skills that he has used to survive past crises. No hospitalization is required.

■ ■ ■

■ ■ ■ VIGNETTE

Jordan S., 31 years old, is taken directly to the psychiatric crisis center by a law enforcement officer. Jordan is nearly mute, so the officer explains to the psychiatric nurse practitioner that Jordan was stopped from jumping off a bridge. After establishing a relationship with Jordan, the nurse determines that he has been treated for a severe and persistent mental disorder for the past 14 years and that, until 3 months ago, he attended a day program at a community mental health cen-

---

TABLE 5-1

Common Nursing Diagnoses with Sample Outcomes and Interventions for Clients During Admission to the Acute Care Hospital

Nursing Diagnoses (NANDA)	Nursing Outcomes Classification (NOC)	Nursing Interventions Classification (NIC)
Risk for other-directed violence: At risk for behaviors in which an individual demonstrates that he or she can be physically, emotionally, and/or sexually harmful to others	*Aggression Self-Control:* Self-restraint of assaultive, combative, or destructive behaviors towards others	*Anger Control Assistance:* Facilitation of the expression of anger in an adaptive, nonviolent manner
Risk for self-directed violence: At risk for behaviors in which an individual demonstrates that he or she can be physically, emotionally, and/or sexually harmful to self	*Suicide Self-Restraint:* Personal actions to refrain from gestures and attempts at killing self	*Behavior Management: Self-Harm:* Assisting the patient to decrease or eliminate self-mutilating or self-abusive behaviors
Disturbed thought processes: Disruption in cognitive operations and activities	*Cognitive Orientation:* Ability to identify person, place, and time accurately	*Reality Orientation:* Promotion of patient's awareness of personal identity, time, and environment
Disturbed sensory perception (auditory): Change in the amount or patterning of incoming stimuli accompanied by a diminished, exaggerated, distorted, or impaired response to such stimuli	*Communication: Receptive:* Reception and interpretation of verbal and/or nonverbal messages	*Hallucination Management:* Promoting the safety, comfort, and reality orientation of a patient experiencing hallucinations

From North American Nursing Diagnosis Association. (2005). *NANDA nursing diagnoses: Definitions and classification 2005-2006.* Philadelphia: Author; Moorhead, S., Johnson, M., & Maas, M. (2004). *Nursing outcomes classification (NOC)* (3rd ed.). St. Louis, MO: Mosby; and Dochterman, J. M., & Bulechek, G. M. (2004). *Nursing interventions classification (NIC)* (4th ed.). St. Louis, MO: Mosby.

ter. He lost contact with his family 2 years ago. Jordan continually states that "God wants me to liquidate myself." After consultation with the attending psychiatrist, the nurse practitioner arranges for voluntary admission, and Jordan agrees.

■ ■ ■

RIGHTS OF THE HOSPITALIZED CLIENT

People who are hospitalized still retain their rights as citizens. The psychiatric team has an obligation to balance the client's needs for safety with his or her rights as a citizen. All mental health facilities provide a written statement of these rights, often with copies of applicable state laws attached. Students are also advised to become familiar with the client's handbook and the policy and procedure manual on the unit. Each student should be familiar with the unit's procedures for (1) suicide precautions, (2) seclusion and restraints, and (3) client elopement (see Chapter 8). Box 5-1 provides a sample list of client's rights.

BOX 5-1

Typical Items Included in Hospital Statements of Client's Rights

1. Right to be treated with dignity.
2. Right to be involved in treatment planning and decisions.
3. Right to refuse treatment, including medications.
4. Right to request to leave the hospital, even against medical advice.
5. Right to be protected against the possible impulse to harm oneself or others that might occur as a result of a mental disorder.
6. Right to the benefit of the legally prescribed process of an evaluation occurring within a limited period (in most states, 72 hours) in the event of a request for discharge against medical advice that may lead to harm to self or others.
7. Right to legal counsel.
8. Right to vote.
9. Right to communicate privately by telephone and in person.
10. Right to informed consent.
11. Right to confidentiality regarding one's disorder and treatment.
12. Right to choose or refuse visitors.
13. Right to be informed of research and to refuse to participate.
14. Right to the least restrictive means of treatment.
15. Right to send and receive mail and to be present during any inspection of packages received.
16. Right to keep personal belongings unless they are dangerous.
17. Right to lodge a complaint through a plainly publicized procedure.
18. Right to participate in religious worship.

■ ■ ■ *VIGNETTE*

Helen Weaver, RN, C, is a certified psychiatric mental health nurse. She has just heard the morning report, learning about the conditions of all the clients on the unit and about the status of the treatment community. When she hears that Jordan S. is to be readmitted to her acute care unit, she volunteers to conduct the admissions process, because Jordan had been one of her primary clients during his previous three hospital admissions. Ms. Weaver proceeds to interview Jordan. Although her assessment priority is his risk for self-harm, she also gathers data regarding his physical, social, cognitive, and emotional status. The physician is contacted for orders based on these data. A plan of care is initiated.

Based on Ms. Weaver's assessment of Jordan's current ability to understand, she ensures that Jordan has freely consented to hospitalization and explains to him his rights as a hospitalized client. He is given a copy of the hospital's Patient's Bill of Rights and is shown where it is displayed on the unit. Jordan is oriented to the unit and to the schedule of activities. With the assistance of a client who is designated the "host," Ms. Weaver introduces Jordan to a few of the other clients. Because of Jordan's risk for self-harm, Ms. Weaver maintains a distance of no more than an arm's length from him during these activities. After Jordan demonstrates some degree of comfort with his new situation, Ms. Weaver delegates responsibility for keeping Jordan under close watch to another staff member. Ms. Weaver then documents her assessment and plan. This initial plan will guide Jordan's care until the treatment team meets to consider his needs.

■ ■ ■

Refer to Chapter 23 for a description of suicide precautions.

INTERDISCIPLINARY TEAMWORK AND CARE MANAGEMENT

The client's care is planned and implemented by a team composed of nurses, social workers, counselors, psychologists, occupational and activity therapists, psychiatrists, medical physicians, mental health workers, pharmacists, and other members of the hospital's health care team, according to the client's needs. In many inpatient settings, nurses convene and lead planning meetings and facilitate planning with assessment data and problem identification obtained via the nursing admission process (Antai-Otong, 2003b; Costell, 2003). This nursing leadership reflects the holistic nature of nursing as well as the fact that nursing is the discipline that is represented on the unit at all times. See Box 5-2 for a brief description of the roles of other members of the health team.

Members of each discipline are responsible for gathering data and participating in the planning of care. For the newly admitted client, this can prove extremely stressful or threatening. The team members, often on the recommendation of the nurse, must consider the need for timing. The scheduling of these as-

BOX 5-2

Other Members of the Health Team

Social workers: Basic level social workers help the client to prepare a support system that will promote mental health on discharge from the hospital. This includes contacts with day treatment centers, employers, sources of financial aid, and landlords. Licensed clinical social workers undergo training in individual, family, and group therapies, and often are primary care providers.

Counselors: Counselors, prepared in disciplines such as psychology, rehabilitation counseling, and addiction counseling, may augment the treatment plan by co-leading groups, providing basic supportive counseling, or assisting in psychoeducational and recreational activities.

Psychologists: In keeping with their master's or doctoral degree preparation, psychologists conduct psychological testing, provide consultation for the team, and offer direct services such as specialized individual, family, or marital therapies.

Occupational, recreational, art, music, and dance therapists: Based on their specialist preparation, these therapists assist clients in gaining skills that help them to cope more effectively, to gain or retain employment, to use leisure time to the benefit of their mental health, and to express themselves in healthy ways.

Psychiatrists: Depending on their specialty of preparation, psychiatrists may provide in-depth psychotherapy or medication therapy or head a team of mental health providers functioning as a private service based in the community. As physicians, psychiatrists may be employed by the hospital or may hold practice privileges in the facility. Because they have the legal power to prescribe and to write orders, psychiatrists often function as the leaders of the teams managing the care of the patients individually assigned to them.

Medical physicians: Medical physicians provide medical diagnosis and treatments on a consultation basis. Occasionally, a physician trained as an addiction specialist may play a more direct role on a unit that offers treatment for addictive disease.

Mental health workers: Like nursing assistants, mental health workers function under the direction and supervision of registered nurses. They provide assistance to clients in meeting basic needs and also help the community to remain supportive, safe, and healthy.

Pharmacists: In view of the intricacies of prescribing, coordinating, and administering combinations of psychotropic and other medications, the consulting pharmacist can offer a valuable safeguard. Physicians and nurses collaborate with the pharmacist regarding new medications, which are proliferating at a steady rate.

who assesses the client and consults with the unit physicians.

Members of the various disciplines meet within 72 hours to formulate or select a plan of care that reflects the consensus of the team. The plan reflects nursing process or an interdisciplinary path-based approach to care. The latter approach may be in the form of a **multidisciplinary treatment plan** or a **clinical pathway**. Clinical pathways, used by some organizations, seek to standardize the daily expected outcomes for clients (Rossi, 2003). The team either composes the plan of care or selects the clinical pathway, revising the plan or making clinical decisions if the client's progress differs from the expected outcomes. In this managed care environment, it is common for a member of the hospital's case management services, often the social worker, to participate in all treatment planning conferences and daily report meetings to monitor client progress. The reduction of overt symptoms and development of an adequate outpatient plan signal that discharge is imminent. However, mental health practitioners find that the influence of managed care on clinical decisions—in particular, length of hospital stay—results in provision of less than optimal inpatient services (Hopko et al., 2001; Jarskog et al., 2000). Thus discharge planning and the role of psychiatric case management in the outpatient setting are significant features in the continuum of care provided for clients with psychiatric disabilities.

Psychiatric Case Management

Psychiatric case management has been defined as any systematic program that coordinates individual patient care throughout the organizationally defined continuum of services and settings (Rossi, 2003, p. 566). In the inpatient setting, case managers on the hospital team communicate daily or weekly with the client's insurer and provide the treatment team with guidance regarding the availability of resources. In the community, multiple levels of intervention are available within case management services, ranging from daily assistance with medications to ongoing resolution of housing and financial issues. Ideally, psychiatric case managers establish enduring relationships with clients, facilitate their involvement in outpatient settings, and access resources, thereby helping to avoid the crises that result in readmission to the acute care hospital. Psychiatric case management fosters success in all aspects of community living by supporting recovery from acute symptoms, reducing recidivism, and enhancing the quality of life for the client with long-term illness (Antai-Otong, 2003a).

■ ■ ■ ■ **VIGNETTE**

Jordan is approached by the nurse on the next shift as that nurse briefly assesses Jordan's mental status and suicide status. He notices that once again he is being asked about

sessments should balance the urgency of the need for data against the client's ability to tolerate the assessments. Often, the assessments of the intake worker and the nurse provide the basis for initial care. In most settings the psychiatrist must assess and provide orders within a limited time. Medical problems are usually referred to a primary care physician or specialist,

thoughts of harming himself. So far he has spoken with the intake nurse, with his primary nurse (Ms. Weaver), with his psychiatrist, with a counselor who conducts a group activity in conjunction with his nurse, and with a social worker who states that he will be meeting with Jordan tomorrow. Jordan has been asked to take a medication that will "help you think more clearly and feel more secure."

After Jordan's admission and assessments by the nurse and the psychiatrist, the treatment team meets to discuss several people under the care of that psychiatrist. Ms. Weaver introduces the team to the data and the initial list of Jordan's identified problems and needs. The case manager reports that Jordan is approved by his MBHO for 5 hospital days. Priorities are set and agreements are reached regarding what further data are needed and which members of the team will obtain these data. They note that Jordan has already progressed in terms of a decreased risk for self-harm but has not yet met the expected criteria for a reduction in psychotic thinking. The team agrees on the use of prn (as needed) medication, as ordered by the psychiatrist, and the gentle guidance of Jordan's thought processes during one-to-one contacts with staff and during simple group activities to reduce psychotic thinking. It is agreed that the nurses will report on Jordan's progress in gaining clarity of thought at the next treatment planning meeting.

■ ■ ■

NURSING ON THE INPATIENT UNIT

Management

Nurses assume the bulk of the management of the daily functioning of the inpatient mental health unit. Organizationally, an arrangement of nursing management with a parallel program manager or a clinical coordinator may exist. The program staff may provide social services, activities, occupational therapy, and specialized counseling services, among others. On the other hand, these services may be managed by a nursing manager.

In either case, the nurse manager is responsible for an awareness of the safety of the unit, its effectiveness in the delivery of services, and the degree to which the components of the health care team are integrating their services well. The nurse manager, in conjunction with the medical director, plans a comprehensive schedule of therapeutic activities. The constraints of an inpatient environment, the physicians' schedules, and the availability of staff influence the composition of the daily program. Nursing management must be able to campaign effectively to gain administrative support for the program's clinical goals.

■ ■ ■ *VIGNETTE*

Consistency and attentiveness are essential to Jordan's safety during the time that he poses a risk to his own safety. The system of staffing and shift-to-shift reporting on Ms.

Weaver's unit provide for continuity of care by overlapping of shifts combined with both a tape-recorded report and an opportunity for face-to-face clarification by nurses and other staff members. By the end of the report, the staff members know their roles and responsibilities for the upcoming shift. During the time Jordan is at risk for self-harm, continuous one-to-one assignment of staff to his care is provided. A documentation sheet is maintained by the assigned staff member to indicate client status at frequent intervals.

Two days after Jordan's admission, a neurologist arrives on the unit to examine him because of neurological symptoms that Ms. Weaver has reported to the psychiatrist. Because the neurologist arrives during a group therapy session in which Jordan is participating, the charge nurse informs the neurologist that Jordan's chart may be reviewed but that the physician must wait until the conclusion of the group session before Jordan can be examined. The neurologist accepts this restriction because of previous negotiations carried out by the nurse manager of the unit with the medical staff.

■ ■ ■

Therapeutic Strategies

Psychiatric mental health nurses implement a major portion of the treatment plan. The plan is partly carried out in formal sessions with the client but is followed more frequently during informal contacts with individuals and with small groups of clients. Often, the informal contacts can be viewed as more significant than the formal ones, because they occur during natural activities of daily and social living and are therefore based on reality.

Appropriate psychological counseling skills are the basis for all nursing interventions. Nurses are prepared educationally with psychosocial communication skills to help clients feel heard and supported, develop trust and increased feelings of safety, receive feedback, and learn more adaptive coping skills. The development of a nurse-client relationship that meets basic human needs continues to be an important paradigm for psychiatric nursing (Raingruber, 2003). Nurses who have furthered their formal education, participated in workshops, and gained recognition as certified psychiatric mental health nurses or nurse specialists can conduct more intensive interpersonal or group therapies. Nurses continue to provide such therapeutic interventions as team members, sharing successes and difficulties with the team to provide for consistency of care and to gain feedback regarding timing and technique. Group work is typically co-led, with at least one of the co-leaders trained in such therapies. The co-leaders plan before sessions and evaluate the group process and their joint efforts afterward.

■ ■ ■ *VIGNETTE*

Jordan continues to experience difficulty trusting and relating to others. The plan is to build trust gradually and to introduce Jordan to increasingly complex interpersonal and group challenges. Ms. Weaver and the other nurses approach Jordan cautiously in a nonthreatening way. They offer empathetic comments regarding his nonverbal messages of distrust and discomfort. As Jordan shows increasing comfort with such one-to-one interactions, the nurses invite him to join in simple social activities on the unit, such as eating and talking with other clients. Ms. Weaver and a social worker co-lead a structured group therapy session for clients, the goals of which include organizing clients' thought processes and allowing socialization at a basic level. Jordan participates in this activity, gradually extending trust to several other clients and permitting himself to laugh and talk briefly about his immediate experiences and thoughts. After the most recent session, Ms. Weaver and the social worker discuss how Ms. Weaver's role with Jordan is purposefully being reduced to encourage Jordan to interact more with others.

Milieu
Group Activities

Experienced mental health nurses conduct specific, structured activities involving the therapeutic community, special groups, or families on most mental health units. Examples of these activities include morning goal-setting meetings and evening goal-review meetings. Community meetings may be held daily or at other scheduled times of the week. At these meetings, new clients are greeted and departing clients are given farewells, ideas for unit activities are discussed, community problems or successes are considered, and other business of the therapeutic community is conducted. Nurses also offer psychoeducational groups for clients and families on topics such as stress management, coping skills, grieving, management of medications, and communication skills. Group therapy addresses communication and sharing, helps clients explore life problems and decrease their isolation and anxiety, and engages clients in the recovery process (Simpson, 2002). For a fuller discussion of unit groups led by nurses, refer to Chapter 35.

■ ■ ■ *VIGNETTE*

Helen Weaver and another nurse are conducting a morning goal-setting meeting of the community. A thought for the day is chosen by the two nurses, who take into account some of the common concerns of a number of the clients. One client volunteers to read the thought from an inspirational book, and Ms. Weaver encourages the clients to discuss the reading briefly. Clients and staff members then introduce themselves, and each states a goal that is specific and can realistically be accomplished that day. The two nurses help each community member to state a realistic goal in measurable, concrete terms. They invite the other members of the community to offer words of encouragement. The meeting ends with the community's choice of another reading or with the ever-popular Serenity Prayer.

Management of Milieu

On an inpatient unit, nursing is the discipline primarily responsible for maintenance of a therapeutic milieu. Each nurse, through the course of a workday, is constantly gathering data about the well-being of the therapeutic community. As noted earlier, reports from shift to shift provide information on the emotional climate and level of tension on the unit.

To maintain an atmosphere in which healing and growth can take place, nurses strive to keep communications and interpersonal feedback open and constructively honest. Verbal messages must be clear or must be clarified as needed. Nonverbal messages must also be congruent with verbal messages. Ideally, staff and clients should be interacting often and be seen as sharing a number of community goals. Clients need to be involved in some decisions and given explanations for those decisions that must be left to the staff. Behavioral limits and rules should be plainly understood and consistently enforced by all staff in order to provide clear boundaries. All clients and staff must be held responsible for their own behavior and for the well-being of the community.

The therapeutic milieu operates on the understanding that the community can serve as a real-life training ground for learning about self and for practicing communication and coping skills in preparation for a return to the community outside the hospital. Even events that seemingly distract from the program of therapies can be turned into valuable learning opportunities for the members of the community.

■ ■ ■ *VIGNETTE*

Sally K., 34 years old, is a client on the unit who is well known to both clients and staff. Her bright, intelligent, and outgoing manner has made her popular. Because of her leadership and knowledge, however, she has prompted a number of clients to begin to question the unit's rules, schedules, and therapies. One of the nurses, Bob Kay, notices that he has begun to feel uncomfortable with several clients with whom he formerly had good rapport. He thinks that they are avoiding him and withholding trust. He mentions this in his shift report. Ms. Weaver validates his feelings by noting that she had also experienced this but had assumed that it may have been her own personal reaction to being a member of a different sociocultural group. The nursing staff consult with the rest of the treatment team and decide to open the community meeting to questions regarding the unit's rules, schedules, and therapies. At the meeting, the airing of issues satisfies the client community. Several of the clients involved ask to speak privately with staff about their feelings of having been influenced by Sally. Sally herself speaks with her nurse about how she realizes that she was using the situation to avoid working on her own painful feelings and decisions.

Safety

The psychiatric mental health nurse assumes a responsibility for ongoing vigilance regarding safety hazards. Today clients on inpatient units have very acute illnesses, which contributes to an increased risk of danger. The nurse carries out a variety of measures designed to reduce this risk on a daily basis. Environmental perils, such as fire, may also occur. Nurses must be able to rapidly isolate or evacuate clients while remaining in control of clients' whereabouts and minimizing their sense of threat.

The nurse must supervise the unit's systems for tracking which clients are on or off the unit and for performing periodic or constant checks on those clients at risk of harming themselves or others. The flow of visitors and of objects being brought onto the unit must be managed. Procedures for the safe control of sharp objects must be implemented. Use of illegal drugs or alcohol and sexual activity between clients must be prevented. Violence and disruption must be minimized while maintaining an atmosphere that promotes healthy and appropriate expression of anger and other feelings. Elopement (escape) of clients must be prevented, but in a way that avoids an atmosphere of imprisonment. Routine nursing concerns related to safety issues such as slippery floors, client falls, and electrical hazards must be addressed.

■ ■ ■ *VIGNETTE*

Helen Weaver has woven concern for safety into her daily nursing practice. As she enters or leaves the unit, she checks the unit's locks. She is alert to any potential electrical or fire hazards. Her eyes routinely scan the unit for possible sharp objects. She tracks the locations of clients as she moves about the unit. If she is aware that staff members have not been present in certain locations, she is sure to include those places in her rounds. Ms. Weaver informs new clients of rules regarding sharp objects, smoking, medications from home, visitors, exit from the unit, and behavioral restrictions. She clearly advises clients against the possession of alcohol and illicit drugs. She supervises inspection of clients' personal items and of any medications brought from home. She will later document her findings in clients' medical records. She participates in community meetings during which staff provide clarification of these rules. When visitors arrive, she teaches them the rules and checks bags and other incoming items.

■ ■ ■

Documentation

Documentation of client progress is the responsibility of the entire mental health team. Although communication among team members and coordination of services are the primary goals when choosing a system for charting, practitioners in the inpatient setting must also consider professional standards, legal issues, requirements for reimbursement by insurers, and accreditation by regulatory agencies. Information must also be in a format that is retrievable for quality assurance monitoring, utilization management, peer review, and research. For nursing, documentation of the nursing process is a guiding concern and is reflected in the different reporting formats that are commonly found in psychiatric hospitals. See Chapter 9 for an overview of documentation options. Computerized clinical documentation is the common trend in inpatient settings today.

Psychopharmacological Responsibilities

Nurses on the inpatient acute care unit are responsible for addressing complex health problems in clients. Medical comorbidity and mortality due to medical illness among clients with psychiatric disabilities is well documented (Cradock-O'Leary et al., 2002; Folsom et al., 2002). Both detection and prevention of medical illnesses are compromised by clients' reluctance to seek treatment, poor communication skills, and denial and lack of awareness of health status (Cradock-O'Leary et al., 2002). General lack of fitness, obesity, poor nutrition, alcohol consumption, and cigarette smoking account for an estimated 60% of premature deaths among clients with schizophrenia (Lambert, Velakoulis, & Pantelis, 2003). In addition, anxiety, lack of trust, or thought impairment may cause clients to resist procedures such as measurement of vital signs, blood glucose monitoring, and insulin administration. As the therapeutic relationship develops, clients become more tolerant of physical interventions, and the nurse may begin to address physical health status.

The safe administration of medications and monitoring of their effects is a 24-hour responsibility for the nurse. Because of their active leadership during treatment planning, nurses often exert great influence on medication decisions on mental health units. Detailed knowledge of psychoactive medications and of the interactions and psychological side effects of other medications is expected of mental health nurses. The nurse's observations of the expected and adverse effects of medications provide data necessary for daily medication decisions by the psychiatrist and treatment team. For example, feedback about a client's excessive sedation or increased agitation will lead to a decision to decrease or increase the dosage of an antipsychotic medication. The legal issues of resistance to taking medication and of noncompliance are dealt with in Chapter 8.

In some hospital settings, clients come to a central location for medication administration. This fosters client responsibility and involvement in the treatment process. Psychiatric mental health nurses often have numerous decisions to make about prn medications. These decisions must be based on a combination of factors: the client's request, the team's plan, attempts to use alternative methods of coping, and the nurse's judgments regarding timing and the client's behavior. Documentation for administering each prn medication must include the rationale for its use and the effects.

▪ ▪ ▪ *VIGNETTE*

Helen Weaver has provided the team with data leading to an accurate diagnosis and choice of medications for Jordan. This choice reflects Ms. Weaver's knowledge of how Jordan responded to medication regimens during previous hospitalizations. His current regimen includes orders for medications that reduce his disorganized thought processes and thereby reduce his risk for self-harm. On Ms. Weaver's day off, the nurse assigned to Jordan assesses that he hears voices "commanding me to cease living." The nurse refers to Jordan's chart. The plan directs the nurse to spend 15 minutes helping Jordan to recall that he has learned to understand that when he hears such voices, it is his mind's way of expressing his feeling of being overwhelmed. He is to use relaxation techniques, but if he does not obtain relief within 20 minutes, he may use his prn medication along with relaxation.

The nurse notes that Jordan has received his oral dose of medication (the same drug as the prn medication) only 10 minutes before her assessment. Based on her knowledge of the time needed for this medication to begin to take effect, she follows the plan of care. The relaxation technique, along with the onset of action of Jordan's usual dose of the drug, leads to relief of his symptoms at this time.

▪ ▪ ▪

Crisis Management

Nurses anticipate, prevent, and manage emergencies and crises on the unit. These crises may be of a medical or behavioral nature. Mental health units, whether situated in a general hospital or independent facilities, must be able to stabilize the condition of a client who experiences a medical crisis. Mental health or addictive disease units that manage detoxification (withdrawal from alcohol or other drugs) must anticipate several common medical crises associated with that process. Mental health units therefore store crash carts containing the emergency medications used to treat shock and cardiorespiratory arrest. Nurses must maintain their cardiopulmonary resuscitation skills and be able to use basic emergency equipment. To be effective and to practice at a high level of competency, nurses are advised to attend inservice sessions and workshops designed to teach and maintain skills. Nurses must be able to alert medical support systems quickly and mobilize transportation to the appropriate medical facility.

▪ ▪ ▪ *VIGNETTE*

Lester D., age 55, a client with acute mania and hypertension, complains of chest pain. The nurse asks Lester to be seated and checks his vital signs, carefully listening to his apical pulse. Noting irregularities that were not observed on previous assessments, the nurse stays with Lester while asking another nurse to notify the physician and to ready the crash cart. The portable electrocardiographic (ECG) monitor is attached and the nurse observes erratic, irregular heart beats. Transportation is arranged, and Lester is transferred after an intravenous line is inserted and ECG monitoring is set up. The emergency is managed within 25 minutes of the client's first complaint.

▪ ▪ ▪

Behavioral crises can lead to client violence toward self or others. Crises are usually, but not always, observed to escalate through fairly predictable stages. Crisis prevention and management techniques are practiced by staff in most mental health facilities. Many psychiatric hospitals have special teams made up of nurses, psychiatric aides, and other professionals who respond to psychiatric emergencies called codes. Each member of the team takes part in the team effort to defuse a crisis in its early stages. If preventive measures fail, each member of the team participates in a rapid, organized movement designed to immobilize, medicate, or seclude a client. The nurse is most often this team's leader, not only organizing the plan but also timing the intervention and managing the concurrent use of prn medications. The nurse can initiate such an intervention in the absence of a physician in most states but must secure a physician's order for restraint or seclusion within a specified time. (Refer to Chapters 8 and 24 for further discussions and protocols for use of restraints and seclusion.)

The nurse also advocates for clients by ensuring that their legal rights are preserved, no matter how difficult their behavior may be for the staff to manage.

Crises on the unit are upsetting and threatening to other clients in the therapeutic community. A staff member is usually reserved to address the needs of the community. This person removes other clients from the area of crisis and helps them express their fears. Clients may be concerned for the involved client and may fear that they, too, might experience such a loss of behavioral control.

▪ ▪ ▪ *VIGNETTE*

Jordan appears upset as he approaches a mental health worker. Jordan reports that Anthony, another client, is angrily throwing objects at the staff person assigned on a one-to-one basis to Anthony. The mental health worker reports this to the charge nurse, who quickly assigns the worker to remove other clients from the area. The nurse organizes other staff and checks Anthony's prn orders. The team gathers at the far area of the day room while the nurse and one other staff person use calm but limit-setting communication techniques: "Anthony, you are not to hurt yourself or anyone here. If you are having trouble controlling your impulses, we will help you." Because Anthony's behavior continues to escalate toward violence, the charge nurse directs another nurse to prepare Anthony's prn medication while the rest of the staff prepares to direct Anthony to the seclusion room. The staff members use their numbers as a "show of force" to convince Anthony of the seriousness of this directive. Anthony agrees and also reluctantly takes the prn medication. The staff remain prepared to intervene safely but decisively to take Anthony to the seclusion room if he cannot agree to the directive. While the charge nurse telephones the physician to report the incident and to obtain orders for seclusion, another nurse gathers the community in the day room to allow for expression of feelings about the situation. The nurse is careful to avoid breaking Anthony's confidentiality during this activity.

Careful, accurate documentation in Anthony's chart demonstrates the need for these measures and describes how the intervention was carried out. While Anthony is in seclusion, he will be monitored at frequent intervals by a staff member.

■ ■ ■

Preparation for Discharge to the Community

As members of the multidisciplinary team, nurses assist clients and their families to prepare for independent or assisted living in the community. Community-based programs provide clients with psychosocial rehabilitation that moves the mentally ill beyond stabilization toward a higher quality of life. This is especially important to the concept and practice of managed behavioral health care, aiming toward the goal of reducing the length and frequency of hospital stays by the client.

Nurses therefore focus on the factors precipitating the crisis that led to hospital admission. Clients are assisted in learning coping skills and behaviors that will help them avert future crises. Psychoeducational groups, individual exploration of options and supports, and on-the-spot instruction (such as during medication administration) offer the client numerous learning opportunities. Nurses encourage clients to use their everyday experiences on the unit to practice newly learned behavior.

The treatment plan or clinical pathway chosen for the client should reflect this discharge planning emphasis as early as the day of admission. The client is expected to begin to progress toward a resolution of acute symptoms, assumption of personal responsibility, and improved interpersonal functioning. Clients with prolonged mental illness benefit most from a seamless transition to community services. This is facilitated by collaboration with community mental health services and the intensive case management programs available there (Antai-Otong, 2003a). Readiness for community reentry should include

preparation by members of the client's support system for their role in enhancing the client's mental health.

■ ■ ■ *VIGNETTE*

The unit's schedule reflects its commitment to success in the community. Once his condition permits, Jordan attends evening group sessions that present information about safe and consistent use of medications, the importance of regular attendance in a community care program, communication skills, cognitive restructuring, self-esteem building, use of spiritual supports, and healthy interaction with one's family. Jordan uses role playing to learn more comfortable communication and assertiveness skills. The social worker invites Jordan's intensive case manager from the community mental health center to attend a treatment team meeting. Jordan agrees to return to daily participation in a day program and have a monthly medication evaluation. An appointment time is scheduled for assessment and readmission to the day program. In the group session, Jordan's peers encourage him to contact his family. He says one morning that his goal for the day is to phone his parents. The group helps him decide how to communicate during the phone conversation and later encourages him to discuss the results.

By the day of his discharge from the hospital, Jordan is arriving for his medications independently, has plans for his follow-up care, is ready to return to his apartment, and has been invited to lunch with his parents.

■ ■ ■

Policy Review and Revision

Mental health nurses are usually expected or invited to participate in decisions about the system of providing care and the working environment. Nurses may address issues such as problems in scheduling of activities, work schedules, assignments, opportunities to expand professional practice, and safety. Nurses may research novel approaches to these or other aspects of delivery of care. Committee work may offer the nurse the chance to participate in the management and future of the unit.

■ ■ ■ *VIGNETTE*

Ms. Weaver collaborates with other nurses and program staff to develop a system for monitoring clinical outcomes. This system, based on the clinical pathways, will enable the staff to argue more persuasively for insurance payments for clients. It will also provide data useful for contracting with large regional employers to provide mental health services for their employees. Ms. Weaver describes her enthusiasm about participating in research and expanding beyond her customary nursing roles.

■ ■ ■

■■■ KEY POINTS to REMEMBER

- ■ Inpatient psychiatric nursing requires strong skills in management, communication, and collaboration.
- ■ The nurse plays a leadership role and also functions as a team member in the multidisciplinary treatment team.
- ■ The nurse advocates for the client and ensures that the client's rights are protected.
- ■ Basic level interventions include counseling, crisis management, milieu therapy, health teaching, and psychobiological interventions.
- ■ The therapeutic milieu depends on client and staff behavior: clear, consistent communication is practiced; physical safety and comfort are maintained; everyone is treated with respect; and all individuals are encouraged to take responsibility for their own decision making and growth.
- ■ Discharge planning begins on the day of admission and requires input from the treatment team and the community mental health provider.
- ■ Documentation is an important form of communication to promote consistency in client care and to justify the client's stay in the hospital.

Visit the Evolve website at **http://evolve.elsevier.com/Varcarolis** for a posttest on the content in this chapter. *evolve*

Critical Thinking and Chapter Review

Visit the Evolve website at **http://evolve.elsevier.com/Varcarolis** for additional self-study exercises. *evolve*

■■■ CRITICAL THINKING

1. How does a nurse decide to place the clients' safety needs before their right to make decisions for themselves?
2. If nurses function as equal members of the multidisciplinary mental health team, what differentiates the nurse from the other members of the team?
3. What effect do MBHOs have on the care of mentally ill clients?
4. How is a community affected when clients with severe and persistent mental illness live in group homes?

■■■ CHAPTER REVIEW

Choose the most appropriate answer.

1. The presence of which symptom will exert the greatest pressure to admit an individual to an inpatient psychiatric unit?
    1. Suicidal ideation
    2. Moderate anxiety
    3. Feelings of sadness
    4. Auditory hallucinations
2. When the mental health team meets initially to plan care for a client on an inpatient unit, the outcome should be
    1. greater team cohesion.
    2. support for the psychiatrist.
    3. equal distribution of responsibility for the client among members of the staff.
    4. an interdisciplinary care plan delineating assessments, interventions, treatments, and outcomes across a time line.
3. Which goal should be evaluated as met prior to a client's discharge from an inpatient psychiatric unit?
    1. Family members are ready to accept the client.
    2. The client can return to productive work.
    3. The admission crisis is resolved.
    4. The client's illness is cured.
4. A therapeutic milieu for an inpatient psychiatric unit is characterized by
    1. few rules.
    2. staff control.
    3. open communication.
    4. conflict suppression.
5. Of the several psychiatric inpatient unit staff activities listed below, which is most characteristically assumed by the discipline of nursing?
    1. Advocating for the legal rights of clients
    2. Complying with documentation standards
    3. Creating an individualized client plan of care
    4. Leading a behavioral crisis management team

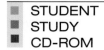

■ **STUDENT**
■ **STUDY**
■ **CD-ROM**

Access the accompanying CD-ROM for animations, interactive exercises, review questions for the NCLEX examination, and an audio glossary.

REFERENCES

Antai-Otong, D. (2003a). Psychosocial rehabilitation. *Nursing Clinics of North America, 38,* 151-160.

Antai-Otong, D. (2003b). Treatment considerations for the patient with borderline personality disorder. *Nursing Clinics of North America, 38,* 101-109.

Costell, S., (2003). Evidence-based treatment of mood disorders. *Nursing Clinics of North America, 38,* 21-33.

Cradock-O'Leary, J., et al. (2002). Use of general medical services by VA patients with psychiatric disorders. *Psychiatric Services, 53*(7), 874-878.

Folsom, D., et al. (2002). Medical comorbidity and receipt of medical care by older homeless people with schizophrenia or depression. *Psychiatric Services, 53*(11), 1456-1460.

Hopko, D., et al. (2001). Assessing predictive factors for extended hospitalization at acute psychiatric admission. *Psychiatric Services, 52*(10), 1367-1373.

Jarskog, L., et al. (2000). First-episode psychosis in a managed care setting: Clinical management and research. *American Journal of Psychiatry, 157*(6), 878-884.

Lambert, T. J., Velakoulis, D., & Pantelis, C. (2003, May). Medical comorbidity in schizophrenia. *Medical Journal of Australia, 178*(9 Suppl. 5), S67-S70.

Raingruber, B. (2003). The fundamental significance of relationship as a paradigm for mental health nursing. *Perspectives in Psychiatric Care, 39*(3), 104-135.

Rossi, P. (2003). Case management in health care (2nd ed.). Philadelphia: Saunders.

Simpson, I. (2002). Inpatient group work for patients with psychosis. *Nursing Times, 98*(41), 33-35.

CHAPTER 6

Mental Health Nursing in Community Settings

NANCY CHRISTINE SHOEMAKER ▪ SUSAN CAVERLY

▪ KEY TERMS and CONCEPTS

The key terms and concepts listed here appear in color where they are defined or first discussed in this chapter.

barriers to treatment, 95

continuum of psychiatric mental health treatment, 90

deinstitutionalization, 86

ethical dilemmas, 95

seriously mentally ill, 86

▪ OBJECTIVES

After studying this chapter, the reader will be able to

1. Explain the evolution of the community mental health movement.
2. Identify elements of the nursing assessment that are critically important to the success of community treatment.
3. Distinguish between the hospital and community settings with regard to characteristics, goals of treatment, and nursing interventions.
4. Compare and contrast the roles of the nurse in community mental health according to the nurse's educational preparation.
5. Explain the role of the nurse as the biopsychosocial care manager in the multidisciplinary team.
6. Discuss the continuum of psychiatric treatment.
7. Describe the role of the psychiatric nurse in four specific settings: partial hospitalization program; psychiatric home care; assertive community treatment; and community mental health center.
8. Identify two resources to assist the community psychiatric nurse in resolving ethical dilemmas.
9. Discuss barriers to mental health treatment.

evolve Visit the Evolve website at **http://evolve.elsevier.com/Varcarolis** for a pretest on the content in this chapter.

The first psychiatric nurses working in the community setting were community health nurses who developed a specialty practice in mental health. They were able to move within the community, were comfortable meeting with clients in the home or neighborhood center, were competent to act independently, used professional judgment in sometimes unanticipated situations, and possessed knowledge of community resources.

The heritage of these nurses can be traced back to the European women who cared for the sick at home and American women who organized into religious and secular societies during the 1800s to visit the sick

in their homes. By 1877, trained nurses worked as public health nurses visiting the homes of the poor in northeastern cities and generalist nurses made community visits to rural areas for health promotion and care of the sick (Smith, 1995).

CONTEXT FOR PSYCHIATRIC NURSING IN THE COMMUNITY

In 1963, President Kennedy signed into law the Community Mental Health Centers Act, thus solidifying the shift of mental health care from the institution to the community and heralding the era of deinstitutionalization. Media focus raising public awareness regarding the horrors of psychiatric institutions, the mental health care needs presented by returning servicemen, and the development of psychopharmacological agents all acted as catalysts for needed change in psychiatric treatment philosophy (Marcos, 1990; Rochefort, 1993).

The 1960s were also the time when federal entitlement programs proliferated: Social Security Disability, Supplemental Security Income, Medicaid, Medicare, housing assistance, and food stamps. These social programs provided the means for moving the mentally ill out of institutions and into the community. Policymakers believed that community care would be more humane and less expensive than the historic hospital-based care.

Caring for seriously mentally ill (also called chronically mentally ill) clients in the community, however, presented many challenges. At the time, there were few choices for outpatient treatment, mainly a community mental health center or therapy in a private office. Government promises to expand funding for community services were not kept, and there were more clients than resources. In addition, many seriously mentally ill clients resisted treatment with available providers, and providers began to use scarce resources for the less disabled but more compliant population. Despite these problems, a second wave of deinstitutionalization took place in the 1980s after President Carter's Commission on Mental Health highlighted the needs of the underserved and unserved seriously mentally ill group.

Over the past 30 years, with advances in psychopharmacology and psychosocial treatments, levels of psychiatric care in the community have multiplied into a continuum with many choices. The role of the community psychiatric registered nurse (RN) has diversified to include providing services in all of these treatment settings. In this chapter, you will learn about the role of the basic level RN in different multidisciplinary treatment teams across this spectrum. Many nontraditional nursing roles have developed outside of the recognized treatment sites. Psychiatric needs are well known in the criminal justice system and in the homeless population. In 1999, the U.S. Department of Justice estimated that 16% of people in jail (those in for short stays as opposed to the long-term prison population) reported a history of an emotional problem (McQuistion et al., 2003, p. 671). Repeated studies since the 1980s suggest that one third to one half of homeless people have severe psychiatric illness (McQuistion et al., 2003, p. 669). Psychiatric RNs are actively involved in forensic settings and in creative outreach efforts in public places.

School-based clinics have increased as communities have recognized the need for early detection and treatment for children. In addition to performing screening and mental health teaching, psychiatric RNs are a part of crisis teams that respond to episodes of school violence, either adolescent suicide or mass homicide. The issue of increasing violence has had great impact on community nurses in all settings, especially with the emergence of terrorism and bioterrorism (see Chapter 14). Educators now believe that all nurses need core competencies in emergency preparedness to be ready for human-created disasters (Gebbie & Qureshi, 2002). One example of this need for quick action was in the aftermath of the September 11, 2001, terrorist attack in New York City. The state department of mental health immediately established a program to provide free crisis counseling services to all city residents (Rudenstine et al., 2003).

As noted earlier, community psychiatric nurses practice in diverse settings among people who may or may not be diagnosed with a mental illness. The principles of the public health concept of prevention are useful to support all of these interventions. Primary prevention activities are directed to healthy populations to provide information and to teach coping skills to reduce stress, with the goal of avoiding mental illness. For example, a nurse may teach parenting skills in a well-baby clinic. Secondary prevention involves the early detection and treatment of psychiatric symptoms with the goal of minimizing impairment. For example, a nurse may conduct screening for depression at a work site. Tertiary prevention involves those services that address residual impairments in psychiatric clients, in an effort to promote the highest level of community functioning. For example, a nurse may provide long-term treatment in a clinic. Box 6-1 presents examples of community practice sites for the psychiatric mental health nurse.

ASPECTS OF COMMUNITY NURSING

Psychiatric nursing in the community setting differs markedly from psychiatric nursing in the hospital. The community setting requires flexibility on the part of the psychiatric nurse and knowledge about a broad array of community resources. Clients need assistance with problems related to individual psychiatric symptoms, family and support systems, and basic living needs such as housing and financial support. Outside of a traditional clinic or office, the setting is the realm of the client rather than of the health care provider. Community treatment hinges on enhancing client strengths in the same environment in which daily life must be maintained, which makes individually tailored psychiatric care imperative. The hospital repre-

Possible Community Mental Health Practice Sites

Primary Prevention
Adult and youth recreational centers
Schools
Day care centers
Churches, temples, synagogues, mosques
Ethnic cultural centers

Secondary Prevention
Crisis centers
Shelters (homeless, battered women, adolescents)
Correctional community facilities
Youth residential treatment centers
Partial hospitalization programs
Chemical dependency programs
Nursing homes
Industry/work sites
Outreach treatment in public places
Hospices and acquired immunodeficiency syndrome programs
Assisted living facilities

Tertiary Prevention
Community mental health centers
Psychosocial rehabilitation programs

Elements of Biopsychosocial Nursing Assessment

Presenting problem and referring party
Psychiatric history, including symptoms, treatments, medications, and most recent service utilization
Health history, including illnesses, treatments, medications, and allergies
Substance abuse history and current use*
Family history, including health and mental health disorders and treatments
Psychosocial history, including:
- Developmental history
- School performance
- Socialization
- Vocational success or difficulty
- Interpersonal skills or deficits
- Income and source of income*
- Housing adequacy and stability*
- Family and support system*
- Level of activity
- Ability to care for needs independently or with assistance
- Religious or spiritual beliefs and practices

Legal history
Mental status examination
Strengths and deficits of the client
Cultural beliefs and needs relevant to psychosocial care

*Strongly related to the probability that the client will experience successful outcomes in the community.

sents a controlled setting and promotes stabilization, but strides made during hospitalization can be lost upon return home. Treatment in the community permits clients and those involved in their support to learn new ways of coping with symptoms or situational difficulties. The result can be one of empowerment and self-management, to the extent possible given the client's disability.

Psychiatric Nursing Assessment Strategies

Assessment of the biopsychosocial needs and capacities of clients living in the community requires expansion of the general psychiatric nursing assessment. For the hospitalized client, the nurse must understand community living challenges and resources to assess presenting problems as well as to plan for discharge. The community psychiatric RN must also develop a comprehensive understanding of the client's ability to cope with the demands of living in the community, to be able to plan and implement effective treatment. Box 6-2 identifies the areas covered in a biopsychosocial assessment.

Four key elements of this assessment are strongly related to the probability that the client will experience successful outcomes in the community. Problems in any of these areas require immediate attention before other treatment goals are pursued.

- Housing adequacy and stability—If a client faces daily fears of homelessness, it is not possible to focus on other treatment issues.
- Income and source of income—A client must have a basic income, whether from an entitlement, a relative, or other sources, to obtain necessary medication and to meet daily needs for food and clothing.
- Family and support system—The presence of a family member, friend, or neighbor supports the client's recovery and also gives the RN a contact person, with the client's consent.
- Substance abuse history and current use—Often hidden or minimized during hospitalization, substance abuse can be a destructive force undermining medication effectiveness and interfering with community acceptance and procurement of housing.

Individual cultural characteristics of clients are also very important to assess. For example, working with a person for whom Spanish is the primary language requires the nurse to consider the implications of language and cultural background. The use of an interpreter or cultural consultant, from the agency or from the family, is essential when the nurse and client speak different languages (see Chapter 7).

Psychiatric Nursing Intervention Strategies

In the hospital setting, the focus of care is on stabilization, as defined by staff. In the community setting, treatment goals and interventions are negotiated rather than imposed on the client. Community psychiatric nurses must approach interventions with flexibility and resourcefulness to meet the broad range of needs of clients. The complexity of navigating the mental health system and the social service funding systems is often overwhelming to clients. Not unexpectedly, client outcomes with regard to mental status and functional level have been found to be more positive and to be achieved with greater cost effectiveness when the community psychiatric RN integrates case management into the professional role (Chan, Mackenzie, & Jacobs, 2000; Chan et al., 2000).

Differences in characteristics, treatment outcomes, and interventions between inpatient and community settings are outlined in Table 6-1. Note that all of these interventions fall within the practice domain of the basic level RN.

ROLES AND FUNCTIONS OF THE COMMUNITY PSYCHIATRIC NURSE

As noted in Chapter 4, psychiatric mental health nurses are educated at a variety of levels: associate, diploma, baccalaureate, masters, and doctoral. Perhaps the most significant distinction among the multiple levels of preparation is the degree to which the nurse acts autonomously and provides consultation to other providers both inside and outside of the particular agency. The nurse practice acts of individual states grant nurses authority to practice, and the standards of psychiatric nursing developed by the American Nurses Association in collaboration with psychiatric groups also define levels of practice. Table 6-2 describes the roles of psychiatric nurses according to level of education.

Member of Multidisciplinary Community Practice Team

The concept of using multidisciplinary treatment teams originated with the Community Mental Health Centers Act of 1963. Psychiatric nursing practice was identified as one of the core mental health disciplines, along with psychiatry, social work, and psychology. This recognition permitted the allocation of resources

TABLE 6-1

Characteristics, Treatment Outcomes, and Interventions by Setting

Inpatient Setting	Community Mental Health Setting
Characteristics	
Unit locked by staff	Home locked by client
24-hour supervision	Intermittent supervision
Boundaries determined by staff	Boundaries negotiated with client
Milieu with food, housekeeping, security services	Client-controlled environment with self-care, safety risks
Treatment Outcomes	
Stabilization of symptoms and return to community	Stable or improved level of functioning in community
Interventions	
Develop short-term therapeutic relationship.	Establish long-term therapeutic relationship.
Develop comprehensive plan of care with attention to sociocultural needs of client.	Develop comprehensive plan of care for client and support system with attention to sociocultural needs.
Enforce boundaries by seclusion or restraint, as needed.	Negotiate boundaries with client.
Administer medication.	Encourage compliance with medication regimen.
Monitor nutrition and self-care with assistance as needed.	Teach and support adequate nutrition and self-care with referrals as needed.
Provide health assessment and intervention as needed.	Assist client in self-assessment with referrals for health needs in community as needed.
Offer structured socialization activities.	Use creative strategies to refer client to positive social activities.
Plan for discharge with family/significant other with regard to housing and follow-up treatment.	Communicate regularly with family/support system to assess and improve level of functioning.

TABLE 6-2

Community Psychiatric Nursing Roles Relevant to Educational Preparation

Role	Advanced Practice (MS, PhD)	Basic Practice (Diploma, AA, BS)
Practice	Nurse practitioner or clinical nurse specialist; manage consumer care and prescribe or recommend interventions independently	Provide nursing care for consumer and assist with medication management as prescribed, under direct supervision
Consultation	Consultant to staff about plan of care, to consumer and family about options for care; collaborate with community agencies about service coordination and planning processes	Consult with staff about care planning and work with nurse practitioner or physician to promote health and mental health care; collaborate with staff from other agencies
Administration	Administrative or contract consultant role within mental health agencies or mental health authority	Take leadership role within mental health treatment team
Research and education	Role as educator or researcher within agency or mental health authority	Participate in research at agency or mental health authority; serve as preceptor to undergraduate nursing students

to educate psychiatric nurses and emphasized their unique contributions to the team.

In team meetings, the individual and discipline-specific expertise of each member is recognized. Generally, the composition of the team reflects the availability of fiscal and professional resources in the area. Similar to the team defined in Chapter 5, the community psychiatric team may include psychiatrists, nurses, social workers, psychologists, dual-diagnosis specialists, and mental health workers. Recognition of the ability of nurses to have an equal voice in team treatment planning with other professionals was novel at the time the team approach was implemented in community mental health practice. This level of professional performance was later used as a model for other nursing specialties.

Some writers believe that the multidisciplinary team approach dilutes the nursing role, because nurses adopt the language of psychiatry and social services. But ideally, the nurse is able to integrate a strong nursing identity into the team perspective. At the basic or advanced practice level, the community psychiatric RN is in a critical position to link the biopsychosocial and spiritual components relevant to mental health care for the individual. The RN also communicates in a manner that the client, significant others, and members of the team can accept and understand. In particular, the management and administration of psychotropic medications have become a significant task the community RN is expected to perform. There is evidence that medications are most effective when the nurse approaches drug therapy seeking to empower the individual client (Marland & Sharkey, 1999).

Biopsychosocial Care Manager

The role of the community psychiatric RN includes the coordination of mental health, physical health, spiritual health, social service, educational service, and vo-

cational realms of care for the mental health client. The reality of community practice in the new millennium is that few clients seeking treatment have uncomplicated symptoms of a single mental illness. The severity of illness, especially in the public sector, has increased and is correlated with increased substance abuse, poverty, and stress. In addition, repeated studies show that the mentally ill have a higher risk for medical disorders than the general population (Dickey et al., 2002).

The 1980s brought increased emphasis on implementing case management as a core service in treating the seriously mentally ill client. In the private domain, case management or care management has also found a niche. The intent is to charge case managers with designing individually tailored treatment services for clients and tracking outcomes of care. Case management includes the following functions: assessing client needs; developing a plan for service; linking the client with necessary services; monitoring the effectiveness of services; and advocating for the client, as needed (Shoemaker, 2000). Nursing and medicine are the only mental health disciplines possessing the knowledge, skill, and legal authority to provide the full range of mental health care interventions. This scope of practice, coupled with issues of personnel cost and availability, underscores the critical need for community psychiatric RNs to participate in coordination of care activities.

A successful life in the community is more likely when medications are taken as prescribed. Nurses are in a position to help the client to manage medication, recognize side effects, and be aware of the interactions among drugs prescribed for physical illness and mental illness. Client-family education and behavioral strategies, in the context of a therapeutic relationship with the clinician, have been shown to significantly increase compliance with the medication regimen (Lacro & Glassman, 2004).

COMMUNITY SETTINGS

Many community psychiatric RNs originally practiced on site at community mental health centers. As financial, health care, regulatory, cultural, and population changes have occurred, the practice locations have changed. Nurses are providing primary mental health care at therapeutic day care centers, schools, partial hospitalization programs, and shelters. In addition to these more traditional environments for care, psychiatric RNs are also entering forensic settings and drug and alcohol treatment centers. Mobile mental health units have been developed in some service areas. In a growing number of communities, mental health programs are collaborating with other health or community services to provide integrated approaches to treatment. A prime example of this is the growth of dual-diagnosis programming at both mental health and chemical dependency clinics. Technology has begun to contribute to the venues for providing community care: telephone crisis counseling, telephone outreach, and even the Internet are being used to enhance access to mental health services (Wilson & Williams, 2000).

In the following sections, you will find descriptions of four different community psychiatric settings, with illustrations of the practice of the basic level RN in each team. Nursing interventions in these settings include most of those defined for basic practice, for example:

- Counseling—assessment interviews, crisis intervention, problem solving in individual, group, or family sessions.
- Promotion of self-care activities—fostering of grooming, instruction in use of public transportation, budgeting; in home settings, the RN may directly assist as necessary.
- Psychobiological interventions—medication administration, teaching of relaxation techniques, promotion of sound eating and sleep habits.
- Health teaching—medication use, illness characteristics, coping skills, relapse prevention.
- Case management—communication with family, significant others, and other health care or community resource personnel to coordinate an effective plan of care.

Figure 6-1 presents the continuum of psychiatric mental health treatment. Movement along the continuum is fluid, from higher to lower levels of intensity, and changes are not necessarily step by step. Upon discharge from acute hospital care or a 24-hour supervised crisis unit, many clients need intensive services to maintain their initial gains or to "step down" in care. Multiple studies show that failure to follow up in outpatient treatment increases the likelihood of rehos-

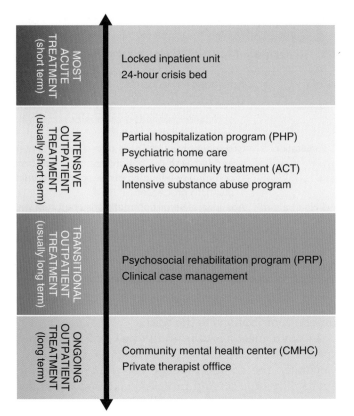

FIGURE 6-1 The continuum of psychiatric mental health treatment.

pitalization and other adverse outcomes (Kruse & Rohland, 2002).

Other clients with a preexisting community treatment team may return directly to their community mental health center or psychosocial rehabilitation program. Homeless clients may be referred to a shelter with linkage to intensive case management or assertive community treatment. Clients with a substantial problem with substance abuse may be transferred directly into a residential substance abuse treatment program (see Chapter 27). It is also notable that clients may pass through the continuum of treatment in the reverse direction; that is, if symptoms exacerbate, a lower intensity service may refer the client temporarily to a higher level of care in an attempt to prevent total decompensation and hospitalization.

Partial Hospitalization Program

Partial hospitalization programs (PHPs) offer intensive, short-term treatment similar to an inpatient level of care, except that the client is able to return home each day. Criteria for referral to a PHP include the need for prevention of hospitalization for serious symptoms *or* step-down from acute inpatient treatment *and* the presence of a responsible relative or caregiver who can assure the client's safety (Shoemaker,

2000). Referrals come from inpatient or outpatient providers. Transportation is usually provided, and clients receive 5 to 6 hours of treatment daily. Programs operate up to 7 days a week, and the length of stay is approximately 1 month. The multidisciplinary team consists of at least a psychiatrist, RN, and social worker. The RN is supervised by the psychiatrist.

Treatment outcomes related to nursing care in a PHP, in the language of the Nursing Outcomes Classification (NOC) may include the following (Moorhead, Johnson, & Maas, 2004):

- Client identifies correct name of medications.
- Client identifies precursors of depression.
- Client exhibits impulse control.
- Client perceives support of health care providers.

The following vignette illustrates the role of the psychiatric RN in a PHP.

■ ■ ■ *VIGNETTE*

Jane Tyson is an RN who works in a PHP in a rural county. The PHP is part of the only community mental health center in this region, which has one state hospital and one private inpatient unit. Jane worked for 3 years in the state hospital before transferring to the PHP. Jane is the nurse member of the team, and today her schedule is as follows.

8:30-9:00: Jane arrives at the PHP and prepares a teaching outline for her coping skills group.

9:00-10:00: Jane meets with eight clients to teach about coping with depression, using a five-page outline to explain steps to decrease negative thinking. All group members have a diagnosis of major depression and are encouraged to ask questions and to give feedback to each other. Throughout the session, Jane assesses each client's changes in mood and behavior since the previous day.

10:00-10:30: Jane briefly checks with all the clients to ensure that they have taken their morning medications. Three clients have brought their medication boxes with them because she needs to directly observe them take their medication.

10:30-11:30: Jane has an intake interview with a newly admitted client. Ms. Brown is a 50-year-old woman with a history of major depression who was hospitalized for 1 week after a drug overdose following an argument with her boyfriend. Jane completes the extensive 10-page standardized interview form, paying extra attention to risk factors for suicide. When asked about substance abuse, Ms. Brown admits that she has been drinking heavily for the past 2 years, including the night that she took a drug overdose. When the interview is completed, the client is referred to the psychiatrist for a diagnostic evaluation.

12:00-1:00: During the client lunch period, Jane meets with the team for daily rounds. She presents the newly admitted client, and the team develops an individual treatment plan. In this treatment plan, the team notes discharge planning needs for referrals to a community mental health center and alcohol treatment program.

1:00-2:00: Jane co-leads a therapy group with the social worker for eight clients with a variety of diagnoses. Due to the short-term nature of the group with almost daily turnover, the leaders take a psychoeducational approach with a defined topic for each session. Today's group focuses on symptoms of psychosis, and members are invited to describe their individual experiences.

2:00-2:30: Next, Jane has a discharge meeting with Mr. Jones. He is a 48-year-old man with a diagnosis of schizophrenia who was referred to the PHP by his clinic therapist to prevent hospitalization due to increasing paranoia and agitation. After 2 weeks in the PHP, he has restabilized and recognizes that he must be 100% compliant with his antipsychotic medication regimen. Jane finalizes his medication teaching and confirms his aftercare appointments with his previous therapist and psychiatrist.

2:30-3:00: Jane meets with Ms. Brown before she goes home to share the individual treatment plan and to begin a discussion of resources for alcohol treatment, including Alcoholics Anonymous.

3:00-4:30: After all clients leave, Jane completes her notes and discharge summary. She also makes case management telephone calls to arrange for community referrals, to communicate with families, and to report to managed behavioral care programs for utilization review.

■ ■ ■

Psychiatric Home Care

Psychiatric home care was defined by Medicare regulations in 1979 as requiring four elements: (1) homebound status of the client, (2) presence of a psychiatric diagnosis, (3) need for the skills of a psychiatric RN, and (4) development of a plan of care under orders of a physician.

"Homebound" refers to the client's inability to leave home independently to access community mental health care because of physical or mental conditions. Psychiatric RNs are defined to include a range of nursing personnel from basic level RNs with a certain number of years of experience to advanced practice RNs (APRNs) (Carson, 1998). Other payers besides Medicare also authorize home care services. Clients are referred to psychiatric home care following an acute inpatient episode, either psychiatric or somatic, or to prevent hospitalization. The psychiatric RN visits the client one to three times per week for approximately 1 to 2 months, and usually sees five or six clients daily.

Family members or significant others are closely involved in most cases. Because many clients are older than 65 years of age, there are usually concurrent somatic illnesses to assess and monitor. The RN acts as case manager to coordinate all specialists involved in the client's care, for example, physical therapist, occupational therapist, and home health aide. The RN is supervised by an APRN team leader, who is always available by telephone.

Boundaries become important in the home setting, where there is inherently a greater degree of intimacy between nurse and client. It may be important for the RN to begin a visit informally, by chatting about client family events or accepting refreshments offered. This interaction can be a strain for the RN who struggles to maintain a professional distance. However, there is great significance to the therapeutic use of self in such circumstances, to establish a level of comfort for the client and family.

Treatment outcomes related to nursing care in psychiatric home care setting, in the language of the NOC, may include the following:

- Client uses relaxation techniques to reduce anxiety.
- Client describes actions, side effects, and precautions for medications.
- Client upholds a suicide contract.
- Client recognizes hallucinations or delusions.

The following vignette illustrates a typical day for the psychiatric home care RN.

■ ■ ■ *VIGNETTE*

Natalie Beaumont is an RN employed by a home care agency in a large rural county. She worked for 2 years in the state psychiatric hospital before joining the psychiatric home care agency. She visits clients in a radius of 50 miles from her home and has daily telephone contact with her supervisor. She stops by the office weekly to drop off paperwork, and she attends the team meeting once a month. The team includes her team leader, other field RNs, team psychiatrist consultant, and social worker. Natalie chooses to make her visits from 8 AM to 3:30 PM and then completes her documentation at home.

8:00-9:00: Her first client is Mr. Johnson, a 66-year-old man with a diagnosis of major depression after a stroke. He was referred by his primary care physician due to suicidal ideation. Natalie has met with him and his wife three times per week for the past 2 weeks. He has contracted for safety and has been compliant in taking his antidepressant. Today she teaches the couple about stress management techniques. Case management responsibilities for Mr. Johnson include supervision of the home health aide who helps him with hygiene and coordination with the physical and occupational therapists who also treat him.

9:30-11:30: Natalie has an intake interview scheduled with Ms. Barker, a 45-year-old single woman with a diagnosis of schizophrenia who lives with her mother. She was referred by the inpatient psychiatrist after an involuntary hospitalization for repeatedly calling 911 with bizarre reports of violence in her back yard. She had not been in the hospital for 5 years but recently had dropped out of treatment when her private psychiatrist of 15 years retired. Natalie completes the extensive structured intake interview, including the mother's feedback. She teaches them about the new antipsychotic medication Ms. Barker is taking and sets up the weekly medication box. Natalie explains that she will visit two times

a week for the next 2 months. Her case management role will include identification of a new community psychiatrist for the client and a possible family support group for the mother.

12:30-1:30: Next, Natalie sees Ms. Graves, a 62-year-old widow diagnosed with major depression after the death of her husband and a move into an assisted living facility. Ms. Graves has diabetes and is wheelchair bound due to an amputation. She was referred by the nurse director of the assisted living facility. Natalie has met with her two times per week for the past 4 weeks, teaching about depression, grief, medications, and coping skills. Today her focus is on identifying a new social system, including increased contact with long-distance relatives, social activities at the facility, and spiritual support. With input from the director, Natalie learns of a grief counseling group at the local church run by a pastoral counselor and she recommends that resource to Ms. Graves.

2:00-3:00: Natalie's last client for the day is Mr. Cooper, a 55-year-old single man with a diagnosis of panic disorder with agoraphobia. Mr. Cooper lives with his older brother and was referred by the brother's primary care physician after the physician found out that the client had not been out of the house for 5 years since the death of his mother. Natalie has been working with Mr. Cooper for 7 weeks and has decreased visits to once a week. She has taught Mr. Cooper about his illness, medication, and relaxation techniques. He has progressed to being able to walk outside for 15 minutes at a time. Today's plan is to attempt riding in the car with his brother for 10 minutes, in preparation for discharge when he will have to ride for 30 minutes to reach the community mental health center.

Following this visit, Natalie returns home to complete documentation, to call in a report to her team leader and the physicians, and to make other case management telephone contacts for community referrals.

■ ■ ■

Assertive Community Treatment

Assertive community treatment (ACT) teams or mobile treatment units have sprung up in various areas throughout the United States to respond to those mentally ill clients who cannot effectively use traditional outpatient mental health services. Professional staff pursue and "woo" clients and support treatment in whatever settings clients find themselves in—at home or in a public place. Clients may be assessed and treated in fast food restaurants, receive one of the decanoate medications (e.g., Haldol, Prolixin) in a restaurant bathroom, and at the close of a "session" be offered a milkshake and a meal as a reward. If adherence to a prescribed medication regimen is a problem related to understanding, medications are packaged and labeled with the time and date they are to be taken. Creative problem solving and interventions are hallmarks of care provided by mobile teams. The Evidence-Based Practice box describes clinical research related to ACT teams.

EVIDENCE-BASED PRACTICE

Assertive Community Treatment

Background
Over the past 20 years since deinstitutionalization, much research has focused on community treatment for schizophrenia and other severe mental illness (SMI). Clients with SMI have significant difficulties with self-care, social relationships, work, and leisure. There is now a body of evidence demonstrating that psychosocial treatment can improve the long-term outcomes for these clients.

Studies
More than 25 controlled studies have evaluated the effects of assertive community treatment (ACT) on clients with SMI. ACT is a model for case management to serve clients who are non-compliant with standard outpatient treatment. Elements of the model include provision of services in the community instead of on site in a clinic, use of multidisciplinary treatment teams with low client-to-staff ratio (10:1) and high frequency of contact (three to five times per week), shared caseloads with clinicians, and 24-hour coverage for emergencies.

Results of Studies
Most of the studies were conducted in urban settings with approximately 100 clients and follow-up over 18 months. ACT was compared to standard case management for effects on housing stability, time spent in the hospital, social adjustment, and cost effectiveness. With regard to housing stability, 12 studies showed positive effects of ACT. Time spent in the hospital was reduced by the use of ACT in 14 studies. Social adjustment was not consistently improved by ACT, with only three studies showing benefits. Because ACT considerably reduced hospital use, it was considered cost effective in the majority of studies.

Implications for Nursing Practice
The nurse is a member of the ACT team and administers medication, teaches skills in self-care and health maintenance, coordinates access to medical care, and makes referrals to community services such as housing. These interventions require the nurse to establish a supportive relationship with the client and to collaborate with the other team members to ensure 24-hour continuity of care.

Mueser, K. T., Bond, G. R., & Drake, R. E. (2001). Community-based treatment of schizophrenia and other severe mental disorders: Treatment outcomes. *Medscape General Medicine* 6(1), 1-31.

Clients are referred to ACT teams by inpatient or outpatient providers because of a pattern of repeated hospitalizations with severe symptoms, along with an inability to participate in traditional treatment. Care is provided by a multidisciplinary team, and the psychiatric RN may manage a caseload of 10 clients whom he or she visits three to five times per week. The RN is supervised by a psychiatrist or APRN. Length of treatment may extend to years, until the client is ready to accept transfer to a more structured site for care. There is a 24-hour on-call system to allow the client to reach the team during an emergency.

Treatment outcomes related to nursing care through an ACT team, in the language of the NOC, may include the following:

- Client avoids alcohol and recreational drugs.
- Client adheres to treatment regimen as prescribed.
- Client uses health services congruent with need.
- Client exhibits reality-based thinking.

The following vignette describes the role of the psychiatric RN on the ACT team.

▩ ▩ ▩ *VIGNETTE*

Susan Green is a nurse who works on an ACT team at a large inner-city university medical center. She had 5 years of inpatient experience before joining the ACT team, and she works with an APRN, two social workers, two psychiatrists, and a mental health worker. She is supervised by the APRN.

8:00-9:00: Susan starts the day at the clinic site with team rounds. Because she was on call over the weekend, she updates the team on three emergency department visits: two clients were able to return home after she met with them and the emergency department physician; one client was admitted to the hospital because he made threats to his caregiver.

9:30-10:30: Her first client is Mr. Donaldson, a 35-year-old man with a diagnosis of bipolar disorder and alcohol dependence. He lives with his mother and has a history of five hospitalizations with noncompliance with outpatient clinic treatment. Except during his manic episodes, he isolates himself at home or visits a friend in the neighborhood at whose house he drinks excessively. Today he is due for his biweekly decanoate injection. Susan goes first to his house and learns that he is not at home. She speaks with his mother about his recent behavior and an upcoming medical clinic appointment. Then she goes to the friend's house and finds Mr. Donaldson playing cards and drinking a beer. He and his friend are courteous to her, and Mr. Donaldson cooperates in receiving his injection. He listens as Susan repeats teaching about the risks of alcohol consumption, and she encourages his attendance at an Alcoholics Anonymous meeting. He reports that he did go to one meeting yesterday. Susan praises him and encourages him and his friend to go again that night.

11:00-1:00: The next client is Ms. Abbott, a 53-year-old single woman with a diagnosis of schizoaffective disorder and hypertension. She lives alone in a senior citizen building and has no contact with family. Ms. Abbott was referred by her clinic team because she experienced three hospitalizations over 1 year for psychotic decompensation, despite receiving monthly decanoate injections. The ACT team is now the payee for her Social Security check. Today, Susan has to take Ms. Abbott out to pay her bills and to go to her primary care physician for a checkup. Ms. Abbott greets Susan warmly at the door, wearing excessive makeup and inappropriate summer clothing. With gentle encouragement, she agrees to wear warmer clothes. She is reluctant to show Susan her medication box and briefly gets irritable when Susan points out that she has not taken her morning medications. As they stop by the apartment office to pay the rent, Susan talks with the manager briefly. This apartment manager is the only contact person for Ms. Abbott, and she calls the team whenever any of the other residents report any unusual behavior. Over the next 1½ hours, Susan and Ms. Abbott drive to various stores and go to Ms. Abbott's somatic appointment.

2:00-4:30: The last client visit for today is with Mr. Hunter, a 60-year-old widowed man diagnosed with schizophrenia and cocaine dependence. Mr. Hunter was referred by the emergency department last year after repeated visits due to psychosis and intoxication. Initially, he was homeless, but he now lives in a recovery house shelter and has been clean of illegal substances for 6 months. He receives a monthly decanoate injection and is socially isolated in the house. Now that he has received his Social Security Disability income, he is seeking an affordable apartment. Today, Susan has two appointments to visit apartments. After greeting him, Susan notes that he is wearing the same clothes that he had on 2 days earlier, and his hair is uncombed. She suggests that he shower and change his clothes before they go out, and he agrees.

At the end of the day, Susan jots down information that she will use to write her progress notes in clients' charts on the next day when she returns to the clinic.

Community Mental Health Center

Community mental health centers were created in the 1960s and have since taken center stage for those who have no access to private care. The range of services available at such centers varies, but generally they provide emergency services, adult services, and children's services. Common components of treatment at community mental health centers include medication administration, individual therapy, psychoeducational and therapy groups, family therapy, and dual-diagnosis treatment. A clinic may also be aligned with a **psychosocial rehabilitation program** that offers a structured day program, vocational services, and residential services. Some community mental health centers have an associated intensive case management service to assist clients in finding housing or obtaining entitlements.

There is a multidisciplinary team, and the psychiatric RN may carry a caseload of 60 clients, whom she sees one to four times per month. The basic level RN is supervised by an APRN. Clients are referred to the clinic for long-term follow-up by inpatient units or other providers of outpatient care at higher intensity levels. Clients may attend the clinic for years or be discharged when they improve and reach desired goals.

Treatment outcomes related to nursing care in a community mental health center, in the language of the NOC, may include the following:

- Client describes self-care responsibility for ongoing treatment.
- Client describes actions to prevent substance abuse.
- Client refrains from responding to hallucinations or delusions.
- Client keeps appointments with health care professionals.

The following vignette provides an example of one work day for the RN in a community mental health center.

■ ■ ■ VIGNETTE

Mary Smith is an RN who works at a community mental health center in a large university hospital in an urban setting. She has been an RN for 10 years and transferred to the clinic 2 years ago from the inpatient unit at the same university. She is a nurse on the adult team and carries a caseload of clients diagnosed with chronic mental illness. She is supervised by an APRN.

8:30-9:00: Upon arriving at the clinic, she finds a voice mail message from Ms. Thompson, who is crying and saying that she is out of medication. Mary consults with the psychiatrist and calls Ms. Thompson to arrange for an emergency appointment later that day.

9:00-9:30: Mary's first client is Mr. Enright, who is a 35-year-old man diagnosed with schizophrenia, in treatment at the clinic for 10 years. During their 30-minute counseling session, she assesses him for any exacerbation of psychotic symptoms (he has a history of grandiose delusions), for eating and sleep habits, and for social functioning in the psychosocial rehabilitation program that he attends 5 days per week. Today he presents as stable. Mary gives him his decanoate injection and schedules a return appointment for 1 month, reminding him of his psychiatrist appointment the following week.

10:00-11:00: Mary co-leads a medication group with a psychiatrist. This group consists of seven clients with chronic schizophrenia who have been compliant in attending biweekly group sessions and receiving decanoate injections for the past 5 years. She leads the group discussion as the psychiatrist writes prescriptions for each client, because most of the members also take oral medication. Today Mary asks the group to explain relapse prevention to a new member. She teaches significant elements, including compliance with the medication regimen and healthy habits. As group members give examples from their own experiences, she assesses each client's mental status. At the end of the group, she administers injections and gives members appointment cards for the next group session. After the clients leave, she meets with the psychiatrist to evaluate the session and to discuss any necessary changes in treatment.

11:00-12:00: Mary documents progress and medication notes, responds to telephone calls, and prepares for the staff meeting.

12:00-2:00: All adult team staff attend the weekly intake meeting, at which new admissions are discussed and individual treatment plans are written with team input. Mary presents a client in intake, reading from the standardized interview form. She also gives nursing input about treatment for the other five newly admitted clients. The new client she presented is assigned to her, and she plans to call him later in the afternoon to set up a first appointment.

2:00-3:00: Mary co-leads a dual-diagnosis therapy group with the dual-diagnosis specialist, who is a social worker. The group is made up of seven clients who have concurrent diagnoses of substance abuse and a major psychiatric illness. The leaders take a psychoeducational approach, and today's planned topic is teaching about the physical effects of alcohol on the body. Mary focuses on risks associated with the interaction between alcohol and medications, and answers the members' specific questions. Because this is an ongoing group, members take a more active role, and discussion may vary according to members' needs instead of following planned topics. After the session, the co-leaders discuss the group dynamics and write progress notes.

3:30-4:00: Mary meets with Ms. Thompson, who arrives at the clinic tearful and agitated. Ms. Thompson says that she missed her appointment this month because her son died suddenly. Mary uses crisis intervention skills to assess Ms. Thompson's status, for example, any risks for her safety related to her history of suicidal ideation. After helping Ms. Thompson clarify a plan to increase support from her family, Mary notes that insomnia is a new problem. She takes Ms. Thompson to the psychiatrist who is covering "emergency prescription time" for that day and explains the change in the client's status. The psychiatrist refills Ms. Thompson's usual antidepressant and adds a medication to aid sleep. Mary makes an appointment for the client to return to see her in 1 week instead of the usual 1 month, and also schedules her to meet with her assigned psychiatrist that same day.

4:00-4:30: Mary completes all notes and makes necessary telephone calls, for example, to other staff in the psychosocial rehabilitation program who are working with her clients and to her new client to schedule an appointment.

ETHICAL ISSUES

As community psychiatric RNs assume greater autonomy and accountability for the care they deliver, ethical concerns become more of an issue. Ethical dilemmas are common in disciplines and specialties that care for the vulnerable and disenfranchised.

Psychiatric RNs have an obligation to develop a model for assessing the ethical implications of their clinical decisions. Each incident requiring ethical assessment is somewhat different, and the individual RN brings personal insights to each situation. The role of the nurse is to act in the best interests of the client and of society, to the degree that this is possible.

In most organizations that employ RNs, there is a designated resource for consultation regarding ethical dilemmas. For example, hospitals (with associated outpatient departments) are required by regulatory bodies to have an ethics committee to respond to clinicians' questions. Home care agencies or other independent agencies may have an ethics consultant in the administrative hierarchy of the organization. Professional nursing organizations and even boards of nursing can be used as a resource by the individual practitioner. Refer to Chapter 8 for more discussion of ethical guidelines for nursing practice.

FUTURE ISSUES

Despite the current availability and variety of community psychiatric treatments in the United States, many clients in this country in need of services still are not receiving them. The National Survey on Drug Use and Health in 2002 estimated that 17.5 million adults had serious mental illness (Aquila & Emanuel, 2003, p. 3). Less than half, however, received treatment in 2001 (Aquila & Emanuel, 2003, p. 6). Barriers to treatment have been identified by many authors and studies. The stigma of mental illness has lessened over the past 40 years; there is increased recognition of symptoms due to brain disorders, and well-known people have come forward to admit that they have received psychiatric treatment. Yet, many people still are afraid to admit to a psychiatric diagnosis (Pardes, 2003). Instead, they seek medical care for vague somatic complaints from primary care providers, who too often fail to diagnose anxiety (or depressive) disorders (Rollman et al., 2003).

In addition to stigma, there are geographic, financial, and systems factors that impede access to psychiatric care. Mental health services are scarce in some rural areas, and many American families cannot afford health insurance even if they are working. President George W. Bush's New Freedom Commission on Mental Health identified national system and policy problems in 2002: fragmented care for children and adults with serious mental illness, high unemployment and disability among the seriously mentally ill, undertreatment of older adults, and lack of national priorities for mental health and suicide prevention (President's commission, 2002).

To meet the challenges of the twenty-first century, Price and Capers (1995, p. 27) suggested that, in training the associate degree nurse, "educators must increase their focus on leadership development, include principles of home health nursing, increase content on gerontology, and introduce basic community health concepts." Those RNs who elect to work with elderly psychiatric clients will be more and more in demand as the population ages, and the health care needs of this subgroup are increasingly complex (Hedelin &

Svensson, 1999). Community psychiatric RNs may collaborate more with primary health care practitioners to fill the gap in existing community services (Walker, Barker, & Pearson, 2000). Certainly, community psychiatric RNs need to be committed to teach the public about resources for mental health care, whether for long-term serious mental illness or for short-term situational stress. More innovative efforts to locate treatment in neutral community sites are still needed. For example, one study offered treatment to depressed women in a supermarket setting using a conference room; participants stated that they preferred that to a clinic because it was more private or convenient (Swartz et al., 2002).

■ ■ ■ KEY POINTS to REMEMBER

- Community mental health nursing has historical roots dating to the 1800s and has been significantly influenced by public policies.
- Deinstitutionalization brought promise and problems for the chronically mentally ill population.

- The basic level community psychiatric nurse practices in many traditional and nontraditional sites.
- There are significant differences between inpatient psychiatric nursing and community psychiatric nursing.
- In the multidisciplinary team, the community mental health nurse functions as a biopsychosocial care manager.
- The continuum of psychiatric treatment includes numerous community treatment alternatives with varying degrees of intensity of care.
- The community psychiatric nurse needs access to resources to address ethical dilemmas encountered in clinical situations.
- There are still barriers to mental health care that the community psychiatric nurse may be able to diminish through daily practice.

Visit the Evolve website at **http://evolve.elsevier.com/Varcarolis** for a posttest on the content in this chapter. *evolve*

Critical Thinking and Chapter Review

Visit the Evolve website at **http://evolve.elsevier.com/Varcarolis** for additional self-study exercises. *evolve*

■ ■ ■ CRITICAL THINKING

1. You are a community psychiatric mental health nurse working at a local mental health center. You are doing an assessment interview with a single male client who is 45 years old. He reports that he has not been sleeping and that his thoughts seem to be "all tangled up." He informs you that he hopes you can help him today because he does not know how much longer he can go on. He does not make any direct reference to suicidal intent. He is disheveled and has been sleeping at shelters. He has little contact with his family and starts to become agitated when you suggest that it might be helpful for you to contact them. He refuses to sign any release of information forms. He admits to recent hospitalization at the local veterans hospital and reports previous treatment at a dual-diagnosis facility even though he denies substance abuse. In addition to his mental health problems, he says that he has tested positive for human immunodeficiency virus and takes multiple medications that he cannot name.

   A. What are your biopsychosocial and spiritual concerns about this client?

   B. What is the highest-priority problem to address before he leaves the clinic today?

   C. Do you feel that you need to consult with any other members of the multidisciplinary team today about this client?

   D. In your role as case manager, what systems of care will you need to coordinate to provide quality care for this client?

   E. How will you start to develop trust with the client to gain his cooperation with the treatment plan?

■ ■ ■ CHAPTER REVIEW

Choose the most appropriate answer.

1. A significant influence allowing psychiatric treatment to move from the hospital to the community was
   1. television.
   2. the discovery of psychotropic medication.
   3. identification of external causes of mental illness.
   4. the use of a collaborative approach by clients and staff focusing on rehabilitation.

2. For psychiatric nurses, a major difference between caring for clients in the community and caring for clients in the hospital is that
   1. treatment is negotiated rather than imposed in the community setting.
   2. fewer ethical dilemmas are encountered in the community setting.
   3. cultural considerations are less important during treatment in the community.
   4. the focus in the community setting is solely on managing symptoms of mental illness.

Critical Thinking and Chapter Review—cont'd

Visit the Evolve website at **http://evolve.elsevier.com/Varcarolis** for additional self-study exercises.

3. A typical treatment goal for a client with mental illness being treated in a community setting is that the client will

   1. experience destabilization of symptoms.

   2. take medications as prescribed.

   3. learn to live with dependency and decreased opportunities.

   4. accept guidance and structure of significant others.

4. Assessment data that would be considered least relevant to developing an understanding of the ability of a persistently mentally ill 65-year-old client to cope with the demands of living in the community are

   1. strengths and deficits of the client.

   2. school and vocational performance.

   3. client health history and current mental status.

   4. client home environment and financial status.

5. Which action on the part of a community psychiatric nurse visiting the home of a client would be considered inappropriate?

   1. Turning off an intrusive TV program without the client's permission

   2. Facilitating the client's access to a community kitchen for two meals a day

   3. Going beyond the professional role boundary to hang curtains for an elderly client

   4. Arranging to demonstrate the use of public transportation to a mental health clinic

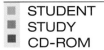

STUDENT STUDY CD-ROM

Access the accompanying CD-ROM for animations, interactive exercises, review questions for the NCLEX examination, and an audio glossary.

REFERENCES

Aquila, R., & Emanuel, M. (2003, September 25). Managing the long-term outlook of schizophrenia. *Medscape Psychiatry & Mental Health,* 1-10.

Carson, V. B. (1998). Designing an effective psychiatric home care program. *Home Healthcare Consultant, 5*(4), 16-21.

Chan, S., Mackenzie, A., & Jacobs, P. (2000). Cost-effectiveness analysis of case management versus a routine community care organization for patients with chronic schizophrenia. *Archives of Psychiatric Nursing, 14*(2), 98-104.

Chan, S., et al. (2000). An evaluation of the implementation of case management in the community psychiatric nursing service. *Journal of Advanced Nursing, 31*(1), 144-156.

Dickey, B., et al. (2002). Medical morbidity, mental illness, and substance use disorders. *Psychiatric Services, 53*(7), 861-867.

Gebbie, K. M., & Qureshi, K. (2002). Emergency and disaster preparedness: Core competencies for nurses. *American Journal of Nursing, 102*(1), 46-51.

Hedelin, B., & Svensson, P. (1999). Psychiatric nursing for promotion of mental health and prevention of depression in the elderly: A case study. *Journal of Psychiatric and Mental Health Nursing, 6*(2), 115-124.

Kruse, G. R., & Rohland, B. M. (2002). Factors associated with attendance at a first appointment after discharge from a psychiatric hospital. *Psychiatric Services, 53*(4), 473-476.

Lacro, J., & Glassman, R. (2004). Medication adherence. *Medscape Psychiatry & Mental Health, 9*(1), 1-4.

Marcos, L. R. (1990). The politics of deinstitutionalization. In N. L. Cohen (Ed.), *Psychiatry takes to the streets: Outreach and crisis intervention for the mentally ill* (pp. 3-15). New York: Guilford Press.

Marland, G. R., & Sharkey, V. (1999). Depot neuroleptics, schizophrenia, and the role of the nurse: Is practice evidence based? A review of the literature. *Journal of Advanced Nursing, 30*(6), 1255-1262.

McQuistion, H. L., et al. (2003). Challenges for psychiatry in serving homeless people with psychiatric disorders. *Psychiatric Services, 54*(5), 669-676.

Moorhead, S., Johnson, M., & Maas, M. (2004). Nursing outcomes classification (NOC) (3rd ed.). St. Louis, MO: Mosby.

Pardes, H. (2003). Psychiatry's remarkable journey: The past 40 years. *Psychiatric Services, 54*(6), 896-901.

President's commission finds fragmented system, outdated treatments, incentives for dependency [Editorial News & Notes]. (2002). *Psychiatric Services, 53*(12), 1644-1645.

Price, C. R., & Capers, E. S. (1995). Associate degree nursing education: Challenging premonitions with resourcefulness. *Nursing Forum, 30*(4), 26-29.

Rochefort, D. A. (1993). *From poorhouses to homelessness: Policy analysis and mental health care.* Westport, CT: Auburn House.

Rollman, B. L., et al. (2003). A contemporary protocol to assist primary care physicians in the treatment of panic and generalized anxiety disorders. *General Hospital Psychiatry, 25,* 74-82.

Rudenstine, S., et al. (2003). Awareness and perceptions of a community wide mental health program in New York

City after September 11. *Psychiatric Services, 54*(10), 1404-1406.

Shoemaker, N. (2000). The continuum of care. In V. B. Carson (Ed.), *Mental health nursing: The nurse-patient journey* (2nd ed., pp. 368-387). Philadelphia: Saunders.

Smith, C. M. (1995). Origins and future of community health nursing. In C. M. Smith & F. A. Maurer (Eds.), *Community health nursing: Theory and practice* (pp. 30-52). Philadelphia: Saunders.

Swartz, H. A., et al. (2002). A pilot study of community mental health care for depression in a supermarket setting. *Psychiatric Services, 53*(9), 1132-1137.

Walker, L., Barker, P., & Pearson, P. (2000). The required role of the psychiatric-mental health nurse in primary health care: An augmented Delphi study. *Nursing Inquiry, 7*(2), 91-102.

Wilson, K., & Williams, A. (2000). Visualism in community nursing: Implications for telephone work with service users. *Qualitative Health Research, 10*(4), 507-520.

CHAPTER 7

Culturally Relevant Mental Health Nursing: A Global Perspective

MARY CURRY NARAYAN

KEY TERMS and CONCEPTS

The key terms and concepts listed here appear in color where they are defined or first discussed in the chapter.

acculturation, 108
assimilation, 108
bicultural, 108
cultural awareness, 110
cultural broker, 106
cultural competence, 110
cultural desire, 112
cultural encounters, 111
cultural imposition, 105
cultural knowledge, 110
cultural pain, 111
cultural skill, 111
culturally relevant nursing, 99
culture, 100
culture shock, 109
culture-bound syndromes, 107
Eastern tradition, 101
enculturation, 103
ethnicity, 100
ethnocentrism, 105
ethnopharmacology, 108
generalizations, 111
immigrants, 108
indigenous cultures, 102

intraethnic diversity, 111
limited English proficiency, 106
minority, 100
preserve-accommodate-restructure framework, 112
race, 100
refugee, 109
somatization, 106
stereotyping, 111
Western tradition, 101
worldview, 100

OBJECTIVES

After studying this chapter, the reader will be able to

1. Describe the importance of culturally relevant care in mental health nursing practice.
2. Discuss potential problems in applying American or Western psychological theory to clients of other cultures.
3. Compare and contrast American nursing beliefs, values, and practices with the beliefs, values, and practices of clients from diverse cultures.
4. Perform a culturally sensitive assessment, including an assessment for risk factors and barriers to quality mental health care that culturally diverse clients frequently encounter.
5. Develop a culturally appropriate nursing care plan for clients of diverse cultures.

evolve Visit the Evolve website at **http://evolve.elsevier.com/Varcarolis** for a pretest on the content in this chapter.

According to a report issued by the U.S. Surgeon General, cultural, racial, and ethnic minorities in America do not have the same access to quality mental health services as do mainstream Americans. The report *Mental Health: Culture, Race, and Ethnicity* (U.S. Department of Health and Human Services, 2001) identifies **culturally inappropriate services** as one of the reasons minority groups in America do not receive and benefit from needed mental health services.

Mental health nurses need to practice **culturally relevant nursing** if they are to meet the needs of their culturally diverse clients. The goal of nursing is to promote health and well-being, but if mental health services are to achieve this goal for culturally diverse populations, the care must be congruent with their cultural beliefs, values, and practices. This kind of care has been given different names—culturally competent care, culturally appropriate care, culturally comfortable care, culturally sensitive care, and culturally congruent care—but whatever the name, effective care adapts psychiatric and mental health nursing assessments and interventions to the client's cultural needs and preferences.

This chapter focuses on culture and how it affects the mental health and care of clients with mental illness. In this chapter you will learn about the following:

- Culture, race, ethnicity, minority status, and how they are related
- Demographic shifts, which make it essential that mental health nurses know how to provide culturally appropriate care
- Impact of cultural worldviews on mental health nursing
- Variations in cultural beliefs, values, and practices that affect mental health and care of clients with mental health problems
- Barriers to providing quality mental health services to culturally diverse clients
- Culturally diverse populations at increased risk of developing mental illness
- Techniques for providing culturally competent care to diverse populations

CULTURE, RACE, ETHNICITY, AND MINORITY STATUS

In his mental health report, the Surgeon General discussed culture, race, and ethnicity in relation to minority groups (U.S. Department of Health and Human Services, 2001). Although the definitions of these terms distinguish them from one another, they are related.

Minority status is connected more to economic and social standing in society than to cultural identity. However, many cultural, racial, and ethnic minority groups are also economically and socially disadvantaged groups.

Culture is the shared beliefs, values, and practices that guide a group's members in patterned ways of thinking and acting. Groups pass these beliefs, values, and practices on to new group members (Leininger, 2002b). Cultural groups can be ethnic, religious, geographic, socioeconomic, occupational, ability or disability related, or sexual orientation related. Each of these groups has cultural beliefs, values, and practices that guide the group's members in ways of thinking and acting. The cultural norms help members of the group make sense of the world around them and make decisions about appropriate ways to relate and behave. Cultural norms prescribe what is "normal" and

"abnormal," and thus culture helps develop concepts of mental health and illness.

Ethnic groups have a common heritage and history (ethnicity). These groups share a worldview, a system for thinking about how the world works and how people should behave in the world and in relationship to one another. From this worldview, they develop beliefs, values, and practices that guide members of the group in how they should think and act in different situations. In this chapter, the terms *cultural groups* and *ethnic groups* are used interchangeably.

Although race has been used to categorize people, there is a growing recognition that race is a social and political construct and not a biological one (Segall, 2002). Acknowledging the inadequacy of race to capture minority groups in America, the U.S. Census Bureau created a combined race-ethnicity categorization system. The federally defined racial-ethnic groups currently are the following (U.S. Census Bureau, 2000):

- American Indian or Alaska Native
- Asian
- Black or African American
- Hispanic or Latino
- Native Hawaiian or Pacific Islander
- White

The purpose of categorizing groups of people into racial-ethnic categories is to help the government know the needs of its citizens. For instance, the Surgeon General used data from this classification system to identify the disparities in mental health care along racial-ethnic lines. These classifications also facilitate knowing when and how the health care needs of these populations are being met.

Despite the benefits of this system, this way of classifying groups of people can be confusing, confounding, or offensive. Consider the following:

- Each racial group contains multiple different ethnic cultures. There are over 560 Native American and Alaskan tribes and over 40 countries in Asia and the Pacific Islands. The cultural norms of blacks or African Americans whose ancestors have been here since slave days are very different from the norms of those who have recently immigrated from Africa or the Caribbean. Americans of European origin are a diverse group, some of whom have been in America for hundreds of years and some of whom are new immigrants.
- The Latino-Hispanic group is a cultural group based on a shared language, but all its members are also members of a racial group or groups (white, black, and/or Native American).
- Some vulnerable cultural groups with a culture very different from that of others of similar race are lost in the categories. (For instance, people from the Middle East and those from the Arabian subcontinent are considered "white" in the classification system.)

- Although children of biracial-bicultural marriages are able to indicate more than one category, their unique identity is not distinguished.

Because there are problems with this system, the mental health nurse can make better decisions on behalf of clients if the focus is on ethnicity rather than race.

DEMOGRAPHIC SHIFTS

Presently, 25%* of the U.S. population self-identifies with one of the federally defined minority groups. Over 10% of the people living in the United States are foreign-born immigrants, with 50% of those coming from Latin America and 25% from Asian countries. Almost 20% of the American population speaks a language other than English as their first language, and for 10% that language is Spanish (U.S. Census Bureau, 2002).

The United States is becoming increasingly more diverse. Shortly after the year 2050, no single racial-ethnic group will hold a majority population position (Table 7-1). With these changing demographics, every mental health nurse will care for culturally diverse clients. Unless nurses know how to provide culturally relevant care, the problem of mental health disparities among culturally diverse populations will become more prevalent.

WORLDVIEWS AND MENTAL HEALTH NURSING

American nursing, psychological theories, and their understanding of mental health and illness have grown out of a Western philosophical and scientific

---

*All statistical percentages from the 2000 census are rounded to the nearest 5%.

TABLE 7-1

Year 2050 Population Projections (in percent)*

	2000	2050
White non-Hispanic	70	50
Black non-Hispanic	13	15
Hispanic (of any race)	13	24
Asian	4	8
All other races	3	5

From U.S. Census Bureau. (March 2004). *U.S. interim projections by age, sex, race, and Hispanic origin.* Retrieved February 11, 2005, from the U.S. Census Bureau website: http://www.census.gov/ipc/www/usinterimproj/.
Shortly after the year 2050, the white non-Hispanic population will comprise less than 50% of the United States population. The Hispanic and Asian populations are growing at the fastest rates.
*Population percentages are rounded to the nearest 1%.

framework. Mental health nurses base their practice on the personality and developmental theories of Freud, Erikson, Maslow, Piaget, and other Europeans and Americans (Saint Arnault, 2002). This framework for mental health and illness is based on Western cultural ideals, beliefs, and values. Because mental health nursing is grounded in Western culture, nurses must question its assumptions about the person, personality development, emotional expression, ego boundaries, and interpersonal relationships when caring for culturally diverse clients.

Western science and European-American norms for mental health have grown out of a long history—the history of Western civilization. Beliefs and values about the person, and how the person is to relate to the world and to other people, are based on Greek, Roman, and Judeo-Christian thought. Other Western scientists and philosophers, such as Descartes (credited with the Western concept of body-mind dualism) have contributed to the Western scientific tradition. Nursing knowledge of psychology, development, and mental health and illness is based on this tradition.

Many people of the world have very different philosophical histories and traditions, however (Table 7-2). The Eastern cultures of Asia are based on the philosophical thought of Chinese and Indian philosophers, and the spiritual traditions of Confucianism, Buddhism, and Taoism. Indigenous cultures, such as diverse cultures found among Native Americans, African tribes, and tribal peoples on other continents, frequently have rich cultural traditions that are based on the person's deep connection to the natural world and the tribe. These traditions have inspired a different view of what it means to be a person and how the person should interact with others.

In the Western tradition, one's identity is found in one's individuality. This inspires the valuing of autonomy, independence, and self-reliance. Mind and body are seen as two separate entities, so that different practitioners treat disorders of the body and the mind. Disease is considered to have a specific, measurable, and observable cause, and treatment is aimed at eliminating the cause. Time is seen as linear, so time always moves forward, and time waits for no one. Success in life is obtained by preparing for the future.

Eastern tradition, however, sees the family as the basis for one's identity, so that family interdependence and group decision making are the norm. Body-mind-spirit are seen as a single entity; there is no sense of separation between a physical illness and a psychological one. Disease is caused by fluctuations in opposing forces—the yin-yang energies. Time is seen as circular and recurring, as in the belief in reincarnation. One is born into a fate, with which one has a duty to comply. It is not for the individual to change that fate (Higgins, 2001).

TABLE 7-2

Worldviews

World cultures have grown out of different worldviews and philosophical traditions. Worldview shapes how cultures perceive reality, the person, and the person in relation to the world and to others. Worldview also shapes perceptions about time, health and illness, and rights and obligations in society. The three worldviews compared here are broad categories and generalizations created to contrast some of the themes found in diverse world cultures. They do not necessarily fit any particular cultural group.

Western (Science)	Eastern (Balance)	Indigenous (Harmony)
Roman, Greek, Judeo-Christian; the Enlightenment; Descartes.	Chinese and Indian philosophers: Buddha, Confucius, Lao-tse.	Deep relationship with nature.
The "real" has form and essence; reality tends to be stable.	The "real" is forces and energy; reality is always changing.	The "real" is multidimensional; reality transcends time and space.
Cartesian dualism: body and mind-spirit.	Mind-body-spirit unity.	Mind, body, and spirit are considered so united that there may not be words to indicate them as distinct entities.
Self is starting point for identity.	Family is starting point for identity.	Community is starting point for identity—a person is only an entity in relation to others. The self does not exist except in relation to others. There may be no concept of person or personal ownership.
Time is linear.	Time is circular, flexible.	Time is focused on the present.
Wisdom: preparation for the future.	Wisdom: acceptance of what is.	Wisdom: knowledge of nature.
Disease has a cause (pathogen, toxin, etc.) that creates the effect; disease can be observed and measured.	Disease is caused by a lack of balance in energy forces (e.g., yin-yang, hot-cold); imbalance between daily routine, diet, and constitutional type (Ayurveda).	Disease is caused by a lack of personal, interpersonal, environmental, or spiritual harmony; thoughts and words can shape reality; evil spirits exist.

Ethics of rights and obligations:
■ Based on the individual's right
■ Value given to
  —Right to decide
  —Right to be informed
  —Open communication
  —Truthfulness
	Ethics of care:
	■ Based on promoting positive relationships
	■ Value given to
	  —Sympathy, compassion, fidelity, discernment
	  —Action on behalf of those with whom one has a relationship
	■ Persons in need of health care considered to be vulnerable and to require protection from cruel truth
		Ethics of community:
		■ Based on needs of the community
		■ Value given to contribution to community

© 2002, 2004 by Mary Curry Narayan.

Indigenous cultures frequently manifest an even more dramatic difference in their understanding of the person and the way the world works. Frequently, the basis of one's identity is the tribe. There may be no concept of person; instead, a person is an entity only in relation to others. The holism of body-mind-spirit may be so complete that there may be no adequate words to describe them as separate entities. Disease is frequently seen as a lack of harmony of the individual with others or the environment (Higgins, 2001).

Mental health nurses must recognize that mental health nursing theories and methods are themselves part of a cultural tradition. Psychiatric nursing care is a culturally derived set of interventions designed to promote verbalization of feelings, teach individually focused coping skills, and assist clients with behavioral and emotional self-control consistent with Western cultural ideals. When a nurse understands that many of the concepts and methods found in psychiatric mental health nursing are based on a different set of assumptions than that of the nurse's culturally diverse clients, the nurse has begun the process of becoming culturally competent.

CULTURE AND MENTAL HEALTH

Diverse cultures have evolved from the three broad categories of worldview described in the previous section. Cultures develop norms to be consistent with their worldviews and to adapt to their historical experiences and the influences of the "outside" world. Cultures are not static; they change and adjust, although usually very slowly. Each culture has different patterns of nonverbal communication (Table 7-3), etiquette norms (Box 7-1), beliefs and values that shape the culture (Table 7-4), and beliefs, values, and practices that influence how the culture understands health and illness (Table 7-5). For instance, in American culture, eye contact is a sign of respectful attention, but in the client's culture, it may be considered arrogant and intrusive. In American culture, emotional expressiveness is valued, but in the client's culture, it may be a sign of immaturity. In American culture, independence and self-reliance are encouraged, whereas the family interdependence valued by another culture may be seen, from an American perspective, as a symbiotic relationship, a pathological *enmeshment*.

Members of the group are introduced to the culture's worldview, beliefs, values, and practices in a process called enculturation. As children, they learn from their parents which behaviors are the "right" ones and which are "wrong." They learn the rules for living within the culture—which beliefs, values, and actions are considered "right." These "right" things include many options, but the options are limited. The individual is free to make choices, but the culture expects these choices to be made from its acceptable range of options (Saint Arnault, 2002).

Deviance from cultural expectations is considered by others within the culture to be a problem and frequently is defined by the cultural group as "illness." Often, mental health is seen as the degree to which a person fulfills the expectations of the culture. The culture defines what types of differences are still within the range of normal (mentally healthy) and which ones are outside the range of normal (mentally ill) (Saint Arnault, 2002).

The same thoughts and behaviors that are considered mentally healthy in one culture can be considered illness in another. For example, many religious traditions view "speaking in tongues" as mentally healthy and a gift from God, whereas a different cultural group might consider this same behavior as psychotic gibberish and a sign of mental illness. This creates challenges for the psychiatric mental health nurse. Another challenge is that, even if the nurse and client agree that the client has a mental health problem, they may advocate very different ways of treating the problem.

According to the American Nurses Association (1991), good nursing care *adapts* care to the client's cul-

TABLE 7-3

Selected Nonverbal Communication Patterns

People perceive very strong messages from nonverbal communication patterns. However, the same nonverbal communication pattern can mean very different things to different cultures, as this table indicates. This table does not provide an exhaustive list of possible differences.

Nonverbal Communication Pattern	Predominate American Patterns	Patterns Seen in Other Cultures
Eye contact	Eye contact is associated with attentiveness, politeness, respect, honesty, self-confidence.	Eye contact is avoided as a sign of rudeness, arrogance, challenge, or sexual interest.
Personal space	▪ Intimate space: 0-1½ ft ▪ Personal space: 1½-3 ft In a personal conversation, if a person enters into the intimate space of the other, the person is perceived as aggressive, overbearing, and offensive. If a person stays more distant than expected, the person is perceived as aloof.	Personal space is significantly closer or more distant than in American culture. ▪ Closer—Middle Eastern, Southern European, and Latin American cultures ▪ Farther—Asian cultures When closer is the norm, standing very close frequently indicates acceptance of the other.
Touch	Moderate touch indicates personal warmth and conveys caring.	Touch norms vary. ▪ Low-touch cultures—Touch may be considered an overt sexual gesture capable of "stealing the spirit" of another or taboo between women and men. ▪ High-touch cultures—People touch one another as frequently as possible (e.g., linking arms when walking or holding hand or arm when talking).
Facial expressions and gestures	▪ A nod means "yes." ▪ Smiling and nodding means "I agree." ▪ Thumbs up means "good job." ▪ Rolling one's eyes while another is talking is an insult.	▪ Raising eyebrows or rolling the head from side to side means "yes." ▪ Smiling and nodding means "I respect you." ▪ Thumbs up is an obscene gesture. ▪ Pointing one's foot at another is an insult.

Norms of Etiquette

People tend to feel offended when their rules for "polite" behavior are violated. However, the rules for polite behavior vary greatly from one culture to another. Unless the nurse is aware of cultural differences in etiquette norms, the nurse could infer rudeness on the part of a client who is operating from a different set of cultural norms and believes that his or her behavior is respectful toward the nurse.

Norms of etiquette that vary across cultures include the following:

- Whether "promptness" is expected and how important it is to be on time
- How formal one should be in addressing others
- Which people deserve recognition and honor and how respect is shown
- Whether shaking hands and other forms of social touch are appropriate
- Whether or not shoes can be worn in the home
- How much clothing must be worn to be "modest"
- What it means to accept or reject offers of food or drink and other gestures of hospitality
- What importance is given to "small talk" and how long it should continue before "getting down to business"
- Whether communication should be direct and forthright or circuitous and subtle
- What the tone of voice and pace of the conversation should be
- Which topics are considered taboo
- Whether or not the children in the home can be touched and admired

Cultural Belief and Value Systems

This table contrasts beliefs and values that are predominant in American culture with those that are common in various other world cultures. Belief and value systems are best viewed as a continuum. The beliefs and values of cultures, and of the individuals within cultures, fall at various points along the continuum.

Predominant Patterns and Concepts in American Culture	Patterns and Concepts in Various Other Cultures
Individualism	Familism
Independence, self-reliance	Interdependence of family
Autonomy, autonomous decision making	Interconnectedness
	Family decision making
Egalitarianism—everyone has an equal voice and deserves equal opportunities.	Social hierarchy—some deserve more honor or power than others because of their age, gender, occupation, or role in the family; family hierarchies can be patriarchal or matriarchal.
Youth	Age
Physical beauty	Wisdom
Competition	Cooperation
Achievement	Relationships
Materialistic orientation	Metaphysical orientation
Possessions	Spirituality, nature, relationships
Reason and logic	Meditation and intuition
Doing and activity	Being and receptivity
Mastery over nature	Harmony with nature
Latest technology	Natural, traditional ways
Master of one's fate—"I am the master of my destiny."	Fate is one's master—"Fate is responsible for my destiny."
Optimism	Fatalism
Internal locus of control: life events and circumstances are the result of one's actions.	External locus of control: life events and circumstances are beyond one's own control and rest in the hands of fate, chance, other people, or God.
Future orientation—"He who prepares for tomorrow will be successful."	Present orientation—"Live for today and let tomorrow take care of itself."
Punctuality ("clock time")—"Time waits for no one." "Time flies." "Time is money."	Past orientation—tradition
Being on time is a sign of courtesy and responsibility.	"People time"—time is flexible, indefinite; "Time starts when the group gathers." "Time walks. *El tiempo anda.*"
	Being on time can be a sign of compulsiveness and disregard for the people one was with before the appointment time.

TABLE 7-5

Cultural Beliefs and Values About Health and Illness

This table contrasts the views typically held by Western nurses and the views about health and illness that their clients from diverse cultures may hold.

	Western Biomedical Perspective	Perspective of Various Other Cultures
Health	■ Absence of disease ■ Ability to function at a high level	■ Being in a state of balance ■ Being in a state of harmony ■ Ability to perform family roles
Disease causation	■ Measurable, observable cause that leads to measurable, observable effect ■ Pathogens, mutant cells, toxins, poor diet	■ Frequently intangible, immeasurable cause ■ Lack of balance (yin and yang) ■ Lack of harmony with environment
Location of disorder	■ Body ■ Mind	■ Whole entity: mind, body, and spirit are completely merged ■ Disorder may be in the family or environment causing disease in the person
Decisions about care	■ Made by client or holder of power of attorney ■ Goals are autonomy and confidentiality ■ Truth telling required so client has information to make decisions	■ Made by the whole family or family head ■ Goals are protection and support of client ■ Hope should be preserved; client should be protected from painful truth
Sick role	■ Sick people should be as independent and self-reliant as possible ■ Self-care is encouraged; one gets better by "getting up and getting going"	■ Sick people should be as passive as possible ■ Family members should "take care of" and "do for" the sick person ■ Passivity stimulates recovery
Best treatments	■ Physician-prescribed drugs and treatments ■ Advanced medical technology	■ Regaining of lost balance or harmony by counteracting of negative forces with positive ones and vice versa ■ Treatment by folk healers and traditional remedies
Pain	■ Stoicism valued ■ Pain described quantitatively ■ Able to pinpoint location of pain ■ In cultures in which negative feelings are not expressed freely, pain is kept as silent as possible: Northern European, Asian, Native American	■ Pain expressed vocally and dramatically ■ Use of quantitative scales to measure pain is difficult ■ Pain experienced globally ■ In cultures in which emotional expression is encouraged, more dramatic pain expression is expected: Southern European, African, Middle Eastern
Ethics	■ Based on bioethical principles of autonomy, beneficence, justice, and confidentiality ■ Informed consent requires truthfulness	■ Based on virtue or community needs ■ Hope should be preserved, painful truth hidden ■ Support and care should be provided ■ Emphasis is on greatest good for the greatest number

© 2002, 2004 by Mary Curry Narayan.

tural needs and preferences. Although nurses may be tempted to think that "good care" is the care that they have learned to believe in, value, and practice, this could lead to ethnocentrism, which carries client risks. Ethnocentrism is the assumption that one's own beliefs, values, and practices are the best, preferred, or only way of being. Everyone has a tendency to be ethnocentric. All people are raised to see the world and everything in it through their own cultural lens—and nurses are no exception.

Ethnocentric care, however, is not good nursing care. Imposing our own cultural norms on members of other cultural groups is known as cultural imposition

(Leininger, 2002b). It is culturally inappropriate care, does not promote health and well-being for diverse people, and is considered to be unethical (American Nurses Association, 1991).

BARRIERS TO QUALITY MENTAL HEALTH SERVICES

The first part of this chapter focused on the impact of culture on mental health and illness in a theoretical way. In this next section, you will learn about some of the practice issues that nurses are likely to encounter when providing care to culturally diverse clients.

Three areas are considered: communication barriers, barriers to appropriate diagnosis, and ethnic differences in pharmacodynamics. You will also learn ways to overcome these barriers.

Communication Barriers

Therapeutic communication is key to the nursing care of clients with mental illness. Yet, many times nurses cannot speak the language of their clients. Clients with limited English proficiency are clients who cannot speak English or do not speak English well enough to meet their communication needs during a health care encounter. According to the Office of Civil Rights (2000), the 1964 Civil Rights Act gives clients with limited English proficiency the right to have a professional medical interpreter at no cost to the client when obtaining care from any service provider who receives federal funds (e.g., Medicare or Medicaid).

When a professional interpreter is engaged to facilitate communication between the nurse and the client, the interpreter should not only share the same language but should also be matched to the client as much as possible in gender, age, social status, and religion. In addition to interpreting the language, the interpreter can alert the nurse to the meaning of nonverbal communication patterns and cultural norms that are relevant to the encounter. In this way, the interpreter acts as a cultural broker, not only interpreting the language, but also the culture.

Clients with limited English proficiency may choose a family member as interpreter, but use of family interpreters has advantages and disadvantages. It may be, because of norms of family interconnectedness, that the family member's ability to support the client is enhanced by participating in the communication process. On the other hand, it may be that the stigma of the mental health problem will prevent the openness needed during the encounter. Also, family members frequently do not have the language skills necessary to meet the demands of interpretation, which is a very complex task. Languages frequently cannot be translated word for word, the literal translations of words in one language can carry many different connotations in the other language, and certain concepts are so culturally linked that an adequate translation is very difficult.

When English is the client's second language, even though the client may speak English very well, the client may have difficulty communicating emotional nuances in English; these may be more accessible to the client in the mother tongue. In addition, misinterpretation of phrases and idioms occurs frequently (Westermeyer, 1993). For instance, the terms *feeling blue* or *feeling down* may have no meaning at all in the client's literal understanding of English.

The nurse must be cautious about interpreting nonverbal communication patterns, such as considering the impassive facial expression of a Native American as a "flat affect" or the downcast eyes of an Asian woman as a sign of "evasiveness." Nonverbal communication patterns must be interpreted from within the client's cultural perspective, not the American-Western medical perspective.

Misdiagnosis

Studies indicate that blacks and African Americans, Asian Americans, and Latino-Hispanic Americans run a significant risk of being misdiagnosed with schizophrenia when the true diagnosis is bipolar disease or an affective disorder (U.S. Department of Health and Human Services, 2001). Why does this happen?

One reason for misdiagnosis is the use of culturally inappropriate psychometric instruments and other diagnostic tools. Most available tools have been validated using subjects of European origin. For instance, Kim (2002) states that, although there are over 40 validated depression scales, they tend to be "linguistically irrelevant and culturally inappropriate" (p. 110) for some groups, and they fail to identify depression in Koreans. Kim argues that the current scales measure "Western" ways of expressing depression by focusing on the affective domain, whereas for Koreans more attention needs to be given to the somatic domain. To rectify this problem, Kim created and validated a depression scale for Korean Americans.

As this inadequacy of diagnostic tools suggests, psychological distress is manifested in different cultures in different ways. In cultures in which the body and mind are seen as one entity, or in cultures in which there is a high degree of stigma associated with mental health problems, people frequently somatize their feelings of psychological distress. In somatization, psychological distress is experienced as physical problems. Instead of perceiving the distress as emotional or affective, the psychological distress is perceived in the body (Ryder, Yang, & Heini, 2002).

Somatization is just one example of a different way of experiencing psychological distress, however. Just as we learn from our parents whether the appropriate way to deal with pain is with dramatic expressiveness or with stoicism and denial, we learn different ways to manifest and express mental pain and pathology. Because of this, many cross-cultural mental health experts (Marsella, 2003) are skeptical about using the criteria of the *Diagnostic and Statistical Manual of Mental Disorders,* fourth edition, text revision *(DSM-IV-TR)* (American Psychiatric Association, 2000) for diagnosing mental illness in culturally diverse populations, because the criteria are based on studies with predominately white American samples.

The Glossary of Culture-Bound Syndromes, added to the *DSM-IV-TR,* acknowledges the limits of the *DSM-IV*'s ability to capture and name the symptoms and pathology of culturally diverse clients. Culture-bound syndromes are sets of symptoms that are common in some cultural groups but virtually nonexistent in most other cultural groups (Box 7-2).

Many culture-bound illnesses—such as *ghost illness* or *hwa-byung*—seem exotic or irrational to American nurses. Many of these illnesses cannot be understood within a Western medical framework. Their causes, manifestations, and treatments do not make sense to nurses whose understanding is limited to a Western conception of disease and illness. However, these illnesses are frequently well understood by the people within the cultural group. They know the name of the problem, its etiology, its course, and the way it should be treated, and frequently when these illnesses are treated in culturally prescribed ways, the remedies are quite effective.

Many culture-bound syndromes have been identified. Some of these syndromes seem to be mental health problems manifest in somatic ways. *Hwa-byung* and *neurasthenia* have many similarities to depression (Park et al., 2001), but because the somatic complaints are so prominent and clients frequently deny feelings of sadness or depression, they may not fit the *DSM-IV* diagnostic criteria for depression.

Another group of culture-bound illnesses is characterized by abnormal behaviors that people in the culture understand as illness but that are not found in other cultures, such as *ataque de nervios* and *ghost sickness*. These types of illness seem to be culturally acceptable ways for clients to indicate that they can no longer endure the stressors in their lives. People in the culture understand that the client is ill and provide support using culturally prescribed treatments, which actually relieve the stresses through cultural remedies that the client finds helpful.

Another kind of cultural-bound illness seems to be merely a cultural explanation of an illness that Western medicine understands as having a biomedical cause. From a Western perspective, the client may be suffering from an infection or inflammation, but the client may describe the cause as *susto* or *wind illness*.

Culture-bound illnesses are frequently thought of as being found only in "other" (i.e., non-Western) cultures. However, some authors have pointed out that anorexia nervosa and bulimia seem to be bound to Western culture, apparently because other cultures do not value the thinness so prized by European and Northern American cultural groups (Marsella, 2003). Some feel that almost all the descriptions of psychological illness in the *DSM-IV* are culture-bound to Western clients because the *DSM-IV* criteria were developed through studies of Western clients (Marsella, 2003).

Clinicians who do not understand the client's culture are likely to see culturally normal behavior as "abnormal" instead of merely "different." For instance, in African American churches, it is common to talk about

---

BOX 7-2

Culture-Bound Syndromes

Because so many culture-bound syndromes have been identified, they cannot all be described in this chapter. However, the list here includes some of the syndromes the mental health nurse might encounter.

Ataque de nervios: Latin American. Characterized by a sudden attack of trembling, palpitations, dyspnea, dizziness, and loss of consciousness. Thought to be caused by an evil spirit and related to intolerable stress. Treated by an *espiritista* (spiritual healer) and by the support of the family and community, who provide aid to the client and consider the client to be calling for help in a culturally acceptable way.

Ghost sickness: Navaho Indian. Characterized by "being out of one's mind," dyspnea, weakness, and bad dreams. Thought to be caused by an evil spirit. Treated by overcoming the evil spirit with a stronger spiritual force that the healer, a "singer," calls forth through a powerful healing ritual.

Hwa-byung: Korean. Characterized by epigastric pain, anorexia, palpitations, dyspnea, and muscle aches and pains. Thought to be caused by a lack of harmony in the body or in interpersonal relationships. Treated by reestablishing harmony. Some researchers feel that it is closely related to depression.

Neurasthenia: Chinese. Characterized by somatic symptoms of depression, such as anorexia, weight loss, fatigue, weakness, trouble concentrating, and insomnia, although feelings of sadness or depression are denied. Thought to be related to a lack of yin-yang balance.

Susto: Latin American. Characterized by a broad range of somatic and psychological symptoms. Thought to be related to a traumatic incident or fright that caused the client's soul to leave the body. Treated by an *espiritista* (spiritual healer).

Wind illness: Chinese, Vietnamese. Characterized by a fear of cold, wind, or drafts. Derived from the belief that ying-yang and hot-cold elements must be in balance in the body, or illness occurs. Treated by keeping very warm and avoiding foods, drinks, and herbs that are cold or considered to have a cold quality, as well as "cold" colors, emotions, and activities. Also treated by a variety of means designed to pull the "cold wind" out of the client, such as by coining (vigorously rubbing a coin over the body) or cupping (applying a heated cup to the skin, creating a vacuum).

---

spiritual experiences in terms a clinician may misinterpret. If the client says, "I was talking to Jesus this morning" to indicate that he was praying, the clinician may misinterpret the client's meaning and think that the client is delusional (Neighbors, 2003). If a Vietnamese father indicates that he tried to take the "wind illness" out of his child by vigorously rubbing a coin down her back, the clinician may believe that the father is delusional and a threat to the child. However, if the clinician understands the Vietnamese cultural perspective, the clinician will recognize that this is a concerned father who is caring for his child in a culturally appropriate way that, from a Western perspective, is not harmful to the child.

When there is a cultural mismatch between the clinician and the client, misdiagnosis and culturally inappropriate treatments frequently result (Kozuki & Kennedy, 2004; Ruiz, 1998). One might be tempted to think that the only way to solve these problems is to ensure that clients have mental health providers who match the client's culture. However, another way to solve the problem is for the nurse to take the time to study the client's culture, to learn from the client the client's cultural perspective, and to adapt care to meet the client's cultural needs.

Ethnic Variation in Pharmacodynamics

A third clinical practice issue, which can cause a barrier to quality mental health services, is genetic variations in drug metabolism. There is a growing realization that many drugs vary in their action and effect along genetic-ethnic lines, and what was found true in drug studies (which were primarily performed with subjects of European origin) may not be true in ethnically diverse populations. Genetic variations in drug metabolism have been documented for several classifications of drugs, including antidepressants and antipsychotics (U.S. Department of Health and Human Services, 2001).

Ethnopharmacology investigates these ethnic variations in drug pharmacokinetics. For example, many drugs are metabolized, at least in part, by the enzyme cytochrome P-450 (Rogers, Nafziger, & Bertino, 2002). Populations of European origin tend to have more of this enzyme than many clients of African or Asian origin. Therefore, clients of African and Asian origin are more likely to metabolize several medications for psychosis and depression at a slower rate than their counterparts of European origin. The result is that drug life is longer in people who lack this enzyme, which causes higher blood levels. This, in turn, leads to an increased incidence of intolerable side effects, which decreases client compliance with the drug regimen (U.S. Department of Health and Human Services, 2001). The dosages of antidepressants and antipsychotics normally prescribed turn out to be too high for many clients of African and Asian origin.

At the same time that this research is occurring, there is also an awareness that these sorts of genetic variations in drug metabolism are found in people of all ethnicities. Although statistically more people of European origin have the cytochrome P-450 enzyme than do those of African and Asian origin, this enzyme is found in people of all ethnicities. So making treatment decisions based on statistical differences among various ethnic groups may increase the odds but does not guarantee an appropriate dosage. The best way to determine ap-

propriate dosage is to determine the underlying phenotype of the client (a capability not yet available in general practice) and treat by phenotype, rather than by current drug dosage charts or by ethnicity.

For now, mental health nurses need to be aware that there are ethnic variations in drug metabolism. When nurses note medication problems, they can question whether the client's genetic ability to metabolize the psychotropic medication could indicate that the drug dosage should be lowered, or raised, to achieve maximal effectiveness with tolerable side effects.

CULTURALLY DIVERSE POPULATIONS AT RISK

Many culturally diverse populations are subject to experiences that challenge their mental health in ways that most Americans of European origin do not have to face. Among these challenges are issues related to the experience of being an immigrant, the socioeconomic disadvantages of minority status, and the severe stigma associated with mental health problems that is found in some cultural groups.

Immigrant Status

Immigrants face many unknowns. Upon arriving in the country, they may not speak English, yet need to learn how to navigate new economic, political, legal, educational, transportation, and health care systems. Many who had status and skills in their homeland—jobs as teachers, administrators, or other professional positions—find that, because of certification requirements or limited English skills, only menial jobs are open to them. After immigration, family roles may be upset, with wives finding jobs before their husbands. Adults discover how very difficult, if not impossible, it is to learn a new language when one is no longer a child. Immigrant families may find the struggle to live successfully in America arduous and wearing. Their long-honored cultural values and traditions, which once provided them with stability, are challenged by new cultural norms. During the period of adjustment, many immigrants find that the hope they felt on first immigrating turns into anxiety and depression (U.S. Department of Health and Human Services, 2001).

Immigrants and their families embark on a process of acculturation. During this process, which sometimes takes several generations, immigrants learn the beliefs, values, and practices of their new cultural setting. Some immigrants adapt to the new culture quickly, absorbing the new worldview, beliefs, values, and practices rapidly, until these are more natural than the ones they learned in their homeland (assimilation). Others attempt to maintain their traditional cultural ways. Some may become bicultural—able to move in and out of their traditional culture and their new culture, depending on where they are and with whom they associate. Some may suffer culture shock, finding the new norms disconcerting or offensive because they contrast so deeply with the immigrants' traditional beliefs, values, and practices.

Many families find that the children assimilate the new culture at a rapid pace, whereas the elders maintain their traditional cultural beliefs, values, and practices. This sets the stage for intergenerational conflict. The traditional status of elders in a hierarchical family may be challenged by children who are assimilating different values about family. Some children may feel lost between two cultures and unsure of where to place their cultural identity.

A refugee is a special kind of immigrant. Whereas the immigrant values the new culture and wishes to enjoy a change in life circumstances, the refugee has left his or her homeland to escape intolerable conditions and would have preferred to stay in his or her own culture if that had been possible. Refugees do not perceive entry into the new culture as an active choice and may experience the stress of adjusting as imposed on them against their will. Many refugees from Southeast Asia, Central America, and Africa have been traumatized by war, genocide, torture, starvation, and other catastrophic events. Many have lost family members, a way of life, and a homeland to which they can never return. The degree of trauma and loss they have experienced make them particularly vulnerable to posttraumatic stress disorder (U.S. Department of Health and Human Services, 2001).

Minority Status

Another difficulty that many culturally diverse people face is the socioeconomic disadvantages of being a "minority." Among these are poverty, limited opportunities for education and jobs, and residence in disadvantaged neighborhoods. In addition, cultural minority groups frequently are the victims of bias, discrimination, and racism.

In the United States, the incidence of various types of mental health disorders among cultural and racial minority groups is similar to that among white Americans *if* the poor and other vulnerable populations (homeless, institutionalized, children in foster care, and victims of trauma) within the minority groups are excluded. However, if those living in poverty and other vulnerable populations are included, the incidence of minority mental health problems increases. Therefore, the higher incidence of mental health problems in minority groups is related to poverty, not to ethnicity (U.S. Department of Health and Human Services, 2001).

People who live in poverty are two to three times more likely to develop mental illness than are those who live above the poverty line. Although only 8% of European American families live in poverty, 11% of

Asian and Pacific Islander Americans, 23% of Latino-Hispanic Americans, 24% of blacks and African Americans, and 26% of Native Americans live below the poverty line. Poverty is highly associated with other disadvantages, such as scarce educational and economic opportunities, which in turn are associated with substance abuse and violent crime. Poor people are subject to a daily struggle for survival, and this takes its toll on their mental health (U.S. Department of Health and Human Services, 2001).

Many people of diverse cultural groups have experienced, and continue to experience, various types of bias, discrimination, and racism. Discrimination and racism leave the victims feeling excluded, diminishing their self-esteem and self-efficacy.

People from cultural minorities have reported that they perceived bias and experienced care from health care providers that was culturally uncomfortable, which made them less likely to seek medical services in the future (U.S. Department of Health and Human Services, 2001). According to a report issued by the Institute of Medicine, *Unequal Treatment: Confronting Racial and Ethnic Disparities in Healthcare,* bias and discrimination infect the health care system, which results in further stresses on the mental health of minority groups, instead of delivery of the help they need (Smedley, Stith, & Nelson, 2002).

Stigma of Mental Illness

Mental illness is a highly stigmatized disorder. Many people, in all sectors of American society, associate mental illness with moral weakness. Others express fear of, or bias against, those with mental health problems. However, in many cultural groups, the stigma of mental illness is more severe and prevalent than it generally is in American society.

In some cultural groups, in which the interdependence and harmony of the family are emphasized, mental illness may be perceived as a failure of the family. Because of this, the stakes in having a mental illness are raised. It is not just the individual who is perceived as ill, but the whole family—and the illness reflects badly on the character of all family members. Stigma and shame can lead to a reluctance to seek help, and so members of these cultural groups may enter the mental health care system at an advanced stage, when the family has exhausted its ability to cope with the problem (Ryder et al., 2002).

CULTURALLY COMPETENT CARE

So far, this chapter has described why the nursing needs of culturally diverse client populations may be different from the needs the nurse might otherwise assume. Mental health and illness are biological, psychological, social, and cultural processes—and the cultural aspect cannot be ignored. Cultural competence is required if nurses are to assist clients in achieving mental health and well-being. But how, exactly, are mental health nurses to practice "culturally competent care"? The remainder of this chapter suggests techniques that answer this question.

The Office of Minority Health (2000) defines culturally competent care as attitudes and behaviors that enable a nurse to work effectively *within* the client's cultural context. Cultural competence means that nurses adjust *their* practices to meet their clients' cultural beliefs and practices, needs, and preferences. Culturally competent care goes beyond culturally sensitive care; it *adapts* care to the client's cultural needs and preferences.

Campinha-Bacote (2002) recommends a blueprint to psychiatric mental health nurses for providing culturally effective care with the Process of Cultural Competence in the Delivery of Health Care Model. In this model, nurses view themselves as *becoming* culturally competent rather than *being* culturally competent. This model suggests that nurses must constantly see themselves as learners throughout their careers—always open to, and learning from, the immense cultural diversity they will see among their clients.

This model consists of five constructs: cultural awareness, cultural knowledge, cultural encounters, cultural skill, and cultural desire. These constructs are the trellis on which cultural competence grows.

Cultural Awareness

Through cultural awareness, the nurse becomes committed to "cultural humility," a lifetime commitment to self-evaluation and self-critique regarding one's level of cultural awareness (Tervalon & Murray-Garcia, 1998, p. 117). The nurse recognizes the enormous impact culture makes on what clients' health values and practices are, how and when clients decide they are ill and need care, and what treatments they will seek when illness occurs (U.S. Department of Health and Human Services, 2001).

Cultural awareness inspires nurses to acknowledge themselves as cultural beings, so close to the norms of their own ethnic and professional cultures that these norms seem to be the "right" ones (ethnocentrism) and not just "cultural." Therefore, in accordance with the demands of cultural awareness, nurses examine their beliefs, values, and practices (Campinha-Bacote, 2002) to ascertain which ones are cultural and which ones could be universally held. Through cultural awareness and cultural humility, nurses discover that many of their norms are cultural, that few are universal, and that, therefore, nurses have an obligation to be open to and respectful of clients' cultural norms.

By practicing cultural awareness, nurses also examine their cultural assumptions and expectations about what constitutes mental health, a "healthy" self-concept, a "healthy" family, and the "right way" to behave in society. Nurses examine their assumptions and expectations about how people manifest psychological distress. The culturally aware nurse questions whether the evidence-based guideline proposed for a particular client (derived from studies involving primarily subjects of European origin) needs to be modified to address the cultural aspects of this client's life and illness (Campinha-Bacote, 2002).

Through cultural awareness, the nurse recognizes that during a cultural encounter three cultures are intersecting: the culture of the client, the culture of the nurse, and the culture of the setting (agency, clinic, hospital) (U.S. Department of Health and Human Services, 2001). In the nurse's role as a client advocate, the nurse negotiates and advocates on behalf of the client's cultural needs and preferences.

Cultural Knowledge

Nurses enhance their cultural knowledge in various ways. Nurses can attend cultural events and programs, forge friendships with members of diverse cultural groups, and participate in in-service programs at which members of diverse groups talk about their cultural norms. Another way to obtain cultural knowledge is to study resources designed for health care providers, such as books and Internet sources; refer to the Evolve website for a list of resources. Cultural knowledge prevents the nurse from assuming that the client's underlying worldview and values are the same as those of the nurse and alerts the nurse to areas in which there may be cultural differences. Cultural knowledge also helps the nurse understand behaviors that might be misinterpreted except for this knowledge. Cultural knowledge helps the nurse establish rapport, ask the right questions, avoid misunderstandings, and identify cultural variables that may need to be considered when planning care (Narayan, 2002).

Cultural guides and resources include information such as the following about various ethnic and religious cultures (Campinha-Bacote, 2002):

- Worldview, beliefs, and values that permeate the culture
- Nonverbal communication patterns, such as the meaning of eye contact, facial expressions, gestures, and touch
- Etiquette norms, such as the importance of punctuality, the pace of conversation, and the way respect and hospitality are shown
- Family roles and psychosocial norms, such as the way decisions are made and the degree of independence versus interdependence of family members
- Cultural views about mental health and illness, such as the degree of stigma, and the nature of the sick role

- Patterns related to health and illness, including culture-bound syndromes, ethnopharmacological variations, and folk and herbal treatments frequently used within the culture

Cultural Encounters

Although obtaining cultural knowledge sets a foundation, cultural guides cannot tell us anything about a particular client. According to Campinha-Bacote (2002), multiple cultural encounters with diverse clients deter nurses from stereotyping. Although generalizations can be made about cultures, stereotyping individuals within the group robs them of the individuality that they deserve.

Each person is a unique blend of the many cultures to which the person belongs: ethnic, religious, socioeconomic, geographic, educational, and occupational cultures. In addition, each person brings a unique personality, life experiences, and creative thought to self-development. Each person makes choices about which cultural norms to adopt or abandon. In the end, each person is a unique individual who never adheres to all, and may not adhere to any, of the norms of his or her culture of origin.

Stereotyping is the tendency to believe that every member of a group is like all other members of the group. However, multiple cultural encounters enable the nurse to experience the intraethnic diversity of cultural groups. The nurse comes to know that, although there are patterns that characterize a culture, individual members of the culture adhere to the culture's norms in diverse ways. The only way to know about the norms of a client's culture is to ask the client.

In addition, cultural encounters help the nurse develop confidence in cross-cultural interactions. The nurse is likely to make cultural blunders and will need to recover from cultural mistakes. Cultural encounters help the nurse develop skill at recognizing, avoiding, and reducing the cultural pain that can occur when the nurse causes the client discomfort or offense by failing to be sensitive to cultural norms (Kavanaugh, 2003). The nurse learns to recognize signs of cultural pain such as the client's discomfort or alienation. The nurse takes measures to recover trust and rapport by asking the client if the nurse has caused offense, apologizing for the lack of sensitivity, and expressing willingness to learn from the client how care can be provided in a culturally sensitive way.

Cultural Skill

Cultural skill is the ability to perform a cultural assessment in a sensitive way (Campinha-Bacote, 2002). The first step is to ensure that meaningful communication can occur. If the client is not proficient in English, a professional medical interpreter needs to be engaged.

Many cultural assessment tools are available (Andrews & Boyle, 2003; Giger & Davidhizar, 2003; Leininger, 2002a; Narayan, 2003; Purnell & Paulanka, 2003; Spector, 2003). An appendix of the *DSM-IV-TR* (American Psychiatric Association, 2000), Outline for Cultural Formulation, recommends cultural assessment areas. A very useful mental health assessment tool is the classic set of questions proposed by Kleinman, Eisenberg, and Good (1978):

- What do you call this illness? *(diagnosis)*
- When did it start? Why then? *(onset)*
- What do you think caused it? *(etiology)*
- How does the illness work? What does it do to you? *(course)*
- How long will it last? Is it serious? *(prognosis)*
- How have you treated the illness? How do you think it should be treated? *(treatment)*

These questions allow the client to feel heard and understood. They also help in eliciting culture-bound syndromes. They can be expanded to include questions such as the following:

- What are the chief problems this illness has caused you?
- What do you fear most about this illness? Do you think it is curable?
- Do you know others who have had this problem? What happened to them? Do you think this will happen to you?

Approaching these questions conversationally is generally more effective than using a direct, formal approach. One indirect technique is to ask the client what another family member thinks is causing the problem. Instead of saying, "What do you call this illness? When did it start and why then?" The nurse can ask, "What does your family think is wrong? Why do they think it started? What do they think you should do about it?" After the client describes what the family thinks, the nurse can simply ask, in a nonjudgmental way, if the client agrees.

Another technique for promoting openness is to first make a declaratory statement before asking the questions. For instance, before asking about cultural treatments the client has tried, the nurse can first say, "Everyone has remedies they find help them when they are ill. Are there any special healers or treatments that you have used or that you think might be helpful to you?"

Some areas that deserve special attention during an assessment interview are the following:

- Ethnicity and religious affiliation, and degree of acculturation to American-Western medical culture
- Spiritual practices that are important to preserve or regain health
- Degree of proficiency in speaking and reading English
- Dietary patterns, including foods prescribed for sick people

- Attitudes about pain and experiences with pain in a Western medical setting
- Attitudes about, and experience with, Western medications
- Cultural remedies, such as healers, herbs, and practices that the client may find helpful
- Who the client considers "family," who should receive health information, and how decisions are made in the family
- Cultural customs that the client feels are essential to preserve and is fearful will be violated in the mental health setting

The purpose of a culturally sensitive assessment is to develop a therapeutic plan that is mutually agreeable, culturally acceptable, and potentially capable of producing positive outcomes. While gathering assessment data, the nurse identifies cultural patterns that may support or interfere with the client's health and recovery process. The nurse uses professional knowledge to categorize the client's cultural norms into three different groups:

1. Those that facilitate the client's health and recovery
2. Those that are harmful to the client's health and well-being
3. Those that are neither helpful nor harmful from the Western medical perspective

Leininger (2002c) suggests a preserve-accommodate-restructure framework for care planning. Using this framework, the nurse **preserves** the aspects of the client's culture that, from a Western perspective, promote health and well-being, such as a strong family support system and traditional values like cooperation and emphasis on relationships.

Cultural values and practices that are neither helpful nor harmful are **accommodated.** The nurse encourages the client to benefit from these neutral values and practices, such as folk remedies and healers. By including these culture-specific interventions in the care as complementary interventions, the nurse builds on the client's own coping and healing systems. For example, Native Americans with substance abuse problems may find tribal healing ceremonies, as a complement to the therapeutic program, to be very helpful.

Finally, when cultural patterns are indeed a problem, the nurse attempts to **restructure** the patterns. For instance, if a client is taking an herb that interferes with the client's medication regimen, the nurse educates and negotiates until a mutually agreeable therapeutic program is developed.

Cultural Desire

The last construct in Campinha-Bacote's cultural competence model for psychiatric mental health nurses (2002) is cultural desire. Although it may be easier to establish a therapeutic relationship when the nurse comes from a similar cultural background, cultural de-

sire enables the nurse to achieve good outcomes with culturally diverse clients.

Cultural desire prompts nurses to have a genuine concern for clients' welfare and a willingness to listen until they truly understand each client's viewpoint. Nurses exhibit cultural desire through patience, consideration, and empathy. They give the impression that they are willing to learn from the client, instead of the impression that they know it all and are going to impose the "correct" treatment on the client. Cultural desire inspires openness and flexibility in applying nursing principles to meet the client's cultural needs.

■ ■ ■ KEY POINTS to REMEMBER

- Mental health and illness are biological, psychological, social, and cultural phenomena.
- As the diversity of the world and America increases, psychiatric mental health nurses will be caring for more and more people of diverse cultural groups.
- Nurses must learn to deliver culturally relevant care—culturally sensitive assessments and culturally congruent interventions.
- Culture is the shared beliefs, values, and practices of a group that shape their thinking and behavior in patterned ways. Cultural groups share these norms with new members of the group through enculturation.
- A group's culture influences its members' worldview, nonverbal communication patterns, etiquette norms, and ways of viewing the person, the family, and the "right" way to think and behave in society.
- The concept of mental health is formed within a culture, and deviance from cultural expectations can be defined as "illness" by other members of the group.
- Psychiatric mental health nursing is based on personality and developmental theories advanced by Europeans and Americans, which are grounded in Western cultural ideals and values.
- Nurses are as influenced by their own professional and ethnic cultures as are clients by their cultures. Nurses must guard against ethnocentric tendencies when caring for clients, because cultural imposition does not promote client health and well-being.
- Barriers to quality mental health care include language barriers, ethnic variations in psychotropic drug metabolism, and culturally inappropriate diagnostic tools.
- Immigrants (especially refugees) and minority groups who suffer from the effects of low socioeconomic status, including poverty and discrimination, are at particular risk for mental illness.
- Cultural competence consists of five constructs: cultural awareness, cultural knowledge, cultural encounters, cultural skill, and cultural desire (Campinha-Bacote, 2002).
- Through cultural awareness, nurses recognize that nurses, as well as clients, have cultural beliefs, values, and practices.
- Cultural knowledge is obtained by seeking cultural information from friends, participating in in-service programs, immersing oneself in the culture, or consulting books and Internet sources.

- Nurses experience intraethnic diversity through multiple cultural encounters, which protect nurses from stereotyping their clients.
- Nurses demonstrate cultural skill by performing culturally sensitive assessment interviews and adapting care to meet clients' cultural needs and preferences.
- Care can be adapted by using the preserve-accommodate-restructure care planning framework of Leininger (2002c) when creating the therapeutic plan.

- Cultural desire enables nurses to provide considerate, flexible, and respectful care to clients of diverse cultures.

Visit the Evolve website at **http://evolve.elsevier.com/Varcarolis** for a posttest on the content in this chapter.   **evolve**

Critical Thinking and Chapter Review

Visit the Evolve website at **http://evolve.elsevier.com/Varcarolis** for additional self-study exercises.   **evolve**

CRITICAL THINKING

1. Describe the cultural factors that have influenced Western mental health nursing practice. Contrast these Western influences with the cultural factors that influence clients who come from an Eastern or indigenous culture.

2. Analyze the effect that ethnocentrism and cultural imposition can have on psychiatric mental health nurses and their clients. Describe several ways nurses can avoid the negative effects of ethnocentrism and cultural imposition.

3. Name three barriers to culturally competent mental health services and identify ways to overcome these barriers.

4. A Chinese woman has recently moved to America. She is a wife and the mother of two small children and lives in a tight-knit Chinese community with her husband's parents. She comes to an emergency department with complaints of fatigue, headache, and stomach pain. Diagnostic tests are unrevealing. Inquiry by the nurse indicates that the woman wants to be more like an American woman but her husband and in-laws view her attempts as "not being a good wife."

   A. Using Campinha-Bacote's five cultural competence constructs, analyze the factors influencing this client's symptoms and the care she should receive.

   B. Crease a culturally competent care plan for this client.

CHAPTER REVIEW

Choose the most appropriate answer.

1. Providing culturally relevant mental health nursing requires the nurse to
   1. assume that Western psychological theories can be applied to non-Western clients.
   2. recognize the superiority of Western cultural values, beliefs about relationships, and worldviews.
   3. understand the values and beliefs embedded within the nurse's own culture and medical practices.
   4. educate clients on language and culture so they are not offended by Western customs and terminology.

2. Use of a cultural handbook by a nurse caring for a client of different cultural background
   1. will prevent stereotyping the client.
   2. is an excellent way to learn about a new culture.
   3. may mislead because of failure to recognize subgroup differences.
   4. will provide understanding of the universality of cultural processes.

3. One possible negative result of applying Western psychological theories when assessing individuals of other cultures is
   1. identifying client idioms of distress.
   2. identifying cognitive deficit where none exists.
   3. recognizing individual variation among group members.
   4. seeing a sociocentric individual as developmentally immature.

4. Culturally relevant psychiatric nursing practice includes
   1. understanding all self-structures, worldviews, and explanatory models of illness.
   2. seeking clarification of the client's health-related beliefs.
   3. applying a standard model of assessment to all clients.
   4. using standard interventions for all clients.

5. Which action on the part of the nurse is least useful in promoting delivery of culturally relevant psychiatric nursing care?
   1. Working within the cultural context of the client
   2. Providing a culturally relevant client assessment
   3. Using direct eye contact and touch to facilitate communication
   4. Bridging the gap between the U.S. health care system and the health belief system of the client

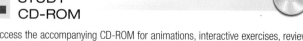

Access the accompanying CD-ROM for animations, interactive exercises, review questions for the NCLEX examination, and an audio glossary. **evolve**

REFERENCES

American Nurses Association. (1991). *Position statement on cultural diversity in nursing practice*. Washington, DC: Author.

American Psychiatric Association. (2000). *Diagnostic and statistical manual of mental disorders (DSM-IV-TR)* (4th ed., text rev.). Washington, DC: Author.

Andrews, M., & Boyle, J. (2003). *Transcultural concepts in nursing care* (4th ed.). Philadelphia: Lippincott.

Campinha-Bacote, J. (2002). Cultural competence in psychiatric nursing: Have you asked the right questions? *Journal of the American Psychiatric Nurses Association, 8*(6), 183-187.

Giger, J. N., & Davidhizar, R. E. (2003). *Transcultural nursing: Assessment and intervention* (3rd ed.). St. Louis: Mosby.

Higgins, K. (2001). *World philosophy*. Chantilly, VA: Teaching Company.

Kavanaugh, K. H. (2003). Transcultural perspectives in mental health nursing. In M. Andrews & J. Boyle, *Transcultural concepts in nursing care*. Philadelphia: Lippincott Williams & Wilkins.

Kim, M. (2002). Measuring depression in Korean Americans: Development of the Kim Depression Scale for Korean Americans. *Journal of Transcultural Nursing, 13*(2), 109-117.

Kleinman, A., Eisenberg, L., & Good, B. (1978). Culture, illness and care: Clinical lessons from anthropologic and cross-cultural research. *Annals of Internal Medicine, 88*, 251-258.

Kozuki, Y., & Kennedy, M. (2004). Cultural incommensurability in psychodynamic psychotherapy in Western and Japanese traditions. *Journal of Nursing Scholarship, 36*(1), 30-38.

Leininger, M. (2002a). Culture care assessments for congruent competency practices. In M. Leininger & M. McFarland (Eds.), *Transcultural nursing: Concepts, theories, research and practice* (3rd ed., pp. 117-144). New York: McGraw-Hill.

Leininger, M. (2002b). Essential transcultural nursing care concepts, principles, examples, and policy statements. In M. Leininger & M. McFarland (Eds.), *Transcultural nursing: Concepts, theories, research and practice* (3rd ed., pp. 45-70). New York: McGraw-Hill.

Leininger, M. (2002c). The theory of culture care and the ethnonursing research method. In M. Leininger & M. McFarland (Eds.), *Transcultural nursing: Concepts, theories, research and practice* (3rd ed., pp. 117-144). New York: McGraw-Hill.

Marsella, A. J. (2003). Cultural aspects of depressive experience and disorders. In W. J. Lonner et al. (Eds.), *Online readings in psychology and culture* (Unit 9, Chapter 4). Retrieved November 17, 2004, from Western Washington University, Center for Cross-Cultural Research website: http://www.ac.wwu.edu/~culture/Marsella.htm.

Narayan, M. C. (2002). Six steps to cultural competence: A clinician's guide. *Home Health Care Management & Practice, 14*(5), 378-386.

Narayan, M. C. (2003). Cultural assessment and care planning. *Home Healthcare Nurse, 21*(9), 611-618.

Neighbors, H. (2003, January 22). *The (mis)diagnosis of African Americans implementing DSM criteria in the hospital and the community*. Retrieved April 4, 2004, from University of Michigan Department of Psychiatry, Psychiatry Grand Rounds website: http://www.med.umich.edu/psych/mlk2003.htm.

Office of Civil Rights, U.S. Department of Health and Human Services. (2000). Policy guidance on Title VI of the Civil Rights Act of 1964: Prohibition against national origin discrimination as it affects persons with limited English proficiency. *Federal Register 65*(169), 52762-52774.

Office of Minority Health, U.S. Department of Health and Human Services. (2000). National standards for culturally and linguistically appropriate services in the delivery of healthcare. *Federal Register 65*(247), 80865-80879.

Park, Y., et al. (2001). A survey of hwa-byung in middle-age Korean women. *Journal of Transcultural Nursing, 12*(2), 115-122.

Purnell, L. D., & Paulanka, B. J. (2003). *Transcultural health care: A culturally competent approach* (2nd ed.). Philadelphia: F. A. Davis.

Rogers, J., Nafziger, A., & Bertino, J. (2002). Pharmacogenetics affects dosing, efficacy, and toxicity of cytochrome P450-metabolized drugs. *American Journal of Medicine, 113*(9), 746-750.

Ruiz, P. (1998). The role of culture in psychiatric care. *American Journal of Psychiatry, 155*, 1763-1765.

Ryder, A. G., Yang, J., & Heini, S. (2002). Somatization vs. psychologization of emotional distress: A paradigmatic example for cultural psychopathology. In W. J. Lonner et al. (Eds.), *Online readings in psychology and culture* (Unit 9, Chapter 3). Retrieved November 17, 2004, from Western Washington University, Center for Cross-Cultural Research website: http://www.ac.wwu.edu/~culture/RyderYangHeine.htm.

Saint Arnault, D. (2002). Culturally relevant mental health nursing. In E. Varcarolis (Ed.), *Foundations of psychiatric mental health nursing* (4th ed.). Philadelphia: Saunders.

Segall, M. H. (2002). Why is there still racism if there is no such thing as "race"? In W. J. Lonner et al. (Eds.), *Online readings in psychology and culture* (Unit 15, Chapter 5). Retrieved November 17, 2004, from Western Washington University, Center for Cross-Cultural Research website: http://www.ac.wwu.edu/~culture/segall.htm.

Smedley, B., Stith, A., & Nelson, A. (2002). *Unequal treatment: Confronting racial and ethnic disparities in healthcare* (Institute of Medicine Report). Washington, DC: National Academy Press.

Spector, R. E. (2003). *Cultural diversity in health and illness*. Upper Saddle River, NJ: Prentice-Hall.

Tervalon, M., & Murray-Garcia, J. (1998). Cultural humility versus cultural competence: A critical distinction in defining physician training outcomes in multicultural education. *Journal of the Poor and Underserved, 9*, 117-125.

U.S. Census Bureau. (2002). *National population projection. I. Summary files*. Retrieved April 4, 2004, from the U.S. Census Bureau website: http://www.census.gov/population/www/projections/natsum-T3.html.

U.S. Census Bureau. (2000). *Racial and ethnic classifications used in census 2000 and beyond*. Retrieved April 4, 2004, from the U.S. Census Bureau website: http://www.census.gov/population/www/socdemo/race/racefactcb.html.

U.S. Department of Health and Human Services. (2001). *Mental health: Culture, race, and ethnicity: A supplement to Mental health: A report of the surgeon general*. Rockville, MD: U.S. Department of Health and Human Services, Substance Abuse and Mental Health Services Administration, Center for Mental Health Services.

Westermeyer, J. (1993). Cross-cultural psychiatric assessment. In A. C. Gaw (Ed.), *Culture, ethnicity, and mental illness*. Washington DC: American Psychiatric Press.

CHAPTER 8

Legal and Ethical Guidelines for Safe Practice

PENNY SIMPSON BROOKE

KEY TERMS and CONCEPTS

The key terms and concepts listed here appear in color where they are defined or first discussed in this chapter.

OBJECTIVES

After studying this chapter, the reader will be able to

1. Compare and contrast the terms *ethics* and *bioethics,* and identify five principles of bioethics.
2. Discuss at least five client rights that come under the Patient's Bill of Rights.
3. Give examples of the client's (a) right to treatment, (b) right to refuse treatment, and (c) right to informed consent.
4. Identify the steps nurses are advised to take if they suspect negligence or illegal activity on the part of a professional colleague or peer.
5. Apply legal considerations of client privilege (a) after a client has died, (b) if the client tests positive for human immunodeficiency virus, or (c) if the client's employer states a "need to know."
6. Provide explanations for situations in which health care professionals have a duty to break client confidentiality.
7. Discuss a client's civil rights and how they pertain to restraint and seclusion.
8. Develop an awareness of the balance between the client's rights and the rights of society with respect to the following legal concepts relevant in nursing and psychiatric nursing: (a) duty to intervene, (b) documentation and charting, and (c) confidentiality.

evolve Visit the Evolve website at **http://evolve.elsevier.com/Varcarolis** for a pretest on the content in this chapter.

This chapter introduces you to current legal and ethical issues that may be encountered in the practice of psychiatric nursing. Because the law is dynamic and evolving, it does not always lend itself to clear answers. Accordingly, in situations in which the law is not clearly stated by statute, regulation, or court decision, the nurse often encounters an ethical dilemma (a situation that requires a choice between morally conflicting alternatives).

The fundamental goal in resolving any legal or ethical issue confronting the nurse in a psychiatric setting is striking a balance between the rights of the individual client and the rights of society at large. This chapter is designed to assist you in identifying competing ethical or legal interests involved in various nursing interventions and to help you consider their impact on decision making.

You are encouraged to be aware of the mental health statutes in your own state. Copies of these state codes can be obtained from the state department of professional licensure through state boards of nursing and often are available on websites. They are also commonly accessible at law school libraries and state agencies such as the attorney general's office.

ETHICAL CONCEPTS

Ethics is the study of philosophical beliefs about what is considered right or wrong in a society. Discussions of ethical practice in nursing involve the topics of morals and values. The term bioethics is used in relation to ethical dilemmas surrounding client care. Bioethics in psychiatric mental health nursing is the application of ethical principles within the scope of the psychiatric nursing practice setting.

The five principles of bioethics are as follows:

1. Beneficence is the duty to act so as to benefit or promote the good of others, for example, making a decision to remain by the bedside of an extremely anxious client to be supportive, even if the shift has ended, until a replacement can be found.
2. Autonomy is the right to make one's own decisions and respect for the rights of others to make their own decisions, for example, acknowledging the client's right to make decisions that do not conform with the recommendation of the staff.
3. Justice is treating others fairly and equally.
4. Fidelity (nonmaleficence) is maintaining loyalty and commitment to the client and doing no wrong to the client, for example, showing a commitment to clinical expertise by participating in continuing education.
5. Veracity refers to one's duty always to tell the truth. Clients have the right to know about their diagnosis, treatment, and prognosis. There are times when limitation of information may be justified (when the truth would be knowingly harmful to a client).

Ethical decisions involve morals and values that may differ widely among decision makers. Therefore, it is important to respect and protect the client's autonomy and the client's right to be the ultimate decision maker about decisions that affect his or her life. You must avoid trying to impose personal values on the client. Your life experiences may be dramatically different from those of the client, and part of becoming a professional is developing the ability to recognize and accept the client's right to have an opinion that differs from your own.

At times, your values may be in conflict with the value system of the institution. This situation further complicates the decision-making process and necessitates careful consideration of the client's desires. For example, you may experience a conflict in a setting in which there is abundant use of tranquilizers for the treatment of elderly or depressed clients. Whenever one's value system is challenged, increased stress results.

With today's technological revolution, nurses and clients have more choices than ever, and ethical decisions are more complex than ever before. When faced with tough ethical decisions, you should use a number of resources to help with the problem-solving process. These resources include the following (Dunn, 1994):

- Legal advice
- Nurse practice acts
- Hospital and organizational policies
- Patient's Bill of Rights
- Colleagues
- Clergy
- Examination of one's own ideals and morals
- *Code of Ethics for Nurses with Interpretive Statements* of the American Nurses Association (ANA, 2001) (Box 8-1)
- Standards of Care from the *Scope and Standards of Psychiatric-Mental Health Nursing Practice* (ANA, American Psychiatric Nurses Association, & International Society of Psychiatric-Mental Health Nurses, 2000) (provided on the inside back cover of this book)

Ethical standards, although lacking the clarity and power of law, do serve as a field guide for decision making. As each generation advances in knowledge and technology, society inherits increased options.

The distinction between legal and ethical issues is often vague. However, there is an important difference between relying on ethical guiding principles and following the guiding principles of law. You are bound to comply with the laws, and even though you may feel morally obligated to follow ethical guidelines, these guidelines should not override laws. For example, if you are aware of a statute or a specific rule or regulation created by the state board of nursing that pro-

Code of Ethics for Nurses

The House of Delegates of the American Nurses Association approved these nine provisions of the new *Code of Ethics for Nurses* at its June 30, 2001, meeting in Washington, DC. In July 2001, the Congress of Nursing Practice and Economics voted to accept the new language of the interpretive statements resulting in a fully approved revised *Code of Ethics for Nurses with Interpretive Statements*.

1. The nurse, in all professional relationships, practices with compassion and respect for the inherent dignity, worth, and uniqueness of every individual, unrestricted by considerations of social or economic status, personal attributes or the nature of health problems.

2. The nurse's primary commitment is to the patient, whether an individual, family, group, or community.

3. The nurse promotes, advocates for, and strives to protect the health, safety, and rights of the patient.

4. The nurse is responsible and accountable for individual nursing practice and determines the appropriate delegation of tasks consistent with the nurse's obligation to provide optimum patient care.

5. The nurse owes the same duties to self as to others, including the responsibility to preserve integrity and safety, to maintain competence, and to continue personal and professional growth.

6. The nurse participates in establishing, maintaining, and improving health care environments and conditions of employment conducive to the provision of quality health care and consistent with the values of the profession through individual and collective action.

7. The nurse participates in the advancement of the profession through contributions to practice, education, administration, and knowledge development.

8. The nurse collaborates with other health professionals and the public in promoting community, national, and international efforts to meet health needs.

9. The profession of nursing, as represented by associations and their members, is responsible for articulating nursing values, for maintaining the integrity of the profession and its practice, and for shaping social policy.

From American Nurses Association. (2001). *Code of ethics for nurses with interpretive statements.* Washington, DC: American Nurses Publishing.

hibits a certain action (e.g., restraining clients against their will) and you feel you have an ethical obligation to protect the client by engaging in such an action (e.g., using restraints), you would be wise to follow the law. Laws override ethical principles, which do not have the same legal strength. However, ethical dilemmas can influence laws when society is concerned enough to take specific ethical issues to the courts or to the legislature.

Ethical issues become legal issues when decisions are made in court cases or when the legislature has heard from many people that a law is needed to protect certain rights.

Mental Illness and the Social Norm

Social norms are known to every society, and most members of society conform to these norms. However, some members of society do not conform. What happens to them? Must all people conform? Does society need the nonconformist (the artist, the scientist, the inventor)? Does the majority have the right to impose its will on the individual?

What about the freedom of individuals to do what they want to do when they want to do it? When is the right of the individual curtailed for the benefit of society? Take, for example, the street lady who for years has been unobtrusively pilfering from trash containers every evening. This behavior, although not desirable, is acceptable. Eventually, she starts rummaging after midnight, and as the noise level escalates, the community responds by notifying authorities of the violation of the peace. What was once tolerable behavior becomes unacceptable. The Surgeon General's 1999 report on mental health (U.S. Department of Health and Human Services, 1999) states that the public perception of people with psychosis as being dangerous is stronger today.

What constitutes desirable or acceptable behavior of the individual is decided by the group (society) that establishes the norms. Methods of changing human behavior include behavior modification techniques and psychotherapy. Psychotropic drugs can also dramatically alter behavior and must therefore be prescribed carefully. Freedom of expression is a fundamental value of our society, a right embodied in the U.S. Constitution. Some hold the view that many psychiatric treatment modalities alter the individual's thought processes and thus challenge our fundamental societal values.

Responsibilities of the Therapeutic Relationship

The psychotherapeutic relationship carries with it serious ethical and legal obligations to the client. The psychotherapist becomes extremely important to the client and must assume this role conscientiously. Termination of the psychotherapeutic relationship can be traumatic to clients if the break is not handled skillfully. Nurse clinicians also have a legal and ethical obligation to the client and to society not to abuse the power that can exist when a client relies on them.

Protection of the client when he or she is in a vulnerable state of mind must be considered. Sadly, many therapeutic relationships are in the news because of sexual abuse of clients by therapists. This misuse of the therapeutic relationship constitutes grounds for losing a license and violates the ethical duty of fidelity to the client. Pennington and associates (1993) reported sexual intimacy to be the primary boundary issue for nurses studied and reported in the literature, although it is not directly addressed in the ANA *Code of Ethics for Nurses*. Boundary issues are covered in more depth in Chapter 10.

Protection of the confidentiality and privacy of the client's disclosures during therapeutic communication is also vitally important. Because of the complexity of human behavior, therapeutic relations may be long-lasting and complicated. Skilled nurse clinicians must have great insight into their own behavior as well as the client's behavior. Without self-awareness, nurses risk imposing their own value system upon the client. Issues of confidentiality are covered in more depth in Chapter 11.

MENTAL HEALTH LAWS

Laws have been enacted in each state to regulate the care and treatment of the mentally ill. Many of these laws have undergone major revision since 1963, which reflects a shift in emphasis from state institutional care of the mentally ill to community-based care. This was heralded by the enactment of the Community Mental Health Center Act of 1963 under President John Kennedy. Outpatient commitment laws exist in 41 states and the District of Columbia. Outpatient treatment is less expensive than hospitalization and provides a less restrictive treatment setting (Pekkanen, 2003).

Along with this shift in emphasis has come the more widespread use of psychotropic drugs in the treatment of mental illness—which has enabled many people to integrate more readily into the larger community—and an increasing awareness of the need to provide the mentally ill with humane care that respects their civil rights.

Civil Rights

Persons with mental illness are guaranteed the same rights under federal and state laws as any other citizen. Most states specifically prohibit any person from depriving an individual receiving mental health services of his or her civil rights, including the right to vote; the right to civil service ranking; the rights related to granting, forfeit, or denial of a driver's license; the right to make purchases and to enter contractual relationships (unless the client has lost legal capacity by being adjudicated incompetent); and the right to press charges against another client or staff. The psychiatric client's rights include the right to humane care and treatment. The medical, dental, and psychiatric needs of the client must be met in accordance with the prevailing standards accepted in these professions. The mentally ill in prisons and jails are afforded the same protections. The right to religious freedom and practice, the right to social interaction, and the right to exercise and recreational opportunities are also protected (see Box 5-1).

Specific Client Rights

Client Consent

Proper orders for specific therapies and treatments are required and must be documented in the client's chart. Consent for surgery, electroconvulsive treatment, or the use of experimental drugs or procedures must be obtained. Clients have the right to refuse participation in experimental treatments or research and the right to voice grievances and recommend changes in policies or services offered by the facility, without fear of punishment or reprisal.

Communication

Clients have the right to communicate fully and privately with those outside the facility. They have a right to receive visitors, to have reasonable access to phones and mail, and to send as well as receive unopened correspondence. Clients may seek, at their own expense, consultation with other mental health professionals or attorneys. Clients may not be forced to work for the hospital, with the exception of being assigned routine duties that are developed to enhance their ability to live outside the facility. The rules and regulations of the hospital need to be explained to the client. For instance, most inpatient facilities have rules against sexual activities between clients because of the risk that their psychiatric illnesses may prevent one or both of the clients from fully giving consent. Clients need access to interpreters for various languages, including sign language, as well as access to communication with persons outside the hospital.

Freedom from Harm

Most state laws also provide for the right to be free from harm, which includes freedom from unnecessary or excessive physical restraint, isolation, and medication, as well as freedom from abuse or neglect. Use of medications for staff convenience, as a punishment, or as a substitute for treatment programs is explicitly prohibited.

Dignity and Respect

Clients in psychiatric hospitals have the right to be treated with dignity and respect. These rights are not only ethically important but also legally protected. Clients have the right to be free from discrimination on the basis of ethnic origin, gender, age, disability, or religion.

Confidentiality

Confidentiality of care and treatment is also an important right for all clients, particularly psychiatric clients. The client's records must be treated as confidential by the staff. Photographs may not be taken without the client's written consent. The client's privacy is protected along with the confidentiality of the treatment. Any discussion or consultation involving a client should be conducted discreetly and only with individuals who have a need and a right to know this privileged information. Discussions about a client in public places such as elevators and the cafeteria, even when the client's name is not mentioned, can lead to disclosures of confidential information and liabilities for you and the hospital. The regulations of the Health Insurance Portability and Accountability Act (HIPAA) must be understood and followed to protect confidentiality of care and the privacy of the client.

The client's permission must be obtained to share information with persons who are not directly involved in his or her care. These protections also apply to the client's medical record, which should be read only by individuals directly involved in the client's treatment or in monitoring of the quality of care given. Clients must issue a written authorization to allow others to read their medical records. They have a right to expect that all communications and other records relating to treatment be handled as confidential. Institutions that use computerized record keeping must safeguard against intrusion into their client record systems. This issue of client confidentiality is discussed in more detail later in the chapter.

Participation in Plan of Care

Additional rights the psychiatric client enjoys include provision of a written individualized treatment plan that is reviewed regularly and that involves the client in the planning decisions. Clients are also entitled to a discharge plan that includes follow-up care or continuing care requirements. The treatment plan needs to include the least restrictive treatment environment that is appropriate. Reasonable safety is an expectation of this environment. The client's family may also be involved in treatment and discharge decisions. If the client is unable to make these decisions, the person legally authorized to act on the client's behalf must be consulted.

Clients have the right to be informed by their physicians of the benefits, risks, and side effects of all medications and treatment procedures used. **They cannot be subjected to any procedure or treatment without their consent, or a battery will have occurred.** (Assault and battery are discussed in greater detail later in this chapter.)

ADMISSION, COMMITMENT, AND DISCHARGE PROCEDURES

Due Process in Civil Commitment

The courts have recognized that involuntary civil commitment to a mental hospital is a "massive curtailment of liberty" (*Humphrey v. Cady,* 1972, p. 509) requiring due process protections in the civil commitment procedure. This right derives from the Fifth Amendment of the U.S. Constitution, which states that "no person shall . . . be deprived of life, liberty, or property without due process of law." The Fourteenth Amendment explicitly prohibits states from depriving citizens of life, liberty, and property without due process of law. State civil commitment statutes, if challenged in the courts on constitutional grounds, must afford minimal due process protections to pass the court's scrutiny (*Zinernon v. Burch*, 1990).

In most states, a client can institute a court proceeding to seek a judicial discharge. This is referred to as a writ of habeas corpus, meaning a writ to "free the person." The writ of habeas corpus is the procedural mechanism used to challenge unlawful detention by the government.

The writ of habeas corpus and the least restrictive alternative doctrine are two of the most important concepts applicable to civic commitment cases. The least restrictive alternative doctrine mandates that the least drastic means be taken to achieve a specific purpose.

Admission to the Hospital

All students are encouraged to become familiar with the important provisions of the laws in their own states regarding admissions, discharges, client's rights, and informed consent.

Neither voluntary nor involuntary admission to a mental facility determines whether clients are capable of making informed decisions about the health care they may need to receive. The involuntarily committed client is considered to be capable of consenting to treatment, unless a judicial determination has been made or the client lacks the capacity to understand the implications of his or her decision. Involuntary commitment also requires that the client retain freedom from unreasonable bodily restraints and the right to refuse medications, including psychotropic or antipsychotic medications.

A medical standard or justification for admission should exist. A well-defined psychiatric problem must be established, based on current illness classifications in the *Diagnostic and Statistical Manual of Mental Disorders,* fourth edition, text revision (American Psychiatric Association, 2000). The presenting illness should also be of such a nature that it causes an immediate crisis situation or that other less restrictive alternatives are inadequate or unavailable. There should also be a reasonable expectation that the hospitalization and treatment will improve the presenting problems.

Voluntary Admission

Generally, voluntary admission is sought by the client or the client's guardian through a written application to the facility. Voluntarily admitted clients have the right to demand and obtain release. If the client is a minor, the release may be contingent on the consent of the parents or guardian. However, few states require voluntarily admitted clients to be notified of the rights associated with their status. In addition, many states require that a client submit a written release notice to the facility staff, who reevaluate the client's condition for possible conversion to involuntary status according to criteria established by state law.

Involuntary Admission (Commitment)

Involuntary admission is made without the client's consent. Generally, involuntary admission is necessary when a person is in need of psychiatric treatment, presents a danger to self or others, or is unable to meet his or her own basic needs. Three different commitment procedures are commonly available: judicial determination, administrative determination, and agency determination. In addition, a specified number of physicians must certify that a person's mental health status justifies detention and treatment.

Involuntary hospitalization can be further categorized by the nature and purpose of the involuntary admission. It may be emergency, observational or temporary, or indeterminate or extended.

Emergency Involuntary Hospitalization. Most states provide for emergency involuntary hospitalization or civil commitment for a specified period (1 to 10 days on average) to prevent dangerous behavior that is likely to cause harm to self or others. Police officers, physicians, and mental health professionals may be designated by statute to authorize the detention of mentally ill persons who are a danger to themselves or others.

Observational or Temporary Involuntary Hospitalization. Civil commitment for observational or temporary involuntary hospitalization is of longer duration than emergency hospitalization. The primary purpose of this type of hospitalization is observation, diagnosis, and treatment for persons who have mental illness or pose a danger to themselves or others. The length of time is specified by statute and varies markedly from state to state. Application for this type of admission can be made by a guardian, family member, physician, or other public health officer. States vary in their procedural requirements for

this type of involuntary admission. Medical certification by two or more physicians that a person is mentally ill and in need of treatment or a judicial or administrative review and order is often required for involuntary admission.

Long-Term or Formal Commitment. Long-term commitment for involuntary hospitalization has as its primary purpose extended care and treatment of the mentally ill. Like clients who undergo observational involuntary hospitalization, those who undergo extended involuntary hospitalization are committed solely through judicial or administrative action or medical certification. States that do not require a judicial hearing before commitment often provide the client with an opportunity for a judicial review after commitment procedures. This type of involuntary hospitalization generally lasts 60 to 180 days, but it may be for an indeterminate period.

Clients who are involuntarily committed do not lose their right of informed consent. Clients must be considered legally competent until they have been declared incompetent through a legal proceeding. Competency is related to the capacity to understand the consequences of one's decisions. The determination of legal competency is not necessarily the function of the psychiatric staff but is made by the courts. Although courts hold a strong presumption of a client's continued competency, the court may appoint a legal guardian or representative who is legally responsible for giving or refusing consent for a person the court has found to be incompetent. Court-appointed guardians must always consider the client's wishes, if they are known when the client was still fully competent. For a legal guardian to be appointed, the court must first declare that the client is incompetent and then appoint a guardian either temporarily or permanently. Guardians are usually selected from among family members. The order of selection is usually (1) spouse, (2) adult children or grandchildren, (3) parents, (4) adult brothers and sisters, and (5) nieces and nephews. This order of selection has been supported by both state laws and court decisions (*Matter of Jobes*, 1987). In the event that a family member is either unavailable or unwilling to serve as guardian, the court may also appoint a social worker representing the county or state or a member of the community who has been trained and approved by the court to function in that capacity.

Involuntary Outpatient Commitment. Beginning in the 1990s, states began to pass legislation that permitted outpatient commitment as an alternative to forced inpatient treatment. Recently states are using involuntary outpatient commitment as a preventive measure, allowing a court order before the onset of a psychiatric crisis that would result in an inpatient commitment. The order for involuntary outpatient commitment is usually tied to receipt of goods and services provided by social welfare agencies, including disability benefits and housing. To access these goods and services the client is mandated to participate in treatment and may face inpatient admission if he or she fails to participate in treatment (Chan, 2003; Monahan, Swartz, & Bonnie, 2003; Rainey, 2001). Forced treatment raises ethical dilemmas regarding autonomy versus paternalism, privacy rights, duty to protect, and right to treatment, and has been challenged on constitutional grounds.

Release from the Hospital

Release from hospitalization depends on the client's admission status. Clients who sought informal or voluntary admission, as previously discussed, have the right to request and receive release. Some states, however, do provide for conditional release of voluntary clients, which enables the treating physician or administrator to order continued treatment on an outpatient basis if the clinical needs of the client warrant further care.

Conditional Release

Conditional release usually requires outpatient treatment for a specified period to determine the client's compliance with medication protocols, ability to meet basic needs, and ability to reintegrate into the community. Generally, a voluntarily hospitalized client who is conditionally released cannot be reinstitutionalized without consent unless the institution complies with the procedures for involuntary hospitalization. However, an involuntarily hospitalized client who is conditionally released may be reinstitutionalized while the commitment is still in effect without recommencement of formal admission procedures.

Discharge

Discharge, or unconditional release, is the termination of a client-institution relationship. This release may be court ordered or administratively ordered by the institution's officials. Generally, the administrative officer of an institution has the discretion to discharge clients.

CLIENT'S RIGHTS UNDER THE LAW

Right to Treatment

With the enactment of the Hospitalization of the Mentally Ill Act in 1964, the federal statutory right to psychiatric treatment in public hospitals was created. The statute requires that medical and psychiatric care and treatment be provided to all persons admitted to a public hospital.

Although state courts and lower federal courts have decided that there may be a federal constitutional right to treatment, the U.S. Supreme Court has never firmly grounded the right to treatment in a constitutional principle. The evolution of these cases in the courts provides an interesting history of the development and shortcomings of our mental health delivery system. Based on the decisions of a number of early court cases, treatment must meet the following criteria:

- The environment must be humane.
- Staff must be qualified and sufficient to provide adequate treatment.
- The plan of care must be individualized.

The initial cases presenting the psychiatric client's right to treatment arose in the criminal justice system. An interesting case regarding a person's right to treatment is *O'Connor v. Donaldson* (1975), described in Box 8-2.

The U.S. Supreme Court, in declining to affirm the lower court's finding of damages and a broad constitutional right to treatment, narrowly defined the issue for consideration: whether or not a finding of mental

---

BOX 8-2

Right to Treatment: *O'Connor v. Donaldson* (1975)

In 1957, Mr. Donaldson was involuntarily committed, on his father's initiation, to a Florida state hospital for care, treatment, and maintenance. For 14 years before his commitment, he was gainfully employed. Despite the fact that Mr. Donaldson posed no danger to himself or others, his requests for ground privileges, occupational training, and an opportunity to discuss his case with the superintendent, Dr. O'Connor, or others were denied. During his 15 years of confinement, he was not provided with any treatment.

Mr. Donaldson frequently requested his release, which the superintendent was authorized to grant even though Mr. Donaldson was lawfully confined, because even if he continued to be mentally ill, he posed no danger to himself or others. Between 1964 and 1968, Mr. Donaldson's friend requested on four separate occasions that Mr. Donaldson be released into his custody. These requests, and requests made by a halfway house on Mr. Donaldson's behalf, were all denied by Dr. O'Connor, who believed that Mr. Donaldson should be released into his parents' custody. Dr. O'Connor further believed that Mr. Donaldson's parents were too old and infirm to care for him adequately.

The court found that Mr. Donaldson's care was merely custodial because he received no treatment. He was not dangerous, community alternatives were available for him, and the physician's refusal to release him was "malicious." The Federal Court of Appeals ruled that Mr. Donaldson had a constitutional right to treatment and awarded him $38,000 in damages.

illness alone can justify the state's indefinite custodial confinement of a mentally ill person against his or her will. The Court held that a "state cannot constitutionally confine a nondangerous individual who is capable of surviving safely in freedom by himself or with the help of willing and responsible family members or friends" (*O'Connor v. Donaldson,* 1975, p. 576).

Right to Refuse Treatment

A corollary to the right to consent to treatment is the right to withhold consent. A client may also withdraw consent at any time. Retraction of consent previously given must be honored, whether it is a verbal or written retraction. However, the mentally ill client's right to refuse treatment with psychotropic drugs has been debated in the courts, based partly on the issue of mental clients' competency to give or withhold consent to treatment and their status under the civil commitment statutes. These early cases, initiated by state hospital clients, considered medical, legal, and ethical considerations, such as basic treatment problems, the doctrine of informed consent, and the bioethical principle of autonomy. For a summary of the evolution of one landmark set of cases regarding the client's right to refuse treatment, see Table 8-1.

In instances in which forcible medication is sought to prevent violence to third persons, to prevent suicide, or to preserve security, the court noted that the medication is being used as a chemical restraint, and the justification for medication thus changes from individual treatment to public protection. Accordingly, the infringement on a person's liberty is at least equal to that with involuntary commitment. In this circumstance, the noninstitutionalized, competent, mentally ill client has the right, through substituted judgment, to determine whether to be involuntarily committed or to be medicated.

In New Jersey, involuntarily committed psychiatric clients also brought a suit in federal court alleging violation of their constitutional rights through forcible administration of antipsychotic drugs. See Table 8-2 for a summary of the evolution of the *Rennie v. Klein* (1979, 1981, 1982, 1983) case.

An interesting study by Schwartz, Vingiano, and Perez (1988) of clients' attitudes after involuntary medication concluded that the decision to refuse treatment was based more on symptoms of the clients' illness rather than on autonomous functioning.

Cases involving the right to refuse psychotropic drug treatment are still evolving. Without clear direction from the Supreme Court, there will be different case outcomes in different jurisdictions.

The numerous cases involving the right to refuse medication have illustrated the complex and difficult task of translating social policy concerns into a clearly articulated legal standard.

Right to Informed Consent

The principle of informed consent is based on a person's right to self-determination, as enunciated in the landmark case of *Canterbury v. Spence* (1972):

TABLE 8-1

Right to Refuse Treatment: Evolution of Massachusetts Case Law to Present Law

Case	Court	Decision
Rogers v. Okin, 478 F. Supp. 1342 (D. Mass. 1979)	Federal district court	Ruled that involuntarily hospitalized clients with mental illness are competent and have the right to make treatment decisions.
		Forcible administration of medication is justified in an emergency if needed to prevent violence and if other alternatives have been ruled out.
		A guardian may make treatment decisions for an incompetent client.
Rogers v. Okin, 634 F.2nd 650 (1st Cir. 1980)	Federal court of appeals	Affirmed that involuntarily hospitalized clients with mental illness are competent and have the right to make treatment decisions.
		The staff has substantial discretion in an emergency.
		Forcible medication is also justified to prevent the client's deterioration.
		A client's rights must be protected by judicial determination of incompetency.
Mills v. Rogers, 457 U.S. 291 (1982)	U.S. Supreme Court	Set aside the judgment of the court of appeals with instructions to consider the effect of an intervening state court case.
Rogers v. Commissioner of the Department of Mental Health, 458 N.E.2d 308 (Mass. 1983)	Massachusetts Supreme Judicial Court answering questions certified by federal court of appeals	Ruled that involuntarily hospitalized clients are competent and have the right to make treatment decisions unless they are judicially determined to be incompetent.

TABLE 8-2

Right to Refuse Treatment: Evolution of New Jersey Case Law to Present Law

Case	Court	Decision
Rennie v. Klein, 476 F. Supp. 1292 (D. N.J. 1979)	Federal district court	Ruled that involuntarily hospitalized clients with mental illness have a qualified constitutional right to refuse treatment with antipsychotic drugs. Voluntarily hospitalized clients have an absolute right to refuse treatment with antipsychotic drugs under New Jersey law.
Rennie v. Klein, 653 F.2d 836 (3d Cir. 1981)	Federal court of appeals	Ruled that involuntarily hospitalized clients with mental illness have a constitutional right to refuse antipsychotic drug treatment. The state may override a client's right when the client poses a danger to self or others. Due process protections must be complied with before forcible medication of clients in nonemergency situations.
Rennie v. Klein, 454 U.S. 1078 (1982)	U.S. Supreme Court	Set aside the judgment of the court of appeals with instructions to consider the case in light of the U.S. Supreme Court decision in *Youngberg v. Romeo.*
Rennie v. Klein, 720 F.2d 266 (3d Cir. 1983)	Federal court of appeals	Ruled that involuntarily hospitalized clients with mental illness have the right to refuse treatment with antipsychotic medication. Decisions to forcibly medicate must be based on "accepted professional judgment" and must comply with due process requirements of the New Jersey regulations.

The root premise is the concept, fundamental in American jurisprudence, that every human being of adult years and sound mind has a right to determine what shall be done with his own body. . . . True consent to what happens to one's self is the informed exercise of choice, and that entails an opportunity to evaluate knowledgeably the options available and the risks attendant on each. (p. 780)

For consent to be effective legally, it must be informed. Generally, the informed consent of the client must be obtained by the physician or other health professional to perform the treatment or procedure. Clients must be informed of the nature of their problem or condition, the nature and purpose of a proposed treatment, the risks and benefits of that treatment, the alternative treatment options, the probability that the proposed treatment will be successful, and the risks of not consenting to treatment. It is important for psychiatric nurses to know that the presence of psychotic thinking does not mean that the client is incompetent or incapable of understanding.

Because psychiatric mental health nursing procedures are generally noninvasive and are commonly understood by the client, the need to obtain informed consent does not occur as frequently for nurses as it does for those providing medical treatment. Many procedures that nurses perform have an element of implied consent attached. For example, if you approach the client with a medication in hand and the client indicates a willingness to receive the medication, implied consent has occurred. A general rule for you to follow is that the more intrusive or risky the procedure, the higher is the likelihood that informed consent must be obtained. The fact that you may not have a legal duty to be the person to inform the client of the associated risks and benefits of a particular medical procedure does not excuse you from clarifying the procedure to the client and ensuring his or her expressed or implied consent.

Rights Surrounding Involuntary Commitment and Psychiatric Advance Directives

Clients concerned that they may be subject to involuntary psychiatric commitment can prepare an advance psychiatric directive document that will express their treatment choices. The advance directive for mental health decision making should be followed by health care providers when the client is not competent to make informed decisions for himself or herself. This document can clarify the client's choice of a surrogate decision maker and instructions about hospital choices, medications, treatment options, and emergency interventions. Clients can, through this document, give their consent to and refuse treatment options, including participation in experimental drug trials. Identification of persons who are to be notified of the client's hospitalization and who may have visitation rights is especially helpful given the privacy demands of HIPAA (Bazelon, 2003).

Rights Regarding Restraint and Seclusion

Legally, behavioral restraint and seclusion are authorized as an intervention under the following circumstances:

- When the particular behavior is physically harmful to the client or a third party
- When alternative or less restrictive measures are insufficient in protecting the client or others from harm
- When a decrease in sensory overstimulation (seclusion only) is needed
- When the client anticipates that a controlled environment would be helpful and requests seclusion

As indicated earlier, most state laws prohibit the use of unnecessary physical restraint or isolation. The use of seclusion and restraint is permitted only under the following circumstances (Simon, 1999):

- On the written order of a physician
- When orders are confined to specific time-limited periods (e.g., 2 to 4 hours)
- When the client's condition is reviewed and documented regularly (e.g., every 15 minutes)
- When the original order is extended after review and reauthorization (e.g., every 24 hours) and specifies the type of restraint

Only in an emergency may the charge nurse place a client in seclusion or restraint and obtain a written or verbal order as soon as possible thereafter. Federal laws require the consent of the client unless an emergency situation exists in which an immediate risk of harm to the client or others can be documented. The client must be removed from restraints when safer and quieter behavior is observed. While in restraints, the client must be protected from all sources of harm. The behavior leading to restraint or seclusion and the time the client is placed in and released from restraint must be documented; the client in restraint must be assessed at regular and frequent intervals (e.g., every 15 to 30 minutes) for physical needs (food, hydration, toileting), safety, and comfort, and these observations must also be documented (every 15 to 30 minutes).

Restraint and seclusion should never be used as punishment or for the convenience of the staff. For example, if the unit is short staffed, restraining clients to protect them while you pass medications is an inappropriate use of restraints.

Use of the least restrictive means of restraint for the shortest duration is always the general rule. Verbal interventions are the first approach; restraints are used only to prevent harm or to provide benefit to the client. Chemical restraints are more subtle than physical restraints but can have a greater impact on the client's ability to relate to the environment. The psychiatric mental health nurse must be aware of the severe and powerful impact of chemical restraints on psychiatric clients. The client's personality and ability to relate to others is greatly controlled by chemical restraints. The practice of secluding a client is comparable with the practice of sedating a client until the client is secluded within himself or herself.

An example of the misuse of chemical restraints is a case in which a verbally abusive or pacing client is deeply sedated and placed in his or her room to control the unit's environment. You must always be able to document professional judgment regarding the use of physical or chemical restraint, as well as the use of seclusion.

With recent changes in the law regarding the use of restraint and seclusion that require a client's consent to be restrained, agencies have revised their policies and procedures, greatly limiting these practices of the past. Most agencies have found no negative impact associated with the reduced use of restraints and seclusion. Alternative methods of therapy and cooperation with the client have been successful.

Nurses also need to know under which circumstances the use of seclusion and restraints is contraindicated (Box 8-3).

MAINTENANCE OF CLIENT CONFIDENTIALITY

Ethical Considerations

The ANA *Code of Ethics for Nurses* (2001) asserts the duty of the nurse to protect confidential client information. Failure to provide this protection may harm the nurse-client relationship, as well as the client's well-being. However, the code clarifies that this duty is not absolute. In some situations disclosure may be mandated to protect the client, other persons, or the public health.

BOX 8-3

Contraindications to Seclusion and Restraint

- Extremely unstable medical and psychiatric conditions*
- Delirium or dementia leading to inability to tolerate decreased stimulation*
- Severe suicidal tendencies*
- Severe drug reactions or overdoses or need for close monitoring of drug dosages*
- Desire for punishment of client or convenience of staff

From Simon, R. I. (2001). *Concise guide to psychiatry and law for clinicians* (3rd ed., p. 117). Washington, DC: American Psychiatric Press. Copyright 2001, American Psychiatric Press.
*Unless close supervision and direct observation are provided.

Legal Considerations

Health Insurance Portability and Accountability Act

The psychiatric client's right to receive treatment and to have medical records kept confidential is legally protected. The fundamental principle underlying the ANA code on confidentiality is a person's constitutional right to privacy. Generally, your legal duty to maintain confidentiality is to act to protect the client's right to privacy. The HIPAA privacy rule became effective on April 14, 2003. Therefore, you may not, without the client's consent, disclose information obtained from the client or information in the medical record to anyone except those persons for whom it is necessary for implementation of the client's treatment plan. Special protection of notes used in psychotherapy that are kept separate from the client's health information was created by this HIPAA rule (2003).

Client's Employer

For example, your release of information to the client's employer about the client's condition, without the client's consent, is a breach of confidentiality that subjects you to liability for the tort of invasion of privacy as well as a HIPAA violation. On the other hand, discussion of a client's history with other staff members to determine a consistent treatment approach is not a breach of confidentiality.

Generally, for a situation to be created in which information is privileged, a client–health professional relationship must exist and the information must concern the care and treatment of the client. The health professional may refuse to disclose information to protect the client's privacy. However, the right to privacy is the client's right, and health professionals cannot invoke confidentiality for their own defense or benefit.

Rights After Death

A person's reputation can be damaged even after death. It is therefore important not to divulge information after a person's death that could not have been legally shared before the death. The Dead Man's Statute protects confidential information about people when they are not alive to speak for themselves.

A legal privilege of confidentiality is enacted legislatively and exists to protect the confidentiality of professional communications (e.g., nurse-client, physician-client, attorney-client). The theory behind such privileged communications is that clients will not be comfortable or willing to disclose personal information about themselves if they fear that nurses will repeat their confidential conversations.

In some states in which the legal privilege of confidentiality has not been legislated for nurses, you must respond to a court's inquiries regarding the client's disclosures even if this information implicates the client in a crime. In these states, the confidentiality of communications cannot be guaranteed. If a duty to report exists, you may be required to divulge private information shared by the client.

Client Privilege and Human Immunodeficiency Virus Status

Some states have enacted mandatory or permissive statutes that direct health care providers to warn a spouse if a partner tests positive for human immunodeficiency virus (Table 8-3). Nurses must understand the laws in their jurisdiction of practice regarding privileged communications and warnings of infectious disease exposure.

Exceptions to the Rule

Duty to Warn and Protect Third Parties

The California Supreme Court, in its 1974 landmark decision *Tarasoff v. Regents of University of California*, ruled that a psychotherapist has a duty to warn a client's potential victim of potential harm. This decision created much controversy and confusion in the psychiatric and medical communities over breach of client confidentiality and its impact on the therapeutic relationship in psychiatric care and over the ability of the psychotherapist to predict when a client is truly dangerous. This trend continues as other jurisdictions have adopted or modified the California rule despite the objections of the psychiatric community. These jurisdictions view public safety to be more important than privacy in narrowly defined circumstances.

The *Tarasoff* case acknowledged that generally there is no common law duty to aid third persons. An exception is when special relationships exist, and the court found the client-therapist relationship sufficient to create a duty of the therapist to aid Ms. Tarasoff, the victim. The duty to protect the intended victim from danger arises when the therapist determines—or, pursuant to professional standards, should have determined—that the client presents a serious danger to another. Any action reasonably necessary under the circumstances, including notification of the potential victim, the victim's family, and the police, discharges the therapist's duty to the potential victim.

In 1976, the California Supreme Court issued a second ruling in the case of *Tarasoff v. Regents of University of California* (now known as *Tarasoff II*). This ruling broadened the earlier ruling, the duty to warn, to include the **duty to protect.**

Most states currently have similar laws regarding the duty to warn third parties of potential life threats. The duty to warn usually includes the following:

- Assessing and predicting the client's danger of violence toward another

TABLE 8-3

Legal Issues Involving Human Immunodeficiency Virus (HIV) Status and Psychiatric Mental Health Nursing

Issue	The Law
Involuntary HIV testing of psychiatric clients	Consent of the psychiatric client must be sought to test blood for HIV. Substitute decision making applies only to children aged 13 years or younger and to involuntarily committed adult psychiatric clients (Lo, 1989).
Involuntary confinement of a psychiatric client who is HIV positive and having sex with other clients	Knowing transmission of HIV through sexual contact is prohibited by law. The institution has the legal means to prohibit such contact. The Illinois Supreme Court held that a statute prohibiting a person from knowingly transmitting HIV was constitutional (*Illinois v. Russel*, 1994).
Duty to warn the partner of a psychiatric client who is HIV positive	In 1988, New York and California enacted laws permitting notification of contacts of HIV persons. These laws require that the informant persuade the client to allow notification without disclosing the identity of the client. Alternatively, public health officials may be asked to notify contacts. Recent statutes, however, do not require notification but encourage voluntary notification (Lo, 1989).
Disclosure of a psychiatric client's HIV status by the nurse to an unauthorized person	The Arkansas Supreme Court held that a nurse's disclosure of information about a man's HIV test result to an unauthorized third party did not constitute medical malpractice (*Wyatt v. St. Paul Fire & Marine Ins. Co.*, 1994).
Psychiatric nurses' refusal to care for an HIV-positive client	In general, nurses have no legal duty to care for HIV-positive psychiatric clients. However, moral obligation, employment contracts, and professional and ethical standards may impose some obligation on the nurse to care for HIV-positive clients.
Psychiatric nurses' duty to inform their employers of their HIV status	While HIV-positive psychiatric nurses have a moral obligation to inform their employers of their HIV status, their right to privacy should be balanced with the risk of infection to co-workers or clients who come under their care.
Nurses' claims based on emotional distress caused by exposure to acquired immunodeficiency syndrome (AIDS) or needlestick	In *Tischler v. DiMenna* (1994), a New York court recognized claims for damages for emotional distress caused by exposure to AIDS. Moreover, the Montana Supreme Court held that the state Worker's Compensation Act provided the exclusive remedy for a former employee who developed a fear of AIDS after being punctured by a needle (*Blythe v. Radiometer America, Inc.*, 1993).

From Constantino, R. E. B. (1996). Legal issues in psychiatric–mental health nursing. In S. Lego (Ed.), *Psychiatric nursing: A comprehensive reference* (2nd ed.). Philadelphia: Lippincott.

- Identifying the specific persons being threatened
- Taking appropriate action to protect the identified victims

Nursing Implications. As this trend toward making it the therapist's duty to warn third persons of potential harm continues to gain wider acceptance, it is important for students and nurses to understand its implications for nursing practice. Although none of these cases has dealt with nurses, it is fair to assume that in jurisdictions that have adopted the *Tarasoff* doctrine, the duty to warn third persons will be applied to advanced practice psychiatric mental health nurses in private practice who engage in individual therapy.

If, however, a staff nurse who is a member of a team of psychiatrists, psychologists, psychiatric social workers, and other psychiatric nurses does not report client threats of harm against specified victims or classes of victims to the team of the client's management psychotherapist for assessment and evaluation, this failure is likely to be considered substandard nursing care.

So, too, the failure to communicate and record relevant information from police, relatives, or the client's old records might also be deemed negligent. Breach of client-nurse confidentiality should not pose ethical or legal dilemmas for nurses in these situations, because a team approach to the delivery of psychiatric care presumes communication of pertinent information to other staff members to develop a treatment plan in the client's best interest.

Child and Elder Abuse Reporting Statutes

Because of their interest in protecting children, all 50 states and the District of Columbia have enacted child abuse reporting statutes. Although these statutes differ from state to state, they generally include a definition of child abuse, a list of persons required or encouraged to report abuse, and the governmental agency designated to receive and investigate the reports. Most statutes include civil penalties for failure to report. Many states specifically require nurses to report cases of suspected abuse.

There is a conflict between federal and state laws with respect to child abuse reporting when the health care professional discovers child abuse or neglect during the suspected abuser's alcohol or drug treatment. Federal laws and regulations governing confidentiality of client records, which apply to almost all drug abuse and alcohol treatment providers, prohibit any disclosure without a court order. In this case, federal law supersedes state reporting laws, although compliance with the state law may be maintained under the following circumstances:

- If a court order is obtained, pursuant to the regulations
- If a report can be made without identifying the abuser as a client in an alcohol or drug treatment program
- If the report is made anonymously (some states, to protect the rights of the accused, do not allow anonymous reporting)

As reported incidents of abuse to other persons in society surface, states may require health professionals to report other kinds of abuse. A growing number of states are enacting elder abuse reporting statutes, which require registered nurses (RNs) and others to report cases of abuse of the elderly. The elderly are defined as adults 65 years of age and older. These laws also apply to dependent adults—that is, adults between 18 and 64 years of age whose physical or mental limitations restrict their ability to carry out normal activities or to protect themselves—when the RN has actual knowledge that the person has been the victim of physical abuse.

Under most state laws, a person who is required to report suspected abuse, neglect, or exploitation of a disabled adult and who willfully does not do so is guilty of a misdemeanor crime. Most state statutes declare that anyone who makes a report in good faith is immune from civil liability in connection with the report.

You may also report knowledge of, or reasonable suspicion of, mental abuse or suffering. Both dependent adults and elders are protected by the law from purposeful physical or fiduciary neglect or abandonment. **Because state laws vary, students are encouraged to become conversant with the requirements of their states.**

TORT LAW APPLIED TO PSYCHIATRIC SETTINGS

Torts are a category of civil law that commonly applies to health care practice. A tort is a civil wrong for which money damages may be collected by the injured party (the plaintiff) from the wrongdoer (the defendant). The injury can be to person, property, or reputation. Because tort law has general applicability to nursing practice, this section may contain a review of material previously covered elsewhere in your nursing curriculum.

Nurses are more likely to encounter provocative, threatening, or violent behavior in a psychiatric setting than in other care settings. Such behavior may require the use of restraint or seclusion until a client demonstrates quieter and safer behavior. Accordingly, the nurse in the psychiatric setting should understand the **intentional torts** of battery, assault, and false imprisonment, described more fully later in this chapter.

Common Liability Issues

Protection of Clients

Legal issues common in psychiatric nursing relate to the failure to protect the safety of clients. If a suicidal client is left alone with the means to harm himself or herself, the nurse who has a duty to protect the client will be held responsible for the resultant injuries. Leaving a suicidal client alone in a room on the sixth floor with an open window is an example of unreasonable judgment on the part of the nurse. Precautions to prevent harm must be taken whenever a client is restrained. Miscommunications and medication errors are common in all areas of nursing, including psychiatric care. A common area of liability in psychiatry is abuse of the therapist-client relationship. Issues of sexual misconduct during the therapeutic relationship have become a source of concern in the psychiatric community. Misdiagnosis is also frequently charged in legal suits.

Defamation of Character

Charges of defamation of character, either written (libel) or oral (slander), can be brought if confidential information regarding a client is divulged that harms his or her reputation. The privacy protections afforded all clients by the law are especially protective of the rights of psychiatric clients.

Supervisory Liability

Supervisory liability may be incurred if nursing duties are delegated to persons who cannot safely perform these duties. The nurse who does not verify that the assistive personnel can safely and appropriately provide the care being delegated will be held vicariously liable for any harm or injury the client suffers. Supervision of assistive personnel is essential.

Short-Staffing Issues

Short-staffing issues have raised concerns about client safety as well as about delegation of care to assistive personnel. A study by the ANA (1996) found that hospitalized clients have better outcomes in hospitals with higher ratios of RNs. The study concluded that care provided by registered nurses makes a significant difference in reducing complications and discharging clients well on the road to recovery.

The Joint Commission on Accreditation of Healthcare Organizations (2004) requires the collection of clinical and human resource indicators for analysis of staffing effectiveness.

In October 1999, California became the first state to mandate nurse/client ratios. ANA supports the approach suggested in a bill proposed in 2003, the Registered Nurse Safe Staffing Act. This act would require input on staffing from RNs and provide whistleblower protection for nurses who report client care issues (Mandatory nurse/client ratios, 2003).

If you believe that a staffing pattern is not allowing appropriate and reasonable care, a written appeal to the nursing supervisor and the institution will document your concerns. Nurses should not perform tasks for which they are not prepared, including the assumption of responsibility for the safety and care of an unreasonable number of clients. If the institution is unwilling to correct an unsafe situation, you must determine whether you wish to remain employed and incur possible liability if a client for whom you are ultimately responsible is injured. Proper channels of appeal must be followed to avoid charges of insubordination and possible firing. Institutional policies should outline the correct procedure for voicing a reasonable grievance.

Note, however, that the ANA believes that nurses should reject assignments that put clients or themselves in serious immediate jeopardy, even when there is not a specific legal protection for rejecting such an assignment (ANA, 1996).

Some guidelines for avoiding liability include the following:

1. Always put the client's rights and welfare first.
2. Comply with the rules and regulations in the hospital's or agency's policy manual.
3. Practice within the scope of the nurse practice act.
4. Maintain current understanding and knowledge of established practice standards.
5. Keep accurate, concise, and timely nursing records.

Intentional Torts

Some torts can also carry criminal penalties. An **intentional tort** is a voluntary act performed with the intent to bring about a physical consequence. In the most basic terms, a voluntary act is a voluntary movement of the body. The requirement for intent is met when the defendant acts purposefully to achieve a result or is substantially certain that the result will occur. If the injured party consents to participate in an act, there can be no intentional tort. Likewise, self-defense and defense of others are privileges that can be used to defend successfully against a court action for intentional tort.

Reckless behavior may be classified as intentional or negligent. Malpractice actions typically result from negligent behavior. For example, the foreseeability that a suicidal client will harm himself or herself if left alone with sharp objects or in a room with an open window is great enough for negligence to be found on the part of the nurse, who has a duty to protect the client. If the nurse left the client alone knowing of the likelihood of self-harm, an intentional act could be argued. It would not be a wise nursing judgment to test the suicidal client's ability to be left alone with dangers in the immediate environment.

Assault and Battery

In legal terms, an **assault** is an act resulting in a person's apprehension of an immediate harmful or offensive touching (battery). In an assault, there is no physical contact. The aggressor's act must amount to a threat to use force, although threatening words alone are not enough. The aggressor must also have the opportunity and the ability to carry out the threatened act immediately. A **battery** is a harmful or offensive touching of another's person. For example, the nurse approaches the client with a restraint in hand. The client's behavior does not pose an immediate danger to self or others, and the client fearfully pleads not to be restrained. If the nurse proceeds to apply the restraints, both an assault and a battery may be charged against the nurse.

False Imprisonment

False imprisonment is an act with the intent to confine a person to a specific area. The use of seclusion or restraint that is not defensible as being necessary and in the client's best interest may result in false imprisonment of the client and liability for the nurse. As another example, if a psychiatric client wants to leave the hospital and the nurse prohibits the client from leaving, the nurse may have falsely imprisoned the client if the client was voluntarily admitted and if there are no agency or legal policies for detaining the client. On the other hand, if the client was involuntarily admitted or had agreed to an evaluation before discharge, the nurse's actions would be reasonable.

Punitive Damages

Punitive damages may be recoverable by an injured party in an intentional tort action. Because these damages are designed to punish and make an example, punitive damage awards can be very large. Often, the actual damages experienced by the plaintiff's are insignificant, and nominal damages may be awarded in the sum of $1.00. Intentional acts are not covered by malpractice insurance, however, and for this reason intentional torts are a less attractive avenue of liability for injured clients to pursue in lawsuits against health professionals and hospitals. The case of *Plumadore v. State* *of New York* (1980), described in Box 8-4, illustrates the use of intentional tort in the psychiatric setting.

Violence

Violent behavior is not acceptable in our society. Nurses must protect themselves in both institutional and community settings. Employers are not typically held responsible for employee injuries due to violent client behavior. Nurses have placed themselves knowingly in the range of danger by agreeing to care for unpredictable clients. It is therefore important for nurses to protect themselves by participating in setting policies that create a safe environment. Good judgment means not placing oneself in a potentially violent situation. Nurses, as citizens, have the same rights as clients not to be threatened or harmed. Appropriate security support should be readily available to the nurse practicing in an institution. When you work in community settings, you must avoid placing yourself unnecessarily in dangerous environments, especially when alone at night. You should use common sense

---

BOX 8-4

False Imprisonment and Negligence: *Plumadore v. State of New York* (1980)

Mrs. Plumadore was admitted to Saranac Lake General Hospital for a gallbladder condition. Her medical workup revealed emotional problems stemming from marital difficulties, which had resulted in suicide attempts several years before her admission. After a series of consultations and tests, she was advised by the attending surgeon that she was scheduled to have gallbladder surgery later that day. After the surgeon's visit, a consulting psychiatrist who examined her directed her to dress and pack her belongings because he had arranged to have her admitted to a state hospital at Ogdensburg.

Subsequently, two uniformed state troopers handcuffed her and strapped her into the back seat of a patrol car. She was also accompanied by a female hospital employee and was transported to the state hospital. On arrival, the admitting psychiatrist recognized that the referring psychiatrist lacked the requisite authority to order her involuntary commitment. He therefore requested that she sign a voluntary admission form, which she refused to do. Despite Mrs. Plumadore's protests regarding her admission to the state hospital, the psychiatrist assigned her to a ward without physical or psychiatric examination and without the opportunity to contact her family or her medical doctor. The record of her admission to the state hospital noted an "informed admission," which is client-initiated voluntary admission in New York.

The court awarded $40,000 to Mrs. Plumadore for false imprisonment, negligence, and malpractice.

---

and enlist the support of local law enforcement officers when needed. A violent client is not being abandoned if placed safely in the hands of the authorities.

The psychiatric mental health nurse must also be aware of the potential for violence in the community when a client is discharged following a short-term stay. The duty of the nurse to protect both the client and others who may be threatened by the violent client is discussed in the section Duty to Warn and Protect Third Parties later in this chapter. The nurse's assessment of the client's potential for violence must be documented and acted on if there is legitimate concern regarding discharge of a client who is discussing or exhibiting potentially violent behavior. The psychiatric mental health nurse must communicate his or her observations to the medical staff when discharge decisions are being considered.

There may be situations in which your duty is to protect not only the client but also, indirectly, third parties, when the client, because of his or her mental or physical condition, presents a risk of harm to that third party.

Negligence

Negligence is an act or an omission to act that breaches the duty of due care and results in or is responsible for a person's injuries. The five elements required to prove negligence are (1) duty, (2) breach of duty, (3) cause in fact, (4) proximate cause, and (5) damages. Foreseeability of harm is also evaluated.

Duty is measured by a standard of care. When nurses represent themselves as being capable of caring for psychiatric clients and accept employment, a duty of care has been assumed. The duty is owed to psychiatric clients to understand the theory and medications used in the specialty care of these clients. Persons who represent themselves as possessing superior knowledge and skill, such as psychiatric nurse specialists, are held to a higher standard of care in the practice of their profession. The staff nurse who is assigned to a psychiatric unit must be knowledgeable enough to assume a reasonable or safe duty of care for the clients.

If you are not capable of providing the standard of care that other nurses would be expected to supply under similar circumstances, you have breached the duty of care. **Breach of duty** is the conduct that exposes the client to an unreasonable risk of harm, through either commission or omission of acts by the nurse. If you do not have the required education and experience to provide certain interventions, you have breached the duty by neglecting or omitting to provide necessary care. You can also act in such a way that the client is harmed and can thus be guilty of negligence through acts of commission.

Cause in fact may be evaluated by asking the question, "Except for what the nurse did, would this injury have occurred?" **Proximate cause,** or legal cause, may be evaluated by determining whether there were any intervening actions or persons that were, in fact, the causes of harm to the client. **Damages** include actual damages (e.g., loss of earnings, medical expenses, and property damage) as well as pain and suffering.

DETERMINATION OF A STANDARD OF CARE

Professional standards of practice determined by professional associations differ from the standards embodied in the minimal qualifications set forth by state licensure for entry into the profession of nursing. The ANA has established standards for psychiatric mental health nursing practice and credentialing for the psychiatric mental health RN and the advanced practice RN in psychiatric mental health nursing (ANA et al., 2000).

Standards for psychiatric mental health nursing practice differ markedly from minimal state requirements because the primary purposes for setting these two types of standards are different. The state's qualifications for practice provide consumer protection by ensuring that all practicing nurses have successfully completed an approved nursing program and passed the national licensing examination. The professional association's primary focus is to elevate the practice of its members by setting standards of excellence. The Standards of Care from the *Scope and Standards of Psychiatric-Mental Health Nursing Practice* are provided on the inside back cover of this book.

Nurses are held to the standard of care provided by other nurses possessing the same degree of skill or knowledge in the same or similar circumstances. In the past, community standards existed for urban and rural agencies. However, with greater mobility and expanded means of communication, national standards have evolved. Psychiatric clients have the right to the standard of care recognized by professional bodies governing nursing, whether they are in a large or a small, a rural or an urban, facility. Nurses must participate in continuing education courses to stay current with existing standards of care.

Hospital policies and procedures set up institutional criteria for care, and these criteria, such as the frequency of rounds for clients in seclusion, may be introduced to prove a standard that the nurse met or failed to meet. The shortcoming of this method is that the hospital's policy may be substandard. For example, the state licensing laws for institutions might set a minimal requirement for staffing or frequency of rounds for certain clients, and the hospital policy might fall below that minimum. **Substandard institutional policies do not absolve the individual nurse of responsibility to practice on the basis of professional standards of nursing care.**

Like hospital policy and procedures, custom can be used as evidence of a standard of care. For example, in the absence of a written policy on the use of restraint, testimony might be offered regarding the customary use of restraint in emergency situations in which the combative, violent, or confused client poses a threat of harm to self or others. Using custom to establish a standard of care may result in the same defect as in using hospital policies and procedures: custom may not comply with the laws, recommendations of the accrediting body, or other recognized standards of care. Custom must be carefully and regularly evaluated to ensure that substandard routines have not developed. Substandard customs do not protect you when a psychiatric client charges that a right has been violated or that harm has been caused by the staff's common practices.

Guidelines for Nurses Who Suspect Negligence

It is not unusual for a student or practicing nurse to suspect negligence on the part of a peer. In most states, as a nurse you have a legal duty to report such risks of harm to the client. It is also important that you document the evidence clearly and accurately before making serious accusations against a peer. If you question a physician's orders or actions, or those of a fellow nurse, it is wise to communicate these concerns directly to the person involved. If the risky behavior continues, you have an obligation to communicate these concerns to a supervisor, who should then intervene to ensure that the client's rights and well-being are protected. If you suspect a peer of being chemically impaired or of practicing irresponsibly, you have an obligation to protect not only the rights of the peer but also the rights of all clients who could be harmed by this impaired peer. If, after you have reported suspected behavior of concern to a supervisor, the danger persists, you have a duty to report the concern to someone at the next level of authority. It is important to follow the channels of communication in an organization, but it is also important to protect the safety of the clients. If the supervisor's actions or inactions do not rectify the dangerous situation, you have a continuing duty to report the behavior of concern to the appropriate authority, such as the state board of nursing.

A useful reference for nurses is the ANA's *Guidelines on Reporting Incompetent, Unethical, or Illegal Practices* (1994).

Duty to Intervene and Duty to Report

The psychiatric mental health nurse has a duty to intervene when the safety or well-being of the client or another person is obviously at risk. A nurse who follows an order that is known to be incorrect or that the nurse believes will harm the client is responsible for the harm that results to the client. **If you have information that leads you to believe that the physician's orders need to be clarified or changed, it is your duty to intervene and protect the client.** It is important that you communicate with the physician who has ordered the treatment to explain the concern. If the treating physician does not appear willing to consider your concerns, you should carry out the duty to intervene through other appropriate channels.

It is important for you to express your concerns to the supervisor to allow the supervisor to communicate with the appropriate medical staff for intervention in the physician's treatment plan. As the client's advocate, you have a duty to intervene to protect the client; at the same time, you do not have the right to interfere with the physician-client relationship.

It is also important to follow agency policies and procedures for communicating differences of opinion. If you fail to intervene and the client is injured, you may be partly liable for the injuries that result because of failure to use safe nursing practice and good professional judgment.

The legal concept of **abandonment** may also arise when a nurse does not leave a client safely back in the hands of another health professional before discontinuing treatment. Abandonment issues arise when accurate, timely, and thorough reporting has not occurred or when follow-through of client care, on which the client is relying, has not occurred. The same principles apply for the psychiatric mental health nurse who is working in a community setting. For example, if a suicidal client refuses to come to the hospital for treatment, you cannot abandon the client but must take the necessary steps to ensure the client's safety. These actions may include enlisting the assistance of the law in temporarily involuntarily committing the client.

The duty to intervene on the client's behalf poses many legal and ethical dilemmas for nurses in the workplace. Institutions that have a chain-of-command policy or other reporting mechanisms offer some assurance that the proper authorities in the administration are notified. Most client care issues regarding physicians' orders or treatments can be settled fairly early in the process by the nurse's discussion of the concerns with the physician. If further intervention by the nurse is required to protect the client, the next step in the chain of command can be followed. Generally, the nurse then notifies the immediate nursing supervisor; the supervisor thereupon discusses the problem with the physician, and then with the chief of staff of a particular service, until a resolution is reached. If there is no time to resolve the issue through the normal process because of the life-threatening nature of the situation, the nurse must act to protect the client's life.

Unethical or Illegal Practices

The issues become more complex when a professional colleague's conduct, including that of a student nurse, is criminally unlawful. Specific examples include the diversion of drugs from the hospital and sexual misconduct with clients. Increasing media attention and the recognition of substance abuse as an occupational hazard for health professionals have led to the establishment of substance abuse programs for health care workers in many states. These programs provide appropriate treatment for impaired professionals to protect the public from harm and to rehabilitate the professional.

The problem previously discussed—of reporting impaired colleagues—becomes a difficult one, particularly when no direct harm has occurred to the client. Concern for professional reputations, damaged careers, and personal privacy rather than public protection has generated a code of silence regarding substance abuse among health professionals.

Several states now require reporting of impaired or incompetent colleagues to the professional licensing boards. In the absence of such a legal mandate, the questions of whether to report and to whom to report become ethical ones. You are again urged to use the ANA's *Guidelines on Reporting Incompetent, Unethical, or Illegal Practices* (1994). Chapter 27 deals more fully with issues related to the chemically impaired nurse.

The duty to intervene includes the duty to report known abusive behavior. Most states have enacted statutes to protect children and the elderly from abuse and neglect. Psychiatric mental health nurses working in the community may be required by law to report unsafe relationships they discover.

DOCUMENTATION OF CARE

Purpose of Medical Records

The purpose of the medical record is to provide accurate and complete information about the care and treatment of clients and to give health care personnel responsible for that care a means of communicating with each other. The medical record allows for continuity of care. A record's usefulness is determined by evaluating, when the record is read later, how accurately and completely it portrays the client's behavioral status at the time it was written. The client has the right to see the chart, but the chart belongs to the institution. The client must follow appropriate protocol to view his or her records.

For example, if a psychiatric client describes to a nurse a plan to harm himself or herself or another person and that nurse fails to document the information, including the need to protect the client or the identified victim, the information will be lost when the nurse leaves work, and the client's plan may be carried out.

The harm caused could be linked directly to the nurse's failure to communicate this important information. Even though documentation takes time away from the client, the importance of communicating and preserving the nurse's memory through the medical record cannot be overemphasized.

Accrediting agencies, such as the Joint Commission on Accreditation of Healthcare Organizations, and state regulatory agencies require health care facilities to maintain records on clients' care and treatment. Noncompliance with record-keeping responsibilities may result in fines, loss of accreditation, or both.

Facility Use of Medical Records

The medical record has many other uses aside from providing information on the course of the client's care and treatment to health care professionals. A retrospective chart review can provide valuable information to the facility on the quality of care provided and on ways to improve that care. A facility may conduct reviews for risk management purposes to determine areas of potential liability for the facility and to evaluate methods used to reduce the facility's exposure to liability. For example, documentation of the use of restraints and seclusion for psychiatric clients may be reviewed by risk managers. Accordingly, the chart may be used to evaluate care for quality assurance or peer review. Utilization review analysts review the chart to determine appropriate use of hospital and staff resources consistent with reimbursement schedules. Insurance companies and other reimbursement agencies rely on the medical record in determining what payments they will make on the client's behalf.

Medical Records as Evidence

From a legal perspective, the chart is a recording of data and opinions made in the normal course of the client's hospital care. It is deemed to be good evidence because it is presumed to be true, honest, and untainted by memory lapses. Accordingly, the medical record finds its way into a variety of legal cases for a variety of reasons. Some examples of its use include determining (1) the extent of the client's damages and pain and suffering in personal injury cases, such as when a psychiatric client attempts suicide while under the protective care of a hospital; (2) the nature and extent of injuries in child abuse or elder abuse cases; (3) the nature and extent of physical or mental disability in disability cases; and (4) the nature and extent of injury and rehabilitative potential in workers' compensation cases.

Medical records may also be used in police investigations, civil conservatorship proceedings, competency hearings, and commitment procedures. In states that mandate mental health legal services or a clients' rights advocacy program, audits may be performed to determine the facility's compliance with state laws or violation of clients' rights. Finally, medical records may be used in professional and hospital negligence cases.

During the discovery phase of litigation, the medical record is a pivotal source of information for attorneys in determining whether a cause of action exists in a professional negligence or hospital negligence case. Evidence of the nursing care rendered will be found in what the nurse charted.

Nursing Guidelines for Computerized Charting

Accurate, descriptive, and legible nursing notes serve the best interests of the client, the nurse, and the institution. As computerized charting becomes more widely available, it will also be important for psychiatric mental health nurses to understand how to protect the confidentiality of these records. Institutions must also protect against intrusions into the privacy of the client record systems.

Computerized charting is becoming common practice across our country. Concerns for the privacy of the legitimate client's records have been addressed legally by federal laws that provide guidelines for agencies that use computerized charting. These guidelines include the recommendation that staff be assigned a password for entering clients' records to identify which staff have gained access to clients' confidential information. There are penalties, including grounds for firing the staff, if they enter a record for which they are not authorized to have access. Only those staff who have a legitimate need to know about the client are authorized to access a client's computerized chart. It is important for you to keep your password private and never to allow someone else to access a record under your password. You are responsible for all entries into records using your password. The various systems used allow specific time frames within which the nurse must make any necessary corrections if a charting error is made.

Any charting method that improves communication between care providers should be encouraged. Courts assume that nurses and physicians read each other's notes on client progress. Many courts take the attitude that, if care is not documented, it did not occur. Your charting also serves as a valuable memory refresher if the client sues years after the care is rendered. In providing complete and timely information on the care and treatment of clients, the medical record enhances communication among health professionals. Internal institutional audits of the record can improve the quality of care rendered. Nurses' charting is improved by following the guidelines in Box 9-5. Chapter 9 describes common charting forms and gives examples as well as the pros and cons of each.

■ ■ ■ KEY POINTS to REMEMBER

- The states' power to enact laws for public health and safety and for the care of those unable to care for themselves often pits the rights of society against the rights of the individual.
- Psychiatric nurses frequently encounter problems requiring ethical choices.
- The nurse's privilege to practice nursing carries with it the responsibility to practice safely, competently, and in a manner consistent with state and federal laws.

- Knowledge of the law and the ANA *Code of Ethics for Nurses* and Standards of Care from the *Scope and Standards of Psychiatric-Mental Health Nursing Practice* are essential to provide safe, effective psychiatric nursing care and will serve as a framework for decision making when the nurse is presented with complex problems involving competing interests.

■ ■ ■

Visit the Evolve website at **http://evolve.elsevier.com/Varcarolis** for a posttest on the content in this chapter.

Critical Thinking and Chapter Review

Visit the Evolve website at **http://evolve.elsevier.com/Varcarolis** for additional self-study exercises.

■ ■ ■ CRITICAL THINKING

1. Two nurses, Joe and Beth, have worked on the psychiatric unit for 2 years. During the past 6 months, Beth has confided to Joe that she has been experiencing a particularly difficult marital situation. Joe has observed that over the 6 months Beth has become increasingly irritable and difficult to work with. He notices that minor tranquilizers are frequently missing from the unit dose cart on the evening shift. He complains to the pharmacy and is informed that the drugs were stocked as ordered. Several clients state that they have not been receiving their usual drugs. Joe finds that Beth has recorded that the drugs have been given as ordered. He also notices that Beth is diverting the drugs.
   A. What action, if any, should Joe take?
   B. Should Joe confront Beth with his suspicions?
   C. If Beth admits that she has been diverting the drugs, should Joe's next step be to report Beth to the supervisor or to the board of nursing?
   D. Should Joe make his concern known to the nursing supervisor directly by identifying Beth, or should he state his concerns in general terms?
   E. Legally, must Joe report his suspicions to the board of nursing?
   F. Does the fact that harm to the clients is limited to increased agitation affect your responses?

2. Nurse A has worked in a psychiatric setting for 5 years, since she was licensed as a registered nurse by the state. She arrives at work on her unit and is informed that the nursing office has requested a nurse from the psychiatric unit to assist the intensive care unit staff in caring for an agitated car accident victim with a history of schizophrenia. Nurse A works with Nurse B in caring for the client. While the client is sleeping, Nurse B leaves the unit for a coffee break. Nurse A, unfamiliar with the telemetry equipment, fails to recognize an arrhythmia, and the client experiences cardiopulmonary arrest. The client is successfully resuscitated after 6 minutes but suffers permanent brain damage.
   A. Can Nurse A legally practice? (That is, does her license permit her to practice in the intensive care unit?)
   B. Does the ability to practice legally in an area differ from the ability to practice competently in that area?
   C. Did Nurse A have any legal or ethical grounds to refuse the assignment to the intensive care unit?
   D. What are the risks in accepting an assignment in an area of specialty in which you are professionally unprepared to practice?
   E. What are the risks in refusing an assignment in an area of specialty in which you are professionally unprepared to practice?
   F. Would there have been any way for Nurse A to minimize the risk of action for insubordination by the employer had she refused the assignment?
   G. What action could Nurse A have taken to protect the client and herself when Nurse B left the unit for a coffee break?
   H. If Nurse A is negligent, is the hospital liable for any harm to the client caused by Nurse A?

3. A 40-year-old man who is admitted to the emergency department for a severe nosebleed has both nares packed. Because of his history of alcoholism and the probability of ensuing delirium tremens, the client is transferred to the psychiatric unit. He is admitted to a private room, placed in restraints, and checked by a nurse every hour per physician's orders. While unattended, the client suffocates, apparently by inhaling the nasal packing, which had become dislodged from the nares. On the next 1-hour check, the nurse finds the client without pulse or respiration.

   A state statute requires that a restrained client on a psychiatric unit be assessed by a nurse every hour for safety, comfort, and physical needs.
   A. If standards are not otherwise specified, do statutory requirements set forth minimal or maximal standards?
   B. Does the nurse's compliance with the state statute relieve him or her of liability in the client's death?
   C. Does the nurse's compliance with the physician's orders relieve him or her of liability in the client's death?

Continued

Critical Thinking and Chapter Review—cont'd

Visit the Evolve website at **http://evolve.elsevier.com/Varcarolis** for additional self-study exercises.

evolve

D. Was the order for the restraint appropriate for this type of client?

E. What factors did you consider in making your determination?

F. Was the frequency of rounds for assessment of client needs appropriate in this situation?

G. Did the nurse's conduct meet the standard of care for psychiatric nurses? Why or why not?

H. What nursing action should the nurse have taken to protect the client from harm?

4. Assume that there are no mandatory reporting laws for impaired or incompetent colleagues in the following clinical situation. In a private psychiatric unit in California, a 15-year-old boy is admitted voluntarily at the request of his parents because of violent, explosive behavior that seems to stem from his father's recent remarriage after his parents' divorce. A few days after admission, while in group therapy, he has an explosive reaction to a discussion about weekend passes for Mother's Day. He screams that he has been abandoned and that nobody cares about him. Several weeks later, on the day before his discharge, he elicits from the nurse a promise to keep his plan to kill his mother confidential.

Consider the ANA *Code of Ethics for Nurses* on client confidentiality, the principles of psychiatric nursing, the statutes on privileged communications, and the duty to warn third parties in answering the following questions:

A. Did the nurse use appropriate judgment in promising confidentiality?

B. Does the nurse have a legal duty to warn the client's mother of her son's threat?

C. Is the duty owed to the client's father and stepmother?

D. Would a change in the admission status from voluntary to involuntary protect the client's mother without violating the client's confidentiality?

E. Would your response be different depending on the state in which the incident occurred? Why or why not?

F. What nursing action, if any, should the nurse take after the disclosure by the client?

■ ■ ■ **CHAPTER REVIEW**

Choose the most appropriate answer.

1. Which resource will provide the least authoritative help for a psychiatric mental health nurse faced with a client care ethical dilemma?

    1. Scope and Standards of Psychiatric-Mental Health Nursing Practice (ANA)

    2. Federal and state laws

    3. Code of Ethics for Nurses (ANA)

    4. Peer opinion

2. The single most important action nurses can take to protect the rights of a psychiatric client is to

    1. be aware of that state's laws regarding care and treatment of the mentally ill.

    2. refuse to participate in imposing restraint or seclusion.

    3. document concerns about unit short staffing.

    4. practice the five principles of bioethics.

3. To provide appropriate care for a client who has been admitted involuntarily to a psychiatric unit, the nurse must be aware of the fact that the client has the right to

    1. refuse psychotropic medications.

    2. be treated by unit staff of his or her choice.

    3. be released within 24 hours of making a written request.

    4. have a consultation with other mental health professionals at the hospital's expense.

4. In which situation might the psychiatric mental health nurse incur liability?

    1. Placing a client with annoying behavior in seclusion

    2. Reporting the substandard practice of a nurse peer

    3. Reporting threats against a third party to the treatment team

    4. Discussing an unclear medical order with the physician

5. Observing the client's right to privacy permits the psychiatric mental health nurse to

    1. freely disclose information in the medical record to the client's employer.

    2. use information about the client when preparing a journal article.

    3. discuss observations about the client with the treatment team.

    4. disclose confidential information after the client's death.

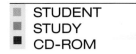

STUDENT
STUDY
CD-ROM

Access the accompanying CD-ROM for animations, interactive exercises, review questions for the NCLEX examination, and an audio glossary.

REFERENCES

American Nurses Association. (1994). *Guidelines for reporting incompetent, unethical, and illegal practices.* Kansas City, MO: Author.

American Nurses Association. (1996). Position statement: The rights to accept or reject an assignment. *Pulse, 33*(1), 4-5, 11.

American Nurses Association. (2001). *Code of ethics for nurses with interpretive statements.* Washington, DC: American Nurses Publishing. Retrieved November 18, 2004, from the American Nurses Association website: http://www.nursingworld.org/ethics/code/ethicscode150.htm.

American Nurses Association, American Psychiatric Nurses Association, & International Society of Psychiatric-Mental Health Nurses. (2000). *Scope and standards of psychiatric-mental health nursing practice.* Washington, DC: American Nurses Publishing.

American Psychiatric Association. (2000). *Diagnostic and statistical manual of mental disorders (DSM-IV-TR)* (4th ed., text rev.). Washington, DC: Author.

Bazelon, D. L. (2003). *Advance psychiatric directives.* Washington, DC: Bazelon Center for Mental Health Law.

Blythe v. Radiometer America, Inc., 866 P.2d 218 (Mont. Sup. Ct. 1993).

Canterbury v. Spence, 464 F.2d 722 (D.C. Cir. 1972), quoting Schloendorf v. Society of N.Y. Hosp., 211 N.Y. 125 105 N.E.2d 92, 93 (1914).

Chan, C. (2003, May 13-18). *Mandatory outclient treatment: Issues to consider.* Paper presented at the 153rd annual meeting of the American Psychiatric Association, Chicago, IL.

Dunn, D. G. (1994). Bioethics in nursing. *Nursing Connections, 7*(3), 43-51.

Health Insurance Portability and Accountability Act, U.S.C.45C.F.R § 164.501 (2003).

Humphrey v. Cady, 405 U.S. 504 (1972).

Illinois v. Russel, 630 N.E.2d 794 (Ill. Sup. Ct. 1994).

Joint Commission on Accreditation of Healthcare Organizations. (2004). *Comprehensive accreditation manual for hospitals: The official handbook (Standard R1.2.30).* Oakbrook Terrace, IL: Author.

Lo, B. (1989). Clinical ethics and HIV-related illnesses: Issues in treatment and health services. In W. Le Vee (Ed.), *New perspectives on HIV-related illnesses: Progress in health services research* (pp. 170-179). Bethesda, MD: U.S. Department of Health and Human Services.

Mandatory nurse/client ratios: A good idea or not? [Editorial] (2003). *Nursing 2003, 33*(10), 46-48.

Matter of Jobes, 108 N.J. 394, 407 (1987).

Monahan, J., Swartz, M., & Bonnie, R. J. (2003). Mandated treatment in the community for people with mental disorders. *Health Affairs, 22*(5), 28-38.

O'Connor v. Donaldson, 422 U.S. 563 (1975).

Pekkanen, J. (2003, December). Dangerous minds. *Readers Digest,* p. 138.

Pennington, S., et al. (1993). Addressing ethical boundaries among nurses. *Nurse Manager, 24*(6), 36-39.

Plumadore v. State of New York, 427 N.Y.S.2d 90 (1980).

Rainey, C. (2001, October 10-14). *Mandated outclient treatment resources and data.* Presented at American Psychiatric Association—53rd Institute on Psychiatric Services, Orlando, FL.

Rennie v. Klein, 476 F. Supp. 1294 (D.N.J. 1979).

Rennie v. Klein, 653 F.2d 836 (3d Cir. 1981).

Rennie v. Klein, 454 U.S. 1078 (1982).

Rennie v. Klein, 720 F.2d 266 (3d Cir. 1983).

Schwartz, H., Vingiano, W., & Perez, C. (1988). Autonomy and the right to refuse treatment: Client's attitudes after involuntary medication. *Hospital & Community Psychiatry, 39,* 1049.

Simon, R. I. (1999). The law and psychiatry. In R. E. Hales, S. C. Yadofsky, & J. A. Talbott (Eds.), *Textbook of psychiatry* (3rd ed.). Washington, DC: American Psychiatric Press.

Tarasoff v. Regents of University of California, 529 P.2d 553, 118 Cal Rptr 129 (1974).

Tarasoff v. Regents of University of California, 551 P.2d 334, 131 Cal Rptr 14 (1976).

Tischler v. DiMenna, 609 N.Y.S.2d 1002 (S.Ct. Westchester Co., March 1, 1994).

U.S. Department of Health and Human Services. (1999). *Mental health: A report of the Surgeon General.* Rockville, MD: U.S. Department of Health and Human Services, Center for Mental Health Services, National Institutes of Health.

Zinernon v. Burch, 494 U.S. 113, 108 L.Ed.2d 100, 110 S. Ct. 975 (1990).

A NURSE SPEAKS

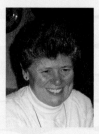

Communication with a psychiatric client that can convey knowledge, caring, encouragement, and support can lead that client along a path that endorses wellness and well-being. This is termed *therapeutic communicating* or *therapeutic relating*. Let me share a story from my own experience that illustrates the power of such communication.

I was working in a psychiatric day treatment program when I met Sue. Sue was brand new to the program. I could see the same confusion and denial in Sue that I so often see in persons newly diagnosed with mental health problems. Sue truly did not believe that she was facing a diagnosis of schizophrenia. She believed she was overly stressed but certainly not mentally ill. If the health care team would just listen to her, believe her, and help her, she could get over this. She described the attacks "they" were making upon her person and her life. "They" followed her, repeated to her segments of conversations she had with her family, invaded the privacy of her home, and harassed her at her job.

As Sue's psychiatric nurse, I perceived that she was experiencing fear, panic, and feelings that her life was totally out of control. I acknowledged the feelings that this frightened woman expressed. I offered Sue support and help as treatment with medications and therapy began. Adjusting to an antipsychotic medication was difficult, especially because Sue really did not think she needed it. After all, she believed that she was just very stressed and talking to someone about it was bound to help.

I provided Sue with some simple explanations about how the antipsychotic medication would work to correct the chemical imbalance that existed in her brain. I was fully aware that these explanations and ongoing teaching would mean nothing if Sue did not feel that I cared and was sincerely interested in her. Sue needed to feel safe, cared about, and protected at a time when her world was so foreboding.

As medication dulled the delusional thoughts that raced through Sue's mind, I could see her transform into a calmer, more trusting person. Sue's gifts became apparent—she was smart and very creative. I acknowledged these gifts and called them into play. This bolstered Sue's self-confidence, which had been badly battered by the symptomatology of the illness.

I was determined to focus on Sue's personal gifts and talents, as well as the evident manifestations of the disease, addressing both as I could. Sue's response to this approach was positive. She began to feel less like a "sick, overwhelmed person." She was encouraged to grasp and hold on to that which had been good and positive in her life before the onset of her illness. I truly believe that reaching out to the well person that Sue could and would become was helpful.

The progress was slow and painstaking. I believed it was worth all of the effort involved. My hope was that Sue would leave treatment stabilized, less stressed, and aware that a nurse she met at the day program believed in her, reached out to her, and walked the road to wellness with her.

Miriam Jacik

PSYCHOSOCIAL NURSING TOOLS

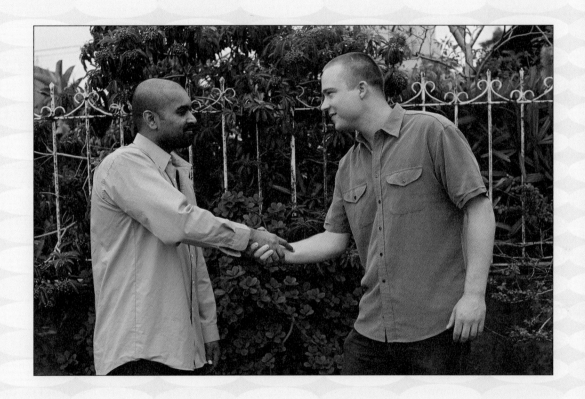

IT IS ONE OF THE MOST BEAUTIFUL COMPENSATIONS OF LIFE THAT NO MAN CAN SINCERELY TRY TO HELP ANOTHER WITHOUT HELPING HIMSELF.

Ralph Waldo Emerson

CHAPTER 9

Assessment Strategies and the Nursing Process

ELIZABETH M. VARCAROLIS

KEY TERMS and CONCEPTS

The key terms and concepts listed here appear in color where they are defined or first discussed in this chapter.

counseling, 148

evidence-based practice (EBP), 147

health teaching, 149

mental status examination (MSE), 141

milieu therapy, 149

Nursing Interventions Classification (NIC), 146

Nursing Outcomes Classification (NOC), 146

outcome criteria, 146

psychosocial assessment, 142

self-care activities, 149

OBJECTIVES

After studying this chapter, the reader will be able to

1. Conduct a mental status examination of a classmate.
2. Perform a psychosocial assessment of a client agreed upon with your instructor.
3. Explain three principles the nurse follows in planning actions to reach agreed-upon outcome criteria.
4. Construct a plan of care for a client with a mental health problem.
5. Identify three advanced practice psychiatric nursing interventions.
6. Demonstrate one of the basic nursing interventions (with your instructor's guidance) and evaluate your care using your stated outcome criteria.
7. Contrast and compare the differences and similarities among the Nursing Interventions Classification, Nursing Outcomes Classification, and evidence-based nursing practice.

evolve Visit the Evolve website at **http://evolve.elsevier.com/Varcarolis** for a pretest on the content in this chapter.

The nursing process continues to be the basic framework for all significant action taken by nurses in providing developmentally and culturally relevant psychiatric mental health care to all patients (American Nurses Association [ANA], American Psychiatric Nurses Association, & International Society of Psychiatric-Mental Health Nurses, 2000). The nursing process is integral to the *Scope and Standards of Psychiatric-Mental Health Nursing Practice* as defined by the ANA (ANA et al., 2000). The **Standards of Care** are the basis for the following:

- Criteria for certification
- Legal definition of nursing, as reflected in many states' nurse practice acts
- National Council of State Boards of Nursing Licensure Examination (NCLEX-RN)

The Standards of Care are found on the inside back cover of this text.

The nursing process is a six-step problem-solving approach intended to facilitate and identify appropriate safe and quality care for clients. A client may be an individual, a family, a group, or a community. Assessment is made on many levels: physical, social, emotional, intellectual, spiritual, and cultural. Psychiatric mental health nursing practice bases nursing judgments and behaviors on an accepted theoretical framework. Whenever possible, interventions are supported by research (evidence based). The importance of a theoretical framework has been supported by the *Scope and Standards of Psychiatric-Mental Health Nursing Practice* (ANA et al., 2000). Figure 9-1 depicts the nursing process in psychiatric mental health nursing.

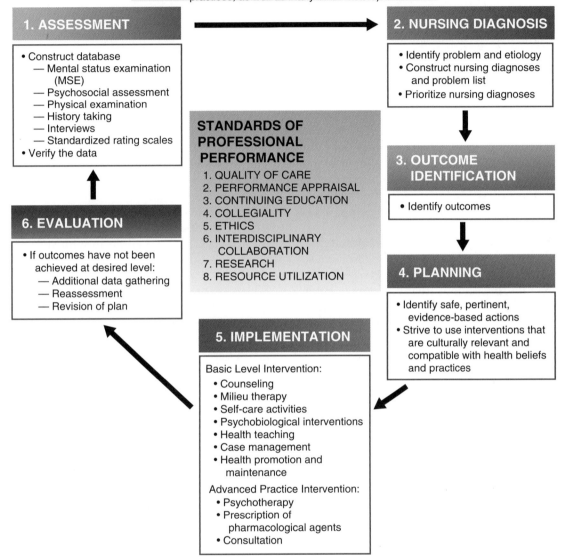

NURSING ASSESSMENT

The assessment interview requires culturally effective communication skills and encompasses a large database (e.g., significant support system; family; cultural and community system; spiritual and philosophical values, strengths, and health beliefs and practices; as well as many other factors).

1. ASSESSMENT

- Construct database
  — Mental status examination (MSE)
  — Psychosocial assessment
  — Physical examination
  — History taking
  — Interviews
  — Standardized rating scales
- Verify the data

2. NURSING DIAGNOSIS

- Identify problem and etiology
- Construct nursing diagnoses and problem list
- Prioritize nursing diagnoses

STANDARDS OF PROFESSIONAL PERFORMANCE

1. QUALITY OF CARE
2. PERFORMANCE APPRAISAL
3. CONTINUING EDUCATION
4. COLLEGIALITY
5. ETHICS
6. INTERDISCIPLINARY COLLABORATION
7. RESEARCH
8. RESOURCE UTILIZATION

3. OUTCOME IDENTIFICATION

- Identify outcomes

6. EVALUATION

- If outcomes have not been achieved at desired level:
  — Additional data gathering
  — Reassessment
  — Revision of plan

4. PLANNING

- Identify safe, pertinent, evidence-based actions
- Strive to use interventions that are culturally relevant and compatible with health beliefs and practices

5. IMPLEMENTATION

Basic Level Intervention:
- Counseling
- Milieu therapy
- Self-care activities
- Psychobiological interventions
- Health teaching
- Case management
- Health promotion and maintenance

Advanced Practice Intervention:
- Psychotherapy
- Prescription of pharmacological agents
- Consultation

FIGURE 9-1 The nursing process in psychiatric mental health nursing.

STANDARD I. ASSESSMENT

A **mental status examination (MSE)** and the assessment of the client's **psychosocial status** are part of any nursing assessment, along with the assessment of the client's physical health.

The assessment interview or intake interview may be conducted in a psychiatric inpatient setting, but most likely, it will take place in a variety of other settings such as emergency care units, medical-surgical units, intensive care units, crisis units, community mental health centers, private practice, homes, and schools. The time required for the interview varies, depending on the clinical setting and the circumstances of the client. During emergencies, immediate intervention is often based on a minimal amount of data. A scheduled MSE and psychosocial assessment in a structured setting allows more time for an elaborate assessment. At times, completing the assessment process may involve many interviews.

The nurse's *primary source* for data collection is the client; however, there may be times when the client is unable to assist with the assessment. For example, if the client is severely delusional, mute, comatose, or extremely confused, *secondary sources* should be used. Such secondary sources include members of the family, friends, neighbors, police, other members of the health team, medical records, and laboratory results. It may be necessary to use both primary and secondary sources to complete the assessment.

Personal Considerations

Both the client and the nurse bring to their relationship their total background experiences. These experiences include cultural beliefs and biases, religious attitudes, educational background, and occupational and life experiences, as well as attitudes regarding sexual roles. These attitudes, beliefs, and values influence the nurse's interactions with clients. It is important for nurses, through examining their personal beliefs and clarifying their values, to be aware of their biases and values and not feel compelled to impose their personal beliefs on others. The process of self-monitoring is part of professional behavior (see Chapter 11).

Although the nurse shares perceptions and alternatives with the client, the goal is to work with the client so that decisions and actions taken are the right ones for the client. Theoretically, this sounds easy, but often it is not. When beginning practitioners share their perceptions and thoughts with a more experienced nurse, unrecognized biases and value judgments often become evident. Countertransference issues may also play a role in the beginning practitioner's perceptions. **Countertransference** is the nurse's reactions to a client that are based on the nurse's unconscious needs, conflicts, problems, or view of the world. These reactions are inappropriate in the nurse-client relationship. Experience and supervision help a nurse separate what is important to the client from any bias that might impede accomplishment of mutually agreed goals. This phenomenon and its effect on a therapeutic relationship are discussed in Chapter 10.

The best atmosphere in which to conduct an assessment is one of minimal anxiety. Therefore, if an individual becomes upset, defensive, or embarrassed regarding any topic, the topic should be abandoned. The nurse can acknowledge that this is a subject that makes the client uncomfortable and can suggest that it would best be discussed when the client feels more comfortable. It is important that the nurse not probe, pry, or push for information that is difficult for the client to discuss. However, it should be recognized that increased anxiety about any subject is data in itself. The nurse can note this in the assessment without obtaining any further information.

Age Considerations

All clients, regardless of age or circumstance, need to undergo a thorough physical examination before a diagnosis is made. See Box 9-1 for examples of physical conditions that may mimic psychiatric disorders.

Assessment of an Elderly Client

Elderly clients often need special attention. The nurse needs to be aware of any physical limitations—that is, any sensory condition (difficulty seeing or hearing), motor condition (difficulty walking or maintaining balance), or medical condition (cardiac or refractory)—that could cause increased anxiety, stress, or physical discomfort for the client.

It is wise to identify any physical needs the client may have at the onset of the intervention and make accommodations for them. For example, if the client is hard of hearing, speak a little more slowly and in clear, louder tones (but not too loud) and seat the client close to you without invading his or her personal space.

Assessment of Children

The assessment of children is covered in depth in Chapter 32. Play serves as an important means of expression and learning for children. Use of storytelling, dolls, drawing, games, and a lot more can be useful in assessing critical concerns and painful issues a child may have. Usually, a clinician with special training in child and adolescent psychiatry works with young children.

Assessment of an Adolescent Client

Assessment tools and strategies for the adolescent are discussed in Chapter 32; however, some points are given here. All people need to feel safe during a psychiatric interview and assessment. This is particularly true for children and adolescents. All clients are concerned with confidentiality. This is especially true for adolescents. Adolescents may fear that anything they say to the nurse will be repeated to their parents. The adolescent needs to know that the nurse will not give out information without informing the adolescent in advance. Discussion about feelings can be kept confidential; however, threats of suicide, homicide, use of illegal drugs, or issues of abuse have to be shared with other professionals as well as with the parents. Because identifying risk factors is one of the key objectives when assessing adolescents, it is helpful to use a brief structured interview technique called the HEADSSS interview (Box 9-2).

Psychiatric Nursing Assessment

The purpose of the psychiatric nursing assessment is to do the following:
- Establish a rapport.
- Obtain an understanding of the current problem.
- Assess for risk factors affecting the safety of the client or others (e.g., suicide or self-harm, assault or violence, substance use withdrawal, allergies).
- Assess for the person's current level of psychological functioning and psychosocial status.

BOX 9-1

Some Medical Conditions That May Mimic Psychiatric Illness

Depression

Neurological disorders
- Cerebrovascular accident (stroke)
- Alzheimer's disease
- Brain tumor
- Huntington's disease
- Epilepsy (seizure disorder)
- Multiple sclerosis
- Parkinson's disease

Cancer

Infections
- Mononucleosis
- Encephalitis
- Hepatitis
- Tertiary syphilis
- Human immunodeficiency virus (HIV) infection

Endocrine disorders
- Hypothyroidism and hyperthyroidism
- Cushing's syndrome
- Addison's disease
- Parathyroid disease

Gastrointestinal disorders
- Liver cirrhosis
- Pancreatitis

Cardiovascular disorders
- Hypoxia
- Congestive heart failure

Respiratory disorders
- Sleep apnea

Nutritional disorders
- Thiamine deficiency
- Protein deficiency
- B_{12} deficiency
- B_6 deficiency
- Folate deficiency

Collagen vascular diseases
- Lupus erythematosus
- Rheumatoid arthritis

Anxiety

Neurological disorders
- Alzheimer's disease
- Brain tumor
- Stroke
- Huntington's disease

Infections
- Encephalitis
- Meningitis
- Neurosyphilis
- Septicemia

Endocrine disorders
- Hypothyroidism and hyperthyroidism
- Hypoparathyroidism
- Hypoglycemia
- Pheochromocytoma
- Carcinoid

Metabolic disorders
- Low calcium
- Low potassium
- Acute intermittent porphyria
- Liver failure

Cardiovascular disorders
- Angina
- Congestive heart failure
- Pulmonary embolus

Respiratory disorders
- Pneumothorax
- Acute asthma
- Emphysema

Drug effects
- Stimulants
- Sedatives (withdrawal)

Lead, mercury poisoning

Psychosis

Medical conditions
- Temporal lobe epilepsy
- Migraine headaches
- Temporal arteritis
- Occipital tumors
- Narcolepsy
- Encephalitis
- Hypothyroidism
- Addison's disease
- HIV infection

Drug effects
- Hallucinogens (e.g., LSD [lysergic acid diethylamide])
- Phencyclidine
- Alcohol (withdrawal)
- Stimulants
- Cocaine
- Corticosteroids

BOX 9-2

The HEADSSS Psychosocial Interview Technique

H   Home environment (e.g., relations with parents and siblings)

E   Education and employment (e.g., school performance)

A   Activities (e.g., sports participation, after-school activities, peer relations)

D   Drug, alcohol, or tobacco use

S   Sexuality (e.g., whether the client is sexually active; whether he or she practices safe sex [uses condoms] or uses contraception)

S   Suicide risk or symptoms of depression or other mental disorder

S   "Savagery" (e.g., violence or abuse in home environment or in neighborhood)

- Perform an MSE.
- Identify what the client and family hope to gain from treatment.
- Identify what behaviors, beliefs, or other areas of client life need to be modified to effect positive change.
- Formulate a plan of care.

Gathering Data

Mental Status Examination. Fundamental to the assessment is a mental status examination (MSE). In fact, an MSE is part of the assessment in all areas of medicine. The MSE in psychiatry is analogous to the physical examination in general medicine. The purpose of the MSE is to evaluate an individual's current cognitive processes. For acutely disturbed clients, it is not unusual for the mental health clinician (psychiatrist, nurse clinician) to administer MSEs every day. Sommers-Flanagan and Sommers-Flanagan (2003) advise anyone seeking employment in the medical–mental health field to be competent in communicating with other professionals via MSE reports. Refer to Box 9-3 for an example of the elements of a basic MSE.

The MSE, by in large, aids in collecting *objective data*. The nurse observes the client's physical behavior, nonverbal communication, appearance, speech patterns, thought content, and cognitive ability.

Psychosocial Nursing Assessment. A psychosocial assessment includes identification of the following information about the client:

- Personal background
- Social background
- Strengths as well as weaknesses
- Usual coping strategies
- Cultural beliefs and practices that may affect implementation of traditional treatment
- Spiritual beliefs or practices that are an integral part of the client's lifestyle

The client's psychosocial history is most often the *subjective* part of the assessment. The focus of the history is the client's perceptions and recollections of current lifestyle, and life in general (family, friends, education, work experience, coping styles, and spiritual and cultural beliefs).

A psychosocial assessment elicits information about the systems in which a person operates. To conduct such an assessment, the nurse should have fundamental knowledge of growth and development and of basic cultural and religious practices, as well as of pathophysiology, psychopathology, and pharmacology. An example of a comprehensive nursing assessment tool that includes both mental status and psychosocial issues is offered as a tear-out card at the front of this book. Terms are defined in the Glossary in the back of the text. A basic psychosocial assessment tool is found in Box 9-4.

Special Note on Spiritual and Cultural Assessment

Spiritual Assessment. The importance of religion and spirituality to the American public has been increasingly highlighted by the media, opinion polls, and empirical studies (Koenig, McCullough, & Larson, 2001). Such observations include all Americans from all cultures, with a wide diversity of religious and spiritual beliefs. It is just as important for nurses to support spiritual aspects of care as to address biophysical elements. Carson and Koenig (2004) highlight the necessity for mental health nurses and allied clinical staff to be conscious that their clients may have spiritual and religious needs. This area of assessment is often overlooked in all fields of health care. It is believed by

---

BOX 9-3

Mental Status Examination

Personal Information
- Age
- Sex
- Marital status
- Religious preference
- Race
- Ethnic background
- Employment
- Living arrangements

Appearance
- Grooming and dress
- Level of hygiene
- Pupil dilation or constriction
- Facial expression
- Height, weight, nutritional status
- Presence of body piercing or tattoos, scars, other
- Relationship between appearance and age

Behavior
- Excessive or reduced body movements
- Peculiar body movements (e.g., scanning of the environment, odd or repetitive gestures, level of consciousness, balance and gait)
- Abnormal movements (e.g., tardive dyskinesia, tremors)
- Level of eye contact *(keep cultural differences in mind)*

Speech
- Rate: slow, rapid, normal
- Volume: loud, soft, normal
- Disturbances (e.g., articulation problems, slurring, stuttering, mumbling)
- Cluttering (e.g., rapid, disorganized, tongue-tied speech)

Affect and Mood
- Affect: flat, bland, animated, angry, withdrawn, appropriate to context
- Mood: sad, labile, euphoric

Thought
- Thought process (e.g., disorganized, coherent, flight of ideas, neologisms, thought blocking, circumstantiality)
- Thought content (e.g., delusions, obsessions, suicidal thought)

Perceptual Disturbances
- Hallucinations (e.g., auditory, visual)
- Illusions

Cognition
- Orientation: time, place, person
- Level of consciousness (e.g., alert, confused, clouded, stuporous, unconscious, comatose)
- Memory: remote, recent, immediate
- Fund of knowledge
- Attention: performance on serial sevens, digit span tests
- Abstraction: performance on tests involving similarities, proverbs
- Insight
- Judgment

BOX 9-4

Psychosocial Assessment

A. Previous hospitalizations
B. Educational background
C. Occupational background
    1. Employed? _____ Where? _____ What length of time? _____
    2. Special skills
D. Social patterns
    1. Describe family.
    2. Describe friends.
    3. With whom does the client live?
    4. To whom does the client go in time of crisis?
    5. Describe a typical day.
E. Sexual patterns
    1. Sexually active? _____ Practices safe sex? _____ Practices birth control? _____
    2. Sexual orientation
    3. Sexual difficulties
F. Interests and abilities
    1. What does the client do in his or her spare time?
    2. What sport, hobby, or leisure activity is the client good at?
    3. What gives the client pleasure?
G. Substance use and abuse
    1. What medications does the client take? _____
       How often? _____ How much? _____
    2. What herbal or over-the-counter drugs does the client take? _____
       How often? _____ How much? _____
    3. What psychotropic drugs does the client take? _____
       How often? _____ How much? _____
    4. How many drinks of alcohol does the client take per day? _____ per week? _____
    5. What recreational drugs does the client take? _____
       How often? _____ How much? _____
    6. Does the client identify the use of drugs as a problem?
H. Coping abilities
    1. What does the client do when he or she gets upset? _____
    2. To whom can the client talk? _____
    3. What usually helps to relieve stress? _____
    4. What did the client try this time? _____
I. Spiritual assessment
    1. What importance does religion or spirituality have in the client's life? _____
    2. Do the client's religious or spiritual beliefs relate to the way the client takes care of himself or herself or of the client's illness? _____ How? _____
    3. Does the client's faith help the client in stressful situations? _____
    4. Whom does the client see when he or she is medically ill? _____
       mentally upset? _____
    5. Are there special health care practices within the client's culture that address his or her particular mental problem? _____
    _____

a growing number of nurses and other health care providers that religious and spiritual needs should be a part of assessments and that multidisciplinary liaison and spiritual and religious resources should be available to all those who need them (Carson & Koenig, 2004). For some clients, prayer or religious or spiritual practices are an important part of the quality of their lives and can give them hope, comfort, and support in healing. As nurses, whatever our personal feelings may be regarding spiritual or religious beliefs, we are wise to support those beliefs in our clients and use appropriate referral services when agreed on by clients. Some questions we can ask to help with a spiritual assessment are the following:

- What role does religion or spirituality play in your life?
- Does your faith help you in stressful situations?
- Do you pray or meditate?
- Who or what supplies you with strength and hope?
- Has your illness affected your religious practices?
- Do you participate in any religious activities?

- Do you have a spiritual advisor or member of the clergy (priest, rabbi, minister) readily available?
- Is there anyone I can contact to help put you back in touch with your church/synagogue/place of worship/practice of prayer?

Cultural and Social Assessment. Because nurses are increasingly faced with caring for culturally diverse populations, there is an increasing need for nursing assessment, nursing diagnoses, and subsequent care to be planned around unique cultural health care beliefs, values, and practices. Kavanaugh (2003) advocates that mental health nurses have a thorough understanding of the complexity of the cultural and social factors that influence health and illness. Awareness of individual cultural beliefs and health care practices can help nurses minimize labeling of clients. Some questions we can ask to help with a cultural and social assessment are the following:

- What is your primary language? Would you like an interpreter?
- How would you describe your cultural background?
- Who are you close to? Who do you seek in times of crisis?
- Who do you live with?
- Who do you seek when you are medically ill? mentally upset or concerned?
- What do you do to get better when you are medically ill? mentally ill?
- What are the attitudes toward mental illness in your culture?
- How is your mental health problem viewed by your culture? Is it seen as a problem to fix? a disease? a taboo? a fault or curse?
- Are there special foods that you eat?
- Are there special health care practices within your culture that address your particular mental health problem?
- What economic resources are available to your family?

After you have concluded the assessment, it is useful to summarize pertinent data with the client. This summary provides the client with reassurance that he or she has been heard and it allows the client the opportunity to clarify any misinformation. The client should be told what will happen next. For example, if the initial assessment takes place in the hospital, you should tell the client who else the client will be seeing. If the initial assessment was conducted by a psychiatric nurse in a mental health clinic, you should let the client know when and how often he or she will meet with the nurse to work on the client's problems. If you believe a referral is necessary (e.g., to a mental health clinician, social worker, or medical physician), you should discuss this with the client.

Verifying Data

It is necessary that you validate data obtained from the client with secondary sources. Whenever possible, family members should be a part of the assessment. Is there anything going on in the family that is affecting the client? How does the family define the problem? How do the client's problems affect the family?

Family, friends, and neighbors may verify or contradict the client's self-perception and actions or may add information. Often, police officers are the ones who bring clients into the psychiatric emergency department. You must know as much as possible about what the client was doing that warranted police intervention.

Other members of the health team are important sources of information and data verification. Many members of the health team will have contact with the client on admission to the hospital. The psychiatrist or psychologist, social worker, psychiatric nurse, recreation therapist, therapy aides, and student nurses can add to your database. If, however, there is no one to verify the client's information, you need to document this.

Old charts and medical records, most now computer accessible, are a great help in validating information you already have or adding new information to your database. Medical history can aid in assessing physical losses and stress and can alert the staff to potential medical problems. If the client has been admitted to a psychiatric unit in the past, information about the client's previous level of functioning and behavior gives you a baseline for making clinical judgments. Consent forms may need to be signed to allow you to obtain information for this purpose.

Laboratory reports can provide useful information. When the body's chemistry is abnormal, personality changes and violent behaviors can result. For example, abnormal liver enzyme levels can explain irritability, depression, and lethargy. People who have chronic renal disease often suffer from the same symptoms when their blood urea nitrogen and electrolyte levels are abnormal. People with endocrine diseases such as diabetes can have changes in mood and level of consciousness related to glucose and insulin levels. Results of a toxicology screen for the presence of either prescription or illegal drugs may also provide useful information.

Using Rating Scales

There are a number of standardized rating scales that are useful for psychiatric evaluation and monitoring. Rating scales are often administered by a clinician (nurse, psychologist, social worker, psychiatrist), but many are self-administered. Table 9-1 lists some of the common ones in use. Many of the clinical chapters in this book include a rating scale.

TABLE 9-1

Standardized Rating Scales*

Use	Scale
Depression	Beck Inventory
	Geriatric Depression Scale (GDS)
	Hamilton Depression Scale
	Zung Self-Report Inventory
Anxiety	Modified Spielberger State Anxiety Scale
	Hamilton Anxiety Scale
Substance use disorders	Addiction Severity Index (ASI)
	Recovery Attitude and Treatment Evaluator (RAATE)
	Brief Drug Abuse Screen Test (B-DAST)
Obsessive-compulsive behavior	Yale-Brown Obsessive-Compulsive Scale (Y-BOCS)
Mania	Mania Rating Scale
Schizophrenia	Scale for Assessment of Negative Symptoms (SANS)
	Brief Psychiatric Rating Scale (BPRS)
Abnormal movements	Abnormal Involuntary Movement Scale (AIMS)
	Simpson Neurological Rating Scale
General psychiatric assessment	Brief Psychiatric Rating Scale (BPRS)
	Global Assessment of Functioning Scale (GAF)
Cognitive function	Mini-Mental State Examination (MMSE)
	Alzheimer's Disease Rating Scale (ADRS)
	Memory and Behavior Problem Checklist
	Functional Assessment Screening Tool (FAST)
	Global Deterioration Scale (GDS)
Family assessment	McMaster Family Assessment Device
Eating disorders	Eating Disorders Inventory (EDI)
	Body Attitude Test
	Diagnostic Survey for Eating Disorders

*These rating scales highlight important areas in psychiatric assessment. Because many of the answers are subjective, experienced clinicians use these tools as a guide when planning care, and also draw on their knowledge of their clients.

STANDARD II. NURSING DIAGNOSIS

Formulating a Nursing Diagnosis

As you have learned, a nursing diagnosis is a clinical judgment about the response of a client (individual, family, community) to actual and potential health problems or life processes. A well-chosen and well-stated nursing diagnosis is the basis for selecting therapeutic outcomes and interventions (North American Nursing Diagnosis Association [NANDA], 2005).

A nursing diagnosis has three structural components:

1. Problem (unmet need)
2. Etiology (probable cause)
3. Supporting data (signs and symptoms)

The *problem*, or unmet need, describes the state of the client at present. Problems that are within the nurse's domain to prescribe for and treat are termed *nursing diagnoses.* The nursing diagnostic title states what should change, for example, *hopelessness.*

Etiology, or probable cause, is linked to the diagnostic title with the words "related to." Stating the etiology or probable cause tells what needs to be done to effect the change and identifies causes that the nurse can treat through nursing interventions. For example:

Hopelessness related to multiple losses

Supporting data, or signs and symptoms, state what the condition is like at present. Supporting data (defining characteristics) that validate the diagnosis include the following:

1. Client's statement "It's no use, nothing will change"
2. Lack of involvement with family and friends
3. Lack of motivation to care for self or environment

Refer to Appendix C for a list of all current NANDA-approved nursing diagnoses.

STANDARD III. OUTCOME CRITERIA

Determining Outcomes

Outcome criteria are the hoped-for outcomes that reflect the maximal level of client health that can realistically be reached by nursing interventions. Outcomes are variable concepts that can be measured along a continuum. Therefore, outcomes are stated as concepts that reflect a client's actual state rather than expected goals (Moorhead, Johnson, & Maas, 2004, p. 20). Outcomes reflect a new language in nursing. Although we are moving away from the use of goal statements to the use of more measurable indicators, the profession is in a transition period. Many schools of nursing as well as health care facilities continue to use behavioral goals to measure the effectiveness of nursing interventions. In recognition of this transitional period, we provide you with both the new language of the Nursing Outcomes Classification (NOC) (Moorhead et al., 2004) as well as the language of goals. In each of the clinical chapters you will encounter outcomes from NOC; you will also encounter short-term behavioral goals in each of the nursing care plans.

The strengths of the NOC system are that outcomes are grounded in clinical practice and research; outcomes are written in clear, clinically useful language; standardized outcomes statements facilitate communication across disciplines; outcomes are easily linked to the language of the NANDA-approved nursing diagnoses and the Nursing Interventions Classification (NIC) (Dochterman & Bulechek, 2004); and the classification is based on an easy-to-use organizing structure.

NOC includes a total of 330 standardized outcomes that provide nursing with a mechanism to communicate the impact of nursing on the well-being of clients, families, and communities. This mechanism is essential for nurses to work effectively with managed care organizations to improve quality and reduce costs and to measure and document client outcomes influenced by nursing care. Each outcome has an associated group of indicators that are used to determine client status in relation to the outcome. These indicators are measured along a five-point Likert-type scale that quantifies a client's status along a continuum from least to most desirable and provides a rating at a point in time. Table 9-2 provides suggested NOC indicators for the outcome of Suicide Self-Restraint along with the Likert scale that quantifies the achievement on each indicator from 1 (never demonstrated) to 5 (consistently demonstrated).

NOC does not distinguish between short- and long-term outcomes. However, in the clinical chapters you will find that we have made a distinction among the outcomes to demonstrate that the achievement of some outcomes is possible in the short term whereas the achievement of others will require more time as you continue to intervene with the client to achieve the overall outcome.

Behavioral goals have different criteria: they must be realistic and acceptable to both client and nurse; they are stated in observable or measurable terms; they indicate client behaviors; they establish a specific time for goal achievement; and they are written in positive terms. Let's look at how a specific outcome criterion and behavioral goals fit together when the nursing diagnosis is *risk for self-directed violence: possible suicide behaviors related to multiple losses.*

OUTCOME CRITERION	SHORT-TERM GOALS
Refrains from attempting suicide.	1. Client will remain free from injury throughout hospital stay.
	2. Client will speak to nurse, spouse, or chaplain when feeling overwhelmed or self-destructive.

STANDARD IV. PLANNING

The Nursing Interventions Classification (NIC) (Dochterman & Bulechek, 2004) is a research-based standardized listing of 514 interventions that the nurse can use to plan care and reflects current clinical practice. In all settings nurses can use NIC's standardized classification of nursing interventions to support quality client care and incorporate evidence-based nursing actions. However, many safe and appropriate interventions may not be included in NIC. NIC is a useful guide for standardized care, but specific interventions that meet a client's special needs should always be part of the planning as well.

More and more units, both inpatient and community-based facilities, are using standardized care plans or clinical pathways for clients with specific diagnoses. Other health care facilities devise individual plans of care. Whatever the care planning procedures in a specific institution, the nurse considers specific principles when planning care. Nursing interventions planned for meeting a specific outcome need to be the following:

- *Safe.* They must be safe for the client as well as for other clients, staff, and family.
- *Appropriate.* They must be compatible with other therapies and with the client's personal goals and cultural values, as well as with institutional rules.
- *Individualized.* They should be realistic: (1) within the client's capabilities given the client's age, physical strength, condition, and willingness to change; (2) based on the number of staff available; (3) reflective of the actual available community resources; and (4) within the student's or nurse's capabilities.
- *Evidence-based.* They should be based on scientific principles.

Evidence-based practice is discussed with increasing frequency in the psychiatric literature (Gray, 2002). David Sackett, one of the founders of evidence-based

TABLE 9-2

Suicide Self-Restraint (NOC)

Definition: Personal actions to refrain from gestures and attempts at killing self
Outcome target rating: Maintain at _____. Increase to _____.

Suicide Self-Restraint Overall Rating	Never Demonstrated 1	Rarely Demonstrated 2	Sometimes Demonstrated 3	Often Demonstrated 4	Consistently Demonstrated 5	
			Indicators			
Expresses feelings	1	2	3	4	5	NA
Expresses sense of hope	1	2	3	4	5	NA
Maintains connectedness in relationships	1	2	3	4	5	NA
Seeks help when feeling self-destructive	1	2	3	4	5	NA
Verbalizes suicidal ideas	1	2	3	4	5	NA
Controls impulses	1	2	3	4	5	NA
Refrains from gathering means for suicide	1	2	3	4	5	NA
Refrains from giving away possessions	1	2	3	4	5	NA
Refrains from inflicting serious injury	1	2	3	4	5	NA
Refrains from using non-prescribed mood-altering substance(s)	1	2	3	4	5	NA
Discloses plan for suicide if present	1	2	3	4	5	NA
Upholds suicide contract	1	2	3	4	5	NA
Maintains self-control without supervision	1	2	3	4	5	NA
Refrains from attempting suicide	1	2	3	4	5	NA
Seeks treatment for depression	1	2	3	4	5	NA
Seeks treatment for substance abuse	1	2	3	4	5	NA
Reports adequate pain control for chronic pain	1	2	3	4	5	NA
Uses suicide prevention resources and social support groups within the community	1	2	3	4	5	NA
Uses available mental health services	1	2	3	4	5	NA
Plans for future	1	2	3	4	5	NA

From Moorhead, S., Johnson, M., & Maas, M. (2004). *Nursing outcomes classification (NOC)* (3rd ed.). St. Louis, MO: Mosby.

medicine, has defined it as "the conscientious, explicit, and judicious use of current best evidence in making decisions about the care of individual patients" (Sackett et al., 1996, p. 71). Evidence-based practice (EBP) for nurses is a combination of clinical skill and the use of clinically relevant research in the delivery of effective client-centered care. Refer to the Evidence-Based Practice box for an example of how research can be used as a guide in nursing practice.

As current today as they were in 1982 are Bower's words that, underlying all of the nurse's actions, there are basic premises:

- Individuals have the right to decide their own destinies and to be involved in decisions that affect them.
- Nursing intervention is designed to help individuals to meet their own needs or to solve their own problems.
- The ultimate goal of all nursing action is to assist individuals in maximizing their independent level of functioning.

When choosing nursing interventions from NIC or other sources, the nurse uses not just ones that fit the nursing diagnosis (e.g., *risk for suicide*) but interven-

EVIDENCE-BASED PRACTICE

Social Supports

Background
The value of social supports for mental and physical health has long been researched and established. Social supports for the elderly are especially important because friends are lost, ability to participate in sports or other activities may be diminished, and often there is loss of a spouse.

More and more research is being conducted on the health benefits of being a social support to others through volunteering and helping others.

Study
Some 423 couples were asked what type of practical support they provided for friends or relatives, whether they could count on help from others when needed, and what emotional support they gave each other. The couples were followed for a period of 5 years during which time 134 people died.

Results of Study
After adjusting for a variety of factors including age, gender, and physical and emotional health, the researchers found that there was an association between reduced risk of dying and giving help, but no association between receiving help and reduced death risk. Even after the researchers controlled for such factors as functional health, health satisfaction, health behaviors, age, income and educational level, they concluded that those who provided no instrumental or emotional support to others were more than twice as likely to die in the 5 years as people who helped spouses, friends, relatives, and neighbors.

Implications for Nursing Practice
Referring clients to supportive community services has long been a nursing function. The authors concluded: "If giving, rather than receiving, promotes longevity, then interventions that are currently designed to help people feel supported may need to be redesigned so that the emphasis is on what people do to help others" (Brown et al., 2003, p. 326).

Brown, S. L., et al. (2003). Providing social support may be more beneficial than receiving it. Results from a prospective study of mortality. *Psychological Science, 14*(4), 320-327.

---

tions that match the defining data. Although the outcome criteria (NOC) might be similar or the same (e.g., Suicide Self-Restraint), the safe and appropriate interventions may be totally different because of the defining data. For example, for the nursing diagnosis

***Risk for suicide* related to feelings of despair** as evidenced by two recent suicide attempts and repeated statements that "I want to die"

the planning of appropriate nursing interventions might include the following:

- Initiate suicide precautions (e.g., ongoing observations and monitoring of the patient, provision of a protective environment) for the person who is at serious risk for suicide.
- Search the newly hospitalized client and personal belongings for weapons or potential weapons during inpatient admission procedure, as appropriate.
- Use protective interventions (e.g., area restriction seclusion, physical restraints) if the client lacks the restraint to refrain from harming self, as needed.
- Assign hospitalized client to a room located near the nursing station for ease in observations, as appropriate.

On the other hand, if the defining data are different, so will be the appropriate interventions. For example:

***Risk for suicide* related to loss of spouse** as evidenced by lack of self-care and statements evidencing loneliness

The community health nurse might choose the following interventions for the client's plan of care:

- Determine the presence and degree of suicidal risk.
- Facilitate support of the client by family and friends.

- Consider strategies to decrease isolation and opportunity to act on harmful thoughts.
- Assist the client in identifying a network of supportive persons and resources within the community (e.g., support groups, clergy, care providers).
- Provide information about what community resources and outreach programs are available.

Refer to Chapter 23 for a comprehensive discussion on suicide.

STANDARD V. IMPLEMENTATION

The *Scope and Standards of Psychiatric-Mental Health Nursing Practice* (ANA et al., 2000) identifies 10 areas for intervention. Seven of these areas of intervention are at the basic level. Recent graduates and practitioners new to the psychiatric setting will participate in many of these activities with the guidance and support of more experienced health care professionals.

Three other areas are specific for the advanced level practitioner who is prepared at the master's level or higher.

Basic Level Practice Interventions
Va. Counseling

Counseling is usually carried out by a nurse minimally prepared at the basic level in psychiatric mental health nursing. The nurse is skilled in basic techniques of therapeutic communication. Some of the interventions include reinforcement of healthy patterns of behavior; application of problem-solving, interviewing, and communication skills; crisis intervention; stress management; instruction in relaxation techniques; conflict resolution; and use of behavior modification.

Vb. Milieu Therapy

Milieu therapy is an extremely important consideration for the nurse working with a client. The client should feel comfortable and safe and be assured that help is available. Milieu management includes familiarizing the client with the physical environment, the norms and rules of the unit that guide behavior and activities of daily living, and the schedule of activities. In addition, the nurse is aware of the effect of the environment on the client and uses this knowledge to guide interventions. In creating a therapeutic environment the nurse draws upon resources in the physical environment, the culture, and social structures. Activities are selected that meet the client's physical and mental health needs. In the hospital setting and day hospital setting, recreational, occupational, and dance therapists are often available to create appropriate activities for clients and give structure to their day. At times, milieu management might mean setting limits (restraints, seclusion, time-out).

Vc. Promotion of Self-Care Activities

Self-care activities assist the client in assuming personal responsibility for activities of daily living (ADLs) and are aimed at improving the client's mental and physical well-being.

Vd. Psychobiological Interventions

One of the nurse's functions is the administration of medications to clients. Nurses need to know the intended action, therapeutic dosage, adverse reactions, and safe blood levels, and to monitor these when appropriate (e.g., blood levels for lithium). The nurse is expected to discuss and provide medication teaching tools to the client and family regarding drug action, adverse side effects, dietary restrictions, and drug interactions, and to provide time for questions. The nurse's observations of the client's response to psychobiological interventions are communicated to other members of the team.

Ve. Health Teaching

Health teaching includes identifying the health education needs of the client and teaching basic principles of physical and mental health, such as giving information about coping, interpersonal relations, social skills, mental disorders, the treatments for such illnesses, and their effects on daily living.

Vf. Case Management

Many clients who come for treatment have a variety of physical, mental, emotional, and social problems. A case manager coordinates health services among a variety of agencies depending on the client's needs and resources. Case management can be done by a variety of health care providers, including nurses, social workers, and others. For example, an individual may have cardiac problems, but he comes into the health care system because of an attempted suicide. Later it is found out that he suffers from severe depression over the recent loss of his job of 20 years. This is an instance in which a case manager would coordinate medical, mental health, and social services to provide comprehensive holistic care for this client.

Vg. Health Promotion and Health Maintenance

Psychiatric mental health nurses employ a variety of health promotion and disease prevention strategies. "These strategies are based on knowledge of health beliefs, practices, evidence-based findings, and epidemiological principles, along with social, cultural, and political issues that affect mental health in an identified community" (ANA et al., 2000, p. 37).

Advanced Practice Interventions

The following interventions are carried out by the advanced practice registered nurse in psychiatric-mental health nursing (APRN-PMH).

Vh. Psychotherapy

The APRN-PMH is educationally and clinically prepared to conduct individual, group, and family psychotherapy, as well as other therapeutic treatments for clients with a variety of mental health disorders. Psychotherapy is helpful in improving mental health status and functional ability and in assisting clients to minimize and/or prevent potential mental illness and disability (ANA et al., 2000, p. 38).

Vi. Prescriptive Authority and Treatment

The APRN-PMH is educated and clinically prepared to prescribe psychopharmacological agents in accordance with state and federal laws and regulations.

Vj. Consultation

The APRN-PMH consults with other clinicians to provide services for clients and effect change within the system.

STANDARD VI. EVALUATION

Sadly, evaluation of client outcomes is often the most neglected part of the nursing process. Evaluation of the individual's response to treatment should be systematic and ongoing (ANA et al., 2000). Ongoing assessment of data allows for revisions of nursing diagnoses, changes to more realistic outcomes, and/or identification of more appropriate interventions when outcomes are not met.

Refer to the Evolve website to follow a client, Mr. Saltzberg, as the nurse proceeds through the steps of the nursing process and Standards of Care. In the counseling section you will see how the nurse applies therapeutic techniques.

DOCUMENTATION

Documentation could be considered the seventh step in the nursing process. Besides the evaluation of stated outcomes, the chart should record changes in client condition, informed consents (for medications and treatments), reaction to medication, documentation of symptoms (verbatim when appropriate), concerns of the client, and any untoward incidents in the health care setting. Documentation of client progress is the responsibility of the entire mental health team.

Although communication among team members and coordination of services are the primary goals when choosing a system for charting, practitioners in all settings must also consider professional standards, legal issues, requirements for reimbursement by insurers, and accreditation by regulatory agencies.

Information must also be in a format that is retrievable for quality assurance monitoring, utilization management, peer review, and research. For nursing, documentation of the nursing process is a guiding concern and is reflected in different formats that are commonly used in health care settings (Table 9-3). Computerized

TABLE 9-3

Charting Methods

	Narrative	Problem-Oriented Charting (SOAPIE)
Characteristics	A descriptive statement of client status written in chronological order throughout a shift. Used to support assessment finding from a flow sheet. In charting by exception, narrative notes are used to indicate significant symptoms, behaviors, or events that are exceptions to norms identified on an assessment flow sheet.	Developed in the 1960s for physicians to reduce inefficient documentation. Intended to be accompanied by a problem list. Originally SOAP, with IE added later. The emphasis is on problem identification, process, and outcome. **S:** Subjective data (patient statement) **O:** Objective data (nurse observations) **A:** Assessment (nurse interprets S and O and describes either a problem or a nursing diagnosis) **P:** Plan (proposed intervention) **I:** Interventions (nurse's response to problem) **E:** Evaluation (client outcome)
Example	Date/time/discipline. Client was agitated in the morning and pacing in the hallway. Blinked eyes, muttered to self and looked off to the side. Stated he heard voices. Verbally hostile to another client. Offered 2 mg haloperidol (Haldol) prn and sat with staff in quiet area for 20 min. Client returned to community lounge and was able to sit and watch television.	Date/time/discipline. **S:** "I'm so stupid. Get away, get away." "I hear the devil telling me bad things." **O:** Client paced the hall, mumbling to self and looking off to the side. Shouted derogatory comments when approached by another client. Watched walls and ceiling closely. **A:** Client was having auditory hallucinations and increased agitation. **P:** Offered client haloperidol prn. Redirected client to less stimulating environment. **I:** Client received 2 mg haloperidol PO prn. Sat with client in quiet room for 20 min. **E:** Client calmer. Returned to community lounge, sat and watched television.
Advantages	Uses a common form of expression (narrative writing). Can address any event or behavior. Explains flow sheet findings. Provides multidisciplinary ease of use.	Structured. Provides consistent organization of data. Facilitates retrieval of data for quality assurance and utilization management. Contains all elements of the nursing process. Minimizes inclusion of unnecessary data. Provides multidisciplinary ease of use.
Disadvantages	Unstructured. May result in different organization of information from note to note. Makes it difficult to retrieve quality assurance and utilization management data. Frequently leads to omission of elements of the nursing process. Commonly results in inclusion of unnecessary and subjective information.	Requires time and effort to structure the information. Limits entries to problems. May result in loss of data about progress. Not chronological. Carries negative connotation.

BOX 9-5

Legal Considerations for Documentation of Care

Do's

- Chart in a timely manner all pertinent and factual information.
- Be familiar with the nursing documentation policy in your facility and make your charting conform to this standard. The policy generally states the method of charting, the frequency, and pertinent assessments, interventions, and outcomes to be recorded. If your agency's policies and procedures do not encourage or allow for quality documentation, bring the need for change to the administration's attention.
- Chart legibly in ink.
- Chart facts fully, descriptively, and accurately.
- Chart what you see, hear, feel, and smell.
- Chart pertinent observations: psychosocial observations, physical symptoms pertinent to the medical diagnosis, and behaviors pertinent to the nursing diagnosis.
- Chart follow-up care provided when a problem has been identified in earlier documentation. For example, if a client has fallen and injured a leg, describe how the wound is healing.
- Chart fully the facts surrounding unusual occurrences and incidents.
- Chart *all* nursing interventions, treatments, and outcomes, including teaching efforts and client responses, and safety and client protection interventions.
- Chart the client's expressed subjective feelings.
- Chart each time you notify a physician and record the reason for notification, the information that was communicated, the accurate time, the physician's instructions or orders, and the follow-up activity.
- Chart physician's visits and treatments.
- Chart discharge medications and instructions given for use, as well as all discharge teaching performed and note which family members were included in the process.

Dont's

- Do *not* chart opinions that are not supported by the facts.
- Do *not* defame clients by calling them names or by making derogatory statements about them (e.g., "an unlikable client who is demanding unnecessary attention").
- Do *not* chart before an event occurs.
- Do *not* chart generalizations, suppositions, or pat phrases (e.g., "client in good spirits").
- Do *not* obliterate, erase, alter, or destroy a record. If an error is made, draw one line through the error, write "mistaken entry" or "error," and initial. Follow your agency's guidelines closely.
- Do *not* leave blank spaces for chronological notes. If you must chart out of sequence, chart "late entry." Identify the time and date of the entry and the time and date of the occurrence.
- If an incident report is filed, do *not note in the chart that one was filed.* This form is generally a privileged communication between the hospital and the hospital's attorney. Describing it in the chart may destroy the privileged nature of the communication.

clinical documentation is increasingly seen in inpatient as well as outpatient settings today. Whatever documentation format is used by a health care facility, it needs to be focused, organized, and pertinent, and to conform to certain legal and other generally accepted principles (Box 9-5).

■ ■ ■ KEY POINTS to REMEMBER

- The nursing process is a six-step problem-solving approach to client care.
- The *primary source* of assessment is the client. *Secondary sources* of information include the family, neighbors, friends, police, and other members of the health team. Both the nurse's and the client's anxiety levels need to be acknowledged, as do personal biases and value judgments.
- The assessment interview includes gathering subjective data (client history) and objective data (mental or emotional status).

- An MSE and psychosocial assessment are basic to a psychiatric nursing assessment. A medical history and examination round out a complete assessment.
- Assessment tools and standardized rating scales that may be used to evaluate and monitor a client's progress are useful and can help the nurse focus the interview.
- When the nurse develops skill and becomes more comfortable in this role, the interview becomes less formal without sacrificing important data.
- Determination of the nursing diagnosis (NANDA) is a crucial phase in the nursing process. The diagnosis performs a number of functions: it defines the practice of nursing, improves communication between staff members, and assists in accountability for care.
- A nursing diagnosis consists of (1) an unmet need or problem, (2) an etiology or probable cause, and (3) supporting data.
- Outcome criteria (NOC) are established that are realistic and within the client's level of ability.

- Outcomes are variable, measurable, and stated in terms that reflect a client's actual state. NOC provides 330 standardized outcomes. Planning involves determining desired outcomes.
- Goals may also be identified as part of the planning process. Goals are measurable, indicate the desired client behavior(s), include a set time for achievement, and must be short and specific.
- Planning nursing actions (NIC or other sources) to achieve the outcomes includes the use of specific principles: the plan should be (1) safe, (2) evidence-based whenever possible, (3) realistic, and (4) compatible with other therapies. NIC provides all nurses with standardized nursing interventions that are applicable for use in all settings.
- Practice in psychiatric nursing encompasses seven basic level interventions: counseling, milieu therapy, promotion of self-care activities, psychobiological interventions, health teaching, case management, and health promotion and maintenance.
- Advanced practice interventions are carried out by a nurse who is educated at the master's level or higher. Nurses certi-fied for advanced practice psychiatric mental health nursing can practice psychotherapy, prescribe certain medications, and perform consulting work.
- The evaluation of care is done by determining to what extent the outcome criteria have been achieved. Supporting data are included to clarify the evaluation. If outcomes have not been achieved, the nurse decides whether priorities in diagnosis need changing; new diagnoses need to be added; new interventions are required to achieve outcomes; and diagnosis, outcomes, interventions, and plans are currently appropriate.
- Documentation of client progress through evaluation of the outcome criteria is crucial. The chart is a legal document and should accurately reflect the client's condition, medications, treatment, tests, responses to these, and any untoward incidents.

Visit the Evolve website at **http://evolve.elsevier.com/Varcarolis** for a posttest on the content in this chapter. *evolve*

Critical Thinking and Chapter Review

Visit the Evolve website at **http://evolve.elsevier.com/Varcarolis** for additional self-study exercises. *evolve*

■ ■ ■ CRITICAL THINKING

Ms. Jamison is a 25-year-old woman who came to the hospital because voices told her to kill herself and she became very frightened. She appears tense. Her posture is rigid, her respiration is rapid, and she says she has not eaten for 3 days. When asked what she usually does when she gets upset, she says that she used to talk to her mother, but her mother died a year ago. Since then, she has been extremely lonely. She tells the nurse she does not have any friends and works part-time as a temporary secretary. She says her voices started a week after her mother died. "They used to be friendly voices, but now they want me to die." She has an aunt and a brother but is hesitant to contact them. She states, "They really don't need my problems; they have busy lives." She says she is frightened about the voices and is afraid she might obey them. She asks the nurse to help her.

Questions 1 to 3 refer to this situation. They are organized according to the steps of the nursing process.

1. There are a number of diagnoses the nurse could choose. Formulate one nursing diagnosis for Ms. Jamison. (Refer to Appendix C for a list of current NANDA-approved nursing diagnoses.) Include the problem statement, probable etiology, and supporting data.

    A. The diagnostic title: What should change? _____

    B. The etiology or possible cause related to _____

    C. Supporting data to validate diagnosis: _____

2. State one outcome criterion and two supporting short-term goals for the diagnosis in question.

    A. *Outcome criterion:* _____

    B. *Short-term goal:* _____

    C. *Short-term goal:* _____

3. When planning nursing care for Ms. Jamison, list four principles you would consider.

    A. _____

    B. _____

    C. _____

    D. _____

4. Discuss three positive reasons for having standardized classification systems of outcomes (NOC) and interventions (NIC). Think in terms of the managed care environment supporting quality care for clients in all settings.

Critical Thinking and Chapter Review—cont'd

Visit the Evolve website at **http://evolve.elsevier.com/Varcarolis/** for additional self-study exercises.

■ ■ ■ CHAPTER REVIEW

Choose the most appropriate answer.

1. Which statement by a nurse suggests an undesirable outcome of a psychiatric assessment interview conducted by the psychiatric nurse?
    1. "I think I was able to establish good rapport with the client."
    2. "I believe the client understands that my values differ from his."
    3. "I was able to obtain a good understanding of the client's current problem."
    4. "I was able to perform a complete assessment of the client's level of psychological functioning."

2. Assessment of an elderly client will be facilitated if the nurse
    1. identifies and accommodates client physical needs early.
    2. pledges complete confidentiality of all topics to the client.
    3. adheres strictly to the order of questions on the standardized assessment tool.
    4. interprets data without regard to the client's spiritual and cultural beliefs and practices.

3. A nurse tells a peer, "I place greatest weight on the subjective data I obtain during client assessment." From this the peer can infer that the nurse depends more on
    1. data obtained from secondary sources than data obtained from the primary source.
    2. the client's perceptions of the presenting problem than on data obtained from the mental status examination.
    3. data obtained from the mental status examination than on information elicited during history taking.
    4. gut-level hunches about client strengths and weaknesses than on data obtained from rating scales.

4. Which statement about nursing diagnosis is correct?
    1. A nursing diagnosis has three structural components: a problem, the etiology of the problem, and supporting data that validate the diagnosis.
    2. A nursing diagnosis is complete when the problem statement reflects an unmet need and the etiology given reflects a probable cause.
    3. An accurate nursing diagnosis requires a problem statement that identifies causes the nurse can treat via nursing interventions.
    4. A nursing diagnosis must always be based on objective data measured by the nurse; subjective data may be used only as supporting data to validate the diagnosis.

5. What is the relationship between evidence-based practice and clinically relevant research?
    1. Evidence-based practice reflects realistic processes for achieving client progress, whereas clinical research suggests best nursing practices.
    2. Evidence-based practice is a set of guidelines for meeting nursing standards and does not relate directly to clinical research.
    3. Evidence-based practice is accomplished by utilizing clinically relevant research.
    4. Evidence-based practice is required as part of interdisciplinary treatment plans, whereas clinically relevant research is specific to the discipline of nursing.

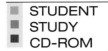

■ STUDENT
■ STUDY
■ CD-ROM

Access the accompanying CD-ROM for animations, interactive exercises, review questions for the NCLEX examination, and an audio glossary.

REFERENCES

American Nurses Association, American Psychiatric Nurses Association, & International Society of Psychiatric-Mental Health Nurses. (2000). *Scope and standards of psychiatric-mental health nursing practice.* Washington, DC: American Nurses Publishing.

Bower, F. L. (1982). *The process of planning nursing care.* St. Louis, MO: Mosby.

Carson, V. B., & Koenig, H. G. (2004). *Spiritual caregiving: Healthcare as a ministry.* Philadelphia: Templeton Foundation Press.

Dochterman, J. M., & Bulechek, G. M. (2004). *Nursing interventions classification (NIC)* (4th ed.). St. Louis, MO: Mosby.

Gray, G. E. (2002). Evidence-based medicine: An introduction for psychiatrists. *Journal of Psychiatric Practice, 8*(1), 5-13.

Kavanaugh, K. H. (2003). Transcultural perspectives in mental health nursing. In M. Andrews & J. Boyle. *Transcultural concepts in nursing care.* Philadelphia: Lippincott Williams & Wilkins.

Koenig, H. G., McCullough, M., & Larson, D. B. (2001). *Handbook of religion and health.* New York: Oxford University Press.

Moorhead, S., Johnson, M., & Maas, M. (2004). *Nursing outcomes classification (NOC)* (3rd ed.). St. Louis, MO: Mosby.

North American Nursing Diagnosis Association. (2005). *NANDA nursing diagnoses: Definitions and classification 2005-2006.* Philadelphia: Author.

Sackett, D. L., et al. (1996). Evidence-based medicine: What it is and what it isn't. *British Medical Journal, 312,* 71-72.

Sommers-Flanagan J., & Sommers-Flanagan, R. (2003). *Clinical interviewing* (3rd ed.). Hoboken, NJ: Wiley.

Developing Therapeutic Relationships

ELIZABETH M. VARCAROLIS

KEY TERMS and CONCEPTS

The key terms and concepts listed here appear in color where they are defined or first discussed in this chapter.

confidentiality, 165

contract, 164

countertransference, 159

empathy, 157

genuineness, 157

intimate relationship, 156

orientation phase, 164

social relationship, 156

termination phase, 167

therapeutic encounter, 163

therapeutic relationship, 156

transference, 159

values, 162

values clarification, 162

working phase, 165

OBJECTIVES

After studying this chapter, the reader will be able to

1. Contrast and compare the purpose, focus, communications styles, and goals for (a) a social relationship, (b) an intimate relationship, and (c) a therapeutic relationship.
2. Define and discuss the role of empathy, genuineness, and positive regard on the part of the nurse in a nurse-client relationship.
3. Identify two attitudes and four actions that may reflect the nurse's positive regard for a client.
4. Analyze what is meant by boundaries and the influence of transference and countertransference on boundary blurring.
5. Contrast and compare the three phases of the nurse-client relationship.
6. Role-play how you would address the four areas of concern during your first interview with a client.
7. Explore aspects that foster a therapeutic nurse-client relationship and those that are inherent in a nontherapeutic nursing interactive process as identified in the research of Forchuk and associates (2000).
8. Describe four testing behaviors a client may demonstrate and discuss possible nursing interventions for each behavior.

evolve Visit the Evolve website at **http://evolve.elsevier.com/Varcarolis** for a pretest on the content in this chapter.

The therapeutic nurse-client relationship is the basis, the very core, of all psychiatric nursing treatment approaches regardless of the specific aim. The very first process between nurse and client is to establish an understanding in the client that the nurse is entering into a relationship with the client that essentially is safe, confidential, reliable, and consistent with appropriate and clear boundaries (LaRowe, 2004). It is true that disorders that have strong biochemical and genetic components such as schizophrenia and major affective disorders cannot be healed through therapeutic means. However, many of the accompanying emotional problems such as poor self-image and low self-esteem can be significantly improved through a thera-peutic nurse-client alliance or relationship (LaRowe, 2004).

Randomized clinical trials have repeatedly found that development of a positive alliance (therapeutic relationship) is one of the best predictors of outcomes in therapy (Kopta et al., 1999). The authors analyzed data from the large-scale National Institute of Mental Health Treatment of Depression Collaborative Research Program that compared treatments for depression. Analysis indicated that the development of a therapeutic alliance (therapeutic relationship) was predictive of treatment success for all conditions.

Establishing a therapeutic alliance or relationship with a client takes time. Skills in this area gradually improve with guidance from those with more skill and experience. When clients do not engage in a therapeutic alliance, chances are that, no matter what plans of care or planned interventions are made, nothing much will happen except mutual frustration and mutual withdrawal.

THERAPEUTIC VERSUS OTHER TYPES OF RELATIONSHIPS

The nurse-client relationship is often loosely defined, but a therapeutic relationship incorporating principles of mental health nursing is more clearly defined and differs from other relationships. A therapeutic nurse-client relationship has specific goals and functions. Goals in a therapeutic relationship include the following:

Facilitating communication of distressing thoughts and feelings

Assisting clients with problem solving to help facilitate activities of daily living

Helping clients examine self-defeating behaviors and test alternatives

Promoting self-care and independence

A relationship is an interpersonal process that involves two or more people. Throughout life, we meet people in a variety of settings and share a variety of experiences. With some individuals we develop long-term relationships; with others the relationship lasts only a short time. Naturally, the kinds of relationships we enter into vary from person to person and from situation to situation. Generally, relationships can be defined as (1) social, (2) intimate, or (3) therapeutic.

Social Relationships

A social relationship can be defined as a relationship that is primarily initiated for the purpose of friendship, socialization, enjoyment, or accomplishment of a task. Mutual needs are met during social interaction (e.g., participants share ideas, feelings, and experiences). Communication skills used in social relationships may include giving advice and (sometimes) meeting basic dependency needs, such as lending money and helping with jobs. Often the content of the communication remains superficial. During social interactions, roles may shift. Within a social relationship, there is little emphasis on the evaluation of the interaction.

Intimate Relationships

An intimate relationship occurs between two or more individuals who have an emotional commitment to each other. Those in an intimate relationship usually react naturally to each other. Often the relationship is a partnership in which each member cares about the other's needs for growth and satisfaction. Within the relationship, mutual needs are met and intimate desires and fantasies are shared. Short- and long-range goals are usually mutual. Information shared between these individuals may be personal and intimate. People may want an intimate relationship for many reasons, such as procreation, sexual and/or emotional satisfaction, economic security, social belonging, and reduced loneliness. Depending on the style, level of maturity, and awareness of both parties, evaluation of the interactions may or may not be ongoing.

Therapeutic Relationships

The therapeutic relationship between nurse and client differs from both a social and an intimate relationship in that the nurse maximizes his or her communication skills, understanding of human behaviors, and personal strengths to enhance the client's growth. The focus of the relationship is on the client's ideas, experiences, and feelings. Inherent in a therapeutic (helping) relationship is the nurse's focus on significant personal issues introduced by the client during the clinical interview. The nurse and the client identify areas that need exploration and periodically evaluate the degree of change in the client. Although the nurse may assume a variety of roles (e.g., teacher, counselor, socializing agent, liaison), **the relationship is consistently focused on the client's problem and needs.** Nurses must get their needs met outside the relationship. When nurses begin to want the client to "like them," "do as they suggest," "be nice to them," or "give them recognition," the needs of the client cannot be adequately met and the interaction could be detrimental (nontherapeutic) to the client. Working under supervision is an excellent way to keep the focus and boundaries clear. Communication skills and knowledge of the stages of and phenomena occurring in a therapeutic relationship are crucial tools in the formation and maintenance of that relationship. Within the context of a helping relationship, the following occur:

- The needs of the client are identified and explored.
- Alternate problem-solving approaches are taken.
- New coping skills may develop.
- Behavioral change is encouraged.

Staff nurses as well as students may struggle with requests by clients to "be my friend." In fact, students often feel more comfortable "being a friend" because it is a more familiar role. However, when this occurs, the nurse or student needs to make it clear that the relationship is a therapeutic (helping) one. This does *not* mean that the nurse is not friendly toward the client at times. It does mean, however, that the nurse follows the stated guidelines regarding a therapeutic relationship; essentially, the focus is on the client, and the relationship is not designed to meet the nurse's needs. The client's problems and concerns are explored, potential solutions are discussed by both client and nurse, and solutions are implemented by the client.

FACTORS THAT ENHANCE GROWTH IN OTHERS

Rogers and Truax (1967) identified three personal characteristics that help promote change and growth in clients which are still valued today as vital components for establishing a therapeutic alliance or relationship: (1) genuineness, (2) empathy, and (3) positive regard.

Genuineness

Genuineness, or self-awareness of one's feelings as they arise within the relationship and the ability to communicate them when appropriate, is a key ingredient in building trust. Essentially, genuineness is the ability to meet person to person in a therapeutic relationship. It is conveyed by actions such as not hiding behind the role of nurse, listening to and communicating with others without distorting their messages, and being clear and concrete in communications with clients. Being genuine in a therapeutic relationship implies the ability to use therapeutic communication tools in an appropriately spontaneous manner, rather than rigidly or in a parrot-like fashion. Genuine helpers do not take refuge in a role such as that of "nurse" or "clinical practitioner."

Empathy

Empathy is a complex multidimensional concept that has moral, cognitive, emotional, and behavioral components (Mercer & Reynolds, 2002). Empathy means that one understands the ideas expressed, as well as the feelings that are present in the other person. Empathy signifies a central focus and feeling with and in the client's world. It involves the following (Mercer & Reynolds, 2002):

- Accurately perceiving the client's situation, perspective, and feelings
- Communicating one's understanding to the client and checking with the client for accuracy
- Acting on this understanding in a helpful (therapeutic) way toward the client

Actually, empathy may even have a new biological dimension as well. Leslie, Johnson-Frey, and Grafton (2004) believe that the discovery of the mirror neuron suggests that the nervous system can map the observed actions of others onto the premotor cortex of the self. The authors suggest that there may be a right hemisphere mirroring system that could provide a neural substrate for empathy.

There is much confusion regarding empathy versus sympathy. Being empathetic and being sympathetic are defined by many as two different things. For example, sympathy is thought to have more to do with feelings of compassion, pity, and commiseration. Although these are human traits, they may not be par-ticularly useful in a counseling situation. However, as Rich (2003) points out, "compassion is central to holistic nursing care, it involves the recognition that all humans desire happiness and not suffering" (p. 203).

When people express sympathy, they express agreement with another, which may in some situations discourage further exploration of a person's thoughts and feelings. Sympathy is the actual sharing of another's feelings and consequently the experiencing of the need to reduce one's own personal distress. When a helping person is feeling sympathy with another, objectivity is lost, and the ability to assist the client in solving a personal problem ceases. For the sake of simplicity, the following two examples are given to clarify the distinction between empathy and sympathy. A friend tells you that her mother was just diagnosed with inoperable cancer. Your friend then begins to cry and pounds the table with her fist.

Sympathetic response: "I know exactly how you feel. My mother was hospitalized last year and it was awful. I was so depressed. I still get upset just thinking about it." You go on to tell your friend about the incident.

Sometimes, when nurses try to be sympathetic, they are apt to project their own feelings onto the client's, which thus limits the client's range of responses. A more useful response might be as follows:

Empathetic response: "How upsetting this must be for you. Something similar happened to my mother last year and I had so many mixed emotions. What thoughts and feelings are you having?" You continue to stay with your friend and listen to his or her thoughts and feelings.

In the practice of psychotherapy or counseling, empathy is an essential ingredient in a therapeutic relationship both for the better-functioning client and for the client who functions at a more primitive level. In a review of the nursing literature from 1992 to 2000, Kunyk and Olson (2001) identified five conceptualizations of empathy: (1) a human trait, (2) a professional state, (3) a communication process, (4) a caring process, and (5) a special relationship. Various nurse authors have approached empathy from a range of perspectives as well. Some looked at empathy from the perspective of time frames, others at measurements of empathy, and still others at outcomes when empathy was evident. Empathy as a concept, then, is maturing and gathering more breadth and depth. Kunyk and Olson view all of these concepts as valuable but state that a more mature concept of empathy will eventually emerge.

Positive Regard

Positive regard implies respect. It is the ability to view another person as being worthy of caring about and as someone who has strengths and achievement potential. Respect is usually communicated indirectly by actions rather than directly by words.

Attitudes

One attitude through which a nurse might convey respect is willingness to work with the client. That is, the nurse takes the client and the relationship seriously. The experience is viewed not as "a job," "part of a course," or "time spent talking" but as an opportunity to work with the client to help him or her develop personal resources and actualize more of his or her potential in living.

Actions

Some actions that manifest an attitude of respect are attending, suspending value judgments, and helping clients develop their own resources.

Attending. Attending behavior is the foundation of interviewing (Ivey & Ivey, 1999). To succeed, nurses must pay attention to their clients in culturally and individually appropriate ways (Sommers-Flanagan & Sommers-Flanagan, 2003). Disturbances in thinking, feeling, and behaving are ways that individuals express themselves. Special expertise in listening (attending) is a vital component in identifying these disturbances. *Attending* refers to an intensity of presence, or being with the client. At times, simply being with another person during a painful time can make a difference. Some nonverbal behaviors that reflect the degree of attending are the following:

- The nurse's body posture (leaning forward toward the client, arms comfortably at sides)
- The nurse's degree of eye contact
- The nurse's body language (e.g., degree of relaxation during the interaction and evaluation of the client's response to nurse behaviors)

It must be noted that body posture, eye contact, and body language are highly culturally influenced and need to be assessed with regard to the client's cultural norms.

Suspending Value Judgments. Nurses are more effective when they guard against using their own value systems to judge clients' thoughts, feelings, or behaviors. For example, if a client is taking drugs or is involved in sexually risky behavior, you might recognize that these behaviors are hindering the client from living a more satisfying life, posing a potential health threat, or preventing the client from developing satisfying relationships. However, labeling these activities as bad or good is not useful. Rather, focus on exploring the behavior of the client and work toward identifying the thoughts and feelings that influence this behavior. Judgmental behavior on the part of the nurse will most likely interfere with further exploration.

The first steps in eliminating judgmental thinking and behaviors are to (1) recognize their presence, (2) identify how or where you learned these responses to the client's behavior, and (3) construct alternative ways to view the client's thinking and behavior. Just denying judgmental thinking will only compound the problem.

Client: I am really sexually promiscuous and I love to gamble when I have money. I have sex whenever I can find a partner and spend most of my time in the casino. This has been going on for at least 3 years.

A judgmental response would be the following:

Nurse A: So your promiscuous sexual and compulsive gambling behaviors really haven't brought you much happiness, have they? You are running away from your problems and could end up with acquired immunodeficiency syndrome and broke.

A more helpful response would be the following:

Nurse B: So, your sexual and gambling activities are part of the picture also. You sound as if these activities are not making you happy.

In this example, Nurse B focuses on the client's behaviors and the possible meaning they might have to the client. Nurse B does not introduce personal value statements or prejudices regarding promiscuous behavior, as does Nurse A. Empathy and positive regard are essential qualities in a successful nurse-client relationship. See the discussion of the results of the study of Forchuk and associates (2000) later in this chapter.

Helping Clients Develop Resources. The nurse becomes aware of clients' strengths and encourages clients to work at their optimal level of functioning. The nurse does not act for clients unless absolutely necessary, and then only as a step toward helping them act on their own. It is important that clients remain as independent as possible to develop new resources for problem solving.

Client: This medication makes my mouth so dry. Could you get me something to drink?

Nurse: There is juice in the refrigerator. I'll wait here for you until you get back.

or

Nurse: I'll walk with you while you get some juice from the refrigerator.

Another example of this follows:

Client: Could you ask the doctor to let me have a pass for the weekend?

Nurse: Your doctor will be on the unit this afternoon. I'll let her know that you want to speak with her.

Consistently encouraging clients to use their own resources helps minimize the clients' feelings of helplessness and dependency and also validates their potential for change.

ESTABLISHING BOUNDARIES

The nurse's role in the therapeutic relationship is theoretically rather well defined. The client's needs are separated from the nurse's needs, and the client's role is different from that of the nurse. Therefore, the boundaries of the relationship seem to be well stated. In reality, boundaries are at risk of blurring, and a shift in the nurse-client relationship may lead to nontherapeutic dynamics. Pilette and associates (1995) described the following two common circumstances that can produce blurring of boundaries:

- When the relationship slips into a social context
- When the nurse's needs are met at the expense of the client's needs

The nursing actions that may be manifested when boundaries are blurred include the following (Pilette et al., 1995):

Overhelping—doing for clients what they are able to do themselves or going beyond the wishes or needs of clients

Controlling—asserting authority and assuming control of clients "for their own good"

Narcissism—having to find weakness, helplessness, and/or disease in clients to feel helpful, at the expense of recognizing and supporting clients' healthier, stronger, and more competent features

Table 10-1 identifies potential client behaviors in response to the overinvolvement or underinvolvement of the nurse. When situations such as these arise, the relationship has ceased to be a helpful one and the phenomenon of control becomes an issue. Role blurring is often a result of unrecognized transference or countertransference.

Transference

Transference is a phenomenon originally identified by Sigmund Freud when he used psychoanalysis to treat clients. Transference is the process whereby a person unconsciously and inappropriately displaces (transfers) onto individuals in his or her current life those patterns of behavior and emotional reactions that originated in relation to significant figures in childhood. Although the transference phenomenon occurs in all relationships, transference seems to be intensified in relationships of authority. Because the process of transference is accelerated toward a person in authority, physicians, nurses, and social workers all are potential objects of transference. It is important to realize that the client may experience thoughts, feelings, and reactions toward a health care worker that are realistic and appropriate; these are *not* transference phenomena.

Common forms of transference include the desire for affection or respect and the gratification of dependency needs. Other transferential feelings the client might experience are hostility, jealousy, competitiveness, and love. Requests for special favors (e.g., cigarettes, water, extra time in the session) are concrete examples of transference phenomena.

Countertransference

Countertransference refers to the tendency of the nurse clinician to displace onto the client feelings related to people in the therapist's past. Frequently, the

TABLE 10-1

Client and Nurse Behaviors That Reflect Blurred Boundaries

When the Nurse Is Overly Involved	When the Nurse Is Not Involved
More frequent requests by the client for assistance, which causes increased dependency on the nurse	Client's increased verbal or physical expression of isolation (depression)
Inability of the client to perform tasks of which he or she is known to be capable prior to the nurse's help, which causes regression	Lack of mutually agreed goals
Unwillingness on the part of the client to maintain performance or progress in the nurse's absence	Lack of progress toward goals
Expressions of anger by other staff who do not agree with the nurse's interventions or perceptions of the client	Nurse's avoidance of spending time with the client
Nurse's keeping of secrets about the nurse-client relationship	Failure of the nurse to follow through on agreed interventions

Data from Pilette, P. C., et al. (1995). Therapeutic management of helping boundaries. *Journal of Psychosocial Nursing and Mental Health Services, 33*(1), 40-47.

client's transference to the nurse evokes countertransference feelings in the nurse. For example, it is normal to feel angry when attacked persistently, annoyed when frustrated unreasonably, or flattered when idealized. A nurse might feel extremely important when depended on exclusively by a client. If the nurse does not recognize his or her own omnipotent feelings as countertransference, encouragement of independent growth in the client might be minimized at best. Recognizing our countertransference reactions maximizes our ability to *empower* our clients. When we fail to recognize our countertransferences toward our clients (and others, for that matter) the therapeutic relationship stalls, and essentially we *disempower* our clients by experiencing them not as individuals but rather as inner projections.

If the nurse feels either a strongly positive or a strongly negative reaction to a client, the feeling most often signals countertransference in the nurse. One common sign of countertransference in the nurse is overidentification with the client. In this situation the nurse may have difficulty recognizing or understanding problems the client has that are similar to the nurse's own. For example, a nurse who is struggling with an alcoholic family member may feel disinterested, cold, or disgusted toward an alcoholic client. Other indications of countertransference occur when the nurse gets involved in power struggles, competition, or argument with the client. Table 10-2 identifies some common countertransferential reactions and gives some suggestions for self-intervention.

Identifying and working through various transference and countertransference issues is crucial if the nurse is to achieve professional and clinical growth and if the possibility is to be created for positive change in the client. These issues are best dealt with through the use of supervision by either the peer group or therapeutic team. Regularly scheduled supervision sessions provide the nurse with the opportunity to increase self-awareness, clinical skills, and growth, as well as allow for continued growth of the client.

Self-Check on Boundary Issues

It is helpful for all of us to take time out to be reflective and to try to be aware of our thoughts and actions with clients, as well as with colleagues, friends, and family. Figure 10-1 is a helpful self-test you can use throughout your career, no matter what area of nursing you choose.

TABLE 10-2

Common Countertransference Reactions

As a nurse, you will sometimes experience countertransference feelings. Once you are aware of them, use them for self-analysis to understand those feelings that may inhibit productive nurse-client communication.

Nurse's Reaction to Client	Characteristic Nurse Behavior	Self-Analysis	Solution
Boredom (indifference)	▪ Showing inattention ▪ Frequently asking the client to repeat statements ▪ Making inappropriate responses	▪ Is the content of what the client presents uninteresting? Or is it the style of communication? Does the client exhibit an offensive style of communication? ▪ Have you anything else on your mind that may be distracting you from the client's needs? ▪ Is the client discussing an issue that makes you anxious?	▪ Redirect the client if he or she provides more information than you need or goes "off the track." ▪ Clarify information with the client. ▪ Confront ineffective modes of communication.
Rescue	▪ Reaching for unattainable goals ▪ Resisting peer feedback and supervisory recommendations ▪ Giving advice	▪ What behavior stimulates your perceived need to rescue the client? ▪ Has anyone evoked such feelings in you in the past? ▪ What are your fears or fantasies about failing to meet the client's needs? ▪ Why do you want to rescue this client?	▪ Avoid secret alliances. ▪ Develop realistic goals. ▪ Do not alter meeting schedule. ▪ Let the client guide interaction. ▪ Facilitate client problem solving.
Overinvolvement	▪ Coming to work early, leaving late ▪ Ignoring peer suggestions, resisting assistance ▪ Buying the client clothes or other gifts ▪ Accepting the client's gifts ▪ Behaving judgmentally at family interventions ▪ Keeping secrets ▪ Calling the client when off-duty	▪ What particular client characteristics are attractive? ▪ Does the client remind you of someone? Who? ▪ Does your current behavior differ from your treatment of similar clients in the past? ▪ What are you getting out of this situation? ▪ What needs of yours are being met?	▪ Establish firm treatment boundaries, goals, and nursing expectations. ▪ Avoid self-disclosure. ▪ Avoid calling the client when off duty.
Overidentification	▪ Having special agenda, keeping secrets ▪ Increasing self-disclosure ▪ Feeling omnipotent ▪ Experiencing physical attraction	▪ With which of the client's physical, emotional, cognitive, or situational characteristics do you identify? ▪ Recall similar circumstances in your own life. How did you deal with the issues now being created by the client?	▪ Allow the client to direct issues. ▪ Encourage a problem-solving approach from the client's perspective. ▪ Avoid self-disclosure.

Data from Aromando, L. (1995). *Mental health and psychiatric nursing* (2nd ed.). Springhouse, PA: Springhouse.

TABLE 10-2

Common Countertransference Reactions—cont'd

Nurse's Reaction to Client	Characteristic Nurse Behavior	Self-Analysis	Solution
Misuse of honesty	■ Withholding information ■ Lying	■ Why are you protecting the client? ■ What are your fears about the client's learning the truth?	■ Be clear in your responses and aware of your hesitation; do not hedge. ■ If you can provide information, tell the client and give your rationale. ■ Avoid keeping secrets. ■ Reinforce the client with regard to the interdisciplinary nature of treatment.
Anger	■ Withdrawing ■ Speaking loudly ■ Using profanity ■ Asking to be taken off the case	■ What client behaviors are offensive to you? ■ What dynamic from your past may this client be re-creating?	■ Determine the origin of the anger (nurse, client, or both). ■ Explore the roots of client anger. ■ Avoid contact with the client if the anger is not understood.
Helplessness or hopelessness	■ Feeling sadness	■ Which client behaviors evoke these feelings in you? ■ Has anyone evoked similar feelings in the past? Who? ■ What past expectations were placed on you (verbally and nonverbally) by this client?	■ Maintain therapeutic involvement. ■ Explore and focus on the client's experience rather than on your own.

NURSING BOUNDARY INDEX SELF-CHECK

Please rate yourself according to the frequency with which the following statements reflect your behavior, thoughts, or feelings within the past 2 years while providing patient care.*

1. Have you ever received any feedback about your behavior being overly intrusive with patients and their families?	Never _____	Rarely _____	Sometimes _____	Often _____
2. Do you ever have difficulty setting limits with patients?	Never _____	Rarely _____	Sometimes _____	Often _____
3. Do you ever arrive early or stay late to be with your patient for a longer period?	Never _____	Rarely _____	Sometimes _____	Often _____
4. Do you ever find yourself relating to patients or peers as you might to a family member?	Never _____	Rarely _____	Sometimes _____	Often _____
5. Have you ever acted on sexual feelings you have for a patient?	Never _____	Rarely _____	Sometimes _____	Often _____
6. Do you feel that you are the only one who understands the patient?	Never _____	Rarely _____	Sometimes _____	Often _____
7. Have you ever received feedback that you get "too involved" with patients or families?	Never _____	Rarely _____	Sometimes _____	Often _____
8. Do you derive conscious satisfaction from patients' praise, appreciation, or affection?	Never _____	Rarely _____	Sometimes _____	Often _____
9. Do you ever feel that other staff members are too critical of "your" patient?	Never _____	Rarely _____	Sometimes _____	Often _____
10. Do you ever feel that other staff members are jealous of your relationship with your patient?	Never _____	Rarely _____	Sometimes _____	Often _____
11. Have you ever tried to "match-make" a patient with one of your friends?	Never _____	Rarely _____	Sometimes _____	Often _____
12. Do you find it difficult to handle patients' unreasonable requests for assistance, verbal abuse, or sexual language?	Never _____	Rarely _____	Sometimes _____	Often _____

* Any item that is responded to with "Sometimes" or "Often" should alert the nurse to a possible area of vulnerability. If the item is responded to with "Rarely," the nurse should determine whether it is an isolated event or a possible pattern of behavior.

FIGURE 10-1 Nursing boundary index self-check. (From Pilette, P., Berck, C., & Achber, L. [1995]. Therapeutic management. *Journal of Psychosocial Nursing, 33*[1], 45.)

UNDERSTANDING SELF AND OTHERS

Relationships are complex. We bring into our relationships a multitude of thoughts, feelings, beliefs, and attitudes—some rational and some irrational. It is helpful, even crucial, that we have an understanding of our own personal values and attitudes so that we may become aware of the beliefs or attitudes we hold that may interfere with the establishment of positive relationships with those under our care.

Values

Increasingly we are working with, living with, and caring for people from diverse cultures and subcultures whose life experiences and life values may be quite different from our own. Values are abstract standards and represent an ideal, either positive or negative. For example, in the United States, to create a social order in which people can live peaceably together and feel secure in their persons and property, society has adopted the two values of respecting one another's liberty and working cooperatively for a common goal. Not all the nation's people live up to these ideals all the time, and there may exist for some a dichotomy between theory and practice. For example, some people may pay lip service to the values of authority, whereas their behavior contradicts these values. They may stress honesty and respect for the law, yet cheat on their taxes and in their business practices. They may love their neighbors on Sunday and demean or downgrade them for the rest of the week. They may declare themselves patriots, but label others traitors or even deny freedom of speech to any dissenters whose concept of patriotism differs from theirs.

A person's value system greatly influences both everyday and long-range choices. Values and beliefs provide a framework for what life goals people develop and for what they want their life to include. Our values are usually culturally oriented and influenced in a variety of ways through our parents, teachers, religious institutions, workplaces, peers, and political leaders as well as through Hollywood and the media. All these influences attempt to instill their values and to form and influence ours (Simon, Howe, & Kirschenbaum, 1995).

We also form our values through the example of others. **Modeling** is perhaps one of the most potent means of value education because it presents a vivid example of values in action (Simon et al., 1995). We all need role models to guide us in negotiating life's many choices. Young people in particular are hungry for role models and will find them among peers as well as adults. As nurses, parents, bosses, co-workers, friends, lovers, teachers, spouses, singles, or whatever, we are constantly (in either a positive or negative manner) providing a role model to others.

One of the steps in the nursing process is to plan outcome criteria. We emphasize that the client and the nurse identify outcomes together. What happens when the nurse's beliefs and values are very different from those of a client? For example, the client wants an abortion, which is against the nurse's values (or vice versa). The client engages in irresponsible sex with multiple partners, and that is against the nurse's values. The client puts material gain and objects far ahead of loyalty to friends and family, in direct contrast with the nurse's values (or vice versa). The client's lifestyle includes taking illicit drugs, and substance abuse is against the nurse's values. The client is deeply religious, and the nurse is a nonbeliever who shuns organized religion. Can a nurse develop a working relationship and help a client solve a problem when the values and goals of the client are so different from his or her own?

As nurses, it is useful for us to understand that our values and beliefs are not necessarily right, and certainly not right for everyone. It is helpful for us to realize that our values (1) reflect our own culture, (2) are derived from a whole range of choices, and (3) are those we have *chosen* for ourselves from a variety of influences and role models. These chosen values guide us in making decisions and taking the actions we hope will make our lives meaningful, rewarding, and full. Personal values may change over time; indeed, personal values may change many times over the course of a lifetime. The values you held as a child are different from those you held as an adolescent and change in young adulthood, and so forth. Self-awareness requires that we understand what we value and those beliefs that guide our behavior. It is critical that as nurses we not only understand and accept our own values but also are sensitive to and accepting of the unique and different values of others.

Values Clarification

Values clarification is a process that helps people understand and build their value systems, addressing some questions in the process. For example, "Where do we learn whether to stick to the old moral and value standards or try new ones? How do we learn to relate to people whose values differ from our own? What do we do when two important values are in conflict?" (Simon et al., 1995).

A popular approach to values clarification was initially formulated by Louis Raths and colleagues (1966). In their framework, a value has three components: emotional, cognitive, and behavioral. We do not just hold our values; we *feel* deeply about them and will stand up for them and affirm them when appropriate. We *choose* our values from a variety of options after weighing the pros and cons, including the consequences of these choices and positions. And, ultimately, *we act* upon our values. Our values determine how we live our lives. Values, according to Raths, Harmin, and Simon (1966), are composed of seven subprocesses:

Prizing one's beliefs and behaviors (emotional)
1. Prizing and cherishing
2. Publicly affirming, when appropriate

Choosing one's beliefs and behaviors (cognitive)
3. Choosing from alternatives
4. Choosing after consideration of consequences
5. Choosing freely

Acting on one's beliefs (behavioral)
6. Acting
7. Acting with a pattern, consistency, and repetition

The suggestion of Sommers-Flanagan and Sommers-Flanagan (2003) for enhancing psychosocial awareness is to reflect intentionally on your own values and career goals:

1. What are my important values?
2. What are my life goals? What do I really want out of life? Does my everyday behavior move me toward my life goals?
3. What are my career goals? If I want to be a nurse, nurse therapist, or other specialist, how will I achieve this? Why do I want to be a nurse or other specialist?
4. How would I describe myself in a few words? How would I describe myself to a stranger? What do I particularly like and what do I dislike about myself?

PHASES OF THE NURSE-CLIENT RELATIONSHIP

The ability of the nurse to engage in interpersonal interactions in a goal-directed manner for the purpose of assisting clients with their emotional or physical health needs is the foundation of the nurse-client relationship.

The nurse-client relationship is synonymous with a professional helping relationship. Behaviors that have relevance to health care workers, including nurses, are as follows:

Accountability. The nurse assumes responsibility for his or her conduct and the consequences of his or her actions.

Focus on client needs. The interest of the client rather than the nurse, other health care workers, or the institution is given first consideration. The nurse's role is that of client advocate.

Clinical competence. The criteria on which the nurse bases his or her conduct are principles of knowledge and those that are appropriate to the specific situation. This involves awareness and incorporation of the latest knowledge made available from research (evidence-based practice).

Supervision. Validation of performance quality is through regularly scheduled supervisory sessions. Supervision is conducted either by a more experienced clinician or, more commonly, through discussion with a therapeutic team (nurses, physician, social worker, etc.).

Nurses interact with clients in a variety of settings, such as emergency departments, medical-surgical units, obstetric and pediatric units, clinics, community settings, schools, and clients' homes. Nurses who are sensitive to clients' needs and have effective assessment and communication skills can significantly help clients confront current problems and anticipate future choices.

Sometimes, the type of relationship that occurs may be informal and not extensive, such as when the nurse and client meet for only a few sessions. However, even though it is brief, the relationship may be substantial, useful, and important for the client. This limited relationship is often referred to as a therapeutic encounter. When the nurse really is concerned with another's circumstances (has positive regard, empathy), even a short encounter with the individual can have a powerful impact on that individual's life.

At other times, the encounters may be longer and more formal, such as in inpatient settings, mental health units, crisis centers, and mental health facilities. This longer time span allows the development of a therapeutic nurse-client relationship.

Hildegard Peplau introduced the concept of the nurse-client relationship in 1952 in her groundbreaking book *Interpersonal Relations in Nursing*. This model of the nurse-client relationship is well accepted in the United States and Canada and has become an important tool for all nursing practice. Peplau (1952) proposed that the nurse-client relationship "facilitates forward movement" for both the nurse and the client (p. 12). Peplau's interactive nurse-client process is designed to facilitate the client's boundary management, independent problem solving, and decision making that promotes autonomy (Haber, 2000).

It is most likely that in the brief period you have for your psychiatric nursing rotation, all the phases of the nurse-client relationship will not have time to develop. However, it is important for you to be aware of these phases because you must be able to recognize and use them later.

Peplau (1952, 1999) described the nurse-client relationship as evolving through interlocking, overlapping phases. The following distinctive phases of the nurse-client relationship are generally recognized:

- Orientation phase
- Working phase
- Termination phase

Although various phenomena and goals are identified for each phase, they often overlap from phase to phase. Even before the first meeting, the nurse may have many thoughts and feelings related to the first clinical session. This is sometimes referred to as the *preorientation phase*.

Preorientation Phase

Beginning health care professionals who are new to the psychiatric setting usually have many concerns and experience a mild to moderate degree of anxiety on their first clinical day. One common concern involves fear of physical harm or violence. Your instructor usually discusses this common concern in your first preconference. There are unit protocols for intervening with clients who have poor impulse control, and staff and unit safeguards should be constantly in place to help clients gain self-control. Although such disruptions are not common, the concern is valid. Most unit staff are trained in and practice interventions for clients who are having difficulty with impulse control. Hospital security is readily available to give the staff support.

Some of you may be concerned with saying the wrong thing, using the client as a guinea pig, feeling inadequate about new and developing communication skills, feeling vulnerable without the uniform as a clear indicator of who is the nurse and who is the client, and feeling exposed as you relate to your own earlier personal experiences or crises. These are universal and valid feelings; if they were not discussed in class, they will be brought up on the first clinical day, either by you or by your instructor. Chapter 11 deals with a variety of clinical concerns student nurses have when beginning their psychiatric nursing rotation (e.g., what to do if clients do not want to talk, if they ask the nurse to keep a secret, if they cry). Usually after the first clinical day your anxiety is much lower, and it is easier to focus on clinical issues with the support of your instructor and classmates. The preorientation phase revolves around planning for the first interaction with the client.

Orientation Phase

The orientation phase can last for a few meetings or can extend over a longer period. This first phase may be prolonged in the case of severely and persistently ill mental health clients.

The first time the nurse and the client meet, they are strangers to each other. When strangers meet, whether or not they know anything about each other, they interact according to their own backgrounds, standards, values, and experiences. This fact—that each person has a unique frame of reference—underlies the need for self-awareness on the part of the nurse.

As the relationship evolves through an ongoing series of reactions, each participant may elicit in the other a wide range of positive and negative emotional reactions. Remember that the projection of feelings in the client to the nurse is referred to as *transference*, and the projection of feelings in the nurse or clinician to the client is referred to as *countertransference*. As discussed earlier, the nurse is responsible for identifying these two phenomena and maintaining appropriate boundaries.

Establishing Trust

A major emphasis during the first few encounters with the client is on providing an atmosphere in which trust can grow. As in any relationship, trust is nurtured by demonstrating genuineness and empathy, developing positive regard, showing consistency, and offering assistance in alleviating the client's emotional pain or problems. This may take only a short period, but in many instances it may be a long time before a client feels free to discuss painful personal experiences and private thoughts.

During the orientation phase, four important issues need to be addressed:

1. Parameters of the relationship
2. Formal or informal contract
3. Confidentiality
4. Termination

Parameters of the Relationship. The client needs to know about the nurse (who the nurse is and what the nurse's background is) and the purpose of the meetings. For example, a student might furnish the following information:

Student: Hello, Mrs. James. I am Nancy Rivera from Orange Community College. I am in my psychiatric rotation, and I will be coming to York Hospital for the next six Thursdays. I would like to spend time with you each Thursday if you are still here. I'm here to be a support person for you as you work on your treatment goals.

Formal or Informal Contract. A contract emphasizes the client's participation and responsibility because it shows that the nurse does something *with* the client rather than *for* the client. The contract, either stated or written, contains the place, time, date, and duration of the meetings. During the orientation phase, the client may begin to express thoughts and feelings, identify problems, and discuss realistic goals. Therefore, the mutual agreement on goals is also part of the contract. If the goals are met, the client's level of functioning will return to a previous level, or at least improve from the present level. If fees are to be paid, the client is told how much they will be and when the payment is due.

Student: Mrs. James, we will meet at 10 AM each Thursday in the consultation room at the clinic for 45 minutes, from September 15th to October 27th. We can use that time for further discussion of your feelings of loneliness and anger you mentioned and explore some things you could do to make the situation better for yourself.

Confidentiality. The client has a right to know who else will be given the information being shared with the nurse. He or she needs to know that the information may be shared with specific people, such as a clinical supervisor, the physician, the staff, or other students in conference. The client also needs to know that the information will *not* be shared with his or her relatives, friends, or others outside the treatment team, except in extreme situations. Extreme situations include those in which (1) the information may be harmful to the client or to others, (2) the client threatens self-harm, or (3) the client does not intend to follow through with the treatment plan. If information must be given to others, this is usually done by the physician, according to legal guidelines (see Chapter 8). The nurse must be aware of the client's right to confidentiality and must not violate that right.

> *Student:* Mrs. James, I will be sharing some of what we discuss with my nursing instructor, and at times I may discuss certain concerns with my peers in conference or with the staff. However, I will *not* be sharing this information with your husband or any other members of your family or anyone outside the hospital without your permission.

Termination. Termination begins in the orientation phase. It may also be mentioned when appropriate during the working phase if the nature of the relationship is time limited (e.g., six or nine sessions). The date of the termination phase should be clear from the beginning. In some situations the nurse-client contract may be renegotiated when the termination date has been reached. In other situations, when the therapeutic nurse-client relationship is an open-ended one, the termination date is not known.

> *Student:* Mrs. James, as I mentioned earlier, our last meeting will be on October 27th. We will have three more meetings after today.

During the orientation phase and later, clients often unconsciously employ behaviors to test the nurse. The client wants to know if the nurse will do the following:

- Be able to set limits when the client needs them.
- Still show concern if the client acts angry, babyish, unlikable, or dependent.
- Still be there if the client is late, leaves early, refuses to speak, or is angry.

Table 10-3 identifies some testing behaviors and possible responses by nurses.

In summary, the initial interview includes the following:

- The nurse's role is clarified and the responsibilities of both the client and the nurse are defined.
- The contract containing the time, place, date, and duration of the meetings is discussed.
- Confidentiality is discussed and assumed.
- The terms of termination are introduced (these are also discussed throughout the orientation phase and beyond).
- The nurse becomes aware of transference and countertransference issues (which will later be discussed in the team conference or peer supervision setting).
- An atmosphere is established in which trust can grow.
- Client problems are articulated and mutually agreed goals are established.

Working Phase

Moore and Hartman (1988) identified specific tasks of the working phase of the nurse-client relationship that are relevant in current practice:

- Maintain the relationship.
- Gather further data.
- Promote the client's problem-solving skills, self-esteem, and use of language.
- Facilitate behavioral change.
- Overcome resistance behaviors.
- Evaluate problems and goals and redefine them as necessary.
- Promote practice and expression of alternative adaptive behaviors.

During the working phase, the nurse and client together identify and explore areas in the client's life that are causing problems. Often, the client's present ways of handling situations stem from earlier means of coping devised to survive in a chaotic and dysfunctional family environment. Although certain coping methods may have worked for the client at an earlier age, they now interfere with the client's interpersonal relationships and prevent him or her from attaining current goals. The client's dysfunctional behaviors and basic assumptions about the world are often defensive, and the client is usually unable to change the dysfunctional behavior at will. Therefore, most of the problem behaviors or thoughts continue because of unconscious motivations and needs that are out of the client's awareness.

The nurse can work with the client to identify these unconscious motivations and assumptions that keep the client from finding satisfaction and reaching potential. Describing, and often reexperiencing, old conflicts generally awakens high levels of anxiety in the client. Clients may use various defenses against anxiety and displace their feelings onto the nurse. Therefore, during the working phase, intense emotions such as anxiety, anger, self-hate, hopelessness, and helplessness may surface. Behaviors such as acting out anger inappropriately, withdrawing, intellec-

TABLE 10-3

Testing Behaviors Used by Clients

Client Behavior	Client Example	Nurse Response	Rationale
Shifts focus of interview *to* the nurse, *off* the client	"Do you have any children?" or "Are you married?"	"This time is for you." If appropriate, the nurse should add: ■ "Do you have any children?" or "What about your children?" ■ "Are you married?" or "What about your relationships?"	1. The nurse refocuses back to the client and the client's concerns. 2. The nurse sticks to the contract.
Tries to get the nurse to take care of him or her	"Could you tell my doctor?"	"I'll leave a message with the unit clerk that you want to see the doctor" or "You know best what you want the doctor to know. I'll be interested in what the doctor has to say."	1. The nurse validates that the client is able to do many things for himself or herself. This aids in increasing self-esteem.
	"Should I take this job?"	"What do you see as the pros and cons of this job?"	2. The nurse always encourages the person to function at the highest level, even if he or she doesn't want to.
Makes sexual advances toward the nurse (e.g., touches the nurse's arm, wants to hold hands with or kiss the nurse)	"Would you go out with me? . . . Why not?" or "Can I kiss you? . . . Why not?"	"I am not comfortable having you touch (kiss) me." The nurse briefly reiterates the nurse's role: "This time is for you to focus on your problems and concerns." If the client stops: "I wonder what this is all about?" 1. Is the client afraid the nurse will not like him or her? 2. Is the client trying to take the focus off the problems? If the client continues: "If you can't stop this behavior, I'll have to leave. I'll be back at (time) to spend time with you then."	1. The nurse needs to set clear limits on expected behavior. 2. Frequently restating the nurse's role throughout the relationship can help maintain boundaries. 3. Whenever possible, the meaning of the client's behavior should be explored. 4. Leaving gives the client time to gain control. The nurse returns at the stated time.
Continues to arrive late for meetings	"I'm a little late because (excuse)."	The nurse arrives on time and leaves at the scheduled time. (The nurse does not let the client manipulate him or her or bargain for more time.) After a couple of such instances, the nurse can explore behavior (e.g., "I wonder if there is something going on that you don't want to deal with?" or "I wonder what these latenesses mean to you?").	1. The nurse keeps the contract. Clients feel more secure when "promises" are kept, even though clients may try to manipulate the nurse through anger, helplessness, and so forth. 2. The nurse does not tell the client what to do, but the nurse and the client need to explore the meaning of the behavior.

tualizing, manipulating, and denying are to be expected.

During the working phase, strong transference feelings may appear. The emotional responses and behaviors in the client may also awaken strong countertransference feelings in the nurse. **The nurse's awareness of personal feelings and reactions to the client is vital for effective interaction with the client.** Common transference feelings, as well as the reactions that nurses experience in response to different client behaviors and situations, are discussed in the planning component of each of the clinical chapters.

The development of a strong working relationship can allow the client to experience increased levels of anxiety and demonstrate dysfunctional behaviors in a safe setting, and try out new and more adaptive coping behaviors.

Termination Phase

Termination is discussed during the first interview. During the working stage, the fact of eventual termination may also be raised at appropriate times. Reasons for terminating the nurse-client relationship include the following:

- Symptom relief
- Improved social functioning
- Greater sense of identity
- Development of more adaptive behaviors
- Accomplishment of the client's goals
- Impasse in therapy that the nurse is unable to resolve

In addition, forced termination may occur, such as when the student completes the course objectives, a nurse clinician leaves the clinical setting, or the insurance coverage runs out and there is a change of staff. The termination phase is the final phase of the nurse-client relationship. Important reasons for the student or nurse counselor to address the termination phase are as follows:

1. Termination is an integral phase of the therapeutic nurse-client relationship, and without it the relationship remains incomplete.
2. Feelings are aroused in both the client and the nurse with regard to the experience they have had; when these feelings are recognized and shared, clients learn that it is acceptable to feel sadness and loss when someone they care about leaves.
3. The client is a partner in the relationship and has a right to see the nurse's needs and feelings about their time together and the ensuing separation.
4. Termination can be a learning experience; clients can learn that they are important to at least one person.
5. By sharing the termination experience with the client, the nurse demonstrates caring for the client.
6. This may be the first successful termination experience for the client.

Termination often awakens strong feelings in both nurse and client. Termination of the relationship between the nurse and the client signifies a loss for both, although the intensity and meaning of termination may be different for each. If a client has unresolved feelings of abandonment or loneliness, or feelings of not being wanted or of being rejected by others, these feelings may be reawakened during the termination process. This process can be an opportunity for the client to express these feelings, perhaps for the first time.

It is not unusual to see a variety of client behaviors that indicate defensive maneuvers against the anxiety of separation and loss. For example, a client may withdraw from the nurse and not want to meet for the final session or may become outwardly hostile and sarcastic—for instance, accusing the student of using the client for personal gains ("like a guinea pig") as a way of deflecting the awakening of anger and pain that are rooted in past separations. Often, a client will deny that the relationship had any impact or that ending the relationship evokes any emotions whatsoever. Regression is another behavioral manifestation; it may be seen as increased dependency on the nurse or a return of earlier symptoms.

It is important for the nurse to work with the client to bring into awareness any feelings and reactions the client may be experiencing related to separations. If a client denies that the termination is having an effect (assuming the nurse-client relationship was strong), the nurse may say something like, "Good-byes are difficult for people. Often they remind us of other good-byes. Tell me about another separation in the past." If the client appears to be displacing anger, either by withdrawing or by being overtly angry at the nurse, the nurse may use generalized statements such as, "People may experience anger when saying goodbye. Sometimes they are angry with the person who is leaving. Tell me how you feel about my leaving." New practitioners as well as students in the psychiatric setting need to give thought to their last clinical experience with their client and work with their supervisor or instructor to facilitate communication during this time.

Summarizing the goals and objectives achieved in the relationship is part of the termination process. Ways for the client to incorporate into daily life any new coping strategies learned during the time spent with the nurse can be discussed. Reviewing situations that occurred during the time spent together and exchanging memories can help validate the experience for both nurse and client and facilitate closure of that relationship.

A common response of beginning practitioners is feeling guilty about terminating the relationship. These feelings may be manifested by the student's giving the client his or her telephone number, making plans to get together for coffee after the client is discharged, continuing to see the client afterward, or exchanging letters. Beginning practitioners need to understand that such actions may be motivated by their own sense of guilt or by misplaced feelings of responsibility, not by concern for the client. Indeed, part of the termination process may be to explore, after discussion with the client's case manager, the client's plans for the future: where the client can go for help in the future, which agencies to contact, and which specific resource persons may be available.

During the student affiliation, the nurse-client relationship exists for the duration of the clinical course only. The termination phase is just that. Thoughts and feelings the student may have about continuing the relationship are best discussed with the instructor or shared in conference with peers, because these are common reactions to the student's experience.

WHAT HINDERS AND WHAT HELPS THE NURSE-CLIENT RELATIONSHIP

Not all nurse-client relationships follow the classic phases as outlined by Peplau. Some nurse-client relationships start in the orientation phase but move to a mutually frustrating phase and finally to mutual withdrawal (Figure 10-2).

Forchuk and associates (2000) conducted a qualitative study of the nurse-client relationship. They examined the phases of both the therapeutic and the nontherapeutic relationship. From this study, they identified certain behaviors that were beneficial to the progression of the nurse-client relationship as well as those that hampered the development of this relationship. The study emphasized the importance of consistent, regular, and private interactions with clients as essential to the development of a therapeutic alliance. Nurses in this study stressed the importance of listening, pacing, and consistency.

Specifically, Forchuk and associates (2000) identified the following factors that were inherent in a nurse-client relationship that progressed in a mutually satisfying manner:

Consistency includes ensuring that a nurse is always assigned to the same client and that the client has a regular routine for activities. Interactions are facilitated when they are frequent and regular in duration, format, and location. Consistency also refers to the nurse's being honest and consistent (congruent) in what is said to the clients.

Pacing includes letting the client set the pace and letting the pace be adjusted to fit the client's moods. A slow approach helps reduce pressure, and at times it is necessary to step back and realize that developing a strong relationship may take a long time.

Listening includes letting the client talk when this is the client's need. The nurse becomes a sounding board for the client's concerns and issues. Listening is perhaps the most important skill for nurses to master. Truly listening to another person, attending to what is behind the words, is a learned skill and is addressed in Chapter 11.

Initial impressions, especially positive initial attitudes and preconceptions, are significant considerations in how the relationship will progress. Preconceived negative impressions and feelings toward the client usually bode poorly for the positive growth of the relationship. In contrast, the nurse's feeling that the client is "interesting" or a "challenge" and a positive attitude about the relationship are usually favorable signs for the developing therapeutic alliance.

Comfort and control, that is, promoting client comfort and balancing control, usually reflect caring behaviors. Control refers to keeping a balance in the relationship: not too strict and not too lenient.

Client factors that seem to enhance the relationship include trust on the part of the client and the client's active participation in the nurse-client relationship.

In relationships that did not progress to therapeutic levels, there seemed to be some specific factors that hampered the development of positive relationships. These included the following:

Inconsistency and unavailability on the part of the nurse or the client or both, as well as lack of contact (infrequent meetings, meetings in the hallway, and client reluctance or refusal to spend time with the nurse), play a key role (mutual avoidance).

The nurse's feelings and awareness are significant factors. Major elements that contributed to the lack of progression of positive relationships were the lack of self-awareness on the part of the nurse and the nurse's own feelings. Negative preconceived ideas about the client and negative feelings (e.g., discomfort, dislike of the client, fear, and avoidance) seem to be a constant in relationships that end in frustration and mutual withdrawal. This is in contrast with more successful relationships in which the nurse's attitude is that of positive regard and interest in understanding the client's story.

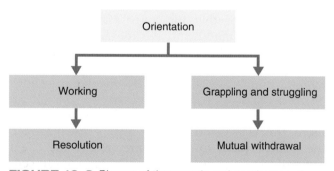

FIGURE 10-2 Phases of therapeutic and nontherapeutic relationships. (From Forchuk, C., et al. [2000]. The developing nurse-client relationship: Nurse's perspectives. *Journal of the American Psychiatric Nurses Association, 6*[1], 3-10.)

■■■ KEY POINTS to REMEMBER

- The nurse-client relationship is well defined, and the roles of the nurse and the client must be clearly stated.
- It is important that the nurse be aware of the differences between a therapeutic relationship and a social or intimate relationship. In a therapeutic nurse-client relationship, the focus is on the client's needs, thoughts, feelings, and goals. The nurse is expected to meet personal needs outside this relationship, in other professional, social, or intimate arenas.
- Genuineness, positive regard, and empathy are personal strengths in the helping person that foster growth and change in others.
- Although the boundaries of the nurse-client relationship generally are clearly defined, these boundaries can become blurred, and this blurring can be insidious and may occur on an unconscious level. Usually, transference and countertransference phenomena are operating when boundaries are blurred. A blurring of boundaries may be indicated when the nurse is too helpful or not helpful enough.
- It is important to have a grasp of common countertransferential feelings and behaviors and of the nursing actions to counteract these phenomena.
- The importance of supervision cannot be overemphasized. Supervision often takes the form of peer or therapeutic team supervision. Supervision aids in promoting the professional growth of the nurse as well as in safeguarding the integrity of the nurse-client relationship. It enhances the progression of the nurse-client relationship, allowing the client's goals to be worked on and met.
- The phases of the nurse-client relationship include the orientation, working, and termination phases.
- At the first interaction of the orientation phase, certain matters need to be addressed: (1) the parameters of the relationship—who the nurse is and the purpose of the meetings; (2) the contract—specifying the who, what, where, when, and how long of the nurse-client meetings; (3) the issue of confidentiality; and (4) the date of termination, if known. During the orientation phase (and at times throughout the relationship), a number of common client testing behaviors may arise that will require specific nursing interventions.
- Forchuk and associates (2000) identified six specific factors that seem to be characteristic of a successful nurse-client relationship and two that may foreshadow an unsuccessful relationship.

■ ■ ■

Visit the Evolve website at **http://evolve.elsevier.com/Varcarolis** for a posttest on the content in this chapter.

Critical Thinking and Chapter Review

Visit the Evolve website at **http://evolve.elsevier.com/Varcarolis** for additional self-study exercises.

■■■ CRITICAL THINKING

1. On your first clinical day you spend time with an older woman, Mrs. Schneider, who is very depressed. Your first impression is "Oh my, she looks like my mean Aunt Helen. She even sits like her." Mrs. Schneider asks you, "Who are you and how can you help me?" She tells you that "a student" could never understand what she is going through. She then says, "If you really wanted to help me you could get me a good job after I leave here."

   A. Identify transference and countertransference issues in this situation. What is your most important course of action? What in the study of Forchuk and associates (2000) indicates that this is a time for you to exercise self-awareness and self-insight to establish the potential for a therapeutic encounter or relationship to occur?

   B. How could you best respond to Mrs. Schneider's question about who you are? What other information will you give her during this first clinical encounter? Be specific.

   C. What are some useful responses you could give her regarding her legitimate questions about ways you could be of help to her?

   D. Analyze Mrs. Schneider's request that you find her a job. How does this request relate to boundary issues, and how can this be an opportunity for you to help Mrs. Schneider develop resources? Keeping in mind the aim of Peplau's interactive nurse-client process, describe some useful ways you could respond to this request.

■■■ CHAPTER REVIEW

Choose the most appropriate answer.

1. Which of the following is an accurate statement about transference?

   1. Transference occurs when the client attributes thoughts and feelings toward the therapist that pertain to a person in the client's past.

   2. Transference occurs when the therapist attributes thoughts and feelings toward the client that pertain to a person in the client's past.

   3. Transference occurs when the therapist understands and builds a value system consistent with the client's value system.

   4. Transference occurs when the therapist recalls circumstances in his or her life similar to those the client is experiencing and shares this with the client.

Continued

Critical Thinking and Chapter Review—cont'd

Visit the Evolve website at **http://evolve.elsevier.com/Varcarolis** for additional self-study exercises.

2. A basic tool the nurse uses when establishing a relationship with a client with a psychiatric disorder is
    1. narcissism.
    2. role blurring.
    3. self-reflection.
    4. formation of value judgments.

3. A nurse behavior that jeopardizes the boundaries of the nurse-client relationship is
    1. focusing on client needs.
    2. suspending value judgments.
    3. recognizing the value of supervision.
    4. allowing the relationship to become social.

4. A nurse behavior that would not be considered a boundary violation is
    1. narcissism.
    2. controlling.
    3. genuineness.
    4. keeping secrets about the relationship.

5. Which statement describes an event that would occur during the working phase of the nurse-client relationship?
    1. The nurse summarizes the objectives achieved in the relationship.
    2. The nurse assesses the client's level of psychological functioning, and mutual identification of problems and goals occurs.
    3. Some regression and mourning occur, although the client demonstrates satisfaction and competence.
    4. The client seeks connections among actions, thoughts, and feelings and engages in problem solving and testing of alternative behaviors.

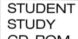

■ **STUDENT**
■ **STUDY**
■ **CD-ROM**

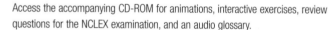

Access the accompanying CD-ROM for animations, interactive exercises, review questions for the NCLEX examination, and an audio glossary.

REFERENCES

Forchuk, C., et al. (2000). The developing nurse-client relationship: Nurse's perspectives. *Journal of the American Psychiatric Nurses Association, 6*(1), 3-10.

Haber, J. (2000). Hildegard E. Peplau: The psychiatric nursing legacy of a legend. *Journal of the American Psychiatric Nursing Association, 6*(2), 56-62.

Ivey, A. E., & Ivey, M. (1999). *Intentional interviewing and counseling* (4th ed.). Pacific Grove, CA: Brooks/Cole.

Kopta, S. M., et al. (1999). Individual psychotherapy outcome and process research: Challenge leading to great turmoil or positive transition? *Annual Review of Psychology, 50,* 441-469.

Kunyk, D., & Olson, J. K. (2001). Classifications on conceptions of empathy. *Journal of Advanced Nursing, 35*(3), 317-325.

LaRowe, K. (2004). *The therapeutic relationship.* Retrieved February 3, 2005, from the Breath of Relief website: http://www.breathofrelief.com/article_12.html.

Leslie, K. R., Johnson-Frey, S. H., & Grafton, S. T. (2004). Functional imaging of face and hand imitation: Towards a motor theory of empathy. *Neuroimage, 21*(2), 601-607.

Mercer, S. W., & Reynolds, W. (2002). Empathy and quality of care. *British Journal of General Practice, 52*(Suppl.), S9-S12.

Moore, J. C., & Hartman, C. R. (1988). Developing a therapeutic relationship. In C. K. Beck, R. P. Rawlins, & S. R. Williams (Eds.), *Mental health–psychiatric nursing.* St. Louis, MO: Mosby.

Peplau, H. E. (1952). *Interpersonal relations in nursing: A conceptual frame of reference for psychodynamic nursing.* New York: Putnam.

Peplau, H. E. (1999). *Interpersonal relations in nursing: A conceptual frame of reference for psychodynamic nursing.* New York: Springer.

Pilette, P. C., et al. (1995). Therapeutic management of helping boundaries. *Journal of Psychosocial Nursing and Mental Health Services, 33*(1), 40-47.

Raths, L., Harmin, M., & Simon, S.B. (1966). *Values and teaching.* Columbus, OH: Merrill.

Rich, I. C. (2003). Revisiting Joyce Travelbee's question: What's wrong with sympathy? *Journal of the American Psychiatric Association, 9*(6), 202-203.

Rogers, C. R., & Truax, C. B. (1967). The therapeutic conditions antecedent to change: A theoretical view. In C. R. Rogers (Ed.), *The therapeutic relationship and its impact.* Madison, WI: University of Wisconsin Press.

Simon, S. B., Howe, L. W., & Kirschenbaum, H. (1995). *Values clarification.* New York: Warner Books.

Sommers-Flanagan, J., & Sommers-Flanagan, R. (2003). *Clinical interviewing* (3rd ed.). Hoboken, NJ: Wiley.

CHAPTER 11

The Clinical Interview and Communication Skills

ELIZABETH M. VARCAROLIS

KEY TERMS and CONCEPTS

The key terms and concepts listed here appear in color where they are defined or first discussed in this chapter.

active listening, 186
clarifying techniques, 189
clinical supervision, 173
cultural filters, 185
double messages, 180
double-bind messages, 181
excessive questioning, 190
exploring, 189
feedback, 178
giving advice, 192
giving approval, 192
nonverbal behaviors, 180
nonverbal communication, 180
obstructive (nontherapeutic) techniques, 185
paralinguistics, 183
paraphrasing, 189
process recordings, 174
reflecting, 189
restating, 189
silence, 186
therapeutic (helpful) techniques, 185
verbal communication, 179
"why" questions, 193

OBJECTIVES

After studying this chapter, the reader will be able to

1. Identify and give rationales for suggested (a) setting, (b) seating, and (c) beginning of the nurse-client interaction.
2. Explain to a classmate the importance of clinical supervision and how it works.
3. Identify four client behaviors a nurse can anticipate and discuss possible nursing interventions for each behavior.
4. Identify three personal factors that can impede accurate communication.
5. Identify two environmental factors that can impede accurate communication.
6. Give a personal example of a recent complementary exchange and a recent symmetrical exchange and explain how the relationship affected the quality of the communication.
7. Discuss the differences between verbal and nonverbal communication and identify five areas of nonverbal communication.
8. Identify two attending behaviors that the nurse might focus on to increase communication skills.
9. Relate potential problems that can arise when nurses are insensitive to cultural differences in clients' communication styles.
10. Compare and contrast the range of nonverbal and verbal behaviors of different cultural groups in the areas of (a) communication style, (b) eye contact, and (c) touch. Give examples.
11. Demonstrate the use of four techniques that can enhance communication, highlighting what makes them effective.
12. Demonstrate the use of four techniques that can obstruct communication, highlighting what makes them ineffective.

evolve Visit the Evolve website at **http://evolve.elsevier.com/Varcarolis** for a pretest on the content in this chapter.

THE CLINICAL INTERVIEW

As part of the nursing process, the clinical interview differs from the intake interview, or the assessment interview, which is described in Chapter 9. In most instances, when a nurse meets a client for the first time, a mental status examination and psychosocial assessment have already been performed and documented. In the hospital setting the mental status examination and psychosocial assessment are often recorded in the chart by a physician or psychiatric mental health nurse. In the community setting the physician or nurse clinician is often the person doing the intake interview. However, during the clinical rotation, it is not uncommon for the student to obtain important data from the client that can be added to the client database.

The content and direction of the clinical interview are decided by the client. The client leads. The nurse employs communication skills and active listening (identifying what the client says as well as what the client does not say) to better understand the client's situation. Active listening includes attention to body language, facial expressions, and vocal tone. The nurse also observes how congruent the content (what the client says) is with the process (what the client does). During the clinical interview, the nurse provides the opportunity for the client to reach specific goals, such as the following:

- To feel understood and comfortable
- To identify and explore problems relating to others
- To discuss healthy ways of meeting emotional needs
- To experience a satisfying interpersonal relationship

Communication and interviewing techniques are acquired skills and basic ingredients of a therapeutic nurse-client relationship. Nurses learn to increase their ability to use communication and interviewing skills through practice, supervision by a more experienced clinician, and/or observation of and modeling by more experienced clinicians. Effective communication skills are integral to the establishment and maintenance of a therapeutic alliance. The second half of this chapter outlines ways you can increase your ability to use communication skills in an effective manner.

Health care practitioners new to the psychiatric setting often say they feel overwhelmed by the severity of some of the clients' problems and that they feel responsible for doing something to positively affect the emotional health of clients. It may help to know that numerous studies show that a strong therapeutic relationship is more important for a successful therapeutic outcome than a variety of other factors. The overall conclusion of research that evaluates variables in counseling situations is that a warm, personable, and confiding relationship is a significant therapeutic factor (Glasser, 2000; Hubble, Duncan, & Miller, 1999); that

is, a good therapeutic relationship is considered a necessary, but in and of itself not always a sufficient, ingredient for both positive development and change (Sommers-Flanagan & Sommers-Flanagan, 2003). Clinical training, skills, and experience are all part of the picture. Research, however, does imply the need for clinicians to convey genuine interest in another human, without being patronizing or condescending. Refer to Chapter 10 for a discussion of the correlation between therapeutic relationship and improved outcomes.

Anxiety during the first interview is to be expected, as in any meeting between strangers. Clients may be anxious about their problems, about the nurse's reaction to them, or about their treatment. Students may be anxious about how the clients will react to them, whether they will be able to provide help, what the instructor will think of them, and how they will do compared with their peers.

Students have many concerns when beginning their psychiatric experience. Two common concerns are (1) how to begin the interview and (2) what to do in response to specific client behaviors. The following section offers some basic guidelines for the first interview, identifies some common problems in clinical situations, and suggests possible solutions.

How to Begin the Interview

Helping a person with an emotional or medical problem is rarely a straightforward task. The goal of assisting a client to regain psychological or physiological stability can be difficult to achieve. Extremely important to any kind of counseling is permitting the client to set the pace of the interview, no matter how slow the progress may be (Arnold & Boggs, 2003).

Setting

Effective communication can take place almost anywhere. However, because the quality of the interaction—whether in a clinic, a clinical unit, an office, or the client's home—depends on the degree to which the nurse and client feel safe, establishing a setting that enhances feelings of security can be important to the helping relationship. A health care setting, a conference room, or a quiet part of the unit that has relative privacy but is within view of others is ideal. When the interview takes place in the home, it offers the nurse a valuable opportunity to assess the person in the context of everyday life.

Seating

In all settings, chairs need to be arranged so that conversation can take place in normal tones of voice and eye contact can be comfortably maintained or avoided. For example, a nonthreatening physical environment for nurse and client would involve the following:

- Assuming the same height, either both sitting or both standing.
- Avoiding a face-to-face stance when possible; a 90- to 120-degree angle or side-by-side position may be less intense, and client and nurse can look away from each other without discomfort.
- Avoiding settings without ready access to a door; the client should not be positioned between the nurse and the door.
- Avoiding a desk barrier between the nurse and the client.

Introductions

In the orientation phase, students tell the client who they are and what is the name of their school, what the purpose of the meetings is, and how long and at what time they will be meeting with the client. As discussed in Chapter 10, the issue of confidentiality is brought up during the initial interview. Please remember that all health care professionals must respect the private, personal, and confidential nature of the client's communication except in specific situations as outlined in Chapter 10 and Chapter 8. What is discussed with staff and your clinical group in conference should not be discussed outside with others, no matter who they are (e.g., client's relatives, news media, friends, etc.). The client needs to know that whatever is discussed will stay confidential unless the client gives permission for it to be disclosed, barring the exceptions outlined in Chapters 10 and 8 (e.g., harm to self or others, child abuse, elder abuse).

The nurse can then ask the client how he or she would like to be addressed. This question accomplishes a number of tasks (Arnold & Boggs, 2003). For example:

- It conveys respect.
- It gives the client direct control over an important ego issue. (Some clients like to be called by their last names; others prefer being on a first-name basis with the nurse.)

How to Start

Once introductions have been made, the nurse can turn the interview over to the client by using one of a number of open-ended statements such as the following:

- "Where should we start?"
- "Tell me a little about what has been going on with you."
- "What are some of the stresses you have been coping with recently?"
- "Tell me a little about what has been happening in the past couple of weeks."
- "Perhaps you can begin by letting me know what some of your concerns have been recently."
- "Tell me about your difficulties."

Communication can be facilitated by appropriately **offering leads** (e.g., "Go on"), making **statements of** acceptance (e.g., "Uh-huh"), or otherwise conveying the nurse's interest.

Tactics to Avoid

The nurse needs to avoid some behaviors (Moscato, 1988). For example:

DO NOT	TRY TO
- Argue with, minimize, or challenge the client.	- Keep focus on facts and the client's perceptions.
- Praise the client or give false reassurance.	- Make observations of the client's behavior. "Change is always possible."
- Interpret to the client or speculate on the dynamics of the client's problem.	- Listen attentively, use silence, clarify.
- Question the client about sensitive areas.	- Pay attention to nonverbal communication. Strive to keep the client's anxiety decreased.
- Try to sell the client on accepting treatment.	- Encourage the client to look at pros and cons.
- Join in attacks the client launches on his or her mate, parents, friends, or associates.	- Focus on facts and the client's perceptions; be aware of nonverbal communication.
- Participate in criticism of another nurse or any other staff member.	- Focus on facts and the client's perceptions.
	- Check out serious accusations with the other nurse or staff member.
	- Have the client meet with the nurse or staff member in question and senior staff or clinician and clarify perceptions.

Helpful Guidelines

Some guidelines for conducting the initial interviews are offered by Meier and Davis (2001), including the following:

- Speak briefly.
- When you don't know what to say, say nothing.
- When in doubt, focus on feelings.
- Avoid advice.
- Avoid relying on questions.
- Pay attention to nonverbal cues.
- Keep the focus on the client.

Clinical Supervision and Process Recordings

Communication and interviewing techniques are acquired skills. Nurses learn to increase their ability to use communication and interviewing skills through practice and through clinical supervision by a more experienced clinician. In clinical supervision, the focus is on the nurse's behavior in the nurse-client relationship. During clinical supervision, the nurse and the supervisor examine and analyze the nurse's feelings and reactions to the client and the way they affect the nurse-client relationship. Farkas-Cameron (1995) stated that "the nurse who does not engage in the clinical supervisory process stagnates both theoretically and clinically, while depriving him- or herself of the opportunity to advance professionally" (p. 44). She went on to observe that clinical supervision can be a therapeutic process for the nurse. During the process, feelings and concerns are ventilated as they relate to the developing nurse-client relationship. The opportunity to examine your interactions, obtain insights, and devise alternative strategies for dealing with various clinical issues enhances your clinical growth and minimizes frustration and burnout. Clinical supervision is a necessary professional activity that fosters professional growth and helps minimize the development of nontherapeutic nurse-client relationships.

The best way to increase communication and interviewing skills is to review clinical interactions exactly as they occur. This process offers students the opportunity to identify themes and patterns in their own, as well as their clients', communications. Students also learn to deal with the variety of situations that arise in the clinical interview.

Many clinicians learn by reviewing their interactions with clients through the use of videotaping, which reveals the nonverbal as well as the verbal communications between the two parties. Another method of capturing the interaction between clinician and client is through an audiotape recording. Such taping is always done with the client's written consent and is confidential. It is often carried out for learning purposes only, in order to advance nurse and clinician skills. However, the most common method of evaluating nurse-client interactions in academic settings is through process recordings.

The use of process recordings is a popular way to identify patterns in the student's and the client's communication. Process recordings are written records of a segment of the nurse-client session that reflects as closely as possible the verbal and nonverbal behaviors of both client and nurse. Process recordings have some disadvantages because they rely on memory and are subject to distortions. However, they can be a useful tool for identifying communication patterns. It is usually best if the student can write notes verbatim (word for word) in a private area immediately after the interaction has taken place. Sometimes, a clinician takes notes during the interview. This practice also has disadvantages. One disadvantage is that it may be distracting for both interviewer and client; another is that some clients (especially those with a paranoid disorder) may resent or misunderstand the nurse's intent. Table 11-1 shows a segment of a process note. Nurses record their words and the client's words, identify whether the responses are therapeutic, and recall their emotions at the time.

TABLE 11-1

Segment of a Process Note

Nurse	Client	Communication Technique	Student's Thoughts and Feelings
"Good morning, Mr. Long."		*Therapeutic.* Giving recognition. Acknowledging a client by name can enhance self-esteem and communicates that the client is viewed as an individual by the nurse.	I was feeling nervous. He had attempted suicide and I didn't know if I could help him. Initially I was feeling somewhat overwhelmed.
	"Who are you and where the devil am I?" *Gazes around with a confused look on his face—quickly sits on the edge of the bed.*		
"I am Ms. Rodriguez. I am a student nurse from [X] college, and you are at Mt. Sinai Hospital. I would like to spend some time with you today."		*Therapeutic.* Giving information. Informing the client of facts needed to make decisions or come to realistic conclusions. *Therapeutic.* Offering self. Making oneself available to the client.	
	"What am I doing here? How did I get here?" *Spoken in a loud, demanding voice.*		I felt a bit intimidated when he raised his voice.

TABLE 11-1

Segment of a Process Note—cont'd

Nurse	Client	Communication Technique	Student's Thoughts and Feelings
"You were brought in by your wife last night after swallowing a bottle of aspirin. You had to have your stomach pumped."		*Therapeutic.* Giving information. Giving needed facts so that the client can orient himself and better evaluate his situation.	
	"Oh . . . yeah." *Silence for 2 minutes. Shoulders slumped, Mr. Long stares at the floor and drops his head and eyes.*		I was uncomfortable with the silence, but since I didn't have anything useful to say, I stayed with him in silence for the 2 minutes.
"You seem upset, Mr. Long. What are you thinking about?"		*Therapeutic.* Making observations. He looks sad.	I began to feel sorry for him; he looked so sad and helpless.
		Therapeutic. Giving broad openings in an attempt to get at his feelings.	
	"Yeah, I just remembered . . . I wanted to kill myself." *Said in a low tone almost to himself.*		
"Oh, Mr. Long, you have so much to live for. You have such a loving family."		*Nontherapeutic.* Defending. *Nontherapeutic.* Introducing an unrelated topic.	I felt overwhelmed. I didn't know what to say—his talking about killing himself made me nervous. I could have said, "You must be very upset" (verbalizing the implied) or "Tell me more about this" (exploring).
	"What do you know about my life? You want to know about my family? . . . My wife is leaving me, that's what." *Faces the nurse with an angry expression on his face and speaks in loud tones.*		Again, I felt intimidated by his anger, but now I linked it with his wife's leaving him, so I didn't take it as personally as I did the first time.
"I didn't know. You must be terribly upset by her leaving."		*Therapeutic.* Reflective. Observing the angry tone and content of the client's message and reflecting back the client's feelings.	I really felt for him, and now I thought that encouraging him to talk more about this could be useful for him.

What to Do in Response to Specific Client Behaviors

Often, students new to the mental health setting are concerned about being in situations that they may not know how to handle. These concerns are universal and often arise in the clinical setting. Table 11-2 identifies common client behaviors (e.g., crying, asking the nurse to keep a secret, threatening to commit suicide, giving a gift). The table gives examples of an appropriate response, the rationale for the response, and a possible verbal statement. Read Table 11-2, paying particular attention to the rationales for responses. The exact words depend on the situation, but understanding the rationale will aid you in applying the information later on.

TABLE 11-2

Common Client Behaviors and Nurse Responses

Possible Reactions by Nurse	Useful Responses by Nurse
What to Do If the Client Cries	
The nurse may feel uncomfortable and experience increased anxiety or feel somehow responsible for making the person cry.	The nurse should stay with the client and reinforce that it is all right to cry. Often, it is at that time that feelings are closest to the surface and can be best identified. ■ "You seem ready to cry." ■ "You are still upset about your brother's death." ■ "What are you thinking right now?" The nurse offers tissues when appropriate.
What to Do If the Client Asks the Nurse to Keep a Secret	
The nurse may feel conflict because the nurse wants the client to share important information but is unsure about making such a promise.	The nurse *cannot* make such a promise. The information may be important to the health or safety of the client or others. ■ "I cannot make that promise. It might be important for me to share it with other staff." The client then decides whether to share the information or not.
What to Do If the Client Leaves Before the Session Is Over	
The nurse may feel rejected, thinking it was something that he or she did. The nurse may experience increased anxiety or feel abandoned by the client.	Some clients are not able to relate for long periods without experiencing an increase in anxiety. On the other hand, the client may be testing the nurse. ■ "I will wait for you here for 15 minutes, until our time is up." During this time, the nurse does not engage in conversation with any other client or even with the staff. When the time is up, the nurse approaches the client, tells him or her the time is up, and restates the day and time the nurse will see the client again.
What to Do If Another Client Interrupts During Time with Your Selected Client	
The nurse may feel a conflict. The nurse does not want to appear rude. Sometimes the nurse tries to engage both clients in conversation.	The time the nurse had contracted with a selected client is that client's time. By keeping his or her part of the contract, the nurse demonstrates that the nurse means what he or she says and views the sessions as important. ■ "I am with Mr. Rob for the next 20 minutes. At 10 AM, after our time is up, I can talk to you for 5 minutes."
What to Do If the Client Says He or She Wants to Kill Himself or Herself	
The nurse may feel overwhelmed or responsible for "talking the client out of it." The nurse may pick up some of the client's feelings of hopelessness.	The nurse assesses whether the client has a plan and the lethality of the plan. The nurse tells the client that this is serious, that the nurse does not want harm to come to the client, and that this information needs to be shared with other staff. ■ "This is very serious, Mr. Lamb. I do not want any harm to come to you. I will have to share this with the other staff." The nurse can then discuss with the client the feelings and circumstances that led up to this decision. (Refer to Chapter 23 for strategies in suicide intervention.)
What to Do If the Client Says He or She Does Not Want To Talk	
The nurse new to this situation may feel rejected or ineffectual.	At first, the nurse might say something to this effect: ■ "It's all right. I would like to spend time with you. We don't have to talk." The nurse might spend short, frequent periods (e.g., 5 minutes) with the client throughout the day. ■ "Our 5 minutes is up. I'll be back at 10 AM and stay with you 5 more minutes." This gives the client the opportunity to understand that the nurse means what he or she says and is back on time consistently. It also gives the client time between visits to assess how he or she feels and what he or she thinks about the nurse, and perhaps to feel less threatened.

TABLE 11-2

Common Client Behaviors and Nurse Responses—cont'd

Possible Reactions by Nurse	Useful Responses by Nurse
What to Do If the Client Seeks to Prolong the Interview	
Sometimes, clients open up dynamic or interesting topics just before the interview time is up. This is often to test or manipulate the nurse. The nurse might feel tempted to extend the scheduled time or might not want to hurt the client's feelings.	The nurse sets limits and restates and reinforces the original contract. The nurse states that they will use the issues for the next session. ■ "Our time is up now, Mr. Jones. This would be a good place to start at our next session, which is Wednesday at 10 AM."
What to Do If the Client Gives the Nurse a Present	
The nurse may feel uncomfortable when offered a gift. The meaning needs to be examined. Is the gift (1) a way of getting better care, (2) a way to maintain self-esteem, (3) a way of making the nurse feel guilty, (4) a sincere expression of thanks, or (5) a cultural expectation?	Possible guidelines: If the gift is expensive, the only policy is to graciously refuse. If it is inexpensive, then (1) if it is given at the end of hospitalization when a relationship has developed, graciously accept; (2) if it is given at the beginning of the relationship, graciously refuse and explore the meaning behind the present. ■ "Thank you, but it is our job to care for our clients. Are you concerned that some aspect of your care will be overlooked?" If the gift is money, it is always graciously refused.
What to Do If the Client Asks You a Personal Question	
The nurse may think that it is rude not to answer the client's question. *or* A new nurse might feel relieved to put off having to start the interview. *or* The nurse may feel put on the spot and want to leave the situation. New nurses are often manipulated by a client into changing roles. This keeps the focus off the client and prevents the building of a relationship.	The nurse may or may not answer the client's query. If the nurse decides to answer a natural question, he or she answers in a word or two, then refocuses back on the client. *Client:* Are you married? *Nurse:* Yes. Do you have a spouse? *Client:* Do you have any children? *Nurse:* This time is for you—tell me about yourself. *Client:* You can just tell me if you have any children. *Nurse:* This is your time to focus on your concerns. Tell me something about your family.

COMMUNICATION

Beginning practitioners who are new to a psychiatric setting are often concerned that they may say the wrong thing, especially when initially learning to apply therapeutic techniques. *Will* you say the wrong thing? The answer is yes, you probably will. That is how we all learn to find more useful and effective ways of helping clients reach their goals. The challenge is to recover from your mistakes and use them for learning and growth (Sommers-Flanagan & Sommers-Flanagan, 2003). Will saying the wrong thing be harmful to the client? This is doubtful, especially if your intent is honest, your approach is respectful, and you have a genuine concern for the client. We know that special skills (e.g., communications skills) and methods that can aid people in becoming more effective helpers have been identified through scientific investigations. However, knowledge of skills and techniques is not enough, as mentioned previously. Being an effective communicator, whether in nursing or in any other area of life, is not just a matter of knowing what techniques to use. Genuine respect for the individual, the ability to listen and to understand the client's concerns, and a desire to work with the individual to help his or her situation are also key factors.

The idea of using techniques is "sometimes met with skepticism because it can imply that someone is deliberately and consciously trying to manipulate someone else" (Myrick & Erney, 1984). Mechanical or forced use of communication skills is not helpful. However, when such skills are a genuine part of the helping process, applied with concern and respect for the other person, communication techniques can be a dynamic tool in working effectively with people in any setting. As you continue to practice and evaluate the use of these techniques, you will develop your own style and rhythm, and eventually they will become a part of the way you communicate with others.

The Communication Process

Communication is the process of sending a message to one or more persons. One way of thinking about the process of communication is to use a basic communication model that identifies the parts of an interaction (Berlo, 1960). Very simply put, then, the basic format is the following:

1. One person has a need to communicate with another **(stimulus).** For example, the stimulus for communication can be a need for information, comfort, or advice. A stimulus in a nurse might be the perception that the client is feeling discomfort or confusion. A stimulus in a client might be the experience of anxiety, despair, or pain.
2. The person sending the message **(sender)** initiates interpersonal contact.
3. The **message** is the information sent or expressed to another. The clearest messages are those that are well organized and expressed in a manner familiar to the receiver.
4. The message can be sent through a variety of **media.** A message can be sent through an auditory (hearing), visual (seeing), tactile (touch), or even smell medium, or any combination of these. For example, a person may send a clear message through silence, body language, or a hug, as well as through the stated word.
5. The person receiving the message **(receiver)** then evaluates and interprets the message. Often the message from the sender may act as a stimulus to the receiver. The person receiving the message may then respond to the sender by giving feedback to the sender. The nature of the feedback often indicates whether the meaning of the message sent by the sender has been correctly interpreted by the receiver. Validating the accuracy of the sender's message is extremely important. An accuracy check may be obtained by simply asking the sender, "Is this what you mean?" or "It seems you are saying . . . ." Feedback in a counseling situation may entail pointing out certain observed behaviors and giving your impression or reaction. "I notice you turn away when we talk about your going back to college. Is there a conflict there?" When the receiver gives feedback to the sender, communication becomes reciprocal. Communication is most effective when the message sent is the same as the message received.

Figure 11-1 shows this simple model of communication along with some of the many factors that affect it. Communication is a complex process. Communication involves a variety of personal and environmental factors that can distort both the sending and the re-

ceiving of messages as shown in Figure 11-1 and discussed in the next section.

Factors That Affect Communication

Personal Factors. Personal factors that can impede accurate transmission or interpretation of messages include emotional factors (e.g., mood, responses to stress, personal bias), social factors (e.g., previous experience, cultural differences, language differences), and cognitive factors (e.g., problem-solving ability, knowledge level, language use).

Environmental Factors. Environmental factors that may affect communication include physical factors (e.g., background noise, lack of privacy, uncomfortable accommodations) and societal determinants (e.g., sociopolitical, historical, and economic factors, the presence of others, expectations of others).

Relationship Factors. Relationship factors refer to whether the participants are equal or unequal. When the two participants are equal, such as friends or colleagues, the relationship is said to be **symmetrical.** However, when there is a difference in status or power, such as between nurse and patient or teacher and student, the relationship is characterized by inequality (one participant is "superior" to the other) and is called a **complementary** relationship (Ellis, Gates, & Kenworthy, 2003).

Effective communication in helping relationships depends on nurses' knowing what they are trying to convey (the purpose of the message), communicating what is really meant to the client, and comprehending the meaning of what the client is intentionally or unintentionally conveying (Arnold & Boggs, 2003). Fundamental to all of this is determining where the client is coming from so that the nurse and client can start on common ground. Peplau (1952) identified two main principles that can guide the communication process during the nurse-client interview: (1) **clarity,** which ensures that the meaning of the message is accurately understood by both parties "as the result of joint and sustained effort of all parties concerned," and (2) **continuity,** which promotes connections among ideas "and the feelings, events, or themes conveyed in those ideas" (p. 290).

Communication consists of verbal and nonverbal elements. Shea (1998), a nationally renowned psychiatrist and communication workshop leader, stated that communication is roughly 10% verbal and 90% nonverbal. Rankin (2001) believes that nonverbal behaviors comprise from 65% to 95% of a sent message. Therefore, learning to be an effective communicator means paying attention to both verbal and nonverbal cues.

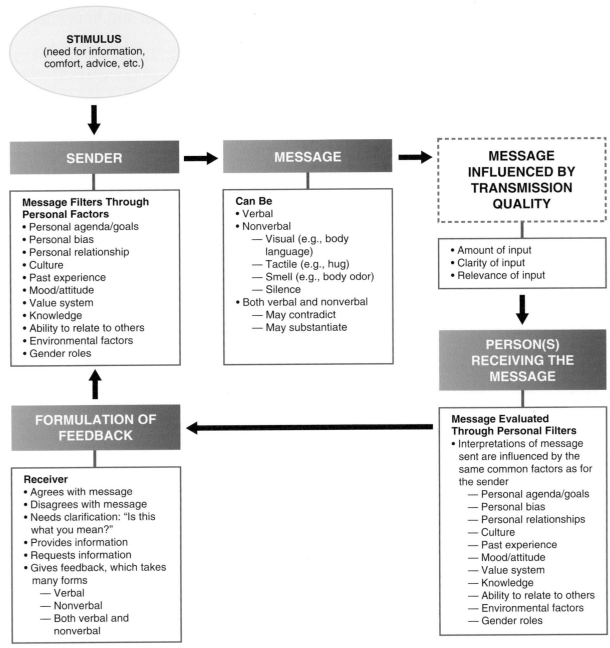

FIGURE 11-1 Operational definition of communication. (Data from Ellis, R., & McClintock, A. [1990]. *If you take my meaning*. London: Arnold.)

Verbal Communication

Verbal communication consists of all words a person speaks. We live in a society of symbols, and our supreme social symbol is words. Talking is our most common activity—our public link with one another, the primary instrument of instruction, a need, an art, and one of the most personal aspects of our private lives. When we speak, we

- Communicate our beliefs and values.
- Communicate perceptions and meanings.

- Convey interest and understanding *or* insult and judgment.
- Convey messages clearly *or* convey conflicting or implied messages.
- Convey clear, honest feelings *or* disguised, distorted feelings.

Even if the nurse and client have the same cultural background, the mental image they have of a given word may not be exactly the same. Although they believe they are talking about the same thing, the nurse and client may actually be talking about two quite different things. Words are the symbols for emotions as well as for mental images.

Nonverbal Communication

Nonverbal behaviors are the behaviors displayed by an individual that are not the actual content of speech. Tone of voice and the manner in which a person paces speech are examples of nonverbal communication. Other common examples of nonverbal communication (often called **cues**) are physical appearance, facial expressions, body posture, amount of eye contact, eye cast (emotion expressed in the eyes), hand gestures, sighs, fidgeting, and yawning. Table 11-3 identifies key components of nonverbal behaviors. Nonverbal behaviors need to be observed and interpreted in light of a person's culture, class, gender, age, sexual orientation, and spiritual norms.

TABLE 11-3

Nonverbal Behaviors

Possible Behaviors	Example
Body Behaviors	
Posture, body movements, gestures, gait	The client is slumped in a chair, puts her face in her hands, and occasionally taps her right foot.
Facial Expressions	
Frowns, smiles, grimaces, raised eyebrows, pursed lips, licking of lips, tongue movements	The client grimaces when speaking to the nurse; when alone, he smiles and giggles to himself.
Eye Cast	
Angry, suspicious, and accusatory looks	The client's eyes harden with suspicion.
Voice-Related Behaviors	
Tone, pitch, level, intensity, inflection, stuttering, pauses, silences, fluency	The client talks in a loud sing-song voice.
Observable Autonomic Physiological Responses	
Increase in respirations, diaphoresis, pupil dilation, blushing, paleness	When the client mentions discharge, she becomes pale, her respirations increase, and her face becomes diaphoretic.
Personal Appearance	
Grooming, dress, hygiene	The client is dressed in a wrinkled shirt and his pants are stained; his socks are dirty and he is unshaven.
Physical Characteristics	
Height, weight, physique, complexion	The client appears grossly overweight and his muscles appear flabby.

Interaction of Verbal and Nonverbal Communication

Communication thus involves two radically different but interdependent kinds of symbols. The first type is the **spoken word,** which represents our public selves. Verbal assertions can be straightforward comments or can be skillfully used to distort, conceal, deny, and generally disguise true feelings. The second type, **nonverbal behaviors,** covers a wide range of human activities, from body movements to responses to the messages of others. How a person listens and uses silence and sense of touch may also convey important information about the private self that is not available from conversation alone, especially when viewed from a cultural perspective.

Some elements of nonverbal communication, such as facial expressions, seem to be inborn and are similar across cultures. Dee (1991) cited studies that found a high degree of agreement in spontaneous facial expressions or emotions across 10 different cultures. In public, however, some cultural groups (e.g., the Japanese) may control their facial expressions when observers are present. Other types of nonverbal behaviors, such as how close people stand to each other when speaking, depend on cultural conventions. Some nonverbal communication is formalized and has specific meanings (e.g., the military salute, the Japanese bow).

Messages are not always simple and can appear to be one thing when in fact they are another (Ellis et al., 2003). An interaction consists of both verbal and nonverbal messages. Often, people have more conscious awareness of their verbal messages and less awareness of their nonverbal behaviors. The verbal message is sometimes referred to as the **content** of the message, and the nonverbal behavior is called the **process** of the message. When the content (verbal message) is congruent with (agrees with) the process (nonverbal behavior), the communication is more clearly understood and is considered healthy. For example, if a student says, "It's important that I get good grades in this class," that is *content*. If the student has bought the books, takes good notes, and has a study buddy, that is *process*. Therefore, the content and process are congruent and straightforward, and there is a "healthy" message. If, however, the verbal message is not reinforced or is in fact contradicted by the nonverbal behavior, the message is confusing. For example, if the student says, "It's important that I get good grades in this class," that is *content*. If the student does not have the books, skips several classes, and does not study, that is *process*. Here the student is sending out two different messages.

Conflicting messages are known as double messages or *mixed messages*. Dee (1991) suggested that one way a nurse can respond to verbal and nonverbal incongruity is to reflect and validate the client's feelings. "You say you are upset that you did not pass this semester, but I notice that you look more relaxed and less conflicted than you have all term. What do you see as some of the pros and cons of not passing the course this semester?"

Bateson and colleagues (1956) coined the term double-bind messages. Messages are sent to create meaning but can also be used defensively to hide what is actually going on, create confusion, and attack relatedness (Ellis et al., 2003). A double-bind message is a mix of content (what is said) and process (what is going on picked up nonverbally) that has both nurturing and hurtful aspects. For example:

A young 17-year-old female student who lives at home with her mother wants to go out for an evening with her friends. She is told by her chronically ill but not helpless mother: "Oh, go ahead, have fun. I'll just sit here by myself, and I can always call 911 if I don't feel well, but you go ahead and have fun." The mother says this while looking sad, eyes cast down, slumped in her chair, while letting her cane drop to the floor.

The recipient of this double-bind message is caught inside contradictory statements so that she cannot do the right thing. If she goes, the implication is that she is being selfish by leaving her sick mother alone, but if she stays, the mother could say, "I told you to go have fun." If she does go, the chances are she won't have much fun. This is a good example of a "damned if you do, damned if you don't" situation.

With experience, nurses become increasingly aware of a client's verbal and nonverbal communication. Nurses can compare clients' dialogue with their nonverbal communication to gain important clues about the real message. What individuals do may either express and reinforce, or contradict, what they say. As in the saying "Actions speak louder than words," actions often reveal the true meaning of a person's intent, whether it is conscious or unconscious.

TOWARD A MORE COMPLEX MODEL OF COMMUNICATION

In actuality, as Watzlawick, Benoin, and Jackson (1967) pointed out long ago, an enormous number of messages flow between two people in a one-to-one communication "in an uninterrupted series of interchanges." Besides the verbal message there are a myriad of nonverbal messages being transmitted between the two participants. Many nonverbal messages include those already mentioned, such as facial expression, tonal quality, appearance, relationship of the individuals, history, cultural filters, and on and on. Some of these messages are given and received on an unconscious level.

Some people consciously (and unconsciously) use language to impress, mystify, dominate, humiliate, or indicate their social position (Ellis et al., 2003). Most of us have been in the company of others who use technical, professional, or social "in-group" talk with the intent of excluding or impressing others. In these situations, multiple messages are sent, and the surface or direct message is secondary to the "disguised" meaning. Ellis et al. (2003) give the example of teenagers who constantly make up "in" words to create boundaries between in groups and out groups.

Ellis and colleagues (2003) state that many of the messages sent never get through to the receiver; some are disregarded when they do get through; and some messages are out of the conscious awareness of one or both of the individuals involved and are perceived only by those outside the interaction. So, a more complete yet complex model of communication could look something like Figure 11-2.

Attending Behaviors: The Foundation of Interviewing

Engaging in attending behaviors and listening well are two key principles of counseling on which just about everyone agree (Sommers-Flanagan & Sommers-Flanagan, 2003). Attending behaviors were addressed in Chapter 10 but are covered more thoroughly here as they relate to the clinical interview. Ivey and Ivey (1999) define attending behaviors as "culturally and individually appropriate . . . eye contact, body language, vocal qualities and verbal tracking" (p. 15). Sommers-Flanagan and Sommers-Flanagan (2003) state that positive attending behaviors can open up communication and encourage free expression. However, negative attending behaviors are more likely to inhibit expression. These behaviors need to be evaluated in terms of cultural patterns and past experiences of both the interviewer and the interviewee. There are no universals; however, there are guidelines that students can follow.

Eye Contact

The cultural variations regarding eye contact are discussed more fully later in this chapter. However, there is also individual variation in what an individual is personally comfortable with in terms of eye contact. For some clients and interviewers, sustained eye contact is normal and comfortable, whereas for other clients and interviewers it may be more comfortable and natural to make brief eye contact but look away or down much of the time. Sommers-Flanagan and Sommers-Flanagan (2003) state that it is appropriate for most nurse clinicians to maintain more eye contact when the client speaks and less constant eye contact when the nurse speaks. However, in general, white

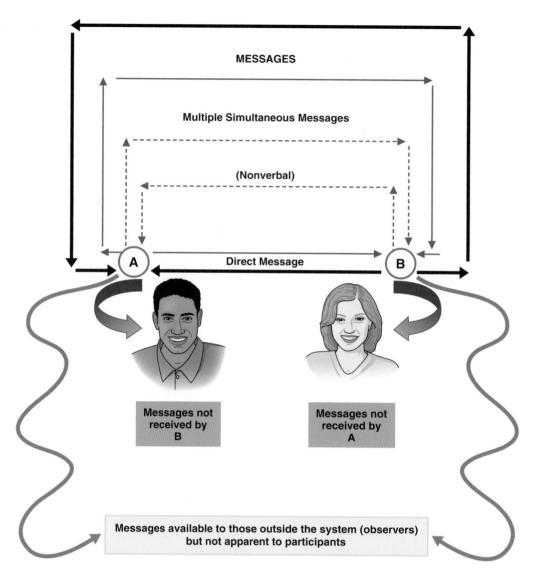

MESSAGES

Multiple Simultaneous Messages

(Nonverbal)

Direct Message

Messages not received by B

Messages not received by A

Messages available to those outside the system (observers) but not apparent to participants

* Additional conscious or unconscious use of language may apply at times (for the purpose of impressing, mystifying, dominating, humiliating, excluding, etc.).

FIGURE 11-2 Toward a more complex model of communication. (Adapted from Ellis, R., & McClintock, A. [1990]. *If you take my meaning*. London: Arnold.)

clients are more comfortable with more sustained eye contact much of the time whereas Native Americans, African Americans, and Asian clients often prefer less eye contact. Refer to the section on culture and eye contact.

Body Language

Body language involves two elements: kinesics and proxemics. *Kinesics* is associated with physical characteristics such as body movements and postures. The way someone holds the head, legs, and shoulders, facial expressions, eye contact or lack thereof, and so on convey a multitude of messages. For example, a person who slumps in a chair, rolls the eyes, and sits with arms crossed in front of the chest can be perceived as resistant and unreceptive to what another wants to communicate.

On the other hand, positive body language may include leaning in slightly toward the speaker, maintaining a relaxed and attentive posture, making direct eye contact, making hand gestures that are unobtrusive and smooth while minimizing the number of other movements, and matching one's facial expressions to one's feelings or to the client's feelings.

Proxemics refers to personal space and what distance between oneself and others is comfortable for an individual. Proxemics takes into account that these distances may be different for different cultural groups. **Intimate distance** in the United States is 0 to 18 inches and is reserved for those we trust most and with whom we feel most safe. **Personal distance** (18 to 40 inches) is for personal communications such as those with friends or colleagues. **Social distance** (4 to 12 feet) is applied to strangers or acquaintances, often in public places or formal social gatherings. **Public distance** (12 feet or more) relates to public space (e.g., public speaking). In public space one may hail another and the parties may move about while communicating with one another.

Vocal Qualities

Vocal quality, or paralinguistics, encompasses voice loudness, pitch, rate, and fluency. Sommers-Flanagan and Sommers-Flanagan (2003) state that "effective interviewers use vocal qualities to enhance rapport, communicate interest and empathy and to emphasize special issues or conflicts" (p. 56). This supports the old adage, "It's not *what* you say, but *how* you say it." Speaking in soft and gentle tones is apt to encourage a person to share thoughts and feelings, whereas speaking in a rapid, high-pitched tone may convey anxiety and create it in the client. Consider, for example, how tonal quality can affect communication in a simple sentence like "I will see you tonight."

1. "*I* will see you tonight." (I will be the one who sees you tonight.)
2. "I *will* see you tonight." (No matter what happens; or could also signify: whether you like it or not, I will see you tonight.)
3. "I will see *you* tonight." (Even though others are present, it is you I want to see.)
4. "I will see you *tonight*." (It is definite, tonight is the night we will meet.)

Verbal Tracking

Verbal tracking is just that: tracking what the client is saying. Individuals cannot know if you are hearing or understanding what they are saying unless you provide them with cues. Verbal tracking is giving neutral feedback in the form of restating or summarizing what the client has already said. It does not include personal or professional opinions of what the client has said (Sommers-Flanagan & Sommers-Flanagan, 2003). For example:

Client: I don't know what the fuss is about. I smoke marijuana to relax and everyone makes a fuss.

Interviewer: You don't see this as a problem.

Client: No, I don't. It doesn't affect my work . . . well, most of the time, anyway. I mean, of course, if I have to think things out and make important decisions, then obviously it can get in the way. But most of the time I'm cool.

Interviewer: So when important decisions have to be made then it interferes; otherwise, you don't see it affecting your functioning.

Client: Yeah . . . most of the time I'm cool.

Meier and Davis (2001) state that verbal tracking involves pacing the interview with the client by sticking closely with the client's speech content (as well as speech volume and tone as discussed earlier). This can be difficult if the client introduces many topics at once so that it is difficult to know which leads to follow.

Negotiating Cultural Communication Barriers

Ethnically diverse populations are a rapidly growing segment of the American population. Health care professionals are gradually becoming aware of the need to become more familiar with the verbal and nonverbal communication characteristics of the diverse multicultural populations now using the health care system.

The nurse's awareness of the cultural meaning of certain verbal and nonverbal communications in initial face-to-face encounters with a client can lead to the formation of positive therapeutic alliances with members of culturally diverse populations (Kavanaugh, 2003).

Unrecognized differences between aspects of the cultural identities of client and nurse can result in assessment and interventions that are not optimally respectful of the client and can be inadvertently biased or prejudiced (Lu et al., 1995). Lu and colleagues further emphasized that health care workers need to have not only knowledge of various clients' cultures but also awareness of their own cultural identities. Especially important are nurses' attitudes and beliefs toward those from ethnically diverse populations, because these will affect their relationships with clients (Kavanaugh, 2003). Four areas that may prove problematic for the nurse interpreting specific verbal and nonverbal messages of the client include the following:

1. Communication styles
2. Use of eye contact
3. Perception of touch
4. Cultural filters

Communication Styles

People from some ethnic backgrounds may communicate in an intense and highly emotional manner. For example, from the perspective of a non-Hispanic person, Hispanic Americans may appear to use dramatic body language when describing their emotional problems. For clinicians from a non-Hispanic background, such behavior may be perceived as out of control and thus viewed as having a degree of pathology that is not actually present. Within the Hispanic culture, however, intensely emotional styles of communication often are culturally appropriate and are to be expected (Kavanaugh, 2003). French and Italian Americans also show animated facial expressions and expressive hand gestures during communication that can be mistakenly interpreted by others.

Conversely, in other cultures, a calm facade may mask severe distress. For example, in Asian cultures, expression of either positive or negative emotions is a private affair, and open expression of emotions is considered to be in bad taste and possibly to be a weakness. A quiet smile by an Asian American may express joy, an apology, stoicism in the face of difficulty, or even anger (U.S. Department of Health and Human Services, 2001). German and British Americans highly value the concept of self-control and may show little facial emotion in the presence of great distress or emotional turmoil.

It is important to understand an ethnic minority in light of the historical context in which it evolved and its relationship to the dominant culture. For example, African Americans, whose historical background in the United States is one of slavery and oppression, are likely to be aware of a basic need for survival. As a result of their experiences, many African Americans have become highly selective and guarded in their communication with those outside their cultural group. Therefore, a tendency toward guarded and selective communication among African American clients may represent a healthy cultural adaptation (Smedley, Stith, & Nelson, 2002; U.S. Department of Health and Human Services, 2001).

Eye Contact

Culture also dictates a person's comfort or lack of comfort with direct eye contact. Some cultures consider direct eye contact disrespectful and improper. For example, Hispanic individuals have traditionally been taught to avoid eye contact with authority figures such as nurses, physicians, and other health care professionals. Avoidance of direct eye contact is seen as a sign of respect to those in authority. To nurses or other health care workers from non-Hispanic backgrounds, however, this lack of eye contact may be wrongly interpreted as disinterest in the interview or even as a lack of respect. Conversely, the nurse is expected to look directly at the client when conducting the interview (Kavanaugh, 2003). Similarly, in Asian cultures, respect is shown by avoiding eye contact. For example, in Japan, direct eye contact is considered to show lack of respect and to be a personal affront; preference is for shifting or downcast eyes. With many Chinese, gazing around and looking to one side when listening to another is considered polite. However, when speaking to the elderly, direct eye contact is used (Kavanaugh, 2003). Philippine Americans may try to avoid eye contact; however, once it is established, it is important to return and maintain eye contact. Many Native Americans also believe it is disrespectful or even a sign of aggression to engage in direct eye contact, especially if the speaker is younger. Direct eye contact by members of the dominant culture in the health care system can and does cause discomfort for some clients (Kavanaugh, 2003).

Among German Americans, direct and sustained eye contact indicates that the person listens, trusts, is somewhat aggressive, or in some situations is sexually interested. Russians also find direct, sustained eye contact the norm for social interactions. In Haiti, it is customary to hold eye contact with everyone but the poor (Kavanaugh, 2003; U.S. Department of Health and Human Services, 2001). French, British, and many African Americans maintain eye contact during conversation; avoidance of eye contact by another person may be interpreted as being disinterested, not telling the truth, or avoiding the sharing of important information. In some Arab cultures, for a woman to make direct eye contact with a man may imply a sexual interest or even promiscuity. In Greece, staring in public is acceptable (Kavanaugh, 2003).

Touch

The therapeutic use of touch is a basic aspect of the nurse-client relationship, and touch is normally perceived as a gesture of warmth and friendship. However, touch can be perceived as an invasion of privacy or an invitation to intimacy by some clients (Dee, 1991). The response to touch is often culturally defined. For example, many Hispanic Americans are accustomed to frequent physical contact. For some Hispanics, holding the client's hand in response to a distressing situation or giving the client a reassuring pat on the shoulder may be experienced as supportive and thus help facilitate openness early in the therapeutic relationship (Kavanaugh, 2003). However, the degree of comfort conveyed by touch in the nurse-client relationship depends on the country of origin. People of Italian and French cultural backgrounds may also be accustomed to frequent touching during conversation (U.S. Department of Health and Human Services, 2001). In the Russian culture, touch is also an important part of nonverbal communication. In other cultures, personal touch within the context of an interview might be experienced as patronizing, intrusive, aggressive, or sexually inviting. For example, among German, Swedish, and British Americans, touch practices are infrequent, although a handshake may be common at the beginning and end of an interaction. In India, men may shake hands with other men but not with women; an Asian Indian man may greet a woman by nodding and holding the palms of his hands together but not touching the woman. In Japan, handshakes are acceptable; however, a pat on the back is not. Chinese Americans may not like to be touched by strangers. Some Native Americans extend their hand and lightly touch the hand of the person they are greeting rather than shake hands (Kavanaugh, 2003). Even among people of the same culture, the use of touch has different interpretations and rules when the touch is between individuals of different genders and classes. **Students are urged to check the policy manual of their facility because some facilities have a "no touch" policy, particularly with adolescents and children who may have experienced inappropriate touch and would not know how to interpret the touch of the health care worker.**

Cultural Filters

It is important for all of us to recognize that it is impossible to listen to people in an unbiased way. In the process of socialization we develop cultural filters through which we listen to ourselves, others, and the world around us (Egan, 2001). Cultural filters are a form of cultural bias or cultural prejudice that determine what we pay attention to and what we ignore.

Egan (1994) stated that we need these cultural filters to provide structure for ourselves and to help us interpret and interact with the world. However, unavoidably, these cultural filters also introduce various forms of bias into our listening, because they are bound to influence our personal, professional, familial, and sociological values and interpretations. Egan also described how strong cultural filters can influence the likelihood of bias with multicultural clients. He used the example of a white, middle-class helper who would tend to use white, middle-class filters when listening. These cultural filters may not interfere with, and could even facilitate, working with someone from a white, middle-class background. However, if our own cultural filters go unacknowledged, the likelihood is great that they will distort our perceptions and interpretations of clients of other ethnicities. Therefore, a white, middle-class helper, if not cognizant of personal cultural biases, can easily introduce bias when working with, for example, a well-to-do Asian client with high social status in the community; an African American mother from the urban ghetto; or a poor white subsistence farmer (Egan, 2001). We all need a frame of reference to help us function in our world. The trick is to understand that other people use many other frames of reference to help them function in their worlds. Acknowledging that others view the world quite differently and trying to understand other people's ways of experiencing and living in the world can go a long way toward minimizing our personal distortions in listening. Building acceptance and understanding of those culturally different from ourselves is a skill, too.

Box 11-1 lists some strategies that may increase nurses' awareness of culturally specific verbal and nonverbal behaviors.

EFFECTIVE COMMUNICATION SKILLS

The art of communication (e.g., interviewing, problem solving, counseling, and health teaching) was emphasized by Peplau to highlight the importance of nursing interventions in facilitating achievement of quality patient care and quality of life (Haber, 2000). Therefore, as previously stated, the goals of the nurse in the mental health setting are to help the client

- Feel understood and comfortable.
- Identify and explore problems relating to others.

BOX 11-1

Strategies to Increase Cultural Awareness

- Engage in personal and professional workshops and training seminars that facilitate awareness of biases and prejudices toward people who are culturally different.
- Once trust has been established in a nurse-client relationship, share your observations with the client. Seek clarification and validate your perceptions with the client.
- Explore the meaning of the behavior with the client, being careful not to inject preconceived notions.
- Acquire knowledge outside your professional practice through participation in culturally diverse activities and through nonprofessional contacts.
- Read history and literature written by members of the cultural group with which you are working.
- Engage in discussion of racial issues when they emerge in the context of your interaction with clients, peers, and others outside your work setting.
- Gain an appreciation of how your own culture communicates and what you observe as different in other cultures (e.g., foods, celebrations, issues of trust, expressions of joy or fear).

Data from Ingram, C. A. (1991). How can we become more aware of culturally specific body language and use this awareness therapeutically? *Journal of Psychosocial Nursing, 29*(11), 40-41.

- Discover healthy ways of meeting emotional needs.
- Experience satisfying interpersonal relationships.

The goal for the nurse is to establish and maintain a therapeutic alliance (relationship) in which the client will feel safe and hopeful that positive change is possible.

Once specific needs and problems have been identified, the nurse can work with the client on increasing problem-solving skills, learning new coping behaviors, and experiencing more appropriate and satisfying ways of relating to others. To do this, the nurse needs to have a sound knowledge of communication skills. Therefore, the nurse must become more aware of his or her own interpersonal methods, eliminating obstructive (nontherapeutic) techniques and developing additional responses that maximize nurse-client interactions and increase the use of therapeutic (helpful) techniques.

Useful tools for nurses when communicating with their clients are (1) the use of silence, (2) active listening, and (3) clarifying techniques.

Use of Silence

Silence can frighten both interviewers and clients (Sommers-Flanagan & Sommers-Flanagan, 2003). In our society, and in nursing, there is an emphasis on action. In communication, we tend to expect a high level of verbal activity. Many students and practicing nurses find that, when the flow of words stops, they become uncomfortable. Silence, on the other hand, can be soothing.

Silence is not the absence of communication; it is a specific channel for transmitting and receiving messages. The practitioner needs to understand that silence is a significant means of influencing and being influenced by others.

In the initial interview the client may be reluctant to speak because of the newness of the situation, the fact that the nurse is a stranger, self-consciousness, embarrassment, or shyness. Talking is highly individualized; some find the telephone a nuisance, whereas others believe they cannot live without their cell phones. The nurse must recognize and respect individual differences in styles and tempos of responding. How else can nurses learn of another's nature and their own but through courtesy, care, and time? People who are quiet, those who have a language barrier or speech impediment, the elderly, and those who lack confidence in their ability to express themselves may be communicating through their silences a need for support and encouragement in acts of self-expression (Collins, 1983; Arnold & Boggs, 2003).

Although there is no universal rule concerning how much silence is too much, silence has been said to be worthwhile only as long as it is serving some function and not frightening the client. Knowing when to speak during the interview is largely dependent on the nurse's perception about what is being conveyed through the silence. Icy silence may be an expression of anger and hostility. Being ignored or given the silent treatment is recognized as an insult and is a particularly hurtful form of communication. Silence among some African American clients may relate to anger, insulted feelings, or acknowledgment of a nurse's lack of cultural sensitivity (Smedley et al., 2002).

On the other hand, silence may provide meaningful moments of reflection for both participants. It gives each an opportunity to contemplate thoughtfully what has been said and felt, to weigh alternatives, to formulate new ideas, and to gain a new perspective on the matter under discussion. If the nurse waits to speak and allows the client to break the silence, the client may share thoughts and feelings that would otherwise have been withheld. Nurses who feel compelled to fill every void with words often do so because of their own anxiety, self-consciousness, and embarrassment. When this occurs, the nurse's need for comfort tends to take priority over the needs of the client.

Conversely, prolonged and frequent silences by the nurse may hinder an interview that requires verbal articulation. Although the untalkative nurse may be comfortable with silence, this mode of communication may make the client feel like a fountain of information to be drained dry. Moreover, without feedback, clients have no way of knowing whether what they said was understood.

Active Listening

People want more than just physical presence in human communication. Most people want the other person to be there for them psychologically, socially, and emotionally (Egan, 2001). Active listening includes the following:

- Observing the client's nonverbal behaviors
- Listening to and understanding the client's verbal message
- Listening to and understanding the person in the context of the social setting of his or her life
- Listening for "false notes" (e.g., inconsistencies or things the client says that need more clarification)
- Providing the client with feedback information about himself or herself of which the client might not be aware

We have already noted that effective interviewers must become accustomed to silence. It is just as important, however, for effective interviewers to learn to become active listeners when the client is talking, as well as when the client becomes silent. During active listening, nurses carefully note what the client is saying verbally and nonverbally, as well as monitoring their own nonverbal responses. Using silence effectively and learning to listen on a deeper, more significant level to the client as well as to your own thoughts and reactions are both key ingredients in effective communications. Both these skills take time to develop but can be learned, and you will become more proficient with guidance and practice.

Some principles important to active listening include the following (Mohl, 2003):

- The answer is always inside the patient.
- Objective truth is never as simple as it seems.
- Everything you hear is modified by the client's filters.
- Everything you hear is modified by your own filters.
- It is okay to feel confused and uncertain.
- Listen to yourself, too.

Active listening helps strengthen the client's ability to solve personal problems. By giving the client undivided attention, the nurse communicates that the client is not alone; rather, the nurse is working along with the client, seeking to understand and help. This kind of intervention enhances self-esteem and encourages the client to direct energy toward finding ways to deal with problems. Serving as a sounding board, the nurse listens as the client tests thoughts by voicing them aloud. This form of interpersonal interaction often enables the client to clarify thinking, link ideas, and tentatively decide what should be done and how best to do it (Collins, 1983; Arnold & Boggs, 2003).

Refer to Table 11-4 for more examples of techniques that enhance communication.

TABLE 11-4

Techniques That Enhance Communication

Discussion	Example

Using Silence

Gives the person time to collect thoughts or think through a point.	Encouraging a person to talk by waiting for the answers.

Accepting

Indicates that the person has been understood. The statement does not necessarily indicate agreement but is nonjudgmental. However, nurses do not imply that they understand when they do not understand.	"Yes." "Uh-huh." "I follow what you say."

Giving Recognition

Indicates awareness of change and personal efforts. Does not imply good or bad, or right or wrong.	"Good morning, Mr. James." "You've combed your hair today." "I notice that you shaved today."

Offering Self

Offers presence, interest, and a desire to understand. Is not offered to get the person to talk or behave in a specific way.	"I would like to spend time with you." "I'll stay here and sit with you awhile."

Offering General Leads

Allows the other person to take direction in the discussion. Indicates that the nurse is interested in what comes next.	"Go on." "And then?" "Tell me about it."

Giving Broad Openings

Clarifies that the lead is to be taken by the client. However, the nurse discourages pleasantries and small talk.	"Where would you like to begin?" "What are you thinking about?" "What would you like to discuss?"

Placing the Events in Time or Sequence

Puts events and actions in better perspective. Notes cause-and-effect relationships and identifies patterns of interpersonal difficulties.	"What happened before?" "When did this happen?"

Making Observations

Calls attention to the person's behavior (e.g., trembling, nail biting, restless mannerisms). Encourages the person to notice the behavior to describe thoughts and feelings for mutual understanding. Helpful with mute and withdrawn persons.	"You appear tense." "I notice you're biting your lips." "You appear nervous whenever John enters the room."

Encouraging Description of Perception

Increases the nurse's understanding of the client's perceptions. Talking about feelings and difficulties can lessen the need to act them out inappropriately.	"What do these voices seem to be saying?" "What is happening now?" "Tell me when you feel anxious."

Encouraging Comparison

Brings out recurring themes in experiences or interpersonal relationships. Helps the person clarify similarities and differences.	"Has this ever happened before?" "Is this how you felt when . . . ?" "Was it something like . . . ?"

Restating

Repeats the main idea expressed. Gives the client an idea of what has been communicated. If the message has been misunderstood, the client can clarify it.	*Client:* I can't sleep. I stay awake all night. *Nurse:* You have difficulty sleeping? *Client:* I don't know . . . he always has some excuse for not coming over or keeping our appointments. *Nurse:* You think he no longer wants to see you?

Reflecting

Directs questions, feelings, and ideas back to the client. Encourages the client to accept his or her own ideas and feelings. Acknowledges the client's right to have opinions and make decisions and encourages the client to think of self as a capable person.	*Client:* What should I do about my husband's affair? *Nurse:* What do you think you should do? *Client:* My brother spends all of my money and then has the nerve to ask for more. *Nurse:* You feel angry when this happens?

Continued

TABLE 11-4

Techniques That Enhance Communication—cont'd

Discussion	Example

Focusing

Concentrates attention on a single point. It is especially useful when the client jumps from topic to topic. If a person is experiencing a severe or panic level of anxiety, the nurse should not persist until the anxiety lessens.

"This point you are making about leaving school seems worth looking at more closely."
"You've mentioned many things. Let's go back to your thinking of 'ending it all.'"

Exploring

Examines certain ideas, experiences, or relationships more fully. If the client chooses not to elaborate by answering no, the nurse does not probe or pry. In such a case, the nurse respects the client's wishes.

"Tell me more about that."
"Would you describe it more fully?"
"Could you talk about how it was that you learned your mom was dying of cancer?"

Giving Information

Makes available facts the person needs. Supplies knowledge from which decisions can be made or conclusions drawn. For example, the client needs to know the role of the nurse; the purpose of the nurse-client relationship; and the time, place, and duration of the meetings.

"My purpose for being here is . . ."
"This medication is for . . ."
"The test will determine . . ."

Seeking Clarification

Helps clients clarify their own thoughts and maximizes mutual understanding between nurse and client.

"I am not sure I follow you."
"What would you say is the main point of what you just said?"
"Give an example of a time you thought everyone hated you."

Presenting Reality

Indicates what is real. The nurse does not argue or try to convince the client, just describes personal perceptions or facts in the situation.

"That was Dr. Todd, not a man from the Mafia."
"That was the sound of a car backfiring."
"Your mother is not here; I am a nurse."

Voicing Doubt

Undermines the client's beliefs by not reinforcing the exaggerated or false perceptions.

"Isn't that unusual?"
"Really?"
"That's hard to believe."

Seeking Consensual Validation

Clarifies that both the nurse and client share mutual understanding of communications. Helps the client become clearer about what he or she is thinking.

"Tell me whether my understanding agrees with yours."

Verbalizing the Implied

Puts into concrete terms what the client implies, making the client's communication more explicit.

Client: I can't talk to you or anyone else. It's a waste of time.
Nurse: Do you feel that no one understands?

Encouraging Evaluation

Aids the client in considering people and events from the perspective of the client's own set of values.

"How do you feel about . . . ?"
"What did it mean to you when he said he couldn't stay?"

Attempting to Translate into Feelings

Responds to the feelings expressed, not just the content. Often termed *decoding*.

Client: I am dead inside.
Nurse: Are you saying that you feel lifeless? Does life seem meaningless to you?

Suggesting Collaboration

Emphasizes working with the client, not doing things for the client. Encourages the view that change is possible through collaboration.

"Perhaps you and I can discover what produces your anxiety."
"Perhaps by working together we can come up with some ideas that might improve your communications with your spouse."

Summarizing

Brings together important points of discussion to enhance understanding. Also allows the opportunity to clarify communications so that both nurse and client leave the interview with the same ideas in mind.

"Have I got this straight?"
"You said that . . ."
"During the past hour, you and I have discussed . . ."

Encouraging Formulation of a Plan of Action

Allows the client to identify alternative actions for interpersonal situations the client finds disturbing (e.g., when anger or anxiety is provoked).

"What could you do to let anger out harmlessly?"
"The next time this comes up, what might you do to handle it?"
"What are some other ways you can approach your boss?"

Clarifying Techniques

Understanding depends on clear communication, which is aided by verifying with a client the nurse's interpretation of the client's messages. The nurse must request feedback on the accuracy of the message received from both verbal and nonverbal cues. The use of clarifying techniques helps both participants identify major differences in their frame of reference, giving them the opportunity to correct misperceptions before these cause any serious misunderstandings. The client who is asked to elaborate on or to clarify vague or ambiguous messages needs to know that the purpose is to promote mutual understanding.

Paraphrasing

For clarity, the nurse might use paraphrasing, which means restating in different (often fewer) words the basic content of a client's message. Using simple, precise, and culturally relevant terms, the nurse may readily confirm interpretation of the client's previous message before the interview proceeds. By prefacing statements with a phrase such as "I'm not sure I understand" or "In other words, you seem to be saying . . . ," the nurse helps the client form a clearer perception of what may be a bewildering mass of details. After paraphrasing, the nurse must validate the accuracy of the restatement and its helpfulness to the discussion. The client may confirm or deny the perceptions through nonverbal cues or by direct response to a question such as, "Was I correct in saying . . . ?" As a result, the client is made aware that the interviewer is actively involved in the search for understanding.

Restating

In restating, the nurse mirrors the client's overt and covert messages; thus, this technique may be used to echo feeling as well as content. Restating differs from paraphrasing in that it involves repetition of the same key words the client has just spoken. If a client remarks, "My life is empty . . . it has no meaning," additional information may be gained by restating, "Your life has no meaning?" The purpose of this technique is to explore more thoroughly subjects that may be significant. However, too frequent and indiscriminate use of restating might be interpreted by clients as inattention, disinterest, or worse. It is easy to overuse this tool so that its application becomes mechanical. Parroting or mimicking what another has said may be perceived as poking fun at the person, so that use of this nondirective approach can become a definite barrier to communication. To avoid overuse of restating, the nurse can combine restatements with direct questions that encourage descriptions: "What does your life lack?" "What kind of meaning is missing?" "Describe one day in your life that appears empty to you."

Reflecting

Reflection is a means of assisting people to better understand their own thoughts and feelings. Reflecting may take the form of a question or a simple statement that conveys the nurse's observations of the client when sensitive issues are being discussed. The nurse might then describe briefly to the client the apparent meaning of the emotional tone of the client's verbal and nonverbal behavior. For example, to reflect a client's feelings about his or her life, a good beginning might be, "You sound as if you have had many disappointments." **Sharing observations** with a client shows acceptance. The nurse helps make the client aware of inner feelings and encourages the client to own them. For example, the nurse may tell a client, "You look sad." Perceiving the nurse's concern may allow a client spontaneously to share feelings. The use of a question in response to the client's question is another reflective technique (Arnold & Boggs, 2003). For example:

Client: Nurse, do you think I really need to be hospitalized?
Nurse: What do you think, Jane?
Client: I don't know; that's why I'm asking you.
Nurse: I'll be willing to share my impression with you at the end of this first session. However, you've probably thought about hospitalization and have some feelings about it. I wonder what they are.

Exploring

A technique that enables the nurse to examine important ideas, experiences, or relationships more fully is exploring. For example, if a client tells the nurse that he does not get along well with his wife, the nurse will want to further explore this area. Possible openers include the following:

- *"Tell me* more about your relationship with your wife."
- *"Describe* your relationship with your wife."
- *"Give me an example* of how you and your wife don't get along."

Asking for an example can greatly clarify a vague or generic statement made by a client.

Client: No one likes me.
Nurse: Give me an example of one person who doesn't like you.

or

Client: Everything I do is wrong.
Nurse: Give me an example of one thing you do that you think is wrong.

Degree of Openness

Any questions or statements can be classified as (1) open-ended verbalizations, (2) focused questions, or (3) closed-ended verbalizations. Furthermore, any questions or statement can be classified along the **continuum of openness.** There are three variables that influence where verbalization sits on this openness continuum (Shea, 1998), including

1. The degree to which the verbalization tends to produce a spontaneous and lengthy response.
2. The degree to which the verbalization does not limit the client's answer set.
3. The degree to which the verbalization facilitates interaction with a client who does not appear to want to talk.

Open-Ended Questions

Open-ended questions require more than one-word answers (i.e., yes or no). Even with a client who is sullen, resistant, or guarded, open-ended questions can encourage lengthy information on experiences, perceptions of events, or responses to a situation. Some examples of open-ended questions are the following:

- "What are some of the stresses you are grappling with?"
- "What do you perceive to be your biggest problem at the moment?"
- "Tell me something about your family."

Open-ended questions or gentle inquiries (e.g., "Tell me about . . ." or "Share with me . . .") are especially helpful when at the beginning of a relationship and in the early interviews. Although the initial responses may be short, over time the responses often become more informative as the client becomes more at ease. This is an especially valuable technique for clients who are resistant or guarded, but it is a good method for the opening phases of any interview, especially in the early phase of establishing a rapport with an individual.

Closed-Ended Questions

Closed-ended questions, in contrast, are questions that ask for specific information (dates, names, numbers, yes or no information). They are closed-ended questions because they limit the client's freedom of choice. For example:

- "Is your mother alive?"
- "When did you first start hearing voices telling you to die?"
- "Did you seek therapy after your first suicide attempt?"
- "Do you think the medication is helping you?"

Closed-ended questions elicit specific information when needed, such as during an initial assessment or intake interview, or ascertain results, as in "Are the medications helping you?" They are usually answered by yes, no, or a short response. When closed-ended questions are used frequently during a counseling session, particularly during an initial interview, they can close an interview down rapidly. This is especially true with a guarded or resistant client.

Indirect or Implied Questions

The use of an indirect or implied question is a good approach when you don't want to pressure an individual to respond but are curious about what a person might be thinking or feeling. Indirect questions should be used sparingly so as to avoid sounding sneaky or manipulative and only when a rapport has been established (Sommers-Flanagan & Sommers-Flanagan, 2003). For example:

- "*It must* have been hard for you not to get that job."
- "*I wonder* what plans you've made now that the divorce is final."
- "*You must* have some thoughts or feelings about having to repeat the semester."

OBSTRUCTIVE TECHNIQUES TO MONITOR AND MINIMIZE

Although people may use these techniques in their daily lives, they can become problematic when one is working with clients who are attempting to cope with disruptions in their lives. Refer to Table 11-5 for samples of obstructive techniques and suggestions for more helpful responses. Two other techniques, excessive questioning and giving approval or disapproval, are discussed in the following sections. Giving advice and "why" questions are discussed in more detail.

Asking Excessive Questions

Excessive questioning, or asking multiple questions at the same time, especially closed-ended questions, casts the nurse in the role of interrogator, raising a demand for information without respect for the client's willingness or readiness to respond. This approach conveys lack of respect for and sensitivity to the client's needs. Excessive questioning or asking multiple questions at the same time controls the range and nature of the response and can easily result in a therapeutic stall or shut down an interview. It is a controlling tactic and may reflect the interviewer's lack of security in letting the client tell his or her own story. It is better to ask more open-ended questions and follow the client's lead. For example:

Excessive questioning:

- "Why did you leave your wife? Did you feel angry at her? What did she do to you? Are you going back to her?"

Better to say:

- "Tell me about the situation between you and your wife."

Giving Approval or Disapproval

"You look great in that dress." "I'm proud of the way you controlled your temper at lunch." "That's a great quilt you made." What could be bad about giving

TABLE 11-5

Obstructive Communications

Technique	Example	Discussion	More Helpful Response
Giving premature advice	"Get out of this situation immediately."	Assumes the nurse knows best and the client can't think for self. Inhibits problem solving and fosters dependency.	"What are the pros and cons of your situation?" "What were some of the actions you thought you might take?" "What are some of the ways you have thought of to meet your goals?" **Encouraging problem solving**
Minimizing feelings	**Client:** I wish I were dead. **Nurse:** "Everyone gets down in the dumps." "I know what you mean." "I know how you feel." "You should feel happy you're getting better." "Things get worse before they get better."	Indicates that the nurse is unable to understand or empathize with the client. Here the client's feelings or experiences are being belittled, which can cause the client to feel small or insignificant.	"You must be feeling very upset. Are you thinking of hurting yourself?" **Empathizing and exploring**
Falsely reassuring	"I wouldn't worry about that." "Everything will be all right." "You will do just fine, you'll see."	Underrates a person's feelings and belittles a person's concerns. May cause the client to stop sharing feelings if the client thinks he or she will be ridiculed or not taken seriously.	"What specifically are you worried about?" "What do you think could go wrong?" "What are you concerned might happen?" **Clarifying the client's message**
Showing nonverbal signs of boredom or resentment	The nurse frequently checks his or her watch, rustles papers, avoids eye contact, does not respond to the client's concerns, looks annoyed at something the client is doing or has said.	Because the client will quickly pick up the nurse's disapproval or boredom, may cause the client to think the nurse disapproves of or is bored with the client. Diminishes the client's self-esteem and may cause the client to feel demeaned.	The nurse needs to be alert to personal feelings toward the client. If the client's behavior is bothering the nurse (e.g., smoking in a nonsmoking room), the nurse needs to deal with the issue and not remain angry. If the nurse is feeling bored, it may be a clue to what is going on with the client that needs exploring. If there is something going on with the nurse, the nurse should make it clear to the client that it is the nurse who is distracted and it has nothing to do with the client. **Performing self-assessment**
Making value judgments	"How come you still smoke when your wife has lung cancer?"	Prevents problem solving. Can make the client feel guilty, angry, misunderstood, not supported, and/or anxious to leave.	"I notice you are still smoking even though your wife has lung cancer. Is this a problem?" **Making observations**
Asking "why" questions	"Why did you stop taking your medication?"	Implies criticism; often has the effect of making the client feel defensive.	"Tell me some of the reasons that led up to your not taking your medications." **Asking open-ended questions—giving a broad opening**
Asking excessive questions	**Nurse:** How's your appetite? Are you losing weight? Are you eating enough? **Client:** No.	Results in the client's not knowing which question to answer and possibly being confused about what is being asked.	"Tell me about your eating habits since you've been depressed." **Clarifying**

Adapted from Hays, J. S., & Larson, K. (1963). *Interacting with patients.* New York: Macmillan. Copyright © 1963 Macmillan Publishing Company.   *Continued*

TABLE 11-5

Obstructive Communications—cont'd

Technique	Example	Discussion	More Helpful Response
Giving approval, agreeing	"I'm proud of you for applying for that job." "I agree with your decision."	Implies that the client is doing the *right* thing—and that not doing it is wrong. May lead the client to focus on pleasing the nurse or clinician; denies the client the opportunity to change his or her mind or decision.	"I noticed that you applied for that job. What factors will lead up to your changing your mind?" **Making observations** "What led up to that decision?" **Asking open-ended questions—giving a broad opening**
Disapproving; disagreeing	"You really should have shown up for the medication group." "I disagree with that."	Can make a person defensive.	"What was going through your mind when you decided not to come to your medication group?" "That's one point of view. How did you arrive at that conclusion?" **Exploring**
Changing the subject	*Client:* I'd like to die. *Nurse:* Did you go to Alcoholics Anonymous like we discussed?	May invalidate the client's feelings and needs. Can leave the client feeling alienated and isolated and increase feelings of hopelessness.	*Client:* I'd like to die. *Nurse:* This sounds serious. Have you thought of harming yourself? **Validating and exploring**

someone a pat on the back once in a while? Nothing, if it is done without carrying a judgment (positive or negative) by the nurse. We often give our friends and family approval when they do something well. However, in a nurse-client situation, giving approval often becomes much more complex. A client may be feeling overwhelmed, be experiencing low self-esteem, be feeling unsure of where his or her life is going, and be very needy for recognition, approval, and attention. Yet, when people are feeling vulnerable, a value comment might be misinterpreted. For example:

Nurse: You did a great job in group telling John just what you thought about how rudely he treated you.

Implied in this message is that the nurse was pleased by the manner in which the client talked to John. The client then sees such a response as a way to please the nurse by doing the right thing. To continue to please the nurse (and get approval), the client may continue the behavior. The behavior might be useful behavior for the client, but when a behavior is being done to please another person, it is not coming from the individual's own volition or conviction. Also, when the other person whom the client needs to please is not around, the motivation for the new behavior might not be there either. Thus, the new response really is not a change in behavior as much as a ploy to win approval and acceptance from another person. Giving approval also cuts off further communication. It is a statement of the observer's (nurse's) judgment about another person's (client's) behavior. A more useful comment would be the following:

Nurse: I noticed that you spoke up to John in group yesterday about his rude behavior. How did it feel to be more assertive?

This opens the way for finding out if the client was scared, was comfortable, wants to work more on assertiveness, or something else. It also suggests that this was a self-choice the client made. The client is given recognition for the change in behavior, and the topic is also opened for further discussion.

Disapproving is moralizing and implies that the nurse has the right to judge the client's thoughts or feelings. Again, an observation should be made instead.

Nurse: You really should not cheat, even if you think everyone else is doing it.

A more useful comment would be the following:

Nurse: Can you give me two examples of how cheating could negatively affect your goal of graduating?

Advising

Although we ask for and give advice all the time in daily life, giving advice to a client is rarely helpful. Often, when we ask for advice, our real motive is to discover if we are thinking along the same lines as someone else or if they would agree with us. When the nurse gives advice to a client who is having trouble assessing and problem solving in conflicted areas of the client's life, the nurse is interfering with the client's ability to make personal decisions. When the nurse offers the client solutions, the client eventually begins to think that the nurse does not view the client as capable of making effective decisions. People often feel inadequate when they are given no choices over decisions in their lives. Giving advice to clients can foster dependency ("I'll have to ask the nurse what to do about . . ."). Giving people advice can undermine their sense of competence and adequacy. It also keeps the nurse in control and feeling like the strong one, although this might be unconscious on the nurse's part. However, people do need information to make informed decisions. Often, the nurse can help the client define a problem and identify what information might be needed to come to an informed decision. A more useful approach would be, "What do you see as some possible actions you can take?" It is much more constructive to encourage problem solving by the client. At times, the nurse can suggest several alternatives that a client might consider (e.g., "Have you ever thought of telling your friend about the incident?"). The client is then free to say yes or no and make his or her own decision from among the suggestions.

Asking "Why" Questions

"Why did you come late?" "Why didn't you go to the funeral?" "Why didn't you study for the exam?" Very often, "why" questions imply criticism. We may ask our friends or family such questions and, in the context of a solid relationship, the "Why?" may be understood more as "What happened?" With people we do not know—especially an anxious person who may be feeling overwhelmed—a "why" question from a person in authority (nurse, physician, teacher) can be experienced as intrusive and judgmental, which serves only to make the person defensive. Most of the time we do not know why we do things, although when confronted by "Why did you . . . ?" we may make up all sorts of responses on the spur of the moment.

It is much more useful to ask *what* is happening rather than *why* it is happening. Questions that focus on who, what, where, and when often elicit important information that can facilitate problem solving and further the communication process.

EVALUATION OF CLINICAL SKILLS

After you have had some introductory clinical experience, you may find the facilitative skills checklist in Figure 11-3 useful for evaluating your progress in developing interviewing skills. Note that some of the items might not be relevant for some of your clients (e.g., numbers 11 through 13 may not be possible to do when a client is highly psychotic). Self-evaluation of clinical skills is a way to focus on therapeutic improvement. Role playing can be a useful tool for preparation for the clinical experience as well as a practice in acquiring more effective and professional communication skills.

FACILITATIVE SKILLS CHECKLIST

Instructions: Periodically during your clinical experience, use this checklist to identify areas where growth is needed and progress has been made. Think of your clinical client experiences. Indicate the extent of your agreement with each of the following statements by marking the scale: *SA*, strongly agree; *A*, agree; *NS*, not sure; *D*, disagree; *SD*, strongly disagree.

1. I maintain good eye contact.	SA	A	NS	D	SD
2. Most of my verbal comments follow the lead of the other person.	SA	A	NS	D	SD
3. I encourage others to talk about feelings.	SA	A	NS	D	SD
4. I am able to ask open-ended questions.	SA	A	NS	D	SD
5. I can restate and clarify a person's ideas.	SA	A	NS	D	SD
6. I can summarize in a few words the basic ideas of a long statement made by a person.	SA	A	NS	D	SD
7. I can make statements that reflect the person's feelings.	SA	A	NS	D	SD
8. I can share my feelings relevant to the discussion when appropriate to do so.	SA	A	NS	D	SD
9. I am able to give feedback.	SA	A	NS	D	SD
10. At least 75% or more of my responses help enhance and facilitate communication.	SA	A	NS	D	SD
11. I can assist the person to list some alternatives available.	SA	A	NS	D	SD
12. I can assist the person to identify some goals that are specific and observable.	SA	A	NS	D	SD
13. I can assist the person to specify at least one next step that might be taken toward the goal.	SA	A	NS	D	SD

FIGURE 11-3 Facilitative skills checklist. (Adapted from Myrick, D., & Erney, T. [2000]. *Caring and sharing* [2nd ed., p. 168]. Copyright © 2000 by Educational Media Corporation, Minneapolis, Minnesota.)

■ ■ ■ KEY POINTS to REMEMBER

- The clinical interview is a key component of psychiatric mental health nursing. Presented are the considerations needed for establishing a safe setting and planning for appropriate seating, introduction, and initiation of the interview.

- Whether you are working in a psychiatric unit, in a clinic, or in the client's home, you will be confronted with an array of behaviors during your student experience. It is useful to be somewhat prepared for specific client behaviors (e.g., clients cry, ask you to keep a secret, or say they want to kill themselves). Potentially problematic client behaviors during the interview, as well as guidelines for nursing interventions, are addressed in Table 11-2.

- A knowledge of communication and interviewing techniques is the foundation for development of any nurse-client relationship. When effective communication skills are a genuine part of the helping process and are applied with concern and respect for the other person, they can be dynamic tools in working effectively with people. Berlo's communication model has five parts: stimulus, sender, message, medium, and receiver.

- Feedback is a vital component of the communication process for validating the accuracy of the sender's message.

- A number of factors can minimize or enhance the communication process. For example, differences in culture, language, and knowledge levels; noise; lack of privacy; the presence of others; and the expectations of others all can influence communication.

- There are verbal and nonverbal elements in communication; the nonverbal elements often play the larger role in conveying a person's message. Verbal communication consists of all words a person speaks. Nonverbal communication consists of the behaviors displayed by an individual, in contrast to the actual content of speech.

- Communication is a complex process, and two models are available that help operationally define some of the dynamics.

- Communication has two levels: the content level (verbal) and the process level (nonverbal behavior). When content is congruent with process, the communication is said to be healthy. When the verbal message is not reinforced by the communicator's actions, the message is ambiguous; we call this a double (or mixed) message.

- Attending behaviors (e.g., eye contact, body language, vocal qualities, and verbal tracking) are a key element in effective communication.

- Cultural background (as well as individual differences) has a great deal to do with what nonverbal behavior means to different individuals. The degree of eye contact and the use of touch are two nonverbal aspects that can be misunderstood by individuals of different cultures.

- There are a number of effective counseling and communication techniques that nurses can use to enhance their nursing practices. Many widely used communication enhancers are cited in Table 11-4.

- There are also a number of obstructive behaviors that nurses can learn to avoid to enhance their effectiveness with people. Some are cited in Table 11-5 along with suggestions for more helpful responses.

- Most nurses are most effective when they use nonthreatening and open-ended communication techniques.

- Effective communication is a skill that develops over time and is integral to the establishment and maintenance of a therapeutic alliance.

■ ■ ■

Visit the Evolve website at **http://evolve.elsevier.com/Varcarolis** for a posttest on the content in this chapter. *evolve*

Critical Thinking and Chapter Review

Visit the Evolve website at **http://evolve.elsevier.com/Varcarolis** for additional self-study exercises.
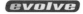

■ ■ ■ CRITICAL THINKING

1. You are attempting to conduct a clinical interview with a very withdrawn client. You have tried silence and open-ended statements to engage the client, but all you get is one-word answers. What other actions could you take at this time?

2. You have been spending time with a client for 5 weeks, twice a week, at a community mental health center. Your client has been upset over the fact that her son has been diagnosed with acquired immunodeficiency syndrome, and you and she have been spending a lot of time discussing many of the painful issues she is presently dealing with. She is going away for 3 weeks to visit her son in Seattle, and she brings

you a brightly covered cloth notebook "to keep your client notes in." How would you handle this situation? If she had brought you the gift during the first week, how would you have handled it?

3. Keep a log for 30 minutes a day of your communication pattern (a tape recorder is ideal). Pick out four effective techniques that you notice you use frequently. Identify two techniques that are obstructive. In your log, rewrite these obstructive communications and replace them with statements that would better facilitate discussion of thoughts and feelings. Share your log and discuss the changes you are working on with one classmate.

Critical Thinking and Chapter Review—cont'd

Visit the Evolve website at **http://evolve.elsevier.com/Varcarolis** for additional self-study exercises.

evolve

■■ ■ CHAPTER REVIEW

Choose the most appropriate answer.

1. Paraphrasing, restating, reflecting, and exploring are techniques used for the purpose of
    1. clarifying.
    2. summarizing.
    3. encouraging comparison.
    4. placing events in time and sequence.

2. Which communication technique would yield positive results within the context of a therapeutic relationship?
    1. Advising
    2. Giving approval
    3. Listening actively
    4. Asking "why" questions

3. When the client makes the statement, "I get all balled up when I try to talk to him," and the nurse responds, "Give me an example of getting all balled up," the nurse is using the technique called
    1. exploring.
    2. reflecting.
    3. interpreting.
    4. paraphrasing.

4. Which advice will be helpful in establishing rapport when the nurse is beginning a relationship with a client?
    1. Fill any silences the client leaves.
    2. When in doubt, focus on feelings.
    3. Rely on direct questions to explore sensitive areas.
    4. Pay more attention to verbal than to nonverbal communication.

5. Which statement by the nurse to a client would be considered nontherapeutic?
    1. "I know exactly how you feel."
    2. "I'm not sure I understand what you mean."
    3. "Tell me more about what happened when you resigned."
    4. "I see that you are wringing your hands as we talk about the job interview."

■ STUDENT
■ STUDY
■ CD-ROM

Access the accompanying CD-ROM for animations, interactive exercises, review questions for the NCLEX examination, and an audio glossary.

REFERENCES

Arnold, E., & Boggs, K. U. (2003). *Interpersonal relationships: Professional communication skills for nurses* (4th ed.). Philadelphia: Saunders.

Bateson, G., et al. (1956). Toward a theory of schizophrenia. *Behavioral Sciences, 1*(4), 251-264.

Berlo, D. K. (1960). *The process of communication.* San Francisco: Reinhart Press.

Collins, M. (1983). *Communication in health care: The human connection in the life cycle* (2nd ed.). St. Louis: Mosby.

Dee, V. (1991). How can we become more aware of culturally specific body language and use this awareness therapeutically? *Journal of Psychosocial Nursing, 29*(11), 39-40.

Egan, G. (1994). The skilled helper: A problem management approach (5th ed.). Pacific Grove, CA: Brooks/Cole.

Egan, G. (2001). *The skilled helper: A systematic approach to effective helping* (7th ed.). Pacific Grove, CA: Wadsworth.

Ellis, R. B., Gates, B., & Kenworthy, N. (2003). *Interpersonal communicating in nursing* (2nd ed.). London: Churchill Livingstone.

Farkas-Cameron, M. M. (1995). Clinical supervision in psychiatric nursing. *Journal of Psychosocial Nursing and Mental Health Services, 33*(2), 40-47.

Glasser, W. (2000). *Counseling with choice theory: The new reality therapy.* New York: HarperCollins.

Haber, J. (2000). Hildegard E. Peplau: The psychiatric nursing legacy of a legend. *Journal of the American Psychiatric Nursing Association, 6*(2), 56-62.

Hubble, M. A., Duncan, B. L., & Miller, S. D. (1999). *The heart and soul of change: What works in therapy.* Washington, DC: American Psychological Association.

Ivey, A. E., & Ivey, M. (1999). *International interviewing and counseling* (4th ed.). Pacific Grove, CA: Brooks/Cole.

Kavanaugh, K. H. (2003). Transcultural perspectives in mental health nursing. In M. Andrews & J. Boyle, *Transcultural concepts in nursing care.* Philadelphia: Lippincott Williams & Wilkins.

Lu, F. G., et al. (1995). Issues in the assessment and diagnosis of culturally diverse individuals. In J. M. Oldhan & M. B. Riba (Eds.), *Review of psychiatry* (Vol. 14, pp. 477-510). Washington, DC: American Psychiatric Press.

Meier, S. T., & Davis, S. R. (2001). *The elements of counseling* (4th ed.). Pacific Grove, CA: Brooks/Cole.

Mohl, P. C. (2003). Listening to the patient. In A. Tasman, J. Kay, & J. A. Lieberman (Eds.), *Psychiatry* (2nd ed.). West Sussex, England: Wiley.

Moscato, B. (1988). The one-to-one relationship. In H. S. Wilson & C. S. Kneisel (Eds.), *Psychiatric nursing* (3rd ed.). Menlo Park, CA: Addison-Wesley.

Myrick, R. D., & Erney, T. (1984). *Caring and sharing.* Minneapolis, MN: Educational Media Corporation.

Peplau, H. E. (1952). *Interpersonal relations in nursing: A conceptual frame of reference for psychodynamic nursing.* New York: Putnam.

Rankin, J. A. (2001). *Body language in negotiations and sales* (2nd ed.) Springfield, VA: Rankin File.

Shea, S. C. (1998). *Psychiatric interviewing: The art of understanding* (2nd ed.). Philadelphia: Saunders.

Smedley, B., Stith, A., & Nelson, A. (2002). *Unequal treatment: Confronting racial and ethnic disparities in healthcare* (Institute of Medicine Report). Washington, DC: National Academy Press.

Sommers-Flanagan, J., & Sommers-Flanagan, R. (2003). *Clinical interviewing* (3rd ed.). Hoboken, NJ: Wiley.

U.S. Department of Health and Human Services. (2001). *Mental health: Culture, race, and ethnicity: Supplement to mental health: A report of the surgeon general.* Rockville, MD: U.S. Department of Health and Human Services, Substance Abuse and Mental Health Services Administration, Center for Mental Health Services.

Watzlawick, P., Benoin, J., & Jackson, D. (1967). *Pragmatics of human communication.* New York: W. W. Norton.

CHAPTER **12**

Understanding Stress and Holistic Approaches to Stress Management

ELIZABETH M. VARCAROLIS

KEY TERMS and CONCEPTS

The key terms and concepts listed here appear in color where they are defined or first discussed in this chapter.

assertiveness training, 207

Benson's relaxation techniques, 204

biofeedback, 206

cognitive reframing, 206

coping styles, 202

distress, 198

eustress, 198

guided imagery, 205

humor, 207

journal keeping, 206

meditation, 204

physical stressors, 200

progressive muscle relaxation (PMR), 206

psychological stressors, 200

psychoneuroimmunology (PNI), 198

restructuring and setting priorities, 206

OBJECTIVES

After studying this chapter, the reader will be able to

1. Recognize the short- and long-term physiological consequences of stress.
2. Contrast and compare Cannon's (fight-or-flight), Selye's (general adaptation syndrome), and psychoneuroimmunological models of stress.
3. Identify the relationship between stress and anxiety.
4. Analyze and give examples of the ways in which culture can affect a person's perception of and reaction to stress.
5. Assess life change units in a client's life using the Life-Changing Events Questionnaire.
6. Differentiate among four categories of coping and give at least two examples of each.
7. Teach a classmate or client two simple behavioral techniques to help lower stress and anxiety.
8. Explain how cognitive techniques can help lower a person's level of stress.

evolve Visit the Evolve website at **http://evolve.elsevier.com/Varcarolis** for a pretest on the content in this chapter.

TOWARD A HOLISTIC MODEL OF STRESS

Initial Alarm Reaction to Stress: Fight or Flight

Walter Cannon (1871-1945), a groundbreaker in the field of stress research, methodically investigated the sympathetic nervous system as a pathway of the response to stress, known more commonly as the flight (withdrawal) or fight (aggression) response. The well known **fight-or-flight response** is the body's way of

preparing for a situation that an individual perceives as a threat to survival. Brigham (1994) operationally defines the steps in the fight-or-flight response as follows:

1. The threat-to-survival message is conveyed to the hypothalamus, which chemically communicates with the pineal or the pituitary gland (considered the master control center of the body).
2. The pituitary begins mobilizing the release of adrenocorticotropic hormone (ACTH) as well as activating hormones for the adrenal medulla.
3. The adrenal medulla pumps adrenaline, noradrenaline, and other catecholamines into the bloodstream, which results in the following:

a. Heart rate and blood pressure rise, which increases circulation of blood (oxygen) to the body.

b. Airways in the lungs dilate to facilitate oxygenation of blood with the increased blood flow.

c. Blood flow shifts from the smooth muscles of the digestive system to the skeletal muscles to enable fight or flight.

d. Plasma levels of glucose, triglycerides, and free fatty acids increase so they may be used by the body as fuel.

e. Platelet aggregation increases to aid blood clotting.

f. Kidney clearance is reduced to prevent loss of water.

Acute and Long-Term Effects of Stress: General Adaptation Theory

Hans Selye (1907-1982), another pioneer in stress research, expanded Cannon's theory of stress in 1956 in his formulation of the **general adaptation syndrome (GAS)**. The GAS occurs in two stages: (1) an initial adaptive response (fight or flight) in the alarm or acute stress phase, and (2) the eventual maladaptive responses to prolonged stress. Stress produces a wide array of psychological and physiological responses. Table 12-1 gives an overview of some of the body's responses to acute stress and prolonged (chronic) stress. The body reacts physiologically in the same manner regardless of whether the stress is a real threat or a situation or object that is only perceived as a threat, and whether the threat is physical, psychological, or social.

The chemicals produced by the stress response (such as cortisol, adrenaline, and other catecholamines) have a profound effect on the systems of the body. Figure 12-1 portrays the initial short-term adaptive fight-or-flight response and the eventual long-term maladaptive **physiological effects** of stress on the hypothalamic (brain)–pituitary (endocrine) and sympathetic–adrenal medullary systems. A variety of chronic physical disorders (e.g., hypertension, diabetes) and numerous physical diseases have been linked to long-term, sustained stress as depicted in Figure 12-1 and discussed further in Chapter 29.

In 1974 Selye distinguished between the psychological reactions of *distress* and *eustress*:

Distress—negative, draining energy (e.g., anxiety, depression, confusion, helplessness, hopelessness, fatigue)

Eustress—positive, beneficial stress that motivates energy (e.g., happiness, hopefulness, peacefulness, purposeful movement); the positive emotions of eustress often serve to replenish damaged resources (Lazarus, Kanner, & Folkman, 1980)

Psychoneuroimmunology: A Biopsychosocial Model

Cannon and Selye focused on the physical and mental responses of the nervous and endocrine systems to acute and chronic stress. The **psychoneuroimmunological model** considers the immune system response, which is an integral part of the acute or alarm phase (Mausch, 2000). Studies in psychoneuroimmunology (PNI) provided evidence that stress, through the

---

TABLE 12-1

Some Reactions to Acute and Prolonged (Chronic) Stress

Acute Stress Can Cause	Prolonged Stress Can Cause
Uneasiness and concern	Anxiety and panic attacks
Sadness	Depression or melancholia
Loss of appetite	Anorexia or overeating
Suppression of the immune system	Lowered resistance to infections, leading to increase in opportunistic viral and bacterial infections
Increased metabolism and use of body fats	Insulin-resistant diabetes
	Hypertension
Infertility	Amenorrhea or loss of sex drive
	Impotence, anovulation
Increased energy mobilization and use	Increased fatigue and irritability
	Decreased memory and learning
Increased cardiovascular tone	Increased risk for cardiac events (e.g., heart attack, angina, and sudden heart-related death)
	Increased risk of blood clots and stroke
Increased cardiopulmonary tone	Increased respiratory problems

THE STRESS RESPONSE

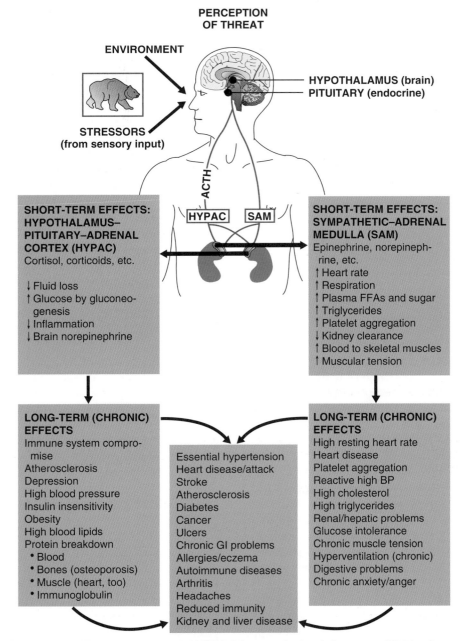

FIGURE 12-1 The stress response. *ACTH*, Adrenocorticotropic hormone; *BP*, blood pressure; *FFAs*, free fatty acids; *GI*, gastrointestinal. (From Brigham, D. D. [1994]. *Imagery for getting well: Clinical applications of behavioral medicine.* New York: W. W. Norton.)

hypothalamic-pituitary-adrenal and sympathetic–adrenal medullary axes, can induce modulation of the immune system (Yang & Glaser, 2002). The activation of the immune system sets up a bilateral process. Once activated by stress, the immune system sends chemical messages (proinflammatory cytokines) to the brain. The brain then releases its own cytokines, which signal the central nervous system to initiate a myriad of responses to help the body adapt to the stress. This process changes neural activity in the brain, which

in turn can alter everything that flows from neural activity—essentially behavior, thought, and mood (Azar, 2001; DeAngelis, 2002). Thus, it seems that immune system responses are regulated by the brain and behavior as well as by the presence of antigens (Lutz, Tarkowski, & Dudek, 2001).

The PNI model helps explain what clinicians and others have believed and witnessed for centuries: that there is a link between stress (biopsychosocial), the immune system, and disease—a very clear mind-body connection that may alter health outcomes. The immune response and the resulting cytokine activity in the brain also raise questions regarding the origins of psychological and cognitive states such as depression and memory dysfunction.

PNI, as a purely biomedical framework, is still limited. There is a long way yet to go to show definite links between PNI variables and disease; however, PNI research is becoming increasingly sophisticated. Investigators are examining how psychosocial factors such as optimism and social support moderate the stress response; they are mapping the biological and cellular mechanisms by which stress affects the immune system as well as testing new theories (DeAngelis, 2002).

STRESSORS AND FACTORS MEDIATING THE STRESS RESPONSE

Stressors

A variety of dissimilar situations (e.g., emotional arousal, fatigue, fear, loss, humiliation, loss of blood, and even great and unexpected success) all are capable of producing stress and triggering the stress response (Selye, 1993). There are no factors that can be singled out as the cause of the stress reaction; however, stressors can be divided into two categories: physical and psychological. Physical stressors include environmental conditions such as trauma and excessive cold or heat, as well as physical conditions such as infection, hemorrhage, hunger, and pain. Psychological stressors include such things as divorce, loss of a job, unmanageable debt, death of a loved one, retirement, and fear of a terrorist attack, as well as changes we might consider to be positive, such as marriage, arrival of a new baby, or unexpected success.

In 1967, Holmes and Rahe published the Social Readjustment Rating Scale. This life-change scale is a means of monitoring the level of stressful life events over a given period (1 year). This questionnaire has been rescaled twice, first in 1978 and again in 1997.

Since Holmes and Rahe's contribution, a variety of scales have been devised to measure stressful life events, which are conceptualized in different ways. Research using these scales also shows stressful life events to be related to a wide variety of physical and mental disorders (Brown & Harris, 1989; Dohrenwend & Dohrenwend, 1974, 1983; Lazarus & DeLongis, 1983).

Researchers have looked at the degree to which various life events upset a specific individual. They have found that it is more the *perception* of a recent life event that determines the person's emotional and psychological reactions to it (Rahe, 1995). For example, a man

in his forties who has a new baby, has just purchased a home, and is laid off with 6 months' severance pay may feel the stress of the event (lost job) more intensely than a man who is 62 years of age, financially secure, and asked to take an early retirement.

Mediating Factors

Responses to stress and anxiety are affected by factors such as age, sex, culture, life experiences, and lifestyle. These all are elements that may work to lessen or increase the degree of emotional or physical influence and the sequelae of stress.

Individual and Social Factors

Social support is one mediating factor that has been heavily researched and has significant implications for nurses and other health care professionals. The fact that strong social support from significant others can enhance mental and physical health and act as a significant buffer against distress has been well documented in the literature. Numerous studies have found a strong correlation between lower mortality rates and intact support systems (Koenig, McCullough, & Larson, 2001).

The proliferation of self-help groups attests to the need people have for social supports, and the explosive growth of a great variety of support groups reflects the effectiveness of such groups for many people. Many of the support groups currently available are for people going through similar stressful life events, such as the prototypical Alcoholics Anonymous, Gamblers Anonymous, Reach for Recovery (for cancer patients), and Parents Without Partners, to note but a few.

It is important, however, to differentiate between social support relationships of high quality and those of low quality. Low-quality support relationships (e.g., living in an abusive home situation or with a controlling and demeaning person) may, and often do, negatively affect a person's coping effectiveness in a crisis. High-quality relationships have been linked to less loneliness, more supportive behavior, and greater life satisfaction (Hobfall & Vaux, 1993). High-quality emotional support is a critical factor in enhancing a person's sense of control and rebuilding feelings of self-esteem and competency. Supportive relationships of high quality have the following characteristics: (1) they are relatively free from conflict and negative interactions, and (2) they are close, confiding, and reciprocal (Hobfall & Vaux, 1993).

Culture

Each culture not only emphasizes certain problems of living more than others but also interprets emotional problems differently from other cultures. For example, the specific characteristics of the dysphoria of depression vary cross-culturally (Kim, 2002; Neighbors, 2003). The Hopi of North America express depressive states through feelings of guilt, shame, and sinfulness. On the other hand, Puerto Ricans and other Latinos describe irritability, rage, and "nervousness" as indicators of a depressive affect.

Although Western European and North American cultures subscribe to a psychophysiological view of stress and somatic distress, this does not hold true cross-culturally. The overwhelming majority of Asians, Africans, and Central Americans "not only express subjective distress in somatic terms, but actually experience this distress somatically, such that psychological interpretations of suffering may not be much use cross-culturally" (Gonzalez, Griffith, & Ruiz, 1995). The following vignette illustrates this point:

▪ ▪ ▪ *VIGNETTE*

A 62-year-old Puerto Rican woman was referred for evaluation of incapacitating abdominal pain present for the previous 9 months, because a medical diagnostic evaluation of this pain gave negative results. The pain had begun approximately 1 month after her substance-abusing son had been jailed for killing his lover, whom the patient loved "like a daughter." The patient expected that the psychiatrist would prescribe medication that would take her pain away, and she was initially distressed to learn that she was expected to talk about her life. Although not ruling out the use of medication, the therapist explained to her that her pain might be related to the wrenching emotional ordeal of the past year. The therapist made it a point to validate her pain and took great care not to imply that the pain was "merely"

the expression of unacknowledged emotion. In particular, he told her that he understood her pain to be very real and that he did not expect her pain to be gone overnight. This approach allowed the patient to engage in a course of brief psychotherapy during which her conflicted feelings about her substance-abusing offspring were examined, although these feelings were never specifically identified as the cause of her pain. Eventually the patient felt strong enough to make drastic changes in her role as enabler of her children, at which point she reported that her pain was much improved (Gonzalez et al., 1995, p. 60).

▪ ▪ ▪

Spirituality and Prayerfulness

There are many religious and spiritual beliefs that are helpful for many people in coping with stress. These deserve closer scientific investigation. Studies have demonstrated that spiritual practices can enhance the immune system and sense of well-being (Koenig et al., 2001). Some scholars propose that spiritual well-being helps people deal with health issues primarily because spiritual beliefs help people cope with issues of living. People who include spiritual solutions to physical or mental distress often gain a sense of comfort and support that can aid in healing and lowering stress. Even prayer, in and of itself, can elicit the relaxation response, discussed later in this chapter, which is known to reduce stress physically and emotionally, and to reduce stress on the immune system.

Figure 12-2 operationally defines the process of stress and the positive or negative results of attempts to relieve stress.

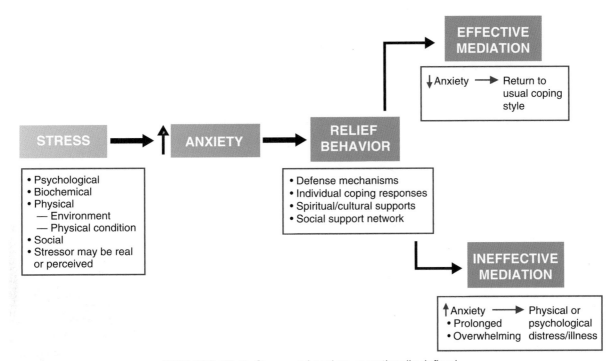

FIGURE 12-2 Stress and anxiety operationally defined.

ASSESSING STRESS AND COPING STYLES

Measuring Stress

An interesting recent finding (Miller & Rahe, 1997) is that life stress appears to have increased markedly over the last 35 years. This finding has significance for modern-day stress and illness research. Another finding of Miller and Rahe's studies (1997) is that there is a gender difference. Women's stress scores, for example, appear significantly higher for financial situation (a growing concern for women), pregnancy, miscarriage or abortion, and death of a child. In fact, women assess and react to life stress events at a higher level than do men. These findings provide support for the more recent interest in assessing and treating women based on findings regarding women's health needs and concerns.

Men, on the other hand, underrate life change units by about 17% in Miller and Rahe's Life-Changing Events Questionnaire. This fact points up the need to break down denial and carefully assess the stress in the life of some male clients (Miller & Rahe, 1997). When individuals experience overwhelming or multiple stressors, and/or use inadequate coping skills, they are at an elevated risk for illness in the near future.

Take a minute to assess your stress level for the past 6 to 12 months using the Life-Changing Events Questionnaire (Table 12-2). However, keep in mind that, when you administer the questionnaire, you must take into account the following:

- Not all events are perceived to have the same degree of intensity or disruptiveness.
- Culture may dictate whether or not an event is stressful, or how stressful it is.
- Different people may have different thresholds beyond which disruptions occur.
- The questionnaire equates change with stress.

Assessing Coping Styles

People use a variety of ways to cope with life stressors, and a number of factors can act as effective mediators to decrease stress in our lives, such as life satisfaction (work, family, hobbies, humor) and social supports. Rahe (1995) identified four discrete personal attributes (coping styles) that people can develop to help them manage stress:

1. Health-sustaining habits (e.g., medical compliance, proper diet, relaxation, pacing one's energy)
2. Life satisfactions (e.g., work, family, humor, spiritual solace, arts, nature)
3. Social supports
4. Effective and healthy responses to stress

TABLE 12-2

Life-Changing Events Questionnaire

Life-Changing Event	Life Change Unit (LCU)
Health	
An injury or illness that:	
Kept you in bed a week or more, or sent you to the hospital	74
Was less serious than above	44
Major dental work	26
Major change in eating habits	27
Major change in sleeping habits	26
Major change in your usual type and/or amount of recreation	28
Work	
Change to a new type of work	51
Change in your work hours or conditions	35
Change in your responsibilities at work:	
More responsibilities	29
Fewer responsibilities	21
Promotion	31
Demotion	42
Transfer	32
Troubles at work:	
With your boss	29
With co-workers	35
With persons under your supervision	35
Other work troubles	28
Major business adjustment	60
Retirement	52
Loss of job:	
Laid off from work	68
Fired from work	79
Correspondence course to help you in your work	18
Home and Family	
Major change in living conditions	42
Change in residence:	
Move within the same town or city	25
Move to a different town, city, or state	47
Change in family get-togethers	25
Major change in health or behavior of family member	55
Marriage	50
Pregnancy	67
Miscarriage or abortion	65
Gain of a new family member:	
Birth of a child	66
Adoption of a child	65
A relative moving in with you	59
Spouse beginning or ending work	46
Child leaving home:	
To attend college	41
Due to marriage	41
For other reasons	45
Change in arguments with spouse	50
In-law problems	38

TABLE 12-2

Life-Changing Events Questionnaire—cont'd

Life-Changing Event	Life Change Unit (LCU)
Change in the marital status of your parents:	
Divorce	59
Remarriage	50
Separation from spouse:	
Due to work	53
Due to marital problems	76
Divorce	96
Birth of grandchild	43
Death of spouse	119
Death of other family member:	
Child	123
Brother or sister	102
Parent	100
Personal and Social	
Change in personal habits	26
Beginning or ending of school or college	38
Change of school or college	35
Change in political beliefs	24
Change in religious beliefs	29
Change in social activities	27
Vacation	24
New close personal relationship	37
Engagement to marry	45
Girlfriend or boyfriend problems	39
Sexual differences	44
"Falling out" of a close personal relationship	47
An accident	48
Minor violation of the law	20
Being held in jail	75
Death of a close friend	70
Major decision regarding your immediate future	51
Major personal achievement	36
Financial	
Major change in finances:	
Increase in income	38
Decrease in income	60
Investment and/or credit difficulties	56
Loss or damage of personal property	43
Moderate purchase	20
Major purchase	37
Foreclosure on a mortgage or loan	58

From Miller, M. A., & Rahe, R. H. (1997). Life changes scaling for the 1990s. *Journal of Psychosomatic Research, 43*(3), 279-292.
Six-month totals ≥300 LCUs or 1-year totals ≥500 LCUs are considered indications of high recent life stress.

Examining these four coping categories can help nurses identify areas to target for improving their clients' and their own quality of life. Table 12-3 presents some positive and some negative responses to stress.

HOLISTIC APPROACHES TO STRESS MANAGEMENT

Poor management of stress has been correlated with an increased incidence of a number of physical and emotional conditions, such as heart disease, poor diabetes control, chronic pain, and significant emotional distress (Slater et al., 2003). PNI provides the foundation for several integrative therapies, also referred to as *mind-body therapies*. There is now considerable evidence that many mind-body therapies can be used as effective adjuncts to conventional medical treatment for a number of common clinical conditions (Astin et al., 2003). A fuller discussion of holistic, mind-body, and integrative therapies is found in Chapter 37.

Many nurses are aware of a variety of stress and anxiety reduction techniques and teach their clients alternative ways of handling anxiety and stress. The following are some of the known benefits of stress reduction:

- Alters the course of certain medical conditions such as high blood pressure, arrhythmias, arthritis, cancer, and peptic ulcers
- Decreases the need for medications such as insulin, analgesics, and antihypertensives
- Diminishes or eliminates the urge for unhealthy and destructive behaviors such as smoking, addiction to drugs, insomnia, and overeating
- Increases cognitive functions such as learning and concentration, and improves study habits
- Breaks up static patterns of thinking and allows fresh and creative ways of perceiving life events
- Increases the sense of well-being through endorphin release
- Treats anxiety, increases comfort, and helps decrease sleep disturbances

Behavioral Approaches

Cognitive-behavioral methods are the most effective ways to reduce stress. There is no one cognitive-behavioral technique that is right for everyone; employing a mixture of cognitive-behavioral techniques brings the best results. All are useful in a variety of situations for specific individuals. Given the fixed nature of many stressors (loss of loved one, chronic illness, pressure at work) cognitive-behavioral therapy, which teaches new ways of responding to stress, may be the most effective method of permanently relieving stress in everyday life (CBS Health Watch, 2000). Essentially there are stress-reducing techniques for every personality type, situation, and level of stress.

Behavioral methods include a number of relaxation techniques (meditation, guided imagery, breathing exercises, and muscle relaxation). Techniques that require special training include progressive muscle

| TABLE 12-3 |

Positive and Negative Responses to Stress

Positive Stress Responses	Negative Stress Responses
1. **Problem solving**—figuring out how to deal with the situation	1. **Avoidance**—choosing not to deal with the situation, letting negative feelings and situations fester and continue to become chronic
2. **Using social support**—calling in others who are caring and may be helpful	2. **Self-blame**—faulting oneself, which keeps the focus on minimizing one's self-esteem and prevents positive action toward resolution or working through of the feelings related to the event
3. **Reframing**—redefining the situation to see the positive as well as the negative sides and the way to use the situation to one's advantage	3. **Wishful thinking**—believing that things will resolve by themselves and that "everything will be fine" (a form of denial)

Adapted from Lazarus, R. S., & Folkman, S. (1984). *Stress, appraisal, and coping.* New York: Springer.

relaxation, eye movement desensitization, and biofeedback.

Relaxation Techniques

Benson's Relaxation Techniques. Herbert Benson (1985, 1996) outlined specific techniques that enable most people to elicit what he referred to as the *relaxation response.* Essentially, Benson's relaxation techniques teach the client how to switch from the sympathetic mode of the autonomic nervous system (fight-or-flight response) to a state of relaxation (the parasympathetic mode). Follow the steps in Box 12-1 to practice the relaxation response.

Benson's relaxation techniques have been combined successfully with meditation and visual imagery to treat numerous disorders, such as diabetes, high blood pressure, migraine headaches, cancer, and peptic ulcers.

Meditation. Meditation follows the basic guidelines described for the relaxation response. It is a discipline for training the mind to develop greater calm and then using that calm to bring penetrative insight into one's experience. Meditation can be used to help people reach their deep inner resources for healing, calm the mind, and operate more efficiently in the world. It can help people develop strategies to cope with stress, make sensible adaptive choices under pressure, and feel more engaged in life (Kabat-Zinn, 1993; Miller, 2000). Meditation elicits a relaxation response by creating a hypometabolic state of quieting the sympathetic nervous system. Some people meditate using a visual object or a sound to help them focus. Others may find it useful to concentrate on their breathing while meditating. There are many meditation techniques, some with a spiritual base, such as Siddha meditation or

prayer. Meditation is easy to practice anywhere. Some students find that meditating the morning of a test helps them focus and lessens anxiety. Keep in mind

| BOX 12-1 |

Benson's Relaxation Technique

The nurse instructs the client as follows:

1. Choose any word or brief phrase that reflects your belief system, such as *love, unity in faith and love, joy, shalom, one God, peace.*
2. Sit in a comfortable position.
3. Close your eyes.
4. Deeply relax all your muscles, beginning at your feet and progressing up to your face. Keep them relaxed.
5. Breathe through your nose. Become aware of your breathing. As you breathe out, say your word or phrase silently to yourself. For example, breathe IN . . . OUT (phrase), IN . . . OUT (phrase), and so forth. Breathe easily and naturally.
6. Continue for 10 to 20 minutes. You may open your eyes and check the time but do not use an alarm. When you finish, sit quietly for several minutes, at first with your eyes closed and then with your eyes open. Do not stand up for a few minutes.
7. Do not worry about whether you are successful in achieving a deep level of relaxation. Maintain a passive attitude and permit relaxation to occur at its own pace. When distracting thoughts occur, try to ignore them by not dwelling on them and return to repeating your word or phrase. With practice, the response should come with little effort. Practice the technique once or twice daily, but not within 2 hours after any meal, because the digestive process seems to interfere with the elicitation of the relaxation response.

From Benson, H. (1985). *The relaxation response* (2nd ed.). New York: William Morrow.

that, to produce the relaxation responses, meditation, like most other skills, must be practiced.

Guided Imagery. Used in conjunction with the relaxation response, guided imagery is a process whereby a person is led to envision images that are both calming and health enhancing. The content of the imagery exercises is shaped by the person helping with the imagery process. If a person has dysfunctional images, he or she can be helped to generate more effective and functional coping images to replace the depression- or anxiety-producing ones (Miller, 2000). For example, athletes have discovered that the use of images of positive coping and success can lead to improvement in performance (Aetna InteliHealth, 2004). Refer to Box 12-2.

Imagery techniques are a useful tool in the management of many medical conditions. They are an effective means of relieving pain for many people. Pain is reduced by producing muscle relaxation and focusing the person away from the pain. For some, imagery techniques are healing exercises in that they not only relieve the pain but in some cases diminish the source of the pain (Koenig et al., 2001). Guided imagery is used with cancer patients to help them reduce their chronic high levels of cortisol, epinephrine, and catecholamines (which prevent the immune system from functioning effectively) and to produce β-endorphins (which increase pain thresholds and enhance lymphocyte proliferation) (Brigham, 1994; Koenig et al., 2001).

Guided imagery is used for all sorts of healing. Often tapes are made specifically for clients and their particular situations. However, many healing tapes are available to clients and health care workers.

Breathing Exercises. Within the past several years, there has been increasing evidence that respiratory retraining, usually in the form of learning abdominal (diaphragmatic) breathing, has some definite merits in the modification of stress and anxiety reactions (Miller, 2000). One breathing exercise that has proved helpful for many clients with anxiety disorders has two parts, as described in Box 12-3. The first part focuses on abdominal breathing. The second part helps clients interrupt trains of thought and thereby quiet mental noise. With increasing skill, this becomes a tool for dampening the cognitive processes likely to set off stress and anxiety reactions. In clinical work with people who have performance anxiety, 50% reported breathing exercises to be useful during the feared situation (Stoyva & Carlson, 1993).

Muscle Relaxation and Exercise

Physical exercise in many forms can lead to protection from the harmful effects of stress on both physical and mental states. Results of cross-sectional and longitudinal studies are consistent in finding exercise to have antidepressant and anxiolytic effects in adults, children, and the elderly (George & Goldberg, 2001; Hassmen, Koivula, & Uutela, 2000; Salmon, 2001; Williamson, Dewey, & Steinberg, 2001). For example, **yoga,** an ancient form of exercise, can reduce stress, relieve muscular tension and pain, and increase one's sense of well-being (Gura, 2002). Other popular forms of exercise that can decrease stress and improve well-being are walking, tai chi, dancing, aerobics, and water exercise.

BOX 12-2

Script for Guided Imagery

Imagine releasing all the tension in your body . . . letting it go.
Now, with every breath you take, feel your body drifting down deeper and deeper into relaxation . . . floating down . . . deeper and deeper.
Imagine a peaceful scene. You are sitting beside a clear, blue mountain stream. You are barefoot, and you feel the sun-warmed rock under your feet. You hear the sound of the stream tumbling over the rocks. The sound is hypnotic, and you relax more and more. You see the tall pine trees on the opposite shore bending in the gentle breeze. Breathe the clean, scented air, with each breath moving you deeper and deeper into relaxation. The sun warms your face.
You are very comfortable. There is nothing to disturb you. You experience a feeling of well-being.
You can return to this peaceful scene by taking time to relax. The positive feelings can grow stronger and stronger each time you choose to relax.
You can return to your activities now, feeling relaxed and refreshed.

BOX 12-3

Deep Breathing Exercise

Find a comfortable position. Relax your shoulders and chest; let your body relax.
First, shift to relaxed, abdominal breathing. Take a deep breath through your mouth, expanding the abdomen. Hold it for 3 seconds and then exhale slowly through the nose; exhale completely, telling yourself to relax.
Second, with every breath, turn attention to the muscular sensations that accompany the expansion of the belly.
As you concentrate on your breathing, you will start to feel focused. Repeat this exercise for 2 to 5 minutes.

Progressive muscle relaxation (PMR) is a technique that can help people achieve deep relaxation, but its use requires special training. The premise behind PMR is that deep relaxation can occur when muscle contraction is almost completely eliminated.

Biofeedback

Biofeedback also requires special training. Biofeedback is usually thought to be most effective in people with low to moderate hypnotic ability. For people with hypnotic ability, meditation, PMR, and other cognitive-behavioral therapy techniques produce the most rapid reduction in clinical symptoms. By using sensitive instrumentation, biofeedback gives a person prompt and exact information, otherwise unavailable, regarding muscle activity, brain waves, skin temperature, heart rate, blood pressure, and other bodily functions. Indicators of the particular internal physiological process are detected and amplified by a sensitive recording device. An individual can achieve greater voluntary control over phenomena once considered to be exclusively involuntary if he or she knows instantaneously, through an auditory or visual signal, whether a somatic activity is increasing or decreasing.

With increasing recognition of the role of stress in a variety of medical illnesses, including diseases affected by immune dysfunction, biofeedback has emerged as one of the strategies used in stress management. Although it is uncertain whether it is necessary to use the complex instrumentation required for proper biofeedback regarding minute levels of muscle tension or certain patterns of electroencephalographic activity, it has been confirmed that teaching people to relax deeply and to apply these skills in response to real-life stressors can be helpful in lowering stress levels.

Cognitive Approaches

A number of cognitive techniques are discussed here: journal keeping and writing, priority restructuring, cognitive reframing, humor, and assertiveness training. Many nurses employ these useful tools in their practices.

Journal Keeping and Writing

Journal keeping is an extremely useful and surprisingly simple initial method of identifying what makes a person feel stressed. Journal keeping is a technique that can ease worry and obsession and help identify hopes and fears as well as increase energy levels and confidence (Cortright, 2003). Grief counselors advocate journal keeping to help heal those suffering painful losses (Cullen, 2004). Keeping an informal diary of daily events and activities can reveal surprising information on sources of daily stress. It need not be a chore or a painstaking exercise, but noting which activities put a strain on energy and time, which trigger anger or anxiety, and which precipitate a negative physical experience (headache, backache, fatigue) can be an important first step in actual stress reduction. Writing down thoughts and feelings is helpful not only in dealing with stress and stressful events but also in healing both physically and emotionally (Cullen, 2004).

Subsequent experiments demonstrate that writing can strengthen the immune system, decrease reliance on pain medication and improve lung function in people with asthma, and reduce symptoms in people with rheumatoid arthritis (Cullen, 2004).

Priority Restructuring

The next step is restructuring and setting priorities, which involves shifting the balance from stress-producing to stress-reducing activities. A recent study indicated that the daily occurrence of pleasant events had a positive effect on the immune system. In fact, adding pleasurable events has more benefit than simply reducing stressful or negative ones (CBS Health Watch, 2000).

Essentially, learn to replace time-consuming chores that are not really necessary with activities that are pleasurable or interesting. Making time for recreation is as essential for healthy living as is paying bills or shopping for groceries.

Cognitive Reframing

Cognitive reframing has been found to be positively correlated with greater positive affect and higher self-esteem (Miller, 2000). Cognitive restructuring includes recasting irrational beliefs and replacing worried self-statements ("I can't pass this course, I can't pass this course") with more positive self-statements ("If I choose to study for this course, I will increase my chances of success"). Cognitive restructuring and cognitive reframing are techniques commonly used in cognitive therapies.

Reframing is a healthy stress reduction tool and a technique used by some counselors for a variety of purposes. Imagery may be used along with cognitive reframing to reduce stress. The goal of reframing is to change the individual's perceptions of stress through cognitive restructuring. Essentially, reframing is reassessing a situation. We can learn from most situations by asking ourselves the following questions:

- "What positive came out of the situation or experience?"
- "What did I learn in this situation?"
- "What would I do in a different way?"

The desired result is to restructure a disturbing event or experience into one that is less disturbing and in which the client can have a sense of control. When the perception of the disturbing event is changed, there is less stimulation to the sympathetic nervous system, which in turn reduces the secretion of cortisol and catecholamines that destroy the balance of the immune system (Miller, 2000).

Cognitive distortions often include overgeneralizations ("He always . . . " or "I'll never . . .") and "should" statements ("I should have done better" or "He shouldn't have said that"). Table 12-4 shows some examples of cognitive reframing of anxiety-producing thoughts. Often, cognitive restructuring is done along with progressive relaxation.

Humor

The use of humor is a good example of how a stressful situation can be "turned upside down" through cognitive restructuring. The intensity attached to a stressful thought or situation can be dissipated when it is made to appear absurd or comical. Essentially, the bee loses its sting.

Assertiveness Training

Assertiveness is a learned behavior that includes standing up for one's rights without violating the rights of others. Assertiveness training has proved to be a successful way of decreasing stress, anxiety, and conflict resulting from stressful interpersonal relationships, although some may find the initial training and practice itself to be somewhat stressful (Beare & Myers, 1998). It has been demonstrated that stress and anxiety are considerably lowered when people openly and honestly express their needs, feelings, and desires while respecting the feelings and rights of others.

The concept of assertiveness is different from that of aggressiveness or passivity. Aggressively expressing feelings is exemplified more by venting frustration on workers or subordinates, boring friends with emotional minutiae, wallowing in self-pity, or driving mindlessly and recklessly and thereby endangering one's own life and the lives of others. When people are aggressive, their behavior escalates; their voices become loud; they interrupt others; and physiologically their heart rate, blood pressure, and levels of certain stress-related hormones are elevated. This sequence, in turn, can increase stress and anxiety in others so that it becomes impossible to problem solve effectively or work together toward a solution in a respectful, understanding manner. In extreme situations, escalating anger can lead to physical violence. On the other hand, when people suppress their feelings or are passive, they may suffer high levels of anxiety, discomfort, and depression or develop physical problems. Brigham (1994) identified four formulas for assertive communications, as outlined in Table 12-5.

More Effective Stress Reducers

Box 12-4 identifies some known stress busters that can be incorporated into our lives with little effort.

TABLE 12-4

Reframing Anxiety-Producing Thoughts

Irrational Beliefs	Positive Statements
1. "I'll never be happy until I am loved by someone I really care about."	1a. "If I do not get love from one person, I can still get it from others and find happiness that way."
	1b. "If someone I deeply care for rejects me, that will seem unfortunate, but I will hardly die."
	1c. "If the only person I truly care for does not return my love, I can devote more time and energy to winning someone else's love and probably find someone better for me."
	1d. "If no one I care for ever cares for me, I can still find enjoyment in friendships, in work, in books, and in other things."
2. "He should treat me better after all I do for him."	2. "I would like him to do certain things to show that he cares. If he chooses to continue to do things that hurt me after he understands what those things are, I am free to make choices about leaving or staying in this hurtful relationship."

Adapted from Ellis, A., & Harper, R. A. (1975). *A new guide to rational living.* North Hollywood, CA: Wilshire.

TABLE 12-5

Formulas for Assertive Communication

Formula	Example
Formula 1 (Simple Assertion)	
a. Simply make an open, honest, direct statement of a request, an opinion, a question, a feeling, or a need.	a. "No, I don't think that is the best plan of action." "Right now, I need some help with this." "Yes, I do like the way she handled that situation."
Formula 2 (Empathetic Assertion)	
a. Show understanding and recognition of the other person's feelings, *yet* b. Assertively state what one needs.	a. "I know you are concerned that I will be hurt by this decision, b. but I need to make this decision myself."
Formula 3 (Feeling Assertion)	
a. Nonaccusingly describe the situation or behavior in question. b. State one's feelings (not opinions), *and* c. Ask for a change.	a. "When I am criticized in front of others, b. I feel embarrassed and hurt. c. I'd prefer that if you need to tell me something, you do it in private."
Formula 4 (Confrontational Assertion)	
a. Ask for private time to talk. b. Point out the facts in a nonaccusing manner. c. Check areas in which you may not understand the situation. d. Ask for the changes you need.	a. "I need to talk to you privately. b. It seems to me that our communication is not what it has been in the past. I notice that you watch TV while I am telling you things that are important to me. c. It seems to me that we just aren't as close. Am I off base? d. I'd like to find out what the problem is so we can get our relationship back on track."

Data from Brigham, D. D. (1994). *Imagery for getting well: Clinical applications of behavioral medicine.* New York: W. W. Norton.

BOX 12-4

More Effective Stress Busters

Sleep
1. Chronically stressed people are often fatigued, so go to sleep 30 to 60 minutes earlier each night for a few weeks.
2. If you are still fatigued, try going to bed another 30 minutes earlier.
3. Sleeping later in the morning is not helpful and can throw off body rhythms.

Exercise (Aerobic)
1. Exercise
   - Can dissipate chronic and acute stress.
   - May decrease levels of anxiety, depression, and sensitivity to stress.
   - Can decrease muscle tension and increase endorphin levels.
2. It is recommended to exercise for at least 30 minutes, three or more times a week.
3. It is best to exercise at least 3 hours before bedtime.

Reduction or Cessation of Caffeine Intake
1. Such a simple thing as lowering or stopping caffeine intake can lead to more energy and fewer muscle aches and help you feel more relaxed.
2. Slowly wean off coffee, tea, colas, and chocolate drinks.

Music (Classical or Soft Melodies of Choice)
1. Listening to music increases your sense of relaxation.
2. Increased healing effects may result.
3. Therapeutically, music can
   - Decrease agitation and confusion in the elderly.
   - Increase quality of life in hospice settings.

Pets
1. Pets can bring joy and stress reduction.
2. They can be an important social support.
3. Pets can alleviate medical problems aggravated by stress.

Massage
1. Massage can slow the heart rate and relax the body.
2. Alertness may actually increase.

■ ■ ■ KEY POINTS to REMEMBER

- Stress is a universal experience. Cannon introduced the fight-or-flight model of stress. Selye popularized the now-famous GAS.
- Stress elicits an initial adaptive response (defense mechanisms or relief actions of some sort), and most of the time these suffice to lower people's stress levels so that they can continue with their lives.
- The PNI model describes the bidirectional response to stress by the immune system and the immune system's effect on neural pathways in the brain.
- Prolonged stress can lead to chronic psychological and physiological responses (eventual maladaptive consequences) when not mitigated at an earlier stage. There are basically two categories of stressors: physical (e.g., heat, hunger, cold, noise, trauma) and psychological (e.g., death of a loved one, loss of job, school, humiliation).
- Age, sex, culture, life experience, and lifestyle all are important in identifying the degree of stress a person is experiencing.
- Perhaps the most important factor to assess is a person's support system. Studies have shown that high-quality social and intimate supports can go a long way toward minimizing the long-term effects of stress.
- Cultural differences exist in the extent to which people perceive an event as stressful and in the behaviors they consider appropriate to deal with a stressful event.
- Spiritual practices have been found to lead to an enhanced immune system and a sense of well-being.
- There are a variety of stress coping models; the one used in this chapter is that developed by Miller and Rahe (1997).
- Stress can be psychological, social, or biological. The body reacts the same regardless of whether the threat is real or perceived.
- Physiologically, the body reacts to anxiety and fear by arousal of the sympathetic nervous system. Specific symptoms include rapid heart beat, increased blood pressure, diaphoresis, peripheral vasoconstriction, restlessness, repetitive questioning, feelings of frustration, and difficulty concentrating.
- Nurses seek training in a great variety of holistic, noninvasive approaches to relieving people's stress and helping to bolster the immune system.
- It is well accepted through replicated studies that the reduction of chronic stress is beneficial in many ways. For example, lowering the effects of chronic stress can alter the course of many physical conditions; decrease the need for some medications; diminish or eliminate the urge for unhealthy and destructive behaviors such as smoking, insomnia, and drug addiction; and increase a person's cognitive functioning.
- Cognitive-behavioral holistic approaches are very effective methods to reduce stress. Ways to implement these techniques for either the self or clients are discussed. Use of some techniques requires special training.

■ ■ ■

Visit the Evolve website at **http://evolve.elsevier.com/Varcarolis** for a posttest on the content in this chapter. **evolve**

Critical Thinking and Chapter Review

Visit the Evolve website at **http://evolve.elsevier.com/Varcarolis** for additional self-study exercises.
evolve

■ ■ ■ CRITICAL THINKING

1. Assess your level of stress using the life events scale found in Table 12-2 and evaluate your potential for illness in the coming year. Identify stress reduction techniques, described toward the end of the chapter, that you think would be useful for you to learn.

2. Teach a classmate the breathing technique identified in this chapter.

3. Assess a classmate's coping styles. Have the same classmate assess yours. Discuss the relevance of both of your findings.

4. Using Figure 12-1, explain to a classmate the short-term effects of stress on the sympathetic–adrenal medulla system and identify three long-term effects if the stress is not relieved. Have the classmate summarize what you have just told him or her.

5. Have a classmate explain to you, using Figure 12-1, the short-term effects of stress on the hypothalamus–pituitary–adrenal cortex and the eventual long-term effects if the stress becomes chronic. Summarize to your classmate your understanding of what was just presented.

6. Discuss in postconference one patient you have cared for in the hospital who had one of the stress-related diseases identified in Figure 12-1. See if you can identify some stressors in that person's life and possible ways that the person could lower his or her chronic stress levels.

Continued

Critical Thinking and Chapter Review—cont'd

Visit the Evolve website at **http://evolve.elsevier.com/Varcarolis** for additional self-study exercises.

■■■■ CHAPTER REVIEW

Choose the most appropriate answer.

1. Which statement best contrasts the short-term and long-term physiological consequences of stress?
    1. Acute stress produces an initial adaptive response and prolonged stress produces maladaptive consequences.
    2. Acute stress produces maladaptive consequences and prolonged stress invokes adaptive responses.
    3. Acute stress produces immune system compromise and prolonged stress results in increased muscular tension and gluconeogenesis.
    4. Acute stress produces hypertension, anxiety, and depression and prolonged stress results in hyperlipidemia, glucose intolerance, and heart disease.

2. Which statement about the influence of culture on stress can serve to guide nursing assessment, planning, and intervention?
    1. Client appraisal of a stressful event is little influenced by culture.
    2. Culture dictates the kind of interventions the client will find helpful.
    3. Culture rarely regulates the expression of emotion produced by a stressful event.
    4. Nursing interventions that promote adaptive behavior are the same across cultures.

3. Which should the nurse assess as being the most beneficial method to reduce stress?
    1. Psychophysiological responses within the client's awareness
    2. Change in diet
    3. Life satisfactions such as work or family
    4. Cognitive-behavioral methods

4. A useful tool for assessing an individual's susceptibility to physical and mental illness is
    1. biofeedback.
    2. Rational Living Survey.
    3. Life-Changing Events Questionnaire.
    4. GAS.

5. Which of the following interventions is considered to be a cognitive-behavioral technique?
    1. Avoidance
    2. Benson's relaxation techniques
    3. Hypnosis
    4. Psychopharmacological interventions

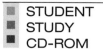

■ STUDENT
■ STUDY
■ CD-ROM

Access the accompanying CD-ROM for animations, interactive exercises, review questions for the NCLEX examination, and an audio glossary.

REFERENCES

Aetna InteliHealth. (2004, May 12). *Guided imagery.* Retrieved February 9, 2005, from the Aetna InteliHealth website: http://www.intelihealth.com.

Astin, J. A., et al. (2003). Mind-body medicine: State of science, implications for practice. *Journal of the American Board of Family Practice, 16*(2), 131-147.

Azar, B. (2001). A new take at psychoneuroimmunology. *Monitor on Psychology, 32*(11), retrieved June 2, 2004, from the American Psychological Association website: http://www.apa.org/monitor/dec01/anewtake.html.

Beare, P. G., & Myers, J. L. (1998). *Adult health nursing* (3rd ed.). St. Louis, MO: Mosby.

Benson, H. (1985). *The relaxation response* (2nd ed.). New York: William Morrow.

Benson, H., & Stark, M. (1996). *Timeless healing.* New York: Scribner.

Brigham, D. D. (1994). *Imagery for getting well: Clinical applications of behavioral medicine.* New York: W. W. Norton.

Brown, G. W., & Harris, T. (1989). *Social origins of depression: A study of psychiatric disorders in women.* New York: Free Press.

CBS Health Watch by Medscape. (2000, March 27). Retrieved from http://cbshealthwatch.health.aol.com.RecId=202426 pluscontenttype=Library.

Cortright, S. M. (2003). *Journaling: A tool for your spirit.* Retrieved February 4, 2005, from the Journal for You website: http://www.journalforyou.com/full_article.php?article_id=7.

Cullen, D. (2004, February 10). *The power of the pen.* Retrieved February 3, 2005, from The Age website: http://www.theage.com.au/articles/2004/02/09/1076175101614.html?.

DeAngelis, T. (2002). A bright future for PNI. *Monitor on Psychology, 33*(6), retrieved June 2, 2004, from the American Psychological Association website: http://www.apa.org/monitor/jun02/brightfuture.html.

Dohrenwend, B. S., & Dohrenwend, B. P. (1974). *Stressful life events: Their nature and effects.* New York: Wiley.

Dohrenwend, B. S., & Dohrenwend, B. P. (1983). Life stress and illness: Formulation of the issues. In B. S. Dohrenwend & B. P. Dohrenwend (Eds.), *Stressful life events and their contexts.* New Brunswick, NJ: Rutgers University Press.

George, B. J., & Goldberg, N. (2001). The benefits of exercise in geriatric women. *American Journal of Geriatric Cardiology, 10*(5), 260-263.

Gonzalez, C. A., Griffith, E. E. H., & Ruiz, P. (1995). Cross-cultural issues in psychiatric treatment. In G. O. Gabbard (Ed.), *Treatment of psychiatric disorders* (2nd ed., Vol. I, pp. 55-74). Washington, DC: American Psychiatric Press.

Gura, S. T. (2002). Yoga for stress reduction and injury prevention at work. *Work, 19*(1), 3-7.

Hassmen, P., Koivula, N., & Uutela, A. (2000). Physical exercise and psychological well-being: A population study in Finland. *Preventive Medicine, 30*(1), 17-25.

Hobfall, S. E., & Vaux, A. (1993). Social support: Social resources and social context. In L. Goldberger & S. Breznitz (Eds.), *Handbook of stress: Theoretical and clinical aspects* (2nd ed., pp. 685-705). New York: Free Press.

Holmes, T. H., & Rahe, R. H. (1967). The social readjustment rating scale. *Journal of Psychosomatic Research, 11,* 213.

Kabat-Zinn, J. (1993). Meditation. In B. Moyers (Ed.), *Healing and the mind* (pp. 115-144). New York: Doubleday.

Kim, M. (2002). Measuring depression in Korean Americans: Development of the Kim Depression Scale for Korean Americans. *Journal of Transcultural Nursing, 13*(2), 109-117.

Koenig, H. G., McCullough, M. E., & Larson, D. B. (2001). *Handbook of religion and health.* New York: Oxford University Press.

Lazarus, R. S., & DeLongis, A. (1983). Psychological stress and coping in aging. *American Psychologist, 38,* 245.

Lazarus, R. S., Kanner, A. D., & Folkman, S. (1980). A cognitive-phenomenological analysis. In R. Pluchik & H. Kellerman (Eds.), *Theories of emotion: Vol. 1. Emotion: Theory, research, and experience.* New York: Academic Press.

Lutz, W., Tarkowski, M., & Dudek, B. (2001). [Psychoneuroimmunology. A new approach to the function of immunological system]. *Medycyna pracy, 52*(3), 203-209.

Mausch, K. (2000). [Main issues of psychoneuroimmunology: Part 2]. *Psychiatria polska, 34*(3), 381-388.

Miller, M. A., & Rahe, R. H. (1997). Life changes scaling for the 1990s. *Journal of Psychosomatic Research, 43*(3), 279-292.

Miller, W. R. (2000). *Integrating spirituality into treatment.* Washington, DC: American Psychological Association.

Neighbors, H. (2003, January 22). *The (mis)diagnosis of African Americans: Implementing DSM criteria in the hospital and community.* Retrieved April 4, 2004, from Psychiatry Grand Rounds, Department of Psychiatry, University of Michigan website: http://www.med.umich.edu/psych/mlk2003.htm.

Rahe, R. H. (1995). Stress and psychiatry. In H. I. Kaplan & B. J. Sadock (Eds.), *Comprehensive textbook of psychiatry/VI* (6th ed., Vol. 2, pp. 1545-1559). Baltimore: Williams & Wilkins.

Salmon, P. I. (2001). Effects of physical exercise on anxiety, depression, and sensitivity to stress: A unifying theory. *Clinical Psychology Review, 21*(1), 33-61.

Selye, H. (1974). *Stress without distress.* Philadelphia: Lippincott.

Selye, H. (1993). History of the stress concept. In L. Goldberger & S. Breznitz (Eds.), *Handbook of stress: Theoretical and clinical aspects* (2nd ed., pp. 7-17). New York: Free Press.

Slater, M. A., et al. (2003). Behavioral medicine. In A. Tasman, J. Kay, & J. A. Lieberman (Eds.), *Psychiatry* (2nd ed.). West Sussex, England: Wiley.

Smyth, J., et al. (1999). Effects of writing about stressful experiences on symptom reduction with asthma or rheumatoid arthritis: A randomized trial. *Journal of the American Medical Association, 281*(14), 1304-1309.

Stoyva, J. M., & Carlson, J. G. (1993). A coping/rest model of relaxation and stress management. In L. Goldberger & S. Breznitz (Eds.), *Handbook of stress: Theoretical and clinical aspects* (2nd ed., pp. 724-756). New York: Free Press.

Williamson, D., Dewey, A., & Steinberg, H. (2001). Mood change through physical exercise in nine- to ten-year-old children. *Perceptual and Motor Skills, 93*(1), 311-316.

Yang, E. V., & Glaser, R. (2002). Stress-associated immunomodulation and its implications for response to vaccination. *Expert Review of Vaccines, 1*(4), 453-459.

CHAPTER 13

Understanding Anxiety and Anxiety Defenses

ELIZABETH M. VARCAROLIS

KEY TERMS and CONCEPTS

The key terms and concepts listed here appear in color where they are defined or first discussed in this chapter.

acting-out behaviors, 219
acute (state) anxiety, 213
altruism, 217
anxiety, 212
chronic (trait) anxiety, 213
denial, 220
devaluation, 219
displacement, 218
dissociation, 219
fear, 213
humor, 218
idealization, 219
mild anxiety, 213
moderate anxiety, 213
normal anxiety, 213
panic level of anxiety, 215
passive aggression, 218
projection, 219
psychotic denial, 220

rationalization, 218
reaction formation, 218
repression, 218
severe anxiety, 214
somatization, 218
splitting, 219
sublimation, 218
suppression, 218
undoing, 218

OBJECTIVES

After studying this chapter, the reader will be able to

1. Explore the difference between normal anxiety, acute anxiety, and chronic anxiety.
2. Contrast and compare the four levels of anxiety in relation to perceptual field, ability to learn, and physical and other defining characteristics.
3. Summarize five properties of the defense mechanisms.
4. Define and give at least two clinical examples of defense mechanisms in each of the following categories: most healthy, intermediate, and immature.

evolve Visit the Evolve website at **http://evolve.elsevier.com/Varcarolis** for a pretest on the content in this chapter.

An understanding of anxiety and anxiety defense mechanisms is basic to the practice of psychiatric nursing. One of the greatest legacies of Hildegard Peplau (1909-1999) in nursing is her operational definition of the four levels of anxiety and suggestions for interventions appropriate to the level of anxiety the person is experiencing.

ABOUT ANXIETY

Stress is a state produced by a change in the environment that is perceived as challenging, threatening, or damaging to a person's well-being (see Chapter 12).

Stress can lead to a variety of psychological responses, the most common of which is anxiety.

Anxiety is a universal human experience that is a stranger to no one. It is the most basic of emotions. Dysfunctional behavior is often a defense against anxiety. When behavior is recognized as dysfunctional, interventions to reduce anxiety can be initiated by the nurse. As anxiety decreases, dysfunctional behavior will frequently decrease, and vice versa.

Anxiety is experienced on four levels: mild, moderate, severe, and panic anxiety. It can be broken down into three categories—normal, acute, and chronic—and it can be operationally defined.

Peplau, who as a nurse theorist had profound impact in shaping the psychiatric mental health nursing profession, identified anxiety as one of the most important concepts in psychiatric nursing. Nurses can use the concept of anxiety to explain many clinical observations. Peplau (1968) developed an anxiety model useful to the practice of nursing. Conceptualization of anxiety using Peplau's model has led to the formulation of principles that serve as guides in nursing intervention. This conceptual basis of anxiety can be used by nurses as a framework to guide therapeutic approaches to clients in any setting.

Anxiety can be defined as a feeling of apprehension, uneasiness, uncertainty, or dread resulting from a real or perceived threat whose actual source is unknown or unrecognized. Fear is a reaction to a specific danger, whereas anxiety is a vague sense of dread relating to an unspecified danger. However, the body reacts in similar ways physiologically to both anxiety and fear.

An important distinction between anxiety and fear is that anxiety attacks us at a deeper level than does fear. Anxiety invades the central core of the personality. It erodes the individual feelings of self-esteem and personal worth that contribute to a sense of being fully human.

Normal anxiety is a healthy life force that is necessary for survival. It provides the energy needed to carry out the tasks involved in living and striving toward goals. Anxiety motivates people to make and survive change. It prompts constructive behaviors, such as studying for an examination, being on time for job interviews, preparing for a presentation, and working toward a promotion.

Acute anxiety is also referred to as state anxiety. Acute (state) anxiety is precipitated by an imminent loss or change that threatens an individual's sense of security. It may be seen in performers before a concert. For example, many entertainers experience acute anxiety before live concerts or theater performances. Students may experience acute anxiety before an examination. Clients preparing for surgery often experience acute anxiety. The death of a loved one can stimulate acute anxiety when there is great disruption in the life of the bereaved person. In general, crisis involves the experience of acute anxiety.

Trait anxiety is another name for chronic anxiety. Chronic (trait) anxiety is anxiety that the person has lived with for a time. Ego psychologists suggest that in a nurturing environment the developing personality incorporates the primary caregivers' positive attributes, which allows the child to tolerate anxiety. When conditions for personality growth are less than adequate, positive values may not be incorporated, and the child may become anxiety ridden, a state that often covers up overwhelming, angry, and hostile impulses (Sullivan, 1953). A child may demonstrate chronic anxiety by a permanent attitude of apprehension or by overreaction to all unexpected environmental stimuli. In adults, chronic anxiety may take the form of chronic fatigue, insomnia, discomfort in daily activities, discomfort in personal relationships, and ineffective job performance. When the subjective feelings of anxiety become too overwhelming, anxiety is unconsciously placed out of awareness (repressed) and is expressed in behavioral characteristics or symptoms.

An understanding of the types, levels, and defensive patterns used in response to anxiety is basic to psychiatric nursing care. This understanding is essential for assessing and planning interventions to lower a client's level of anxiety, as well as one's own, effectively. With practice, one becomes more skilled both at identifying levels of anxiety and the defenses used to alleviate it, and at evaluating the possible stressors contributing to increases in a person's level of anxiety.

LEVELS OF ANXIETY

Levels of anxiety range from mild to moderate to severe to panic. Peplau's classic delineation of these four levels of anxiety (1968) is based on Sullivan's work (refer to Chapter 2 for more on Peplau and anxiety). Assessment of a client's level of anxiety is basic to therapeutic intervention in any setting—psychiatric, hospital, or community. Identification of a specific level of anxiety can be used as a guideline in selecting interventions (Table 13-1). Although four levels of anxiety from mild to panic have been defined, the boundaries between these levels are not distinct, and the behaviors and characteristics shown by individuals experiencing anxiety can and often do overlap these categories. Use Table 13-1 as a guide for making observations.

Mild Anxiety

Mild anxiety occurs in the normal experience of everyday living. The person's ability to perceive reality is brought into sharp focus. A person sees, hears, and grasps more information, and problem solving becomes more effective. A person may display physical symptoms such as slight discomfort, restlessness, irritability, or mild tension-relieving behaviors (e.g., nail biting, foot or finger tapping, fidgeting).

Moderate Anxiety

As anxiety escalates, the perceptual field narrows, and some details are excluded from observation. The person experiencing moderate anxiety sees, hears, and grasps less information than someone who is not in that state. Individuals may demonstrate **selective inattention,** in which only certain things in the environ-

TABLE 13-1

Anxiety Levels

Mild	Moderate	Severe	Panic
Perceptual Field			
May have heightened perceptual field	Has narrow perceptual field; grasps less of what is going on	Has greatly reduced perceptual field	Unable to focus on the environment
Is alert and can see, hear, and grasp what is happening in the environment	Can attend to more *if pointed out by another* (selective inattention)	Focuses on details or one specific detail Attention scattered	Experiences the utmost state of terror and emotional paralysis; feels he or she "ceases to exist"
Can identify things that are disturbing and are producing anxiety		Completely absorbed with self	In panic, may have hallucinations or delusions that take the place of reality
		May not be able to attend to events in environment *even when pointed out by others*	
		In severe to panic levels of anxiety, the environment is blocked out. It is as if these events are not occurring.	
Ability to Learn			
Able to work effectively toward a goal and examine alternatives	Able to solve problems but not at optimal ability	Unable to see connections between events or details	May be mute or have extreme psychomotor agitation leading to exhaustion
	Benefits from guidance of others	Has distorted perceptions	Shows disorganized or irrational reasoning
Mild and moderate levels of anxiety can alert the person that something is wrong and can stimulate appropriate action.		**Severe and panic levels prevent problem solving and discovery of effective solutions. Unproductive relief behaviors are called into play, thus perpetuating a vicious cycle.**	
Physical or Other Characteristics			
Slight discomfort Attention-seeking behaviors Restlessness Irritability or impatience Mild tension-relieving behavior: foot or finger tapping, lip chewing, fidgeting	Voice tremors Change in voice pitch Difficulty concentrating Shakiness Repetitive questioning Somatic complaints, (e.g., urinary frequency and urgency, headache, backache, insomnia) Increased respiration rate Increased pulse rate Increased muscle tension More extreme tension-relieving behavior; pacing, banging of hands on table	Feelings of dread Ineffective functioning Confusion Purposeless activity Sense of impending doom More intense somatic complaints (e.g., dizziness, nausea, headache, sleeplessness) Hyperventilation Tachycardia Withdrawal Loud and rapid speech Threats and demands	Experience of terror Immobility or severe hyperactivity or flight Dilated pupils Unintelligible communication or inability to speak Severe shakiness Sleeplessness Severe withdrawal Hallucinations or delusions; likely out of touch with reality

ment are seen or heard unless they are pointed out to the person. The ability to think clearly is hampered, but learning and problem solving can still take place, although not at an optimal level. At the moderate level of anxiety, the person's ability to solve problems is greatly enhanced by the supportive presence of another. Physical symptoms include tension, pounding heart, increased pulse and respiration rate, perspiration, and mild somatic symptoms (gastric discomfort, headache, urinary urgency). Voice tremors and shaking may be noticed. Mild or moderate anxiety levels can be con-

structive, because anxiety can be viewed as a signal that something in the person's life needs attention.

Severe Anxiety

The perceptual field of a person experiencing severe anxiety is greatly reduced. A person with severe anxiety may focus on one particular detail or many scattered details. The person may have difficulty noticing what is going on in the environment, even when it is pointed out by another. Learning and problem solving are not possible at this level, and the person may be dazed and confused. Behavior is automatic and aimed at reducing or relieving anxiety. The person may complain of increased severity of somatic symptoms (headache, nausea, dizziness, insomnia), trembling, and pounding heart. The person may also experience hyperventilation and a sense of impending doom or dread.

Panic Level of Anxiety

The panic level of anxiety is the most extreme form and results in markedly disturbed behavior. The person is not able to process what is going on in the environment and may lose touch with reality. The behavior that results may be manifested by confusion, shouting, screaming, or withdrawal. Hallucinations, or false sensory perceptions such as seeing people or objects that are not there, may be experienced by people at panic levels of anxiety. Physical behavior may be erratic, uncoordinated, and impulsive. Automatic behaviors are used to reduce and relieve anxiety, although such efforts may be ineffective. Acute panic may lead to exhaustion. Review Table 13-1 to identify the levels of anxiety through their effects on (1) perceptual field, (2) ability to learn, and (3) physical and other defining characteristics.

INTERVENTIONS

Mild to Moderate Levels of Anxiety

A person experiencing a mild to moderate level of anxiety is still able to solve problems; however, the ability to concentrate decreases as anxiety increases. You can help the client focus and solve problems with the use of specific communication techniques, such as employing open-ended questions, giving broad openings, and exploring and seeking clarification. These techniques can be useful to a client experiencing mild to moderate anxiety. Closing off topics of communication and bringing up irrelevant topics can increase a person's anxiety and are tactics that usually make the *nurse,* not the client, feel better.

Reducing the anxiety level and preventing escalation of anxiety to more distressing levels can be aided by providing a calm presence, recognizing the anxious person's distress, and being willing to listen. Evaluation of effective past coping mechanisms is useful. Often the nurse can help the client consider alternatives to problem situations and offer activities that may temporarily relieve feelings of inner tension. Table 13-2 identifies counseling techniques useful in

TABLE 13-2

Interventions for Mild to Moderate Levels of Anxiety

Nursing diagnosis: *Anxiety (moderate)* related to situational event or psychological stress, as evidenced by increase in vital signs, moderate discomfort, narrowing of perceptual field, and selective inattention

Intervention	Rationale
1. Help the client identify anxiety. "Are you comfortable right now?"	1. It is important to validate observations with the client, name the anxiety, and start to work with the client to lower anxiety.
2. Anticipate anxiety-provoking situations.	2. Escalation of anxiety to a more disorganizing level is prevented.
3. Use nonverbal language to demonstrate interest (e.g., lean forward, maintain eye contact, nod your head).	3. Verbal and nonverbal messages should be consistent. The presence of an interested person provides a stabilizing focus.
4. Encourage the client to talk about his or her feelings and concerns.	4. When concerns are stated aloud, problems can be discussed and feelings of isolation decreased.
5. Avoid closing off avenues of communication that are important for the client. Focus on the client's concerns.	5. When staff anxiety increases, changing the topic or offering advice is common but leaves the person isolated.
6. Ask questions to clarify what is being said. "I'm not sure what you mean. Give me an example."	6. Increased anxiety results in scattering of thoughts. Clarifying helps the client identify thoughts and feelings.
7. Help the client identify thoughts or feelings before the onset of anxiety. "What were you thinking right before you started to feel anxious?"	7. The client is assisted in identifying thoughts and feelings, and problem solving is facilitated.
8. Encourage problem solving with the client.*	8. Encouraging clients to explore alternatives increases sense of control and decreases anxiety.
9. Assist in developing alternative solutions to a problem through role play or modeling behaviors.	9. The client is encouraged to try out alternative behaviors and solutions.
10. Explore behaviors that have worked to relieve anxiety in the past.	10. The client is encouraged to mobilize successful coping mechanisms and strengths.
11. Provide outlets for working off excess energy (e.g., walking, playing ping-pong, dancing, exercising).	11. Physical activity can provide relief of built-up tension, increase muscle tone, and increase endorphin levels.

*Clients experiencing mild to moderate anxiety levels can problem solve.

assisting people experiencing mild to moderate levels of anxiety.

Severe to Panic Levels of Anxiety

A person experiencing a severe to panic level of anxiety is unable to solve problems and may have a poor grasp of what is happening in the environment. Unproductive relief behaviors may take over and the person may not be in control of his or her actions. Extreme regression and running about aimlessly are behavioral manifestations of a person's intense psychic pain. The nurse is concerned with the client's safety and, at times, with the safety of others. Physical needs (e.g., for fluids and rest) must be met to prevent exhaustion. Anxiety reduction measures may take the form of removing the person to a quiet environment in which there is minimal stimulation and providing gross motor activities to drain off

some of the tension. The use of medications may have to be considered, but both medications and restraints should be used only after other more personal and less restrictive interventions have failed to decrease anxiety to safer levels. Although communication may be scattered and disjointed, themes can often be heard, and the nurse can address these themes. The feeling that one is understood can decrease the sense of isolation and also reduce anxiety.

Because individuals experiencing severe to panic levels of anxiety are unable to solve problems, techniques suggested for communicating with persons with mild to moderate levels of anxiety are not always effective. Clients experiencing severe to panic anxiety levels are out of control, so they need to know that they are safe from their own impulses. **Firm, short, and simple statements are useful.** Reinforcing commonalities in the environment and pointing out reality

TABLE 13-3

Interventions for Severe to Panic Levels of Anxiety

Nursing diagnosis: *Anxiety (severe, panic)* related to severe threat (biochemical, environmental, psychosocial), as evidenced by verbal or physical acting out, extreme immobility, sense of impending doom, inability to differentiate reality (possible hallucinations or delusions), and inability to problem solve

Intervention	Rationale
1. Maintain a calm manner.	1. Anxiety is communicated interpersonally. The quiet calm of the nurse can serve to calm the client. The presence of anxiety can escalate anxiety in the client.
2. Always remain with the person experiencing an acute severe to panic level of anxiety.	2. Alone with immense anxiety, a person feels abandoned. A caring face may be the client's only contact with reality when confusion becomes overwhelming.
3. Minimize environmental stimuli. Move to a quieter setting and stay with the client.	3. Helps minimize further escalation of client's anxiety.
4. Use clear and simple statements and repetition.	4. A person experiencing a severe to panic level of anxiety has difficulty concentrating and processing information.
5. Use a low-pitched voice; speak slowly.	5. A high-pitched voice can convey anxiety. Low pitch can decrease anxiety.
6. Reinforce reality if distortions occur (e.g., seeing objects that are not there or hearing voices when no one is present).	6. Anxiety can be reduced by focusing on and validating what is going on in the environment.
7. Listen for themes in communication.	7. In severe to panic levels of anxiety, verbal communication themes may be the only indication of the client's thoughts or feelings.
8. Attend to physical and safety needs when necessary (e.g., need for warmth, fluids, elimination, pain relief, family contact).	8. High levels of anxiety may obscure the client's awareness of physical needs.
9. Because safety is an overall goal, physical limits may need to be set. Speak in a firm, authoritative voice: "You may not hit anyone here. If you can't control yourself, we will help you."	9. A person who is out of control is often terrorized. Staff must offer the client and others protection from destructive and self-destructive impulses.
10. Provide opportunities for exercise (e.g., walk with nurse, punching bag, ping-pong game).	10. Physical activity helps channel and dissipate tension and may temporarily lower anxiety.
11. When a person is constantly moving or pacing, offer high-calorie fluids.	11. Dehydration and exhaustion must be prevented.
12. Assess need for medication or seclusion after other interventions have been tried and not been successful.	12. Exhaustion and physical harm to self and others must be prevented.

when there are distortions can also be useful interventions for severely anxious persons. Table 13-3 suggests some basic nursing interventions for clients with severe to panic levels of anxiety.

Refer to Case Study 13-1 at the end of the chapter for a demonstration of how many of these techniques can be used with a person experiencing severe anxiety. Chapter 12 offers many cognitive and behavioral strategies for decreasing stress and anxiety, and Chapter 14 identifies cognitive-behavioral techniques used in treating anxiety disorders.

DEFENSES AGAINST ANXIETY

Defense mechanisms protect people from painful awareness of feelings and memories that can provoke overwhelming anxiety (Sonnenberg, Ursano, & Ursano, 2003). Adaptive use of defense mechanisms helps people lower anxiety to achieve goals in acceptable ways. Figure 13-1 operationally defines anxiety and shows how defenses come into play.

Defense mechanisms operate all the time. However, when an individual is faced with a situation that triggers high anxiety, the person may become more rigid in the use of defense mechanisms and may revert to using less mature defenses (Sonnenberg et al., 2003). Defense mechanisms may be more or less mature. However, the degree of distortion of reality and disruption in interpersonal relationships determines if the use of a defense mechanism is adaptive (healthy) or not (Vaillant, 1994).

Sigmund Freud and his daughter Anna Freud outlined most of the defense mechanisms that we recognize today. Vaillant (1994) summarized five of the most important properties of defense mechanisms:

1. Defenses are a major means of managing conflict and affect.
2. Defenses are relatively unconscious.
3. Defenses are discrete from one another.
4. Although defenses are often the hallmarks of major psychiatric syndromes, they are reversible.
5. Defenses are adaptive as well as pathological.

All defense mechanisms except sublimation and altruism can be used in both healthy and not-so-healthy ways. (Sublimation and altruism are always healthy coping mechanisms.) Most people use a variety of defense mechanisms but not always at the same level. Keep in mind that whether the use of defense mechanisms is adaptive or maladaptive is determined for the most part by their *frequency*, *intensity*, and *duration* of use.

The defense mechanisms are discussed in the following sections starting with the most mature and healthy, followed by those that are less healthy and then by those that result in a greater degree of reality distortion and disruption in relationships and personal functioning.

Most Healthy Defenses

Altruism. In altruism, emotional conflicts and stressors are dealt with by meeting the needs of others. Unlike in self-sacrificing behavior, in altruism the person receives gratification either vicariously or from the response of others (American Psychiatric Association [APA], 2000). For example, six months after losing her

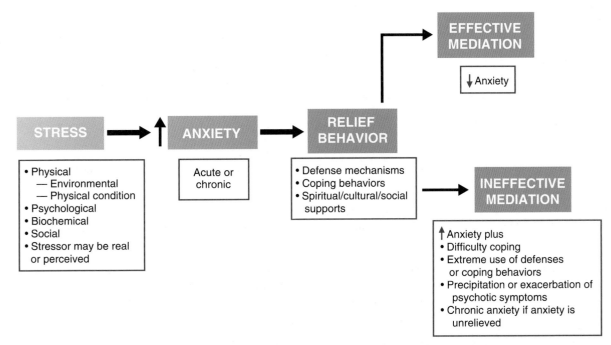

FIGURE 13-1 Anxiety, operationally defined.

husband in a car accident, Jeanette began to spend one day a week doing grief counseling with families who had lost a loved one. She found that she was effective in helping others in their grief, and she obtained a great deal of satisfaction and pleasure from helping others work through their pain.

Sublimation. Sublimation is an unconscious process of substituting constructive and socially acceptable activity for strong impulses that are not acceptable in their original form. Often, these impulses are sexual or aggressive. A man with strong hostile feelings may choose to become a butcher, or he may be involved in rough contact sports. A person who is unable to experience sexual activity may channel this energy into something creative, such as painting or gardening.

Humor. An individual may deal with emotional conflicts or stressors by emphasizing the amusing or ironic aspects of the conflict or stressor through humor (APA, 2000). For example, a man goes to an interview that means a great deal to him. He is being interviewed by the top executives of the company. He has recently had foot surgery and, on entering the interview room, he stumbles and loses his balance. There is a stunned silence, and then the man states calmly, "I was hoping I could put my best foot forward." With everyone laughing, the interview continues in a relaxed manner.

Suppression. Suppression is the conscious denial of a disturbing situation or feeling. For example, a student who has been studying for the state board examinations says, "I can't worry about paying my rent until after my exam tomorrow."

Intermediate Defenses

Repression. Repression is the exclusion of unpleasant or unwanted experiences, emotions, or ideas from conscious awareness. Forgetting the name of a former husband and forgetting an appointment to discuss poor grades are examples. Repression is considered the cornerstone of the defense mechanisms, and it is the first line of psychological defense against anxiety.

Displacement. Transfer of emotions associated with a particular person, object, or situation to another person, object, or situation that is nonthreatening is called displacement. The frequently cited example in which the boss yells at the man, the man yells at his wife, the wife yells at the child, and the child kicks the cat demonstrates the successive use of displaced hostility.

The use of displacement is common but not always adaptive. Spousal, child, and elder abuse are often cases of displaced hostility.

Reaction Formation. In reaction formation (also termed **overcompensation**), unacceptable feelings or behaviors are kept out of awareness by developing the opposite behavior or emotion. For example, a person who harbors hostility toward children becomes a Boy Scout leader.

Somatization. Transforming anxiety on an unconscious level into a physical symptom that has no organic cause is a form of somatization. Often the symptom functions as an attention getter or as an excuse.

▪ ▪ ▪ *VIGNETTE*

A professor develops laryngitis on the day he is scheduled to defend a research proposal to a group of peers.

A woman who does not want to go out with her boss's brother calls to say "her back went out" and she cannot make the date (and, in fact, her back is sore).

▪ ▪ ▪

Undoing. Undoing makes up for an act or communication (e.g., giving a gift to undo an argument). A common behavioral example of undoing is compulsive hand washing. This can be viewed as cleansing oneself of an act or thought perceived as unacceptable.

Rationalization. Rationalization consists of justifying illogical or unreasonable ideas, actions, or feelings by developing acceptable explanations that satisfy the teller as well as the listener. Common examples are, "If I had Lynn's brains, I'd get good grades, too," or "Everybody cheats, so why shouldn't I?" Rationalization is a form of self-deception.

Immature Defenses

Passive Aggression. A passive-aggressive individual deals with emotional conflict or stressors by indirectly and unassertively expressing aggression toward others. On the surface, there is an appearance of compliance that masks covert resistance, resentment, and hostility (APA, 2000). In passive aggression, aggression toward others is expressed through procrastination, failure, inefficiency, passivity, and illnesses that affect others more than oneself. Such passive-aggressive behaviors occur especially in response to assigned tasks or demands for independent action, responsibilities, or obligations (Widiger & Mullins, 2003).

▪ ▪ ▪ *VIGNETTE*

Sam promises his boss that he is working on the presentation for important clients, even though he constantly "forgets" to bring in samples of the presentation. The day of the presentation, Sam calls in sick with the flu.

▪ ▪ ▪

Acting-Out Behaviors. In acting out, an individual deals with emotional conflicts or stressors by actions rather than reflections or feelings (APA, 2000). For example, a person may lash out in anger verbally or physically to distract the self from threatening thoughts or feelings (e.g., powerlessness). The verbal or physical expression of anger can make a person feel temporarily less helpless or vulnerable (i.e., more powerful and more in control). By lashing out at others, an individual can transfer the focus from personal doubts and insecurities to some other person or object. Acting-out behaviors are a destructive coping style.

■ ■ ■ *VIGNETTE*

When Harry was turned down a third time for a promotion, he went to his office and tore apart every client file in his file cabinet. His initial feelings of worthlessness and lowered self-esteem related to the situation were interpreted by Harry to mean "I am no good." This thinking resulted in Harry's quickly transforming these painful feelings into actions of anger and destruction. Temporarily, Harry felt more powerful and less vulnerable.

■ ■ ■

Dissociation. A disruption in the usually integrated functions of consciousness, memory, identity, or perception of the environment is known as dissociation.

■ ■ ■ *VIGNETTE*

A young mother who saw her son run over by a car was taken to a neighbor's house while the police dealt with the accident. Later she told the policeman, "I really don't remember what happened. The last thing I remember is going out the door to check on Johnny." At that moment, to protect herself from an unbearable situation, she split off the threatening event from awareness until she could begin to deal with her feelings of devastation.

■ ■ ■

Devaluation. Devaluation occurs when emotional conflicts or stressors are dealt with by attributing negative qualities to self or others (APA, 2000). When devaluing another, the individual then appears good by contrast.

■ ■ ■ *VIGNETTE*

A woman who is very jealous of a co-worker says, "Oh, yes, she won the award. Those awards don't mean anything anyway, and I wonder what she had to do to be chosen." In this way she minimizes the other's accomplishments and keeps her own fragile self-esteem intact.

■ ■ ■

Idealization. In idealization, emotional conflicts or stressors are dealt with by attributing exaggerated positive qualities to others (APA, 2000). Idealization is an important aspect of the development of the self. Children who grow up with parents they can respect and idealize develop healthy standards of conduct and morality (Merikangas & Kupfer, 1995).

When people idealize and overvalue a person in a new relationship, they are sure to be disappointed when the object of the idealization turns out to be human. This leads to a great deal of disappointment and painful lowering of self-esteem. Such individuals may then end up devaluing and rejecting the object of their affection to protect their own self-esteem. This pattern can be repeated over and over on a job, in friendships, and in marriage.

■ ■ ■ *VIGNETTE*

Mary met the most "wonderful and perfect" man. No one could tell Mary that Jim was nice but had some quirks, like everyone else. Mary wouldn't listen. When Jim failed to live up to Mary's expectations of giving her constant attention, adoration, and gifts, Mary was devastated. Shortly thereafter, she started saying that Jim was, like all men, a brute, and that she wanted no more to do with such an insensitive person.

■ ■ ■

Splitting. Splitting is the inability to integrate the positive and negative qualities of oneself or others into a cohesive image. Aspects of the self and of others tend to alternate between opposite poles; for example, either good, loving, worthy, and nurturing, or bad, hateful, destructive, rejecting, and worthless (APA, 2000). Use of this defense mechanism is prevalent in personality disorders, especially the borderline ones.

■ ■ ■ *VIGNETTE*

Alice viewed her therapist as the most wonderful, loving, and insightful therapist she had ever had. When her therapist refused to write her a prescription for Valium, Alice shouted at her that she was the "stupidest, most uncaring, and thickheaded person" and she demanded another therapist "right away."

■ ■ ■

Projection. A person unconsciously rejects emotionally unacceptable personal features and attributes them to other people, objects, or situations through projection. This is the hallmark of blaming or scapegoating, which is the root of prejudice. People who always feel that others are out to deceive or cheat them may be projecting onto others those characteristics in themselves that they find distasteful and cannot consciously accept.

Projection of anxiety can often be seen in systems (family, hospital, school, business). In a family in which there are problems, the child is often scapegoated, and the pain and anxiety within the family are projected onto the child: "the problem is Tommy." In a larger system in which anxiety and conflict are present, the weakest members are scapegoated: "the problem is the nurses' aides . . . the students . . . the new salesman." When pain and anxiety exist within a system, projection can be an automatic relief behavior. Once the cause of the anxiety is identified, changes in relief behavior can ensue, and the system can become more functional and productive.

Denial. Denial involves escaping unpleasant realities by ignoring their existence. For example, a man believes that physical limitations reflect negatively on one's manhood. Thus, he may deny chest pains, even though heart attacks run in his family, because of a threat to his self-image as a man. A woman whose health has deteriorated because of alcohol abuse denies she has a problem with alcohol by saying she can stop drinking whenever she wants.

The term psychotic denial is used when there is gross impairment in reality testing. A schizophrenic man who says he wants to stay out of the hospital tells the nurse it is his medication, not the cocaine, that makes him frankly psychotic and aggressive.

Table 13-4 presents examples of adaptive and nonadaptive use of some common defense mechanisms.

TABLE 13-4

Defense Mechanisms

Adaptive	Nonadaptive
Repression	
Man forgets his wife's birthday after a marital fight.	Woman is unable to enjoy sex after having pushed out of awareness a traumatic sexual incident from childhood.
Sublimation	
Woman who is angry with her boss writes a short story about a heroic woman. By definition, use of sublimation is always constructive.	None.
Regression	
Four-year-old boy with a new baby brother starts sucking his thumb and wanting a bottle.	Man who loses a promotion starts complaining to others, hands in sloppy work, misses appointments, and comes in late for meetings.
Displacement	
Client criticizes a nurse after his family fails to visit.	Child who is unable to acknowledge fear of his father becomes fearful of animals.
Projection	
Man who is unconsciously attracted to other women teases his wife about flirting.	Woman who has repressed an attraction toward other women refuses to socialize. She fears another woman will make homosexual advances toward her.
Compensation	
Short man becomes assertively verbal and excels in business.	Individual drinks alcohol when self-esteem is low to diffuse discomfort temporarily.
Reaction Formation	
Recovering alcoholic constantly preaches about the evils of drink.	Mother who has an unconscious hostility toward her daughter is overprotective and hovers over her to protect her from harm, interfering with her normal growth and development.
Denial	
Man reacts to news of the death of a loved one by saying, "No, I don't believe you. The doctor said he was fine."	Woman whose husband died 3 years earlier still keeps his clothes in the closet and talks about him in the present tense.
Conversion	
Student is unable to take a final examination because of a terrible headache.	Man becomes blind after seeing his wife flirt with other men.
Undoing	
After flirting with her male secretary, a woman brings her husband tickets to a show.	Man with rigid and moralistic beliefs and repressed sexuality is driven to wash his hands to gain composure when around attractive women.
Rationalization	
Employee says, "I didn't get the raise because the boss doesn't like me."	Father who thinks his son was fathered by another man excuses his malicious treatment of the boy by saying, "He is lazy and disobedient," when that is not the case.

TABLE 13-4

Defense Mechanisms—cont'd

Adaptive	Nonadaptive
Identification	
Five-year-old girl dresses in her mother's shoes and dress and meets her father at the door.	Young boy thinks a neighborhood pimp with money and drugs is someone to look up to.
Introjection	
After his wife's death, husband has transient complaints of chest pains and difficulty breathing—the symptoms his wife had before she died.	Young child whose parents were overcritical and belittling grows up thinking that she is not any good. She has taken on her parent's evaluation of her as part of her self-image.
Suppression	
Businessman who is preparing to make an important speech later in the day is told by his wife that morning that she wants a divorce. Although visibly upset, he puts the incident aside until after his speech, when he can give the matter his total concentration.	A woman who feels a lump in her breast shortly before leaving for a 3-week vacation puts the information in the back of her mind until after returning from her vacation.

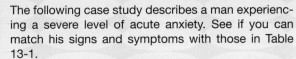

CASE STUDY and NURSING CARE PLAN 13-1   Severe Level of Anxiety

The following case study describes a man experiencing a severe level of acute anxiety. See if you can match his signs and symptoms with those in Table 13-1.

Tom Michaels, a 63-year-old man, comes into the emergency department (ED) with his wife Anne, who has taken an overdose of sleeping pills and antidepressant medications. Ten years earlier, Anne's mother died, and since that time Anne has suffered several episodes of severe depression with suicide attempts. She has needed hospitalization during these episodes. Anne Michaels had been released from the hospital 2 weeks earlier after treatment for depression and threatened suicide.

Tom has a long-established routine of giving his wife her antidepressant medications in the morning and her sleeping medication at night and keeping the bottles hidden when he is not at home. Today, he had forgotten to hide the medications before he went to work. His wife had taken the remaining pills from both bottles with large quantities of alcohol. When Tom returned home for lunch, Anne was comatose.

In the ED, Anne suffers cardiac arrest and is taken to the intensive care unit (ICU).

Tom appears very jittery. He moves about the room aimlessly. He drops his hat, a medication card, and his keys. His hands are trembling, and he looks around the room, bewildered. He appears unable to focus on any one thing. He says over and over, in a loud, high-pitched voice, "Why didn't I hide the bottles?" He is wringing his hands and begins stomping his feet, saying, "It's all my fault. Everything is falling apart."

Other people in the waiting room appear distracted and alarmed by his behavior. Tom seems to be oblivious to his surroundings.

■ ASSESSMENT

Russell Brown, the psychiatric nurse clinician working in the ED, comes into the waiting room and assesses Tom's behavior as indicative of a severe anxiety level. After talking with Tom briefly, Mr. Brown believes nursing intervention is indicated.

Mr. Brown bases his conclusion on the following assessment of the client.

Objective Data

- Unable to focus on anything
- Engaging in purposeless activity (walking around aimlessly)
- Oblivious to his surroundings
- Confused and bewildered
- Showing unproductive relief behavior (stomping, wringing hands, dropping things)

Subjective Data

- "Everything is falling apart."
- "Why didn't I hide the bottles?"
- "It's all my fault."

Continued

■ NURSING DIAGNOSIS (NANDA)

Mr. Brown formulates the following nursing diagnosis:

Anxiety (severe) related to the client's perception of responsibility for his wife's coma and possible death, as evidenced by inability to focus, confusion, and the feeling that "everything is falling apart"

■ OUTCOME CRITERIA (NOC)

Client will demonstrate effective coping strategies.*

■ PLANNING

Mr. Brown thinks that if he can lower Tom's anxiety to a moderate level, he can work with Tom to get a clear picture of his situation and place the events in a more realistic perspective. He also thinks that Tom needs to talk to someone and share some of his pain and confusion in order to sort out his feelings. Mr. Brown identifies two short-term goals:

1. Client's anxiety will decrease from severe to moderate by 4 PM.
2. Client will verbalize his feelings and a need for assistance by 4 PM.

■ INTERVENTION (NIC)

Mr. Brown takes Tom to a quiet room in the back of the ED. He introduces himself to Tom and comments that he notices Tom is upset. He says, "I will stay with you." At first, Tom finds it difficult to sit down and continues pacing around the room. Mr. Brown sits quietly and calmly, listening to Tom' self-recriminations. He attends carefully to what Tom is saying and what he is not saying, to identify themes.

After a while, Tom becomes calmer and is able to sit next to Mr. Brown. Mr. Brown offers him orange juice, which he accepts and holds tightly.

Mr. Brown speaks calmly, using simple, clear statements. He uses communication tools that are helpful to Tom in sorting out his feelings and naming them.

Dialogue	Therapeutic Tool/Comment
Tom: Yes . . . yes . . . I forgot to hide the bottles. She usually tells me when she feels bad. Why didn't she tell me?	
Nurse: You think that if she had told you she wanted to kill herself you would have hidden the pills?	The nurse asks for clarification on Tom's thinking.
Tom: Yes, if I had only known, this wouldn't have happened.	
Nurse: It sounds as if you believe you should have known what your wife was thinking without her telling you.	Here the nurse clarifies Tom's expectations that he should be able to read his wife's mind.
Tom: Well . . . yes . . . when you put it that way . . . I just don't know what I'll do if she dies.	

When Mr. Brown thinks that Tom has discussed his feelings of guilt sufficiently, he asks Tom to clarify his thinking about his wife's behavior. Tom is able to place his feelings of guilt in a more realistic perspective. Next, Mr. Brown brings up another issue—the question of whether Tom's wife will live or die.

Dialogue	Therapeutic Tool/Comment
Nurse: You stated that if your wife dies, you don't know what you will do.	The nurse reflects Tom's feelings back to him.
Tom: Oh, God *(he begins to cry)*, I can't live without her . . . she's all I have in the world.	
Silence	
Nurse: She means a great deal to you.	The nurse reflects Tom's feelings back to him.
Tom: Everything. Since her mother died, we are each other's only family.	
Nurse: What would it mean to you if your wife died?	The nurse asks Tom to evaluate his feelings about his wife.
Tom: I couldn't live by myself, alone. I couldn't stand it. *(Starts to cry again.)*	
Nurse: It sounds as if being alone is very frightening to you.	The nurse restates in clear terms Tom's experience and feelings.
Tom: Yes . . . I don't know how I'd manage by myself.	
Nurse: A change like that could take time to adjust to.	The nurse validates that if Tom's wife died it would be very painful. At the same time, he implies hope that Tom could work through the death in time.
Tom: Yes . . . it would be very hard.	

*The expected outcome will be evaluated on a 5-point Likert scale ranging from 1 (never demonstrated) to 5 (consistently demonstrated).

Again, Mr. Brown gives Tom a chance to sort out his feelings and fears. Mr. Brown helps him focus on the reality that his wife may die and encourages him to express fears related to her possible death. After a while, Mr. Brown offers to go up to the ICU with Tom to see how his wife is doing. When they arrive at the ICU, although Anne is still comatose, her condition has stabilized and she is breathing on her own.

After his arrival at the ICU, Tom starts to worry about whether he had locked the door at home. Mr. Brown encourages him to call neighbors and ask them to check the door. At this time, Tom is able to focus on everyday things. Mr. Brown makes arrangements to see Tom the next day when he comes in to visit his wife.

The next day, Anne has regained consciousness. She is discharged 1 week later. At the time of discharge, Tom and Anne Michaels are considering family therapy with the psychiatric nurse clinician once a week in the outpatient department.

■ EVALUATION

The first short-term goal is to lower anxiety from severe to moderate. Mr. Brown can see that Tom has become more visibly calm: his trembling, wringing of hands, and stomping of feet have ceased, and he is able to focus on his thoughts and feelings with the aid of Mr. Brown.

The second short-term goal established for Tom is that he will verbalize his feelings and need for assistance. Tom is able to identify and discuss with the nurse his feelings of guilt and fear of being left alone in the world if his wife should die. Both these feelings are overwhelming him. He is also able to state that he needs assistance in coping with these feelings in order to make tentative plans for the future.

evolve Visit the Evolve website at **http://evolve.elsevier.com/Varcarolis** for more case studies.

■■■ KEY POINTS to REMEMBER

- Stress is a state produced by change in the environment that is perceived as challenging, threatening, or damaging to a person's well-being. Stress can lead to a variety of psychological and psychobiological responses, the most common of which is anxiety.
- The basic emotion of anxiety is differentiated from fear in that anxiety has an unknown or unrecognized source, whereas fear is a reaction to a specific threat.
- Anxiety can be normal, acute, or chronic.
- Peplau operationally defined four levels of anxiety. The client's perceptual field, ability to learn, and physical and other characteristics are different at each level (see Table 13-1).
- Effective psychosocial interventions are different for persons experiencing mild to moderate levels of anxiety and individuals experiencing severe to panic levels of anxiety. Effective psychosocial nursing approaches are suggested in Tables 13-2 and 13-3. Case Study 13-1 gives good examples of how these interventions can be incorporated when working with individuals experiencing severe to panic levels of anxiety.
- Defenses against anxiety can be adaptive or maladaptive. Defenses are presented in a hierarchy from healthy to intermediate to immature. Table 13-4 provides examples of adaptive and maladaptive use of many of the more common defense mechanisms.

■■■

Visit the Evolve website at **http://evolve.elsevier.com/Varcarolis** for a posttest on the content in this chapter.   **evolve**

Critical Thinking and Chapter Review

Visit the Evolve website at **http://evolve.elsevier.com/Varcarolis** for additional self-study exercises.
evolve

■■■ CRITICAL THINKING

1. Tom La Rue is a senior at college and is taking his final examinations for an engineering course. He is caught looking on and copying from the examination of his willing partner, June. Tom's paper is taken away, and he is asked to see the professor after the examinations are all in. His heart starts to pound, his pulse and respiration rates increase, and he has to wipe perspiration from his hand and face several times. He feels as if he has to vomit and has a throbbing in his head. When speaking to the professor after the examination, he initially has difficulty focusing, and when he starts to speak his voice trembles. Tom says that June convinced him that cheating was done all the time and, in fact, it was her

Continued

Critical Thinking and Chapter Review—cont'd

Visit the Evolve website at **http://evolve.elsevier.com/Varcarolis** for additional self-study exercises.

idea. Tom goes on to say that this "silly little exam" doesn't mean anything anyway, that he already passed the important courses. He tells the professor, "I thought you were the greatest, and now I see that you are a fool." The professor remains calm and explains that, regardless of Tom's thoughts on this matter, Tom was caught cheating, he will have to take responsibility for his actions, and the choice to cheat was his. The professor will have Tom go before the disciplinary board, which is the well-known procedure when one is caught cheating. When Tom realizes that this incident could affect his graduating on time, he begins to yell at the professor and call him unflattering names. Another professor who has come in to take the examination papers to the grading machine witnesses this encounter.

A. Identify the level of anxiety Tom was experiencing once he was caught cheating and describe all of the signs and symptoms that helped you determine the correct level.

B. Identify and define five defense mechanisms that Tom used to lessen his anxiety.

C. Given the circumstances, once Tom was caught, how could he have reacted in a manner that would have reflected more self-responsibility using healthier coping defenses?

D. If at a later date Tom were to use the defense mechanism of altruism, in light of this situation, what are some of the ways he could do this?

▪ ▪ ▪ CHAPTER REVIEW

Choose the most appropriate answer.

1. Shortly after being told that he has 90% blockage of three major coronary arteries and needs emergency coronary artery bypass surgery, Paul is noted by the nurse to appear dazed. His thoughts are scattered, as evidenced by the fact that his conversation jumps from topic to topic. He frequently states, "I'm overwhelmed. I don't know what to do." He is un-

able to give direction to his wife when she asks him whom he wants her to notify. His pulse rate rises 15 points. The nurse can assess the type of anxiety Paul is experiencing as

1. normal anxiety.
2. sublimated anxiety.
3. acute (state) anxiety.
4. chronic (trait) anxiety.

2. In the scenario described in Question 1, the nurse can assess Paul's level of anxiety as

1. mild.
2. moderate.
3. severe.
4. panic.

3. Nursing interventions that are helpful in lowering a client's level of anxiety from severe to moderate include

1. speaking rapidly in a high-pitched voice.
2. permitting the existence of reality distortions.
3. listening for themes the client expresses.
4. providing solitude for client.

4. Defense mechanisms are

1. a means of managing conflict.
2. predominantly conscious.
3. entirely pathological.
4. irreversible.

5. Which characteristic is true of mature ego defenses that is not true of ego defenses at the other levels?

1. Mature defenses arise from experiencing panic-level anxiety.
2. Mature defenses do not distort reality to a significant degree.
3. Mature defenses disguise reality to make it less threatening.
4. Mature defenses are exclusively maladaptive.

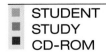

STUDENT
STUDY
CD-ROM

Access the accompanying CD-ROM for animations, interactive exercises, review questions for the NCLEX examination, and an audio glossary.

REFERENCES

American Psychiatric Association. (2000). *Diagnostic and statistical manual of mental disorders* (4th ed., text rev.). Washington, DC: Author.

Merikangas, K. R., & Kupfer, D. J. (1995). Mood disorders: Genetic aspects. In H. I. Kaplan & B. J. Sadock (Eds.), *Comprehensive textbook of psychiatry/VI* (6th ed., Vol. 1, pp. 1102-1115). Baltimore: Williams & Wilkins.

Peplau, H. E. (1968). A working definition of anxiety. In S. F. Burd & M. A. Marshall (Eds.), *Some clinical approaches to psychiatric nursing.* New York: Macmillan.

Sonnenberg, S. M., Ursano, A. M., & Ursano, R. J. (2003). Physician-patient relationship. In A. Tasman, J. Kay, & J. A. Lieberman (Eds.). *Psychiatry* (2nd ed.). West Sussex, England: Wiley.

Sullivan, H. S. (1953). *The interpersonal theory of psychiatry.* New York: W. W. Norton.

Vaillant, G. E. (1994). Ego mechanisms of defense and personality psychopathology. *Journal of Abnormal Psychology, 103*(1), 44.

Widiger, T. A., & Mullins, S. (2003). Personality disorders. In A. Tasman, J. Kay, & J. A. Lieberman (Eds.). *Psychiatry* (2nd ed.). West Sussex, England: Wiley.

A CLIENT SPEAKS

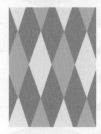

I am a 48-year-old woman, and I was born and raised in Maryland. I grew up with my parents and my older brother. I quit school in the twelfth grade when I had my first daughter. I have been married twice, and I am a widow. I have two daughters who are 30 and 26 years old. I have worked taking care of children and doing housekeeping. I first became aware of my obsessions and compulsions at the age of 12. I was cleaning my body all the time and always thinking of germs; it caused me a lot of stress. My hands used to get red, and touching things was awful for me. I went to a hospital to get help, but they did not know what it was; they just said that I was clean.

In my teens, I became depressed all the time. I went to the hospital again, but it did not seem to help. I know that my state of mind and OCD played a great part in my two marriages. I used to make my children clean up all the time, and I was always checking behind them. My husband did the same thing. They say, "Cleanliness is next to godliness." Drugs became a part of my life in my 30s and caused me great pain. I started to use cocaine after my husband died, and I used for 12 years. Two years ago, I was hospitalized for depression, and I was homeless. The hospital referred me to a 28-day drug rehabilitation program. The drug program referred me to a women's recovery house shelter. I lived there for 6 months while I attended an outpatient mental health center. I got treatment for depression, hallucinations, OCD, and substance use. I had a therapist and psychiatrist in the clinic, along with dual-diagnosis group therapy. I also attended an intensive outpatient drug program right down the hall in the clinic. I worked on my OCD with my therapist, gradually touching on things that made me anxious. In the beginning, I could not stand to touch people or any of their belongings; I had to cover my hand to touch doorknobs. I learned to tolerate my anxiety about being around people.

After being drug-free for 6 months, I was eligible for an independent apartment in a group of apartments supervised by case managers. I love my own apartment. I even got a part-time job as a receptionist at the YWCA. My life is good now that I am clean. My children are still in my life, and we get along better. I have great friends, and I am setting goals. I help my daughter take care of my mother, who has Alzheimer's disease. When I am nervous, the voices do come back, and I start to clean too much. But I take my medicine regularly, and I usually can calm myself with the help of my family. I still go to the clinic once a month.

PSYCHOBIOLOGICAL DISORDERS
Moderate to Severe

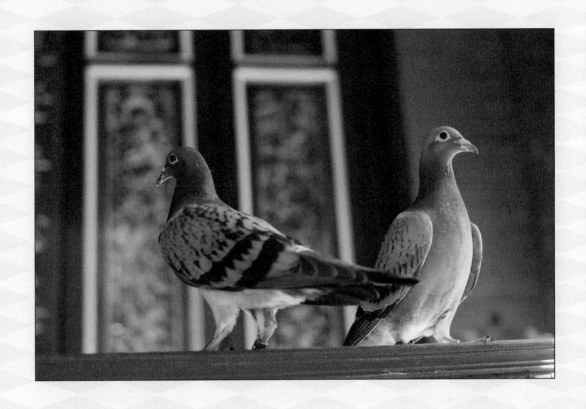

PEOPLE CHANGE AND THEN FORGET TO TELL EACH OTHER.

Lillian Hellman

Anxiety Disorders

NANCY CHRISTINE SHOEMAKER ■ ELIZABETH M. VARCAROLIS

KEY TERMS and CONCEPTS

The key terms and concepts listed here appear in color where they are defined or first discussed in this chapter.

acute stress disorder, 236

agoraphobia, 233

anxiolytic drugs, 246

behavioral therapy, 244

cognitive restructuring, 244

cognitive therapy, 244

cognitive-behavioral therapy, 244

compulsions, 234

flashbacks, 236

flooding, 244

generalized anxiety disorder (GAD), 235

modeling, 244

obsessions, 234

panic attack, 232

panic disorder, 232

phobia, 234

posttraumatic stress disorder (PTSD), 236

relaxation training, 244

response prevention, 244

social anxiety disorder, 234

social phobia, 234

specific phobias, 234

systematic desensitization, 244

thought stopping, 244

OBJECTIVES

After studying this chapter, the reader will be able to

1. Identify genetic, biological, psychological, and cultural factors leading to anxiety disorders.
2. Describe clinical manifestations of each anxiety disorder.
3. Formulate four appropriate nursing diagnoses that can be used in treating a person with an anxiety disorder.
4. Name three defense mechanisms commonly found in clients with anxiety disorders.
5. Describe feelings that may be experienced by nurses caring for clients with anxiety disorders.
6. Propose realistic outcome criteria for a client with (a) generalized anxiety disorder, (b) panic disorder, and (c) posttraumatic stress disorder.
7. Describe five basic nursing interventions used with clients with anxiety disorders.
8. Discuss three classes of medication appropriate for anxiety disorders.
9. Define two advanced practice interventions for anxiety disorders.

evolve Visit the Evolve website at **http://evolve.elsevier.com/Varcarolis** for a pretest on the content in this chapter.

As noted in Chapters 12 and 13, anxiety is a normal response to threatening situations, and everyone experiences occasional distress. Anxiety becomes a problem when it interferes with adaptive behavior, causes physical symptoms, or exceeds a tolerable level.

Individuals with anxiety disorders use rigid, repetitive, and ineffective behaviors to try to control anxiety. The common element of these disorders is that individuals experience a degree of anxiety that is so high that it interferes with personal, occupational, or social functioning. Recent studies also suggest that the presence of chronic anxiety disorders may increase the rate of cardiovascular system–related deaths. Anxiety disorders tend to be persistent and often disabling. The

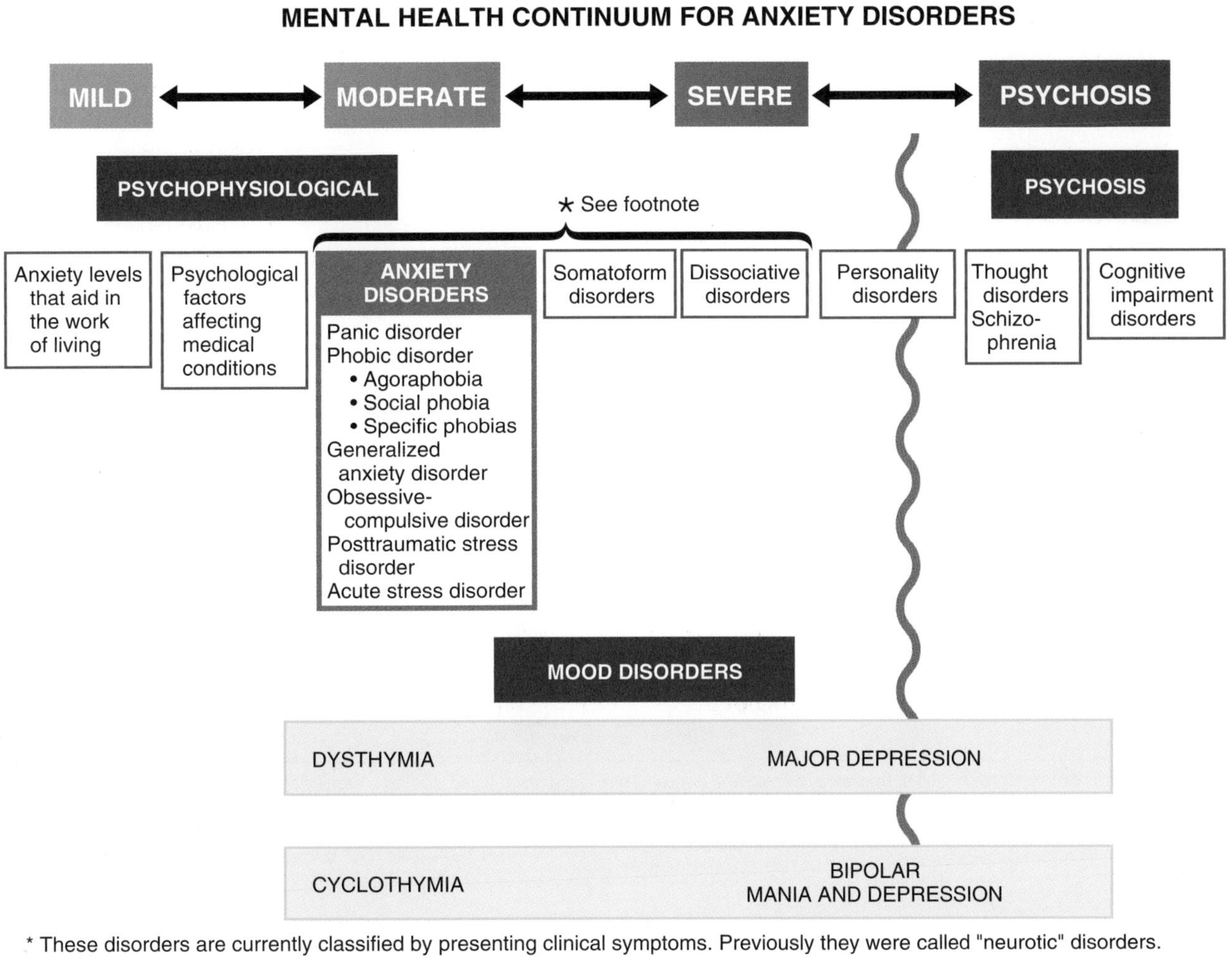

MENTAL HEALTH CONTINUUM FOR ANXIETY DISORDERS

FIGURE 14-1 Mental health continuum for anxiety disorders.

placement of these disorders on the mental health continuum can be seen in Figure 14-1.

PREVALENCE

Anxiety disorders are the most common form of psychiatric disorder in the United States, affecting up to 13.3% of the adult population. People with anxiety disorders frequently seek health care services for relief of physical symptoms, at a cost of approximately $22 billion per year. Women are affected more frequently than men (Anxiety Disorders Association of America, 2003). Refer to Table 14-1 for 1-year prevalence rates for specific anxiety disorders in the United States.

COMORBIDITY

Clinicians and researchers have clearly shown that anxiety disorders frequently co-occur with other psychiatric problems. Several studies suggest that 90% of people with an anxiety disorder develop another psychiatric disorder during their lifetime (Overbeek, 2002). Major depression often co-occurs and produces

a greater impairment with poorer response to treatment (Simon & Rosenbaum, 2003). Substance abuse is also frequently encountered and has a similar negative impact on treatment (Myrick & Brady, 2003). Table 14-1 identifies common comorbid conditions for each of the anxiety disorders.

THEORY

There is no longer any doubt that biological correlates predispose some individuals to pathological anxiety states (e.g., phobias, panic attacks). By the same token, traumatic life events, psychosocial factors, and sociocultural factors are also etiologically significant.

Genetic Correlates

Numerous studies substantiate that anxiety disorders tend to cluster in families. Twin studies indicate the existence of a genetic component to both panic disorder and obsessive-compulsive disorder (OCD) (American Psychiatric Association [APA], 2000). First-degree biological relatives of persons with OCD and persons

TABLE 14-1

Anxiety Disorders

Disorder	Prevalence (%)	Age of Onset	Gender Predilection	Comorbidities
Panic disorder	0.5-1.7	Adolescence to mid-thirties	Two to three times more frequent in women	Major depression Generalized anxiety disorder Substance abuse
Generalized anxiety disorder	2.8-3.0	Childhood to adolescence	Two times more frequent in women	Major depression Panic disorder Substance abuse
Phobias (specific)	4.8-8.0	Childhood to adolescence	Two times more frequent in women	Other anxiety disorders Mood disorders Substance abuse
Social anxiety disorder	3.7-13.0	Adolescence	Equal prevalence in men and women	Other anxiety disorders Mood disorders Substance abuse
Obsessive-compulsive disorder	0.5-2.3	Childhood for males Adulthood for females	Equal prevalence in men and women	Major depression Other anxiety disorders Eating disorders Tourette's disorder
Posttraumatic stress disorder	3.6-8.0	Any age; triggered by trauma	Women more likely affected (rape is a major trigger)	Major depression Other anxiety disorders Substance abuse

Data from American Psychiatric Association. (2000). *Diagnostic and statistical manual of mental disorders* (4th ed., text rev.). Washington, DC: Author; and Anxiety Disorders Association of America. (2003). *Statistics and facts about anxiety disorders.* Retrieved December 29, 2004, from http://www.adaa.org/mediaroom/index.cfm.

with phobias have a higher frequency of these disorders than exists in the general population. First-degree biological relatives of people with panic disorder are up to eight times more likely to experience panic attacks (Brown, 2003). Even for posttraumatic stress disorder (PTSD) and generalized anxiety disorder (GAD), there is evidence of inherited components (APA, 2000).

Biological Findings

Certain anatomic pathways (the limbic system) provide the transmission structure for the electrical impulses that occur when anxiety-related responses are sent or received. Neurons release chemicals (neurotransmitters) that convey these messages. The neurochemicals that regulate anxiety in clients include epinephrine, norepinephrine, dopamine, serotonin, and γ-aminobutyric acid (GABA).

There are various theories regarding the causes of anxiety disorders. One is the GABA benzodiazepine theory. Recently discovered benzodiazepine receptors are linked to a receptor that inhibits the activity of the neurotransmitter GABA. The release of GABA slows neural transmission, which has a calming effect. Binding of the benzodiazepine medications to the benzodiazepine receptors facilitates the action of GABA (Brown, 2003). This theory proposes that abnormalities

of these benzodiazepine receptors may lead to unregulated anxiety levels.

Numerous studies of people with panic disorder have linked sodium lactate infusions and carbon dioxide inhalation with the precipitation of panic attacks. One theory suggests that both of these substances warn the brain of impending suffocation. People with panic disorder overreact to this warning signal compared with control subjects. Likewise, other studies using a stimulant drug show that an area of the brainstem which releases norepinephrine is more sensitive in people with panic attacks, so that they experience the fight-or-flight response more readily than controls (Brown, 2003).

Studies of clients with PTSD suggest that the stress response of the hypothalamus-pituitary-adrenal system is abnormal in these individuals. Repeated trauma or stress not only alters the release of neurotransmitters but also changes the anatomy of the brain—neuroimaging shows that the size of the hippocampus is actually reduced (Gorman, 2000). Refer to Chapters 3 and 12 for information related to the anatomy and physiology of anxiety disorders.

Psychological Factors

Early theories about the development of anxiety disorders centered around the idea that unconscious childhood conflicts are the basis for symptom development.

Sigmund Freud taught that anxiety resulted from the threatened breakthrough of repressed ideas or emotions from the unconscious into consciousness. Freud also suggested that ego defense mechanisms are used by the individual to keep anxiety at manageable levels. Later in this chapter, Table 14-7 defines and gives examples of defense mechanisms commonly used by individuals with anxiety disorders. The use of defense mechanisms results in behavior that is not wholly adaptive because of its rigidity and repetitive nature. Chapters 2 and 13 provide the reader with more details on the dynamics of defense mechanisms.

Harry Stack Sullivan placed anxiety in an interpersonal context. He believed that all anxiety is linked either to the emotional distress caused when early needs go unmet or to the anxiety transmitted to the infant from the caregiver through the process of empathy. Thus, the anxiety experienced early in life becomes the prototype for that experienced when unpleasant events occur later in life.

Learning theories provide another view. Behavioral psychologists conceptualize anxiety as a learned response that can be unlearned. Some individuals may learn to be anxious from the modeling provided by parents or peers. For example, a mother who is fearful of thunder and lightning and who hides in closets during storms may transmit her anxiety to her children, who continue to adopt her behavior even into adult life. Such individuals can unlearn this behavior by observing others who react normally to a storm.

Cognitive theorists take the position that anxiety disorders are caused by distortions in an individual's thinking and perceiving. Because individuals with such distortions believe that any mistake they make will have catastrophic results, they experience acute anxiety.

Cultural Considerations

Reliable data on the incidence of anxiety disorders in this and other cultures are sparse, but sociocultural variation in symptoms of anxiety disorders has been noted. In some cultures, individuals express anxiety through somatic symptoms, whereas in other cultures, cognitive symptoms predominate. Panic attacks in Latin Americans and Northern Europeans often involve sensations of choking, smothering, numbness, or tingling, as well as fear of dying. In other cultural groups, panic attacks involve fear of magic or witchcraft. Social phobias in Japanese and Korean cultures may relate to a belief that the individual's blushing, eye contact, or body odor is offensive to others (APA, 2000).

The *Diagnostic and Statistical Manual of Mental Disorders,* fourth edition, text revision *(DSM-IV-TR)* (APA, 2000) notes cultural aspects of each psychiatric disorder to alert the clinician to consider cultural context before making a psychiatric diagnosis. The Culturally Speaking box discusses factors relevant to one anxiety disorder. Also review Chapter 7 for more discussion of cultural issues.

CLINICAL PICTURE

The term *anxiety disorders* refers to a number of disorders, including the following:
- Panic disorders
- Phobias
- OCD
- GAD
- PTSD
- Acute stress disorder
- Anxiety due to substance use
- Anxiety due to medical conditions
- Anxiety not otherwise specified

■■■ **CULTURALLY SPEAKING**

Posttraumatic Stress Disorder

Cultural and social factors play a major role in posttraumatic stress disorder (PTSD). Minority groups in the United States have much higher rates of PTSD than do non-Hispanic white persons. African Americans of all ages have a high risk of exposure to violent crime. One study found PTSD in 25% of African American youth who were victims of violence. Likewise, American Indians and Alaska Natives have an increased risk of victimization. This higher rate of trauma results in a 22% prevalence rate of PTSD in these groups compared to 8% in the general population.

Refugees are another group at higher risk of PTSD. Central American Hispanics often fled their homelands during civil wars, and rates of PTSD range from 33% to 60% in this refugee group. Similarly, many Asian Americans from Laos, Vietnam, and Cambodia were severely traumatized before they left their native lands. One study of Southeast Asia refugees seeking mental health care showed that 70% met the criteria for PTSD.

U.S. Department of Health and Human Services. (2001). *Mental Health: Culture, race and ethnicity: A supplement to mental health: A report of the surgeon general.* Rockville, MD: U.S. Department of Health and Human Services, Substance Abuse and Mental Health Services Administration, Center for Mental Health Services.

Figure 14-2 presents the *DSM-IV-TR* criteria for various anxiety disorders.

Panic Disorders

Panic Disorder Without Agoraphobia

The panic attack is the key feature of panic disorder. See the following vignette for an example of a client with signs and symptoms of panic attack. Panic disorder without agoraphobia is characterized by recurrent unexpected panic attacks, about which the individual is persistently concerned (APA, 2000).

A panic attack is the sudden onset of extreme apprehension or fear, usually associated with feelings of impending doom. The feelings of terror present during a panic attack are so severe that normal function is suspended, the perceptual field is severely limited, and misinterpretation of reality may occur. Severe personality disorganization is evident. People experienc-

ing panic attacks may believe that they are losing their minds or are having a heart attack. The attacks are often accompanied by highly uncomfortable physical symptoms, such as palpitations, chest pain, breathing difficulties, nausea, feelings of choking, chills, and hot flashes. Typically, panic attacks come "out of the blue" (i.e., suddenly and not necessarily in response to stress), are extremely intense, last a matter of minutes, and then subside. Refer to Table 14-2 for a generic care plan for panic disorder.

■ ■ ■ *VIGNETTE*

Dora, a 30-year-old pharmacist, lives at home and cares for her mother. After her mother's death from heart disease, Dora begins to experience tension, irritability, and sleep disturbance. On several occasions, Dora awakens gasping for breath. Her heart pounds, and she feels a tight sensation, like a band around her chest. Her pulse typically increases to more than 110 beats per minute, and she experiences dizzi-

DSM-IV-TR CRITERIA FOR ANXIETY DISORDERS

ANXIETY DISORDERS

Panic Disorder	**Phobias**	**Obsessive-Compulsive Disorder (OCD)**	**Generalized Anxiety Disorder (GAD)**

1. Both A and B
  A. Recurrent episodes of panic attacks
  B. At least one of the attacks has been followed by 1 month (or more) of the following:
    1. Persistent concern about having additional attacks
    2. Worry about consequences ("going crazy," having a heart attack, losing control)
    3. Significant change in behavior
 	
2. A. Absence of agoraphobia = **Panic disorder without agoraphobia**
  B. Presence of agoraphobia = **Panic disorder with agoraphobia**
	1. Irrational fear of an object or situation that persists although the person may recognize it as unreasonable
	
	2. Types include:
	  • **Agoraphobia**: Fear of being alone in open or public places where escape might be difficult; may not leave home
	  • **Social phobia**: Fear of situations where one might be seen and embarrassed or criticized (e.g., speaking to authority figures, public speaking, or performing)
	  • **Specific phobia**: Fear of a single object, activity, or situation (e.g., snakes, closed spaces, flying)
	
	3. Anxiety is severe if the object, situation, or activity cannot be avoided.
		1. Either obsessions or compulsions
		  A. Preoccupation with persistent intrusive thoughts, impulses, or images (obsession)
		  or
		  B. Repetitive behaviors or mental acts that the person feels driven to perform in order to reduce distress or prevent a dreaded event or situation (compulsion)
		
		2. Person knows the obsessions/compulsions are excessive and unreasonable.
		
		3. The obsession/compulsion can cause increased distress and is time-consuming.
			1. A. Excessive anxiety or worry more days than not over 6 months
			  B. Inability to control the worrying
			
			2. Anxiety and worry associated with three or more of the following symptoms:
			  A. Restless, keyed-up
			  B. Easily fatigued
			  C. Difficulty concentrating, mind goes blank
			  D. Irritability
			  E. Muscle tension
			  F. Sleep disturbance
			
			3. Anxiety or worry or physical symptoms cause significant impairment in social, occupational, or other areas of important functioning.

FIGURE 14-2 Diagnostic criteria for anxiety disorders. (Adapted from American Psychiatric Association. [2000]. *Diagnostic and statistical manual of mental disorders* [4th ed., text rev.]. Washington, DC: Author.)

TABLE 14-2

Generic Care Plan for Panic Disorder

Nursing diagnosis: *Anxiety* as evidenced by sudden onset of fear of impending doom or dying; increased pulse and respirations, shortness of breath, possible chest pain, dizziness, abdominal distress, panic attacks

Outcome criteria: Panic attacks will become less intense and time between episodes will lengthen so that client can function comfortably at the usual level.

Short-Term Goal	Intervention	Rationale
1. Client's anxiety will decrease to moderate by (date).	1a. If hypercapnia occurs, instruct client to take slow, deep breaths. Breathe with the client to obtain cooperation.	1a. Focus is shifted away from distressing symptoms.
	1b. Keep expectations minimal and simple.	1b. Anxiety limits ability to attend to complex tasks.
2. Client will gain mastery over panic episodes by (date).	2a. Help client connect feelings before attack with onset of attack: ▪ "What were you thinking about just before the attack?" ▪ "Can you identify what you were feeling just before the attack?"	2a. Physiological symptoms of anxiety usually appear first as the result of a stressor. They are immediately followed by automatic thoughts, such as "I'm dying" or "I'm going crazy," which are distorted assessments.
	2b. Help client recognize symptoms as resulting from anxiety, not from a catastrophic physical problem. For example: ▪ Explain physical symptoms of anxiety. ▪ Discuss the fact that anxiety causes sensations similar to those of physical events, such as a heart attack.	2b. Factual information and alternative interpretations can help client recognize distortions in thought.
	2c. Identify for client effective therapies for panic episodes.	2c. Cognitive-behavioral treatment is highly effective. Antipanic medication is highly appropriate.
	2d. Teach client abdominal breathing, to be used immediately when anxiety is detected.	2d. Breathing exercises break the cycle of escalating symptoms of anxiety.
	2e. Teach client to use positive self-talk, such as "I can control my anxiety."	2e. Cognitive restructuring is an effective way to replace negative self-talk.
	2f. Teach client and family about any medication ordered for client's panic attacks.	2f. Client and family need to know what the medication can do, what the side effects and toxic effects are, and whom to call if untoward reactions occur.

ness. She fears that she is going to die. On these occasions, Dora telephones a friend to come over. The friend finds Dora wringing her hands, moaning, and appearing totally disorganized. In each instance, the friend takes Dora to the emergency department, where Dora remains overnight for observation and tests. All diagnostic test results are normal. The physician suggests that, because no apparent organic basis exists for the episodes, they likely are panic attacks.

■ ■ ■

Panic Disorder with Agoraphobia

Panic disorder with agoraphobia is a combination of the above symptoms and agoraphobia. Agoraphobia is intense, excessive anxiety or fear about being in places or situations from which escape might be difficult or embarrassing, or in which help might not be available if a panic attack occurred (APA, 2000). The feared places are avoided by the individual in an effort to control anxiety.

Examples of situations that are commonly avoided by clients with agoraphobia are being alone outside; being alone at home; traveling in a car, bus, or airplane; being on a bridge; and riding in an elevator. Avoidance behaviors can be debilitating and life constricting. Consider the effect on a father whose avoidance renders him unable to leave home and who thus cannot see his child's high school graduation, or the businesswoman whose avoidance of flying prevents her from attending distant business conferences. Refer to Figure 14-2 for the *DSM-IV-TR* criteria for panic disorders.

■ ■ ■ *VIGNETTE*

Jim is a 28-year-old man who suffers from panic attacks with agoraphobia. He once lived a very active life, often participating in thrill-seeking activities like bungee jumping and skydiving. Jim's father, who had severe cardiovascular disease, died 2 years previously on his way to work. Since that time, Jim has become increasingly fearful of the outdoors. He has gradually stopped leaving the family home because he experiences panic attacks; he fears that he will die if he leaves home.

■ ■ ■

Simple Agoraphobia

Agoraphobia without a history of panic disorder (i.e., unaccompanied by panic attacks) occurs only rarely, and it occurs early in the client's history. Over time, agoraphobia with panic attacks usually develops (APA, 2000).

Phobias

A phobia is a persistent, irrational fear of a specific object, activity, or situation that leads to a desire for avoidance, or actual avoidance, of the object, activity, or situation (APA, 2000).

Specific phobias are characterized by the experience of high levels of anxiety or fear in response to specific objects or situations, such as dogs, spiders, heights, storms, water, blood, closed spaces, tunnels, and bridges (APA, 2000). Specific phobias are common and usually do not cause much difficulty because people can contrive to avoid the feared object. Clinical names for common phobias are given in Table 14-3.

■ ■ ■ *VIGNETTE*

Tran, who lives and works in Philadelphia, developed a morbid fear of closed spaces, such as elevators, after he read about the bombing of the World Trade Center in New York, even though he was not directly affected by the attack. As his fear and anxiety intensified, it became necessary for him to use only stairs or escalators. Tran even became anxious if he had to enter closets or small storage rooms. Claustrophobia (fear of closed spaces) had developed.

■ ■ ■

TABLE 14-3

Clinical Names for Common Phobias

Clinical Name	Feared Object or Situation
Acrophobia	Heights
Agoraphobia	Open spaces
Astraphobia	Electrical storms
Claustrophobia	Closed spaces
Glossophobia	Talking
Hematophobia	Blood
Hydrophobia	Water
Monophobia	Being alone
Mysophobia	Germs or dirt
Nyctophobia	Darkness
Pyrophobia	Fire
Xenophobia	Strangers
Zoophobia	Animals

Social phobia, or social anxiety disorder, is characterized by severe anxiety or fear provoked by exposure to a social situation or a performance situation (e.g., fear of saying something that sounds foolish in public, not being able to answer questions in a classroom, eating in public, and performing on stage). Fear of public speaking is the most common social phobia.

Characteristically, phobic individuals experience overwhelming and crippling anxiety when they are faced with the object or situation provoking the phobia. Phobic people go to great lengths to avoid the feared object or situation. A phobic person may not be able to think about or visualize the object or situation without becoming severely anxious. The life of a phobic person becomes more restricted as activities are given up so that the phobic object can be avoided. All too frequently, complications ensue when people try to decrease anxiety through self-medication with alcohol or drugs. Figure 14-2 lists the *DSM-IV-TR* criteria for phobias.

■ ■ ■ *VIGNETTE*

Tim, a 22-year-old music theater major, develops a fear of performing on stage. He suffers severe anxiety attacks whenever he is scheduled to appear in a student production. Recently, he has become severely anxious when he is faced with giving classroom readings or singing solo in music class. He is thinking about changing his major.

■ ■ ■

Obsessive-Compulsive Disorder

Obsessions are defined as thoughts, impulses, or images that persist and recur, so that they cannot be dismissed from the mind. Obsessions often seem senseless (ego-dystonic) to the individual who experiences them, although they still cause the individual to experience severe anxiety.

Compulsions are ritualistic behaviors that an individual feels driven to perform in an attempt to reduce anxiety. Performing the compulsive act temporarily reduces high levels of anxiety. Primary gain is achieved by compulsive rituals, but because the relief is only temporary, the compulsive act must be repeated again and again.

Although obsessions and compulsions can exist independently of each other, they most often occur together. Examples of common obsessions and compulsions are given in Table 14-4. OCD behavior exists along a continuum. "Normal" individuals may experience mildly obsessive-compulsive behavior. Nearly everyone has had the experience of having a tune run persistently through the mind, despite attempts to push it away. Many people have had nagging doubts as to whether a door is locked or the stove is turned off. These doubts require the person to go back to

TABLE 14-4

Common Obsessions and Compulsions

Type of Obsession	Example	Accompanying Compulsion
Doubt, need to check	"Did I turn off the stove?" repeatedly intrudes on the thinking of a woman who has recently gone from being a housewife to holding a secretarial position.	Checks to see if appliance is turned off, returning home several times each workday.
Sexual imagery or ideation	Young woman has recurrent thought "Pat his buttocks" when in presence of a man.	Avoids the presence of men if possible; if with men, excuses self to wash hands every 10-15 minutes.
Need for order	"Everything must be in its place" is the recurrent thought.	Arranges and rearranges items.
Violence	Man repeatedly has the thought "I should kill her" when he sees a blonde woman.	Abruptly turns head away from women and squints eyes to try to avoid seeing blondes.
Germs or dirt	Woman ruminates, "Everything is contaminated."	Avoids touching all objects. Scrubs hands if forced to touch any object.

check the door or stove. Minor compulsions, such as touching a lucky charm, knocking on wood, and making the sign of the cross upon hearing disturbing news, are not harmful to the individual. Mild compulsions about timeliness, orderliness, and reliability are valued traits in U.S. society.

At the pathological end of the continuum are obsessive-compulsive symptoms that typically involve issues of sexuality, violence, contamination, illness, or death. These obsessions or compulsions cause marked distress to the individual. People often feel humiliation and shame regarding these behaviors. The rituals are time consuming and interfere with normal routine, social activities, and relationships with others. Severe OCD consumes so much of the individual's mental processes that the performance of cognitive tasks may be impaired. Figure 14-2 identifies the *DSM-IV-TR* criteria for OCD.

Generalized Anxiety Disorder

Generalized anxiety disorder (GAD) is characterized by excessive anxiety or worry about numerous things that lasts for 6 months or longer (APA, 2000). The individual with GAD also displays many of the following symptoms:

- Restlessness
- Fatigue
- Poor concentration
- Irritability
- Tension
- Sleep disturbance

The individual's worry is out of proportion to the true impact of the event or situation about which the individual is worried. Examples of worries typical in GAD are inadequacy in interpersonal relationships, job responsibilities, finances, health of family members, household chores, and lateness for appointments. Sleep disturbance is common because the individual worries about the day's events and real or imagined mistakes, reviews past problems, and anticipates future difficulties. Decision making is difficult, owing to poor concentration and dread of making a mistake. See Figure 14-2 for the *DSM-IV-TR* criteria for GAD and refer to Table 14-5 for a generic care plan for GAD. The Evidence-Based Practice box discusses research concerning effective treatment.

■ ■ ■ VIGNETTE

June is a 49-year-old legal secretary. She comes to the clinic complaining of feeling "so anxious I could jump out of my skin." She is shaky and diaphoretic; she has dilated pupils, an elevated pulse, and a quivering voice. She tells the nurse, "It was probably foolish to come here. Nobody understands me." June's only daughter is expecting her first child. Although the pregnancy is going well, June worries that something is wrong with the baby. "What if it's premature? What if it's deformed?"

June describes herself as tense and irritable. She has difficulty initiating sleep and cannot concentrate at her job. She worries about making mistakes at work, about being fired from her position, and about the financial problems that could result. She often says, "I just can't cope." Her daughter has begun calling several times a day to reassure her that all is well with the pregnancy and to try to decrease June's worry over other matters. The daughter has also begun shopping and housecleaning for June "to help her get some rest."

■ ■ ■

Treatment of Generalized Anxiety Disorder

Background

Generalized anxiety disorder (GAD) has a high prevalence rate, results in many visits to primary care providers for somatic complaints, and has an impact on workplace absenteeism. Studies over the past 20 years provide evidence of the benefits of cognitive-behavioral therapy (CBT) in the treatment of GAD.

Studies

Sixteen experimental studies have been reported and were analyzed as a group. The client population was two-thirds women, with an average age of 40 years, average GAD duration of 7 years, and average length of treatment of 11 sessions. CBT included teaching clients to engage in self-monitoring and observe their anxiety triggers, relaxation training, cognitive therapy to reduce expectation of negative events, and rehearsal of coping responses to graduated exposure to stressful situations. CBT was compared to low-dose diazepam therapy, placebo, supportive listening, and no treatment.

Results of Studies

CBT showed superior results compared with control treatments in the majority of studies, as measured by improved scores on standardized anxiety questionnaires. Clients receiving CBT also maintained or increased their degree of improvement at 6-month and 12-month follow-up.

Implications for Nursing Practice

Nurses need to teach clients with GAD that there are effective psychotherapy treatments for this disorder. Nurses may refer clients to appropriate resources in the community. Also, it is beneficial to teach anxious clients about the benefits of relaxation exercises whenever possible.

Borkovec, T. D., Newman, M. G., & Castonguay, L. G. (2003). Cognitive-behavioral therapy for generalized anxiety disorder with integrations from interpersonal and experiential therapies. *CNS Spectrums, 8*(5), 382-389.

Posttraumatic Stress Disorder

Posttraumatic stress disorder (PTSD) is characterized by repeated reexperiencing of a highly traumatic event that involved actual or threatened death or serious injury to self or others, to which the individual responded with intense fear, helplessness, or horror (APA, 2000). PTSD may occur after any traumatic event that is outside the range of usual experience. Examples are military combat; detention as a prisoner of war; natural disasters such as floods, tornadoes, and earthquakes; human disasters such as plane and train accidents; crime-related events such as bombing, assault, mugging, rape, and being taken hostage; or diagnosis of a life-threatening illness. PTSD symptoms often begin within 3 months after the trauma, but a delay of months or years is not uncommon (Figure 14-3). The major features of PTSD are the following:

- Persistent reexperiencing of the trauma through recurrent intrusive recollections of the event, through dreams, and through flashbacks. (Flashbacks are dissociative experiences during which the event is relived and the person behaves as though he or she is experiencing the event at that time.)
- Persistent avoidance of stimuli associated with the trauma, which results in the individual's avoiding talking about the event or avoiding activities, people, or places that arouse memories of the trauma.
- After the trauma, experience of persistent numbing of general responsiveness, as evidenced by the individual's feeling detached or estranged from others, feeling empty inside, or feeling turned off to others.

- After the trauma, experiencing of persistent symptoms of increased arousal, as evidenced by irritability, difficulty sleeping, difficulty concentrating, hypervigilance, or exaggerated startle response.

Difficulty with interpersonal, social, or occupational relationships nearly always accompanies PTSD, and trust is a common issue of concern. Child and spousal abuse may be associated with hypervigilance and irritability. Chemical abuse may begin as an attempt to self-medicate to relieve anxiety.

It is important for health care workers to realize that exposure to stimuli reminiscent of those associated with the original trauma may cause an exacerbation of the trauma. For example, one nurse therapist observed that the attack on the World Trade Center on September 11, 2001, caused an exacerbation of PTSD symptoms in veterans of World War II (Kaiman, 2003). See Case Study and Nursing Care Plan 14-1 at the end of the chapter, which describes a client with PTSD.

Acute Stress Disorder

Acute stress disorder occurs within 1 month after exposure to a highly traumatic event, such as those listed in the section on PTSD. To be diagnosed with acute stress disorder, the individual must display at least three dissociative symptoms either during or after the traumatic event: a subjective sense of numbing, detachment, or absence of emotional responsiveness; a reduction in awareness of surroundings; derealization (a sense of unreality related to the environment); depersonalization (experience of a sense of unreality or self-estrangement); or dissociative amnesia (loss of memory) (APA, 2000). By definition, acute stress disorder resolves within 4 weeks.

TABLE 14-5

Generic Care Plan for Generalized Anxiety Disorder

Nursing diagnosis: *Ineffective coping* related to persistent anxiety, fatigue, difficulty concentrating
Outcome criteria: Client will maintain role performance.

Short-Term Goal	Intervention	Rationale
1. Client will state that immediate distress is relieved by end of session.	1a. Stay with client. 1b. Speak slowly and calmly. 1c. Use short, simple sentences. 1d. Assure client that you are in control and can assist him or her. 1e. Give brief directions. 1f. Decrease excessive stimuli; provide quiet environment. 1g. After assessing level of anxiety, administer appropriate dose of anxiolytic agent, if warranted. 1h. Monitor and control own feelings.	1a. Conveys acceptance and ability to give help. 1b. Conveys calm and promotes security. 1c. Promotes comprehension. 1d. Counters feeling of loss of control that accompanies severe anxiety. 1e. Reduces indecision. Conveys belief that client can respond in a healthy manner. 1f. Reduces need to focus on diverse stimuli. Promotes ability to concentrate. 1g. Reduces anxiety and allows client to use coping skills. 1h. Anxiety is transmissible. Displays of negative emotion can cause client anxiety.

2. Client will be able to identify source of anxiety by (date).	2a. Encourage client to discuss preceding events.
	2b. Link client's behavior to feelings.
	2c. Teach cognitive therapy principles:
	  ■ Anxiety is the result of a dysfunctional appraisal of a situation.
	  ■ Anxiety is the result of automatic thinking.
	2d. Ask questions that clarify and dispute illogical thinking:
	  ■ "What evidence do you have?"
	  ■ "Explain the logic in that."
	  ■ "Are you basing that conclusion on fact or feeling?"
	  ■ "What's the worst thing that could happen?"
	2e. Have client give an alternative interpretation.
		2a. Promotes future change through identification of stressors.
		2b. Promotes self-awareness.
		2c. Provides a basis for behavioral change.
		
		2d. Helps promote accurate cognition.
		
		2e. Broadens perspective. Helps client think in a new way about problem or symptom.

3. Client will identify strengths and coping skills by (date).	3a. Provides awareness of self as individual with some ability to cope. 3b. Have client write assessment of strengths. 3c. Reframe situation in ways that are positive.	3a. Identify what has provided relief in the past. 3b. Increases self-acceptance. 3c. Provides a new perspective and converts distorted thinking.

■ ■ ■ *VIGNETTE*

Barbara, a 22-year-old college student, is sexually assaulted by a family friend. In the emergency department, she describes feeling detached from her body and being unaware of her surroundings during the assault, "as though it took place in a vacuum." She displays virtually no affect (i.e., she does not cry or appear anxious, angry, or sad). Barbara finds it difficult to concentrate on the examiner's questions. Three days later, Barbara still feels as though her mind is detached from her body; she reports having difficulty sleeping, not being able to concentrate, and startling whenever anyone touches her. When she sees the nurse 4 weeks after the event, Barbara expresses feelings of anger and sadness over the assault, displays the ability to concentrate, and states that she no longer feels as though her mind and body are detached. She describes being able to "sleep better" and "not being so jittery and easily startled."

■ ■ ■

Substance-Induced Anxiety Disorder

Substance-induced anxiety disorder is characterized by symptoms of anxiety, panic attacks, obsessions, and compulsions that develop with the use of a substance or within a month of stopping use of the substance

DSM-IV-TR CRITERIA FOR ANXIETY DISORDERS: STRESS RELATED

ANXIETY DISORDERS: STRESS RELATED

Posttraumatic Stress Disorder

1. The person experienced, witnessed, or was confronted with an event that involved actual, threatened death to self or others, responding in fear, helplessness, or horror.

2. The event is persistently reexperienced by:
   (a) Recurrent and intrusive recollections of the event, including images, thoughts, or perceptions
   (b) Distressing dreams or images
   (c) Reliving the event through flashbacks, illusions, hallucinations

3. Persistent avoidance of stimuli associated with trauma:
   (a) Avoidance of thoughts, feelings, conversations
   (b) Avoidance of people, places, activities
   (c) Inability to recall aspects of trauma
   (d) Decreased interest in usual activities
   (e) Feelings of detachment, estrangement from others
   (f) Restriction in feelings (love, enthusiasm, joy)
   (g) Sense of shortened feelings

4. Persistent symptoms of increased arousal (two or more):
   (a) Difficulty falling/staying asleep
   (b) Irritability/outbursts of anger
   (c) Difficulty concentrating

5. **Duration more than 1 month:**
   • Acute: duration less than 3 months
   • Chronic: duration 3 months or more
   • Delayed: onset of symptoms is at least 6 months after stress

Acute Stress Disorder

1. The person experienced, witnessed, or was confronted with an event that involved actual, threatened death to self or others, responding in fear, helplessness, or horror.

2. Three or more of the following dissociative symptoms:
   (a) Sense of numbing, detachment, or absence of emotional response
   (b) Reduced awareness of surroundings (e.g., "in a daze")
   (c) Derealization
   (d) Depersonalization
   (e) Amnesia for an important aspect of the trauma

3. The event is persistently reexperienced by:
   (a) Distressing dreams or images
   (b) Reliving the event through flashbacks, illusions, hallucinations
   (c) Distress on exposure to reminders of the traumatic event

4. Marked avoidance of stimuli that arouse memory of trauma (thoughts, feelings, people, places, activities, conversations).

5. Marked symptoms of anxiety:
   (a) Difficulty falling/staying asleep
   (b) Irritability/outbursts of anger
   (c) Difficulty concentrating

6. Causes impairment in social, occupational, and other functioning, or impairs ability to complete some memory tasks.

7. **Not due to drug abuse/medications or medical condition.**

8. **Lasts from 2 days to 4 weeks and occurs within 4 weeks of the traumatic event.**

FIGURE 14-3 Diagnostic criteria for anxiety disorders related to stress. (Adapted from American Psychiatric Association. [2000]. *Diagnostic and statistical manual of mental disorders* [4th ed., text rev.]. Washington, DC: Author.)

(APA, 2000). Evidence needs to be obtained through the history, physical examination, or laboratory findings that a substance is involved (e.g., alcohol, cocaine, heroin, hallucinogens).

Anxiety Due to Medical Conditions

In anxiety due to medical conditions, the individual's symptoms of anxiety are a direct physiological result of a medical condition, such as hyperthyroidism, pulmonary embolism, or cardiac dysrhythmias (APA, 2000). To determine whether the anxiety symptoms are due to a medical condition, a careful and comprehensive assessment of multiple factors is necessary. Once again, evidence must be present in the history, physical examination, or laboratory findings to diagnose the medical condition. Refer to Table 14-6 for a list of medical disorders that may contribute to anxiety symptoms.

Anxiety Disorder Not Otherwise Specified

Anxiety disorder not otherwise specified is a diagnosis used for disorders in which anxiety or phobic avoidance predominates but the symptoms do not

TABLE 14-6

Medical Causes of Anxiety

System	Disorders
Respiratory	Chronic obstructive pulmonary disease
	Pulmonary embolism
	Asthma
	Hypoxia
	Pulmonary edema
Cardiovascular	Angina pectoris
	Arrhythmias
	Congestive heart failure
	Hypertension
	Hypotension
	Mitral valve prolapse
Endocrine	Hyperthyroidism
	Hypoglycemia
	Pheochromocytoma
	Carcinoid syndrome
	Hypercortisolemia
Neurological	Delirium
	Essential tremor
	Complex partial seizures
	Parkinson's disease
	Akathisia
	Otoneurological disorders
	Postconcussion syndrome
Metabolic	Hypercalcemia
	Hyperkalemia
	Hyponatremia
	Porphyria

meet full diagnostic criteria for a specific anxiety disorder.

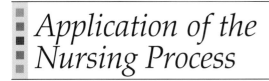

Application of the Nursing Process

■ ASSESSMENT
Overall Symptoms of Anxiety

People with anxiety disorders rarely need hospitalization unless they are suicidal or have compulsions causing injury (cutting self, banging a body part). Therefore, most clients prone to anxiety are encountered in a variety of community settings. A common example is an individual who is taken to an emergency department to rule out a heart attack when, in fact, the individual is experiencing a panic attack. Therefore, one of the first things that may need to be determined is whether the anxiety is due to a secondary source

(medical condition or substances) or due to a primary source, as in an anxiety disorder.

As previously described, the main symptoms of anxiety disorders are panic attacks, excessive anxiety, severe reactions to stress or trauma, phobias, obsessions, and compulsions.

Defenses Used in Anxiety Disorders

People use a variety of ego defenses and behaviors to lessen the uncomfortable levels of anxiety. Psychodynamic theorists believe that people who suffer from anxiety disorders employ specific defenses (Table 14-7). There is a simple preliminary screening test for anxiety disorders (Box 14-1). For cases in which a more comprehensive and sophisticated assessment is needed, the Hamilton Rating Scale for Anxiety is a popular tool (Table 14-8). See how you rate on either or both these tools. *A word of caution:* The Hamilton Rating Scale highlights important areas in the assessment of anxiety. Because many answers are subjective, experienced clinicians use this tool as a guide when planning care and also draw on their knowledge of their clients.

Self-Assessment

When working with an individual with an anxiety disorder, the nurse may experience uncomfortable personal reactions. Often, anxiety originating in the client is experienced by the nurse empathetically. The nurse may experience feelings of frustration or anger while working with the client with anxiety disorder. The rituals of the client with OCD may frustrate the nurse's need to accomplish certain tasks within a given time. Communication with the client with OCD can also be frustrating. Such a client corrects and clarifies repeatedly, as though the client cannot let go of any topic. If the nurse uses therapeutic communication techniques such as reflecting and paraphrasing, the client repeats the material, often angrily implying that the nurse has not understood. Communication requires much patience and the ability to provide clear structure.

In caring for the phobic client, the nurse may become frustrated after realizing that both client and nurse regard the fear as exaggerated and unrealistic, yet the client is still unable to overcome the avoidant behavior. Behavioral change is often accomplished slowly. The process of recovery is different from that seen in a client with an infection, who is given antibiotics and demonstrates improvement within 24 hours. Nurses tend to become impatient with the anxious client and may feel angry when the client does not make rapid progress. Negative feelings are easily transmitted to the client, who then feels increasingly anxious.

TABLE 14-7

Defenses Used in Anxiety Disorders

Phenomenon	Defense	Purpose	Example
Phobia	Displacement	In phobias, anxiety is reduced when strong feelings about the original object are directed at a less threatening object and that object is avoided.	Client has abnormal fear of cats. In therapy, it is discovered that the client unconsciously links cats to a feared and cruel mother.
Compulsion	Undoing	Performing a symbolic act cancels out an unacceptable act or idea.	Client performs symbolic rituals (e.g., hand washing, cleaning, and checking). Hand washing removes guilt. Cleaning removes dirty thoughts. Checking protects against hostile thoughts.
Obsession	Reaction-formation	Anxiety-producing unacceptable thoughts or feelings are kept out of awareness by the opposite feeling or idea.	Client with strong aggressive feelings toward husband repeatedly thinks the opposite ("I love him with all my heart") to keep hostile feelings out of awareness.
	Intellectualization	Excessive use of reasoning, logic, or words prevents the person from experiencing associated feelings.	Person talks in detail about parents' funeral but is unable to feel the associated pain of loss.
Posttraumatic stress disorder	Isolation	Facts associated with anxiety-laden events remain conscious, but associated painful feelings are separated from the experience.	Client describes feeling "numb and empty inside."
	Repression		Client is unable to trust authority figures at work after taking orders from commanding officer to kill civilians while in combat.

BOX 14-1

Preliminary Screening for Assessing Anxiety Symptoms

1. Do you ever experience a sudden unexplained attack of intense fear, anxiety, or panic?
2. Have you been afraid of not being able to get help or not being able to escape in certain situations, such as being on a bridge, in a crowded store, or in a similar situation?
3. Do you find it difficult to control your worrying?
4. Do you spend more time than is necessary doing things over and over again, such as washing your hands, checking things, or counting items?
5. Do you either avoid or feel very uncomfortable in situations involving people, such as parties, weddings, dating, dances, or other social events?
6. Have you ever had an extremely frightening, traumatic, or horrible experience such as being a victim of a crime, seriously injured in a car accident, sexually assaulted, or seeing someone injured or killed?

From Screening for Mental Health, Inc. (1999). *National Anxiety Disorders Screening Day: Sample test for anxiety disorder screening.* http://www.mentalhealthscreening.org.

The nurse who feels anger or frustration may withdraw from the client both emotionally and physically. As a result, the client feels increasingly anxious and also withdraws. Staging outcomes in small, attainable steps can help prevent the nurse from feeling overwhelmed by the client's slow progress and can help the client gain a sense of control.

At the very least, the nurse often experiences increased tension and fatigue from mental strain when working with anxious clients. Unlike the client whose dressing needs to be changed several times a week, the client with anxiety requires emotional bandaging many times a week.

By having a clear understanding of the emotional pitfalls of working with clients who have anxiety disorders, the nurse is more prepared to minimize and avoid guilt associated with strong negative feelings. By examining personal feelings, the nurse is better able to understand their origin and to act objectively and constructively.

TABLE 14-8

Hamilton Rating Scale for Anxiety

Max Hamilton designed this scale to help clinicians gather information about anxiety states. The symptom inventory provides scaled information that classifies anxiety behaviors and assists the clinician in targeting behaviors and achieving outcome measures. Provide a rating for each indicator based on the following scale: 0 = none; 1 = mild; 2 = moderate; 3 = disabling; 4 = severe, grossly disabling.

Item	Symptoms	Rating
1. Anxious mood	Worries, anticipation of the worst, fearful anticipation, irritability	_____
2. Tension	Feelings of tension, fatigability, startle response, moved to tears easily, trembling, feelings of restlessness, inability to relax	_____
3. Fear	Fearful of dark, strangers, being left alone, animals, traffic, crowds	_____
4. Insomnia	Difficulty in falling asleep, broken sleep, unsatisfying sleep and fatigue on waking, dreams, nightmares, night terrors	_____
5. Intellectual (cognitive) manifestations	Difficulty in concentration, poor memory	_____
6. Depressed mood	Loss of interest, lack of pleasure in hobbies, depression, early waking, diurnal swings	_____
7. Somatic (sensory) symptoms	Tinnitus, blurring of vision, hot and cold flushes, feelings of weakness, picking sensation	_____
8. Somatic (muscular) symptoms	Pains and aches, twitchings, stiffness, myoclonic jerks, grinding of teeth, unsteady voice, increased muscular tone	_____
9. Cardiovascular symptoms	Tachycardia, palpations, pain in chest, throbbing of vessels, fainting feelings, missing beat	_____
10. Respiratory symptoms	Pressure of constriction in chest, choking feelings, sighing, dyspnea	_____
11. Gastrointestinal symptoms	Difficulty in swallowing, wind, abdominal pain, burning sensations, abdominal fullness, nausea, vomiting, borborygmi, looseness of bowels, loss of weight, constipation	_____
12. Genitourinary symptoms	Frequency of micturition, urgency of micturition, amenorrhea, menorrhagia, development of frigidity, premature ejaculation, loss of libido, impotence	_____
13. Autonomic symptoms	Dry mouth, flushing, pallor, tendency to sweat, giddiness, tension headache, raising of hair	_____
14. Behavior at interview	Fidgeting, restlessness or pacing, tremor of hands, furrowed brow, strained face, sighing or rapid respiration, facial pallor, swallowing, belching, brisk tendon jerks, dilated pupils, exophthalmos	_____

Adapted from Hamilton, M. (1959). The assessment of anxiety states by rating. *British Journal of Medical Psychology, 32,* 50-55.

Assessment Guidelines Anxiety Disorders

1. Ensure that a sound physical and neurological examination is performed to help determine whether the anxiety is primary or is secondary to another psychiatric disorder, a medical condition, or substance use.
2. Assess for potential for self-harm and suicide, because it is known that people suffering from high levels of intractable anxiety may become desperate and attempt suicide.
3. Perform a psychosocial assessment. Always ask the person, "Why do you think you are so anxious?" The client may identify a problem that should be addressed by counseling (stressful marriage, recent loss, stressful job or school situation).
4. *Note:* Differences in culture can affect how anxiety is manifested.

■ NURSING DIAGNOSIS

The North American Nursing Diagnosis Association (NANDA) (2005) provides many nursing diagnoses that can be considered for clients experiencing anxiety and anxiety disorders. The "related-to" component will vary with the individual client. Table 14-9 identifies potential nursing diagnoses for the anxious client. Included are the signs and symptoms that might be found on assessment that support the diagnoses.

■ OUTCOME CRITERIA

The Nursing Outcomes Classification (NOC) identifies desired outcomes for clients with anxiety or anxiety-related disorders (Moorhead, Johnson, & Maas, 2004). Each outcome contains a definition and rating scale to measure the severity of the symptom or frequency of

TABLE 14-9

Potential Nursing Diagnoses for the Anxious Client

Signs and Symptoms	Nursing Diagnoses
■ Concern that a panic attack will occur ■ Exposure to phobic object or situation ■ Presence of obsessive thoughts ■ Recurrent memories of traumatic event ■ Fear of panic attacks	**Anxiety (moderate, severe, panic)** **Fear**
■ High levels of anxiety that interfere with the ability to work, disrupt relationships, and change ability to interact with others ■ Avoidance behaviors (phobia, agoraphobia) ■ Hypervigilance after a traumatic event ■ Inordinate time taken for obsession and compulsions	**Ineffective coping** **Deficient diversional activity** **Social isolation** **Ineffective role performance**
■ Difficulty with concentration ■ Preoccupation with obsessive thoughts ■ Disorganization associated with exposure to phobic object ■ Intrusive thoughts and memories of traumatic event ■ Excessive use of reason and logic associated with overcautiousness and fear of making a mistake	**Disturbed thought processes** **Posttrauma syndrome**
■ Inability to go to sleep related to intrusive thoughts, worrying, replaying of a traumatic event, hypervigilance, fear	**Disturbed sleep pattern** **Sleep deprivation** **Fatigue**
■ Feelings of hopelessness, inability to control one's life, low self-esteem related to inability to have some control in one's life	**Hopelessness** **Chronic low self-esteem** **Spiritual distress**
■ Inability to perform self-care related to rituals ■ Skin excoriation related to rituals of excessive washing or excessive picking at the skin	**Self-care deficit** **Impaired skin integrity**
■ Inability to eat because of constant ritual performance ■ Feeling of anxiety or excessive worrying that overrides appetite and need to eat	**Imbalanced nutrition: less than body requirements**
■ Excessive overeating to appease intense worrying or high anxiety levels	**Imbalanced nutrition: more than body requirements**

TABLE 14-10

NOC Outcomes for Anxiety Disorders

Nursing Outcome and Definition	Intermediate Indicators	Short-Term Indicators
Anxiety Self-Control: Personal actions to eliminate or reduce feelings of apprehension, tension, or uneasiness from an unidentifiable source*	Controls anxiety response Maintains role performance	Monitors intensity of anxiety Uses relaxation techniques to decrease anxiety Decreases environmental stimuli when anxious Maintains adequate sleep
Coping: Personal actions to manage stressors that tax an individual's resources*	Identifies multiple coping strategies Modifies lifestyle as needed	Reports decrease in physical symptoms of stress Identifies ineffective coping patterns Verbalizes need for assistance Seeks information concerning illness and treatment
Self-Esteem: Personal judgment of self-worth†	Describes pride in self Describes success in social groups	Maintenance of eye contact Maintenance of grooming/hygiene Acceptance of self-limitations Acceptance of compliments from others
Knowledge: Disease Process: Extent of understanding conveyed about a specific disease process‡	Describes usual disease course	Description of signs and symptoms Description of cause or contributing factors Description of signs and symptoms of complications Description of precautions to prevent complications

From Moorhead, S., Johnson, M., & Maas, M. (2004). *Nursing outcomes classification (NOC)* (3rd ed.). St. Louis, MO: Mosby.
*Indicators measured on a five-point Likert scale ranging from 1 (never demonstrated) to 5 (consistently demonstrated).
†Indicators measured on a five-point Likert scale ranging from 1 (never positive) to 5 (consistently positive).
‡Indicators measured on a five-point Likert scale ranging from 1 (none) to 5 (extensive).

the desired response. This rating scale enables the nurse to evaluate outcomes in the nursing care plan. Some of the NOC-recommended outcomes related to anxiety include the following: *Anxiety Self-Control, Anxiety Level, Stress Level, Coping, Social Interaction Skills,* and *Symptom Control.* Refer to Table 14-10 for examples of intermediate and short-term indicators related to NOC outcomes.

■ PLANNING

Anxiety disorders are encountered in numerous settings. Nurses care for people with concurrent anxiety disorders in medical-surgical units and in outpatient settings, such as homes, day programs, and clinics. Usually clients with anxiety disorders do not require admission to inpatient psychiatric units. Therefore, planning for care usually involves selecting interventions that can be implemented in a community setting.

Whenever possible, the client should be encouraged to participate actively in planning. By sharing decision making with the client, the nurse increases the likelihood that positive outcomes will be attained. Shared planning is especially appropriate for a client with mild or moderate anxiety. When the client is experiencing severe levels of anxiety, the client may be unable to participate in planning, which requires the nurse to take a more directive role.

Earlier in this chapter you were given examples of care plans for clients with panic disorder and GAD. Also refer to Case Study and Nursing Care Plan 14-1 involving a client with PTSD.

■ INTERVENTION

The nurse uses the *Scope and Standards of Psychiatric-Mental Health Nursing Practice* (American Nurses Association, American Psychiatric Nurses Association, & International Society of Psychiatric-Mental Health Nurses, 2000) when intervening with clients. The Nursing Interventions Classification (NIC) offers pertinent interventions in the behavioral and safety domains (Dochterman & Bulechek, 2004). Refer to Box 14-2 for potential nursing interventions.

Overall guidelines for basic nursing interventions are as follows:

1. Identify community resources that can offer the client specialized treatment which is proven to be highly effective for people with a variety of anxiety disorders.
2. Identify community support groups for people with specific anxiety disorders and their families.
3. Use counseling, milieu therapy, promotion of self-care activities, and psychobiological and health teaching interventions as appropriate.

BOX 14-2

NIC Interventions for Anxiety Disorders

Anxiety Reduction

Definition: Minimizing apprehension, dread, foreboding, or uneasiness related to an unidentified source of anticipated danger

Activities*:
- Observe for verbal and nonverbal signs of anxiety.
- Instruct the patient in the use of relaxation techniques.
- Create an atmosphere to facilitate trust.
- Use a calm, reassuring approach.

Coping Enhancement

Definition: Assisting a patient to adapt to perceived stressors, changes, or threats that interfere with meeting life demands and roles

Activities*:
- Provide an atmosphere of acceptance.
- Encourage verbalization of feelings, perceptions, and fears.
- Acknowledge the patient's spiritual/cultural background.
- Discourage decision making when the patient is under severe stress.

Hope Instillation

Definition: Facilitation of the development of a positive outlook in a given situation

Activities*:
- Assist the patient to identify areas of hope in life.
- Demonstrate hope by recognizing the patient's intrinsic worth and viewing the patient's illness as only one facet of the individual.
- Avoid masking the truth.
- Help the patient expand spiritual self.

Self-Esteem Enhancement

Definition: Assisting a patient to increase his or her personal judgment of self-worth

Activities*:
- Make positive statements about the patient.
- Monitor frequency of self-negating verbalizations.
- Explore previous achievements.
- Explore reasons for self-criticism or guilt.

Simple Relaxation Therapy

Definition: Use of techniques to encourage and elicit relaxation for the purpose of decreasing undesirable signs and symptoms such as pain, muscle tension, or anxiety

Activities*:
- Demonstrate and practice the relaxation technique with the patient.
- Provide written information about preparing and engaging in relaxation techniques.
- Anticipate the need for the use of relaxation.
- Evaluate and document the response to relaxation therapy.

From Dochterman, J. M, & Bulechek, G. M. (2004). *Nursing interventions classification (NIC)* (4th ed.). St. Louis, MO: Mosby.
*Partial list.

Counseling

Basic level psychiatric mental health nurses use counseling to assist clients with anxiety disorders to reduce anxiety, enhance coping and communication skills, and intervene in crises. When clients request or prefer to use integrative therapies, the nurse performs assessment and teaching as appropriate.

Advanced practice nurses use treatment approaches that include cognitive or cognitive-behavioral therapy, relaxation training, and the behavioral techniques of modeling, systematic desensitization, flooding, and response prevention. Refer to Box 14-3 for a description of these specialized treatments. Also refer to Table 14-11 for a description of medications and psychotherapy for specific disorders.

Milieu Therapy

As mentioned earlier, most clients who demonstrate anxiety disorders can be treated successfully as outpatients. Hospital admission is necessary only if severe anxiety or symptoms that interfere with the individual's health are present, or if the individual is suicidal. When hospitalization is necessary, the following features of the therapeutic milieu can be especially helpful to the client:

- Structuring the daily routine to offer physical safety and predictability, thus reducing anxiety over the unknown
- Providing daily activities to promote sharing and cooperation
- Providing therapeutic interactions, including one-on-one nursing care and behavior contracts

---

BOX 14-3

Advanced Practice Interventions for Anxiety Disorders

Cognitive Therapy

Cognitive therapy is based on the belief that clients make errors in thinking that lead to mistaken negative beliefs about self and others. For example, "I have to be perfect or my husband will not love me." Through a process called cognitive restructuring, the therapist helps the client to identify automatic negative beliefs that cause anxiety, to explore the basis for these thoughts, to reevaluate the situation realistically, and to replace negative self-talk with supportive ideas.

Behavioral Therapy

Behavioral therapy uses various techniques that involve teaching and physical practice of activities to decrease anxious or avoidant behavior.

- Relaxation training—Relaxation exercises for breathing or muscle groups are taught. The relaxation response is the opposite of the stress response, for example, slowed heart rate and breathing, relaxed muscles. Refer to Chapter 12 for a description of different approaches.
- Modeling—The therapist or significant other acts as a role model to demonstrate appropriate behavior in a feared situation and then the client imitates it. For example, the role model rides in an elevator with a claustrophobic client.
- Systemic desensitization—Graduated exposure is used in which the client is gradually introduced to a feared object or experience through a series of steps, from the least frightening to the most frightening. The client is taught to use a relaxation technique at each step when anxiety gets too overwhelming. For example, a client with agoraphobia would start with opening the door to the house to go out on the steps and advance to attending a movie in a theater. The therapist may start with imagined situations in the office before moving on to in vivo (live) exposures.

- Flooding—Unlike gradual desensitization, this method exposes the client to a large amount of an undesirable stimulus in an effort to extinguish the anxiety response. The client learns through a prolonged exposure that survival is possible and that anxiety diminishes spontaneously. For example, an obsessive client who usually touches objects with a paper towel may be forced to touch objects with a bare hand for 1 hour. By the end of that period, the anxiety level is lower.
- Response prevention—In this method, which is used for compulsive behavior, the therapist does not allow the client to perform the compulsive ritual (e.g., hand washing) and the client learns that anxiety does subside even when the ritual is not completed. After trying this in the office, the client learns to set time limits at home to gradually lengthen the time between rituals until the urge fades away.
- Thought stopping—In this technique a negative thought or obsession is interrupted. The client may be instructed to say "Stop!" out loud when the idea comes to mind or to snap a rubber band worn on the wrist. This distraction briefly blocks the automatic undesirable thought and cues the client to select an alternative, more positive idea. (After learning the exercise, the client gives the command silently.)

Cognitive-Behavioral Therapy

Cognitive-behavioral therapy combines cognitive therapy with specific behavioral therapies to reduce the anxiety response. Cognitive-behavioral therapy includes cognitive restructuring, psychoeducation, breathing restraining and muscle relaxation, teaching of self-monitoring for panic and other symptoms, and in vivo exposure to feared objects or situations.

TABLE 14-11

Medications and Psychotherapy for Anxiety Disorders

Disorder	Pharmacotherapy	Psychotherapy
Generalized anxiety disorder	Selective serotonin reuptake inhibitors (SSRIs) Tricyclic antidepressants (TCAs) Buspirone (BuSpar) Serotonin-norepinephrine reuptake inhibitor (SNRI) Valproic acid (Depakene)	Cognitive-behavioral therapy
Obsessive-compulsive disorder	SSRIs, especially fluvoxamine (Luvox) TCAs, especially clomipramine (Anafranil)	Behavioral therapy
Panic disorder	SSRIs Benzodiazepines TCAs Monoamine oxidase inhibitors (MAOIs) β-blockers Valproic acid (Depakote)	Cognitive-behavioral therapy
Posttraumatic stress disorder	SSRIs TCAs Benzodiazepines SNRI MAOIs β-blockers Carbamazepine (Tegretol)	Cognitive-behavioral therapy Family therapy Group therapy with survivors
Social phobia or social anxiety disorder	SSRIs Benzodiazepines Buspirone β-blockers Gabapentin (Neurontin)	Cognitive-behavioral therapy

Data from Brown, A. B. (2003). Panic disorder: Highly disabling, yet treatable. *NARSAD Research Newsletter, 15*(3), 24-28; Hambrick, J. P., et al. (2003). Cognitive-behavioral therapy for social anxiety disorder: Supporting evidence and future directions. *CNS Spectrums, 8*(5), 373-381; Myrick, H., & Brady K. (2003). Editorial review: Current review of the comorbidity of affective, anxiety, and substance use disorders. *Current Opinions in Psychiatry 16*(3), 261-270; Overbeek, T., et al. (2002). Comorbidity of obsessive-compulsive disorder and depression: Prevalence, symptom severity, and treatment effect. *Journal of Clinical Psychiatry, 63*(12), 1106-1112; Perugi, G., et al. (2002). *Journal of Clinical Psychiatry, 63*(12), 1129-1134; Resick, P. A., et al. (2003). How well does cognitive-behavioral therapy treat symptoms of complex PTSD? *CNS Spectrums, 8*(15), 340-342, 351-355; Simon, N. M., & Rosenbaum, J. F. (2003). Anxiety and depression comorbidity: Implications and intervention. *Medscape Psychiatry & Mental Health, 8*(1), 2003. Retrieved May 13, 2003, from Medscape website: http://www.medscape.com/viewarticle/474626.

- Including the client in decisions about his or her own care

Promotion of Self-Care Activities

Clients with anxiety disorders are usually able to meet their own basic physical needs. Self-care activities that are most likely to be affected are discussed in the following sections.

Nutrition and Fluid Intake

Clients who engage in ritualistic behaviors may be too involved with their rituals to take time to eat and drink; some phobic clients may be so afraid of germs that they cannot eat. In general, nutritious diets with snacks should be provided. Adequate intake should be firmly encouraged, but a power struggle should be avoided. Weighing clients frequently (e.g., three times a week) is useful in assessing nutrition.

Personal Hygiene and Grooming

Some clients, especially those with OCD and phobias, may be excessively neat and may engage in time-consuming rituals associated with bathing and dressing. Hygiene, dressing, and grooming may take many hours. Maintenance of skin integrity may become a problem when the rituals involve excessive washing and the skin becomes excoriated and infected.

Some clients are indecisive about bathing or about what clothing should be worn. For the latter, limiting choices to two outfits is helpful. In the event of severe indecisiveness, simply presenting the client with the clothing to be worn may be necessary. The nurse may also need to remain with the client to give simple directions: "Put on your shirt . . . now, put on your slacks." Matter-of-fact support is effective in assisting the client to perform as much of the task as possible. The client should be encouraged to express thoughts and feelings about self-care. This communication can provide a basis for later health teaching or for ongoing dialogue about the client's abilities.

Elimination

Clients with OCD may be so involved with the performance of rituals that they may suppress the urge to void and defecate. Constipation and urinary tract infections may result. Interventions may include creating a regular schedule for taking the client to the bathroom.

Sleep

Anxious clients frequently have difficulty sleeping. Ritualistic clients may perform their rituals to the exclusion of resting and sleeping. Physical exhaustion may occur in highly ritualistic clients. Clients with GAD, PTSD, and acute stress disorder often experience sleep disturbance from nightmares. Teaching clients ways to promote sleep (e.g., warm bath, warm milk, relaxing music) and monitoring sleep through a sleep record are useful interventions. Refer to Chapter 33 for an in-depth discussion of sleep disturbances.

Psychobiological Interventions

Psychobiological interventions include use of simple relaxation exercises and administration of medications. Several classes of medication have been found to be effective in the treatment of anxiety disorders. Refer to Table 14-12 for names and dosages of common medications, and to Table 14-11 for medications used to treat specific disorders. Also, review Chapter 3 for more detailed explanation of the actions of psychotropic medications.

Antidepressants

Selective serotonin reuptake inhibitors (SSRIs) are the first-line treatment for anxiety disorders (Simon & Rosenbaum, 2003). They are preferable to the tricyclic antidepressants (TCAs) because they have more rapid onset of action and fewer problematic side effects. Monoamine oxidase inhibitors (MAOIs) are reserved for treatment-resistant conditions because of the risk of life-threatening hypertensive crisis if the client does not follow dietary restrictions (clients cannot eat foods containing tyramine and must be given specific dietary instructions). Venlafaxine (Effexor) is a serotonin-norepinephrine reuptake inhibitor (SNRI) that is also useful for treatment of anxiety disorders.

Antidepressants have the secondary benefit of treating comorbid depressive disorders in clients. However, there are three notes of caution (Simon & Rosenbaum, 2003). When treatment is started, low doses of SSRIs must be used because of the activating effect, which temporarily increases anxiety symptoms. Also, in clients with co-occurring bipolar disorder, use of an antidepressant may cause a manic episode, which requires

TABLE 14-12

Medications for Anxiety Disorders

Generic Name (Trade Name)	Usual Daily Dose (mg/day)
Antidepressants	
Selective Serotonin Reuptake Inhibitors	
Citalopram (Celexa)	20-40
Escitalopram (Lexapro)	10-20
Fluoxetine (Prozac)	20-80
Fluvoxamine (Luvox)	50-300
Paroxetine (Paxil)	20-60
Sertraline (Zoloft)	50-200
Tricyclics	
Amitriptyline (Elavil)	50-150
Clomipramine (Anafranil)	50-125
Imipramine (Tofranil)	150-500
Nortriptyline (Aventyl, Pamelor)	75-125
Monoamine Oxidase Inhibitor	
Phenelzine (Nardil)	30-90
Serotonin-Norepinephrine Reuptake Inhibitor	
Venlafaxine (Effexor)	37.5-225.0
Anxiolytics	
Benzodiazepines	
Alprazolam (Xanax)	0.25-4.0
Chlordiazepoxide (Librium)	15-75
Clonazepam (Klonopin)	0.5-4.0
Diazepam (Valium)	4-40
Lorazepam (Ativan)	0.5-6.0
Nonbenzodiazepine	
Buspirone (BuSpar)	30-60
Other Classes	
Antihistamines	
Hydroxyzine hydrochloride (Atarax)	100-300
Hydroxyzine pamoate (Vistaril)	100-300
β-Blocker	
Propranolol (Inderal)	15-40
Anticonvulsants	
Carbamazepine (Tegretol)*	400-1200
Gabapentin (Neurontin)	300-1800
Valproic acid (Depakote)*	500-1000

*Based on therapeutic blood levels.

the addition of mood stabilizers or even antipsychotic agents. Further, use of MAOIs is contraindicated in clients with comorbid substance abuse because of the risk of hypertensive crisis with use of stimulant drugs.

Anxiolytics

Anxiolytic drugs (also called *antianxiety drugs*) are often used to treat the somatic and psychological symptoms of anxiety disorders. When moderate or severe anxiety is reduced, clients are better able to participate in treatment directed at their underlying problems. Benzodiazepines are most commonly used because they have a quick onset of action. Because of the potential for dependence, however, these medications should ideally be used for short periods only until other medication or treatment reduces symptoms. It is important for the nurse to monitor for side effects of the benzodiazepines, including sedation, ataxia, and decreased cognitive function. Benzodiazepines are not recommended for clients with a known substance use problem and should not be given to women during pregnancy or breast feeding. Refer to Box 14-4 for important information for client teaching.

Buspirone (BuSpar) is an alternative anxiolytic medication that does not cause dependence, but 2 to 4 weeks are required for it to reach full effects. The drug may be used for long-term treatment and must be taken regularly.

Other Classes of Medication

Other classes of medication sometimes used to treat anxiety disorders include β-blockers, antihistamines, and anticonvulsants. These agents are often added if the first course of treatment is ineffective. The β-blockers have been used to treat panic disorder and social anxiety disorder (SAD) (Simon & Rosenbaum,

---

BOX 14-4

Client and Family Medication Teaching: Anxiety Disorders

1. Caution the client
   - Not to increase dose or frequency of ingestion without prior approval of therapist.
   - That these medications reduce the ability to handle mechanical equipment (e.g., cars, saws, and machinery).
   - Not to drink alcoholic beverages or take other antianxiety drugs because depressant effects of both would be potentiated.
   - To avoid drinking beverages containing caffeine because they decrease the desired effects of the drug.
2. Recommend that the client taking benzodiazepines avoid becoming pregnant because these drugs increase the risk of congenital anomalies.
3. Advise the client not to breast-feed because these drugs are excreted in the milk and would have adverse effects on the infant.
4. Teach a client who is taking monoamine oxidase inhibitors about the details of a tyramine-restricted diet (see Chapter 18).
5. Teach the client that
   - Cessation of benzodiazepine use after 3 to 4 months of daily use may cause withdrawal symptoms such as insomnia, irritability, nervousness, dry mouth, tremors, convulsions, and confusion.
   - Medications should be taken with, or shortly after, meals or snacks to reduce gastrointestinal discomfort.
   - Drug interactions can occur: Antacids may delay absorption; cimetidine interferes with metabolism of benzodiazepines, causing increased sedation; central nervous system depressants, such as alcohol and barbiturates, cause increased sedation; serum phenytoin concentration may build up because of decreased metabolism.

2003). Anticonvulsants have shown some benefit in management of GAD, SAD, and comorbid depression with SAD or panic disorder (Myrick, 2003). They are also useful for treatment of clients with comorbid substance dependence, because use of benzodiazepines is discouraged for such clients. Antihistamines are a safe, nonaddictive alternative to benzodiazepines to lower anxiety levels and again are helpful in treating clients with substance use problems.

Health Teaching

Health teaching is a significant nursing intervention for clients with anxiety disorders. Clients may conceal symptoms for years before seeking treatment and often come to the attention of the nurse due to a co-occurring problem. For example, one study found that only 60% of people who experience panic attacks seek medical treatment (Katerndahl, 2002, p. 464). Teaching about the specific disorder and available effective treatments is a major step to improving the quality of life of these clients.

In the community or hospital setting, the nurse teaches the client about signs and symptoms of the disorder; theory regarding causes or risk factors; risk of co-occurrence with other disorders, especially substance abuse; medication use; use of relaxation exercises; and availability of specialized treatment such as cognitive-behavioral therapy.

Integrative Therapy

Chapter 12 identified a number of complementary practices or integrative therapies that people use to cope with stress in their lives. Herbal therapy is very popular, and Americans spend an estimated $2 billion to $5 billion annually for these products (Hatcher, 2001). However, herbs and dietary supplements are not subject to the same rigorous testing as prescription medications. Also, herbs and dietary supplements are not required to be uniform, and there is no guarantee of bioequivalence of the active compound across preparations (McEnany, 2000). Problems that can occur with the use of psychotropic herbs include toxic side effects and herb-drug interactions. It is important for nurses and other health care providers to improve their knowledge of these products so that they can discuss them with their clients and provide reliable information. The Integrative Therapy box discusses kava kava. Also refer to Chapter 37 for more information.

■ EVALUATION

Identified outcomes serve as the basis for evaluation. Each NOC outcome has a built-in rating scale that helps the nurse to measure improvement. In general, evaluation of outcomes for clients with anxiety disorders deals with questions such as the following:

INTEGRATIVE THERAPY

Kava kava

Kava kava is prepared from a South Pacific plant *(Piper methysticum)* and is used as an herbal sedative with antianxiety effects. Before seeking psychiatric treatment, clients with anxiety disorders may try kava kava in the belief that herbs are safer than medications. But kava kava may interact with any drugs metabolized by the liver, especially central nervous system depressants such as the benzodiazepines. There are reports of elevated liver enzyme levels in clients taking kava kava and one documented case of liver failures in a client who took this herb for 2 months.

Before administering medications to clients with anxiety disorders, the nurse must assess for the use of kava kava or other herbal supplements to avoid toxic effects.

Dasgupta, A. (2003). Review of abnormal laboratory test results and toxic effects due to herbal medicines. *American Journal of Clinical Pathology, 120*(1), 127-137.

- Is the client experiencing a reduced level of anxiety?
- Does the client recognize symptoms as anxiety related?
- Does the client continue to display obsessions, compulsions, phobias, worrying, or other symptoms of anxiety disorders? If still present, are they more or less frequent? more or less intense?
- Is the client able to use newly learned behaviors to manage anxiety?
- Can the client adequately perform self-care activities?
- Can the client maintain satisfying interpersonal relations?
- Can the client assume usual roles?

CASE STUDY and NURSING CARE PLAN 14-1 — Posttraumatic Stress Disorder

Mr. Blake is brought to the emergency department by his wife after she finds him writing a suicide note and planning to take a bottle of prescription sleeping pills.

Mr. Blake is subdued, shows minimal affect, and has the odor of alcohol on his breath. When asked about his suicidal thoughts, he states that he is worthless and that his wife and family would be better off if he were dead. He refuses to contract for safety. The decision is made to hospitalize him to protect him from danger to self.

Mr. Blake's wife gives further history. Her husband is a 50-year-old retired firefighter who was part of the emergency team that responded to the World Trade Center terrorist attack on September 11, 2001. He lost half of his crew members in the fire. A few months later, he decided to take an early retirement so that he and his wife could move south to be near their daughter's family. Initially, he showed no signs of anxiety and refused offers of crisis treatment: "I was in Vietnam, I can handle stress." But 6 months later, Ms. Blake noticed that he had trouble sleeping, his mood was irritable or withdrawn, he avoided news reports on television, and he started drinking daily. He complained of nightmares but would not talk to her about his fears. He only agreed to go to the primary care physician to request sleeping medication.

Mr. Blake is admitted to the psychiatric unit and is assigned to a nurse, Ms. Dawson. He is passive as she orients him to the unit, but she observes that he looks all around carefully and is easily startled by sounds on the unit.

Self-Assessment

Ms. Dawson is a registered nurse with an AA degree and 3 years of experience on this unit. Initially, she feels sympathy for Mr. Blake, and he reminds her of her Uncle James, who also served in Vietnam. She is concerned because his suicide plan was lethal and he is guarded in his speech, not revealing his thoughts or feelings. She realizes that as she implements suicide precautions, she must demonstrate an attitude of hope and acceptance to encourage him to develop trust. Also, she must stay neutral and not convey any pity or sympathy. As a firefighter, Mr. Blake was once a care provider, and he already feels like a failure because he could not save his friends or prevent his own symptoms.

■ ASSESSMENT

Objective Data

- Sleep difficulty, nightmares
- Hypervigilance
- Alcohol use
- Withdrawn mood
- Guarded affect
- Avoidance of news coverage with potential for emergency reports
- Refusal of treatment and safety contract
- Plan for suicide

Subjective Data

- "I don't deserve to live, I should have died with the others."
- "You can't stop me."

■ NURSING DIAGNOSIS (NANDA)

Risk for suicide related to anger and hopelessness due to severe trauma, as evidenced by suicidal plan and verbalization of intent

- Lethal plan with saved prescription medication and alcohol
- Refusal to contract for safety
- Emotional withdrawal from wife

■ OUTCOME CRITERIA (NOC)

Client will consistently refrain from attempting suicide.

■ PLANNING

The initial plan is to maintain safety for Mr. Blake while encouraging him to express feelings and recognize that his situation is not hopeless.

■ INTERVENTION (NIC)

Mr. Blake's plan of care is personalized as follows:

Short-Term Goal	Intervention	Rationale	Evaluation
1. Client will speak to staff whenever experiencing self-destructive thoughts.	**1a.** Administer medications with mouth checks. **1b.** Provide ongoing surveillance of client and environment. **1c.** Contract for "no self-harm" for specified periods. **1d.** Use direct, nonjudgmental approach in discussing suicide. **1e.** Provide illness teaching regarding PTSD.	**1a.** Addresses risk of hiding medications. **1b.** Provides one-to-one monitoring for safety. **1c.** Encourages increased self-control. **1d.** Shows acceptance of client's situation with respect. **1e.** Offers reality of treatment.	GOAL MET After 8 hours, client contracts for safety every shift and starts to discuss feelings of self-harm.
2. Client will express feelings by the third day of hospitalization.	**2a.** Interact with client at regular intervals to convey caring and openness and to provide an opportunity to talk. **2b.** Use silence and listening to encourage expression of feelings. **2c.** Be open to expressions of loneliness and powerlessness. **2d.** Share observations or thoughts about client's behavior or response.	**2a.** Encourages development of trust. **2b.** Shows positive expectation that client will respond. **2c.** Allows client to voice these uncomfortable feelings. **2d.** Directs attention to here-and-now treatment situation.	GOAL MET By second day, client occasionally answers questions about feelings and admits to anger and grief.
3. Client will express will to live by discharge from unit.	**3a.** Listen to expressions of grief. **3b.** Encourage client to identify own strengths and abilities. **3c.** Explore with client previous methods of dealing with life problems. **3d.** Assist in identifying available support systems. **3e.** Refer to spiritual advisor of individual's choice.	**3a.** Supports client that such feelings are natural. **3b.** Affirms client's worth and potential to survive. **3c.** Reinforces client's past coping skills and ability to problem-solve now. **3d.** Addresses fact that anxiety has narrowed client's perspective, distorting reality about loved ones. **3e.** Allows opportunity to explore spiritual values and self-worth.	GOAL MET By third day, client becomes tearful and states that he does not want to hurt his wife and daughter.

■ EVALUATION

See individual outcomes and evaluation within the care plan.

evolve Visit the Evolve website at **http://evolve.elsevier.com/Varcarolis** for a full case study of this client and more case studies and nursing care plans.

■ ■ ■ KEY POINTS to REMEMBER

- Anxiety disorders are the most common psychiatric disorders in the United States and frequently co-occur with depression or substance abuse.
- Research has identified genetic and biological factors in the etiology of anxiety disorders.
- Psychological theories and cultural influences are also pertinent to the understanding of anxiety disorders.
- Clients with anxiety disorders suffer from panic attacks, irrational fears, excessive worrying, uncontrollable rituals, or severe reactions to stress.

- People with anxiety disorders are often too embarrassed or ashamed to seek psychiatric help. Instead, they go to primary care providers with multiple somatic complaints.
- Psychiatric treatment is effective for anxiety disorders.
- Basic level nursing interventions include counseling, milieu therapy, promotion of self-care activities, psychobiological intervention, and health teaching.
- Advanced practice nursing interventions include cognitive and behavioral therapy.

Visit the Evolve website at **http://evolve.elsevier.com/Varcarolis** for a posttest on the content in this chapter.

Critical Thinking and Chapter Review

Visit the Evolve website at **http://evolve.elsevier.com/Varcarolis** for additional self-study exercises.

■ ■ ■ CRITICAL THINKING

1. Ms. Smith, a client with OCD, washes her hands until they are cracked and bleeding. Your nursing goal is to promote healing of her hands. What interventions will you plan?

2. This is Mr. Olivetti's third emergency department visit in a week. He is experiencing severe anxiety accompanied by many physical symptoms. He clings to you, desperately crying, "Help me! Help me! Don't let me die!" Diagnostic tests have ruled out a physical disorder. The client outcome has been identified as "Client anxiety level will be reduced to moderate/mild within 1 hour." What interventions should you use?

   Mr. Olivetti is given an appointment at the anxiety disorders clinic. How will you explain the importance of keeping the clinic appointment?

3. Mrs. Zeamans is a client with GAD. She has a history of substance abuse and is now a recovering alcoholic. During a clinic visit, she tells you she plans to ask the psychiatrist to prescribe diazepam (Valium) to use when she feels anxious. She asks whether you think this is a good idea. How would you respond? What action could you take?

4. You are to perform a nursing assessment of Ms. Lee, a Southeast Asian refugee. What cultural considerations might be pertinent in conducting the assessment?

■ ■ ■ CHAPTER REVIEW

Choose the most appropriate answer.

1. Interventions that would be helpful in caring for clients with anxiety disorders include the following:
   1. Help the client link feelings and behaviors.
   2. Leave the anxious client alone as much as possible.
   3. Advise the client to minimize daily exercise to conserve endorphins.
   4. Teach the client the importance of maintaining caffeine intake at 750 mg or more daily.

2. One possible reason for panic disorder may be
   1. faulty learning.
   2. dopamine deficiency.
   3. inhibition of GABA.
   4. clomipramine (Anafranil) excess.

3. Mrs. T. is preoccupied with persistent intrusive thoughts and impulses and performs ritualistic acts repetitively. She expresses distress that her attention is so consumed that she cannot accomplish her usual daily activities. These symptoms are most consistent with the *DSM-IV-TR* diagnosis of
   1. panic disorder.
   2. social phobia.
   3. GAD.
   4. OCD.

4. In addition to prescribing SSRIs to treat Mr. G.'s panic disorder, the nurse psychotherapist is likely to recommend
   1. family therapy.
   2. psychoanalysis.
   3. vocational rehabilitation.
   4. cognitive-behavioral therapy.

5. A strategy nurses can employ to help clients with anxiety disorders replace negative self-talk is
   1. systematic desensitization and graduated exposure.
   2. counseling to promote cognitive restructuring.
   3. relaxation training.
   4. implosion therapy.

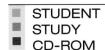

■ STUDENT
■ STUDY
■ CD-ROM

Access the accompanying CD-ROM for animations, interactive exercises, review questions for the NCLEX examination, and an audio glossary.

■ NURSE,
■ CLIENT, AND
■ FAMILY RESOURCES

For suggested readings, information on related associations, and Internet resources, go to **http://evolve.elsevier.com/Varcarolis.** *evolve*

REFERENCES

American Nurses Association, American Psychiatric Nurses Association, & International Society of Psychiatric-Mental Health Nurses. (2000). *Scope and standards of psychiatric-mental health nursing practice*. Washington, DC: American Nurses Publishing.

American Psychiatric Association. (2000). *Diagnostic and statistical manual of mental disorders (DSM-IV-TR)* (4th ed., text rev.). Washington, DC: Author.

Anxiety Disorders Association of America. (2003). *Statistics and facts about anxiety disorders*. Retrieved December 29, 2004, from http://www.adaa.org/mediaroom/index.cfm.

Brown, A. B. (2003). Panic disorder: Highly disabling, yet treatable. *NARSAD Research Newsletter, 15*(3), 24-28.

Dochterman, J. M., & Bulechek, G. M. (2004). Nursing interventions classification (NIC) (4th ed.). St. Louis, MO: Mosby.

Gorman, J. M. (2000). Anxiety disorders: Introduction and overview. In B. J. Sadock & V. A. Sadock (Eds.), *Comprehensive textbook of psychiatry* (7th ed., Vol. 1, pp. 1441-1444). Philadelphia: Lippincott Williams & Wilkins.

Hatcher, T. (2001). The proverbial herb. *American Journal of Nursing, 101*(2), 36-43.

Kaiman, C. (2003). PTSD in the World War II combat veteran. *American Journal of Nursing, 103*(11), 32-40.

Katerndahl, D. A. (2002). Factors influencing care seeking for a self-defined worst panic attack. *Psychiatric Services, 53*(4), 464-470.

McEnany, G. (2000). Herbal psychotropics: III. Focus on kava, valerian, and melatonin. *Journal of the American Psychiatric Nurses Association, 6*(4), 126-132.

Moorhead, S., Johnson, M., & Maas, M. (2004). Nursing outcomes classification (NOC) (3rd ed.). St. Louis, MO: Mosby.

Myrick, H., & Brady, K. (2003). Editorial review: Current review of the comorbidity of affective, anxiety, and substance use disorders. *Current Opinions in Psychiatry, 16*(3), 261-270.

North American Nursing Diagnosis Association. (2005). *NANDA nursing diagnoses: Definitions and classification 2005-2006*. Philadelphia: Author.

Overbeek, T., et al. (2002). Comorbidity of obsessive-compulsive disorder and depression: Prevalence, symptom severity, and treatment effect. *Journal of Clinical Psychiatry, 63*(12), 1106-1112.

Simon, N. M., & Rosenbaum, J. F. (2003). Anxiety and depression comorbidity: Implications and intervention. *Medscape Psychiatry & Mental Health, 8*(1), 2003. Retrieved May 13, 2003, from Medscape website: http://www.medscape.com/viewarticle/474626.

CHAPTER 15

Somatoform and Dissociative Disorders

NANCY CHRISTINE SHOEMAKER ▪ ELIZABETH M. VARCAROLIS

■ KEY TERMS and CONCEPTS

The key terms and concepts listed here appear in color where they are defined or first discussed in this chapter.

alternate personality (alter) or subpersonality, 267

body dysmorphic disorder, 259

conversion disorder, 259

depersonalization disorder, 265

dissociative amnesia, 265

dissociative disorders, 264

dissociative fugue, 266

dissociative identity disorder (DID), 266

factitious disorder, 253

hypochondriasis, 258

la belle indifférence, 259

malingering, 253

pain disorder, 259

psychosomatic illness, 253

secondary gains, 260

somatization, 253

somatization disorder, 258

somatoform disorders, 252

■ OBJECTIVES

After studying this chapter, the reader will be able to

1. Compare and contrast essential characteristics of the somatoform and the dissociative disorders.
2. Differentiate symptoms of somatoform disorders from (a) malingering, (b) factitious disorder, and (c) psychosomatic illness.
3. Give a clinical example of what would be found in each of the somatoform disorders.
4. Describe five psychosocial interventions that would be appropriate for a client with somatic complaints.
5. Plan interventions for a client with conversion disorder who is receiving a great deal of secondary gain from his or her "blindness." Include self-care and family teaching.
6. Explain the key symptoms of the four dissociative disorders.
7. Compare and contrast dissociative amnesia and dissociative fugue.
8. Identify three specialized elements in the assessment of a client with a dissociative disorder.

evolve Visit the Evolve website at **http://evolve.elsevier.com/Varcarolis** for a pretest on the content in this chapter.

As noted in the previous chapter, anxiety exerts a powerful influence on the mind and may lead to clinical conditions known as anxiety disorders. Although clients with anxiety disorders often have some somatic symptoms, the predominant complaint is mental or emotional distress. This chapter introduces the somatoform and dissociative disorders, in which anxiety has a major impact on the body with secondary but significant effects on the mind. These disorders are relatively rare in the psychiatric setting, but the nurse may encounter clients with these disorders in the general medical setting or in specialized units. The placement of these disorders on the mental health continuum can be seen in Figure 15-1.

Somatoform Disorders

Somatoform disorders are defined in the *Diagnostic and Statistical Manual of Mental Disorders*, fourth edi-

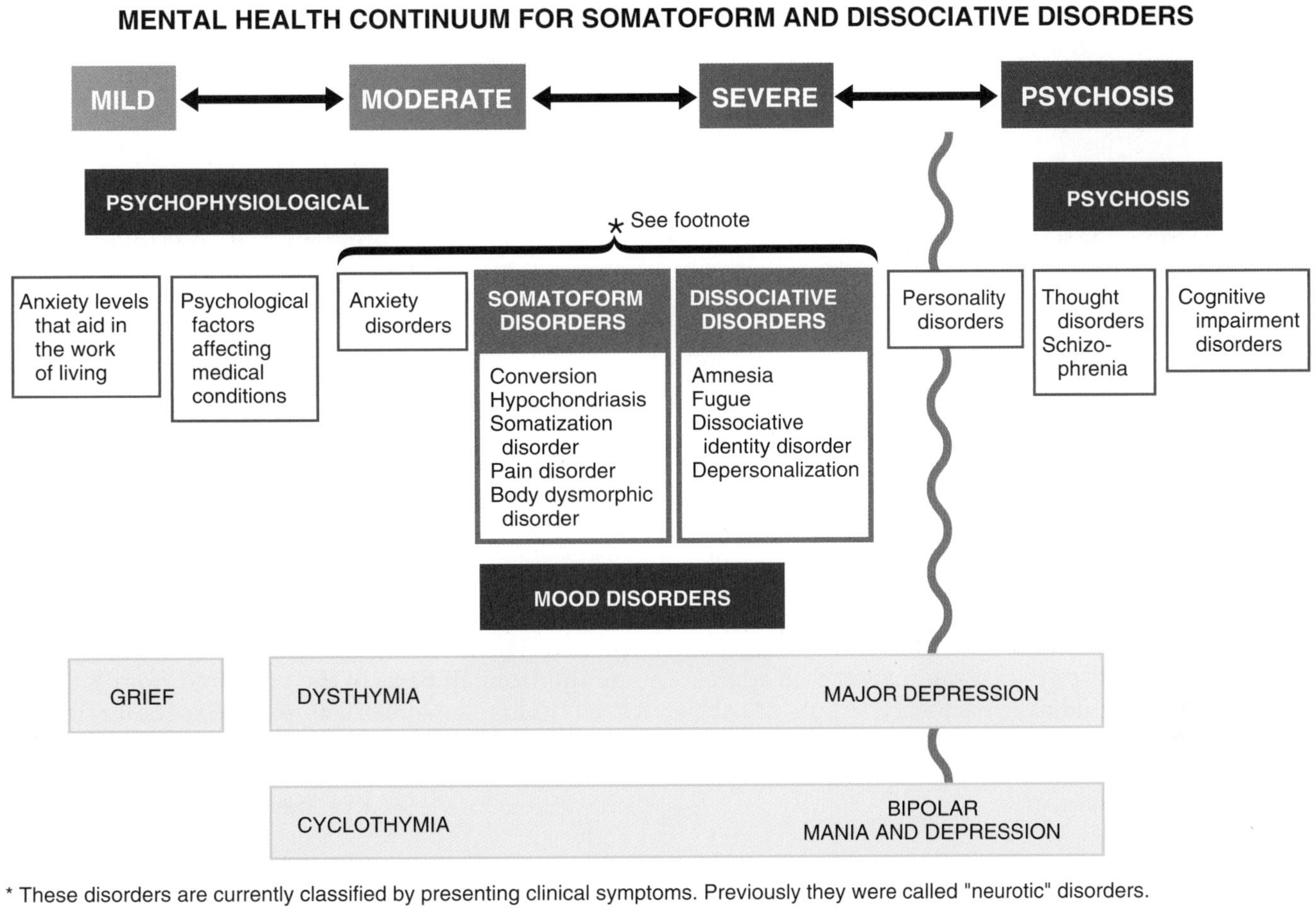

MENTAL HEALTH CONTINUUM FOR SOMATOFORM AND DISSOCIATIVE DISORDERS

MILD	⟷	MODERATE	⟷	SEVERE	⟷	PSYCHOSIS

PSYCHOPHYSIOLOGICAL

* See footnote

PSYCHOSIS

| Anxiety levels that aid in the work of living | Psychological factors affecting medical conditions | Anxiety disorders | **SOMATOFORM DISORDERS** Conversion Hypochondriasis Somatization disorder Pain disorder Body dysmorphic disorder | **DISSOCIATIVE DISORDERS** Amnesia Fugue Dissociative identity disorder Depersonalization | Personality disorders | Thought disorders Schizo-phrenia | Cognitive impairment disorders |

MOOD DISORDERS

GRIEF	DYSTHYMIA	MAJOR DEPRESSION

CYCLOTHYMIA	BIPOLAR MANIA AND DEPRESSION

* These disorders are currently classified by presenting clinical symptoms. Previously they were called "neurotic" disorders.

FIGURE 15-1 Mental health continuum for somatoform and dissociative disorders.

tion, text revision *(DSM-IV-TR)* (American Psychiatric Association [APA], 2000) as a group in which

- Physical symptoms suggest a physical disorder for which there is no demonstrable base.
- There is a strong presumption that the symptoms are linked to psychobiological factors.

Soma is the Greek word for body, and somatization is defined as the expression of psychological stress through physical symptoms. It is important to know that these disorders are grouped together merely because of their similarities in presentation and not because of any sound underlying theory or laboratory findings (Guggenheim, 2000). Somatoform disorders demonstrate complex mind-body interactions, and they cause real distress to the client with significant impairment in social and occupational functioning. Often, the client has another psychiatric disorder as well. (Refer to Chapter 3 to review the biology of the brain to better understand the varied symptoms of these disorders.)

The nurse needs to recognize that in somatoform disorders symptoms are not intentional or under the conscious control of the client, unlike in malingering or factitious disorders. Malingering involves a conscious process of intentionally producing symptoms for an obvious environmental goal; for example, an employee complains of back pain to get disability income. Factitious disorder refers to deliberate fabrication of symptoms or self-inflicted injury with the goal of assuming the sick role; for example, a client injects saliva into the skin to form an abscess (APA, 2000). *Munchausen syndrome by proxy* is the most severe form of factitious disorder, in which a caregiver injures a victim to get attention or sympathy for himself or herself.

The somatoform disorders are also differentiated from psychosomatic illness, in which there is evidence of a general medical condition that may be affected by stress or psychological factors (e.g., ulcerative colitis or essential hypertension).

PREVALENCE AND COMORBIDITY

The somatoform disorders currently recognized by the *DSM-IV-TR* include the following:

- Somatization disorder
- Undifferentiated somatoform disorder
- Conversion disorder
- Pain disorder
- Hypochondriasis
- Body dysmorphic disorder
- Somatoform disorder not otherwise specified

This chapter addresses the five main diagnoses presented in Figure 15-2.

Prevalence rates for these disorders in the general population are unknown. Instead, the literature describes their occurrence in the population of individuals who seek medical care. Differentiating somatoform disorders from physical disorders and identifying comorbid conditions are significant issues for the primary care provider. Research shows that half of all frequent users of medical care have psychological problems. One study identified depression, anxiety, and somatoform disorders as the top three psychiatric diagnoses in this group (Gallagher & Cariati, 2002).

A comprehensive physical examination with appropriate diagnostic studies is necessary to rule out the following medical conditions, which can be confused with somatoform disorders:

- Multiple sclerosis
- Brain tumor

- Hyperthyroidism
- Hyperparathyroidism
- Lupus erythematosus
- Myasthenia gravis

Also, a thorough psychosocial history is required to clarify a somatoform diagnosis as well as comorbid psychiatric disorders. Refer to Table 15-1 for detailed information on the prevalence of somatoform disorders in the general medical population, the age of onset and gender predilection, and comorbidity with other psychiatric disorders.

THEORY

Biological Factors

One way to understand the biology of somatoform disorders is to consider the two main functions of the brain: (1) as an organizer of stimuli from inside and outside of the body, and (2) as an interpreter of experiences. The brain "filters, amplifies or dampens . . . stimuli from all parts of the body and from the brain itself" (Guggenheim, 2000, p. 1505). The brain then creates a message to explain the stimulus, on the basis of past experiences. This message then gets communicated to the rest of the brain and also to the body.

TABLE 15-1

Somatoform Disorders

Disorder	Prevalence	Age of Onset	Gender Predilection	Comorbidities
Conversion disorder	5%-16% of consults in general hospital	Any age	Twice as frequent in women	Major depression Dissociative disorder Personality disorder
Somatization disorder	9% in general hospital	Adolescence to thirties	Women 80%, men 20%	Major depression Panic disorder Personality disorder Substance dependence
Hypochondriasis	2%-7% in general medical population	20-30 years of age	Equal prevalence in women and men	Depressive disorder Anxiety disorder Other somatoform disorders
Pain disorder	8%-13% in general medical population	Any age	Twice as frequent in women	Anxiety disorder Depressive disorder Substance dependence
Body dysmorphic disorder	Unknown	Adolescence to thirties	Equal prevalence in women and men	Major depression Obsessive-compulsive disorder Social phobia

Data from Guggenheim, F. G. (2000). Somatoform disorders. In B. J. Sadock & V. A. Sadock (Eds.), *Comprehensive textbook of psychiatry* (7th ed., Vol. 1, pp. 1504-1532). Philadelphia: Lippincott Williams & Wilkins; and American Psychiatric Association. (2000). *Diagnostic and statistical manual of mental disorders (DSM-IV-TR)* (4th ed., text rev.). Washington, DC: Author.

DSM-IV-TR CRITERIA FOR SOMATOFORM DISORDERS

SOMATOFORM DISORDERS

Somatization Disorder

1. History of many physical complaints beginning before 30 years of age, occurring over a period of years and resulting in impairment in social, occupational, or other important areas of functioning.

2. Complaints must include all of the following:
   - History of pain in at least **four** different sites or functions
   - History of at least **two** gastrointestinal symptoms other than pain
   - History of at least **one** sexual or reproduction symptom
   - History of at least **one** symptom defined as or suggesting a neurological disorder

Conversion Disorder

1. Development of one or more symptoms or deficits suggesting a neurological disorder (blindness, deafness, loss of touch) or general medical condition.

2. Psychological factors are associated with the symptom or deficit because the symptom is initiated or exacerbated by psychological stressors.

3. Not due to malingering or factitious disorder and not culturally sanctioned.

4. Cannot be explained by general medical condition or effects of a substance.

5. Causes impairment in social or occupational functioning, causes marked distress, or requires medical attention.

Hypochondriasis

For at least 6 months:

1. Preoccupation with fears of having, or the idea that one has, a serious disease.

2. Preoccupation persists despite appropriate medical tests and reassurances.

3. Other disorders are ruled out (e.g., somatic delusional disorders).

4. Preoccupation causes significant impairment in social or occupational functioning or causes marked distress.

Pain Disorder

1. Pain in one or more anatomical sites is a major part of the clinical picture.

2. Causes significant impairment in occupational or social functioning or causes marked distress.

3. Psychological factors thought to cause onset, severity, or exacerbation. **Pain associated with psychological factors.**

4. Symptoms not intentionally produced or feigned. If medical condition present, it plays minor role in accounting for pain.

5. **Pain may be associated with a psychological and/or medical condition.** Both factors are judged to be important in onset, severity, exacerbation, and maintenance of pain.

Body Dysmorphic Disorder (BDD)

1. Preoccupation with some imagined defect in appearance. If the defect is present, concern is excessive.

2. Preoccupation causes significant impairment in social or occupational functioning or causes marked distress.

3. Preoccupation not better accounted for by another mental disorder.

FIGURE 15-2 Diagnostic criteria for somatoform disorders. (Adapted from American Psychiatric Association. [2000]. *Diagnostic and statistical manual of mental disorders* [4th ed., text rev.]. Washington, DC: Author.)

Any abnormality in the structure of the brain or in the function of the neurotransmitters can lead to a misinterpretation of ordinary events. For example, the brain may misunderstand (or amplify) a stimulus, identifying a minor gas pain as a serious abdominal injury (somatization); or the brain may overreact in its analysis of the stimulus, deciding that the same minor gas pain is a sign of colon cancer (hypochondriasis).

Remember that research into anxiety disorders has demonstrated structural changes in the brain resulting from prolonged stress or trauma, as well as imbalances in neurotransmitters. Chapters on other disorders will discuss similar evidence. In the case of anxiety disorders, these abnormalities create altered feeling and thinking processes, whereas the processes of perception and interpretation of bodily sensations are fairly intact.

It is theorized that structural or functional abnormalities of the brain also lead to the somatoform disorders. However, in these conditions, the feeling and thinking processes appear to be normal, but the processes of perception and interpretation related to the body are disturbed. It is not known why some clients develop an anxiety disorder whereas others develop a somatoform disorder. Many clients suffer from both: clients with anxiety or depressive disorders are at high risk for unexplained medical symptoms, because of a tendency to amplify physiological events (Katon, Sullivan, & Walker, 2001).

Serotonin and norepinephrine are closely involved in depression and anxiety, but they are also critical components of the internal pain-modulating system. When levels of these neurotransmitters are abnormal, the person experiences more severe pain. Furthermore, chronic pain actually causes changes in the nerve pathways, sensitizing the individual to the next pain episode (Gallagher & Cariati, 2002). It is supposed that the beneficial effect of antidepressants on pain is due to the correction of altered serotonin or norepinephrine levels.

Genetic Factors

The *DSM-IV-TR* notes that somatoform disorders may have a genetic component. Somatization disorder tends to run in families, occurring in 10% to 20% of first-degree female relatives of women with somatization disorder. Twin studies show an increased risk of conversion disorder in monozygotic twin pairs. First-degree biological relatives of people with chronic pain disorder are more likely to have chronic pain, depressive disorder, and alcohol dependence.

Cultural Factors

The *DSM-IV-TR* provides information about the role of culture in somatoform disorders and states that the type and the frequency of somatic symptoms vary across cultures. Burning hands and feet or the sensa-

tion of worms in the head or ants under the skin is more common in Africa and southern Asia than in North America. Alteration of consciousness with falling is a symptom commonly associated with culture-specific religious and healing rituals. Somatization disorder, which is rarely seen in men in the United States, is more often reported in Greek and Puerto Rican men, which suggests that cultural mores may permit these men to use somatization as an acceptable approach to dealing with life stress.

In some cultures, certain physical symptoms are believed to result from the casting of spells on the individual. Spellbound individuals often seek the help of traditional healers in addition to modern medical staff. The medical provider may diagnose a non–life-threatening somatoform disorder, whereas the traditional healer may offer an entirely different explanation and prognosis. The individual may not show improvement until the traditional healer removes the spell. The Culturally Speaking box provides an example of cultural influence on a client with pain disorder.

Psychosocial Factors
Psychoanalytic Theory

Psychoanalytic theorists believe that psychogenic complaints of pain, illness, or loss of physical function are related to repression of a conflict (usually of an aggressive or sexual nature) and transformation of anxiety into a physical symptom that is symbolically related to the conflict. For example, in conversion disorder, conversion symptoms allow a forbidden wish or urge to be partly expressed but sufficiently disguised so that the individual does not have to face the unacceptable wish. The symptoms also permit the individual to communicate a need for special treatment or consideration from others.

Hypochondriasis is considered by many clinicians to have psychodynamic origins. These clinicians suggest that anger, aggression, or hostility that had its source in past losses or disappointments is expressed as a need for help and concern from others. Other clinicians suggest that hypochondriasis is a defense against guilt or low self-esteem. In their view, the somatic symptoms serve as deserved punishment. In pain disorder, the individual's pain may serve an unconscious function, such as a means of obtaining the love and concern of others, or a punishment for real or imagined wrongdoing.

In body dysmorphic disorder, according to some theorists, the individual invests a part of the body with special meaning that may be traceable to some event that occurred at an earlier stage of psychosexual development. The original event is repressed, and the attachment of special meaning to a part of the body comes about through symbolization. Projection is used when the individual makes statements such as, "It makes everyone look at me with horror." Table 15-2

The following account, based on a first-person description by the individual, illustrates cultural influences on the development of a pain disorder.

Dr. A., an African immigrant, attended medical school in the United States and became a psychiatrist. After graduation, he took a teaching job in the same hospital where he had trained. He wanted to perform well to please his former instructors, who were now his colleagues. After 6 months of teaching, he started to feel low back pain, which gradually worsened. He became anxious and preoccupied with the pain, which did not respond to bedrest or pain medication. He was diagnosed with a lumbar disc protrusion, but he realized that the pain fluctuated in areas beyond the disc. For a year, he went to different chiropractors and physical therapists. He could not work full time and he could not carry out his usual activities with his wife and daughter.

After 6 more months without relief, he was preparing for surgery when a colleague offered him a book about the mind-body connection. He read that unconscious feelings, especially anger, could affect the sympathetic nervous system, leading to constriction of blood vessels. Vasoconstriction in back muscles can lead to ischemia, causing pain and spasms.

He began to explore his feelings about his life. He did not recall any abuse as a child, but his father had been autocratic and informed him at an early age that he would become a doctor. In his culture, the male figure was expected to work hard to provide for the family and to solve all problems without showing any fear or anxiety. As an immigrant, Dr. A. always felt that he had to work harder than his peers to be accepted. Now he realized that he was anxious to be liked and respected by his colleagues in the school. Recognizing that he did feel angry and scared gave him insight into the function of his pain. The pain problem allowed him to be a patient and to be taken care of, while at the same time it distracted his attention from uncomfortable feelings.

After redefining the pain in this way, he became less obsessed with his symptoms and started to resume his usual activities. He told himself, "I am not afraid to face my feelings. . . . The pain is a distraction." He allowed himself to be more open in communicating his feelings to family and friends. Within several months, the pain was considerably reduced and he felt more confident in his role at work and with his family.

Alao, A. (2002). Anatomy of the mind. *Psychiatric Services, 53*(6), 665-666.

TABLE 15-2

Examples of Somatoform Disorders and Associated Defense Mechanisms

Defense Mechanism	Example
Conversion Disorder	
Conversion	Jan, a 28-year-old former secretary, awakens one morning to find that she has a tingling in both hands and cannot move her fingers. Two days earlier, her husband had told her that he wanted a separation and that she would have to go back to work to support herself. The conversion of anxiety relates the separation and increase in dependency needs to "paralysis of her fingers" so that she is unable to work.
Pain Disorder	
Displacement	Henry, 47, a laborer, "pulled a muscle" in his back a year ago. Two weeks before this, his wife, a waitress, told him that she wanted to go back to school to get her bachelor's degree. He suffers severe, constant pain, despite negative results from myelography, computed tomography, magnetic resonance imaging, and neurological examinations. He watches television all day and collects disability. His wife, unable now to go back to school, waits on him and has assumed his home responsibilities. Henry displaces his anxiety over the threat to his own self-esteem by his wife's potential change of status onto "pain in his back." The focus of his anxiety is now on his back and not on his threatened self-esteem.
Body Dysmorphic Disorder	
Symbolism and projection	Michele, a young, attractive woman, is preoccupied with her nose, which she considers too long and "ugly." She is constantly concerned by and distressed over her perception. Two plastic surgeons she consulted are hesitant to reshape her nose, but this has not altered her thinking that her nose makes her ugly.
Somatization Disorder	
Somatization	Deanna, 27, presents at the physician's office with excessively heavy menstruation. She tells the nurse that recently she experienced pain "first in my back and then going to every part of my body." She states that she is often bothered by constipation and vomiting when she "eats the wrong food." She says that she was "unwell" and had suffered from seizures and still has them occasionally. The nurse becomes confused, not knowing what symptoms Deanna wants the physician to evaluate. Deanna tells the nurse that she lives at home with her parents because her poor health makes it hard for her to hold a job.
Hypochondriasis	
Denial and somatization	Julio, 52, lost his wife to colon cancer 5 months earlier, which he "took very well." Recently, he saw a sixth physician with the same complaint. He believes that he has liver cancer, despite repeated and extensive diagnostic tests, results of which are all negative. He has ceased seeing his friends, has dropped his hobbies, and spends much of his time checking his sclera and "resting his liver." His son finally demands that he see a doctor.

provides clinical examples of each of the somatoform disorders and the associated defense mechanisms.

Behavioral Theory

Behaviorists suggest that somatoform symptoms are learned ways of communicating helplessness and that they allow the individual to manipulate others. The symptoms become more intense when they are reinforced by attention from others. In the United States, physicians and nurses are taught to be attentive and responsive to a client's reports of pain. Other reinforcers include avoiding activities that the individual considers distasteful, obtaining financial benefit, or gaining some advantage in interpersonal relationships due to the symptom.

Cognitive Theory

Cognitive theorists believe that the client with somatoform symptoms focuses on body sensations, misinterprets their meaning, and then becomes excessively alarmed by them.

DSM-IV-TR CRITERIA AND THE CLINICAL PICTURE OF SOMATOFORM DISORDERS

The five main somatoform disorders identified by the *DSM-IV-TR* are reviewed in this section. Refer back to Figure 15-2 for the specific symptoms of each disorder.

Somatization Disorder

The diagnosis of somatization disorder requires the presence of a certain number of symptoms accompanied by significant functional impairment. The most frequent symptoms are pain (head, chest, back, joints, pelvis), dysphagia, nausea, bloating, constipation, palpitations, dizziness, and shortness of breath (Looper & Kirmayer, 2002). Clients report significant distress and seek out multiple providers for medical care. Anxiety and depression are common comorbid conditions.

The following socioeconomic attributes often characterize individuals who meet full criteria for somatization disorder: unmarried, nonwhite, poorly educated, and from a rural area (Guggenheim, 2000). The course of the illness is chronic and relapsing, with most clients developing a new symptom at least once a year. Suicide threats and gestures are common, but attempts are rarely lethal (Guggenheim, 2000). The Evidence-Based Practice box describes research related to cognitive-behavioral therapy for somatization disorders.

Hypochondriasis

Hypochondriasis is a widespread phenomenon: it is estimated that 1 out of 20 people who seek outpatient medical attention suffer from this disorder (APA, 2002). Clients with this disorder misinterpret innocent physical sensations as evidence of a serious illness.

 EVIDENCE-BASED PRACTICE

Treatment of Somatoform Disorders

Background
Somatoform disorders and other medically unexplained somatic complaints account for approximately 133 million clinic visits in the United States each year. Half of these clients may be diagnosed with anxiety or depression, and they benefit from successful treatment of the comorbid condition. But for the other half of this group, there is no specific treatment that has been proven effective. Research during the 1990s tried to identify helpful treatment approaches.

Studies
Researchers conducted a critical review of all controlled studies of cognitive-behavioral therapy (CBT) for somatoform disorders and specific somatic symptoms. From 1966 to 1999, there were 31 controlled trials: 25 studies focused on specific symptoms (e.g., pain, irritable bowel syndrome); 6 studies focused on general somatization.

The symptoms were chronic, and the average age of subjects was 35 to 45 years. The majority were women, but men comprised at least one third of the sample in 19 studies. The studies were conducted in six different countries, and the study population was drawn from mental health or specialty clinics. CBT was compared to placement on a waiting list,

usual care, behavioral therapy, or miscellaneous forms of supportive attention.

Results of Studies
Three main outcomes were evaluated in the 31 studies: severity of physical symptoms; psychological distress; and functional status. For physical symptoms, 20 studies showed more benefit from CBT than from control conditions. For psychological distress, only 12 studies showed a benefit for CBT. For functional status, improvement with CBT was noted in 14 studies. Twelve studies performed a follow-up of 1 to 24 months, and in all but one, the initial benefits from treatment continued.

Implications for Nursing Practice
Nurses need to be alert to the needs of medical clients with somatoform disorders and other medically unexplained symptoms. The majority of these clients will initially refuse a referral to psychiatric treatment, because of fear that their symptoms are being dismissed or because of the stigma of mental illness. The nurse can teach clients about the benefits of CBT and psychotropic medication, reducing fears about mental health treatment by demonstrating the belief that these interventions are just as acceptable as standard somatic treatments.

Kroenke, K., & Swindle, R. Cognitive-behavioral therapy for somatization and symptom syndromes: A critical review of controlled clinical trials. *Psychotherapy and Psychosomatics, 69*, 205-215.

They cannot be reassured by negative diagnostic test findings and they seek extensive medical care with frustrating results (Barsky, 2001). Most clients refuse referral to a psychiatrist. Approximately two-thirds of the clients with hypochondriasis have a comorbid psychiatric disorder of depression or anxiety disorder (APA, 2002, p. 383).

No specific socioeconomic factors are associated with this disorder (Barsky, 2001). However, many clients have a history of sexual or physical trauma, parental upheaval, or absence from school during childhood for health reasons. The course of the illness is chronic and relapsing, with symptoms exacerbated during times of stress (Guggenheim, 2000). Yet improvement is noted in up to 50% of clients.

Pain Disorder

Pain is one of the most frequent reasons people seek medical attention. When testing rules out any organic cause for the pain and the discomfort leads to significant impairment, pain disorder is diagnosed. Although most pain can be reduced, chronic pain results in significant disability and high costs for health care. In 2000, it was estimated that 7 million Americans suffered from low back pain. Suicide is a serious risk in clients with chronic pain: the suicide rate is nine times higher in such clients than in the general population (Guggenheim, 2000).

Pain is difficult to measure objectively, and individuals react differently to the same injury. Pain thresholds vary among individuals. Typical sites of pain include the head, face, lower back, and pelvis (Guggenheim, 2000). Frequent comorbid conditions include depression, substance dependence, and personality disorders. These clients are at risk for excessive use of narcotic or sedative medications (Guggenheim, 2000). Some research suggests that a background of sexual abuse or trauma is common in women with pain disorder.

The course of pain disorder varies according to the acuity of the symptoms. Acute pain can often be helped, especially with treatment of a comorbid psychiatric condition and family involvement. Chronic pain is more difficult to treat.

Body Dysmorphic Disorder

Clients with body dysmorphic disorder usually have a normal appearance, although a small number do show minor defects (Guggenheim, 2000). Preoccupation with an imagined defective body part results in obsessional thinking and compulsive behavior such as mirror checking and camouflaging. Normal social activities related to academic or occupational functioning are impaired (Carroll, Scahill, & Phillips, 2002). Clients are frequently concerned with the face, skin, genitalia, thighs, hips, and hair. In one study, women were found to be more focused on weight and hips, whereas men were found to be concerned about body build and genitalia (Carroll et al., 2002).

Common comorbid diagnoses include major depression, obsessive-compulsive disorder, and social phobia (Guggenheim, 2000). The disorder is often kept secret for many years, and the client does not respond to reassurance. Even when cosmetic surgery is sought, there is no relief of symptoms (Guggenheim, 2000). The disorder is chronic and the response to treatment is limited.

Conversion Disorder

Conversion disorder is marked by the presence of deficits in voluntary motor or sensory functions (Roelofs et al., 2002). The dysfunction does not correspond to current scientific understanding of the nervous system. Many clients show a lack of emotional concern about the symptoms (la belle indifférence), although others are quite distressed (Guggenheim, 2000). Common symptoms are involuntary movements, seizures, paralysis, abnormal gait, anesthesia, blindness, and deafness (Guggenheim, 2000).

Conversion disorder is the most common somatoform disorder. Socioeconomic factors that seem to be related are lower education and income levels, residence in a rural area, and military service, especially in combat zones (Guggenheim, 2000). Some studies have found an association between childhood physical or sexual abuse and conversion disorder (Roelofs et al., 2002). Common comorbid psychiatric conditions include depression, anxiety, other somatoform disorders, and personality disorders. There are also cases in which a comorbid medical or neurological condition exists and the conversion symptom is an exaggeration of the original problem.

The course of the disorder is related to its acuity: in cases with acute onset during stressful events, remission rate is high; in cases with a more gradual onset, the disorder is not readily treated. About 25% of clients will develop another episode in the 6 years following the first one (Guggenheim, 2000). Refer to the case study at the end of the chapter for a description of a client with conversion disorder.

Application of the Nursing Process

ASSESSMENT

Assessment of clients with somatoform disorders is a complex process that requires careful and complete documentation. This section outlines several areas that are not normally included in a nursing assessment but are of considerable importance in the assessment of a client with suspected somatoform disorder.

Overall Assessment

Symptoms and Unmet Needs

Assessment should begin with collection of data about the nature, location, onset, character, and duration of the symptom or symptoms. Often, clients with conversion disorder report having a sudden loss in function of a body part. "I woke up this morning and couldn't move my arm." Clients with somatization disorder, hypochondriasis, or somatoform pain disorder usually discuss their symptoms in dramatic terms. They may use colorful metaphors and exaggerations: "The pain was searing, like a hot sword drawn across my forehead" or "My symptoms are so rare that I've stumped hundreds of doctors." Individuals with body dysmorphic disorder are concerned about only one part of the body and seek cosmetic surgery; they display disgust with the offending body part.

Information should be sought about clients' ability to meet their own basic needs. Common problems connected with the need for oxygen include tachypnea and tachycardia associated with anxiety. Nutrition, fluid balance, and elimination needs should be evaluated, because clients with somatization disorders often complain of gastrointestinal distress, diarrhea, constipation, and anorexia. The physiological need for sex may be altered by client experiences of painful intercourse, pain in another part of the body, or lack of interest in sex.

Rest, comfort, activity, and hygiene needs may be altered as a result of client problems such as fatigue, weakness, insomnia, muscle tension, pain, and avoidance of diversional activity. Safety and security needs may be threatened by client experiences of blindness, deafness, loss of balance and falling, and anesthesia of various parts of the body.

Voluntary Control of Symptoms

During assessment, it is important to determine if the symptoms are under the client's voluntary control. Somatoform symptoms are not under the individual's voluntary control. The client cannot see the relationship between symptoms and interpersonal conflicts that may be obvious to others.

Secondary Gains

The nurse tries to identify secondary gains the client may be receiving from the symptoms. Secondary gains are those benefits derived from the symptoms alone; for example, in the sick role, the client is not able to perform the usual family, work, and social functions, and receives extra attention from loved ones. If a client derives personal benefit from the symptoms, giving up the symptoms is more difficult. The clinician works

with the client to achieve the same benefits through healthier avenues (e.g., assertiveness training). One approach to identifying the presence of secondary gains is to ask the client questions such as the following:

- What can't you do now that you used to be able to do?
- How has this problem affected your life?

Cognitive Style

In general, clients with these disorders misinterpret physical stimuli and distort reality regarding their symptoms. For example, sensations a normal individual might interpret as a headache might suggest a brain tumor to a client with hypochondriasis. Exploring the client's cognitive style is helpful in distinguishing between hypochondriasis and somatization disorder. The client with hypochondriasis exhibits more anxiety and an obsessive attention to detail, along with a preoccupation with the fear of serious illness. The client with somatization disorder is often rambling and vague about the details of his or her many symptoms and gives a disorganized history.

Ability to Communicate Feelings and Emotional Needs

Clients with somatoform disorders have difficulty communicating their emotional needs. Although they are able to describe their physical symptoms, they cannot verbalize feelings, especially those related to anger, guilt, and dependence. The somatic symptom may be the client's chief means of communicating emotional needs. Psychogenic blindness or hearing loss may represent the symbolic statement, "I can't face this knowledge." For example, after a wife overheard friends discussing her husband's sexual infidelity, she developed total deafness.

Dependence on Medication

Individuals experiencing many somatic complaints often become dependent on medication to relieve pain or anxiety or to induce sleep. Physicians prescribe anxiolytic agents for clients who seem highly anxious and concerned about their symptoms. Clients often return to the physician for prescription renewal or seek treatment from numerous physicians. It is important that the nurse assess the type and the amount of medications being used.

Self-Assessment

Nurses and other health care workers often find working with clients with somatoform disorders to be difficult and unsatisfying. The nurse notes objective data that indicate a lack of physiological basis for the client's symptoms. The nurse then wonders why this client who is "not sick" is taking up valuable time that might better be spent on a "sick" client. The tendency, at times, is for the nurse to feel resentment or anger toward such a client. These negative feelings occur whether the client is being cared for by medical-surgical staff, who tend to prefer working with clients who have physical illnesses, or by psychiatric staff, who often prefer to work with psychotic clients. It is helpful to remember that the symptom the client is experiencing is real to him or her, even though the objective data do not substantiate a physiological basis.

Anger may also rise when staff members find themselves dealing with a client who uses somatic symptoms to manipulate the environment and the people in the environment. In addition, health care workers may experience feelings of helplessness over not being able to make the client realize that his or her symptom has no organic basis. Clients who use somatization exhibit remarkable resistance to change. They cling to their unrealistic beliefs about the origin of the somatic symptoms, despite objective evidence to the contrary. Setting goals that have staged outcomes (i.e., outcomes occurring in small, attainable steps) helps the nurse avoid feelings of helplessness.

Clients with somatoform disorders should be discussed in conferences with other health care members to allow for expression of feelings and consistency of care.

Assessment Guidelines Somatoform Disorders

1. Assess for nature, location, onset, characteristics, and duration of the symptom(s).
2. Assess the client's ability to meet basic needs.
3. Assess risks to safety and security needs of the client as a result of the symptom(s).
4. Determine whether the symptoms are under the client's voluntary control.
5. Identify any secondary gains that the client is experiencing from symptom(s).
6. Explore the client's cognitive style and ability to communicate feelings and needs.
7. Assess type and amount of medication the client is using.

■ NURSING DIAGNOSIS

Clients with somatoform disorders present various nursing problems. *Ineffective coping* is frequently diagnosed. Causal statements might include the following:
- Distorted perceptions of body functions and symptoms
- Chronic pain of psychological origin
- Dependence on pain relievers or anxiolytics

Table 15-3 identifies potential nursing diagnoses for clients with somatoform disorders.

■ OUTCOME CRITERIA

Identifying client outcomes should be a process in which the client participates; shared decision making promotes goal attainment. Outcome criteria must be realistic and attainable. Structuring outcomes in small steps helps the client see concrete evidence of progress. Pertinent Nursing Outcomes Classification (NOC) categories for outcomes for somatoform clients include *Body Image, Coping, Identity, Role Performance, Social Interaction Skills, Family Coping,* and *Self-Esteem* (Moorhead, Johnson, & Maas, 2004). The following are examples of possible indicators related to NOC:
- Client will exhibit sensitivity to others.
- Client will resume performance of work role behaviors.

TABLE 15-3

Potential Nursing Diagnoses for Somatoform Disorders

Signs and Symptoms	Nursing Diagnoses
■ Inability to meet occupational, family, or social responsibilities because of symptoms	Ineffective coping
■ Inability to participate in usual community activities or friendships because of psychogenic symptoms	Ineffective role performance
	Impaired social interaction
■ Dependence on pain relievers	Powerlessness
■ Distortion of body functions and symptoms	Disturbed body image
■ Presence of secondary gains by adoption of sick role	Pain, acute or chronic
■ Inability to meet family role function and need for family to assume role function of the somatic individual	Interrupted family processes
	Ineffective sexuality pattern
■ Assumption of some of the roles of the somatic parent by the children	Impaired parenting
■ Shifting of the sexual partner's role to that of caregiver/parent and of the client's role to that of recipient of care	Risk for caregiver role strain
■ Feeling of inability to control symptoms or understand why he or she cannot find help	Chronic low self-esteem
■ Development of negative self-evaluation related to losing body function, feeling useless, or not feeling valued by significant others	Spiritual distress
■ Inability to take care of basic self-care needs related to conversion symptom (paralysis, seizures, pain, fatigue)	Self-care deficit
	Disturbed sleep pattern
■ Inability to sleep due to psychogenic pain	

- Client will identify ineffective coping patterns.
- Client will make realistic appraisal of strengths and weaknesses.
- Client will verbalize feelings such an anger, shame, or guilt.
- Client will allow family to be involved in decision making.

■ PLANNING

Because clients with somatoform disorders are seldom admitted to psychiatric units specifically because of these disorders, long-term interventions usually take place on an outpatient basis or in the home. Short-term planning may be initiated if the client is admitted to a medical-surgical unit. Such a stay is usually short, and discharge will occur as soon as diagnostic tests are completed and negative results are received.

Nursing interventions should focus initially on establishing a helping relationship with the client. The therapeutic relationship is vital to the success of the care plan, given the client's resistance to the concept that no physical cause for the symptom exists and the client's tendency to go from caregiver to caregiver.

To be successful, therapeutic interventions must address ways to help the client get needs met without resorting to somatization. The secondary gains the client has derived from illness behaviors become less important to the client when underlying needs can be met directly. Collaboration with family or significant others is essential for success.

Case Study and Nursing Care Plan 15-1 at the end of the chapter gives the plan of care for a client with conversion disorder.

■ INTERVENTION
Basic Level Interventions

Generally, for clients with somatoform disorders, nursing interventions take place in the home or clinic setting. Basic level nursing interventions include promotion of self-care activities, health teaching, case management, and psychobiological interventions. The nurse attempts to help the client improve overall functioning through the development of effective coping strategies. The Nursing Interventions Classification (NIC) offers several categories pertinent to caring for clients with somatoform disorders: *Assertiveness Training, Body Image Enhancement, Family Involvement Promotion, Limit Setting, Self-Awareness Enhancement,* and *Self-Esteem Enhancement* (Dochterman & Bulechek, 2004). Refer to Table 15-4 for examples of basic interventions.

Promotion of Self-Care Activities

When somatization is present, the client's ability to perform self-care activities may be impaired, and nursing intervention is necessary. In general, interventions involve the use of a matter-of-fact approach to support the highest level of self-care of which the client is capable. For clients manifesting paralysis, blindness, or severe fatigue, an effective nursing approach is to support clients while expecting them to feed, bathe, or groom themselves. For example, the client who demonstrates paralysis of an arm can be expected to eat using the other arm. The client who is experiencing blindness can be told at what numbers on an imaginary clock the food is located on the plate and encouraged to feed himself or herself. These strategies are effective in reducing secondary gain.

Health Teaching

Some clients who use somatization as a way of coping with anxiety have little formal education. Therefore, teaching these clients basic information about body functions is often warranted. Pictures and charts can be helpful. It is useful to review the same information with the family because their knowledge may also be faulty.

Assertiveness training (see Chapter 12) is often identified as appropriate to teach clients with somatoform disorders. Use of assertiveness techniques gives clients a direct means of getting needs met and thereby decreases the need for somatic symptoms. Teaching an exercise regimen, such as doing range-of-motion exercises for 15 to 20 minutes daily, can help the client feel in control, increases endorphin levels, and may help decrease anxiety.

Case Management

"Doctor shopping" is common among clients with somatoform disorders. The client goes from physician to physician, clinic to clinic, or hospital to hospital, hoping to establish a physical basis for distress. Repeated computed tomographic scans, magnetic resonance images, and other diagnostic tests are often documented in the medical record. Case management can help limit health care costs associated with such visits. The case manager can recommend to the physician that the client be scheduled for brief appointments every 4 to 6 weeks at set times rather than on demand and that laboratory tests be avoided unless they are absolutely necessary. The client who establishes a relationship with the case manager often feels less anxiety because the client has someone to contact and knows that someone is "in charge."

Psychobiological Interventions

Presently, the antidepressants, specifically the selective serotonin reuptake inhibitors, show the greatest promise for helping clients with somatoform disorders (Phillips, Albertini, & Rasmussen, 2002; Stahl, 2003). Clients may also benefit from short-term use of antianxiety medication, which must be monitored carefully because of the risk of dependence. The nurse may

TABLE 15-4

Basic Level Interventions and Rationales for Somatoform Disorders

Intervention	Rationale
1. Offer explanations and support during diagnostic testing.	1. Reduces anxiety while ruling out organic illness
2. After physical complaints have been investigated, avoid further reinforcement (e.g., do not take vital signs each time client complains of palpitations).	2. Directs focus away from physical symptoms
3. Spend time with client at times other than when client summons nurse to voice physical complaint.	3. Rewards non–illness-related behaviors and encourages repetition of desired behavior
4. Observe and record frequency and intensity of somatic symptoms. (Client or family can give information.)	4. Establishes a baseline and later enables evaluation of effectiveness of interventions
5. Do not imply that symptoms are not real.	5. Acknowledges that psychogenic symptoms are real to the client
6. Shift focus from somatic complaints to feelings or to neutral topics.	6. Conveys interest in client as a person rather than in client's symptoms; reduces need to gain attention via symptoms
7. Assess secondary gains that "physical illness" provides for client (e.g., attention, increased dependency, and distraction from another problem).	7. Allows these needs to be met in healthier ways and thus minimizes secondary gains
8. Use matter-of-fact approach to client exhibiting resistance or covert anger.	8. Avoids power struggles; demonstrates acceptance of anger and permits discussion of angry feelings
9. Have client direct all requests to case manager.	9. Reduces manipulation
10. Help client look at effect of illness behavior on others.	10. Encourages insight; can help improve intrafamily relationships
11. Show concern for client while avoiding fostering dependency needs.	11. Shows respect for client's feelings while minimizing secondary gains from "illness"
12. Reinforce client's strengths and problem-solving abilities.	12. Contributes to positive self-esteem; helps client realize that needs can be met without resorting to somatic symptoms
13. Teach assertive communication.	13. Provides client with a positive means of getting needs met; reduces feelings of helplessness and need for manipulation
14. Teach client stress reduction techniques, such as meditation, relaxation, and mild physical exercise.	14. Provides alternate coping strategies; reduces need for medication

administer these medications in certain settings, but teaching about the medication to clients and families is helpful in all settings. Also, teaching of relaxation techniques is useful for the client to learn a means of controlling symptoms.

Advanced Practice Interventions

Advanced practice nurses may use various types of psychotherapy or consultation with the primary care provider in the treatment of somatoform disorders. Refer to Table 15-5 for a summary of the somatoform disorders along with a description of the illness course and enumeration of specific therapeutic approaches.

▪ EVALUATION

Evaluation of clients with somatoform disorders is a simple process when measurable behavioral outcomes have been written clearly and realistically. For these clients, nurses often find that goals and outcomes are only partially met. This should be considered a positive finding, because these clients often exhibit remarkable resistance to change. Clients are likely to re-

port the continuing presence of somatic symptoms, but they often say that they are less concerned about the symptoms. Families are likely to report relatively high satisfaction with outcomes, even without total eradication of the client's symptoms.

Dissociative Disorders

This section describes another group of disorders with altered mind-body connections that are also believed to be related to stress or anxiety: the dissociative disorders. In these conditions, however, a different level of impairment is noted. As previously discussed, the client with an anxiety disorder complains of uncomfortable feelings and thoughts but perceives most body sensations within a normal range. The client with a somatoform disorder complains of somatic distress but retains normal patterns of thinking and feeling overall. Clients in both of these groups are fully oriented and conscious of their identities with relatively unimpaired memory. For dissociative clients, consciousness itself is altered in a dramatic way, whereas thinking, feeling, and perceptions are less im-

TABLE 15-5

Course of and Advanced Practice Interventions for Somatoform Disorders

Disorder	Course	Advanced Practice Interventions
Conversion disorder	Usually acute onset; resolves quickly	Behavioral therapy Family therapy Hypnosis Anxiolytics
Somatization disorder	Chronic and relapsing	Consultation with primary care provider to arrange regular client visits, limited tests Group therapy Cognitive-behavioral therapy
Hypochondriasis	Chronic and relapsing but 50% of clients improve	Cognitive group therapy Antidepressants Stress management
Pain disorder	If acute onset, may improve; risk of suicide	Group therapy Family therapy Cognitive-behavioral therapy Hypnosis Antidepressants
Body dysmorphic disorder	Limited response to treatment	Cognitive-behavioral therapy Antidepressants

Data from Guggenheim, F. G. (2000). Somatoform disorders. In B. J. Sadock & V. A. Sadock (Eds.), *Comprehensive textbook of psychiatry* (7th ed., Vol. 1, pp. 1504-1532). Philadelphia: Lippincott Williams & Wilkins; Looper, K. J., & Kirmayer, L. J. (2002). Behavioral medicine approaches to somatoform disorders. *Journal of Consulting and Clinical Psychology, 70*(3), 810-827; Phillips, K. A., Albertini, R. S., & Rasmussen, S. A. (2002). A randomized placebo-controlled trial of fluoxetine in body dysmorphic disorder. *Archives of General Psychiatry, 59,* 381-388; and Stahl, S. M. (2003). Antidepressants and somatic symptoms: Therapeutic actions are expanding beyond affective spectrum disorders to functional somatic syndromes. *Journal of Clinical Psychiatry, 64*(7), 745-746.

paired. Refer again to Figure 15-1 to recall that these disturbances are moving toward the severe end of the mental health continuum.

The *DSM-IV-TR* defines dissociative disorders as disturbances in the normally well-integrated continuum of consciousness, memory, identity, and perception. Dissociation is an unconscious defense mechanism to protect the individual against overwhelming anxiety. When the ability to integrate memories is impaired, the individual has *dissociative amnesia.* When the ability to maintain one's identity is affected, the individual may develop a *dissociative fugue* or *dissociative identity disorder (DID)* in which aspects of the self may emerge as distinct personalities. (DID was previously referred to as *multiple personality disorder.*) When there is a persistent or recurrent disruption in perception, the individual has *depersonalization disorder,* with a feeling of detachment from the mind or body. Clients with dissociative disorders have intact reality testing; that is, they are not delusional or hallucinating. Mild, fleeting dissociative experiences are relatively common to all of us; for example, we say we are on "automatic pilot" when we drive home from work but cannot recall the last 15 minutes before reaching the house. But research shows that these common experiences are distinctly different from the processes of pathological dissociation (Simeon et al., 2001).

PREVALENCE

There are no clear data regarding the prevalence of dissociative disorders. Overall, these conditions are considered rare. Dissociative amnesia may occur in any age group from children to adults. The amnesia is often related to trauma, and memory returns spontaneously after the individual is removed from the stressful situation (APA, 2000). The dissociative fugue is also related to trauma and occurs mostly in adults. The occurrence of fugue is known to increase in times of stress, such as during war or natural disasters (APA, 2000). DID may occur at any age, but it is diagnosed three to nine times more frequently in adult females than in adult males. There is often a childhood history of severe physical or sexual abuse. Depersonalization disorder is found in adolescents and adults, often in response to acute stress. Clients with this disorder usually seek treatment for another problem, such as anxiety or depression.

COMORBIDITY

Mood disorders and substance-related disorders are commonly associated with all of the dissociative disorders. In addition, dissociative amnesia may be comorbid with conversion disorder or personality disorder. Dissociative fugue may co-occur with posttraumatic stress disorder (PTSD). DID clients may also have PTSD, borderline personality disorder, or sexual, eating, or sleep disorders. Depersonalization disorder occurs with hypochondriasis, anxiety disorder, and personality disorder (APA, 2000).

THEORY

The actual cause of dissociative disorders is unknown. However, childhood physical, sexual, or emotional abuse and other traumatic life events are associated with adult dissociative symptoms. Several factors related to etiology are reviewed in the following sections.

Biological Factors

Current research suggests that the limbic system is involved in the development of dissociative disorders. Traumatic memories are processed in the limbic system, and the hippocampus stores this information. Animal studies show that early prolonged detachment from the caretaker negatively affects the development of the limbic system. For humans, early trauma or detachment from the caregiver could impair memory processing, leading to dissociation (Kreidler et al., 2000). Significant early trauma and lack of attachment have also been demonstrated to have effects on neurotransmitters, specifically on serotonin.

Depersonalization disorder and dissociative fugue have a possible neurological link. Altered perceptions of self and fugue states occur with neurological diseases such as brain tumors and epilepsy, especially complex partial seizure disorder (Coons, 2000). Depersonalization is also experienced by individuals under the influence of certain drugs, such as alcohol, barbiturates, and hallucinogens (Steinberg, 2000a).

Genetic Factors

Several studies suggest that DID is more common among first-degree biological relatives of individuals with the disorder than in the population at large.

Cultural Factors

Certain culturally bound disorders exist in which there is a high level of activity, a trancelike state, and running or fleeing, followed by exhaustion, sleep, and amnesia regarding the episode. These syndromes include *piblokto,* seen in native people of the Arctic, Navajo *frenzy* witchcraft, and *amok* among Western Pacific natives. These syndromes, if observed in individuals native to the corresponding geographical areas, must be differentiated from dissociative disorders.

Psychosocial Factors

Learning theory suggests that dissociative disorders can be explained as learned methods for avoiding stress and anxiety. The pattern of avoidance occurs when an individual deals with an unpleasant event by consciously deciding not to think about it. The more anxiety-provoking the event, the greater the need not to think about it. The more this technique is used, the more likely it is to become automatically invoked as dissociation. When stress is intolerable—for example, in an abused child—the individual develops dissociation to defend against pain and the memory of it.

DSM-IV-TR CRITERIA AND THE CLINICAL PICTURE OF DISSOCIATIVE DISORDERS

The *DSM-IV-TR* lists four major dissociative disorders: (1) depersonalization disorder, (2) dissociative amnesia, (3) dissociative fugue, and (4) DID. Refer to Figure 15-3 for the diagnostic criteria for each disorder.

Depersonalization Disorder

The *DSM-IV-TR* describes depersonalization disorder as a persistent or recurrent alteration in the perception of the self while reality testing remains intact. The person experiencing depersonalization may feel mechanical, dreamy, or detached from the body. These experiences of feeling a sense of deadness of the body, of seeing oneself from a distance, or of perceiving the limbs to be larger or smaller than normal are described by clients as being very disturbing. In some cases, depersonalization may be preceded by severe stress; in other cases, there may be an association with childhood emotional abuse (Simeon et al., 2001).

■ ■ ■ *VIGNETTE*

Margaret describes becoming very distressed at perceiving changes in her appearance when she looks in a mirror. She thinks that her image looks wavy and indistinct. Soon after, she describes feeling as though she is floating in a fog with her feet not actually touching the ground. Questioning reveals that Margaret's son has recently confided to her that he tested positive for human immunodeficiency virus.

■ ■ ■

Dissociative Amnesia

Dissociative amnesia is marked by the inability to recall important personal information, often of a traumatic or stressful nature, that is too pervasive to be explained by ordinary forgetfulness. A client with generalized amnesia is unable to recall information about his or her entire lifetime. The amnesia may also be localized (the client is unable to remember all events

DSM-IV-TR CRITERIA FOR DISSOCIATIVE DISORDERS

DISSOCIATIVE DISORDERS

Dissociative Amnesia*	Dissociative Fugue*	Dissociative Identity Disorder* (DID)	Depersonalization Disorder*
1. One or more episodes of inability to recall important information — usually of a traumatic or stressful nature. 2. Causes significant distress or impairment in social, occupational, or other important areas of functioning.	1. Sudden, unexpected travel away from home or one's place of work with inability to remember past. 2. Confusion about personal identity or assumption of new identity. 3. Symptoms cause significant distress or impairment in social, occupational, or other important areas of functioning.	1. Existence of two or more distinct subpersonalities, each with its own patterns of relating, perceiving, and thinking. 2. At least two of these subpersonalities take control of the person's behavior. 3. Inability to recall important information too extensive to be explained by ordinary forgetfulness.	1. Persistent or recurrent experience of feeling detached from and outside of one's mental processes or body. 2. Reality testing remains intact. 3. The experience causes significant impairment in social or occupational functioning or causes marked distress.
*Not due to substance, medical, neurological, or other psychiatric disorder.	*Not due to substance, medical, neurological, or other psychiatric disorder.	*Not due to substance, medical, neurological, or other psychiatric disorder.	*Not due to substance, medical, neurological, or other psychiatric disorder.

FIGURE 15-3 Diagnostic criteria for dissociative disorders. (Adapted from American Psychiatric Association. [2000]. *Diagnostic and statistical manual of mental disorders* [4th ed., text rev.]. Washington, DC: Author.)

in a certain period) or selective (the client is able to recall some but not all events in a certain period).

▪ ▪ ▪ *VIGNETTE*

A young woman, found wandering in a Florida park, is partly dressed and poorly nourished. She has no knowledge of who she is. Her parents identify her 2 weeks later when she appears in an interview on a national television show. She had just broken up with her boyfriend of 3 years.

▪ ▪ ▪

Dissociative Fugue

Dissociative fugue is characterized by sudden, unexpected travel away from the customary locale and inability to recall one's identity and information about some or all of the past. In rare cases, an individual with dissociative fugue assumes a whole new identity. During a fugue state, individuals tend to lead rather simple lives, rarely calling attention to themselves. After a few weeks to a few months, they may remember their former identities and become amnesic for the time spent in the fugue state. Usually a dissociative fugue is precipitated by a traumatic event.

▪ ▪ ▪ *VIGNETTE*

A middle-aged woman awakens one morning and notices snow outside the window, swirling around unfamiliar buildings and streets. The radio tells her it is December. She is perplexed to find herself in a residential hotel in Chicago with no idea of how she got there. She feels confused and shaken. As she leaves the hotel, she is surprised to find that strangers recognize her and say, "Good morning, Sally." The name Sally does not seem right, but she cannot remember her true identity. She finds her way to a hospital, where she is evaluated and referred to the psychiatric nurse in the emergency department. A day later, "Sally" is able to remember her true identity, Mary Hunt. She tells the nurse tearfully that she can now recall that her husband came home one day and "out of the blue" told her he wanted a divorce to marry a younger woman. Mary calls her sister in New York, who comes to Chicago to take her home.

▪ ▪ ▪

Dissociative Identity Disorder

The essential feature of dissociative identity disorder (DID) is the presence of two or more distinct personality states that recurrently take control of behavior.

Each alternate personality (alter) or subpersonality has its own pattern of perceiving, relating to, and thinking about the self and the environment. It is believed that severe sexual, physical, or psychological trauma in childhood predisposes an individual to the development of DID. The steps in the development of a dissociated identity are theorized to be as follows (McAllister, 2000):

1. The child being harmed by a trusted caregiver splits off the awareness and memory of the traumatic event to survive in the relationship (e.g., "This is not happening to me").
2. The memories and feelings go into the subconscious and are experienced later as a separate personality.
3. This process happens repeatedly at different times so that different personalities develop, containing different memories and performing different functions that are helpful or destructive.
4. Dissociation becomes a coping mechanism for the individual when faced with further stressful situations.

Each alternate personality or subpersonality is a complex unit with its own memories, behavior patterns, and social relationships that dictate how the person acts when that personality is dominant. Often, the original or primary personality is religious and moralistic, and the subpersonalities are pleasure seeking and nonconforming. The alters may behave as individuals of a different sex, race, or religion. The dominant hand and the voice may be different; intelligence and electroencephalographic findings may also be altered. Subpersonalities often exhibit signs of emotional disturbance: common ones are a fearful child and a persecutor who inflicts pain and may try to kill the individual (Putnam & Loewenstein, 2000).

Typical **cognitive distortions** include the insistence that alternate personalities inhabit separate bodies and are unaffected by the actions of one another. The primary personality or host is usually not aware of the subpersonalities and is perplexed by lost time and unexplained events. Experiences such as finding unfamiliar clothing in the closet, being called a different name by a stranger, or not having childhood memories are characteristic of DID. Subpersonalities are often aware of the existence of each other to some degree. Transition from one personality to another occurs during times of stress and may range from a dramatic to a barely noticeable event. Some clients experience the transition when awakening. Shifts may last from minutes to months, although shorter periods are more common.

The student is encouraged to see the film *Sybil* (1976), which is an actual case study of a person with DID, or *The Three Faces of Eve* (1957).

■ ■ ■ ■ **VIGNETTE**

Andrea, a conservative 28-year-old electrical engineer, is the primary personality. Three alternate personalities coexist and vie for supremacy.

Michele is a 5 year old who is sometimes playful and sometimes angry. She speaks with a slight lisp and with the facial expressions, voice inflections, and vocabulary of a precocious child. She likes to play on swings, draw with a crayon, and eat ice cream. She likes to cuddle a teddy bear and occasionally sucks her thumb. Her favorite outfit is jeans and a Mickey Mouse sweatshirt.

Ann is an accomplished ballet dancer. She is shy but firm about needing time to practice. When she is dominant, she likes to wear white and fixes her hair in a severe, pulled-back style. She does little but dance when she is in control.

Bridget is near Andrea's age, although she says a lady never tells her age. She dresses seductively in bright colors, wears her hair tousled, and likes to frequent bars and stay out late. She often drinks to excess and has several male admirers. Bridget has many moods. She states that she would like to get rid of Ann and Andrea because they're such "goody-goodies."

Andrea does not drink, hates ice cream, and sees herself as somewhat awkward. She does not dance. She is a paid soloist in a church choir. Andrea takes public transportation, but Ann and Bridget have driver's licenses. Andrea goes to bed and arises early, but Bridget and Michele like to stay up late.

Andrea seeks treatment when she finds herself behind the wheel of a moving car and realizes that she does not know how to drive. She has been concerned for some time because she has found strange clothes in her closet. She has also received phone calls from men who insist that she has flirted with them in bars. She sometimes misses appointments and cannot account for periods of time. Although she goes to bed early, she is often unaccountably tired in the morning.

■ ■ ■

Application of the Nursing Process

■ ASSESSMENT

For a diagnosis of dissociative disorder to be made, medical and neurological illnesses, substance use, and other coexisting psychiatric disorders must be ruled out as the cause of the client's symptoms. Medical personnel collect objective data from physical examination, electroencephalography, imaging studies, and specific questionnaires designed to identify dissociative symptoms, such as the Structured Clinical Interview for *DSM-IV* Dissociative Disorders—

Revised (SCID-D-R) (Steinberg, 2000b). Most of the time the DID client is treated in the community. However, a client with DID is admitted to a psychiatric unit when suicidal or in need of crisis stabilization. At that time, the nurse gathers specific information about identity, memory, consciousness, life events, mood, suicide risk, and the impact of the disorder on the client and the family.

Overall Assessment

Identity and Memory

Assessing clients' ability to identify themselves requires more than asking clients to state their names. Changes in client behavior, voice, and dress might signal the presence of an alternate personality. Referring to self by another name or in the third person and using the word *we* instead of *I* are indications that the client may have assumed a new identity. The nurse should consider the following when assessing memory:

- Can the client remember recent and past events?
- Is the client's memory clear and complete or partial and fuzzy?
- Is the client aware of gaps in memory, such as lack of memory for events such as a graduation or a wedding?
- Do the client's memories place the self with a family, in school, in an occupation?

Clients with amnesia and fugue may be disoriented with regard to time and place as well as person. Relevant assessment questions include the following:

- Do you ever lose time or have blackouts?
- Do you find yourself in places with no idea how you got there?

Client History

The nurse must gather information about events in the person's life. Has the client sustained a recent injury, such as a concussion? Does the client have a history of epilepsy, especially temporal lobe epilepsy? Does the client have a history of early trauma, such as physical, mental, or sexual abuse? If DID is suspected, pertinent questions include the following:

- Have you ever found yourself wearing clothes that you can't remember buying?
- Have you ever had strange people greet and talk to you as though they were old friends?
- Does your ability to engage in things such as athletics, artistic activities, or mechanical tasks seem to change?
- Do you have differing sets of memories about childhood?

Mood

Is the individual depressed, anxious, or unconcerned? Many clients with DID seek help when the primary personality is depressed. The nurse also observes for mood shifts. When subpersonalities of DID take control, their predominant moods may be different from that of the principal personality. If the subpersonalities shift frequently, marked mood swings may be noted.

Use of Alcohol and Other Drugs

Specific questions should be asked to identify drug or alcohol use. Dissociative episodes may be associated with recent use of alcohol or other substances—cocaine, opioids, sedatives, or stimulants (Steinberg, 2000b).

Impact on Client and Family

Has the client's ability to function been impaired? Have disruptions in family functioning occurred? Is secondary gain evident? In fugue states, individuals often function adequately in their new identities by choosing simple, undemanding occupations and having few intimate social interactions. The families of clients in fugue states report being highly distressed over the client's disappearance. Clients with amnesia may be more dysfunctional. Their perplexity often renders them unable to work, and their memory loss impairs normal family relationships. Families often direct considerable attention toward the client but may exhibit concern over having to assume roles that were once assigned to the client. Clients with DID often have both family and work problems. Families find it difficult to accept the seemingly erratic behaviors of the client. Employers dislike the lost time that may occur when subpersonalities are in control. Clients with depersonalization disorder are often fearful that others may perceive their appearance as distorted and may avoid being seen in public. If they exhibit high anxiety, the family is likely to find it difficult to keep relationships stable.

Suicide Risk

Whenever a client's life has been substantially disrupted, the client may have thoughts of suicide. The nurse gathering data should be alert for expressions of hopelessness, helplessness, or worthlessness and for verbalization or other behavior of a subpersonality that indicates the intent to engage in self-destructive or self-mutilating behaviors.

Self-Assessment

Nurses may experience feelings of skepticism while caring for clients with dissociative disorders. They may find it difficult to believe in the authenticity of the symptoms the client is displaying.

Feeling confused and bewildered by the presence of multiple identities is not unusual. Anger is commonly experienced in reaction to a subpersonality of a client with DID if one personality is perceived as immature, challenging, or unpleasant. Some nurses experience feelings of fascination and are caught up in the intrigue of caring for a client with multiple identities. A sense of inadequacy may accompany the need to be ready to interact in a therapeutic way with whichever personality is in control at the moment.

Similarly, the nurse may feel inadequate when establishment of a trusting relationship occurs slowly. It is important for the nurse to remember that the client with a dissociative disorder has often experienced relationships in which trust was betrayed. When subpersonalities vie for control and attempt to embarrass or harm each other, crises are common. The nurse must be alert and ready to intervene and must always be prepared for the unexpected, including the possibility of a suicide attempt. Continuing hypervigilance by staff can eventually lead to feelings of fatigue. Anxiety may also be experienced by the nurse caring for a client with dissociative disorder in any of the following situations:

- When a client who has regained memory develops panic level anxiety related to guilt feelings
- When a client becomes assaultive because of extreme confusion or panic level anxiety
- When a client attempts self-harm by acting out against the primary personality or other personalities

If the client manifesting symptoms of a dissociative disorder has been involved in the commission of a crime, the nurse may experience concern over the fact that the medical record is likely to be a court exhibit. Nurses may feel anger in this situation if they believe that the client is faking illness to avoid being found guilty of the crime.

Supervision should always be available for nursing staff and clinicians caring for a client with a dissociative disorder. By discussing feelings as well as the plan of care with the treatment team or peers, the nurse can better ensure objective and appropriate care for the client.

> ### Assessment Guidelines Dissociative Disorders
>
> 1. Assess for a history of a similar episode in the past with benign outcomes.
> 2. Establish whether the person suffered abuse, trauma, or loss as a child.
> 3. Identify relevant psychosocial distress issues by performing a basic psychosocial assessment (refer to Chapter 9).

■ NURSING DIAGNOSIS

Nursing diagnoses for clients with dissociative disorders are suggested in Table 15-6.

■ OUTCOME CRITERIA

Outcomes must be established for each nursing diagnosis. General goals are to develop trust, to correct faulty perceptions, and to encourage the client to live in the present instead of dissociating (Kreidler et al., 2000). NOC outcomes potentially appropriate for clients with dissociative disorders include *Identity, Role Performance, Coping, Anxiety Self-Control, Self-Mutilation Restraint,* and *Aggression Self-Control.* Specific examples of indicators that the outcomes are being achieved are the following:

- Client will verbalize clear sense of personal identity.
- Client will report decrease in stress.
- Client will report comfort with role expectations.

TABLE 15-6

Potential Nursing Diagnoses for Dissociative Disorders

Signs and Symptoms	Nursing Diagnoses
■ Amnesia or fugue related to a traumatic event	**Disturbed personal identity**
■ Symptoms of depersonalization; feelings of unreality and/or body image distortions	**Disturbed body image**
■ Alterations in consciousness, memory, or identity	**Ineffective coping**
■ Abuse of substances related to dissociation	**Ineffective role performance**
■ Disorganization or dysfunction in usual patterns of behavior (absence from work, withdrawal from relationships, changes in role function)	
■ Disturbances in memory and identity	**Interrupted family processes**
■ Interrupted family processes related to amnesia or erratic and changing behavior	**Impaired parenting**
■ Feeling of being out of control of memory, behaviors, and awareness	**Anxiety**
■ Inability to explain actions or behaviors when in altered state	**Spiritual distress**
	Risk for other-directed violence
	Risk for self-directed violence

- Client will plan coping strategies for stressful situations.
- Client will refrain from injuring self.

■ PLANNING

The planning of nursing care for the client with a dissociative disorder is influenced by the setting and presenting problem. The basic level nurse will encounter such a client in times of crisis, when the client is admitted to the hospital for suicidal or homicidal behavior. The care plan will focus on safety and crisis intervention. The client may also come for treatment of a comorbid depression or anxiety disorder in the community setting. Planning will address the major complaint with appropriate referrals for treatment of the dissociative disorder.

■ INTERVENTION
Basic Level Interventions

Basic level interventions are aimed at offering emotional presence during the recall of painful experiences, providing a sense of safety, and encouraging an optimal level of functioning. NIC topics that offer relevant interventions include *Anxiety Reduction, Coping Enhancement, Self-Awareness Enhancement, Self-Esteem Enhancement,* and *Emotional Support.* Refer to Table 15-7 for examples of basic level interventions. The fol-

lowing sections describe milieu therapy, health teaching, and psychobiological interventions.

Milieu Therapy

When the client is in a crisis that requires hospitalization, providing a safe environment is fundamental. Other desirable characteristics of the environment are that it be quiet, simple, structured, and supportive. Confusion and noise increase anxiety and the potential for depersonalization, delayed memory return, or shifts among subpersonalities. Inpatient group therapy is not as helpful as task-oriented therapy, such as occupational and art therapy, which give an opportunity for self-expression. Attendance at community or unit milieu meetings relieves feelings of isolation.

Health Teaching

Clients with dissociative disorders need teaching about the illness and instruction in coping skills and stress management. They may need to develop a plan to interrupt a dissociative episode, such as singing or doing a specific activity. Staff and significant others are made aware of the plan in order to foster their cooperation. Clients should also be taught to keep a daily journal to increase their awareness of feelings and to identify triggers to dissociation. If a client has never written a journal, the nurse should suggest beginning with a 5- to 10-minute daily writing exercise.

TABLE 15-7

Basic Level Interventions and Rationales for Dissociative Disorders

Intervention	Rationale
1. Ensure client safety by providing safe, protected environment and frequent observation.	1. Sense of bewilderment may lead to inattention to safety needs; some subpersonalities may be thrill seeking, violent, or careless
2. Provide nondemanding, simple routine.	2. Reduces anxiety
3. Confirm identity of client and orientation to time and place.	3. Supports reality and promotes ego integrity
4. Encourage client to do things for self and make decisions about routine tasks.	4. Enhances self-esteem by reducing sense of powerlessness and reduces secondary gain associated with dependence
5. Assist with other decision making until memory returns.	5. Lowers stress and prevents client from having to live with the consequences of unwise decisions
6. Support client during exploration of feelings surrounding the stressful event.	6. Helps lower the defense of dissociation used by client to block awareness of the stressful event
7. Do not flood client with data regarding past events.	7. Memory loss serves the purpose of preventing severe to panic levels of anxiety from overtaking and disorganizing the individual
8. Allow client to progress at own pace as memory is recovered.	8. Prevents undue anxiety and resistance
9. Provide support during disclosure of painful experiences.	9. Can be healing while minimizing feelings of isolation
10. Help client see consequences of using dissociation to cope with stress.	10. Increases insight and helps client understand own role in choosing behaviors
11. Accept client's expression of negative feelings.	11. Conveys permission to have negative or unacceptable feelings
12. Teach stress reduction methods.	12. Provides alternatives for anxiety relief
13. If client does not remember significant others, work with involved parties to reestablish relationships.	13. Helps client experience satisfaction and relieves sense of isolation

Psychobiological Interventions

There are no specific medications for dissociative disorders, but appropriate antidepressants or anxiolytic medications are given for comorbid conditions. Substance use disorders and suicidal risk, which are common, must be assessed carefully if medication is to be used. In the acute setting, the nurse may witness dramatic memory retrieval in clients with dissociative amnesia or fugue after treatment with intravenous benzodiazepines (Ballew et al., 2003).

Advanced Practice Interventions

Advanced practice nurses may use cognitive-behavioral therapy or psychodynamic psychotherapy to treat dissociative disorders. Cognitive-behavioral group therapy has also proven to be helpful for female sexual abuse survivors (Kreidler et al., 2000).

■ EVALUATION

Treatment is considered successful when outcomes are met. In the final analysis, the evaluation is positive when

- Client safety has been maintained.
- Anxiety has been reduced and the client has returned to a functional state.
- Conflicts have been explored.
- New coping strategies have permitted the client to function at a better level.
- Stress is handled adaptively, without the use of dissociation.

CASE STUDY and NURSING CARE PLAN 15-1   Conversion Disorder

Ms. Andrews is a single female admitted to the neurological unit of a general hospital for evaluation of sudden onset of seizures. It is the eve of her thirtieth birthday, and she is an attractive fashion model who quickly begins to flirt with the male nursing staff and physicians. Her first seizure after admittance occurs during morning rounds just as the staff enter her room. She arches her back and begins pelvic thrusting motions while thrashing her arms and legs about in the bed. She has no loss of consciousness and she is not incontinent. Similar seizures occur over the next 2 days, always witnessed by staff or visitors. Ms. Andrews does not seem concerned about the impact of her symptoms on her career (la belle indifférence). She remains calm and is playful with the male staff. When she is told that her diagnostic test results are negative, she agrees to transfer to the psychiatric unit for further evaluation.

On the psychiatric unit, Ms. Andrews is observed behaving in a more helpless, dependent manner. She will not come out of her room for fear of a seizure, and her father refers to her as his "little girl."

Self-Assessment

Ms. D'Angelo is a registered nurse with an AA degree and 2 years of experience on the psychiatric unit. She recognizes mixed feelings toward Ms. Andrews. On the one hand, the client is interesting and charming as she relates stories of her glamorous career. On the other hand, she is demanding and childish, expecting special privileges on the unit. Ms. Andrews quickly becomes a favorite topic during nursing report, with staff comparing notes on her attention-seeking behaviors. Ms. D'Angelo realizes that she has to carefully monitor her emotional reactions to Ms. Andrews. The nurse will need to adopt a matter-of-fact approach to reduce secondary gains and to encourage the client to resume her independence.

■ ASSESSMENT

Objective Data

- Results of all diagnostic tests for seizure disorder are negative.
- Sudden onset of symptoms coincides with the client's thirtieth birthday.
- The symptoms interrupt the client's career.
- There is no prior history of somatoform or psychiatric disorders.

Subjective Data

- "I don't know what I'm doing here with all of these mental patients."
- "Can my daddy bring in my birthday cake? I never got to celebrate on the other unit."

Continued

■ NURSING DIAGNOSIS (NANDA)

Ineffective coping: related to low self-esteem and unmet needs for recognition and attention, as evidenced by use of conversion symptoms (seizures)

Supporting Data
- No incontinence or injury; seizures vary and occur only in the presence of others
- Relates with seductive behavior toward men
- Bland affect regarding personal problems (la belle indifférence)

■ OUTCOME CRITERIA (NOC)

Client will consistently identify effective coping patterns without using conversion (long-term goal).

■ PLANNING

The initial plan is to maintain safety for Ms. Andrews while encouraging her to explore recent stressful events.

■ INTERVENTION (NIC)

The plan of care for Ms. Andrews is personalized as follows:

Short-Term Goal	Intervention	Rationale	Evaluation
1. Client will perform all activities of daily living (ADLs) by the end of the second day.	1. Explain routine. Establish expectations regarding unit routines; do not allow special privileges. Expect client to eat in dining room, perform ADLs, attend activities.	1. Reduces anxiety; reduces secondary gain and manipulation	GOAL MET Client initially refuses to leave room for meals. Misses one meal. Goes to dining room thereafter. Performs all ADLs, with special attention to applying make-up.
2. Client will remain free of injury throughout the hospitalization.	2. Provide safety measures during seizures but limit attention and discussion about seizures afterward. Monitor physical condition unobtrusively.	2. Prevents harm; reduces secondary gain; minimizes secondary gain while condition is assessed	GOAL MET Client does not sustain injury during seizures. States, "I guess my seizures don't interest staff. No one will talk to me about them." Client has no seizures after day 3 on the psychiatric unit.
3. Client will express feelings about self-worth by the end of the second day.	3. Encourage exploration of feelings about life, work, loved ones.	3. Conveys interest, and uncovers sources of stress	GOAL MET Client states she is scared of losing her glamorous appearance and her job because of age. Demonstrates appropriate affect.
4. Client will verbalize optimism about future by discharge.	4. Focus on alternatives available to client to earn a living when modeling is no longer an option.	4. Encourages problem solving	GOAL MET Client shows fashion sketches to nurse and reveals that she had once thought that she might be a good designer. With encouragement, she decides to explore evening classes in illustration and design to prepare for second career.
5. Client will allow family involvement in decision making by the end of the second day.	5. Identify family's perceptions of the situation, precipitating events, and client's feelings and behaviors.	5. Encourages realistic feedback to client; reduces secondary gain	GOAL MET Family supports plan to study fashion design.

■ EVALUATION

See individual outcomes and evaluation in the care plan.

■■■ KEY POINTS to REMEMBER

- Somatoform disorders are characterized by the presence of multiple real physical symptoms for which there is no evidence of medical illness.
- Dissociative disorders involve a disruption in consciousness with a significant impairment in memory, identity, or perceptions of self.
- Somatoform and dissociative disorders are believed to be responses to psychological stress, although the client shows no insight into the potential stressors.
- Clients with somatoform and dissociative disorders often have comorbid psychiatric illness, primarily depression, anxiety, or substance abuse.
- The course of these disorders may be brief, with acute onset and spontaneous remission, or chronic, with a gradual onset and prolonged impairment.

- Because these clients may not seek psychiatric treatment, the nurse does not usually see them in the acute psychiatric setting, except during a period of crisis such as suicidal risk.
- The nursing assessment is especially important to clarify the history and course of past symptoms, as well as to obtain a complete picture of the current physical and mental status.
- Although these clients do respond to crisis intervention, they usually require referral for psychotherapy to attain sustained improvement in level of functioning.

■■■

Visit the Evolve website at **http://evolve.elsevier.com/Varcarolis** for a posttest on the content in this chapter.   *evolve*

Critical Thinking and Chapter Review

Visit the Evolve website at **http://evolve.elsevier.com/Varcarolis** for additional self-study exercises.
evolve

■■■ CRITICAL THINKING

1. A client with suspected somatization disorder has been admitted to the medical-surgical unit after an episode of chest pain with possible electrocardiographic changes. While on the unit, she frequently complains of palpitations, asks the nurse to check her vital signs, and begs staff to stay with her. Some nurses take her pulse and blood pressure when she asks. Others evade her requests. Most staff try to avoid spending time with her. Consider why staff wish to avoid her. Design interventions to cope with the client's behaviors. Give rationales for your interventions.

2. A client with body dysmorphic disorder talks incessantly about how big her nose is, how those around her are offended by her appearance, and how her appearance has negatively affected her employment and her social life. What interventions could you make to reduce her anxiety?

3. A client with DID has been admitted to the crisis unit for a short-term stay after a suicide threat. On the unit, the client has repeated the statement that she will kill herself to get rid of "all the others," meaning her subpersonalities. The client refuses to sign a "no harm" contract. Design a care plan to meet her safety and security needs.

■■■ CHAPTER REVIEW

Choose the most appropriate answer.

1. Nurses working with clients with somatization and dissociative disorders can expect that these clients will fit on the continuum of psychobiological disorders at the
    1. mild level.
    2. moderate to severe level.
    3. severe to psychotic level.
    4. They do not belong on the continuum, because anxiety has been reduced by ego defense mechanisms.

2. Mr. R. presents with a history of having assumed a new identity in a distant locale and of having no recollection of his former identity. Which *DSM-IV-TR* diagnosis can the nurse expect the psychiatrist to make?
    1. Hypochondriasis
    2. Conversion disorder
    3. Dissociative fugue
    4. Depersonalization disorder

3. The information that is least relevant when assessing a client with a suspected somatoform disorder is
    1. determination of whether the symptom is under voluntary control.
    2. results of diagnostic workups.
    3. limitations in activities of daily living.
    4. potential for violence.

4. A suitable outcome criterion for the nursing diagnosis *ineffective coping* related to dependence on pain relievers to treat chronic pain of psychological origin is which of the following?
    1. Client will resume preillness roles.
    2. Client will cope adaptively as evidenced by use of alternative coping strategies.
    3. Client will demonstrate improved self-esteem as evidenced by focusing less on weaknesses.
    4. Client will replace demanding, manipulative behaviors with more socially acceptable behavior.

5. Which nursing diagnosis would be least likely to be used for a client with hypochondriasis?
    1. Disturbed personal identity
    2. Ineffective denial
    3. Disturbed body image
    4. Interrupted family processes

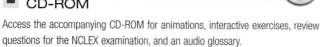

■ **STUDENT**
■ **STUDY**
■ **CD-ROM**

Access the accompanying CD-ROM for animations, interactive exercises, review questions for the NCLEX examination, and an audio glossary.

■ **NURSE,**
■ **CLIENT, AND**
■ **FAMILY RESOURCES**

For suggested readings, information on related associations, and Internet resources, go to **http://evolve.elsevier.com/Varcarolis.** *evolve*

REFERENCES

American Psychiatric Association. (2000). *Diagnostic and statistical manual of mental disorders (DSM-IV-TR)* (4th ed., text rev.). Washington, DC: Author.

American Psychiatric Association. (2002). Consumer and family information: Hypochondriasis. *Psychiatric Services, 53*(4), 383.

Ballew, L., et al. (2003). Intravenous diazepam for dissociative disorder: Memory lost and found. *Psychosomatics, 44,* 346-347.

Barsky, A. J. (2001). The patient with hypochondriasis. *New England Journal of Medicine, 345*(19), 1395-1399.

Carroll, D. H., Scahill, L., & Phillips, K. A. (2002). Current concepts in body dysmorphic disorder. *Archives of Psychiatric Nursing, 16*(2), 72-79.

Coons, P. M. (2000). Dissociative fugue. In B. J. Sadock & V. A. Sadock (Eds.), *Comprehensive textbook of psychiatry* (7th ed., Vol. 1, pp. 1549-1552). Philadelphia: Lippincott Williams & Wilkins.

Dochterman, J. M., & Bulechek, G. M. (2004). *Nursing interventions classification (NIC)* (4th ed.). St. Louis, MO: Mosby.

Gallagher, R. M., & Cariati, S. (2002, October 2). *Clinical update: The pain-depression conundrum: Bridging the body and mind.* Retrieved January 4, 2005, from Medscape website: http://www.medscape.com/viewprogram/2030.

Guggenheim, F. G. (2000). Somatoform disorders. In B. J. Sadock & V. A. Sadock (Eds.), *Comprehensive textbook of psychiatry* (7th ed., Vol. 1, pp. 1504-1532). Philadelphia: Lippincott Williams & Wilkins.

Katon, W., Sullivan, M., & Walker, E. (2001). Medical symptoms without identified pathology: Relationship to psychiatric disorders, childhood and adult trauma, and personality traits. *Annals of Internal Medicine, 134,* 917-925.

Kreidler, M. C., et al. (2000). Trauma and dissociation: Treatment perspectives. *Perspectives in Psychiatric Care, 36*(3), 77-85.

Looper, K. J., & Kirmayer, L. J. (2002). Behavioral medicine approaches to somatoform disorders. *Journal of Consulting and Clinical Psychology, 70*(3), 810-827.

McAllister, M. M. (2000). Dissociative identity disorder: A literature review. *Journal of Psychiatric and Mental Health Nursing, 7,* 25-33.

Moorhead, S., Johnson, M., & Maas, M. (2004). *Nursing outcomes classification (NOC)* (3rd ed.). St. Louis, MO: Mosby.

Phillips, K. A., Albertini, R. S., & Rasmussen, S. A. (2002). A randomized placebo-controlled trial of fluoxetine in body dysmorphic disorder. *Archives of General Psychiatry, 59,* 381-388.

Putnam, F. W., & Loewenstein, R. J. (2000). Dissociative identity disorder. In B. J. Sadock & V. A. Sadock (Eds.), *Comprehensive textbook of psychiatry* (7th ed., Vol. 1, pp. 1552-1563). Philadelphia: Lippincott Williams & Wilkins.

Roelofs, K., et al. (2002). Childhood abuse in patients with conversion disorder. *American Journal of Psychiatry, 159*(11), 1908-1913.

Simeon, D., et al. (2001). The role of childhood interpersonal trauma in depersonalization disorder. *American Journal of Psychiatry, 158*(7), 1027-1033.

Stahl, S. M. (2003). Antidepressants and somatic symptoms: Therapeutic actions are expanding beyond affective spectrum disorders to functional somatic syndromes. *Journal of Clinical Psychiatry, 64*(7), 745-746.

Steinberg, M. (2000a). Depersonalization disorder. In B. J. Sadock & V. A. Sadock (Eds.), *Comprehensive textbook of psychiatry* (7th ed., Vol. 1, pp. 1564-1570). Philadelphia: Lippincott Williams & Wilkins.

Steinberg, M. (2000b). Dissociative amnesia. In B. J. Sadock & V. A. Sadock (Eds.), *Comprehensive textbook of psychiatry* (7th ed., Vol. 1, 1544-1549). Philadelphia: Lippincott Williams & Wilkins.

CHAPTER 16

Personality Disorders

NANCY CHRISTINE SHOEMAKER ▪ ELIZABETH M. VARCAROLIS

KEY TERMS and CONCEPTS

The key terms and concepts listed here appear in color where they are defined or first discussed in this chapter.

antisocial personality disorder, 282

avoidant personality disorder, 284

borderline personality disorder, 282

dependent personality disorder, 284

dialectical behavior therapy (DBT), 295

entitlement, 282

histrionic personality disorder, 282

manipulative, 282

narcissistic personality disorder, 284

obsessive-compulsive personality disorder, 285

paranoid personality disorder, 280

personality, 275

personality disorder (PD), 276

schizoid personality disorder, 280

schizotypal personality disorder, 280

splitting, 279

OBJECTIVES

After studying this chapter, the reader will be able to

1. Analyze the interaction of biological determinants and psychodynamic factors in the etiology of personality disorders.
2. Identify the three clusters of personality disorders.
3. Describe the main characteristic of one personality disorder from each cluster and give an example.
4. Formulate two nursing diagnoses for cluster B personality disorders.
5. Discuss the nature and importance of crisis intervention for people with personality disorders.
6. Describe the feelings that are experienced by nurses and others when working with people with personality disorders.
7. Discuss two realistic nursing outcomes for clients with borderline personality disorder.
8. Plan basic interventions for an impulsive, aggressive, or manipulative client.

evolve Visit the Evolve website at **http://evolve.elsevier.com/Varcarolis** for a pretest on the content in this chapter.

This chapter provides an overview of the 11 personality disorders (PDs) as defined by the *Diagnostic and Statistical Manual of Mental Disorders*, fourth edition, text revision *(DSM-IV-TR)* (American Psychiatric Association [APA], 2000). Ten of the disorders are grouped into three clusters because they are characterized by similar behavior patterns. People with PDs have problematic personalities that stand out from those of the majority of individuals in their own culture. **Personality** is defined as "an enduring pattern of behavior that is considered to be both conscious and unconscious and reflects a means of adapting to a particular environment and its cultural, ethnic and community standards" (Carson, 2000, p. 181). An individ-

ual with a healthy personality has the following characteristics (Marcus, 2000):

- Sees his or her own strengths and weaknesses
- Identifies his or her own boundaries
- Recognizes interactions and thoughts that lead to strong emotions such as joy or anger
- Interacts with others without expecting them to meet all needs
- Seeks a balance of work and play
- Accomplishes goals
- Defines and expresses spirituality

In contrast, **personality disorder (PD)** is defined as "an enduring pattern of inner experience and behavior that deviates markedly from the expectation of the individual's culture, is pervasive and inflexible, has an onset in adolescence or early adulthood, is stable over time, and leads to distress or impairment" (APA, 2000, p. 685). A person with a PD exhibits long-term maladaptive behavior that prevents him or her from accomplishing desired goals in relationships and other endeavors. These behaviors are not experienced as uncomfortable or disorganized by the individual, as are the symptoms of clients with anxiety, mood, or psychotic disorders. It is important to note that some areas of personal functioning may be very adequate; for example, the individual may live independently. The predominant maladaptive behavior may affect only one aspect of the person's life, such as intimate relationships. Therefore, many individuals with PDs do not seek treatment unless there is a crisis or a comorbid diagnosis that causes distress. Refer to Box 16-1 for the *DSM-IV-TR* general criteria for a personality disorder.

All of the PDs have four characteristics in common: (1) inflexible and maladaptive response to stress; (2) disability in working and loving; (3) ability to evoke interpersonal conflict; and (4) capacity to "get under the skin" of others.

1. **Inflexible and maladaptive response to stress.** Personality patterns persist unmodified over long periods of time. Certain patterns and traits may be acceptable within societal norms and are valued by the culture or occupation. For instance, an engineer or administrator needs to possess some compulsive traits, such as the ability to organize complex details and meet deadlines. At other times, these same compulsive traits, when too rigid and limited, may interfere with personal or social functioning. This rigid behavior serves the function of controlling deep anxiety for the person.

2. **Disability in working and loving, which is generally more serious and pervasive than the similar disability found in other disorders.** Certain characteristics observed in people with PDs are similar to those seen in people with mood disorders and schizophrenic disorders (e.g., withdrawal, grandiosity, and suspiciousness). The difference is that, for the most part, individuals with PDs have normal ego functioning and reality testing. There are, however, great disturbances in their ability to find intimate and satisfactory interpersonal relationships or to function at their optimum creative level. All individuals with personality disorders have self-esteem issues, despite any outward appearance of confidence.

3. **Ability to evoke interpersonal conflict.** In individuals with PDs, intense emotional upheavals and hostility lead to frequent interpersonal conflicts. People with PDs lack the ability to see themselves objectively. Therefore, they lack the desire to alter aspects of their behavior to enrich or maintain important relationships. Their inability to take responsibility for their own behavior creates strong negative reactions in others. In essence, they cannot trust others and are constantly fearful of being hurt.

4. **Capacity to "get under the skin" of others.** Getting under the skin of others refers to the uncanny ability of people with PDs to merge personal boundaries with others. This merging is manifested by the intense effect they have on others. The process is often unconscious and the result undesirable.

Judgments about an individual's personality functioning must take into account the person's ethnic, cultural, and social background. Because PDs are often overdiagnosed in clients who are ethnically and culturally different from the health care provider, it is important for the clinician to obtain additional information from others from the individual's cultural background (APA, 2000).

BOX 16-1

DSM-IV-TR Criteria for a Personality Disorder

A. An enduring pattern of inner experience and behavior that deviates markedly from the expectations of the individual's culture. This pattern is manifested in two (or more) of the following areas:
  (1) Cognition (i.e., ways of perceiving and interpreting self, other people, and events)
  (2) Affectivity (i.e., range, intensity, lability, and appropriateness of emotional response)
  (3) Interpersonal functioning
  (4) Impulse control
B. The enduring pattern is inflexible and pervasive across a broad range of personal and social situations.
C. The enduring pattern leads to clinically significant distress or impairment in social, occupational, or other important areas of functioning.
D. The pattern is stable and of long duration, and its onset can be traced back at least to adolescence or early adulthood.
E. The enduring pattern is not better accounted for as a manifestation or consequence of another mental disorder.
F. The enduring pattern is not due to the direct physiological effects of a substance (e.g., a drug of abuse, a medication) or a general medical condition (e.g., head trauma).

From American Psychiatric Association. (2000). *Diagnostic and statistical manual of mental disorders* (4th ed., text rev.). Washington, DC: Author.

Individuals with PDs tend to be less educated or unemployed. They frequently are single or, if married, have marital difficulties. They often have comorbid substance use disorders and may commit violent and nonviolent crimes, including sex offenses (APA, 2000). People with PDs evoke emotional reactions in health care providers. They may be aggravating and demanding, or seductive and dependent; staff may react with inappropriate responses such as sexual interest, the urge to rescue, or the desire to withdraw (Munich & Allen, 2003).

Yet, these clients do suffer real distress and many seek help. They are more difficult to engage in treatment because of the problem with trust. "They are profoundly impaired in their ability to make use of potentially healing attachment relationships" (Munich & Allen, 2003, p. 149). With a high level of motivation, some may show sustained improvement, especially with cognitive-behavioral therapy as described later.

They may seek help from primary care physicians for physical complaints, rather than seeking help in the mental health arena. Under stress, some people with PDs may become psychotic; therefore, PD is positioned toward the severe–psychosis end of the mental health continuum (Figure 16-1).

PREVALENCE AND COMORBIDITY

The prevalence of PDs in the general population ranges from 10% to 15% and is higher in certain settings (Widiger & Mullins, 2003). PDs are predisposing factors for many other psychiatric disorders and often co-occur with depression and anxiety. By definition, their onset usually predates the onset of a major mental disorder, and they have a significant effect on the course of treatment. In addition, various PDs often co-exist, presenting a challenge for diagnosis and treat-

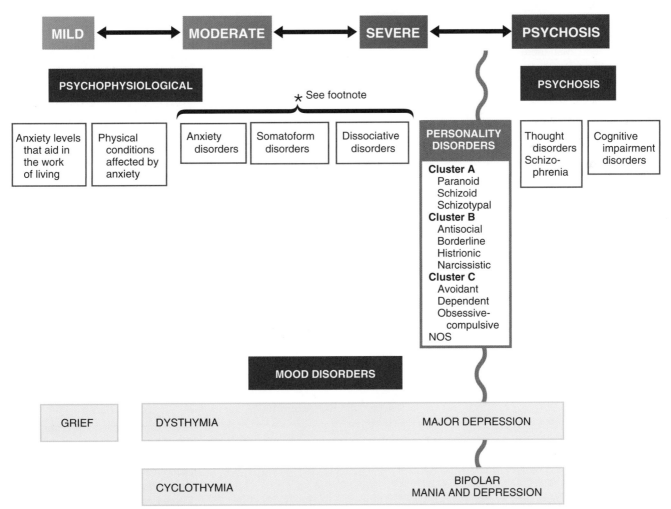

MENTAL HEALTH CONTINUUM FOR PERSONALITY DISORDERS

* These disorders are currently classified by presenting clinical symptoms. Previously they were called "neurotic" disorders.

FIGURE 16-1 The mental health continuum for personality disorders. *NOS,* Not otherwise specified.

ment. Refer to Tables 16-1, 16-2, and 16-3 for a summary of prevalence, gender predilection, and co-morbidities of the major mental disorders in each PD cluster.

THEORY

The answer to the question of what causes PDs is that there is unlikely to be any single cause for a discrete PD. Environmental influences (e.g., child abuse) and biological influences (e.g., genetic factors) as well as psychological factors all seem to come into play. There has not been as much research into the biological and psychosocial causes of PDs as into the causes of affective, anxiety, and psychotic disorders.

Biological Determinants

Research in infant and cross-cultural studies has led to several models of the inheritance of personality characteristics. It is proposed that certain traits are present at birth and that there is a continuum from normal to excessive levels of a given tendency associated with some underlying neurobiological mechanism. PDs may represent an extreme variation of a natural tendency resulting from genetic alterations and/or unfavorable environmental conditions (Widiger & Mullins, 2003). The following nine personality traits have been identified as potentially inherited:
1. Novelty seeking
2. Harm avoidance

TABLE 16-1

Cluster A Personality Disorders

Disorder	Gender Predilection	Prevalence in General Population	Prevalence in Clinical Setting	Comorbidities
Paranoid	Men more than women	0.5%-2.5%	2%-30%	Major depressive disorder Agoraphobia Obsessive-compulsive disorder Substance use disorders
Schizoid	Men more than women	0.4%-4.1%	Uncommon	Major depressive disorder
Schizotypal	Men more than women	3%	No data	Major depressive disorder

Data from American Psychiatric Association. (2000). *Diagnostic and statistical manual of mental disorders* (4th ed., text rev.). Washington, DC: Author; and Widiger, T. A., & Mullins, S. (2003). Personality disorders. In A. Tasman, J. Kay, & J. A. Lieberman (Eds.). *Psychiatry* (2nd ed., Vol. 2). London: Wiley.

TABLE 16-2

Cluster B Personality Disorders

Disorder	Gender Predilection	Prevalence in General Population	Prevalence in Clinical Setting	Comorbidities
Antisocial	Men more than women	Males, 3%; females, 1%	3%-30%	Anxiety disorders Depressive disorders Substance use disorders Somatization disorder
Borderline	Women more than men	2%	10%-20%	Mood disorders Substance use disorders Eating disorders Posttraumatic stress disorder Attention deficit hyperactivity disorder
Histrionic	Women more than men	2%-3%	10%-15%	Major depressive disorder Somatization disorder Conversion disorder
Narcissistic	Men more than women	1%	2%-16%	Depressive disorders Substance use disorders Anorexia nervosa

Data from American Psychiatric Association. (2000). *Diagnostic and statistical manual of mental disorders* (4th ed., text rev.). Washington, DC: Author.

TABLE 16-3

Cluster C Personality Disorders

Disorder	Gender Predilection	Prevalence in General Population	Prevalence in Clinical Setting	Comorbidities
Avoidant	Equal prevalence in men and women	0.5%-1.0%	10%	Mood disorders Anxiety disorders
Dependent	Women more than men	0.1%-10.0%	Most frequently reported personality disorder	Mood disorders Anxiety disorders Adjustment disorder
Obsessive-compulsive	Men more than women	1%	3%-10%	Anxiety disorders Mood disorders Eating disorders

Data from American Psychiatric Association. (2000). *Diagnostic and statistical manual of mental disorders* (4th ed., text rev.). Washington, DC: Author.

3. Reward dependence
4. Persistence
5. Neuroticism (negative affect) versus emotional stability
6. Introversion versus extraversion
7. Conscientiousness versus undependability
8. Antagonism versus agreeableness
9. Closedness versus openness to experiences

Exaggerations of any of these tendencies may predispose someone to the development of a PD; for example, extreme introversion may predispose to the development of schizoid PD; excessive antagonism and undependability, to antisocial PD; and high levels of neuroticism and extraversion, to histrionic PD.

Family and twin studies also suggest genetic factors or linkages between PDs and other mental illnesses (Widiger & Mullins, 2003). Schizotypal PD is frequently seen in first-degree relatives of persons with schizophrenia. There is a definite genetic influence in antisocial PD: biological children of parents with antisocial PD have a higher risk for developing the disorder, even if they are adopted by outsiders. Individuals with borderline PD often have family members with mood or impulse control disorders.

Some people with PDs have a history of repeated psychological, physical, or sexual trauma during childhood. Thus, the neurobiological research related to chronic stress may also be relevant to PDs. As noted in the two previous chapters on anxiety and dissociative disorders, repeated trauma leads to altered neurotransmitter systems and overuse of primitive defense mechanisms. PDs may be another, less disabling expression of these biological and psychological changes.

Psychosocial Factors

Several psychological theories may help to explain the development of PDs. Learning theory emphasizes that the child developed maladaptive responses based on modeling or reinforcement by significant others. Cognitive theory explains the excessive anxiety of clients as caused by a distortion in thinking that is amenable to correction. Psychoanalytic theory focuses on the use of primitive defense mechanisms by these clients.

Several environmental factors are theorized to influence the development of each disorder. It is believed that persons with paranoid PD had parents who were excessively critical or who role-modeled projection of anger and resentment onto an external group. In the case of schizoid PD, the child may have suffered from emotional isolation because the parents were indifferent or detached.

For persons with antisocial PD, histories often reveal excessively harsh or erratic discipline, along with encouragement of aggression. In clients with borderline PD, there is consistent evidence of childhood trauma, including physical and/or sexual abuse, and significant parental conflict or loss. This early distress associated with relationships is theorized to be the reason for the excessive concern with abandonment. For individuals with histrionic PD, there may have been excessive family reinforcement of attention-seeking behavior. For narcissistic PD, there is speculation that parents were neglectful or inconsistent in rewarding the child, alternating between bestowing excessive praise for accomplishments and giving harsh criticism for minor mistakes.

In avoidant PD, it is believed that parents were overprotective. As with dependent PD, there may have been parental overprotection or excessive clinging to the child, which interfered with normal development and separation. Persons with obsessive-compulsive PD may have copied the behavior of authoritarian parents, but psychoanalytic theory suggests issues with unconscious shame or guilt.

The defense mechanisms used by people with PDs include repression, suppression, regression, undoing, and splitting (Kernberg, 1985). Splitting is the inability to incorporate positive and negative aspects of oneself or others into a whole image. For example, the individual may tend to idealize another person (friend, lover, health care professional) at the start of a new relationship, hoping that this person will meet all of his or her needs. But at the first disappointment or frustration, the individual quickly shifts to devaluation, despising the other person. The individual often threatens abandonment or actually leaves the person, which results in unstable relationships and low self-esteem. Splitting is the primary defense used by individuals with borderline PD. (Refer to Chapter 13 for a review of immature defense mechanisms.)

DSM-IV-TR AND THE CLINICAL PICTURE OF CLUSTER A DISORDERS (ODD, ECCENTRIC)

Persons with cluster A PDs are described as odd or eccentric. Refer to Figure 16-2 for the diagnostic criteria for each disorder in this group. In general, these individuals avoid interpersonal relationships, have unusual beliefs, and may be indifferent to the reactions of others to their views. They seldom seek psychiatric treatment, believing firmly in their interpretation of the world. However, they may be seen in acute care settings if they develop brief psychotic symptoms under stress or require treatment of a comorbid psychiatric disorder. Predominant features of each disorder are described in the following sections (Kay, Tasman, & Lieberman, 2000) and are illustrated in the accompanying vignettes.

Paranoid Personality Disorder

Paranoid personality disorder is characterized by distrust and suspiciousness toward others, based on the belief (unsupported by evidence) that others want to exploit, harm, or deceive the person. These individuals are hypervigilant, anticipate hostility, and may provoke hostile responses by initiating a "counterattack." They demonstrate jealousy, controlling behaviors, and unwillingness to forgive. Paranoid persons are difficult to interview because they are reluctant to share information about themselves. Underneath the guarded surface, these persons are actually quite anxious about being harmed.

■ ■ ■ VIGNETTE

Mr. Alonzo is a 54-year-old unemployed male who comes to a mental health clinic complaining of depression and pain. He walks stiffly and uses two old, broken canes. He provides elaborate details about "nerve pain" all over his body resulting from an accident 5 years earlier. He states that multiple doctors refused to help him due to instructions from his insurance company. He believes that his health maintenance organization has circulated his medical record to all health care providers in the region to prevent him from being treated. He refuses to give any social history and is reluctant to share his telephone number. When the nurse indicates that the psychiatrist will not prescribe pain medications, he smiles bitterly and says, "So they already got to you."

■ ■ ■

Schizoid Personality Disorder

Schizoid personality disorder has the primary feature of emotional detachment. The person with this disorder does not seek out or enjoy close relationships. This individual may be able to function in a solitary occupation but shows indifference to praise or criticism from others. Schizoid PD can be a precursor to schizophrenia or delusional disorder. There is increased prevalence of the disorder in families with schizophrenia or schizotypal PD.

■ ■ ■ VIGNETTE

Mr. Gray is a 30-year-old single male who is a graduate student in mathematics at a large state university. He lives alone and has never been married. He works as an assistant in a math classroom in which the professor teaches the course via television. He wears thick eyeglasses and his clothing is inconspicuous. He rarely smiles and seldom looks directly at the students, even when answering questions. He does get somewhat animated when he writes lengthy solutions to math problems on the blackboard. He is content with his low-paying job and has never been in psychiatric treatment.

■ ■ ■

Schizotypal Personality Disorder

Schizotypal personality disorder has the central characteristic of odd beliefs leading to interpersonal difficulties. The individual has an eccentric appearance and shows evidence of magical thinking or perceptual distortions that are not clear delusions or hallucinations. The client's speech may be difficult to follow, because the individual develops a personalized style with vague associations. The person cannot understand the usual interpersonal cues in social situations and thus relates to others inappropriately. In contrast to persons with schizoid PD, the individual with schizotypal PD may seek psychiatric help because of the intense anxiety felt in social relationships.

■ ■ ■ VIGNETTE

Ms. Reese is a 50-year-old single female who lives with her older brother in their family home. A home care registered nurse (RN) meets Ms. Reese when she is assigned to care

DSM-IV-TR CRITERIA FOR CLUSTER A PERSONALITY DISORDERS

CLUSTER A (Odd or Eccentric)

Paranoid Personality Disorder	Schizoid Personality Disorder	Schizotypal Personality Disorder
A. A pervasive distrust and suspiciousness of others such that their motives are interpreted as malevolent, beginning by early adulthood and present in a variety of contexts, as indicated by four or more of the following: (1) Suspects, without sufficient basis, that others are exploiting, harming, or deceiving self (2) Is preoccupied with unjustified doubts about the loyalty or trustworthiness of friends or associates (3) Is reluctant to confide in others because of unwarranted fear that the information will be used maliciously against self (4) Reads hidden demeaning or threatening meanings into benign remarks or events (5) Persistently bears grudges (i.e., is unforgiving of insults, injuries, or slights) (6) Perceives attacks on his or her character or reputation that are not apparent to others and is quick to react angrily or to counterattack (7) Has recurrent suspicions, without justification, regarding fidelity of spouse or sexual partner	A. A pervasive pattern of detachment from social relationships and a restricted range of expression in interpersonal settings, beginning by early adulthood and present in a variety of contexts, as indicated by four or more of the following: (1) Neither desires nor enjoys close relationships, including being part of a family (2) Almost always chooses solitary activities (3) Has little, if any, interest in having sexual experiences with another person (4) Takes pleasure in few, if any, activities (5) Lacks close friends or confidants other than first-degree relatives (6) Appears indifferent to the praise or criticism of others (7) Shows emotional coldness, detachment, or flattened affect	A. A pervasive pattern of social and interpersonal deficits marked by acute discomfort with, and reduced capacity for, close relationships as well as by cognitive or perceptual distortions and eccentricities of behavior, beginning by early adulthood and present in a variety of contexts, as indicated by five or more of the following: (1) Ideas of reference (excluding delusions of reference) (2) Odd beliefs or magical thinking that influence behavior and are inconsistent with subcultural norms (e.g., superstitiousness, belief in clairvoyance, telepathy, or "sixth sense"; in children or adolescents, bizarre fantasies or preoccupations) (3) Unusual perceptual experiences, including bodily illusions (4) Odd thinking and speech (e.g., vague, circumstantial, metaphorical, overelaborate, or stereotyped) (5) Suspiciousness or paranoid ideation (6) Inappropriate or constricted affect (7) Behavior or appearance that is odd, eccentric, or peculiar (8) Lack of close friends or confidants other than first-degree relatives (9) Excessive social anxiety that does not diminish with familiarity and tends to be associated with paranoid fears rather than negative judgments about self

FIGURE 16-2 Diagnostic criteria for cluster A personality disorders. (Adapted from American Psychiatric Association. [2000]. *Diagnostic and statistical manual of mental disorders* [4th ed., text rev.]. Washington DC: Author.)

for the brother's leg wound. Ms. Reese wears all black clothing every day and usually sits quietly on the sofa holding her black cat while the RN visits her brother. She is a writer and goes to the library weekly for research. After several visits, Ms. Reese shyly asks the RN if she would like to read her book. Her story is about the special power of cats and

proves that all humans are descended from them. It gives extensive detail about different breeds and notes that black cats are the most intelligent. After that day, she excitedly talks to the RN at each visit about her ongoing research.

DSM-IV-TR AND THE CLINICAL PICTURE OF CLUSTER B DISORDERS (DRAMATIC, EMOTIONAL, ERRATIC)

Individuals with cluster B PDs are described as dramatic, emotional, or erratic. Refer to Figure 16-3 for the diagnostic criteria for each disorder in this group. In general, individuals with these disorders seek out interpersonal relationships but cannot maintain them because of excessive demands and emotional instability. They are manipulative in their interactions; that is, although they demonstrate charm and superficial warmth for others, their main goal is to use others to meet their own needs. They often display a sense of entitlement: they unconsciously feel that their needs are more important than the needs of others, and they deny the negative effects of hurting others (Kerr, 2002). Many individuals with cluster B disorders receive psychiatric care, either voluntarily because of affective distress, or involuntarily because of illegal behavior. Key attributes for each disorder are described in the following sections (Kay et al., 2000) and are illustrated in the vignettes.

Antisocial Personality Disorder

Antisocial personality disorder has the main features of consistent disregard for others with exploitation and repeated unlawful actions. Persons with antisocial PD were previously called psychopaths or sociopaths. There is a clear history of conduct disorder in childhood (see Chapter 32), and the individuals show no remorse for hurting others. They repeatedly neglect responsibilities, tell lies, and perform destructive or illegal acts, without developing any insight into predictable consequences. This disorder may be underdiagnosed in women and overdiagnosed in clients of lower socioeconomic status. These individuals do not voluntarily seek psychiatric care, but they are often seen for court-referred evaluation or treatment.

■ ■ ■ *VIGNETTE*

Mr. Rouse is a 25-year-old divorced cab driver who is referred to the hospital by the court for competency evaluation after an assault charge. He told the arresting officer that he has bipolar disorder. He has a history of substance abuse and multiple arrests for disorderly conduct or assault. During his intake interview he is polite and even flirtatious with the female RN. He insists that he is not responsible for his behavior because he is manic. The only symptom that he describes is irritability. He points out that he cannot tolerate any psychotropic medications because of the side effects. He also notes that he has dropped out of three clinics after several visits because "the staff don't understand me."

■ ■ ■

Borderline Personality Disorder

Borderline personality disorder has the central characteristic of instability in affect, identity, and relationships. Individuals with borderline PD desperately seek relationships to avoid feeling abandoned. But they often drive others away because of their excessive demands, impulsive behavior, or uncontrolled anger. Their frequent use of the defense of splitting strains personal relationships and creates turmoil in health care settings. Borderline PD is one of the most common PDs seen in psychiatric treatment settings. Under stress, these clients may show psychosis-like symptoms, and they may demonstrate chronic depression or self-destructive behavior. Clients with borderline PD may have a history of multiple or dramatic suicidal gestures, and there is a significant risk of suicide: one in ten clients can be expected to complete suicide (Paris, 2002).

■ ■ ■ *VIGNETTE*

Ms. Bracey is a 28-year-old divorced female who attends the dual diagnosis group at a mental health clinic. She has a history of five hospitalizations for suicidal ideation and self-mutilation. Her main theme in the group involves repeated failures in intimate relationships. In each case, she initially describes a warm, supportive person who will be her "soul mate." But within several months, she reports episodes of disappointment seemingly related to minor events. She then breaks off the relationship, concluding that the boy friend is "just another loser." When a peer in the group suggests that there is a pattern to her behavior, she bursts into tears and runs out of the meeting.

■ ■ ■

Histrionic Personality Disorder

Histrionic personality disorder has the key ingredient of emotional attention-seeking behavior, in which the person needs to be the center of attention. The histrionic person is impulsive and melodramatic, and may act flirtatious or provocative to get the spotlight. Relationships do not last because the partner often feels smothered or reacts to the insensitivity of the histrionic person. The individual with histrionic PD does not have insight into his or her role in breaking up relationships and may seek treatment for depression or another comorbid condition. In the treatment setting, the person demands "the best of everything" and can be very critical.

■ ■ ■ *VIGNETTE*

Ms. Lombard is a 35-year-old twice-divorced female admitted to an inpatient unit after an overdose of asthma medications and antibiotics. She took all of her pills after her primary care doctor refused to order a sleeping pill for her. On the first night, she is withdrawn and tearful in her room. But

DSM-IV-TR CRITERIA FOR CLUSTER B PERSONALITY DISORDERS

CLUSTER B (Dramatic, Emotional, or Erratic)

Antisocial Personality Disorder

A. A pervasive pattern of disregard for and violation of the rights of others occurring since age 15, as indicated by three or more of the following:

(1) Failure to conform to social norms with respect to lawful behaviors as indicated by repeatedly performing acts that are grounds for arrest
(2) Deceitfulness, as indicated by repeatedly lying, using aliases, or conning others for personal profit or pleasure
(3) Impulsivity or failure to plan ahead
(4) Irritability and aggressiveness, as indicated by repeated physical fights or assaults
(5) Reckless disregard for safety of self or others
(6) Consistent irresponsibility, as indicated by repeated failure to sustain consistent work behavior or honor financial obligations
(7) Lack of remorse, as indicated by being indifferent to, or rationalizing, having hurt, mistreated, or stolen from another

B. The individual is at least 18 years of age.

C. There is evidence of conduct disorder with onset before age 15 years.

Borderline Personality Disorder

A. A pervasive pattern of instability of interpersonal relationships, self-image, and affects, and marked impulsivity beginning in early adulthood and present in a variety of contexts, as indicated by five or more of the following:

(1) Frantic efforts to avoid real or imagined abandonment. *Note:* Do not include suicidal or self-mutilating behavior covered in criterion 5.
(2) A pattern of unstable and intense interpersonal relationships characterized by alternating between extremes of idealization and devaluation
(3) Identity disturbance: markedly and persistently unstable self-image or sense of self
(4) Impulsivity in at least two areas that are potentially self-damaging (e.g., spending, sex, substance abuse, reckless driving, binge eating). *Note:* Do not include suicidal or self-mutilating behavior covered in criterion 5.
(5) Recurrent suicidal behavior, gestures, or threats, or self-mutilating behavior
(6) Affective instability due to a marked reactivity of mood (e.g., intense episodic dysphoria, irritability, or anxiety, usually lasting a few hours and rarely more than a few days)
(7) Chronic feelings of emptiness
(8) Inappropriate intense anger or difficulty controlling anger (e.g., frequent displays of temper, constant anger, recurrent physical fights)
(9) Transient, stress-related paranoid ideation or severe dissociative symptoms

Narcissistic Personality Disorder

A. A pervasive pattern of grandiosity (in fantasy and behavior), need for admiration, and lack of empathy, beginning in early adulthood and present in a variety of contexts, as indicated by five or more of the following:

(1) Has a grandiose sense of self-importance (e.g., exaggerates achievements and talents, expects to be recognized as superior without commensurate achievements)
(2) Is preoccupied with fantasies of unlimited success, power, brilliance, beauty, or ideal love
(3) Believes that he or she is "special" and unique and can only be understood by, or should associate with, other special or high-status people (or institutions)
(4) Requires excessive admiration
(5) Has sense of entitlement (i.e., unreasonable expectations of especially favorable treatment or automatic compliance with personal expectations)
(6) Is interpersonally exploitative (i.e., takes advantage of others to achieve personal ends)
(7) Lacks empathy: is unwilling to recognize or identify with the feelings and needs of others
(8) Is often envious of others or believes that others are envious of self
(9) Shows arrogant, haughty behaviors or attitudes

Histrionic Personality Disorder

A. A pervasive pattern of excessive emotionality and attention seeking, beginning in early adulthood and present in a variety of contexts, as indicated by five or more of the following:

(1) Is uncomfortable in situations in which self is not the center of attention
(2) Interaction with others is often characterized by inappropriate sexually seductive or provocative behavior
(3) Displays rapidly shifting and shallow expression of emotions
(4) Consistently uses physical appearance to draw attention to self
(5) Has a style of speech that is excessively impressionistic and lacking in detail
(6) Shows self-dramatization, theatricality, and exaggerated expression of emotion
(7) Is suggestible (i.e., easily influenced by others or circumstances)
(8) Considers relationships to be more intimate than they actually are

FIGURE 16-3 Diagnostic criteria for cluster B personality disorders. (Adapted from American Psychiatric Association. [2000]. *Diagnostic and statistical manual of mental disorders* [4th ed., text rev.]. Washington DC: Author.)

the next morning, she is neatly groomed, even wearing makeup, and socializes with everyone. She denies thoughts of self-harm. Over the next 2 days, she monopolizes the community meetings by talking about how unappreciated she is by her family and physician. She seeks special attention from an evening shift male RN, asking if he can stay late after his shift to sit with her. When he refuses, she demands to be placed back on one-to-one precautions because she suddenly feels suicidal again.

■ ■ ■

Narcissistic Personality Disorder

Narcissistic personality disorder has the primary feature of arrogance, with a grandiose view of self-importance. The individual with this disorder has a need for constant admiration along with a lack of empathy for others that strains most relationships. Underneath the surface of arrogance, narcissistic persons feel intense shame and fear that if they are "bad," they will be abandoned. They are afraid of their own mistakes, as well as the mistakes of others. Narcissistic individuals may seek help for depression, feeling that loved ones do not show enough appreciation of their special qualities.

■ ■ ■ VIGNETTE

Dr. Brightner is a 40-year-old female attending psychiatrist at a university outpatient center. She is twice divorced and has no children. Her grooming and makeup are impeccable, and she likes to chat about her expensive shopping habits. She is quite intelligent and is the only doctor on the staff trained in psychoanalysis. In clinical team meetings, she often discusses this fact, repeatedly telling others that psychoanalysis is the best treatment for mental illness. She frequently makes derogatory remarks to psychiatric residents if they suggest alternative treatment approaches for new cases. She is usually late to staff meetings, and when she is not speaking, she yawns and shifts noisily in her seat. She has a reputation for exhibiting angry outbursts at therapists in the hallway for minor mistakes, such as a scheduling error for a client. She underwent 7 years of psychoanalysis but does not consider it to have been therapy—it was only for training purposes.

■ ■ ■

DSM-IV-TR AND THE CLINICAL PICTURE OF CLUSTER C DISORDERS (ANXIOUS, FEARFUL)

Persons with cluster C PDs are described as anxious or fearful. Refer to Figure 16-4 for the diagnostic criteria for each disorder in this group. In general, individuals with these disorders feel insecure or inadequate, depending on others for reassurance or isolating themselves for fear of rejection. They often come into psychiatric care for treatment of anxiety, related to fear of relationships or the loss of a relationship. The main features of each disorder are summarized in the following sections (Kay et al., 2000), and illustrative vignettes are provided.

Avoidant Personality Disorder

Avoidant personality disorder has the central characteristic of social inhibition and avoidance of all situations that require interpersonal contact. Individuals with this disorder want to have close relationships, but they are preoccupied with fear of rejection. Because in their social presentation they appear timid and inept, with low self-esteem and poor self-care, they are often mistreated in groups. If they do develop relationships, they cling to their partners in a dependent way. They are seen in treatment for symptoms of anxiety, especially social anxiety disorder.

■ ■ ■ VIGNETTE

Ms. Lowell is a 35-year-old single female who works for a computer repair company. As a child she had few friends and never participated in extracurricular activities. She lives alone in her own apartment and has never had an adult intimate relationship. On the job, she rarely talks to co-workers and prefers to work alone. If she has any questions, she asks the supervisor and carefully follows directions. Although she has 7 years of experience and a good work record, she refuses the offer of a promotion because it would require her to interact with customers.

■ ■ ■

Dependent Personality Disorder

Dependent personality disorder has the primary feature of extreme dependency in a close relationship, with an urgent search to find a replacement when one relationship ends. Individuals with dependent PD have difficulty making independent decisions and are constantly seeking reassurance. Their submissiveness makes them vulnerable to abusive relationships. They have a deeply held conviction of personal incompetence, with the fear that they cannot survive on their own. They frequently seek treatment for anxiety or mood disorders related to a loss. In fact, dependent PD is the most frequently seen PD in the clinical setting. It also occurs in clients with a medical disability that requires them to depend on others for care.

■ ■ ■ VIGNETTE

Ms. Shaker is a 45-year-old single unemployed housekeeper who comes to the mental health clinic complaining of anxiety. She had to quit her job recently to stay home full time after her mother was diagnosed with cancer. Ms.

DSM-IV-TR CRITERIA FOR CLUSTER C PERSONALITY DISORDERS

CLUSTER C (Anxious or Fearful)

Dependent Personality Disorder	Obsessive-Compulsive Personality Disorder	Avoidant Personality Disorder
A. A pervasive and excessive need to be taken care of that leads to submissive and clinging behavior and fear of separation, beginning by early adulthood and present in a variety of contexts, as indicated by five or more of the following: (1) Has difficulty making everyday decisions without an excessive amount of advice and reassurance from others (2) Needs others to assume responsibility for most major areas of life (3) Has difficulty expressing disagreement with others because of fear of loss of support or approval. *Note:* Does not include realistic fears of retribution. (4) Has difficulty initiating projects or doing things on own (because of a lack of self-confidence in judgment or abilities rather than a lack of motivation or energy) (5) Goes to excessive lengths to obtain nurturance and support from others, to the point of volunteering to do things that are unpleasant (6) Feels uncomfortable or helpless when alone because of exaggerated fears of being unable to care for self (7) Urgently seeks another relationship as a source of care and support when a close relationship ends (8) Is unrealistically preoccupied with fears of being left to take care of self	A. A pervasive pattern of preoccupation with orderliness, perfectionism, and mental and interpersonal control, at the expense of flexibility, openness, and efficiency, beginning by early adulthood and present in a variety of contexts, as indicated by four or more of the following: (1) Is preoccupied with details, rules, lists, order, organization, or schedules to the extent that the major point of the activity is lost (2) Shows perfectionism that interferes with task completion (e.g., is unable to complete a project because overly strict personal standards are not met) (3) Is excessively devoted to work and productivity to the exclusion of leisure activities and friendships (not accounted for by obvious economic necessity) (4) Is overconscientious, scrupulous, and inflexible about matters of morality, ethics, or values (not accounted for by cultural or religious identification) (5) Is unable to discard worn-out or worthless objects even when they have no sentimental value (6) Is reluctant to delegate tasks or to work with others unless they submit exactly to own way of doing things (7) Adopts a miserly spending style toward both self and others; money is viewed as something to be hoarded for future catastrophes (8) Shows rigidity and stubbornness	A. A pervasive pattern of social inhibition, feelings of inadequacy, and hypersensitivity to negative evaluation, beginning by early adulthood and present in a variety of contexts, as indicated by four or more of the following: (1) Avoids occupational activities that involve significant interpersonal contact, because of fears of criticism, disapproval, or rejection (2) Is unwilling to get involved with people unless certain of being liked (3) Shows restraint within intimate relationships because of fear of being shamed or ridiculed (4) Is preoccupied with being criticized or rejected in social situations (5) Is inhibited in new interpersonal situations because of feelings of inadequacy (6) Views self as socially inept, personally unappealing, or inferior to others (7) Is unusually reluctant to take personal risks or to engage in any new activities because they may prove embarrassing

FIGURE 16-4 Diagnostic criteria for cluster C personality disorders. (Adapted from American Psychiatric Association. [2000]. *Diagnostic and statistical manual of mental disorders* [4th ed., text rev.]. Washington DC: Author.)

Shaker is an only child and has always lived with her mother. She describes their relationship as very close: "she is my best friend." Even prior to her mother's illness, they were constant companions. When Ms. Shaker was working, she called her mother daily on her lunch break. When the psychiatrist suggests starting medication, Ms. Shaker says that she will have to talk it over with her mother first.

■ ■ ■

Obsessive-Compulsive Personality Disorder

Obsessive-compulsive personality disorder has the key characteristic of perfectionism with a focus on orderliness and control. Individuals with this disorder become so preoccupied with details and rules that they may not be able to accomplish a given task.

Although a degree of obsessive-compulsive behavior can be productive in some occupations, it creates tension in close relationships, in which the person tries to control the partner. Persons with obsessive-compulsive PD feel genuine affection for friends and family, and do not have insight about their own difficult behavior. Internally, they are fearful of imminent catastrophe; they rehearse over and over how they will respond in social situations. These individuals do not have full-blown obsessions or compulsions but may seek treatment for anxiety or mood disorders.

■ ■ ■ VIGNETTE

Mr. Wright is a 45-year-old single male postal worker who is assigned to a post office in a small town. He lives alone and has never married. His is well groomed and wears a clean, neatly ironed uniform every day. He carefully follows all policies and procedures and is quite resistant whenever there is any update or change. He frequently challenges the supervisor about policy details and has been referred to the regional personnel office countless times for resolution of these conflicts. In staff meetings, he gives excessive circumstantial details and writes extra material on the back of any required report form. When dealing with the public, he sometimes gets into arguments with customers about postal rules or the schedule. The other staff do not consider him to be a team player, because he seldom volunteers to help others. Even if he is asked to help someone, he is quick to criticize his peer's performance. Although he has worked in the same office for 10 years, he has never advanced beyond the front-line position. He is fairly content with his work and has never been in psychiatric treatment.

■ ■ ■

PERSONALITY DISORDER NOT OTHERWISE SPECIFIED

Finally, there is a diagnostic category called *personality disorder not otherwise specified (NOS)*. This diagnosis is used when an individual meets some but not all criteria for a given disorder or else has a mixture of features from several disorders. In every study in which it is included, this diagnosis is the one most commonly selected by clinicians to describe clients with PDs.

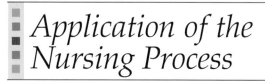

Application of the Nursing Process

■ ASSESSMENT

Assessment Tools

Several structured interview tools are used to diagnose the PDs. These tools are not used in all clinical settings because of the need for lengthy interviews (2 hours or longer) and evaluation. The Minnesota Multiphasic Personality Inventory (MMPI) is the best-known standardized test for evaluating personality.

Assessment of History

Taking a full medical history can help determine if the problem is a psychiatric one, a medical one, or both. Medical illness should never be ruled out as the cause for problem behavior until the data support this conclusion. Important issues in assessment for PDs include the following: a history of suicidal or aggressive ideation or actions; current use of medicines and illegal substances; ability to handle money; and legal history.

Important areas about which further details must be obtained include current or past physical, sexual, or emotional abuse, and level of current risk of harm from self or others. At times, immediate interventions may be needed to ensure the safety of the client or others. Information regarding prior use of any medication, including psychopharmacological agents, is important. This information gives evidence of other contacts the client has made for help and indicates how the health care provider found the client at that time.

Self-Assessment

Finding an approach for helping clients with PDs who have overwhelming needs can be overwhelming for caregivers as well. The intense feelings evoked in the nurse often mirror the feelings being experienced by the client. Caregivers may feel confused, helpless, angry, and frustrated. These clients tell the nurse that the nurse is inadequate, incompetent, and abusive of authority. Clients with PD are often successful in using splitting behaviors with the staff by praising or disparaging the nurse to peers in such a way that the peers begin to react negatively. Usually, this is the peers' attempt to defend against their own feelings of frustration and powerlessness, but the result is that substantial conflict can ensue in the treatment team. For example, a female client with borderline PD may briefly idealize her male nurse on the inpatient unit, telling staff and clients alike that she is "the luckiest client because she has the best nurse in the hospital." The rest of the team initially realizes that this behavior is an exaggeration, and they have a neutral response. But after days of constant dramatic praise (with subtle insults to the rest of the staff), some members of the team may start to feel inadequate and jealous of the nurse. They begin to make critical remarks about minor events to prove that the nurse is not perfect. A similar scenario can occur if the client constantly complains about one staff member; some staff are torn between defending and criticizing the targeted staff member. Open communication in staff meetings and ongoing clinical supervision are important aspects of self-care for the nurse working with these clients to aid in maintaining objectivity.

Assessment Guidelines Personality Disorders

1. Assess for suicidal or homicidal thoughts. If these are present, the client will need immediate attention.
2. Determine whether the client has a medical disorder or another psychiatric disorder that may be responsible for the symptoms (especially a substance use disorder).
3. View the assessment about personality functioning from within the person's ethnic, cultural, and social background.
4. Ascertain whether the client experienced a recent important loss. PDs are often exacerbated after the loss of significant supporting people or in a disruptive social situation.
5. Evaluate for a change in personality in middle adulthood or later, which signals the need for a thorough medical workup or assessment for unrecognized substance use disorder.

■ NURSING DIAGNOSIS

People with PDs are usually admitted to psychiatric institutions because of symptoms of comorbid disorders, dangerous behavior, or court order for treatment. Borderline PD and antisocial PD both present a challenge for health care providers. Because the behaviors central to these disorders often cause disruption in psychiatric and medical-surgical settings, nursing care for clients with these two disorders is emphasized. Emotions such as anxiety, rage, and depression and behaviors such as withdrawal, paranoia, and manipulation are among the most frequent that health care workers need to address. See Table 16-4 for common potential nursing diagnoses.

■ OUTCOME CRITERIA

Realistic outcomes are established for individuals with PDs based on the perspective that personality change occurs one behavioral solution and one learned skill at a time. This can be expected to take much time and repetition. In the acute care setting, the focus is on the presenting problem, which may be depression or severe anxiety. The chronic behavior problems of clients with PDs are not expected to be resolved but rather to be met with appropriate therapeutic feedback. Pertinent categories of nursing outcomes based on the Nursing Outcomes Classification (NOC) include *Aggression Self-Control, Impulse Self-Control, Social Interaction Skills, Fear Level, Abusive Behavior Self-Restraint*, and *Self-Mutilation Restraint* (Moorhead, Johnson, & Maas, 2004). Refer to Table 16-5 for examples of potential nursing outcomes for manipulative, aggressive, and impulsive behaviors.

■ PLANNING

It is often difficult to create a therapeutic relationship with clients who have antisocial or borderline PDs because most of them have experienced failed relationships, including therapeutic alliances. Their distrust and hostility can be a setup for failure. When clients blame and attack others, the nurse needs to understand the context of their complaints; that is, these attacks spring from the feeling of being threatened, and the more intense the complaints, the greater the fear of potential harm or loss. Lacking the ability to trust, clients with PDs require a sense of control over what is happening to them. Giving them realistic choices (e.g., selection of a particular group activity) may enhance compliance with treatment. Refer to Tables 16-6, 16-7, and 16-8 for guidelines for nursing care for each PD cluster and also review the care plan at the end of the chapter in Case Study and Nursing Care Plan 16-1 for a client with borderline PD.

TABLE 16-4

Potential Nursing Diagnoses for Personality Disorders

Signs and Symptoms	Nursing Diagnoses
Crisis, high levels of anxiety	**Ineffective coping**
	Anxiety
	Self-mutilation
Anger and aggression; child, elder, or spouse abuse	**Risk for other-directed violence**
	Ineffective coping
	Impaired parenting
	Disabled family coping
Withdrawal	**Social isolation**
Paranoia	**Fear**
	Disturbed sensory perception
	Disturbed thought processes
	Defensive coping
Depression	**Hopelessness**
	Risk for suicide
	Self-mutilation
	Chronic low self-esteem
	Spiritual distress
Difficulty in relationships, manipulation	**Ineffective coping**
	Impaired social interaction
	Defensive coping
	Interrupted family processes
	Risk for loneliness
Failure to keep medical appointments, late arrival for appointments, failure to follow prescribed medical procedure or medication regimen	**Ineffective therapeutic regimen management**
	Noncompliance

TABLE 16-5

NOC Outcomes for Manipulative, Aggressive, and Impulsive Behaviors

Nursing Outcome and Definition	Intermediate Indicators	Short-Term Indicators
Social Interaction Skills: Personal behaviors that promote effective relationships*	Uses conflict resolution methods	Exhibits receptiveness Exhibits sensitivity to others Cooperates with others Uses assertive behaviors as appropriate Uses confrontation as appropriate
Motivation: Inner urge that moves or prompts an individual to positive action(s)*	Accepts responsibility for actions	Develops an action plan Obtains needed support Self-initiates goal-directed behavior Expresses belief in ability to perform action Expresses that performance will lead to desired outcome
Aggression Self-Control: Self-restraint of assaultive, combative, or destructive behaviors toward others*	Communicates needs appropriately	Identifies when frustrated Identifies when angry Identifies responsibility to maintain control Identifies alternatives to aggression Identifies alternatives to verbal outbursts Vents negative feelings appropriately Refrains from striking others Refrains from harming others
Impulse Self-Control: Self-restraint of compulsive or impulsive behaviors*	Controls impulses	Identifies harmful impulsive behaviors Identifies feelings that lead to impulsive actions Identifies consequences of impulsive actions to self or others Avoids high-risk environments and situations Seeks help when experiencing impulses

From Moorhead, S., Johnson, M., & Maas, M. (2004). *Nursing outcomes classification (NOC)* (3rd ed.). St. Louis, MO: Mosby.
*Measured on a five-point Likert scale from 1 (never demonstrated) to 5 (consistently demonstrated).

TABLE 16-6

Nursing and Therapy Guidelines for Cluster A Disorders (Odd or Eccentric)

Personality Disorder	Characteristics	Nursing Guidelines	Suggested Therapies
Schizotypal	▪ Manifests ideas of reference ▪ Shows cognitive and perceptual distortions ▪ Socially inept ▪ Anxious	1. Respect client's need for social isolation. 2. Be aware of client's suspiciousness and employ appropriate interventions. 3. As with schizoid client, perform careful diagnostic assessment as needed to uncover any other medical or psychological symptoms that may need intervention (e.g., suicidal thoughts).	1. Skills-oriented psychotherapy 2. Cognitive and behavioral measures 3. Highly structured group therapy 4. **Low-dose antipsychotics**
Paranoid	▪ Projects blame ▪ Suspicious ▪ Hostile and violent ▪ Shows cognitive and perceptual distortions	1. Avoid being too "nice" or "friendly." 2. Give clear and straightforward explanations of tests and procedures beforehand. 3. Use simple, clear language; avoid ambiguity. 4. Project a neutral but kind affect. 5. Warn about any changes, side effects of medication, and reasons for delay. Such interventions may help allay anxiety and minimize suspiciousness. A written plan may help encourage cooperation.	1. Supportive psychotherapy, later cognitive-behavioral techniques 2. **Low-dose antipsychotics** if cognitive and perceptual problems chronic 3. **Antidepressant or anxiolytics** as needed
Schizoid	▪ Reclusive ▪ Avoidant ▪ Uncooperative	1. Avoid being too "nice" or "friendly." 2. Do not try to increase socialization. 3. Perform thorough diagnostic assessment as needed to identify symptoms or disorders that the client is reluctant to discuss.	1. Supportive psychotherapy 2. Group therapy 3. **Antipsychotics, antidepressants, anxiolytics** as needed

Data from American Psychiatric Association. (2000). *Diagnostic and statistical manual of mental disorders* (4th ed., text rev.). Washington, DC: Author; Cloninger, C. R., & Svrakic, D. M. (1999). Personality disorders. In B. J. Sadock & V. A. Sadock (Eds.), *Comprehensive textbook of psychiatry* (7th ed.). Philadelphia: Lippincott Williams & Wilkins; Gunderson, J. G., & Phillips, K. A. (1995). Personality disorders. In H. I. Kaplan & B. J. Sadock (Eds.), *Comprehensive textbook of psychiatry/VI* (6th ed., Vol. 2, pp. 1425-1462). Baltimore: Williams & Wilkins; and Widiger, T. A., & Mullins, S. (2003). Personality disorders. In A. Tasman, J. Kay, & J. A. Lieberman (Eds.), *Psychiatry* (2nd ed., Vol. 2, pp. 1603-1637). London: Wiley.

TABLE 16-7

Nursing and Therapy Guidelines for Cluster B Disorders (Dramatic, Emotional, Erratic)

Personality Disorder	Characteristics	Nursing Guidelines	Suggested Therapies
Borderline	■ Shows separation anxiety ■ Manifests ideas of reference ■ Impulsive (suicide, self-mutilation) ■ Engages in splitting (adoring then devaluing persons)	1. Set realistic goals, use clear action words. 2. Be aware of manipulative behaviors (flattery, seductiveness, instilling of guilt). 3. Provide clear and consistent boundaries and limits. 4. Use clear and straightforward communication. 5. When behavioral problems emerge, calmly review the therapeutic goals and boundaries of treatment. 6. Avoid rejecting or rescuing. 7. Assess for suicidal and self-mutilating behaviors, especially during times of stress.	1. Dialectical behavior therapy 2. **SSRIs** for anger and depression 3. **Carbamazepine (Tegretol) (anticonvulsant)** for lack of control and self-harm 4. **Low-dose antipsychotics** for cognitive disturbance (paranoia, magical thinking, illusions)

Antisocial	■ Manipulative
	■ Exploitive of others
	■ Aggressive
	■ Callous towards others
		1. Try to prevent or reduce untoward effects of manipulation (flattery, seductiveness, instilling of guilt):
		  ■ Set clear and realistic limits on specific behavior.
		  ■ Ensure that all limits are adhered to by all staff involved.
		  ■ Carefully document objective physical signs of manipulation or aggression when managing clinical problems.
		  ■ Document behaviors objectively (give times, dates, circumstances).
		  ■ Provide clear boundaries and consequences.
		2. Be aware that antisocial clients can instill guilt when they are not getting what they want. Guard against being manipulated through feelings of guilt.
		3. Treatment of substance abuse is best handled through a well-organized treatment program before counseling and other forms of therapy are started.
			1. Cognitive approach
			2. Structured community residential program
			3. Pharmacologic agents for aggression **(lithium, anticonvulsants, SSRIs)**

Narcissistic	■ Exploitive ■ Grandiose ■ Disparaging ■ Rageful ■ Very sensitive to rejection, criticism	1. Remain neutral; avoid engaging in power struggles or becoming defensive in response to the client's disparaging remarks, no matter how provocative the situation may be. 2. Convey unassuming self-confidence.	1. Cognitive and behavioral measures 2. Group therapy 3. No specific medication
Histrionic	■ Seductive ■ Flamboyant ■ Attention seeking ■ Shallow ■ Depressive and suicidal when admiration withdrawn	1. Understand seductive behavior as a response to distress. 2. Keep communication and interactions professional, despite temptation to collude with the client in a flirtatious and misleading manner. 3. Encourage and model the use of concrete and descriptive rather than vague and impressionistic language. 4. Teach and role-model assertiveness.	1. Group therapy 2. Treatment of comorbid personality disorders 3. **Antidepressants** as needed

Data from American Psychiatric Association. (2000). *Diagnostic and statistical manual of mental disorders* (4th ed., text rev.). Washington, DC: Author; Cloninger, C. R., & Svrakic, D. M. (1999). Personality disorders. In B. J. Sadock & V. A. Sadock (Eds.), *Comprehensive textbook of psychiatry* (7th ed.). Philadelphia: Lippincott Williams & Wilkins; Philips, K. A., & Gunderson, J. G. (1999). Personality disorders. In R. E. Hales, S. C. Yudofsky, & J. A. Talbott (Eds.), *The American Psychiatric Press textbook of psychiatry* (3rd ed.). Washington, DC: American Psychiatric Press; and Widiger, T. A., & Mullins, S. (2003). Personality disorders. In A. Tasman, J. Kay, & J. A. Lieberman (Eds.), *Psychiatry* (2nd ed., Vol. 2, pp. 1603-1637). London: Wiley.
SSRIs, Selective serotonin reuptake inhibitors.

TABLE 16-8

Nursing and Therapy Guidelines for Cluster C Disorders (Anxious or Fearful)

Personality Disorder	Characteristics	Nursing Guidelines	Suggested Therapies
Dependent	■ Excessively clinging ■ Self-sacrificing, submissive ■ Needy, gets others to care for him or her	1. Identify and help address current stresses. 2. Try to satisfy client's needs at the same time that limits are set up in such a manner that client does not feel punished and withdraw. 3. Be aware that strong countertransference often develops in clinicians because of client's excessive clinging (demands of extra time, nighttime calls, crisis before vacations); therefore, supervision is well advised. 4. Teach and role-model assertiveness.	1. Supportive therapy or cognitive-behavioral therapy 2. Group therapy
Obsessive-compulsive	■ Perfectionistic ■ Has need for control ■ Inflexible, rigid ■ Preoccupied with details ■ Highly critical of self and others	1. Guard against engaging in power struggles with client. Need for control is very high in these clients. 2. Intellectualization, rationalization, and reaction formation are the most common defense mechanisms.	1. Supportive or insightful psychotherapy, also cognitive-behavioral therapy 2. **Clomipramine (Anafranil) (tricyclic antidepressant) and SSRIs** for obsessional thinking and depression
Avoidant	■ Excessively anxious in social situations ■ Hypersensitive to negative evaluation	1. A friendly, gentle, reassuring approach is the best way to treat clients. 2. Being pushed into social situations can cause extreme and severe anxiety.	1. Desensitization, social skills training, or other cognitive-behavioral techniques to treat social phobia 2. Group therapy 3. **MAOIs and anxiolytics**

Data from American Psychiatric Association. (2000). *Diagnostic and statistical manual of mental disorders* (4th ed., text rev.). Washington, DC: Author; Cloninger, C. R., & Svrakic, D. M. (1999). Personality disorders. In B. J. Sadock & V. A. Sadock (Eds.), *Comprehensive textbook of psychiatry* (7th ed.). Philadelphia: Lippincott Williams & Wilkins; Philips, K. A., & Gunderson, J. G. (1999). Personality disorders. In R. E. Hales, S. C. Yudofsky, & J. A. Talbott (Eds.), *The American Psychiatric Press textbook of psychiatry* (3rd ed.). Washington, DC: American Psychiatric Press; and Widiger, T. A., & Mullins, S. (2003). Personality disorders. In A. Tasman, J. Kay, & J. A. Lieberman (Eds.), *Psychiatry* (2nd ed., Vol. 2, pp. 1603-1637). London: Wiley.
MAOIs, Monoamine oxidase inhibitors; SSRIs, selective serotonin reuptake inhibitors.

CASE STUDY and NURSING CARE PLAN 16-1 — Borderline Personality Disorder

Mary Drake is a 24-year-old single secretary who lives alone. She has been seen in the emergency department several times for superficial suicide attempts. She is admitted because she has cut her wrists, ankles, and vagina with glass and has lost a lot of blood. This event is precipitated by her graduation from a community college.

Upon admission she is sweet, serene, and grateful to all the nurses, calling them "angels of mercy." Within 1 week she is angry at half of the nurses and demands a new primary nurse, saying that the one she has (to whom she had grown attached) hates her. She has a history of heavy drinking and has managed to sneak alcohol onto the unit. She has been found in bed with a young male client. She continually breaks unit rules and then pleads to have this behavior forgiven and forgotten. When angry, she threatens to cut herself again. When asked why she cut herself, Ms. Drake states, "I was tired." She appears restless and tense and frequently asks for antianxiety medication. When asked what she is anxious about, she says, "Uh . . . I don't know . . . I feel so empty inside." Ms. Drake frequently paces up and down the halls looking both angry and bored.

Her admitting diagnoses include substance abuse disorder and borderline personality disorder.

Self-Assessment

Ms. McCarthy, a recent graduate and Ms. Drake's primary nurse, talks to Ms. Drake's therapist twice a week in staff meetings. The therapist impresses upon Ms. McCarthy the difficulty health care workers have in dealing effectively with people with borderline PDs. These clients constantly act out their feelings in self-destructive and maladaptive ways. They usually are not aware of their feelings or what triggered their actions.

The most difficult area for many health care workers is dealing with the intense feelings and reactions these clients can provoke in others. Ms. McCarthy sets a time twice a week for supervision with Ms. Drake's therapist. At the next meeting, common goals and intervention strategies are discussed.

■ ASSESSMENT

Ms. McCarthy organizes the data into subjective and objective components.

Objective Data	**Subjective Data**
■ Makes frequent, superficial suicide attempts	■ Initially "loved" her primary nurse, now "hates" her and wants another nurse
■ Requests antianxiety medication frequently	■ States she is restless and tense
■ Paces up and down the hall much of the day	■ Complains of feeling empty inside
■ Threatens self-mutilation when anxious	■ Describes self as angry and bored much of the time
■ Brings alcohol onto the unit after pass	
■ Is found in bed with male client	

■ NURSING DIAGNOSIS (NANDA)

Ms. McCarthy formulates two initial nursing diagnoses that have the highest priority during this time:

1. *Ineffective coping* related to inadequate psychological resources, as evidenced by self-destructive behaviors
   - ■ After stating that she feels frustrated, client goes on pass and comes back with alcohol.
   - ■ After stating that she is in love with her therapist, client is found in bed with a male client.
   - ■ After stating that she hates her primary nurse, client demands a new primary nurse.

2. *Self-mutilation* related to anxiety and emptiness, as evidenced by suicidal gestures and poor impulse control
   - ■ Is admitted following self-mutilation
   - ■ Threatens self-mutilation when anxious
   - ■ Threatens self-mutilation on unit

■ OUTCOME CRITERIA (NOC)

1. Client will consistently demonstrate the use of effective coping strategies.
2. Client will refrain from injuring self.

■ PLANNING

The initial plan is to maintain client safety and to encourage verbalization of feelings and impulses instead of action.

■ INTERVENTION (NIC)

Ms. Drake's plan of care is personalized as follows.

Nursing diagnosis: *Ineffective coping* related to inadequate psychological resources, as evidenced by self-destructive behaviors
Outcome criteria: Client will consistently demonstrate the use of effective coping strategies.

Short-Term Goal	**Intervention**	**Rationale**	**Evaluation**
Ms. Drake will consistently demonstrate a decrease in stress as evidenced by talking about feelings with staff every day and an absence of acting out behaviors.	1. Encourage verbalization of feelings, perceptions, and fears. 2. Support the use of appropriate defense mechanisms.	1. Discussing and understanding the dynamics of frustration help to reduce the frustration by helping client take positive action. 2. Discussing and understanding the meaning of defenses help to reduce the potential for acting out.	GOAL MET Ms. Drake was able to experience problems and deal with them appropriately. Acting out was minimal or absent. For example, client had an appointment for a job interview. She wanted to stay in bed and avoid the interview. Instead she talked with the nurse about her fear of "growing up" and was able to get up and go to the interview.

■ INTERVENTION (NIC)

Nursing diagnosis: *Self-mutilation* related to anxiety and emptiness, as evidenced by suicidal gestures and poor impulse control
Outcome criteria: Client will refrain from injuring self.

Continued

Short-Term Goal	Intervention	Rationale	Evaluation
Ms. Drake will consistently demonstrate that she will seek help when feeling urge to injure self as evidenced by the absence of self-injurious behaviors and talking to staff about her troubling feelings on a daily basis.	1. Assist client to identify situations and/or feelings that may prompt self-harm. 2. Instruct client in coping strategies. 3. Provide ongoing surveillance of client and environment.	1. Observing, describing, and analyzing thoughts and feelings reduce the potential for acting them out destructively. 2. Alternative behaviors are offered that can be more satisfying and growth promoting. 3. Times of increased anxiety, frustration, or anger without external controls could increase probability of client self-mutilating behaviors.	GOAL MET Ms. Drake was able to experience troubling thoughts and feelings without self-mutilation. Stated, "I was mad at my therapist today and decided to cut my arms after the session. Instead, I told her I was angry and together we figured out why."

■ **EVALUATION**

See individual outcomes and evaluation in the care plan.

evolve Visit the Evolve website at **http://evolve.elsevier.com/Varcarolis** for a full case study of this client and more case studies and nursing care plans.

■ INTERVENTION
Basic Level Interventions

Basic level nursing interventions for clients with PDs include milieu therapy, psychobiological interventions, and case management. People with borderline PD are impulsive (e.g., suicidal, self-mutilating), aggressive, manipulative, and even psychotic during periods of stress. Persons with antisocial PD are often involuntary clients and are also manipulative, aggressive, and impulsive. Refer to Boxes 16-2, 16-3, and 16-4 for interventions to address these behaviors based on the Nursing Interventions Classification (NIC) (Dochterman & Bulechek, 2004).

Milieu Therapy

When individuals with PDs are in hospital, partial hospitalization, or day treatment settings, milieu therapy is a significant part of treatment. The primary goal of milieu therapy is affect management in a group context. Community meetings, coping skills groups, and socializing groups are all helpful for these clients. They have the opportunity to interact with peers and staff to discuss goals and to learn problem-solving skills. Dealing with emotional issues that arise in the milieu requires a calm, united approach by the staff to maintain safety and to enhance self-control.

There are several successful features of milieu treatment for PD clients. Common problems resulting from splitting can be minimized if the unit leaders hold weekly staff meetings at which staff are allowed to ventilate their feelings about conflicts with clients and each other. Clients take more responsibility for themselves if they are actively involved in treatment plans, for example, by including them in daily staff rounds to set goals and to evaluate progress (Munich & Allen,

2003). Limit setting and confrontation about negative behavior is better accepted by the client if the staff first employ empathic mirroring (i.e., reflecting back to the client an understanding of the client's distress without a value judgment). For example, the nurse can listen to a client's emotional complaints about the staff and the

---

BOX 16-2

NIC Interventions for Manipulative Behavior

Limit Setting
Definition: Establishing the parameters of desirable and acceptable patient behavior
Activities*:
- Discuss concerns about behavior with patient.
- Identify (with patient input, when appropriate) undesirable patient behavior.
- Discuss with patient, when appropriate, what is desirable behavior in a given situation or setting.
- Establish consequences (with patient input, when appropriate) for occurrence or nonoccurrence of desired behaviors.
- Communicate established behavioral expectations and consequences to patient in language that is easily understood and nonpunitive.
- Refrain from arguing or bargaining with patient about established behavioral expectations and consequences.
- Monitor patient for occurrence or nonoccurrence of desired behaviors.
- Modify behavioral expectations and consequences, as needed, to accommodate reasonable changes in patient's situation.

From Dochterman, J. M., & Bulechek, G. M. (2004). *Nursing interventions classification (NIC)* (4th ed.). St. Louis, MO: Mosby.
*Partial list.

BOX 16-3

NIC Interventions for Aggressive Behavior

Anger Control Assistance

Definition: Facilitation of the expression of anger in an adaptive, nonviolent manner

Activities*:

- Determine appropriate behavioral expectations for expression of anger, given patient's level of cognitive and physical functioning.
- Limit access to frustrating situations until patient is able to express anger in an adaptive manner.
- Encourage patient to seek assistance from nursing staff during periods of increasing tension.
- Monitor potential for inappropriate aggression and intervene before its expression.
- Prevent physical harm if anger is directed at self or others (e.g., restraint and removal of potential weapons).
- Provide physical outlets for expression of anger or tension (e.g., punching bag, sports, clay, journal writing).
- Provide reassurance to patient that nursing staff will intervene to prevent patient from losing control.
- Assist patient in identifying source of anger.
- Identify function that anger, frustration, and rage serve for patient.
- Identify consequences of inappropriate expression of anger.

From Dochterman, J. M., & Bulechek, G. M. (2004). *Nursing interventions classification (NIC)* (4th ed.). St. Louis, MO: Mosby.
*Partial list.

BOX 16-4

NIC Interventions for Impulsive Behavior

Impulse Control Training

Definition: Assisting the patient to mediate impulsive behavior through application of problem-solving strategies to social and interpersonal situations

Activities*:

- Assist patient to identify the problem or situation that requires thoughtful action.
- Assist patient to identify courses of possible action and their costs and benefits.
- Teach patient to cue himself or herself to "stop and think" before acting impulsively.
- Assist patient to evaluate the outcome of the chosen course of action.
- Provide positive reinforcement (e.g., praise and rewards) for successful outcomes.
- Encourage patient to self-reward for successful outcomes.
- Provide opportunities for patient to practice problem solving (role playing) within the therapeutic environment.
- Encourage patient to practice problem solving in social and interpersonal situations outside the therapeutic envi-

From Dochterman, J. M., & Bulechek, G. M. (2004). *Nursing interventions classification (NIC)* (4th ed.). St. Louis, MO: Mosby.
*Partial list.

---

hospital without correcting any errors but rather by simply noting that the client truly feels hurt. Showing empathy may also decrease aggressive outbursts if the client feels that staff are trying to understand feelings of frustration (Kerr, 2002). See Table 16-9 for an example of a nurse-client interaction after an antisocial client initiates a fight with a peer in an inpatient unit. A final approach that is useful for clients with borderline PD relates to the response to superficial self-destructive behaviors. Acting in accordance with unit policies, the nurse remains neutral and dresses the wound matter of factly. Then the client is instructed to write down the sequence of events leading up to the injury, as well as the consequences, before staff will discuss the event. This cognitive exercise encourages the client to independently think about his or her own behavior, instead of merely ventilating feelings. It facilitates the discussion with staff about alternative actions (Alper & Peterson, 2001).

Psychobiological Interventions

Clients with PDs may be helped by a broad array of psychotropic agents, all geared toward maintaining cognitive function and relieving symptoms. Depending on the chief complaint, antidepressant, anxiolytic, or antipsychotic medication may be ordered. Clients with PDs usually do not like taking medicine unless it calms them down; they are fearful about taking something over which they have no control. They worry if they do not have an adequate supply but have difficulty organizing themselves to fill a prescription. Sometimes they panic and get preoccupied with side effects, then stop taking the medication.

Refer to Tables 16-6, 16-7, and 16-8 for recommended pharmacological treatments.

Case Management

Many clients with PDs function at a high level, but a significant number need assistance to maintain their independence. Case management is helpful for clients with PDs who are persistently and severely impaired. These clients often have had multiple hospitalizations, have been unable to maintain work or personal relationships, and are relatively alone in their attempts to care for themselves. In the acute care setting, case management focuses on three goals: to gather pertinent history from current or previous providers; to support reintegration with family or loved ones as appropriate; and to ensure appropriate referrals to outpatient care, including substance disorder treatment if needed. In

TABLE 16-9

Dialogue with a Client with Manipulative, Aggressive, and Impulsive Traits

Dialogue	Therapeutic Tool/Comment
Nurse: Donald, I would like to talk with you about what happened this morning. *Donald:* OK, shoot.	Be clear as to purpose of interview.
Nurse: Tell me what started the incident.	Use open-ended statements. Maintain a nonjudgmental attitude.
Donald: Well, as I told you before, I always had to fight to get what I wanted in life. My father and mother abandoned me emotionally when I was a child. *Nurse:* Yes, but tell me about this morning.	Redirect client to present problem or situation.
Donald: OK. I disliked Richard from the first. He has it in for me, I just know it. He doesn't get along with anyone here. Just 2 days ago, he almost had a fight. *Nurse:* Donald, what do you mean, Richard has it in for you?	Explore situation.
Donald: When I'm talking to one of the nurses, he stares and makes comments under his breath. *Nurse:* What does he say?	Encourage description.
Donald: How I'm "in" with the nurses. I'm just trying to do what is expected of me here. *Nurse:* You mean that Richard is envious of your relationship with the nurses?	Validate client's meaning.
Donald: Right. He really doesn't want to be here. He doesn't care about all that therapeutic junk. *Nurse:* You seem to know a lot about how Richard thinks. I wonder how that is.	Assist client to make association to present situation.
Donald: He reminds me of someone I knew when I was young. His name was Joe. We called him "Bones." *Nurse:* Tell me more about Bones.	Explore situation further.
Donald: We called him Bones because he was skinny. He was into drugs and never ate. He was also called Bones because he was selfish. He never shared anything. He never even had a girl that I knew about. *Nurse:* So Richard reminds you of someone who is selfish and lonely?	Make interpretation of information. Note increasing anxiety.
Donald: That's right. I've had three marriages and girlfriends on the side. No one can take them away from me. *(Angrily.)* Just let them try! *Nurse:* What makes you so angry now?	Identify feelings and explore threat or anxiety.
Donald: Richard! I know he wants to be like me, but he can't. I'll hurt him if he makes any more comments about me. *Nurse:* Donald, you will *not* hurt anyone here on the unit.	Set limits on, and expectations of, client's behavior.
Donald: I'm sorry, I didn't mean that. *Nurse:* It's important that we examine your part in the incident this morning and ways to cope without threats or violence.	Focus on client's responsibility and suggest alternative methods of coping with situation.
Donald: Listen, I know I've gotten into trouble because I can't control my temper, but that's because I won't get any respect until I can show them I don't fear them.	Client exhibits rationalization.
Nurse: Who are "they"? *Donald:* People like Richard.	Clarify pronoun.
Nurse: You've told me that fighting was a way of survival as a child, but as an adult, there are other ways of handling situations that make you angry.	Show understanding and suggest other means of coping.
Donald: You're right. I've thought about this. Do you think it would help if you give me some meds to control my anger?	Client exhibits superficial and concrete thinking—possible manipulation.
Nurse: I wasn't thinking of medications but of a plan for being aware of your anger and talking it out instead of fighting it out.	Clarify meaning toward behavior change. Start to explore alternatives Donald can use when angry instead of fighting.
Donald: I told you before, I have to fight. *Nurse:* Have you thought about the consequences of your fighting?	Identify results of impulsive behavior.
Donald: I feel bad afterwards. Sometimes I wish it hadn't happened.	Client continues to explore.

the long-term outpatient setting, case management objectives include reducing hospitalization by providing resources for crisis services and enhancing the social support system.

Advanced Practice Interventions

The advanced practice nurse (APRN) treats clients with PDs in a variety of inpatient and community settings. Research shows that treatment can be effective for many of these persons, especially when a comorbid major mental disorder is targeted. Refer to Tables 16-6 through 16-8 for a summary of psychotherapy approaches used by the APRN.

In the case of clients with borderline PD, the decision to hospitalize or not is a complex one for the nurse therapist. Much effort has gone into the study of behavior patterns and treatment for borderline PD. As noted earlier, people with borderline PD are at serious risk for suicide (see Chapter 23). But assessment of acute suicidal risk is difficult because of the chronic nature of suicidal behavior in this population. Hospitalization is usually recommended if the client is acutely psychotic or makes a life-threatening suicide attempt. In the case of self-mutilation or suicide threats, however, hospitalization may actually reinforce the behavior rather than help to reduce it. Instead, overnight emergency department stays or partial hospitalization day programs, arranged in combination with the outpatient therapist, may be more effective (Paris, 2002).

The high use of inpatient services by clients with PDs has been well documented. One study noted three factors that seem to differentiate clients with borderline PD who were repeatedly hospitalized from those who were not: history of suicidal behavior in the previous 2 years; presence of a comorbid anxiety disorder; and lower cognitive functioning (Comtois et al., 2003). These findings reinforce the importance of addressing comorbid symptoms and ensuring that communication is at the client's level of understanding.

Additional data are being collected by the ongoing Collaborative Longitudinal Personality Disorders Study, which is a large, prospective, multisite research program funded by the National Institute of Mental Health since 2000. For a sample of 621 participants with PDs who were followed for the first year, the following factors showed significant associations with suicide attempts: diagnoses of borderline PD and substance abuse disorder with increased use in the month before the attempt; and comorbid major depression with increased symptoms in the month before the attempt. Thus, the therapist needs to pay close attention to these two variables over the course of treatment for clients with borderline PD (Yen et al., 2003).

Another early report from this long-range study describes factors associated with sudden and sustained improvement in clients with borderline PD (Gunderson et al., 2003). A sample of 160 clients with borderline PD was evaluated every 6 months for 2 years, and it was found that 18 of these clients showed dramatic improvement in the first 6 months. The two main factors explaining this improvement were remission of coexisting major disorders and reduced stress due to situational change (e.g., divorce or other relationship changes). These findings offer hope for treatment of individuals with borderline PD, suggesting that therapists need to actively treat comorbid disorders as well as advocate for action in stressful relationships.

Specifically for borderline PD, one cognitive-behavioral approach has been found to be more effective than other treatments. Known as dialectical behavior therapy (DBT), this treatment is a structured, long-term approach that provides significant teaching for clients, along with a support system for therapists (Linehan, 1993). The name of the therapy is derived from dialectics, a method of argument that examines contradictory facts or ideas in an effort to resolve the differences into a united whole. The client receives individual therapy, group skills training, and crisis telephone access to the therapist. At the same time, all therapists involved receive training and weekly consultation for peer support. The use of DBT with other populations is also being studied, as in the Veterans Administration program for treating male and female veterans with PTSD and comorbid PDs (Spoont et al., 2003). DBT can be considered as an evidence-based practice for the treatment of clients with borderline PD (see the Evidence-Based Practice box).

■ EVALUATION

Evaluating treatment effectiveness in this client population is difficult. Nurses may never know the real results of their interventions, particularly in acute care settings. Even in long-term outpatient treatment, many PD clients find the relationship too intimate an experience to remain long enough for successful treatment. As noted earlier, however, some motivated clients may be able to learn to change their behavior, especially if positive experiences are repeated. Each therapeutic episode offers an opportunity for the client to observe himself or herself interacting with caregivers who consistently try to teach positive coping skills. Perhaps effectiveness can be measured by how successfully the nurse is able to be genuine with the client, to maintain a helpful posture, to offer substantial instruction, and still to care for himself or herself. Specific short-term outcomes may be accomplished, and overall, the client can be given the message of hope that quality of life can always be improved.

EVIDENCE-BASED PRACTICE

Dialectical Behavior Therapy in Treatment of Borderline Personality Disorder

Background

Borderline personality disorder (BPD) constitutes a public health problem, leading to high use of inpatient and outpatient services, and multiple hospitalizations for crises. Up to 80% of the population with BPD show suicidal behavior, with an eventual suicide completion rate of 10%. Despite abundant literature about the disorder, few treatments have proven effective in reducing self-destructive behavior.

Studies

Dialectical behavior therapy (DBT) is the only treatment approach for clients with BPD that has been shown to be effective in controlled studies. DBT is a form of cognitive-behavioral therapy that focuses on gradual behavior change within a context of acceptance and validation for the client. It has four essential clinical components over the course of 1 year: (1) weekly individual psychotherapy sessions; (2) weekly group social skills training sessions using a structured manual; (3) telephone access to the therapist for coaching during crisis events; and (4) weekly consultation group for all therapists involved in the treatment. Five randomized clinical trials and other experimental studies have demonstrated that DBT can reduce hospitalizations and suicidal behavior. It is also notable that clients do not usually drop out of treatment.

Results of Studies

The original study by Linehan (1993) focused on women with BPD who had a history of suicide attempts with a recent attempt. DBT was compared with standard individual psychotherapy for 1 year. Follow-up 6 months and 1 year after treatment showed that clients undergoing DBT had significantly fewer suicidal episodes and spent fewer days in the psychiatric hospital. A second study involving the Veterans Administration system reported similar findings for female vet-

erans diagnosed with BPD, but these clients were not required to have shown recent suicidal behavior for admission to the study. DBT was adapted to a 6-month course of treatment and compared with individual cognitive-behavioral therapy. At the end of treatment, clients receiving DBT reported less suicidal ideation, depression, and anger than those in the comparison group. Linehan and colleagues (1999) later adapted DBT for a sample of women with a dual diagnosis of BPD and substance use disorder. The changes to DBT included a focus on drug use and case management services. The control group received multiple referrals to community treatment. At the end of treatment, the DBT group had significantly less drug abuse and more gains in social adjustment. But there was no significant difference in number of psychiatric hospital days. In a fourth study, DBT was modified for a small sample of female clients with bulimia nervosa and results were compared with those for a client group on the waiting list. The changes to DBT involved a shorter treatment period of 20 weeks, focus on eating patterns, and combining of skills training with individual therapy sessions. The clients undergoing DBT showed a significant decrease in binging-purging behaviors. Finally, DBT was compared with a client-centered approach in treatment of men and women in a community mental health clinic. The same therapists delivered treatment to both groups over the course of 1 year. DBT was modified by including the skills training in individual sessions, so that the total number of treatment hours was equal for both groups. The DBT clients showed significant decreases in suicidal behavior and a reduced number of psychiatric hospital days.

Implications for Nursing Practice

Nurses need to be aware of DBT as a hopeful treatment approach for difficult-to-treat clients with BPD. Clients may need referrals to centers that offer this specialty. If training opportunities are available for the nurse, he or she may be able to support implementation of this treatment in the work setting. Even if the full treatment protocol is not adopted, principles from DBT can be applied to help the nurse develop realistic nursing care plans for clients with BPD.

Swenson, C. R., Torrey, W. C., & Koerner, K. (2002). Implementing dialectical behavior therapy. *Psychiatric Services, 53*(2), 171-178.

▪ ▪ ▪ KEY POINTS to REMEMBER

- All PDs share the characteristics of inflexibility and difficulties in interpersonal relationships that impair social or occupational functioning.
- PDs are most likely caused by a combination of biological and psychosocial factors.
- The *DSM-IV-TR* organizes PDs into three clusters based on similarities in behavior patterns.
- Clients with PDs often enter psychiatric treatment because of distress from a comorbid major mental illness.

- Nurses may experience intense emotional reactions to clients with PDs and need to make use of clinical supervision to maintain objectivity.
- Despite the relatively fixed patterns of maladaptive behavior, some clients with PDs are able to change their behavior over time as a result of treatment.

▪ ▪ ▪

Visit the Evolve website at **http://evolve.elsevier.com/Varcarolis** for a posttest on the content in this chapter. **evolve**

Critical Thinking and Chapter Review

Visit the Evolve website at **http://evolve.elsevier.com/Varcarolis** for additional self-study exercises.

▪ ▪ ▪ CRITICAL THINKING

1. Mr. Rogers is undergoing surgery for a broken leg. He is very suspicious of the staff and believes that everyone is trying to harm him and to "do him in." He scans his environment constantly for danger (hypervigilance) and speaks very little to the nurses or the other clients. He has a paranoid PD.

   A. Explain why being friendly and outgoing may be threatening to Mr. Rogers.

   B. Explain how being matter of fact and neutral, and sticking to the facts would be the most useful to Mr. Rogers.

   C. What could be done to give Mr. Rogers some control over his situation in a hospital setting?

   D. How would you best handle his sarcasm and hostility so that both you and he would feel most comfortable?

2. Ms. Pemrose is brought to the emergency department after slashing her wrist with a razor. She has previously been in the emergency department for drug overdose and has a history of addictions. Ms. Pemrose can be sarcastic, belittling, and aggressive to those who try to care for her. She has a history of difficulty with interpersonal relationships at her job. When the psychiatric triage nurse comes in to see her, Ms. Pemrose is at first adoring and compliant, telling him, "You are the best nurse I've ever seen, and I truly want to change." But when he refuses to support her request for diazepam (Valium) and meperidine (Demerol) for "pain," she yells at him, "You are a stupid excuse for a nurse. I want a doctor immediately." Ms. Pemrose has borderline PD.

   A. What defense mechanism is Ms. Pemrose using?

   B. How could the nurse best handle this situation in keeping with setting limits and offering concern and useful interventions?

▪ ▪ ▪ CHAPTER REVIEW

Choose the most appropriate answer.

1. Which of the following best describes people with PDs?
   1. Readily assume the roles of compromiser and harmonizer
   2. Often seek help to change maladaptive behaviors
   3. Have the ability to tolerate high levels of anxiety
   4. Have difficulty working and loving

2. For which client is the nurse most likely to need to plan interventions to minimize overtly manipulative behavior?
   1. Mr. A, who has been diagnosed with obsessive-compulsive PD
   2. Ms. B, who has been diagnosed with borderline PD
   3. Mr. C, who has been diagnosed with paranoid PD
   4. Ms. D, who has been diagnosed with schizoid PD

3. A priority nursing intervention undertaken by the nurse dealing with clients with PDs is
   1. offering advice.
   2. probing for etiological factors.
   3. encouraging diversional activity.
   4. setting limits.

4. Which statement will provide a foundation for understanding clients with PDs?
   1. The backgrounds of clients with PDs are usually trouble free.
   2. The tendency to develop a PD may have biological determinants.
   3. Clients with PDs are best treated in the inpatient setting.
   4. PDs are more amenable to treatment than are anxiety disorders.

5. Which of the emotional states listed below is the nurse caring for a client with a PD is most likely to experience?
   1. Anger
   2. Depression
   3. Pleasure
   4. Spiritual distress

▪ **STUDENT**
▪ **STUDY**
▪ **CD-ROM**

Access the accompanying CD-ROM for animations, interactive exercises, review questions for the NCLEX examination, and an audio glossary.

▪ **NURSE,**
▪ **CLIENT, AND**
▪ **FAMILY RESOURCES**

For suggested readings, information on related associations, and Internet resources, go to **http://evolve.elsevier.com/Varcarolis**.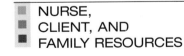

REFERENCES

Alper, G., & Peterson, S. J. (2001). Dialectical behavior therapy for patients with borderline personality disorder. *Journal of Psychosocial Nursing, 39*(10), 38-45.

American Psychiatric Association. (2000). *Diagnostic and statistical manual of mental disorders (DSM-IV-TR)* (4th ed., text rev.). Washington, DC: Author.

Carson, V. B. (2000). *Mental health nursing: The nurse-patient journey* (2nd ed.). Philadelphia: Saunders.

Comtois, K. A., et al. (2003). Factors associated with high use of public mental health services by persons with borderline personality disorder. *Psychiatric Services, 54*(8), 1149-1154.

Dochterman, J. M., & Bulechek, G. M. (2004). *Nursing interventions classification (NIC)* (4th ed.). St. Louis, MO: Mosby.

Gunderson, J. G., et al. (2003). Plausibility and possible determinants of sudden "remissions" in borderline patients. *Psychiatry, 66*(2), 111-118.

Kay, J., Tasman, A., & Lieberman, J. A. (2000). *Psychiatry: Behavioral science and clinical essentials* (pp. 480-498). Philadelphia: Saunders.

Kernberg, O. (1985). *Internal world and external reality.* London: Aronson.

Kerr, N. (2002). Clinical management of "entitled" clients. *Journal of Psychosocial Nursing, 40*(12), 41-45.

Linehan, M. M. (1993). *Skills training manual for treating borderline personality disorder.* New York: Guilford Press.

Linehan, M. M., et al. (1999). Dialectical behavior therapy for patients with borderline personality disorder and drug dependence. *American Journal of Addictions, 8,* 279-292.

Marcus, P. (2000). Behavioral disorders. In V. B. Carson (Ed.), *Mental health nursing: The nurse-patient journey* (2nd ed.). Philadelphia: Saunders.

Moorhead, S., Johnson, M., & Maas, M. (2004). *Nursing outcomes classification (NOC)* (3rd ed.). St. Louis, MO: Mosby.

Munich, R. L., & Allen, J. G. (2003). Psychiatric and sociotherapeutic perspectives on the difficult-to-treat patient. *Psychiatry, 66*(4), 346-356.

Paris, J. (2002). Chronic suicidality among patients with borderline personality disorder. *Psychiatric Services, 53*(6), 738-742.

Spoont, M. R., et al. (2003). Adaptation of dialectical behavior therapy by a VA medical center. *Psychiatric Services, 54*(5), 627-629.

Widiger, T. A., & Mullins, S. (2003). Personality disorders. In A. Tasman, J. Kay, & J. A. Lieberman (Eds.), *Psychiatry* (2nd ed., Vol. 2, pp. 1603-1637). London: Wiley.

Yen, S., et al. (2003). Axis I and axis II disorders as predictors of prospective suicide attempts: Findings from the collaborative longitudinal personality disorders study. *Journal of Abnormal Psychology, 112*(3), 375-381.

CHAPTER 17

Eating Disorders

KATHLEEN IBRAHIM

KEY TERMS and CONCEPTS

The key terms and concepts listed here appear in color where they are defined or first discussed in this chapter.

OBJECTIVES

After studying this chapter, the reader will be able to

1. Discuss the four theories of eating disorder discussed in this chapter.

2. Compare and contrast the signs and symptoms (clinical picture) of anorexia nervosa and bulimia nervosa.

3. Identify three life-threatening conditions, stated in terms of nursing diagnoses, for a client with an eating disorder.

4. Identify three realistic outcome criteria for (a) a client with anorexia nervosa and (b) a client with bulimia nervosa.

5. Recognize which therapeutic interventions are appropriate for the acute phase of anorexia nervosa and which are appropriate for the long-term phase of treatment.

6. Explain the basic premise of cognitive-behavioral therapy in the treatment of anorexia nervosa and bulimia nervosa.

7. Empathize with and describe in the reader's own words the possible thoughts and feelings of a young anorectic girl during the acute phase of her illness.

8. Distinguish between the needs of and treatment(s) for clients with acute bulimia and bulimic individuals in long-term therapy.

9. Differentiate between the long-term prognosis of anorexia nervosa, bulimia nervosa, and binge eating disorder.

evolve Visit the Evolve website at **http://evolve.elsevier.com/Varcarolis** for a pretest on the content in this chapter.

For the majority of people, eating provides nourishment for the body as well as the soul. Families and friends gather together around the table to break bread as they celebrate, mourn, laugh, cry, share, and demonstrate love. For some, however, eating is a totally different experience, failing to nourish either body or soul but providing instead a way of controlling a life that is totally out of control. For these individuals, eating loses its communal value and becomes secretive, hidden, shrouded in secrecy and shame. Eating in these circumstances is disordered, and those who experience eating disorders have real, treatable medical illnesses that not only cause extreme psychic pain but also can be life threatening.

The main types of eating disorder are anorexia nervosa, bulimia nervosa, and eating disorder not otherwise specified (NOS). A fourth disorder, binge eating disorder, is mentioned in the *Diagnostic and Statistical Manual of Mental Disorders,* fourth edition, text revision *(DSM-IV-TR),* as a diagnosis requiring additional research (American Psychiatric Association [APA], 2000a). Individuals with anorexia nervosa refuse to maintain a minimally normal weight for height and express intense fear of gaining weight. The term *anorexia* is a misnomer, because loss of appetite is rare. Some anorectics restrict their intake of food; others engage in binge eating and purging. Individuals with bulimia nervosa engage in repeated episodes of binge eating followed by inappropriate compensatory behaviors such as self-induced vomiting; misuse of laxatives, diuretics, or other medications; fasting; or excessive exercise. Eating disorder NOS is a category that includes disorders of eating that do not meet the criteria for either anorexia nervosa or bulimia nervosa. Each of these disorders is characterized by a significant disturbance in the perception of body shape and weight (APA, 2000a). Individuals with binge eating disorder engage in repeated episodes of binge eating, after which they experience significant distress. These individuals do not regularly use the compensatory behaviors such as self-induced vomiting, misuse of laxatives and other medications, fasting, and excessive exercise that are seen in clients with bulimia nervosa. Each of these disorders is discussed in the following sections.

PREVALENCE

Eating disorders are on the increase. The adage "You can never be too rich or too thin" seems to have become part of the American consciousness. The National Eating Disorders Association (2002) reports that 80% of American women are dissatisfied with their appearance. Many women diet relentlessly to achieve the body of the average American model, even though most fashion models are thinner than 80% of American women (National Eating Disorders Association, 2002). The desire to be thin is not exclusive to older women but also grabs the very young: 42% of first- to third-grade girls express this desire and 81% of 10 year olds express fear of becoming fat (National Eating Disorders Association, 2002). On any given day 45% of American women and 25% of American men are on a diet, and over $40 billion is spent on dieting and diet-related products annually. Estimates are that 35% of normal dieters progress to pathological dieting and, of those, 20% to 25% progress to partial- or full-syndrome eating disorders. Clearly a great deal of energy is expended not only in worrying about weight but also in trying to control and lose weight.

Eating disorders are more common in women than in men. The estimated lifetime prevalence of anorexia nervosa among women is approximately 0.5% (APA, 2000a); among men the prevalence is approximately one tenth that among women. Female athletes, especially those in sports that emphasize thinness (i.e., gymnastics, ballet dancing, figure skating, and distance running), demonstrate an increase in eating disorders. A higher rate of anorexia nervosa (2.8%) was found among male bodybuilders than among the general American male population (0.02%) (APA, 2000b).

The lifetime prevalence of bulimia nervosa among women ranges from 1% to 3%, and again the preva-lence among men is approximately one tenth that among women.

Community surveys estimate that between 2% and 5% of Americans deal with a binge eating disorder, with women approximately 1.5 times more likely to engage in this eating pattern than men.

Eating disorders are increasing not only in the United States but in other industrialized countries as well. A survey in 1998 in Fiji conducted after 3 years of Western influence showed a marked increase in eating disorder symptoms compared with results of a 1995 survey. Chinese women in Hong Kong and Australia are showing increased rates of eating-disordered behaviors, as are adolescents in Iran (Miller & Pumariega, 2001). Women are particularly at risk in industrialized nations, where there is an abundance of food and physical attractiveness is linked with being thin (APA, 2002a).

COMORBIDITY

The incidence of comorbid psychiatric illness is high in clients with eating disorder who seek treatment. Major depressive disorder or dysthymia is diagnosed in 50% to 75% of clients with anorexia nervosa and bulimia nervosa (APA, 2000a). Dysthymia in adolescents was predictive of eating disorder symptoms in a study by Zaider, Johnson, and Cockell (2000). Bipolar disorder is found in 4% to 6%, but some report a rate as high as 13%. The incidence of obsessive-compulsive disorder has been reported to be as high as 25%, and this disorder is common among patients with anorexia nervosa. Most clients with anorexia nervosa are preoccupied with food; some of them collect cookbooks, plan and prepare elaborate meals for others, and hoard food. Anxiety disorders, particularly social phobia, are also common. In addition, substance abuse coexists in as many as 30% to 37% of those with bulimia nervosa and 12% to 18% of those with anorexia nervosa, occurring primarily with binge-purge subtype (APA, 2000b).

The pattern of comorbid psychiatric illness is the same in men as in women. Male veterans with eating disorders have a high rate of comorbid substance use and mood disorders, including those with anorexia nervosa, who appear to be at high risk for schizophrenia or another psychotic disorder. Males with bulimia nervosa are at risk for comorbid organic mental disorder, schizophrenia, and psychotic disorders (APA, 2000b).

Estimates of comorbid personality disorder range from 42% to 75%. There is a noted association between bulimia nervosa and cluster B and C personality disorders, especially borderline personality disorder and avoidant personality disorder, and between anorexia nervosa and the cluster C disorders of avoidant personality disorder and obsessive-compulsive personality disorder. Obsessive-compulsive personality disorder predicted eating disorder symptoms in adolescents in a study of a community sample. Obsessive-compulsive features are often prominent, both food related and not food related. Personality disorders are more common among individuals with the binge-purge subtype of anorexia nervosa than among those with the restricting type or normal-weight clients with bulimia nervosa (APA, 2000b).

A history of sexual abuse is more common in those with eating disorders than in the general population. Women with a history of eating disorders and sexual abuse have a higher rate of other comorbid psychiatric illnesses than women diagnosed solely with eating disorders (APA, 2000b).

THEORY

The eating disorders—anorexia nervosa, bulimia nervosa, and eating disorder NOS, which includes binge eating disorder—are actually entities or syndromes and are not considered to be specific diseases. It is not known if they share a common cause and pathology. It is more appropriate to conceptualize them as syndromes on the basis of the cluster of symptoms they present (Halmi, 2003). A number of theories attempt to explain eating disorders.

Neurobiological and Neuroendocrine Models

Individuals with eating disorders present with symptoms that manifest along a continuum between anorexia nervosa and bulimia nervosa, with many displaying a mixture of anorectic and bulimic behaviors. The comorbidity of eating disorders and depression has received considerable focus in the literature. In depression, as in eating disorders, there are complex interrelationships of altered neurotransmitters, as well as abnormal patterns involving multiple systems and pathways. However, one is cautioned against assuming similar pathological features in eating disorders and depression based on the treatment response to antidepressant medication in the two groups. There is no clear evidence that antidepressant medication is of significant usefulness in the treatment of anorexia nervosa. In bulimia nervosa antidepressant medications are somewhat effective in reducing the symptoms. These improvements seem to be independent of an improvement in symptoms of a mood disturbance (Zhu & Walsh, 2002).

Similar neuroendocrine abnormalities are noted in both anorexia nervosa and bulimia nervosa (Brambilla & Monteleone, 2003). Whether the relationships are causal or result from starvation or abnormal eating behaviors is not clear. Serotonin activity is decreased in low-weight individuals with anorexia; cholecystokinin, an intestinal hormone, is present at low levels in bulimic persons. Endogenous opioids, gastrointestinal hormones, and vasopressin have received attention, but the findings are not clear. The aforementioned findings represent the biological abnormalities observed in people with eating disorders and may help to explain the drive toward dieting, hunger, preoccupation with food, and tendency toward binge eating.

Psychological Models

Anorexia nervosa results in amenorrhea and physiological changes that interfere with the development of an age-appropriate sexual role. Psychoanalytical theorists long believed that conflict over one's sexual role was primary for anorectic persons. The work of Bruch (1973) on anorexia in women failed to prove these theoretical assumptions but postulated developmental factors that led to anorexia nervosa. According to Bruch, girls who develop anorexia experience themselves as ineffectual, passive, and unable to assert their will. Misguided efforts to separate and establish an autonomous adult existence lead to self-starvation and a distorted sense of being special and powerful. People with anorexia are anxious about losing control over their eating and do not accurately experience hunger or satiety. They feel powerless and are unable to identify what they need. Outwardly they may be defiant about their eating, displaying a veneer of competence. However, internally they are afraid and fear losing control.

The "core psychopathology" in both anorexia and bulimia includes low self-esteem and self-doubts about personal worth. These feelings produce harsh self-judgment focused solely on the issue of weight. The overvalued ideas about weight, shape, and control are critical to maintaining the eating-disordered behaviors (Fairburn, 2002).

Sociocultural Models

In countries participating in the global economy, the media promote the body as a commodity, and bodily preoccupation is an acceptable form of self-promotion. Although the number of individuals who are overweight continues to increase, many individuals with eating disorders have internalized the societal ideal to be thin (Davis, Claridge, & Fox, 2000; Wiederman & Pryor, 2000). In modernizing countries such as China and India, anorectic behavior does not include the pursuit of thinness or fear of being fat. In these countries, the self-imposed weight restriction may represent control over one's life circumstances or grow out of spiritual or ascetic values (Miller & Pumariega, 2001).

The Western ideal for women who are at risk is to be competent in both traditional and nontraditional ways. For some women, being a mother and homemaker as well as a career woman may produce conflict. It is interesting to note that eating disorders do not flourish in male-dominated societies in which women are forced into a stereotypical nurturing role; rather, the incidence of eating disorders increases in societies in which women have a choice in social roles (Miller & Pumariega, 2001). The increase in eating disorders in non-Western women assimilating into a Western society may be due either to the conflict of acculturation or identification with the new culture and its emphasis on a thin ideal female body (Lake, Staiger, & Glowinski, 2000).

Genetic Models

There is a strong genetic link for eating disorders. In fact, in many twin studies this link approaches that seen in studies of bipolar disorder and schizophrenia (Klump, Kaye, & Strober, 2001). By comparing identical (monozygotic) and fraternal (dizygotic) twins it is possible to differentiate genetic from environmental effects. One study that looked for genetic factors found a 56% concordance rate for anorexia nervosa in monozygotic twins. The genetic vulnerability that might be responsible for the development of anorexia nervosa might lead to poor affect and impulse control or to an underlying neurotransmitter dysfunction. A family history of affective disorder and alcohol abuse was found to be common in sets of monozygotic twins of which one was diagnosed with bulimia nervosa. A 22.9% concordance rate was found for bulimia in monozygotic twins compared with an 8.7% rate in dizygotic twins.

FUNDAMENTAL ASSESSMENT OF ANOREXIA NERVOSA AND BULIMIA NERVOSA

Anorexia nervosa and bulimia nervosa are two separate syndromes and, as such, present two clinical pictures on assessment. Table 17-1 identifies the clinical features, potential laboratory results, and possible behaviors found on assessment.

TABLE 17-1

Possible Signs and Symptoms of Anorexia and Bulimia

Phenomena Associated with Anorexia Nervosa

- Terror of gaining weight
- Preoccupation with thoughts of food
- View of self as fat even when emaciated
- Peculiar handling of food
  - —Cutting food into small bits
  - —Pushing pieces of food around plate
- Possible development of rigorous exercise regimen
- Possible self-induced vomiting, use of laxatives and diuretics
- Cognition so disturbed that individual judges self-worth by his or her weight

Clinical Presentation	Cause
Low weight	Caloric restriction, excessive exercising
Amenorrhea	Low weight
Yellow skin	Hypercarotenemia
Lanugo	Starvation
Cold extremities	Starvation
Peripheral edema	Hypoalbuminemia and refeeding
Muscle weakening	Starvation, electrolyte imbalance
Constipation	Starvation
Abnormal laboratory values	Starvation
■ Low triiodothyronine, thyroxine levels	
Abnormal computed tomographic scans, electroencephalographic changes	Starvation
Cardiovascular abnormalities	Starvation, dehydration
■ Hypotension	Electrolyte imbalance
■ Bradycardia	
■ Heart failure	

TABLE 17-1

Possible Signs and Symptoms of Anorexia and Bulimia—cont'd

Clinical Presentation—cont'd	Cause—cont'd
Impaired renal function	Dehydration
Hypokalemia (low potassium)	Starvation
Anemic pancytopenia	Starvation
Decreased bone density	Estrogen deficiency, low calcium intake

Phenomena Associated with Bulimia Nervosa

- Binge eating behaviors
- Often self-induced vomiting (or laxative or diuretic use) after bingeing
- History of anorexia nervosa in one fourth to one third of individuals
- Depressive signs and symptoms
- Problems with
  - Interpersonal relationships
  - Self-concept
  - Impulsive behaviors
- Increased levels of anxiety and compulsivity
- Possible chemical dependency
- Possible impulsive stealing

Clinical Presentation	Cause
Normal to slightly low weight	Excessive caloric intake with purging, excessive exercising
Dental caries, tooth erosion	Vomiting (HCl reflux over enamel)
Parotid swelling	Increased serum amylase levels
Gastric dilation, rupture	Binge eating
Calluses, scars on hand (Russell's sign)	Self-induced vomiting
Peripheral edema	Rebound fluid, especially if diuretic used
Muscle weakening	Electrolyte imbalance
Abnormal laboratory values	Purging: vomiting, laxative and/or diuretic use
■ Electrolyte imbalance	
■ Hypokalemia	
■ Hyponatremia	
Cardiovascular abnormalities	Electrolyte imbalance—**can lead to death**
■ Cardiomyopathy	
■ Electrocardiographic changes	
Cardiac failure (cardiomyopathy)	Ipecac intoxication

Eating disorders are serious and in extreme cases can lead to death. Box 17-1 identifies a number of complications that can occur and the laboratory findings that may result in individuals with eating disorders. Because the eating behaviors in these conditions are so extreme, hospitalization may become necessary. Box 17-2 identifies when an individual should be hospitalized; often hospitalization is via the emergency department. Table 17-2 provides the reader with a clinical tool and identifies some of the behaviors and thoughts that, when extreme in intensity or duration, may signal the need for health intervention.

Fundamental to the care of individuals with eating disorders is the establishment and maintenance of a therapeutic alliance. This will take time as well as diplomacy on the part of the nurse.

In treating clients who have been sexually abused or who have otherwise been the victim of boundary violations, it is critical that the nurse and other health care workers maintain and respect clear boundaries (APA, 2000b).

Figure 17-1 identifies the diagnostic criteria for anorexia nervosa, bulimia nervosa, and eating disorders NOS.

Some Medical Complications of Anorexia Nervosa and Bulimia Nervosa

Anorexia Nervosa

- Bradycardia
- Orthostatic changes in pulse or blood pressure
- Cardiac murmur—one third with mitral valve prolapse
- Sudden cardiac arrest due to profound electrolyte disturbances
- Prolonged QT interval on electrocardiogram
- Acrocyanosis
- Symptomatic hypotension
- Leukopenia
- Lymphocytosis
- Carotenemia (elevated carotene levels in blood), which produces skin with yellow pallor
- Hypokalemic alkalosis (with self-induced vomiting or use of laxatives and diuretics)
- Elevated serum bicarbonate levels, hypochloremia, and hypokalemia
- Electrolyte imbalances, which lead to fatigue, weakness, and lethargy
- Osteoporosis, indicated by decrease in bone density
- Fatty degeneration of liver, indicated by elevation of serum enzyme levels
- Elevated cholesterol levels
- Amenorrhea
- Abnormal thyroid functioning
- Hematuria
- Proteinuria

Bulimia Nervosa

- Cardiomyopathy from ipecac intoxication (medical emergency that usually results in death)
- Cardiac arrhythmias
- Sinus bradycardia
- Sudden cardiac arrest due to profound electrolyte disturbances
- Orthostatic changes in pulse or blood pressure
- Cardiac murmur; mitral valve prolapse
- Electrolyte imbalances
- Elevated serum bicarbonate levels (although can be low, which indicates a metabolic acidosis)
- Hypochloremia
- Hypokalemia
- Dehydration, which results in volume depletion, leading to stimulation of aldosterone production, which in turn stimulates further potassium excretion from kidneys; thus there can be an indirect renal loss of potassium as well as a direct loss through self-induced vomiting
- Severe attrition and erosion of teeth producing irritating sensitivity and exposing the pulp of the teeth
- Loss of dental arch
- Diminished chewing ability
- Parotid gland enlargement associated with elevated serum amylase levels
- Esophageal tears caused by self-induced vomiting
- Severe abdominal pain indicative of gastric dilation
- Russell's sign (callus on knuckles from self-induced vomiting)

Data from Halmi, K. A. (2004). Eating disorders. In R. E. Hales & S. C. Yudofsky (Eds.), *Essentials of clinical psychiatry* (2nd ed., pp. 762, 769-770). Washington, DC: American Psychiatric Publishing; and Dixon-Works, D., Nenstiel, R. O., & Aliabadi, Z. (2003). Common eating disorders: A primer for primary care physicians. *Clinical Reviews, 13*(9), 45-51.

Criteria for Hospital Admission of Clients with Eating Disorders

Physical Criteria

- Weight loss over 30% over 6 months
- Rapid decline in weight
- Inability to gain weight with outpatient treatment
- Severe hypothermia due to loss of subcutaneous tissue or dehydration (temperature lower than 36° C or 96.8° F)
- Heart rate less than 40 beats per minute
- Systolic blood pressure less than 70 mm Hg
- Hypokalemia (less than 3 mEq/L) or other electrolyte disturbances not corrected by oral supplementation
- Electrocardiographic changes (especially arrhythmias)

Psychiatric Criteria

- Suicidal or severely out-of-control, self-mutilating behaviors
- Out-of-control use of laxatives, emetics, diuretics, or street drugs
- Failure to comply with treatment contract
- Severe depression
- Psychosis
- Family crisis or dysfunction

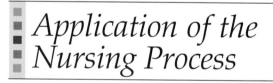

Anorexia Nervosa

Application of the Nursing Process

■ ASSESSMENT

Overall Assessment

Individuals with the binge-purge type of anorexia nervosa may present with severe electrolyte imbalance as a result of purging and enter the health care system through admission to an intensive care unit.

The nurse assessing the anorectic client observes a severely underweight male or female who may have growth of fine, downy hair (lanugo) on the face and back; mottled, cool skin on the extremities; and low blood pressure, pulse, and temperature readings, consistent with a malnourished, dehydrated state. Refer to

TABLE 17-2

The Body Shape Questionnaire

We would like to know how you have been feeling about your appearance over the *past 4 weeks*. Please read the questions and circle the appropriate number to the right. Please answer all questions.

Over the Past 4 Weeks:	Never	Rarely	Sometimes	Often	Very Often	Always
1. Has feeling bored made you brood about your shape?	1	2	3	4	5	6
2. Have you ever been so worried about your shape that you have been feeling you ought to diet?	1	2	3	4	5	6
3. Have you ever thought that your thighs, hips, or bottom is too large for the rest of you?	1	2	3	4	5	6
4. Have you ever been afraid that you might become fat (or fatter)?	1	2	3	4	5	6
5. Have you ever worried about your flesh not being firm enough?	1	2	3	4	5	6
6. Has feeling full (e.g., after eating a large meal) made you feel fat?	1	2	3	4	5	6
7. Have you ever felt so bad about your shape that you have cried?	1	2	3	4	5	6
8. Have you avoided running because your flesh might wobble?	1	2	3	4	5	6
9. Has being with thin women made you feel self-conscious about your shape?	1	2	3	4	5	6
10. Have you worried about thighs spreading out when sitting down?	1	2	3	4	5	6
11. Has eating even a small amount of food made you feel fat?	1	2	3	4	5	6
12. Have you noticed the shape of other women and felt that your own shape compared unfavorably?	1	2	3	4	5	6
13. Has thinking about your shape interfered with your ability to concentrate (e.g., while watching TV, reading, listening to conversation)?	1	2	3	4	5	6
14. Has being naked, such as when taking a bath, made you feel fat?	1	2	3	4	5	6
15. Have you avoided wearing clothes which make you particularly aware of the shape of your body?	1	2	3	4	5	6
16. Have you ever imagined cutting off fleshy areas of your body?	1	2	3	4	5	6
17. Has eating sweets, cakes, or other high-calorie food made you feel fat?	1	2	3	4	5	6
18. Have you not gone out to social occasions (e.g., parties) because you have felt bad about your shape?	1	2	3	4	5	6
19. Have you felt excessively large and rounded?	1	2	3	4	5	6
20. Have you felt ashamed of your body?	1	2	3	4	5	6
21. Has worry about your shape made you diet?	1	2	3	4	5	6
22. Have you felt the happiest about your shape when your stomach has been empty?	1	2	3	4	5	6
23. Have you thought that you are the shape you are because of lack of self-control?	1	2	3	4	5	6
24. Have you worried about other people seeing rolls of flesh around your waist and stomach?	1	2	3	4	5	6
25. Have you felt that it is not fair that other women are thinner than you?	1	2	3	4	5	6
26. Have you vomited in order to feel thinner?	1	2	3	4	5	6
27. When in company, have you worried about taking up too much room (e.g., sitting on a sofa or a bus seat)?	1	2	3	4	5	6
28. Have you worried about your flesh being dumpy?	1	2	3	4	5	6
29. Has seeing your reflection (e.g., in a mirror or shop window) made you feel bad about your shape?	1	2	3	4	5	6
30. Have you pinched areas of your body to see how much fat there is?	1	2	3	4	5	6
31. Have you avoided situations in which people could see your body (e.g., communal changing rooms)?	1	2	3	4	5	6
32. Have you taken laxatives to feel thinner?	1	2	3	4	5	6
33. Have you been particularly self-conscious about your shape when in the company of other people?	1	2	3	4	5	6
34. Has worry about your shape made you feel you ought to exercise?	1	2	3	4	5	6

From Cooper, P. J., et al. (1987). The development and validation of the Body Shape Questionnaire. *International Journal of Eating Disorders, 6*(4), 485-494.

DSM-IV-TR CRITERIA FOR EATING DISORDERS

EATING DISORDERS

Anorexia Nervosa

A. Refusal to maintain body weight at or above a minimally normal weight for age and height (e.g., weight loss leading to maintenance of body weight less than 85% of that expected) or failure to make expected weight gain during period of growth, leading to body weight less than 85% of that expected.

B. Intense fear of gaining weight or becoming fat, even though underweight.

C. Disturbance in the way in which one's body weight or shape is experienced, undue influence of body weight or shape on self-evaluation, or denial of the seriousness of the current low body weight.

D. In females, postmenarcheal amenorrhea (i.e., the absence of at least three consecutive menstrual cycles). (A woman is considered to have amenorrhea if her periods occur only after hormone [e.g., estrogen] administration.)

Specify type:

Binge eating/purging type: During the episode of anorexia nervosa, the person engages in recurrent episodes of binge eating or purging behaviors.

Restricting type: During the episode of anorexia nervosa, the person does *not* engage in recurrent episodes of binge eating or purging behaviors.

Bulimia Nervosa

A. Recurrent episodes of binge eating. An episode of binge eating is characterized by both of the following:

(1) Eating in a discrete period (e.g., within any 2-hour period) an amount of food that is definitely larger than most people would eat during a similar period and under similar circumstances.
(2) A sense of lack of control over eating during the episode (e.g., a feeling that one cannot stop eating or control what or how much one is eating).

B. Recurrent inappropriate compensatory behavior to prevent weight gain such as self-induced vomiting; misuse of laxatives, diuretics, enemas, or other medications; fasting; or excessive exercise.

C. The binge eating and inappropriate compensatory behavior both occur on average at least twice a week for 3 months.

D. Self-evaluation is unduly influenced by body shape and weight.

E. The disturbance does not occur exclusively during episodes of anorexia nervosa.

Specify type:

Purging type: During the current episode of bulimia nervosa, the person has regularly engaged in self-induced vomiting or the misuse of laxatives, diuretics, or enemas.

Nonpurging type: During the current episode of bulimia nervosa, the person has used other inappropriate compensatory behaviors such as fasting or excessive exercise but has not regularly engaged in self-induced vomiting or the misuse of laxatives, diuretics, or enemas.

Eating Disorder Not Otherwise Specified (NOS)

The eating disorder not otherwise specified category is for disorders of eating that do not meet the criteria for any specific eating disorder. Examples include:

1. For females, all the criteria for anorexia nervosa are met except that the individual has regular menses.

2. All the criteria for anorexia nervosa are met except that despite significant weight loss, the individual's current weight is in the normal range.

3. All the criteria for bulimia nervosa are met except that the binge eating and inappropriate compensatory mechanisms occur at a frequency of less than twice a week for a duration of less than 3 months.

4. The regular use of inappropriate compensatory behavior by an individual of normal body weight after eating small amounts of food (i.e., self-induced vomiting after the consumption of two cookies).

5. Repeatedly chewing and spitting out, but not swallowing, large amounts of food.

6. Binge eating disorder: recurrent episodes of binge eating in the absence of the regular use of inappropriate compensatory behaviors characteristic of bulimia nervosa.

FIGURE 17-1 Diagnostic criteria for eating disorders. (Adapted from American Psychiatric Association. [2000]. *Diagnostic and statistical manual of mental disorders* [4th ed., text rev.]. Washington, DC: Author.)

Table 17-1 for the signs and symptoms of anorexia and bulimia.

On admission to an eating disorder unit for inpatient treatment of anorexia nervosa, Tina, a 16-year-old young woman at 60% of ideal body weight, appears cachectic. She has lanugo over most of her body and prominent parotid glands. She is further assessed to be hypotensive (86/50 mm Hg) and dehydrated. In addition, she has a low serum potassium level and dysrhythmias that appear on an electrocardiogram (ECG). A decision is made to transfer her to the intensive care unit until she is medically stabilized. As an intravenous catheter is inserted, her severe weight phobia and fear of fat are underscored when she cries, "There's not going to be sugar in the IV, is there?" The nurse responds, "I hear how frightened you are. We need to do what's necessary to get you past this crisis."

■ ■ ■

As with any comprehensive psychiatric nursing assessment, a complete evaluation of biopsychosocial function is mandatory. The areas to be covered include the following client characteristics:

- Perception of the problem
- Eating habits
- History of dieting
- Methods used to achieve weight control (restricting, purging, exercising)
- Value attached to a specific shape and weight
- Interpersonal and social functioning
- Mental status and physiological parameters

Self-Assessment

The nurse caring for the anorectic client may find it difficult to appreciate the compelling force of the illness, regarding it as trivial (compared to a mental illness such as schizophrenia), incorrectly believing that weight restriction, bingeing, and purging are self-imposed. The nurse may believe that the client "chooses" to engage in behaviors that are risky and blame the client for her or his health problems. In addition, the common personality traits of these clients, including perfectionism, obsessive thoughts and actions relating to food, the need to be people pleasers, and the need to control their therapy in such a way that they are in almost constant conflict with their caregivers, pose challenges to the nurse.

In the effort to motivate the client and take advantage of the decision to seek help and be healthier, the nurse must take care not to allow encouragement to cross the line toward authoritarianism and assumption of a parental role. As the nurse struggles to build a therapeutic alliance and be empathetic, the client's terror at gaining weight and resistance to nursing interventions may engender significant frustration. Nurses must guard against any tendency to be coer-

cive in their approach and must be aware that one of the primary goals of treatment—weight gain—is the very thing the client fears. Frequent acknowledgment of the difficulty of the situation for the client and of the constant struggle that so characterizes the treatment will help during times of extreme resistance.

▶ Assessment Guidelines   Anorexia Nervosa

Determine whether
1. The client has a medical or psychiatric condition that warrants hospitalization (see Box 17-2).
2. The family has information about the disease and knows where to get support.
3. The client is amenable to receiving or compliant with appropriate therapeutic modalities.
4. Family counseling has been offered to the family or individual family members to provide support or to identify a family problem that may be contributing to the client's eating disorder.
5. A thorough physical examination with appropriate blood work has been done.
6. Other medical conditions have been ruled out.
7. The family and client need further teaching or information regarding the client's treatment plan (e.g., psychopharmacological interventions, behavioral therapy, cognitive therapy, family therapy, individual psychotherapy).
8. The client and family desire to participate in a support group.
9. The client and family have been provided referral to a support group.

■ NURSING DIAGNOSIS

Imbalanced nutrition: less than body requirements is usually the most compelling nursing diagnosis initially for individuals with anorexia. *Imbalanced nutrition: less than body requirements* generates further nursing diagnoses, for example, *decreased cardiac output, risk for injury* (electrolyte imbalance), and *risk for imbalanced fluid volume*, which would have first priority when problems are addressed. Other nursing diagnoses include *disturbed body image, anxiety, chronic low self-esteem, deficient knowledge, ineffective coping, powerlessness,* and *hopelessness.*

■ OUTCOME CRITERIA

To evaluate the effectiveness of treatment, outcome criteria are established to measure treatment results. Relevant categories of the Nursing Outcomes Classification (NOC) (Moorhead, Johnson, & Maas, 2004) include *Weight: Body Mass, Weight Control, Appetite, Nutritional Status: Nutrient Intake,* and *Body Image.* Refer to Table 17-3 for examples of intermediate and short-term indicators for the client with anorexia nervosa.

TABLE 17-3

NOC Outcomes for Anorexia Nervosa

Nursing Outcome and Definition	Intermediate Indicators	Short-Term Indicators
Nutritional Status: Nutrient Intake: Adequacy of usual pattern of nutrient intake*		Caloric intake Protein intake Fat intake Carbohydrate intake
Weight: Body Mass: Extent to which body weight, muscle, and fat are congruent to height, frame, gender, and age†		Weight Body fat percentage Waist/hip circumference ratio (women) Neck/waist circumference ratio (men)
Body Image: Perception of own appearance and body functions‡	Congruence between body reality, body ideal, and body presentation Satisfaction with body appearance	Willingness to touch affected body part Willingness to use strategies to enhance appearance Willingness to use strategies to enhance function

From Moorhead, S., Johnson, M., & Maas, M. (2004). *Nursing outcomes classification (NOC)* (3rd ed.). St. Louis, MO: Mosby.
*Indicators measured on a five-point Likert scale ranging from 1 (not adequate) to 5 (totally adequate).
†Indicators measured on a five-point Likert scale ranging from 1 (severe deviation from normal range) to 5 (no deviation from normal range).
‡Indicators measured on a five-point Likert scale ranging from 1 (never positive) to 5 (consistently positive).

■ PLANNING

Planning is affected by the acuity of the client's situation. In the case of an anorectic client who is experiencing extreme electrolyte imbalance or whose weight is below 75% of ideal body weight, the plan is to provide immediate stabilization, most likely in an inpatient unit (APA, 2000b). Inpatient hospitalization is usually brief, attempts only limited weight restoration, and addresses only the acute complications such as electrolyte imbalance and dysrhythmias, and acute psychiatric symptoms such as significant depression. Some hospitalized clients experience the **refeeding syndrome,** a potentially catastrophic treatment complication in which the demands of a replenished circulatory system overwhelm the capacity of a nutritionally depleted cardiac muscle, which results in cardiovascular collapse (APA, 2000b).

Once a client is medically stable, then the plan begins to address the issues underlying the eating disorder. These issues are usually addressed on an outpatient basis.

Because anorexia nervosa is a chronic illness, the plan will most likely require both inpatient and outpatient management, with the bulk of care provided on an outpatient basis. The plan will include individual, group, and family therapy as well as psychopharmacological therapy during different phases of the illness. The nature of the treatment is determined both by the intensity of the symptoms, which may vary over time, and by the experienced disruption in the client's life.

■ INTERVENTION
Basic Level Interventions: Acute Care

Typically, when the client with an eating disorder is admitted to the inpatient psychiatric facility, the client is in a crisis state. The nurse is challenged to establish trust and monitor the eating pattern. Weight restoration and weight monitoring create opportunities to counter the distorted ideas that maintain the illness (Bowers, 2001). The basic level registered nurse (RN) provides milieu therapy, counseling, health teaching, and medication management.

Milieu Therapy

Clients who are admitted to an inpatient unit designed to treat eating disorders participate in a treatment program provided by an interdisciplinary team and consisting of a combination of therapeutic modalities. These modalities are designed to normalize eating patterns and to begin to address the issues raised by the illness. The milieu of an eating disorder unit is purposefully organized to assist the client in establishing more adaptive behavioral patterns, including normalization of eating. The highly structured milieu includes precise meal times, adherence to the selected menu, observation during and after meals, and regularly scheduled weighings. Close monitoring of clients includes monitoring of all trips to the bathroom after eating to ensure that there is no self-induced vomiting. Clients may also need monitoring on bathroom trips after seeing visitors and after any hospital pass. The latter is to ensure that the client has not had access to and ingested any laxatives or diuretics. Therapy groups are led by nurses and other interdisciplinary team members and are tailored to the issues of clients with eating disorders. Client privileges are linked to weight gain and treatment plan compliance.

Counseling

The basic level nurse on an inpatient unit may operate as both primary nurse and group leader. The initial focus depends on the results of a comprehensive assessment. Any acute psychiatric symptoms, such as suicidal ideation, are addressed immediately. At the same time, the anorectic client begins a weight restoration program that allows for incremental weight gain. Based on the client's height, a treatment goal is set at 90% of ideal body weight, the weight at which most women are able to menstruate.

As clients begin to refeed, they ideally begin to participate in the milieu therapy, in which the cognitive distortions that perpetuate the illness are consistently confronted by all members of the interdisciplinary team. Box 17-3 identifies some common types of cognitive distortion characteristic of people with eating disorders. Although the eating behavior is targeted, the underlying emotions of anxiety, dysphoria, low

---

BOX 17-3

Cognitive Distortions

Overgeneralization: A single event affects unrelated situations.
- "He didn't ask me out. It must be because I'm fat."
- "I was happy when I wore a size 6. I must get back to that weight."

All-or-nothing thinking: Reasoning is absolute and extreme, in mutually exclusive terms of black or white, good or bad.
- "If I have one popsicle, I must eat five."
- "If I allow myself to gain weight, I'll blow up like a balloon."

Catastrophizing: The consequences of an event are magnified.
- "If I gain weight, my weekend will be ruined."
- "When people say I look better, I know they think I'm fat."

Personalization: Events are overinterpreted as having personal significance.
- "I know everybody is watching me eat."
- "I think people won't like me unless I'm thin."

Emotional reasoning: Subjective emotions determine reality.
- "I know I'm fat because I feel fat."
- "When I'm thin, I feel powerful."

Adapted from Bowers, W. A. (2001). Basic principles for applying cognitive-behavioral therapy to anorexia nervosa. *Psychiatric Clinics of North America, 24*(2), 293-303.

---

self-esteem, and feelings of lack of control are also addressed through counseling.

▪ ▪ ▪ VIGNETTE

In a multifamily group on an inpatient unit, Mrs. Demi (who last saw her anorectic daughter before she had gained 40 lb) is asked by the group leader how she regards her daughter Lila. Mrs. Demi replies, "She looks healthy." Her daughter responds with an angry, sullen look. She ultimately verbalizes that she experiences comments about her "healthy" appearance as "You look fat." The group leader points out that it is interesting that Lila equates "healthy" with "fat." In the multifamily group, there is a commonly expressed view that the illness "is not about weight" but that thinness confers a feeling of being special and that being at a normal weight (healthy) means this special status is lost.

▪ ▪ ▪

Health Teaching

Self-care activities are an important part of the treatment plan. These activities include learning more constructive coping skills, improving social skills, and developing problem-solving and decision-making skills. The skills become the focus of both therapy sessions and supervised food shopping trips. As the client approaches the goal weight, he or she is encouraged to expand the repertoire to include eating out in a restaurant, preparing a meal, and eating forbidden foods. The following vignette illustrates some of the issues that may complicate discharge.

▪ ▪ ▪ VIGNETTE

Alice, a 35-year-old woman with a long history of refractoriness to treatment for anorexia, wants to leave the hospital on reaching 75% of her ideal body weight (regarded as the minimum weight at which an individual may be considered medically stable). Discharge is feasible for this client only if her mother agrees to take Alice home. Initially, the mother allies herself with the treatment team and refuses to go along with Alice's decision to leave at this low weight. The mother relents when Alice becomes threatening and angry, saying, "I won't love you anymore." Although the mother fears for Alice's life, the perceived emotional abandonment and separation from her seem more real and threatening. The hastily arranged discharge plan for outpatient follow-up includes a counseling referral for this mother.

▪ ▪ ▪

Discharge planning is a critical component in treatment and, as the aforementioned vignette demonstrates, can be complex. Often, family members benefit from counseling. The discharge planning process must address living arrangements, school, and work, as well as the feasibility of independent financial status, applications for state and/or federal program assistance (if needed), and follow-up outpatient treatment.

Advanced Practice Interventions: Long-Term Treatment

Anorexia nervosa is a chronic illness that waxes and wanes. Recovery is evaluated as a stage in the process rather than a fixed event. Factors that influence the stage of recovery include percentage of ideal body weight that has been achieved, the extent to which self-worth is defined by shape and weight, and the amount of disruption existing in the client's personal life. The client will require long-term treatment that might include periodic brief hospital stays, outpatient psychotherapy, and pharmacological interventions. The combination of individual, group, couples, and family therapy (especially for the younger client) provides the anorectic client with the greatest chance for a successful outcome.

Psychotherapy

The advanced practice nurse provides individual, group, or family therapy to the eating disorder client in a variety of settings, including a partial hospitalization program, community mental health center, psychiatric home care program, or more traditional outpatient treatment. Regardless of the setting, the goals of treatment remain the same: weight restoration with normalization of eating habits and initiation of the treatment of the psychological, interpersonal, and social issues that are integral to the experience of the client.

The advanced practice nurse may work in an outpatient partial hospitalization program designed to treat eating disorders. These programs are structured to achieve outcomes comparable to those of inpatient eating disorder units. The nurse, along with other therapists, might contract with anorectic clients regarding the terms of treatment. For example, outpatient treatment can continue only if the client maintains an agreed-on weight. If weight falls below the goal, other treatment arrangements must be made until the client returns to the goal weight. This highly structured approach to treatment of clients whose weight is below 75% of ideal body weight is necessary, even for therapists who are psychodynamically oriented. Techniques such as assisting the client with a daily meal plan, reviewing a journal of meals and dietary intake maintained by the client, and providing for weekly weighings (ideally two to three times a week) are essential if the client is to reach a medically stable weight.

Families often report feeling powerless in the face of behavior that is mystifying. For instance, clients are often unable to experience compliments as supportive and therefore are unable to internalize the support. They often seek attention from others but feel scrutinized when they receive it. Clients express that they want their families to care for and about them but are unable to recognize expressions of care. When others do respond with love and support, clients do not per-ceive this as positive. The following two vignettes demonstrate this phenomenon.

■ ■ ■ VIGNETTE

In a family session, a grandmother says to Gina (her 18-year-old anorectic granddaughter), "Gina, you're young, you're smart, you're beautiful. You can do anything." When the client does not react to the statement by feeling praised, the grandmother looks bewildered. After exploring what Gina is feeling, it becomes clear that such statements result in her feeling guilty and more ineffectual because she does not perceive herself as either beautiful or smart but feels that she should be acting both smart and beautiful.

■ ■ ■

■ ■ ■ VIGNETTE

In a multifamily group setting, Terri's mother tells a poignant story of concern for her anorectic daughter. She describes lying awake at night, afraid that in the morning she will find her daughter dead. Although it seems to the group that this expressed sentiment is genuine, the daughter appears to be unmoved. It is later pointed out by the group and the group leader that although Terri often verbalizes that her mother does not care, she is actually unable to receive expressions of concern for her health as caring.

■ ■ ■

Often, family members and significant others seek ways to communicate clearly with the anorectic client but find that they are frequently misunderstood and that overtures of concern are misinterpreted. Consequently, families experience the tension of saying or doing the wrong thing and then feeling responsible if a setback occurs. Psychiatric nurse clinicians have an important role in assisting families and significant others to develop strategies for improved communication and to search for ways to be comfortably supportive to the client.

The following vignette demonstrates a young anorectic client's awareness of how she has been communicating and a breakthrough in her treatment.

■ ■ ■ VIGNETTE

Harriet, an anorectic client, has made significant strides in her treatment and comes to recognize that her emotions are being expressed through her eating behaviors. In the presence of her family, she says, "It's up to me. Only I can do it." This is said with fierce pride. The issue of control, which is commonly expressed by clients with eating disorders, is highlighted in this exchange. Harriet and other clients like her frequently find it difficult to ask for appropriate help.

■ ■ ■

Psychopharmacology

As with most other psychiatric diagnoses, psychopharmacological treatment is an important component of the successful treatment of anorexia nervosa. The selective serotonin reuptake inhibitors (SSRIs), such as fluoxetine (Prozac), are useful in reducing the occurrence of relapse in anorexia nervosa when the client has reached a maintenance weight and is taking in adequate dietary tryptophan, the precursor for serotonin. Atypical antipsychotic agents such as olanzapine (Zyprexa) are helpful in improving mood and in decreasing obsessional behaviors and resistance to weight gain (Mitchell et al., 2001).

■ EVALUATION

The process of evaluation is built into the outcomes specified by NOC. Evaluation is ongoing, and short-term and intermediate indicators are revised as necessary to achieve the treatment outcomes established. The indicators provide a daily guide for evaluating success and must be continually reevaluated for their appropriateness.

Generally the long-term outcome for anorexia nervosa in terms of symptom recovery is less favorable than that for bulimia nervosa (Bowers, 2001).

See Case Study and Nursing Care Plan 17-1 later in the chapter.

Bulimia Nervosa

Bulimia first entered the *DSM* as a diagnosis in the third edition in 1980 but without purging or inappropriate compensatory behaviors as a criterion. The diagnosis became *bulimia nervosa* with the addition of the preceding criterion in 1987. Currently, in the *DSM-IV-TR* (APA, 2000a), it is further subcategorized as purging or nonpurging type (see Figure 17-1).

Application of the Nursing Process

■ ASSESSMENT
Overall Assessment

Clients with bulimia nervosa may not initially appear to be physically or emotionally ill. They are often at or slightly above or below ideal body weight. However, as the assessment continues and the nurse makes further observations, the physical and emotional problems of the client become apparent. On inspection, the client demonstrates enlargement of the parotid glands with dental erosion and caries if the client has been inducing vomiting. The disclosed history may reveal great difficulties with impulsivity as well as compulsivity. Family relationships are frequently chaotic and reflect a lack of nurturing. Clients' lives reflect instability and troublesome interpersonal relationships as well. It is not un-

common for clients to have a history of impulsive stealing of items such as food, clothing, or jewelry (Halmi, 2003). Refer back to Table 17-1 for a comparison of the characteristics of bulimia nervosa and anorexia nervosa.

■ ■ ■ *VIGNETTE*

Jenny is being admitted to an inpatient eating disorder unit. During the initial assessment, the nurse wonders if Jenny is actually in need of hospitalization. The nurse is struck by how well the client appears, seeming healthy, well dressed, and articulate. As Jenny continues to relate her history, she tells of restricting her intake all day until early evening, when she buys her food and begins to binge as she is shopping. She arrives home and immediately induces vomiting. For the remainder of the evening and into the early morning hours, she "zones out" while watching television and binge eating. Periodically, she goes to the bathroom to vomit. She does this about 15 times during the evening. The nurse admitting Jenny to the unit reminds her of the goals of the hospitalization, including interrupting the binge-purge cycle and normalizing eating. The nurse further explains to Jenny that she has the support of the eating disorder treatment team and the milieu of the unit to assist her toward recovery.

■ ■ ■

Self-Assessment

In working with the bulimic client, the nurse needs to be aware that the client is very sensitive to the perceptions of others regarding his or her illness. The client may feel significant shame and may feel totally out of control. In building a therapeutic alliance, the nurse needs to empathize with the bulimic's feelings of low self-esteem, unworthiness, and dysphoria. The nurse may believe that the client is not being honest when the client does not report actively bingeing or purging or that the client is being manipulative. An accepting, nonjudgmental approach along with a comprehensive understanding of the subjective experience of the client with bulimia will help to build trust.

Assessment Guidelines   Bulimia Nervosa

1. Medical stabilization is the first priority. Problems resulting from purging are disruptions in electrolyte and fluid balance and cardiac function. Therefore, a thorough medical examination is vital.
2. Medical evaluation usually includes a thorough physical examination as well as pertinent laboratory testing:
   - Electrolyte levels
   - Glucose level
   - Thyroid function tests
   - Complete blood count
   - ECG
3. Psychiatric evaluation is advised because treatment of psychiatric comorbidity is important to outcome.

▪ NURSING DIAGNOSIS

The assessment of the client with bulimia nervosa yields nursing diagnoses that result from the disordered eating and weight control behaviors. Problems resulting from purging are a first priority because electrolyte and fluid balance and cardiac function are affected. Common nursing diagnoses include *decreased cardiac output, disturbed body image, powerlessness, chronic low self-esteem, anxiety,* and *ineffective coping* (substance abuse, impulsive responses to problems).

▪ OUTCOME CRITERIA

Relevant NOC outcomes include *Vital Signs, Circulation Status, Electrolyte and Acid/Base Balance, Body Image, Self-Esteem, Hope,* and *Coping.* See Table 17-4 for selected intermediate and short-term indicators for clients with bulimia nervosa.

▪ PLANNING

The criteria for inpatient admission of a client with bulimia nervosa are included in the criteria for inpatient admission of a client with an eating disorder presented in Box 17-2. Like the client with anorexia nervosa, the client with bulimia may be treated for life-threatening complications, such as gastric rupture (rare), electrolyte imbalance, and cardiac dysrhythmias, in an acute care unit of a hospital. If the client is admitted to a general inpatient psychiatric unit because of acute suicidal risk, only the acute psychiatric manifestations are addressed short term. Planning will also include appropriate referrals for continuing outpatient treatment.

▪ ▪ ▪ *VIGNETTE*

Iris weighs 85% of her ideal body weight. She has a history of diuretic abuse, and she becomes very edematous when she stops their use and enters treatment. The nurse informs Iris that the edema is related to the use of diuretics and thus is transient, and that it will resolve after Iris begins to eat normally and discontinues the diuretics. Iris cannot tolerate the weight gain and the accompanying edema that occurs when she stops taking diuretics. She restarts the diuretics, perpetuating the cycle of fluid retention and the risk of kidney damage. The nurse empathizes with Iris's inability to tolerate the feelings of anxiety and dread that she experiences because of her markedly swollen extremities.

▪ ▪ ▪

▪ INTERVENTION
Basic Level Interventions: Acute Care

A client who is medically compromised as a result of bulimia nervosa is referred to an inpatient eating disorder unit for comprehensive treatment of the illness.

TABLE 17-4

NOC Outcomes for Bulimia Nervosa

Nursing Outcome and Definition	Intermediate Indicators	Short-Term Indicators
Vital Signs: Extent to which temperature, pulse, respiration, and blood pressure are within normal range*		Body temperature Apical heart rate Apical heart rhythm Respiratory rate Blood pressure
Circulation Status: Unobstructed, unidirectional blood flow at an appropriate pressure through large vessels of the systemic and pulmonary circuits†		Blood pressure Pulse pressure Oxygen saturation Skin temperature Urinary output
Body Image: Perception of own appearance and body functions‡	Congruence between body reality, body ideal, and body presentation Satisfaction with body appearance	Willingness to touch affected body part Willingness to use strategies to enhance appearance Willingness to use strategies to enhance function
Hope: Optimism that is personally satisfying and life-supporting§	Expresses expectation of a positive future	Consistently expresses faith Consistently expresses will to live Consistently expresses optimism Consistently sets goals

From Moorhead, S., Johnson, M., & Maas, M. (2004). *Nursing outcomes classification (NOC)* (3rd ed.). St. Louis, MO: Mosby.
*Indicators measured on a five-point Likert scale ranging from 1 (severe deviation from normal range) to 5 (no deviation from normal range).
†Indicators measured on a five-point Likert scale ranging from 1 (severely compromised) to 5 (not compromised).
‡Indicators measured on a five-point Likert scale ranging from 1 (never positive) to 5 (consistently positive).
§Indicators measured on a five-point Likert scale ranging from 1 (never demonstrated) to 5 (consistently demonstrated).

The cognitive-behavioral model of treatment is highly effective and frequently serves as the cornerstone of the therapeutic approach. Inpatient units designed to treat eating disorders are especially structured to interrupt the cycle of binge eating and purging and to normalize eating habits. Therapy is begun to examine the underlying conflicts and distorted perceptions of shape and weight that sustain the illness. Evaluation for treatment of comorbid disorders, such as major depression and substance abuse, is also undertaken. In most cases of substance dependence, the treatment of the eating disorder must occur after the substance dependence is treated.

The basic level nurse provides milieu therapy, counseling, and health teaching.

Milieu Therapy

The highly structured milieu of an inpatient eating disorder unit has as its primary goals the interruption of the binge-purge cycle and the prevention of the disordered eating behaviors. Interventions such as observation during and after meals to prevent purging, normalization of eating patterns, and maintenance of appropriate exercise are integral elements of such a unit. The interdisciplinary team of the unit uses a comprehensive treatment approach to address the emotional and behavioral problems that arise when the client is no longer binge eating or purging. The interruption of the binge-purge pattern allows underlying feelings to come to the surface and to be examined.

Counseling

Compared with the food-restricting anorectic client, the client with bulimia nervosa often more readily establishes a therapeutic alliance with the nurse because the eating-disordered behaviors are so ego-dystonic. The therapeutic alliance allows the basic level nurse, along with other members of the interdisciplinary team, to provide counseling that gives the client useful feedback regarding the distorted beliefs held by the client.

Health Teaching

Health teaching focuses not only on the eating disorder but also on meal planning, use of relaxation techniques, maintenance of a healthy diet and exercise, coping skills, the physical and emotional effects of bingeing and purging, and the impact of cognitive distortions. This preparation lays the foundation for the second phase of treatment, in which there are carefully planned challenges to the client's newly developed skills. For instance, the client is expected to have a meal while on pass outside the hospital or to plan an overnight pass with meals at home. On return to the unit, the client shares the experience.

On discharge from the hospital, the client is referred for long-term care to solidify the goals that have been achieved and to address both the attitudes and the perceptions that maintain the eating disorder, and the psychodynamic issues that attend the illness.

Advanced Practice Interventions: Long-Term Treatment

Psychotherapy

Cognitive-behavioral therapy is the most effective treatment for bulimia nervosa, and the advanced practice nurse is able to provide this intervention. Agras and colleagues (2000) developed outcome predictors for identifying those best suited for cognitive behavior treatment. Reduction in purging by the sixth session predicted a successful outcome. Clients with bulimia nervosa, because of possible coexisting depression, substance abuse, and personality disorders, are often undergoing various therapies. Although the specific eating-disordered behaviors may not be targeted specifically in some therapies, it is those very behaviors that are responsible for much of the client's emotional distress. It is imperative that irrational attitudes and perceptions of weight and shape be addressed. Therefore, restructuring faulty perceptions and helping individuals develop accepting attitudes toward themselves and their bodies is a primary focus of therapy. When clients do not indulge in these bulimic behaviors, issues of self-worth and interpersonal functioning become more prominent.

■ ■ ■ *VIGNETTE*

Patty, a 23-year-old client with a 6-year history of bulimia nervosa, struggles with issues of self-esteem. She expresses much guilt about "letting her father down" in the past by drinking alcohol excessively and binge eating and purging. She is determined that this time she is not going to fail at treatment. After her initial success in stopping the aforementioned behaviors, she says defiantly, "I'm doing this for me." Patty experiences her behavior as either pleasing or disappointing to others. She begins to realize that her feeling of self-worth is very much dependent on how others see her and that she needs to develop a better sense of herself.

■ ■ ■

Psychopharmacology

Antidepressant medication along with psychotherapy has been shown to bring about improvement in bulimic symptoms. The use of fluoxetine in addition to cognitive-behavioral treatment produced a modest gain in the treatment benefit. Fluoxetine treatment reduced the number of binge eating and vomiting episodes in patients with and without comorbid depression (Mitchell et al., 2001).

Also refer to Box 17-4 for relevant Nursing Interventions Classification (NIC) interventions for the management of eating disorders (Dochterman & Bulechek, 2004).

Eating Disorders Management (NIC)

Definition: Prevention and treatment of severe diet restriction and overexercising or bingeing and purging of foods and fluids

Activities:

- Collaborate with other members of health care team to develop treatment plan; involve patient and/or significant others as appropriate.
- Confer with team and patient to set a target weight if patient is not within a recommended weight range for age and body frame.
- Establish the amount of daily weight gain that is desired (not exceeding 1 lb per week for outpatients and 2 to 3 lb per week for inpatients).
- Confer with dietitian to determine daily caloric intake necessary to attain and/or maintain target weight.
- Teach and reinforce concepts of good nutrition with patient (and significant others as appropriate).
- Encourage patient to discuss food preferences with dietitian.
- Develop a supportive relationship with patient.
- Monitor physiological parameters (vital signs, electrolyte levels) as needed.
- Weigh patient on a routine basis (e.g., at same time of day and after voiding).
- Monitor intake and output of fluids, as appropriate.
- Monitor daily caloric intake.
- Encourage patient self-monitoring of daily food intake and weight gain or maintenance, as appropriate.
- Establish expectations for appropriate eating behaviors, intake of food and fluid, and amount of physical activity.
- Use behavioral contracting with patient to elicit desired weight gain or maintenance behaviors.
- Restrict food availability to scheduled, pre-served meals and snacks.
- Observe patient during and after meals and snacks to ensure that adequate intake is achieved and maintained.
- Accompany patient to the bathroom during designated observation times following meals and snacks.
- Limit time patient spends in bathroom during periods when patient is not under direct supervision.
- Monitor patient for behaviors related to eating, weight loss, and weight gain.
- Use behavior modification techniques to promote behaviors that contribute to weight gain and to limit weight loss behaviors, as appropriate.
- Provide reinforcement for weight gain and behaviors that promote weight gain.
- Provide remedial consequences in response to weight loss, weight loss behaviors, or lack of weight gain.
- Provide support (e.g., relaxation therapy, desensitization exercises, opportunities to talk about feelings) as patient integrates new eating behaviors, changing body image, and lifestyle changes.
- Encourage patient to use daily logs to record feelings as well as circumstances surrounding urge to purge, vomit, or overexercise.
- Limit physical activity as needed to promote weight gain.
- Provide a supervised exercise program when appropriate.
- Allow opportunity to make limited choices about eating and exercise as weight gain progresses in desirable manner.
- Assist patient (and significant others, as appropriate) to examine and resolve personal issues that may contribute to eating disorder.
- Assist patient to develop self-esteem that is compatible with a healthy body weight.
- Confer with health care team on routine basis about patient's progress.
- Initiate maintenance phase of treatment when patient has achieved target weight and has consistently shown desired eating behaviors for designated period of time.
- Monitor patient's weight on routine basis.
- Determine acceptable range of weight variation in relation to target range.
- Place responsibility for choices about eating and physical activity with patient, as appropriate.
- Provide support and guidance as needed.
- Assist patient to evaluate the appropriateness and consequences of choices about eating and physical activity.
- Reinstitute weight gain protocol if patient is unable to remain within target weight range.
- Institute a treatment program and follow-up care (medical, counseling) for home management.

From Dochterman, J. M., & Bulechek, G. M. (2004). *Nursing interventions classification (NIC)* (4th ed., pp. 301-302). St. Louis, MO: Mosby.

■ EVALUATION

Evaluation of treatment effectiveness is ongoing and built into the NOC categories. Outcomes are revised as necessary to reach the desired outcomes. See Case Study and Nursing Care Plan 17-2 later in the chapter.

Binge Eating Disorder

Binge eating disorder as a variant of compulsive overeating is described here. Although considerable controversy exists over whether this proposed diagnosis constitutes a separate eating disorder, 20% to 30% of obese individuals seeking treatment report binge eating as a pattern of overeating (APA, 2000b). In the *DSM-IV-TR* appendix, research criteria are listed for further study of binge eating disorder (Figure 17-2). Because the individual engages in no compensatory behaviors (purging, exercise) in an attempt to control weight in this disorder, it is currently diagnosed as *eating disorder NOS.*

Overeating is frequently noted as a symptom of an affective disorder (i.e., atypical depression). Higher

DSM-IV-TR CRITERIA FOR BINGE EATING DISORDER

Binge Eating Disorder (Compulsive Overeating)

A. Recurrent episodes of binge eating. An episode of binge eating is characterized by both of the following:
1. Eating, in a discrete period (e.g., within any 2-hour period), an amount of food that is definitely larger than most people would eat in a similar period under similar circumstances.
2. A sense of lack of control over eating during the episode (e.g., a feeling that one cannot stop eating or control what or how much one is eating).

B. The binge eating episodes are associated with three or more of the following:
1. Eating much more rapidly than normal
2. Eating until feeling uncomfortably full
3. Eating large amounts of food when not feeling physically hungry
4. Eating alone because of being embarrassed by how much one is eating
5. Feeling disgusted with oneself, depressed, or very guilty after overeating

C. Marked distress regarding binge eating is present.

D. The binge eating occurs, on average, at least 2 days a week for 6 months.

Note: The method of determining frequency differs from that used for bulimia nervosa; future research should address whether the preferred method of setting a frequency threshold is counting the number of days on which binges occur or counting the number of episodes of binge eating.

E. The binge eating is not associated with the regular use of inappropriate compensatory behaviors (e.g., purging, fasting, excessive exercise) and does not occur exclusively during the course of anorexia nervosa or bulimia nervosa.

FIGURE 17-2 Diagnostic criteria for binge eating disorder. (Adapted from American Psychiatric Association. [2000]. *Diagnostic and statistical manual of mental disorders* [4th ed., text rev.]. Washington, DC: Author.)

rates of affective and personality disorders are found among binge eaters. Binge eaters report a history of major depression significantly more often than non–binge eaters. They further report that binge eating is soothing and helps to regulate their moods. Although dieting is almost always an antecedent of binge eating in bulimia nervosa, in approximately 50% of a sample of obese binge eaters, no attempt to restrict dietary intake occurred prior to bingeing (APA, 2000a).

An effective program for those with binge eating disorder must integrate modification of the disordered eating and the depressive symptoms with the ultimate goal of a more appropriate weight for the individual. Fairburn and associates (2000) found the course of binge eating disorder to be different from that of bulimia nervosa and the outcome to be better. The overwhelming majority of individuals with binge eating disorder recover. Peterson and colleagues (2000) found that the frequency of binge eating episodes prior to intervention was predictive of treatment outcome.

The use of SSRIs to treat binge eating disorder has been studied. The use of sertraline (Zoloft) reduced the frequency of binges and the overall severity of the illness (Mitchell et al., 2001). Devlin and colleagues (2000) added phentermine (Adipex-P) and fluoxetine (Prozac) treatment to cognitive-behavioral therapy; however, patients regained significant weight after discontinuance of medication. These researchers concluded that there was no advantage to adding the medication to the cognitive-behavioral therapy.

Cognitive-behavioral therapy programs are at present the most effective treatment for individuals with binge eating disorders (Wilson, 2003). Many advanced practice nurses are qualified to provide cognitive-behavioral therapy.

See Case Study and Nursing Care Plan 17-3.

CASE STUDY and NURSING CARE PLAN 17-1 Anorexia Nervosa

Cindy is a 20-year-old woman who is brought to the inpatient eating disorder unit of a psychiatric research hospital by two older brothers, who support her on ei- *ther side. She is profoundly weak, holding her head up with her hands.*

Self-Assessment

Mindy Jacobs, RN, is assigned to care for Cindy. Although Mindy is a young nurse, she has spent the last 3 years working on the eating disorders unit. When she began working on the unit, she had difficulty with overidentifying with clients. During college Mindy struggled with bulimia, but with treatment she has done well. She seeks guidance from her nursing supervisor as well as the interdisciplinary team. This support allows her to maintain appropriate boundaries while creating a therapeutic alliance with clients.

Continued

ASSESSMENT

Objective Data

- Height: 62 inches (5 feet 2 inches)
- Weight: 58 lb—50% of ideal body weight
- Blood pressure: 74/50 mm Hg
- Pulse: 54 beats per minute
- Anemic—hemoglobin: 9 g/dl
- Cachectic appearance, pale, with fine lanugo
- Sad facial expression

Subjective Data

- Denies being underweight: "I need treatment because I get fatigued so easily."
- "I check my legs every night. I'm so afraid of getting fat. I hate it if my legs touch each other."
- Depressed mood

NURSING DIAGNOSIS (NANDA)

1. *Imbalanced nutrition: less than body requirements* related to restriction of caloric intake, secondary to extreme fear of weight gain

2. *Disturbed body image* related to fear of being fat even though she weighs 58 lb

The first nursing diagnosis with interventions is developed in the text. Please refer to the Evolve website for the interventions for disturbed body image.

OUTCOME CRITERIA (NOC)

Client will reach 75% of ideal weight (92 lb) by discharge.

PLANNING

The initial plan is to address Cindy's unstable physiological state.

INTERVENTION (NIC)

Cindy's care plan is personalized as follows:

Short-Term Goal	Intervention	Rationale	Evaluation
1. Client will gain a minimum of 2 lb and a maximum of 3 lb weekly through inpatient stay.	**1a.** Acknowledge the emotional and physical difficulty client is experiencing. Use client's extreme fatigue to engage her cooperation in the treatment plan.	**1a.** A first priority is to establish a therapeutic alliance.	WEEK 1: Client increases caloric intake with liquid supplement only. Client unable to eat solid food. Client does not gain weight.
	1b. Weigh client daily for the first week, then three times a week. Client should be weighed in bra and panties only. There should be no oral intake, including a drink of water, before the early morning weigh-in.	**1b.** These measures ensure that weight is accurate.	Client remains hypotensive, bradycardic, anemic (hemoglobin [HGB] = 9 g/dl). WEEK 2: Client gains 2 lb drinking liquid supplement—minimal solid food.
	1c. Do not negotiate weight with client or reweigh client. Client may choose not to look at the scale or request that she not be told the weight.	**1c.** Client may try to control and sabotage treatment.	Client remains hypotensive, bradycardic (HGB = 10 g/dl). WEEK 3: Client gains 3 lb drinking liquid supplement. Client selects meal plan but is unable to eat most of solid food.
	1d. Measure vital signs tid until stable, then daily. Repeat ECG and laboratory tests until stable.	**1d.** As client begins to increase in weight, cardiovascular status improves to within normal range and monitoring is less frequent.	Client's blood pressure (BP) = 84/60 mm Hg; pulse = 68 beats per minute, regular; HGB = 11 g/dl. WEEKS 4-6: Client gains an average of 2.5 lb/wk.
	1e. Provide a pleasant, calm atmosphere at mealtimes. Client should be told the specific times and duration (usually a half hour) of meals.	**1e.** Mealtimes become episodes of high anxiety, and knowledge of regulations decreases tension in the milieu, particularly when client has given up so much control by entering treatment.	Client samples more of solid food selected from meal plan. Client's BP = 90/60 mm Hg; pulse = 68 beats per minute, regular; HGB = 11.5 g/dl.

Short-Term Goal	Intervention	Rationale	Evaluation
	1f. Administer liquid supplement as ordered.	**1f.** Client may be unable to eat solid food at first.	WEEK 7: Client weighs 71 lb (almost 60% of ideal body weight); calories are mostly from liquid supplement.
	1g. Observe client during meals to prevent hiding or throwing away of food and for at least 1 hour after meals and snacks to prevent purging.	**1g,h.** The compelling force of the illness is such that these behaviors are difficult to stop. A power struggle between staff and client may emerge in which client appears to comply but defies the rules (appearing to eat but throwing away food).	Client selects balanced meals, eating more varied solid food: turkey, carrots, lettuce, fruit. Client's HGB = 12.5 g/dl; normal range of BP and pulse are maintained.
	1h. Encourage client to try to eat some solid food. Preparation of client's meals should be guided by likes and dislikes list, because client is unable to make own selections to complete menu.		Client continues to increase participation in social aspects of eating.
	1i. Be empathetic with client's struggle to give up control of her eating and her weight as she is expected to make minimum weight gain on a regular basis. Permit client to verbalize feelings at these times.	**1i.** Client is expected to gain at least 0.5 lb on a specific schedule, usually three times a week (Monday, Wednesday, Friday).	WEEKS 8-12: Client gains an average of 2.5 lb/wk and weighs 82 lb (approx. 68% of ideal body weight). Client is eating more varied solid food, but most caloric intake is still from liquid supplement. Client maintains normal vital signs and HGB levels. Client maintains social interaction during mealtimes and snacks.
	1j. Monitor client's weight gain. A weight gain of 2 to 3 lb/wk is medically acceptable.	**1j.** Weight gain of more than 5 lb in 1 week may result in pulmonary edema.	WEEKS 13-16: Client has reached medically stable weight at the end of 16th week—92 lb (75% of ideal body weight).
	1k. Provide teaching regarding healthy eating as the basis of a healthy lifestyle.	**1k.** Healthy aspects of eating (e.g., increased energy, rather than gaining weight) are reinforced.	Client continues to eat more solid food with relatively less liquid supplement.
	1l. Use a cognitive-behavioral approach to address client's expressed fears regarding weight gain. Identify and examine dysfunctional thoughts; identify and examine values and beliefs that sustain these thoughts.	**1l.** Confronting irrational thoughts and beliefs is crucial to changing eating behaviors.	Client is not able to participate in planned exercise program until client reaches 85% of ideal body weight.
	1m. As client approaches her target weight, there should be encouragement to make her own choices for menu selection.	**1m.** Client can assume more control of her meals, which is empowering for the anorectic client.	
	1n. Emphasize social nature of eating. Encourage conversation that does not have the theme of food during mealtimes.	**1n.** Eating as a social activity, shared with others and with participation in conversation, serves as both a distraction from obsessional preoccupations and a pleasurable event.	
	1o. Focus on the client's strengths, including her good work in normalizing her weight and eating habits.	**1o.** Client who is beginning to normalize weight and eating behaviors has achieved a major accomplishment, of which she should be proud. Noneating activities are explored as a source of gratification.	
	1p. Provide for a planned exercise program when client reaches target weight.	**1p.** Client experiences a strong drive to exercise; this measure accommodates this drive by planning a reasonable amount.	
	1q. Encourage client to apply all the knowledge, skills, and gains made from the various individual, family, and group therapy sessions.	**1q.** Client has been receiving intensive therapy and education, which have provided tools and techniques that are useful in maintaining healthy behaviors.	

Continued

■ EVALUATION

By the end of the sixteenth week, Cindy has achieved a stable weight of 92 lb. This weight is approaching congruency with Cindy's height, frame, and age. Her vital signs and hemoglobin levels are consistently demonstrated as normal. She is participating in therapy and consistently communicating satisfaction with her body appearance.

evolve Visit the Evolve website at **http://evolve.elsevier.com/Varcarolis** for a full case study of this client and more case studies and nursing care plans.

CASE STUDY and NURSING CARE PLAN 17-2 Bulimia Nervosa

Sally is a 30-year-old college graduate who reports that she is an aspiring actress. She is being admitted to a partial hospitalization program designed for clients with eating disorders. Sally has bulimia nervosa.

Self-Assessment

Matthew, a seasoned nurse in the area of eating disorders, is assigned to care for Sally. Matthew enjoys working with clients with bulimia because he believes he can help clients move toward health. When he first encounters Sally, he experiences an immediate negative response that surprises him. He speaks to his supervisor about these feelings and raises the question of whether or not he is the appropriate nurse to care for Sally. As he and the supervisor discuss his feelings, Matthew is able to recognize that Sally reminds him of a girlfriend he had many years earlier. The relationship ended badly. Matthew experiences an emotional release with this realization and believes that he will be able to separate his earlier negative experience from his work with Sally.

■ ASSESSMENT

Objective Data

- Height: 65 inches (5 feet 5 inches)
- Weight: 127 lb—95% of ideal body weight
- Blood pressure: 120/80 mm Hg sitting; 90/60 mm Hg standing
- Pulse: 70 beats/min sitting; 96 beats/min standing
- Potassium level of 2.7 mmol/L (normal range, 3.3 to 5.5 mmol/L)
- ECG: abnormal—consistent with hypokalemia
- Erosion of enamel, enlarged parotid gland consistent with a history of binge eating/purging.

Subjective Data

- "I can't stand to be fat."
- "I'm ashamed that I can't control my bingeing and vomiting—I know it's not good."

■ NURSING DIAGNOSIS (NANDA)

1. *Risk for injury* related to low potassium and other physical changes secondary to binge eating and purging

2. *Powerlessness* related to inability to control bingeing and vomiting cycles

■ OUTCOME CRITERIA (NOC)

Sally will demonstrate ability to regulate eating patterns resulting in consistently normal electrolyte balance.

■ PLANNING

Sally is admitted to a partial hospitalization program designed for clients with eating disorders. She attends the program 3 or 4 days a week and participates in individual and group therapy. She will continue to work as a "temp" for a publishing house.

■ INTERVENTION (NIC)

Sally's care plan is personalized as follows:

Short-Term Goal	Intervention	Rationale	Evaluation
1. Client will identify signs and symptoms of low potassium (K⁺) level and K⁺ level will remain within the normal limits throughout hospitalization.	1a. Educate client regarding the ill effects of self-induced vomiting, low K⁺ level, dental erosion.	1a. Health teaching is crucial to treatment. The client needs to be reminded of the benefits of normalization of eating behavior.	WEEK 1: Client begins to select balanced meals. Client demonstrates knowledge of untoward effects of vomiting and K⁺ deficiency. Client begins to demonstrate understanding of repetitive nature of binge-purge cycle.
	1b. Educate client about binge-purge cycle and its self-perpetuating nature. 1c. Teach client that fasting sets one up to binge eat.	1b,c. The compulsive nature of the binge-purge cycle is maintained by the sequence of intake restriction, hunger, bingeing, and purging accompanied by feelings of guilt, and then repetition of the cycle over and over.	
	1d. Explore ideas about trigger foods.	1d. Client needs to understand beliefs about trigger foods to challenge irrational thoughts.	WEEK 2: Client begins to challenge irrational thoughts and beliefs. Client continues to plan nutritionally balanced meals, including dinner at home. Client begins to sample "forbidden foods" and discuss thoughts and attitudes about same.
	1e. Challenge irrational thoughts and beliefs about "forbidden" foods.	1e. Challenge forces client to examine own thinking and beliefs.	WEEK 3: Client discusses triggers to binge and resultant behavior. Client continues to challenge irrational thoughts and beliefs in individual and group sessions. Client plans meals, including "forbidden foods."
	1f. Teach client to plan and eat regularly scheduled, balanced meals.	1f. This teaching helps to ensure success in maintaining abstinence from binge-purge activity.	WEEK 4: Client reports no binge-purge behaviors at day program or outside. Client demonstrates understanding of repetitive nature of binge-purge cycle. Client continues to challenge irrational thoughts and beliefs.

■ EVALUATION

At the end of 4 weeks Sally reports no binge-purge cycles and her potassium level remains consistently within normal limits. She is beginning to plan meals as well as challenge irrational thoughts and beliefs.

evolve Visit the Evolve website at **http://evolve.elsevier.com/Varcarolis** for a full case study of this client and more case studies and nursing care plans.

CASE STUDY and NURSING CARE PLAN 17-3 Compulsive Overeating (Eating Disorder Not Otherwise Specified)

Phyllis is a 25-year-old schoolteacher who gives a history of overeating since the age of 10 years. She seeks treatment at a community mental health center because she has recently felt more depressed.

Continued

Self-Assessment

The nurse assigned to Phyllis is Bernice. Bernice is new to the community mental health center, and her experience as a psychiatric nurse is primarily with the seriously mentally ill. She has never worked with a client with an eating disorder. During Bernice's initial contact with Phyllis, Bernice feels revulsion with regard to Phyllis's weight. Bernice speaks to her nurse supervisor about this feeling.

Bernice is not able to identify where this feeling comes from and is not sure she can control it. The supervisor recognizes that Bernice's feelings will get in the way of creating a therapeutic alliance with Phyllis and decides to reassign Bernice and provide her with additional support and education regarding the care of the client with an eating disorder.

■ ASSESSMENT

Objective Data

- Height: 61 inches (5 feet 1 inch)
- Weight: 200 lb—180% of ideal weight
- Uncontrollable eating pattern
- Sad facial expression
- Minimal success with participation in Weight Watchers and Overeating Anonymous programs

Subjective Data

- "I'll eat anything in sight."
- "I wish I wouldn't wake up in the morning."
- "I once showed promise and look at me now."
- "I don't take laxatives or diuretics and I don't vomit."
- "I am not suicidal."

■ NURSING DIAGNOSIS (NANDA)

Imbalanced nutrition: more than body requirements related to compulsive overeating including episodes of bingeing

■ OUTCOME CRITERIA (NOC)

Client will normalize eating pattern and achieve a specific target weight according to a predetermined plan.

■ INTERVENTION (NIC)

Phyllis's care plan is personalized as follows:

Short-Term Goal	Intervention	Rationale	Evaluation
1. Client will demonstrate at least two coping strategies that result in adhering to a structured meal schedule.	1a. Clinical nurse specialist can use many techniques of cognitive-behavioral therapy in addressing the issues of overweight and disordered eating. Client should begin a journal.	1a. Cognitive-behavioral techniques can be useful in addressing automatic behaviors. Recording what, when, and where one eats begins to identify patterns that can be modified.	WEEK 1: Client selects a meal plan with structured times and places; begins journal and maintains it consistently. Client begins to relate feelings about eating.
	1b. Teach the client to structure and plan ahead for times and places where she will have her meals and snacks for the day.	1b. Organization and structure can allow for a different choice.	WEEK 2: Client is able to adhere to structured meal schedule approximately 25% of the time. Client expresses the struggle and feelings of tension around implementing structured meal schedule; some modifications are made to allow the client to be more successful. Client shares contents of journal, which she consistently maintains. Client reports weight is unchanged; client was unable to change pattern of exercise.
	1c. Teach client not to abstain from eating for longer periods of time than planned to avoid rebound binge eating. 1d. Review the nutritional content of dietary intake to ensure consumption of a balanced diet.	1c,d. Extended periods of abstinence, restrictive dietary intake, or very low calorie diet can result in rebound overeating.	WEEK 3: Client is adhering to schedule 50% of the time. Client shares journal entries and relates thoughts and feelings concerning eating. Client reports 0.5-lb weight loss. Client is beginning to walk for a half-hour as part of her daily routine.

Short-Term Goal	Intervention	Rationale	Evaluation
	1e. Review journal with client to identify areas for improvement in adhering to the treatment plan.	**1e.** The journal is an important tool in modifying eating behaviors.	WEEK 4: Client continues to adhere to structured schedule approximately 75% of the time.
	1f. Explore with client the thoughts and feelings she is experiencing about this new regimen.	**1f,g.** Nurse must be empathetic and supportive of client's experience, which is one of struggle accompanied by feelings of tension.	Client walks regularly, experiencing a better sense of well-being. Client thinks she is up to the challenge of continuing the plan to normalize her eating pattern and increase her energy expenditure.
	1g. Identify thoughts and beliefs and underlying assumptions that reinforce disordered eating patterns.		Client's weight is 196 lb (−4 lb); she acknowledges that progress has and will continue to be slow.
	1h. Establish a once-a-week schedule of weighing.	**1h.** From day to day, there may be minimal or no weight reduction, which can lead to discouragement.	

■ EVALUATION

At the end of 4 weeks, Phyllis's weight is 196 lb. She adheres to a structured meal plan 75% of the time and has increased her exercise by incorporating daily walks into her routine.

evolve Visit the Evolve website at **http://evolve.elsevier.com/Varcarolis** for a full case study of this client and more case studies and nursing care plans.

■■■ KEY POINTS to REMEMBER

- A number of theoretical models help explain the origins of eating disorders.
- Neurobiological theories identify an association between eating disorders, depression, and neuroendocrine abnormalities.
- Psychological theories explore issues of control in anorexia and affective instability and poor impulse control in bulimia.
- Genetic theories postulate the existence of vulnerabilities that may predispose people toward eating disorders, and increasingly twin studies confirm genetic liability, which perhaps interacts with environmental mechanisms.
- Sociocultural models look at both our present societal ideal of being thin and the ideal feminine role model in general.
- Men with eating disorders share many of the characteristics of women with eating disorders.
- In populations in which eating disorders had been rare and are now appearing, the dynamics—the stress of acculturation versus identification with the new culture—are being examined.
- Anorexia nervosa is a possibly life-threatening eating disorder that includes severe underweight; low blood pressure, pulse, and temperature; dehydration; and low serum potassium level and dysrhythmias.
- Anorexia may be treated in an inpatient treatment setting, in which milieu therapy, psychotherapy (cognitive), development of self-care skills, and psychobiological interventions can be implemented.
- Long-term treatment is provided on an outpatient basis and aims to help clients maintain healthy weight; it includes treatment modalities such as individual therapy, family therapy, group therapy, psychopharmacology, and nutrition counseling.
- Clients with bulimia nervosa are typically within the normal weight range, but some may be slightly below or above ideal body weight.
- Assessment of the bulimic client may show enlargement of the parotid glands, dental erosion, and caries if the client has induced vomiting.
- Acute care may be necessary when life-threatening complications are present, such as gastric rupture (rare), electrolyte imbalance, and cardiac dysrhythmias.
- The goal of interventions is to interrupt the binge-purge cycle.
- Psychotherapy as well as self-care skill training is included.
- Long-term treatment focuses on therapy aimed at addressing any coexisting depression, substance abuse, and/or personality disorders that are causing the client distress and interfering with the client's quality of life. Self-worth and interpersonal functioning eventually become issues that are useful for the client to target.
- Eating disorders NOS include a variety of patterns, and in this chapter binge eating disorder was examined.
- Binge eaters report a history of major depression significantly more often than non–binge eaters.
- Effective treatment for obese binge eaters integrates modification of the disordered eating, improvement of depressive symptoms, and achievement of an appropriate weight for the individual.

Visit the Evolve website at **http://evolve.elsevier.com/Varcarolis** for a posttest on the content in this chapter. ***evolve***

Critical Thinking and Chapter Review

Visit the Evolve website at **http://evolve.elsevier.com/Varcarolis** for additional self-study exercises.

evolve

■ ■ ■ CRITICAL THINKING

1. Tom Shift, a 19-year-old male model, has experienced a rapid decrease in weight over the last 4 months, after his agent told him he would have to lose some weight or lose a coveted account. Tom is 6 feet 2 inches tall and presently weighs 132 lb, down from his usual 176 lb. He is brought to the emergency department with a pulse of 40 beats per minute and severe arrhythmias. His laboratory workup reveals severe hypokalemia. He has become extremely depressed, saying, "I'm too fat. . . . I won't take anything to eat. . . . If I gain weight my life will be ruined. There is nothing to live for if I can't model." Tom's parents are startled and confused, and his best friend, Dick Lamb, is worried and feels powerless to help Tom. "I tell Tom he needs to eat or he will die. . . . I tell him he is a skeleton, but he refuses to listen to me. I don't know what to do."

   A. Which physical and psychiatric criteria suggest that Tom should be immediately hospitalized? What other physical signs and symptoms may be found on assessment?

   B. What are some of the questions you would eventually ask Tom when evaluating his biopsychosocial functioning?

   C. What are your feelings toward someone with anorexia? Can you make a distinction between your thoughts and feelings toward women with anorexia and toward men with anorexia?

   D. What are some things you could do for Tom's parents and Tom's friend Dick in terms of offering them information, support, and referrals? Identify specific referrals.

   E. Explain the kinds of interventions or restrictions that may be used while Tom is hospitalized (e.g., weighing, observation after eating or visits, exercise, therapy, self-care).

   F. How would you describe partial hospitalization programs or psychiatric home care programs when asked if Tom will have to be hospitalized for a long time?

   G. What are some of Tom's cognitive distortions that would be a target for therapy?

   H. Identify at least five criteria that, if met, would indicate that Tom was improving.

2. You and your close friend Mary Alice have been together since nursing school and you are now working on the same surgical unit. Mary Alice told you that in the past she has made several suicide attempts. Today you accidentally come upon her bingeing off unit, and she looks embarrassed and uncomfortable when she sees you. Several times you notice that she spends time in the bathroom and you hear sounds of retching. In response to your concern, she admits that she has been binge-purging for several years but that now she is getting out of control and feels profoundly depressed.

   A. Although Mary Alice doesn't show any physical signs of bulimia nervosa, what would you look for when assessing an individual with bulimia?

   B. What kinds of emergencies could result from bingeing and purging?

   C. What would be the most useful type of psychotherapy for Mary Alice initially and what issues would need to be addressed?

   D. What kinds of new skills does a person with bulimia need to learn to lessen the compulsion to binge and purge?

   E. What would be some signs that Mary Alice is recovering?

■ ■ ■ CHAPTER REVIEW

Choose the most appropriate answer.

1. Which of the following is the most pervasive cognitive distortion nurses will identify among clients with eating disorders?
   1. Thinness equates with self worth.
   2. "I'm unpopular because I'm fat."
   3. Being thin is being powerful.
   4. Being fat is more harmful than being thin.

2. During the weight-restoration phase, a client with anorexia nervosa should not gain more than 5 lb per week to avoid
   1. liver dysfunction.
   2. endocrine imbalance.
   3. pulmonary edema.
   4. compromised kidney function.

3. Which client with an eating disorder would be at greatest risk for hypokalemia?
   1. A client with anorexia who loses weight by restricting food intake
   2. A client with anorexia who purges to promote weight loss
   3. A client with bulimia (nonpurging)
   4. A client with an eating disorder who is at risk for hyponatremia

4. Which medication is likely to be used in the treatment of clients with eating disorders?
   1. An SSRI such as fluoxetine
   2. A neuroleptic such as risperidone
   3. An anxiolytic such as alprazolam
   4. An anticonvulsant such as carbamazepine

5. Which risk factor for eating disorders is most commonly identified in the histories of adolescents with eating disorders?
   1. Dieting
   2. Purging
   3. Overeating
   4. Excessive exercise

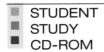
REFERENCES

Agras, W. S., et al. (2000). Outcome predictors for the cognitive behavior treatment of bulimia nervosa: Data from a multi-site study. *American Journal of Psychiatry, 157*(9), 1302-1308.

American Psychiatric Association. (2000a). *Diagnostic and statistical manual of mental disorders (DSM-IV-TR)* (4th ed., text rev.). Washington, DC: Author.

American Psychiatric Association. (2000b). *Practice guidelines for the treatment of psychiatric disorders: Compendium 2000.* Washington, DC: Author.

Bowers, W. A. (2001). Basic principles for applying cognitive-behavioral therapy to anorexia nervosa. *Psychiatric Clinics of North America, 24*(2), 293-303.

Brambilla, F., & Monteleone, P. (2003). Physical complications and physiological aberrations in eating disorders: A review. In M. Maj et al. (Eds.), *Eating disorders* (pp. 139-192). West Sussex, England: Wiley.

Bruch, H. (1973). *Eating disorders: Obesity, anorexia, and the person within.* New York: Basic Books.

Davis, C., Claridge, G., & Fox, J. (2000). Not just a pretty face: Physical attractiveness and perfectionism in the risk for eating disorders. *International Journal of Eating Disorders, 27*, 67-73.

Devlin, M. J., et al. (2000). Open treatment of overweight binge eaters with phentermine and fluoxetine as an adjunct to cognitive behavioral therapy. *International Journal of Eating Disorders, 28*(3), 325-332.

Dochterman, J. M., & Bulechek, G. M. (2004). *Nursing interventions classification (NIC)* (4th ed.). St. Louis, MO: Mosby.

Fairburn, C. G. (2002). Cognitive-behavioral therapy for bulimia nervosa. In C. G. Fairburn & K. D. Brownell (Eds.), *Eating disorders and obesity* (2nd ed., pp. 302-333). New York: Guilford Press.

Fairburn, C. G., et al. (2000). The natural course of bulimia nervosa and binge eating disorder in young women. *Archives of General Psychiatry, 57*, 659-665.

Halmi, K. A. (2003). Classification, diagnosis and comorbidities of eating disorders. In M. Maj et al. (Eds.), *Eating disorders* (pp. 315-338). West Sussex, England: Wiley.

Klump, K. L., Kaye, W. H., & Strober, M. (2001). The evolving genetic foundations of eating disorders. *Psychiatric Clinics of North America, 24*(2), 215-225.

Lake, A. J., Staiger, P. K., & Glowinski, H. (2000). Effect of Western culture on women's attitudes to eating and perceptions of body shape. *International Journal of Eating Disorders, 27*, 83-89.

Miller, M. N., & Pumariega, A. J. (2001). Culture and eating disorders: A historical and cross-cultural review. *Psychiatry, 64*(2), 93-110.

Mitchell, J. E., et al. (2001). Combining pharmacotherapy and psychotherapy in the treatment of patients with eating disorders. *Psychiatric Clinics of North America, 24*(2), 315-323.

Moorhead, S., Johnson, M., & Maas, M. (2004). *Nursing Outcomes Classification (NOC)* (3rd ed.). St. Louis, MO: Mosby.

National Eating Disorders Association. (2002). *Statistics: Eating disorders and their precursors.* Retrieved August 16, 2004, from http://www.NationalEatingDisorders.org/p.asp?WebPage_ID=286&Profile_ID=41138.

Peterson, C. B., et al. (2000). Predictors of treatment outcome for binge eating disorder. *International Journal of Eating Disorders, 28*(2), 131-138.

Wiederman, M. S., & Pryor, T. L. (2000). Body dissatisfaction, bulimia, and depression among women: The mediating role of drive for thinness. *International Journal of Eating Disorders, 27*, 90-95.

Wilson, G. T. (2003). Psychological interventions for eating disorders: A review. In M. Maj et al. (Eds.), *Eating disorders* (pp. 315-338). West Sussex, England: Wiley.

Zaider, T. I., Johnson, J. G., & Cockell, S. J. (2000). Psychiatric comorbidity associated with eating disorder symptomatology among adolescents in the community. *International Journal of Eating Disorders, 28*(1), 58-67.

Zhu, A. J., & Walsh, B. T. (2002). Pharmacologic treatment of eating disorders. *Canadian Journal of Psychiatry, 47*(3), 227-234.

A CLIENT SPEAKS

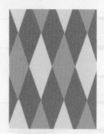

I am a 62-year-old single woman who was born in South Carolina. I grew up with my two lovely parents and seven brothers and sisters. I did not finish high school. I have two grown kids, one boy and one girl. I have never drunk alcohol or taken drugs. I am blind in one eye, and I have a bad heart.

I got sick for the first time when I was 23 years old. I cannot recall the details, but I felt it was a nervous breakdown. I went to the hospital, and I took medication, but I did not go to outpatient treatment. I took a 6-month clerical course after discharge.

Looking back, I feel that medication played a big part in helping me. Time after time I've been in and out of the hospital. I used to feel that I did not want to stay on medication; I felt like a drug addict. But now I realize that if I don't take my medicine, I will get sick again.

After my last hospitalization in 2001, I was referred to an outpatient mental health center. My counselor and my doctor encouraged me to attend a day program. It was hard for me at first. I shed tears. I kept trying because I had goals to meet. One of my goals was to return to church. It took me a long time before I made up my mind to go to church. I worried about how I would be accepted because of my mental illness. When I finally did go to church, I found that it gave me more courage to set new goals.

At the day program, I studied in GED classes to get my high school diploma. I worked in a thrift store for 2 months. Before my 2 months were up, I started seeking another position. I went into training to work as a receptionist. Now I work in a paid position as the substitute for a young lady. This is a challenge for me. It gives me a chance to meet and work with people. Each day I pray and ask God to help me to be a blessing to someone.

I live with my son, and I keep in touch with the rest of my family. I would describe my relationship with my family as good. I read the Bible every day and attend church every Sunday. My future goal is to find a part-time job in the community.

PSYCHOBIOLOGICAL DISORDERS
Severe to Psychotic

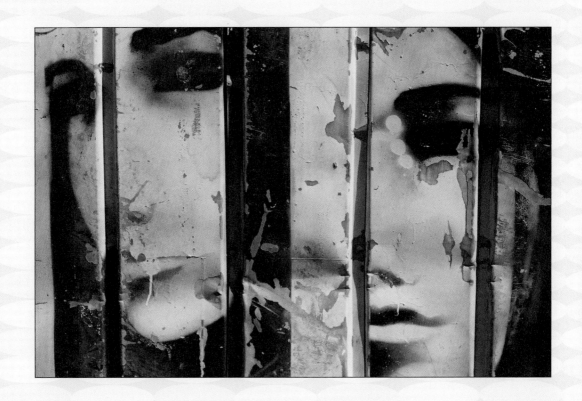

HOLD FAST TO DREAMS
FOR IF DREAMS DIE
LIFE IS A BROKEN-WINGED BIRD
THAT CANNOT FLY.

Langston Hughes

CHAPTER 18

Mood Disorders: Depression

ELIZABETH M. VARCAROLIS

KEY TERMS and CONCEPTS

The key terms and concepts listed here appear in color where they are defined or first discussed in this chapter.

anergia, 331

anhedonia, 331

dysthymic disorder (DD), 328

hypersomnia, 336

light therapy, 352

major depressive disorder (MDD), 327

mood, 328

novel antidepressants, 344

psychomotor agitation, 334

psychomotor retardation, 334

selective serotonin reuptake inhibitors (SSRIs), 343

St. John's wort, 352

transcranial magnetic stimulation (TMS), 352

tricyclic antidepressants (TCAs), 345

vegetative signs of depression, 334

OBJECTIVES

After studying this chapter, the reader will be able to

1. Compare and contrast major depressive disorder with dysthymia.

2. Discuss the links between the stress model of depression and the biological model of depression.

3. Assess behaviors in a depressed individual at the reader's clinical site with regard to each of the following areas: (a) affect, (b) thought processes, (c) feelings, (d) physical behavior, and (e) communication.

4. Formulate five nursing diagnoses for a client who is depressed and include outcome criteria.

5. Name unrealistic expectations that a nurse may have while working with a depressed person and compare them with the reader's personal reactions.

6. Role-play six principles of communication that are useful with depressed clients.

7. Evaluate the advantages of the selective serotonin reuptake inhibitors over the tricyclic antidepressants.

8. Explain the unique attributes of two of the newer atypical antidepressants for use in specific circumstances.

9. Write a medication teaching plan for clients taking the tricyclic antidepressants, including (a) adverse effects, (b) toxic reactions, and (c) other drugs that can trigger an adverse reaction.

10. Discuss two common adverse reactions to the monoamine oxidase inhibitors, state one serious toxic reaction, and identify the appropriate medical intervention.

11. Write a medication teaching plan for a client taking a monoamine oxidase inhibitor, including foods and drugs that are contraindicated.

12. Describe the types of depression for which electroconvulsive therapy is most helpful.

evolve Visit the Evolve website at **http://evolve.elsevier.com/Varcarolis** for a pretest on the content in this chapter.

No amount of information can adequately convey the personal pain and suffering experienced by the individual with depression (Young, Weinberger, & Beck, 2001). All races, all ages, both males and females are susceptible to depressive episodes, although some individuals are more susceptible than others.

PREVALENCE

Depression is the fourth leading cause of disability in the United States, and it is projected to be the second leading cause of disability by 2020 (Montano, 2003).

The lifetime prevalence of a major depressive episode is 17%, up from 10% to 12% a few years ago (Jain & Russ, 2003). Most studies find that major depressive disorder (MDD) is twice as common in women (12.0%) as in men (6.6%) (National Institute of Mental Health [NIMH], 2001a, 2001b). The prevalence rates for MDD appear unrelated to ethnicity, education, income, or marital status (American Psychiatric Association [APA], 2000a). Dysthymic disorder (DD) (chronic mild depression) occurs in about 5.1% of the population during their lifetimes. About 40% of people with DD also meet the criteria for MDD or bipolar disorder (BD) in any given year (NIMH, 2001b).

Children and Adolescents

Children as young as 3 years of age have been diagnosed with depression. MDD is said to occur in as many as 18% of preadolescents, which is perhaps a low estimate because depression in this age group is often underdiagnosed. Children and adolescents between 9 and 17 years of age have a 6% prevalence of depression, and 4.9% have MDD (NIMH, 2000b). Girls 15 years and older are twice as likely to experience a major depressive episode than boys (NIMH, 2000a). Major depression among adolescents is often associated with substance abuse and antisocial behavior, both of which can obscure accurate diagnosis (Dubovsky, Davies, & Dubovsky, 2004).

MDD in children has a high recurrence rate of up to 70% within 5 years. The appearance of MDD in adolescence heralds a severe disorder with a recurrent course (Gruenberg & Goldstein, 2003). Children in families with other depressed members seem to become depressed earlier (age 12 to 13 years) than children in families with no other depressed members (16 to 17 years) (Dubovsky et al., 2004). Even before adolescence, girls are more vulnerable to depression than boys.

Elderly

Depression in the elderly is a major health problem. Depression occurs in 1% or 2% of people younger than 65 years of age but at higher rates in elderly medical populations (NIMH, 2002; Serby & Yu, 2003). For example, among the elderly, depression ranges from 3.5% among community dwellers to 16% among those medically hospitalized and 15% to 20% among the nursing home population (Dubovsky et al., 2004). Depression can be as high as 40% in some older adult populations (Fuller & Sajatovic, 2000). In fact, a disproportionate number of depressed elderly Americans are likely to die by suicide (NIMH, 2003b). Unfortunately, the symptoms of geriatric depression often go unrecognized, although the elderly make frequent medical visits. Thus, elderly individuals suffering

from depression are at risk for being untreated (Guerrero-Berroa & Phillips, 2001).

COMORBIDITY

A depressive syndrome frequently accompanies other psychiatric disorders such as anxiety disorders, schizophrenia, substance abuse, eating disorders, and schizoaffective disorder. People with anxiety disorders (e.g., panic disorder, generalized anxiety disorder, obsessive-compulsive disorder) commonly present with depression, as do people with personality disorders (particularly borderline personality disorder), adjustment disorder, and brief depressive reactions.

Mixed anxiety-depression is perhaps one of the most common psychiatric presentations. Symptoms of anxiety occur in an average of 70% of cases of major depression. The presence of comorbid anxiety disorder and depression has a negative impact on the disease course. Comorbidity has been shown to result in a higher rate of suicide, greater severity of depression, greater impairment in social and occupational functioning, and poorer response to treatment (Simon & Rosenbaum, 2003). This is especially true in elderly depressed individuals with concurrent symptoms of anxiety or an anxiety disorder (Lenze, 2003).

The incidence of major depression greatly increases among people with a medical disorder. People with chronic medical problems are at a higher risk for depression than those in the general population. Depression is often secondary to a medical condition (Table 18-1). Depression may also be secondary to use of substances such as alcohol, cocaine, marijuana, heroin, and even anxiolytics and other prescription medications (Table 18-2). Depression can also be a sequela of bereavement and grief. See Chapter 30 for end-of-life issues and bereavement.

DEPRESSIVE DISORDERS AND CLINICAL PRESENTATIONS

Figure 18-1 presents diagnostic criteria for MDD and DD, the two depressive disorders defined by the *Diagnostic and Statistical Manual of Mental Disorders*, fourth edition, text revision (APA, 2000a). Depression can be manifested in a variety of other symptoms that are called specifiers. Other subgroups are currently being researched as well (Table 18-3).

Major Depressive Disorder

Clients with a major depressive disorder (MDD) experience substantial pain and suffering, as well as psychological, social, and occupational disability, during the depression. A client with MDD presents with a history of one or more major depressive episodes

TABLE 18-1

Medical Disorders Associated with Depressive Syndromes

Type	Disorders
Neurological	Dementias, hydrocephalus, Huntington's chorea, infections (including human immunodeficiency virus infection, neurosyphilis), migraine, multiple sclerosis, myasthenia gravis, Parkinson's disease, seizure disorders, stroke, trauma, tumors, vasculitis, Wilson's disease
Endocrine	Addison's disease, Cushing's syndrome, diabetes mellitus, hyperparathyroidism, hyperthyroidism, hypoparathyroidism, hypothyroidism, menses-related depression, postpartum depression
Metabolic or nutritional	Folate deficiency, hypercalcemia, hypocalcemia, hyponatremia, pellagra, porphyria, uremia, vitamin B_{12} deficiency
Infectious or inflammatory	Influenza, hepatitis, mononucleosis, pneumonia, rheumatoid arthritis, Sjögren's disease, systemic lupus erythematosus, tuberculosis
Other	Anemias, cardiopulmonary disease, neoplasms (including gastrointestinal, lung, pancreatic), sleep apnea

Data from Milner, K. K., Florence, T., & Glick, R. L. (1999). Mood and anxiety syndromes in emergency psychiatry. *Psychiatric Clinics of North America, 22*(4), 761.

TABLE 18-2

Medications and Substances Associated with Depressive Syndromes

Class	Medications and Substances
Neurological, psychiatric	Amantadine, anticholinesterases, antipsychotics, baclofen, barbiturates, benzodiazepines, bromocriptine, carbamazepine, chloral hydrate, disulfiram, ethosuximide, levodopa, phenytoin
Antibacterial, antifungal	Ampicillin, griseofulvin, metronidazole, nalidixic acid, trimethoprim
Antiinflammatory, analgesic	Corticosteroids, indomethacin, opiates, sulindac
Antineoplastic	Asparaginase, azathioprine, bleomycin, hexamethylamine, vincristine, vinblastine
Cardiovascular	Clonidine, digitalis, guanethidine, methyldopa, propranolol, reserpine
Gastrointestinal	Cimetidine, ranitidine
Other	Alcohol, caffeine, oral contraceptives, stimulant withdrawal

Data from Mulner, K. K., Florence, T., & Glick, R. L. (1999). Mood and anxiety syndromes in emergency psychiatry. *Psychiatric Clinics of North America, 22*(4), 761.

and no history of manic or hypomanic episodes. In MDD, the symptoms often interfere with the person's social or occupational functioning and in some cases may include psychotic features. Delusional or psychotic major depression is a severe form of mood disorder that is characterized by delusions or hallucinations. For example, clients might have delusional thoughts that interfere with their nutritional status (e.g., "God put snakes in my stomach and told me not to eat").

The emotional, cognitive, physical, and behavioral symptoms an individual exhibits during a major depressive episode represent a change in the person's usual functioning.

The course of MDD is variable. At least 60% of people can expect to have a second episode. Individuals who have experienced two episodes of major depression have a 70% chance of having a third. Those who have had three episodes have a 90% chance of future episodes (APA, 2000).

Dysthymia

Dysthymic disorder (DD) often has an early and insidious onset and is characterized by a chronic depressive syndrome that is usually present for most of the day, more days than not, for at least 2 years (APA, 2000b). The depressive mood disturbance, because of its chronic nature, cannot be distinguished from the person's usual pattern of functioning ("I've always been this way") (APA, 2000b). Although people with dysthymia suffer from social and occupational distress, it is not usually severe enough to warrant hospitalization unless the person becomes suicidal. The age of onset is usually from early childhood and teenage years to early adulthood. Clients with DD are at risk for developing major depressive episodes as well as other psychiatric disorders.

Differentiating MDD from DD can be difficult, because the disorders have similar symptoms. The main differences are in the duration and the severity of the symptoms (APA, 2000b).

DSM-IV-TR CRITERIA FOR DEPRESSIVE DISORDERS

DEPRESSIVE DISORDERS

Major Depressive Disorder

1. Represents a change in previous functions.

2. Symptoms cause clinically significant distress or impair social, occupational, or other important areas of functioning.

3. **Five or more** of the following occur nearly every day for most waking hours over the same 2-week period:
   - Depressed mood most of day, nearly every day
   - Anhedonia
   - Significant weight loss or gain (more than 5% of body weight in 1 month)
   - Insomnia or hypersomnia
   - Increased or decreased motor activity
   - Anergia (fatigue or loss of energy)
   - Feelings of worthlessness or inappropriate guilt (may be delusional)
   - Decreased concentration or indecisiveness
   - Recurrent thoughts of death or suicidal ideation (with or without plan)

Dysthymia

1. Occurs over a 2-year period (1 year for children and adolescents), depressed mood.

2. Symptoms cause clinically significant distress in social, occupational, and other important areas of functioning.

3. **Two or more** of the following are present:
   - Decreased or increased appetite
   - Insomnia or hypersomnia
   - Low energy or chronic fatigue
   - Decreased self-esteem
   - Poor concentration or difficulty making decisions
   - Feelings of hopelessness or despair

Specifiers Describing Most Recent Episode

1. Chronic

2. Atypical features

3. Catatonic features

4. Melancholic features

5. Postpartum onset

Specify If

1. Early onset (before 21 years of age)

2. Late onset (21 years of age or older)

3. Atypical features

FIGURE 18-1 Diagnostic criteria for major depression and dysthymia. (Adapted from American Psychiatric Association. [2000]. *Diagnostic and statistical manual of mental disorders* [4th ed., text rev.]. Washington, DC: Author.)

Subtypes

The diagnosis for MDD may include a specifier in clients with specific symptoms. Specifiers include the following:

Psychotic features (breaks with reality [e.g., hallucinations, delusions])

Catatonic features (e.g., peculiar voluntary movement, echopraxia or echolalia, and negativism)

Melancholic features (e.g., anorexia or weight loss, diurnal variations with symptoms worse in the morning, early morning awakening)

Postpartum onset (within 4 weeks postpartum [e.g., severe anxiety, possible psychotic features])

Seasonal features (seasonal affective disorder, or SAD) (e.g., generally occurring in fall or winter and remitting in the spring)

TABLE 18-3

Depressive Disorders: Specifiers and Clinical Phenomena

Disorder	*DSM-IV-TR* Status	Symptoms and Comments
Major depression (MDD)	Disorder	Specific *DSM-IV-TR* criteria are outlined in Figure 18-1. Symptoms represent a change from usual functioning. Associated with high mortality rate. Impairment in physical, social, and role functioning, as well as increased potential for pain and physical illness.
with psychotic features	Specifier	Indicates the presence of delusions (e.g., delusions of guilt or being punished for sins, somatic delusions of horrible disease or body rotting, delusions of poverty or going bankrupt), or hallucinations (usually auditory, voices berating person for sins or shortcomings).
with postpartum onset	Specifier	Indicates onset within 4 weeks after childbirth. Can present with or without psychotic features. **Severe ruminations or delusional thoughts about infant signify increased risk of harm to infant.**
with seasonal characteristics (SAD)	Specifier	Indicates that episodes mostly begin in fall or winter and remit in spring. Characterized by anergia, hypersomnia, overeating, weight gain, and a craving for carbohydrates. Responds to light therapy.
with chronic features	Specifier	Indicates MDD lasting 2 years or longer.
Dysthymic disorder (DD)	Disorder	Specific *DSM-IV-TR* criteria are presented in Figure 18-1. Has an early and insidious onset (childhood to early adulthood). Shows a chronic course. Some 75% of people with DD go on to develop MDD. When dysthymia is superimposed on a major depression, it is called **double depression.**
DD and MDD with atypical features	Specifier	Indicates mood reactivity (can be cheered with positive events) and rejection sensitivity (pathological sensitivity to perceived interpersonal rejection) that are present through life and result in functional impairment. Other symptoms include hypersomnia, hyperphagia (overeating), leaden paralysis (feeling weighed down in extremities), etc.
Mixed anxiety-depression	RDC	Prevalence of 5%. Characterized by significant functional disability. Criteria include at least 1 month of persistent dysphoric mood, with possible hypervigilance, difficulty concentrating, fatigue, low self-esteem, irritability, and more, all causing **significant distress or impairment in functioning.**
Recurrent brief depression	RDC	Meets criteria for depressive episode, but episodes last 1 day to 1 week. Depressive episode must recur at least once per month over 12 months or more. **Carries a high risk for suicide.**
Premenstrual dysphoric disorder	RDC	Characterized by more severe symptoms than premenstrual syndrome. Symptoms begin toward last week of luteal phase and are absent in the week following menses. Symptoms include depressed mood, anxiety, affective lability, or persistent and marked anger or irritability. Other symptoms include anergia, overeating, difficulty concentrating, feeling of being out of control or overwhelmed, and more.
Minor depression	RDC	Characterized by sustained depressed mood without the full depressive syndrome. Pessimistic attitude and self-pity are required for the diagnosis (Dubovsky & Buzan, 1999). May be chronic and may be complicated by a superimposed major depressive episode.

RDC, Research diagnostic category; *SAD*, seasonal affective disorder.

Atypical features (e.g., appetite changes or weight gain, hypersomnia, extreme sensitivity to perceived interpersonal rejection)

THEORY

Although many theories attempt to explain the cause of depression, the many psychological, biological, and cultural variables make identification of any one cause difficult. It is unlikely that there is a single cause for depression. It is becoming evident that depression is a heterogeneous systemic illness involving an array of different neurotransmitters, neurohormones, and neuronal pathways (Sadek & Nemeroff, 2000). The idea that depression is the result of a simple hereditary process or traumatic life event that ultimately leads to a single neurotransmitter deficiency is simply unsubstantiated by the evidence (Sadek & Nemeroff, 2000). The high variability in symptoms, response to treatment, and course of the illness supports the supposition that depression may result from a complex interaction of causes. For example, genetic predisposition to the illness combined with childhood stress may lead to significant changes in the central nervous system (CNS) that result in depression.

There are, however, 10 common risk factors for depression that may signal the presence of this common and serious psychiatric illness (Gruenberg & Goldstein, 2003) (Box 18-1).

Four common theories of depression are discussed here: (1) biological theories, (2) psychodynamic influences and life events, (3) cognitive theories, and (4) learned helplessness.

Biological Theories

Genetic Factors

Twin studies consistently show that genetic factors play a role in the development of depressive disorders. Various studies reveal that the average concordance rate for mood disorders among monozygotic twins (twins sharing the same genetic constitution) is 45% to 60%. That is, if one twin is affected, the second has a 45% to 60% chance of being affected. The percentage for dizygotic twins (different genetic complement) is 12%. Thus, identical twins (monozygotic) have a five-fold greater concordance rate than dizygotic twins (Dubovsky et al., 2004).

Mood disorders are heritable for some people. Increased heritability is associated with an earlier age of onset, greater rate of comorbidity, and increased risk of recurrent illness. However, any genetic factors that are present must interact with environmental factors for depression to develop (Dubovsky et al., 2004).

Biochemical Factors

The brain is a highly complex organ that contains billions of neurons. There is much evidence to support the concept that depression is a biologically heteroge-

neous disorder; that is, many CNS neurotransmitter abnormalities can probably cause clinical depression. These neurotransmitter abnormalities may be the result of inherited or environmental factors, or even of other medical conditions, such as cerebral infarction, hypothyroidism, acquired immunodeficiency syndrome, or drug use. Specific neurotransmitters in the brain are believed to be related to altered mood states. Initially it was believed that the two main neurotransmitters involved were **serotonin** (5-hydroxytryptamine, or 5-HT) and **norepinephrine.** Serotonin is an important regulator of sleep, appetite, and libido. A serotonin circuit dysfunction can result in poor impulse control, low sex drive, decreased appetite, and irritability (Sadek & Nemeroff, 2000). Decreased levels of norepinephrine in the medial forebrain bundle may account for anergia (reduction in or lack of energy), anhedonia (an inability to find meaning or pleasure in existence), decreased concentration, and diminished libido in depression (Dubovsky et al., 2004).

Serotonin and norepinephrine are also involved in the perception of pain. Serotonin and norepinephrine modify the effects of substance P, glutamate, γ-aminobutyric acid (GABA), and other pain mediators (Montano, 2003). In fact, one study demonstrated that 43% of people with major depression had at least one chronic painful condition. This was four times the rate in those without MDD (Montano, 2003). There is considerable evidence of overlap in the physiology of pain and mood disorders (Kramer, 2004).

At present, however, research suggests that depression results from the dysregulation of a number of neurotransmitter systems in addition to serotonin and norepinephrine. The dopamine, acetylcholine, and GABA systems are also believed to be involved in the pathophysiology of a major depressive episode (APA, 2000). It is now considered unlikely that a catecholamine deficiency alone is the actual cause of depression (Gruenberg & Goldstein, 2003).

Stressful life events, especially losses, seem to be a significant factor in the development of depression. Norepinephrine, serotonin, and acetylcholine play a role in stress regulation. When these neurotransmitters become overtaxed through stressful events, neurotransmitter depletion may occur. There is evidence that people who possess a "short" gene, or stress-sensitive version of the serotonin transporter gene, are at a higher risk of depression if they have been abused as children and/or if they have been exposed to multiple stressful life events (NIMH, 2003a). People with the "long" or protected version of the gene who underwent multiple life stresses, on the other hand, experienced no more depression than people who were totally spared life stresses (NIMH, 2003a).

At this time, no unitary mechanism of depressant action has been found. The relationships among the serotonin, norepinephrine, dopamine, acetylcholine,

---

BOX 18-1

Primary Risk Factors for Depression

- History of prior episodes of depression
- Family history of depressive disorder, especially in first-degree relatives
- History of suicide attempts and/or family history of suicide
- Female gender
- Age 40 years or younger
- Postpartum period
- Medical illness
- Absence of social support
- Negative, stressful life events
- Active alcohol or substance abuse

From Gruenberg, A. M., & Goldstein, R. D. (2003). Mood disorders: Depression. In A. Tasman, J. Kay, & J. A. Lieberman (Eds.). *Psychiatry* (2nd ed., p. 1210). West Sussex, England: Wiley.

and GABA systems are complex and need further assessment and study. However, treatment with medication that helps regulate these neurotransmitters has proved empirically successful in the treatment of many clients. Figure 18-2 shows a positron emission tomographic (PET) scan of the brain of a woman with depression before and after taking medication. Refer also to Figure 3-7 for PET scans comparing brain activity in an individual with depression and in a nondepressed individual.

Alterations in Hormonal Regulation

Although neuroendocrine findings are as yet inconclusive, the neuroendocrine characteristic most widely studied in relation to depression has been hyperactivity of the hypothalamic-pituitary-adrenal cortical axis. Evidence of increased cortisol secretion is apparent in 20% to 40% of depressed outpatients and 40% to 60% of depressed inpatients (Dubovsky et al., 2004). Dexamethasone, an exogenous steroid that suppresses cortisol, is used in the dexamethasone suppression test for depression. Results of the dexamethasone suppression test are abnormal in about 50% of clients with depression, which indicates hyperactivity of the hypothalamic-pituitary-adrenal cortical axis. However, the findings of this test may also be abnormal in people with obsessive-compulsive disorders and other medical conditions. Significantly, clients with psychotic major depression are among those with the highest rates of nonsuppression of cortisol on the dexamethasone suppression test.

Sleep Abnormalities

Sleep electroencephalogram abnormalities may be evident in 40% to 60% of outpatients and up to 90% of inpatients during a major depressive episode (APA, 2000). People prone to depression tend to have a premature loss of deep, slow (delta)–wave sleep and altered rapid eye movement (REM) latency. The phase of REM sleep associated with dreaming occurs earlier in two thirds of clients with bipolar and major depressive illnesses. This sign is referred to as **reduced REM latency** and is consistent with the expected manifestation of an inherited trait. Reduced REM latency and deficits in slow-wave sleep typically persist following recovery from a depressed episode (Dubovsky et al., 2004). Data also suggest that depressed clients *without* this sign are not likely to respond to treatment with tricyclic antidepressants (TCAs), which suppress early REM sleep.

Psychodynamic Influences and Life Events

The stress-diathesis model of depression in contemporary psychodynamic approaches to mood disorders takes into account the strong biological underpinnings of depression and bipolar disorders (Dubovsky et al., 2004). What is almost certain is that psychosocial stressors and interpersonal events trigger certain neurophysical and neurochemical changes in the brain (NIMH, 2002). Early life trauma may result in long-term hyperactivity of the CNS corticotropin-releasing

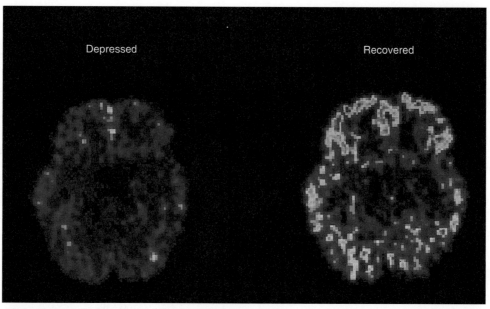

FIGURE 18-2 Positron emission tomographic (PET) scans of a 45-year-old woman with recurrent depression. The scan on the left was taken when the client was on no medication and very depressed. The scan on the right was taken several months later when the client was well, after she had been treated with medication for her depression. Note that her entire brain, particularly the left prefrontal cortex, is more active when she is well. (Courtesy Mark George, MD, Biological Psychiatry Branch, National Institute of Mental Health.)

factor (CRF) and norepinephrine systems with a consequent neurotoxic effect on the hippocampus that leads to neuronal loss. These changes could cause sensitization of the CRF circuits to even mild stress in adulthood, leading to an exaggerated stress response (Heim & Nemeroff, 1999). With exposure to repeated stress in adulthood, these already stress-sensitive pathways become "markedly hyperactive leading to a persistent increase in CRF and cortisol secretion, which causes alterations in the glucocorticoid receptors and thus forms the basis for the development of mood and anxiety disorders" (Sadek & Nemeroff, 2000).

These stressors and life events may lead to a depressive syndrome in some individuals, particularly those who are biologically vulnerable to depression, such as those with the short or stress-sensitive version of the serotonin transporter gene mentioned earlier. Therefore, life events (psychosocial stressors and interpersonal events) may influence the development and recurrence of depression through the psychological and biological experience of stress in some people, which results in changes in the connections among nerve cells in the brain.

Cognitive Theory

Aaron T. Beck, one of the early proponents of cognitive therapy, applied cognitive-behavioral theory to depression. Beck proposed that people acquire a psychological predisposition to depression through early life experiences. These experiences contribute to negative, illogical, and irrational thought processes that may remain dormant until they are activated during times of stress (Beck & Rush, 1995).

Beck found that depressed persons process information in negative ways, even in the midst of positive factors that affect the person's life. Beck believed that three automatic negative thoughts are responsible for the development of depression. These three thoughts are called **Beck's cognitive triad.** They are

1. A negative, self-deprecating view of self
2. A pessimistic view of the world
3. The belief that negative reinforcement (or no validation for the self) will continue in the future

The phrase *automatic negative thoughts* refers to thoughts that are repetitive, unintended, and not readily controllable. This cognitive triad seems to be consistent in all types of depression, regardless of clinical subtype.

The goal of cognitive-behavioral therapy (CBT) is to change the way clients think and thus relieve the depressive syndrome. This is accomplished by assisting the client in the following:

1. Identifying and testing negative cognition
2. Developing alternative thinking patterns
3. Rehearsing new cognitive and behavioral responses

Learned Helplessness

One of the most popular theories of the cause of depression is Martin Seligman's theory of learned helplessness. Seligman (1973) stated that, although anxiety is the initial response to a stressful situation, anxiety is replaced by depression if the person feels that the self has no control over the outcome of a situation. A person who believes that an undesired event is his or her fault and that nothing can be done to change it is prone to depression. The theory of learned helplessness has been used to explain the development of depression in certain social groups, such as the aged, people living in ghettos, and women.

Behavioral therapeutic approaches help individuals gain a sense of control and mastery of the environment by teaching depressed individuals new and more effective coping skills and ways to increase their self-confidence.

Application of the Nursing Process

■ ASSESSMENT

Undiagnosed and untreated depression is often associated with more severe presentation of depression, greater suicidality, somatic problems, and severe anxiety or anxiety disorders. Depression in the elderly is often missed, especially if there are coexisting medical problems. Depression in children and adolescents may go undiagnosed when attention is focused on behavioral problems ("just a stage"). Racial disparities in health care, among other things, allow for underdiagnosing and undertreating African Americans, Hispanics, and some other minorities (Agency for Healthcare Research and Quality, 2004).

A study by Bijl and associates (2004) concluded that depressed individuals who came for treatment manifesting psychological symptomatology were recognized as depressed 90% of the time, in contrast to those who showed somatic symptoms (e.g., chronic pain, insomnia), who were recognized as depressed 50% of the time, and those who had a medical disorder, in whom depression was identified 20% of the time.

Overall Assessment

Because depression can mean so many different things, Goldberg (1998) suggested an evaluation starting with depressive symptoms, then assessing possible cause and past episodes. Goldberg suggested using the assessment tool shown in Figure 18-3 when assessing depressive symptoms.

INITIAL ASSESSMENT GUIDE

Depressive symptoms	Duration
Depressed mood	_____
Decreased energy	_____
Poor concentration	_____
Sleep change	_____
Appetite change	_____
Psychomotor change	_____
Guilt, poor self-esteem	_____
Anhedonia	_____
Suicidality	_____
Chronic pain	_____
Poor functional level	_____
Somatized symptoms	_____

Accompanying symptoms

Delusions	Panic attacks	Mania
Hallucinations	Generalized anxiety	

Possible precipitants

_____

_____

_____

Possible medical causes

_____

_____

_____

Past episodes

_____

_____

_____

FIGURE 18-3 Initial assessment guide. (From Goldberg, R. J. [1998]. *Practical guide to the care of the psychiatric patient* [2nd ed.]. St. Louis, MO: Mosby.)

Assessment Tools

Numerous standardized screening instruments are available that help the clinician assess the type of depression a person may be experiencing. For example, the Beck Depression Inventory, the Hamilton Depression Scale, and the Geriatric Depression Scale all are valuable tools. The Zung Depression Scale is a short inventory that highlights predominant symptoms seen in depressed individuals; it is presented here because of its ease of use (Figure 18-4).

The National Mental Health Association (NMHA) has a website (http://www.depression-screening.org) that enables people to take a confidential screening test for depression on-line and find reliable information on the illness. The website's mission is threefold:

1. To educate people about depression
2. To offer a simple and confidential way for people to get screened for the illness
3. To guide people toward appropriate professional help when necessary

Safety First: Assessment of Suicide Potential

The client should be evaluated for suicidal or homicidal ideation. About 10% to 15% of depressed people eventually commit suicide (Fuller & Sajatovic, 2000). Initial suicide evaluation might include the following statements or questions:

- "You have said you are depressed. Tell me what that is like for you."
- "When you feel depressed, what thoughts go through your mind?"
- "Have you gone so far as to think about taking your own life? Do you have a plan? Do you have the means to carry out your plan? Is there anything that would prevent you from carrying out your plan?"

Refer to Chapter 23 for a detailed discussion of suicide and strategies for suicide prevention, critical risk factors, and warning signs.

Key Findings

A depressed mood and anhedonia are the key symptoms in depression. Almost 97% of people with depression have anergia. **Anxiety,** a common symptom in depression, is seen in about 60% to 90% of depressed clients.

When people are depressed, their thinking is slow, and their memory and concentration are usually affected. Depressed people dwell on and exaggerate their perceived faults and failures and are unable to focus on their strengths and successes. A person with major depression may experience delusions of being punished for doing bad deeds or being a terrible person. Feelings of worthlessness, guilt, anger, and helplessness are common. Psychomotor agitation may be evidenced by constant pacing and wringing of hands. The slowed movements of psychomotor retardation, however, are more common. Somatic complaints (headaches, malaise, backaches) are also common. Vegetative signs of depression (change in bowel movements and eating habits, sleep disturbances, and disinterest in sex) are usually present. Stuart (2003) reports that over two thirds of people suffering from depression complain of **pain** with or without reporting psychological symptoms. People who suffer from **chronic pain** need careful assessment for possible depression.

Areas to Assess

Affect. A person who is depressed sees the world through gray-colored glasses. Posture is poor, and the client may look older than the stated age. Facial expressions convey sadness and dejection, and the client

ZUNG'S SELF-RATING DEPRESSION SCALE				
	None or Little of the Time	Some of the Time	A Good Part of the Time	Most or All of the Time
1. I feel down-hearted, blue, and sad.	1	2	3	4
2. Morning is when I feel the best.	4	3	2	1
3. I have crying spells or feel like it.	1	2	3	4
4. I have trouble sleeping through the night.	1	2	3	4
5. I eat as much as I used to.	4	3	2	1
6. I enjoy looking at, talking to, and being with attractive women/men.	4	3	2	1
7. I notice that I am losing weight.	1	2	3	4
8. I have trouble with constipation.	1	2	3	4
9. My heart beats faster than usual.	1	2	3	4
10. I get tired for no reason.	1	2	3	4
11. My mind is as clear as it used to be.	4	3	2	1
12. I find it easy to do the things I used to do.	4	3	2	1
13. I am restless and can't keep still.	1	2	3	4
14. I feel hopeful about the future.	4	3	2	1
15. I am more irritable than usual.	1	2	3	4
16. I find it easy to make decisions.	4	3	2	1
17. I feel that I am useful and needed.	4	3	2	1
18. My life is pretty full.	4	3	2	1
19. I feel that others would be better off if I were dead.	1	2	3	4
20. I still enjoy the things I used to do.	4	3	2	1

* A raw score of 50 or above is associated with depression requiring hospital treatment.

FIGURE 18-4 Nursing assessment: Zung's Self-Rating Depression Scale. (From Zung, W. K. [1965]. A self-rating depression scale. *Archives of General Psychiatry, 12*, 63. Copyright 1965, American Medical Association.)

may have frequent bouts of weeping. Conversely, the client may say that he or she is unable to cry. Feelings of **hopelessness** and **despair** are readily reflected in the person's affect. For example, the client may not make eye contact, may speak in a monotone, may show little or no facial expression (flat affect), and may make only yes or no responses. Frequent sighing is common.

Thought Processes. As mentioned, identifying the presence of suicidal thoughts and suicide potential has the highest priority in the initial assessment. Approximately two thirds of depressed people contemplate suicide, and up to 15% of untreated or inadequately treated clients give up hope and kill themselves (Dubovsky et al., 2004). Refer to Chapter 23.

During the time a person is depressed, the person's ability to solve problems and think clearly is negatively affected. Judgment is poor, and indecisiveness is common. The individual may claim that the mind is slowing down. Memory and concentration are poor. Evidence of delusional thinking may be seen in a person with major depression. Common statements of delusional thinking are "I have committed unpardonable sins," "God wants me dead," and "I am wicked and should die."

Feelings. Feelings frequently reported by depressed people include anxiety, worthlessness, guilt, helplessness and hopelessness, and anger. As previously men-

tioned, **anxiety** is present in about 60% of depressed persons. Feelings of **worthlessness** range from feeling inadequate to having an unrealistic evaluation of self-worth. These feelings reflect the low self-esteem that is a painful partner to depression. Statements such as "I am no good, I'll never amount to anything" are common. Themes of one's inadequacy and incompetence are repeated relentlessly.

Guilt is a common accompaniment to depression. A person may ruminate over present or past failings. Extreme guilt can assume psychotic proportions: "I have committed terrible sins. God is punishing me for my evil ways."

Helplessness is evidenced by the inability to carry out the simplest tasks. Everything is too difficult to accomplish (e.g., grooming, doing housework, working, caring for children). With feelings of helplessness come feelings of **hopelessness.** Even though most depressive states are usually time limited, during a depressed period, people believe that things will never change. This feeling of utter hopelessness can lead people to look at suicide as a way out of constant mental pain. Hopelessness is one of the core characteristics of depression and suicide, as well as a characteristic of schizophrenia, alcoholism, and physical illness. Hopelessness is a cognitive as well as emotional state that includes the following attributes:

- Negative expectations for the future
- Loss of control over future outcomes

- Passive acceptance of the futility of planning to achieve goals
- Emotional negativism, as expressed in despair, despondency, or depression

Anger and **irritability** are natural outcomes of profound feelings of helplessness. Anger in depression is often expressed inappropriately. For example, anger may be expressed in destruction of property, hurtful verbal attacks, or physical aggression toward others. However, in people who are depressed, anger may be directed toward the self in the form of suicidal or sub-suicidal behaviors (alcohol abuse, substance abuse, overeating, smoking, etc.). These behaviors often result in feelings of low self-esteem and worthlessness.

Physical Behavior. Lethargy and fatigue can result in psychomotor retardation. Movements are extremely slow, facial expressions are decreased, and gaze is fixed. The continuum in **psychomotor retardation** may range from slowed and difficult movements to complete inactivity and incontinence. At other times, the nurse may note **psychomotor agitation.** For example, clients may constantly pace, bite their nails, smoke, tap their fingers, or engage in some other tension-relieving activity. At these times, clients commonly feel fidgety and unable to relax.

Grooming, dress, and personal hygiene are markedly neglected. People who usually take pride in their appearance and dress may be poorly groomed and allow themselves to look shabby and unkempt.

Vegetative signs of depression are universal. Vegetative signs refer to alterations in those activities necessary to support physical life and growth (eating, sleeping, elimination, sex). For example, **changes in eating patterns** are common. About 60% to 70% of people who are depressed report having anorexia; overeating occurs more often in dysthymia.

Changes in sleep patterns are a cardinal sign of depression. Often, people have **insomnia,** waking at 3 or 4 AM and staying awake, or sleeping only for short periods. The light sleep of a depressed person tends to prolong the agony of depression over a 24-hour period. Deep stages of sleep (stages 3 and 4) are usually decreased or totally absent (Dubovsky et al., 2004).

For some, sleep is increased (hypersomnia) and provides an escape from painful feelings. This is more common in young depressed individuals or those with bipolar tendencies. In any event, sleep is rarely restful or refreshing.

Changes in bowel habits are common. Constipation is seen most frequently in clients with psychomotor retardation. Diarrhea occurs less frequently, often in conjunction with psychomotor agitation.

Interest in sex declines (loss of libido) during depression. Some men experience impotence, and a declining interest in sex often occurs among both men and women, which can further complicate marital and social relationships.

Communication. A person who is depressed may speak as well as comprehend very slowly. The lack of an immediate response by the client to a remark does not mean that the client has not heard or chooses not to reply: the client just needs a little more time to compose a reply. In extreme depression, however, a person may be mute.

Self-Assessment

Depressed clients often reject the overtures of the nurse and others. When people are depressed, they do not appear to respond to nursing interventions and seem resistant to change. When this occurs, nurses can experience feelings of frustration, hopelessness, and annoyance. Nurses can alter these problematic responses by

- Recognizing any unrealistic expectations they have of themselves or the client.
- Identifying feelings they are experiencing that originate with the client.
- Understanding the part that neurotransmitters play in the precipitation and maintenance of a depressed mood.

Refer to the Evidence-Based Practice box.

Unrealistic Expectations of Self

Nursing students as well as health care workers new to working with depressed individuals may have expectations of themselves and their clients that are not realistic, and problems result when these expectations are not met. Unmet expectations usually result in the nurse's feeling anxious, hurt, angry, helpless, or incompetent. Unrealistic expectations of self and others may be held even by experienced health care workers, and this phenomenon contributes to staff burnout. Many of the nurse's expectations may not be conscious. However, when these expectations are made conscious and worked through with peers and more experienced clinicians (supervisors), more realistic expectations can be formed and attainable outcomes identified. Realistic expectations of self and the client can decrease feelings of helplessness and can increase the nurse's self-esteem and therapeutic potential.

Client Feelings Experienced by the Nurse

Intense feelings of anxiety, frustration, annoyance, and helplessness may be experienced by the nurse as well as other health care professionals, although the feelings may originate in the client. These feelings can be important diagnostic clues to the client's experience. Often, the nurse senses what the client is feeling through empathy.

EVIDENCE-BASED PRACTICE

Stigma and Help Seeking Related to Depression

Background

The Surgeon General and the President's New Freedom Commission on Mental Health have identified the stigmatization of people with mental illnesses and the effect of this stigmatization on health-seeking behaviors as a significant issue on the nation's health care agenda. It is thought by many that negative perceptions regarding depression and the treatment of depression contribute to the 30,000 suicides that occur in the United States every year.

Study

Nurses enrolled in both a basic and degree-completion baccalaureate program were chosen to help identify the influence of the education process on changes in stigmatizing attitudes and help-seeking intention.

The study was a descriptive correlational study that measured attitudes toward an individual with depression as described in a vignette, as well as personal health-seeking behaviors. The purpose was to examine the effects of personal variables on help-seeking behaviors.

Results of Study

"Students who believed that depression was not under personal control were more likely to endorse help-seeking behaviors for themselves. Individuals who were women, older, upperclassmen, and Catholic reported greater acceptance of seeking psychological help. The psychiatric mental health nursing class and rotation were identified as improving stigmatizing attitudes and increasing help-seeking intention" (p. 42).

Implications for Nursing Practice

As the National Alliance for Research on Schizophrenia and Depression in Great Neck, New York, pointed out, "Mood disorders are caused by a flaw in chemistry, not character" (VanScoy, 2001). Nurses have the potential to exert tremendous influence by educating others regarding the causes of depression and the fact that depression is a treatable disease. The implication of this study is that, when people understand that depression has a physical cause and is not something within a person's control, stigmatizing behavior may decrease and seeking help and counseling is more accepted.

Halter, M. J. (2004). Stigma and help seeking related to depression: A study of nursing students. *Journal of Psychosocial Nursing and Mental Health Services, 42*(2), 42-51.

When the nurse's feelings of annoyance, hopelessness, and anxiety are the result of empathetic communications with the client, the nurse can discuss these feelings with peers and supervisors to separate personal feelings from those originating in the client. If personal feelings are not recognized, named, and examined, withdrawal by the nurse is likely to occur. People naturally stay away from situations and persons that arouse feelings of frustration, annoyance, or intimidation. If the nurse has unresolved feelings of anger and depression, the complexity of the situation is compounded. There is no substitute for competent and supportive supervision to facilitate growth, both professionally and personally. Supervision by a more experienced clinician and sharing with peers help minimize feelings of confusion, frustration, and isolation and can increase therapeutic potential and self-esteem in the nurse.

Assessment Guidelines Depression

1. Always evaluate the client's risk of harm to self or others. Overt hostility is highly correlated with suicide (see Chapter 23).
2. A thorough medical and neurological examination helps determine if the depression is primary or secondary to another disorder. Depression is a mood that can be secondary to a host of medical or other psychiatric disorders, as well as medications. Essentially, evaluate whether
   - The client is psychotic.
   - The client has taken drugs or alcohol.
   - Medical conditions are present.
   - The client has a history of a comorbid psychiatric syndrome (eating disorder, borderline or anxiety disorder).
3. Assess past history of depression and determine what happened as well as what worked and did not work.
4. Assess support systems, family and significant others, and need for information and referrals.

■ NURSING DIAGNOSIS

Depression is complex, and depressed individuals have a variety of needs. Therefore, nursing diagnoses are many. However, during the initial assessment, a high priority for the nurse is identification of the presence of suicide potential. Therefore, the nursing diagnosis of *risk for suicide* is always considered. Refer to Chapter 23 for assessment and interventions for suicidal individuals. Other key targets for nursing interventions are represented by the diagnoses of *hopelessness, ineffective coping, social isolation, spiritual distress,* and *self-care deficit.* Table 18-4 identifies signs and symptoms commonly experienced in depression and offers potential nursing diagnoses.

TABLE 18-4

Potential Nursing Diagnoses for Depression

Signs and Symptoms	Potential Nursing Diagnoses
Previous suicidal attempts, putting affairs in order, giving away prized possessions, suicidal ideation (has plan, ability to carry it out), overt or covert statements regarding killing self, feelings of worthlessness, hopelessness, helplessness	Risk for suicide Risk for self-mutilation
Lack of judgment, memory difficulty, poor concentration, inaccurate interpretation of environment, negative ruminations, cognitive distortions	Disturbed thought processes
Difficulty with simple tasks, inability to function at previous level, poor problem solving, poor cognitive functioning, verbalizations of inability to cope	Ineffective coping Interrupted family processes Risk for impaired parent/infant/child attachment Ineffective role performance
Difficulty making decisions, poor concentration, inability to take action	Decisional conflict
Feelings of helplessness, hopelessness, powerlessness	Hopelessness Powerlessness
Questioning of meaning of life and own existence, inability to participate in usual religious practices, conflict over spiritual beliefs, anger toward spiritual deity or religious representatives	Spiritual distress Impaired religiosity Risk for impaired religiosity
Feelings of worthlessness, poor self-image, negative sense of self, self-negating verbalizations, feeling of being a failure, expressions of shame or guilt, hypersensitivity to slights or criticism	Chronic low self-esteem Situational low self-esteem
Withdrawal, noncommunicativeness, speech that is only in monosyllables, avoidance of contact with others	Impaired social interaction Social isolation Risk for loneliness
Vegetative signs of depression: changes in sleeping, eating, grooming and hygiene, elimination, sexual patterns	Self-care deficit (bathing/hygiene, dressing/grooming) Imbalanced nutrition: less than body requirements Disturbed sleep pattern Constipation Sexual dysfunction

■ OUTCOME CRITERIA

When possible, the nurse and client discuss desired outcomes of health care interventions. Realistic outcome criteria are identified, and concrete, measurable steps are formulated as short-term and intermediate indicators. Each client is different, and indicators are selected according to each person's individual needs.

Table 18-5 presents some outcome criteria from the Nursing Outcomes Classification (NOC) (Moorhead, Johnson, & Maas, 2004).

Indicators for the outcomes of the vegetative or physical signs of depression (e.g., *reports adequate sleep*) are formulated to show, for example, evidence of weight gain, return to normal bowel activity, sleep duration of 6 to 8 hours per night, or return of sexual desire.

TABLE 18-5

NOC Outcomes for Depression

Nursing Outcome and Definition	Intermediate Indicators	Short-Term Indicators
Depression Self-Control: Personal actions to minimize melancholy and maintain interest in life events*	Reports improved mood Adheres to therapy schedule Takes medication as prescribed Follows treatment plan	Monitors intensity of depression Identifies precursors of depression Plans strategies to reduce effects of precursors Reports changes in symptoms to health care provider

From Moorhead, S., Johnson, M., & Maas, M. (2004). *Nursing outcomes classification (NOC)* (3rd ed.). St. Louis, MO: Mosby.
*Indicators measured on a five-point Likert scale ranging from 1 (never demonstrated) to 5 (consistently demonstrated).

■ PLANNING

The planning of care for clients with depression is geared toward the phase of depression the person is in and the particular symptoms the person is exhibiting. At all times, the nurse and members of the health care team are cognizant of the potential for suicide, and assessment of risk for self-harm (or harm to others) is ongoing during the care of the depressed person. We know that a combination of therapy (cognitive, behavioral, interpersonal, and other) and psychopharmacology is an effective approach to the treatment of depression. The nurse is aware that the vegetative signs of depression (changes in eating, sleeping, sexual satisfaction, etc.) as well as changes in concentration, activity level, social interaction, care for personal appearance, and so on, often need targeting. Therefore, the planning of care for a client who is depressed is based on the individual's symptoms and attempts to encompass a variety of areas in the person's life. Safety is always the highest priority.

Refer to Case Study and Nursing Care Plan 18-1 at the end of the chapter.

■ INTERVENTION

Recovery from depression can be conceptualized as a process. There are three phases in the treatment of and recovery from major depression (Gruenberg & Goldstein, 2003):

1. Acute (6 to 12 weeks)
2. Continuation (4 to 9 months)
3. Maintenance (1 or more years)

According to Gruenberg and Goldstein (2003),

- The **acute phase** is directed at reduction of depressive symptoms and restoration of psychosocial and work function. Hospitalization may be required.
- The **continuation phase** is directed at prevention of relapse through pharmacotherapy, education, and depression-specific psychotherapy.
- The **maintenance phase** of treatment is directed at prevention of further episodes of depression.

Basic Level Interventions

The basic level nurse engages in counseling, health teaching, promotion of self-care activities, and milieu management.

Counseling and Communication Strategies

Nurses often have great difficulty communicating with clients without talking. However, some depressed clients are so withdrawn that they are unwilling or unable to speak. Just sitting with a client in silence may seem like a waste of time to the nurse.

Often, the nurse becomes uncomfortable not doing something, and, as anxiety increases, the nurse may start daydreaming, feel bored, remember something that "must be done now," and so on. It is important to be aware that this time spent together can be meaningful to the depressed person, especially if the nurse has a genuine interest in learning about the depressed individual.

■ ■ ■ *VIGNETTE*

Doris, a senior nursing student, is working with a depressed, suicidal, withdrawn woman. The instructor notices in the second week that Doris spends a lot of time talking with other students and their clients and little time with her own client. In postconference, Doris acknowledges feeling threatened and useless and says that she wants a client who will interact with her. After reviewing the symptoms of depression, its behavioral manifestations, and the needs of depressed persons, Doris turns her attention back to her client and spends time rethinking her plan of care. After 4 weeks of sharing her feelings in postconferences, working with her instructor, and trying a variety of approaches with her client, Doris is rewarded. On the day of discharge, the client tells Doris how important their time together was for her: "I actually felt someone cared."

■ ■ ■

It is difficult to say when a withdrawn or depressed person will be able to respond. However, certain techniques are known to be useful in guiding effective nursing interventions. Some communication techniques to use with a severely withdrawn client are listed in Table 18-6. Counseling guidelines for work with depressed persons are offered in Table 18-7.

Health Teaching

It is important for both clients and their families to understand that depression is a legitimate medical illness over which the client has no voluntary control. Depressed clients and their families need to learn about the biological symptoms of depression, as well as about the psychosocial and cognitive changes in depression. Review of the medications and their adverse reactions helps families evaluate clinical changes and stay alert for reactions that might affect client compliance. The section on psychopharmacology provides information on adverse reactions to antidepressants and specific areas to be covered in client and family teaching.

When a client is being discharged from the hospital, predischarge counseling should be carried out with the client and the client's relatives. One purpose of this counseling is to clarify the interpersonal stresses and discuss steps that can alleviate tension in the family system. Including families in discharge planning facilitates progress in the following ways:

- Increases the family's understanding and acceptance of the depressed family member during the aftercare period

TABLE 18-6

Guidelines for Communication with Severely Withdrawn Persons

Intervention	Rationale
1. When a client is mute, use the technique of *making observations:* "There are many new pictures on the wall" or "You are wearing your new shoes."	1. When a client is not ready to talk, direct questions can raise the client's anxiety level and frustrate the nurse. Pointing to commonalities in the environment draws the client into, and reinforces, reality.
2. Use simple, concrete words.	2. Slowed thinking and difficulty concentrating impair comprehension.
3. Allow time for the client to respond.	3. Slowed thinking necessitates time to formulate a response.
4. Listen for covert messages and ask about suicide plans.	4. People often experience relief and decrease in feelings of isolation when they share thoughts of suicide.
5. Avoid platitudes, such as "Things will look up" or "Everyone gets down once in a while."	5. Platitudes tend to minimize the client's feelings and can increase feelings of guilt and worthlessness because the client cannot "look up" or "snap out of it."

- Increases the client's use of aftercare facilities in the community
- Contributes to higher overall adjustment in the client after discharge

Self-Care Activities

In addition to experiencing intense feelings of hopelessness, despair, low self-worth, and fatigue, the depressed person may also report having many physical complaints. Therefore, signs and symptoms of physical neglect may be apparent. Nursing measures for improving physical well-being and promoting adequate self-care are initiated. Some effective interventions targeting the physical needs of the depressed client are listed in Table 18-8. Nurses in the community can work with family members to encourage a depressed family member to perform and maintain his or her self-care activities.

Milieu Therapy

When a person is acutely and severely depressed, the structure of the hospital setting may be indicated. The depressed person needs protection from suicidal acts, a supervised environment for regulating antidepressant medications, and, when indicated, a course of electroconvulsive therapy (ECT). Often, being removed from a stressful interpersonal situation in itself has therapeutic value. Hospitals have protocols re-

TABLE 18-7

Guidelines for Counseling Depressed Persons

Intervention	Rationale/Comment
1. Help the client question underlying assumptions and beliefs and consider alternate explanations to problems.	1. Reconstructing a healthier and more hopeful attitude about the future can alter depressed mood.
2. Work with the client to identify cognitive distortions that encourage negative self-appraisal. For example: a. Overgeneralizations b. Self-blame c. Mind reading d. Discounting of positive attributes	2. Cognitive distortions reinforce a negative, inaccurate perception of self and world. a. The client takes one fact or event and makes a general rule out of it ("He always . . . "; "I never . . . "). b. The client consistently blames self for everything perceived as negative. c. The client assumes others don't like him or her, and so forth, without any real evidence that assumptions are correct. d. The client focuses on the negative.
3. Encourage activities that can raise self-esteem. Identify need for (a) problem-solving skills, (b) coping skills, and (c) assertiveness skills.	3. Many depressed people, especially women, are not taught a range of problem solving and coping skills. Increasing social, family, and job skills can change negative self-assessment.
4. Encourage exercise, such as running and/or weight lifting.	4. Exercise can improve self-concept and potentially shift neurochemical balance.
5. Encourage formation of supportive relationships, such as through support groups, therapy, and peer support.	5. Such relationships reduce social isolation and enable the client to work on personal goals and relationship needs.
6. Provide information referrals, when needed, for religious or spiritual information (e.g., readings, programs, tapes, community resources).	6. Spiritual and existential issues may be heightened during depressive episodes—many people find strength and comfort in spirituality or religion.

TABLE 18-8

Interventions Targeting the Vegetative Signs of Depression

Intervention	Rationale
Nutrition—Anorexia	
1. Offer small high-calorie and high-protein snacks frequently throughout the day and evening.	1. Low weight and poor nutrition render the client susceptible to illness. Small, frequent snacks are more easily tolerated than large plates of food when the client is anorexic.
2. Offer high-protein and high-calorie fluids frequently throughout the day and evening.	2. These fluids prevent dehydration and can minimize constipation.
3. When possible, encourage family or friends to remain with the client during meals.	3. This strategy reinforces the idea that someone cares, can raise the client's self-esteem, and can serve as an incentive to eat.
4. Ask the client which foods or drinks he or she likes. Offer choices. Involve the dietitian.	4. The client is more likely to eat the foods provided.
5. Weigh the client weekly and observe the client's eating patterns.	5. Monitoring the client's status gives the information needed for revision of the intervention.
Sleep—Insomnia	
1. Provide periods of rest after activities.	1. Fatigue can intensify feelings of depression.
2. Encourage the client to get up and dress and to stay out of bed during the day.	2. Minimizing sleep during the day increases the likelihood of sleep at night.
3. Encourage the use of relaxation measures in the evening (e.g., tepid bath, warm milk).	3. These measures induce relaxation and sleep.
4. Reduce environmental and physical stimulants in the evening—provide decaffeinated coffee, soft lights, soft music, and quiet activities.	4. Decreasing caffeine and epinephrine levels increases the possibility of sleep.
Self-Care Deficits	
1. Encourage the use of toothbrush, washcloth, soap, makeup, shaving equipment, and so forth.	1. Being clean and well groomed can temporarily increase self-esteem.
2. When appropriate, give step-by-step reminders such as "Wash the right side of your face, now the left."	2. Slowed thinking and difficulty concentrating make organizing simple tasks difficult.
Elimination—Constipation	
1. Monitor intake and output, especially bowel movements.	1. Many depressed clients are constipated. If the condition is not checked, fecal impaction can occur.
2. Offer foods high in fiber and provide periods of exercise.	2. Roughage and exercise stimulate peristalsis and help evacuation of fecal material.
3. Encourage the intake of fluids.	3. Fluids help prevent constipation.
4. Evaluate the need for laxatives and enemas.	4. These measures prevent fecal impaction.

garding the care and protection of the suicidal client (see Chapter 23).

Advanced Practice Interventions

The advanced practice nurse is qualified to provide psychotherapy, social skills training, and group therapy.

Psychotherapy

Psychotherapy works by changing the way the brain functions. Psychotherapy and learning are similar in that both involve the formation of new connections between nerve cells in the brain (NIMH, 2002). CBT, interpersonal therapy (IPT), time-limited focused psychotherapy, and behavioral therapy all are especially effective in the treatment of depression. However, only CBT and IPT demonstrate superiority in the maintenance phase. CBT helps people change their negative styles of thinking and behaving, whereas IPT focuses on working through personal relationships that may contribute to depression (NIMH, 2002). Outcome research has consistently found that CBT is at least as effective as medication, with clients undergoing CBT showing a lower relapse rate (Young et al., 2001).

A review of several studies (Young et al., 2001) showed apparent prophylactic effects of cognitive therapy in depressed clients, especially those with unipolar depression; that is, people seem to learn something in cognitive therapy that is helpful after the acute phase of treatment, and this knowledge may help prevent a relapse.

Social Skills Training

Social skills training is also helpful in treating depression. The training focuses on assertiveness and coping skills that lead to an increase in positive reinforcement from other people and the environment. Depressed children also benefit from CBT and social skills training. The goals are the same as for adults, that is, to decrease depressive thinking, enhance social skills, and increase pleasant activities (Agras & Berkowitz, 1999).

Group Treatment

Group treatment is a widespread modality for the treatment of depression; it increases the number of people who can receive treatment at a decreased cost per individual. Another advantage is that groups offer clients an opportunity to socialize and to share common feelings and concerns, which decreases feelings of isolation as well as feelings of hopelessness, helplessness, and alienation.

Psychopharmacology

Because mood disorders are caused by "a flaw in chemistry, not character," it follows that medications that alter brain chemistry are an important component in the treatment of mood disorders (VanScoy, 2001). Antidepressant therapy benefits about 65% to 80% of people with nondelusional unipolar depression (Maxmen & Ward, 2002). ECT has a 75% to 85% efficacy rate for those clients who are delusional or melancholic (Maxmen & Ward, 2002). It should be noted, however, that the combination of specific psychotherapies (e.g., CBT, IPT, behavioral) and antidepressant therapy is superior to either psychotherapy or psychopharmacological treatment alone (Sutherland, Sutherland, & Hoehns, 2003). The core symptoms of depression improve with antidepressant therapy, and quality-of-life measures improve with certain psychotherapies (Culpepper et al., 2003).

What Antidepressants Can Do

Antidepressant drugs can positively alter poor self-concept, degree of withdrawal, vegetative signs of depression, and activity level. Target symptoms include the following:

- Sleep disturbance
  - Early morning awakening
  - Frequent awakening
  - Hypersomnia (excessive sleeping)
- Appetite disturbance (decreased or increased)
- Fatigue
- Decreased sex drive
- Psychomotor retardation or agitation
- Diurnal variations in mood (often worse in the morning)
- Impaired concentration or forgetfulness
- Anhedonia (loss of ability to experience joy or pleasure in living)

One drawback to the use of antidepressant medication is that improvement in mood may take 1 to 3 weeks or longer. If a client is acutely suicidal, this may be too long to wait. At these times, ECT can be reliably and effectively used.

Concern has recently been expressed over the need for physicians and clinicians to monitor clients more carefully for worsening depression or suicidal thoughts or behaviors, especially at the beginning of antidepressant drug therapy. This concern applies especially to pediatric clients, as well as to adults and elderly clients.

On March 22, 2004, the Food and Drug Administration (FDA) requested that certain drug manufacturers change the labels of ten antidepressant drugs to include stronger warning statements and cautions about the need to monitor clients for the emergence of suicidal ideation and the worsening of depression.

These antidepressant drugs include fluoxetine (Prozac), sertraline (Zoloft), paroxetine (Paxil), fluvoxamine (Luvox), citalopram (Celexa), escitalopram (Lexapro), bupropion (Wellbutrin), venlafaxine (Effexor), and mirtazapine (Remeron) (U.S. FDA, 2004a).

This action on the part of the FDA does not mean that these drugs cause worsening of depression or suicidality; rather, health care providers should be alert to the fact that an increase in the severity of depression or suicidal thoughts or behaviors can be due to the underlying disease or can be a result of drug therapy (U.S. FDA, 2004b).

Factors Considered in Choosing a Specific Antidepressant

All antidepressants work equally well. However, a variety of antidepressants or a combination of antidepressants may need to be tried before the most effective regimen is found. The antidepressants all have different adverse effects, costs, safety features, and maintenance considerations. Gitlin (1999) proposed the following as the primary and secondary considerations when choosing a specific antidepressant:

Primary considerations:
- Side effect profile (e.g., sexual dysfunction, weight gain)
- Ease of administration
- History of past response
- Safety and medical considerations
- Specific subtype of depression (if applicable)

Secondary considerations:
- Neurotransmitter specificity
- Family history of response
- Blood level considerations
- Cost

It is the neurotransmitters and receptor sites in the brain that are the targets of pharmacological intervention (Table 18-9). While reading the following section, see if you can identify potential side effects caused by the blockage of the given neurotransmitter.

TABLE 18-9

Potential Effects of Receptor Blockade

Receptor Blocked		Potential Effects
NE	Norepinephrine	▪ Decreased depression ▪ Tremors ▪ Tachycardia ▪ Erectile and/or ejaculatory dysfunction
α_1	Specific receptor for epinephrine	▪ Antipsychotic effect ▪ Postural hypotension ▪ Dizziness ▪ Reflux tachycardia ▪ Ejaculatory dysfunction and/or impotence ▪ Memory dysfunction
α_2	Specific receptor for norepinephrine	▪ Priapism
5-HT	Serotonin	▪ Decreased depression ▪ Antianxiety effects ▪ Gastrointestinal disturbance ▪ Sexual dysfunction
5-HT_2	Serotonin	▪ Decreased depression ▪ Decreased suicidal behavior ▪ Antipsychotic effects ▪ Hypotension ▪ Ejaculatory dysfunction ▪ Weight gain and carbohydrate craving
DA	Dopamine reuptake blocked	▪ Decreased depression ▪ Psychomotor agitation ▪ Antiparkinson effect
ACh	Acetylcholine	▪ Anticholinergic effects
H_1	Histamine	▪ Sedation ▪ Orthostatic hypotension ▪ Weight gain ▪ Cognitive impairment

Psychopharmacological and Other Somatic Treatments

Basic antidepressant classes include the following:
First-line agents:
- Selective serotonin reuptake inhibitors (SSRIs)
- The newer atypical antidepressants
- Cyclic antidepressants (e.g., tricyclic antidepressants [TCAs])

Second-line interventions:
- Monoamine oxidase inhibitors (MAOIs)
- Electroconvulsive therapy (ECT)

Selective Serotonin Reuptake Inhibitors. The selective serotonin reuptake inhibitors (SSRIs) represent an important advance in pharmacotherapy. They are neither TCAs nor MAOIs. Essentially, the SSRIs selectively block the neuronal uptake of serotonin (e.g., 5-HT, 5-HT_1 receptors). Through blockade of the reuptake process, serotonergic neurotransmission is enhanced, because serotonin is able to act for an extended period at the synaptic binding sites in the brain. Chapter 3 provides more information on how the SSRIs work.

SSRIs are recommended as first-line therapy for all types of depression *except* for the following: psychotic depression (in which ECT may be the first choice), melancholic depression, and mild depression.

SSRI antidepressant drugs have a lower incidence of anticholinergic side effects (dry mouth, blurred vision, urinary retention), less cardiotoxicity, and faster onset of action than the TCAs. Clients are more likely to comply with a regimen of SSRIs than of TCAs, and compliance is a crucial step toward recovery or remission. The SSRIs seem to be effective in depression with anxiety features as well as in depression with psychomotor agitation.

Because the SSRIs cause fewer adverse effects and have low cardiotoxicity, they are less dangerous when they are taken in overdose. The SSRIs, selective serotonin-norepinephrine reuptake inhibitors (SNRIs), and newer atypical antidepressants have a low lethality risk in suicide attempts compared with the TCAs, which have a very high potential for lethality with overdose.

Indications. The SSRIs have a broad base of clinical use. In addition to their use in treating depressive disorders, the SSRIs have been prescribed with success to treat some of the anxiety disorders, in particular, obsessive-compulsive disorder and panic disorder (see Chapter 14). Fluoxetine has been found to be effective in treating some women who suffer from late luteal phase dysphoric disorder and bulimia nervosa.

Common Adverse Reactions. Agents that selectively enhance synaptic serotonin within the CNS may induce agitation, anxiety, sleep disturbance, tremor, sexual dysfunction (primarily anorgasmia), or tension headache. The effect of the SSRIs on sexual performance may be the most significant undesirable outcome reported by clients.

Autonomic reactions (e.g., dry mouth, sweating, weight change, mild nausea, and loose bowel movements) may also be experienced with the SSRIs. See Table 18-10 for a general side effect profile of the SSRIs, specific SSRIs, and dosage.

Potential Toxic Effects. One rare and life-threatening event associated with the SSRIs is the **central serotonin syndrome.** This is thought to be related to overactivation of the central serotonin receptors, caused by either too high a dose or interaction with other drugs. Symptoms include abdominal pain, diarrhea, sweating, fever, tachycardia, elevated blood pressure, altered mental state (delirium), myoclonus (muscle spasms), increased motor activity, irritability, hostility, and mood change. Severe manifestation can induce hyperpyrexia (excessively high fever), cardiovascular shock, or death. The risk of this syndrome

seems to be the greatest when an SSRI is administered in combination with a second serotonin-enhancing agent, such as an MAOI. For example, a person taking fluoxetine would have to be medication free for a full 5 weeks before being switched to an MAOI (5 weeks is the half-life for fluoxetine). If a client is already taking an MAOI, the person should wait at least 2 weeks before starting fluoxetine therapy. Other SSRIs have shorter periods of activity; for example, sertraline and paroxetine have half-lives of 2 weeks, so there would need to be a 2-week gap between different medications. Box 18-2 lists the signs and symptoms of central serotonin syndrome and gives emergency treatment guidelines. Box 18-3 is a useful tool for client and family teaching about the SSRIs.

New Atypical (Novel) Antidepressants. A newer group of antidepressants has come along, and more continue to be released. The latest at the time of publication of this book is duloxetine (Cymbalta). These novel antidepressants are all effective agents. However, because each of these drugs affects the reuptake of different neurotransmitters, they do not have similar effects nor do they have the same side effect profiles, unlike the SSRIs, TCAs, or MAOIs. Table 18-11 introduces these newer atypical antidepressants and identifies the main neurotransmitters involved. Each of these agents blocks different neurotransmitters and transmitter subtypes, which accounts for their strengths in targeting unique populations of depressed individuals as well as for their efficacy in treating other conditions. Table 18-12 lists the usual maintenance daily dose and presents some of the advantages and disadvantages of each of these atypical

TABLE 18-10

Selective Serotonin Reuptake Inhibitors (SSRIs): Overview of Adverse Reactions and Dosage Range

	Sedation	Weight Gain	Sexual Dysfunction	Other Key Adverse Reactions
SSRIs	Minimal	Rare	Yes	▪ Initial: nausea, loose bowel movements, headache, insomnia ▪ Toxic effects (rare): serotonin syndrome

Generic Name	Trade Name	Initial Dosage (mg/day)	Dosage After 4-8 Weeks (mg/day)	Maximum Dosage (mg/day)
Citalopram	Celexa	10-20	20-60	—
Fluoxetine	Prozac	10-20	20-80	80
Fluvoxamine*	Luvox	50-100	100-200	300
Paroxetine	Paxil	10-20	20-50	50
Sertraline	Zoloft	50	50-200	200
Escitalopram†	Lexapro	10	10-20	20

*Elderly clients and those with hepatic disease should start at 50% less than the standard dosages listed in the table. This applies to clients with coexisting panic or anxiety symptoms.
†Escitalopram is the single active isomer of citalopram, which gives it some advantages in the treatment of depression.

BOX 18-2

Symptoms and Interventions for Central Serotonin Syndrome

Symptoms
- Hyperactivity or restlessness
- Tachycardia → cardiovascular shock
- Fever → hyperpyrexia
- Elevated blood pressure
- Altered mental states (delirium)
- Irrationality, mood swings, hostility
- Seizures → status epilepticus
- Myoclonus, incoordination, tonic rigidity
- Abdominal pain, diarrhea, bloating
- Apnea → death

Emergency Measures
1. Remove offending agent(s)
2. Initiate symptomatic treatment:
   a. Serotonin receptor blockade: cyproheptadine, methysergide, propranolol
   b. Cooling blankets, chlorpromazine for hyperthermia
   c. Dantrolene, diazepam for muscle rigidity or rigors
   d. Anticonvulsants
   e. Artificial ventilation
   f. Paralysis

BOX 18-3

Client and Family Teaching About Selective Serotonin Reuptake Inhibitors (SSRIs)

- SSRIs may cause sexual dysfunction or lack of sex drive. Inform nurse or physician.
- SSRIs may cause insomnia, anxiety, and nervousness. Inform nurse or physician.
- SSRIs may interact with other medications. Be sure physician knows other medications client is taking (digoxin, warfarin). SSRIs should not be taken within 14 days of the last dose of a monoamine oxidase inhibitor.
- No over-the-counter drug should be taken without first notifying physician.
- Common side effects include fatigue, nausea, diarrhea, dry mouth, dizziness, tremor, and sexual dysfunction or lack of sex drive.
- Because of the potential for drowsiness and dizziness, client should not drive or operate machinery until these side effects are ruled out.
- Alcohol should be avoided.
- Liver and renal function tests should be performed and blood counts checked periodically.
- Medication should not be discontinued abruptly. If side effects become bothersome, client should ask physician about changing to a different drug. Abrupt cessation can lead to serotonin withdrawal.
- Any of the following symptoms should be reported to a physician immediately:
  - Increase in depression or suicidal thoughts
  - Rash or hives
  - Rapid heartbeat
  - Sore throat
  - Difficulty urinating
  - Fever, malaise
  - Anorexia and weight loss
  - Unusual bleeding
  - Initiation of hyperactive behavior
  - Severe headache

agents. Drug monographs for each of these newer antidepressants are found on the Evolve website.

Alprazolam. Alprazolam (Xanax) is a benzodiazepine anxiolytic (see Chapter 14). Although it is an effective drug for the management of anxiety disorders (e.g., panic disorders, agoraphobia), it is also as effective as the TCAs for the treatment of mild to moderate depression with anxiety features. Its side effect profile (sedation, minimal cardiovascular effects, lack of anticholinergic activity) can be advantageous for some individuals (Golden et al., 2004). The downside, however, is that the benzodiazepines can cause dependence and potentially severe withdrawal reactions after abrupt discontinuation.

Tricyclic Antidepressants. The tricyclic antidepressants (TCAs) inhibit the reuptake of norepinephrine and serotonin by the presynaptic neurons in the CNS. Therefore, the amount of time that norepinephrine and serotonin are available to the postsynaptic receptors is increased. This increase in norepinephrine and serotonin in the brain is believed to be responsible for mood elevations when TCAs are given to depressed persons.

The sedative effects of the TCAs are attributed to antihistamine (H₁ receptor) actions and somewhat to anticholinergic actions (Maxmen & Ward, 2002). Clients must take therapeutic doses of TCAs for 10 to 14 days or longer before these agents start to work.

The full effects may not be seen for 4 to 8 weeks. An effect on some symptoms of depression, such as insomnia and anorexia, may be noted earlier. Currently, a person who has had a positive response to TCA therapy would probably be maintained on that medication for 6 to 12 months to prevent an early relapse. Choice of TCA is based on the following:
- What has worked for the client or a family member in the past
- The drug's adverse effects

For example, for a client who is lethargic and fatigued, a more stimulating TCA, such as desipramine (Norpramin) or protriptyline (Vivactil) may be best. If a more sedating effect is needed for agitation or restlessness, drugs such as amitriptyline (Elavil) and doxepin (Sinequan) may be more appropriate choices.

TABLE 18-11

Newer Atypical (Novel) Antidepressants

Agent	Neurotransmitters Affected	May Help People with:
Bupropion (Wellbutrin, Zyban)	Blocks norepinephrine (NE) and dopamine (DA) reuptake (NDRI)	<ul><li>ADHD</li><li>Chronic fatigue syndrome</li><li>Rapid cycling bipolar II disorder</li><li>Sexual side effects from use of other antidepressants</li><li>Anxiety disorders (GAD, OCD, phobic disorders, PTSD, panic disorders)</li><li>Nicotine addiction (Zyban)</li></ul>
Trazodone (Desyrel)	Shows selective but moderate blockage of serotonin (5-HT2 receptor) (only used in conjunction with other drugs)	<ul><li>Elderly clients</li><li>SSRI-induced insomnia</li></ul>
Dual-Action Reuptake Inhibitors—SNRIs (Serotonin and Norepinephrine)		
Venlafaxine (Effexor)	Inhibits reuptake of serotonin (5-HT) and norepinephrine (NE) Inhibits dopamine (DA) to a lesser extent	<ul><li>Treatment-resistant depression</li><li>Chronic depression</li><li>Bipolar depression</li><li>Depression with ADHD</li><li>Medical illness and depression</li><li>Anxiety</li><li>Geriatric depression</li></ul>
Mirtazapine (Remeron)	Blocks serotonin (5-HT, 5-HT$_2$, 5-HT$_3$, 5-HT$_4$ receptors), is an α_2-adrenoreceptor antagonist (ACh), and blocks histamine (H$_1$) (enhances both nonadrenergic and serotonergic transmitters)	<ul><li>Sleep disturbances</li><li>Poor appetite</li><li>Pain</li><li>Medical illness with depression</li><li>Anxiety</li><li>SSRI-induced sexual dysfunction</li></ul>
Duloxetine (Cymbalta)	Inhibits reuptake of serotonin (5-HT) and norepinephrine (NE) (SNRI) Inhibits dopamine (DA) to a lesser extent	<ul><li>Major depression</li><li>Geriatric depression</li></ul>
Selective Norepinephrine Reuptake Inhibitors (NRIs)		
Roboxetine (Vestra, Edronax)*	A selective norepinephrine reuptake inhibitor (NE, ACh)	<ul><li>SSRI-related sexual dysfunction</li><li>Lethargy secondary to depression</li><li>Cognitive difficulties secondary to depression</li><li>Impaired social functioning</li><li>Anxiety disorders (panic attacks)</li></ul>

ACh, Acetylcholine; *ADHD*, attention deficit hyperactivity disorder; *GAD*, generalized anxiety disorder; *OCD*, obsessive-compulsive disorder; *PTSD*, posttraumatic stress disorder; *SSRI*, selective serotonin reuptake inhibitor.
*Roboxetine is not yet approved for the U.S. market. It is available in Europe.

Regardless of which TCA is given, the dosage should always be low initially and should be increased gradually. Caution should be used, especially in elderly persons, for whom slow drug metabolism may be a problem. Trimipramine (Surmontil) is a good choice for the elderly because of its low side effects and its rapid effects in promoting sleep. The rule of thumb for the elderly is always, **"Start low, go slow."**

Common Adverse Reactions. The chemical structure of the TCAs is similar to that of the antipsychotic medications. Therefore, the **anticholinergic** actions are similar (e.g., dry mouth, blurred vision, tachycardia, constipation, urinary retention, and esophageal reflux). These side effects are both more common and more severe in clients taking antidepressants. These adverse effects are usually not serious and are often transitory, but **urinary retention and severe constipation warrant immediate medical attention.**

The α-adrenergic blockade of the TCAs can produce postural-orthostatic hypotension and tachycardia. Postural hypotension can lead to dizziness and increase the risk of falls.

Administering the total daily dose of TCA at night is beneficial for two reasons. First, most TCAs have sedative effects and thereby aid sleep. Second, the minor side effects occur during sleep, which increases compliance with drug therapy. Table 18-13 reviews the

TABLE 18-12

Newer Atypical Agents: Dosages and Effects

Agent	Usual Dosage (mg/day)	Advantages	Adverse Effects
Bupropion (Wellbutrin) (Zyban)	200-450 150-300	■ Sexual dysfunction rare ■ No weight gain ■ Stimulant properties ■ Antianxiety properties	■ Medication-induced seizures if over 300 mg ■ High seizure risk in "at risk" individuals ■ Some nausea
Trazodone (Desyrel)	150-400	■ No anticholinergic side effects,* low potential for cardiac effects ■ In conjunction with other anti-depressants, can aid sleep	■ Possible priapism† ■ Postural hypotension ■ Weight gain ■ Memory dysfunction
Dual-Action Reuptake Inhibitors—SNRIs (Serotonin and Norepinephrine)			
Venlafaxine (Effexor)	25-375	■ Useful for treatment-resistant chronic depression ■ Low potential for drug interaction	■ Possible increase in blood pressure (10-15 mm Hg) ■ Possible somnolence, dry mouth, and dizziness
Mirtazapine (Remeron)	15-45	■ Antidote to SSRI sexual dysfunction ■ Noninterference with sleep ■ Low interference with metabolism of other drugs ■ Anxiolytic properties	■ Strong sedating effect ■ Possible increased appetite, weight gain, and cholesterol elevation
Duloxetine (Cymbalta)	30-60 mg bid	■ Response to medication within 1-4 weeks ■ Mild side effects	■ Nausea ■ Somnolence ■ Dry mouth ■ Constipation ■ Decreased appetite ■ Increased sweating ■ Fatigue ■ Twice-a-day dosing
Selective Norepinephrine Reuptake Inhibitors (NRIs)			
Roboxetine (Vestra, Edronax)‡	2-8	■ Anticataleptic effects§ ■ Nonsedating	■ Anticholinergic side effects ■ Decreased libido ■ Potential for drug interactions ■ Twice-a-day dosing ■ Half dose with hepatic disease

*Anticholinergic side effects include dry mouth, blurred vision, constipation, urinary retention, tachycardia, and possible confusion.
†Priapism is prolonged painful penile erection that may warrant surgery.
‡Not yet approved by the U.S. Food and Drug Administration.
§Catalepsy is characterized by a trancelike state of consciousness and a posture in which the limbs hold any position (waxy flexibility). An anticataleptic agent helps minimize/prevent this phenomenon in clients with schizophrenia.

common side effects, TCAs in common use, and dosage range.

Potential Toxic Effects. The most serious effects of the TCAs are cardiovascular: dysrhythmias, tachycardia, myocardial infarction, and heart block have been reported. Because the cardiac side effects are so serious, TCA use is considered a risk in clients with cardiac disease and in the elderly. Clients should have a thorough cardiac workup before beginning TCA therapy.

Adverse Drug Interactions. Individuals taking TCAs can have adverse reactions to numerous other medications. For example, use of an MAOI along with a TCA is contraindicated. A few of the more common

medications usually *not* given while TCAs are being used are listed in Box 18-4. Any client who is taking any of these medications along with a TCA should have medical clearance, because some of the reactions can be fatal.

Use of antidepressants may precipitate a psychotic episode in a person with schizophrenia. An antidepressant can precipitate a manic episode in a client with bipolar disorder. Depressed clients with bipolar disorder often receive lithium along with the antidepressant.

Contraindications. People who have recently had a myocardial infarction (or other cardiovascular problems), those with narrow-angle glaucoma or a his-

TABLE 18-13

Tricyclic Antidepressants (TCAs): Overview of Adverse Reactions and Dosage Range

	Sedation	Weight Gain	Sexual Dysfunction	Other Key Adverse Reactions
TCAs	Minimal	Rare	Yes	▪ Anticholinergic side effects* ▪ Orthostasis ▪ CHF effects (tachycardia, arrhythmias, ECG changes, heart failure) ▪ Lethal in overdose

Generic Name	Trade Name	Initial Dosage (mg/day)	Therapeutic Dosage Range (mg/day)	Maximum Dosage (mg/day)
Amitriptyline	Elavil, Endep	25-50	150-300	300
Amoxapine	Asendin	50-100	150-450	400
Desipramine	Norpramin, Pertofrane	25-50	75-200	300
Doxepin	Adapin, Sinequan	25-50	150-300	300
Imipramine	Tofranil	25-50	150-300	300
Nortriptyline	Aventyl, Pamelor	10-25	50-150	150
Protriptyline	Vivactil	10	15-45	60
Trimipramine	Surmontil	25-50	100-250	300
Maprotiline	Ludiomil	25-50	100-150	225

*Anticholinergic side effects include dry mouth, blurred vision, constipation, urinary retention, tachycardia, and possible confusion.
CHF, Congestive heart failure; *ECG,* electrocardiograph.

BOX 18-4

Drugs to Be Used with Caution in Clients Taking a Tricyclic Antidepressant

▪ Phenothiazines
▪ Barbiturates
▪ Monoamine oxidase inhibitors
▪ Disulfiram (Antabuse)
▪ Oral contraceptives (or other estrogen preparations)
▪ Anticoagulants
▪ Some antihypertensives (clonidine, guanethidine, reserpine)
▪ Benzodiazepines
▪ Alcohol
▪ Nicotine

BOX 18-5

Client and Family Teaching About Tricyclic Antidepressants (TCAs)

▪ The client and family should be told that mood elevation may take from 7 to 28 days. Up to 6 to 8 weeks may be required for the full effect to be reached and for major depressive symptoms to subside.
▪ The family should reinforce this frequently to the depressed family member, because depressed people have trouble remembering and respond to ongoing reassurance.
▪ The client should be reassured that drowsiness, dizziness, and hypotension usually subside after the first few weeks.
▪ When the client starts taking TCAs, the client should be cautioned to be careful working around machines, driving cars, and crossing streets because of possible altered reflexes, drowsiness, or dizziness.
▪ Alcohol can block the effects of antidepressants. The client should be told to refrain from drinking.
▪ If possible, the client should take the full dose at bedtime to reduce the experience of side effects during the day.
▪ If the client forgets the bedtime dose (or the once-a-day dose), the client should take the dose within 3 hours; otherwise the client should wait until the usual medication time the next day. The client should *not* double the dose.
▪ Suddenly stopping TCAs can cause nausea, altered heartbeat, nightmares, and cold sweats in 2 to 4 days. The client should call the physician or take one dose of TCA until the physician can be contacted.

tory of seizures, and pregnant women should not be treated with TCAs, except with extreme caution and careful monitoring.

Client Teaching. Teaching clients and their family members about medications is an expected nursing responsibility. Medication teaching is begun in the hospital. The nurse or another qualified health care provider needs to review with the client and, whenever possible, one or more family members the client's medications, expected side effects, and necessary client precautions. Areas for the nurse to discuss when teaching clients and their families about TCA therapy are presented in Box 18-5. Clients and family members need to have written information for all medications that will be taken at home.

Monoamine Oxidase Inhibitors. The enzyme monoamine oxidase is responsible for inactivating certain brain amines such as norepinephrine, serotonin, dopamine, and tyramine. When a person ingests an MAOI, these amines do not get inactivated, or broken down, and there is an increase of these amines available for synaptic release in the brain. This increase in norepinephrine, serotonin, and dopamine is the desired effect because these neurotransmitters can raise the mood of depressed persons. The increase in tyramine, on the other hand, poses a problem. When the level of the amine tyramine increases and it is not broken down by monoamine oxidase, this increase can lead to high blood pressure, hypertensive crisis, and eventually to a cerebrovascular accident. Therefore, people taking these drugs must reduce their intake of tyramine, so that tyramine does not rise to dangerous levels. For that reason, foods and drugs that are high in tyramine have to be curtailed or the depressed individual can experience a hypertensive crisis. See Table 18-14 for foods and Box 18-6 for medications that are high in tyramine and that need to be avoided or restricted.

Because people who are depressed are often lethargic, confused, and apathetic, adhering to strict dietary limitations may not be feasible. That is why MAOIs,

---

BOX 18-6

Drugs That Can Interact with Monoamine Oxidase Inhibitors

Use of the following drugs should be restricted in clients taking monoamine oxidase inhibitors:

- Over-the-counter medications for colds, allergies, or congestion (any product containing ephedrine, phenylephrine hydrochloride, or phenylpropanolamine)
- Tricyclic antidepressants (imipramine, amitriptyline)
- Narcotics
- Antihypertensives (methyldopa, guanethidine, reserpine)
- Amine precursors (levodopa, L-tryptophan)
- Sedatives (alcohol, barbiturates, benzodiazepines)
- General anesthetics
- Stimulants (amphetamines, cocaine)

TABLE 18-14

Foods That Can Interact with Monoamine Oxidase Inhibitors

	Foods That Contain Tyramine	
Category	**Unsafe Foods (High Tyramine Content)**	**Safe Foods (Little or No Tyramine)**
Vegetables	Avocados, especially if overripe; fermented bean curd; fermented soybean; soybean paste; sauerkraut	Most vegetables
Fruits	Figs, especially if overripe; bananas, in large amounts	Most fruits
Meats	Meats that are fermented, smoked, or otherwise aged; spoiled meats; liver, unless very fresh; beef and chicken liver	Meats that are known to be fresh (exercise caution in restaurants; meats may not be fresh)
Sausages	Fermented varieties; bologna, pepperoni, salami, others	Nonfermented varieties
Fish	Dried, pickled, or cured fish; fish that is fermented, smoked, or otherwise aged; spoiled fish	Fish that is known to be fresh; vacuum-packed fish, if eaten promptly or refrigerated only briefly after opening
Milk, milk products	Practically all cheeses	Milk, yogurt, cottage cheese, cream cheese
Foods with yeast	Yeast extract (e.g., Marmite, Bovril)	Baked goods that contain yeast
Beer, wine	Some imported beers, Chianti	Major domestic brands of beer; most wines
Other foods	Protein dietary supplements; soups (may contain protein extract); shrimp paste; soy sauce	

Foods That Contain Other Vasopressors	
Food	**Comments**
Chocolate	Contains phenylethylamine, a pressor agent; large amounts can cause a reaction.
Fava beans	Contain dopamine, a pressor agent; reactions are most likely with overripe beans.
Ginseng	Headache, tremulousness, and manialike reactions have occurred.
Caffeinated beverages	Caffeine is a weak pressor agent; large amounts may cause a reaction.

From Lehne, R. A., et al. (2001). *Pharmacology for nursing* (4th ed.). Philadelphia: Saunders.

although highly effective, are not often given as a first-line treatment.

MAOIs are particularly effective for people with atypical depression as well as some other disorders (e.g., panic disorder, social phobia, generalized anxiety disorder, obsessive-compulsive disorder, posttraumatic stress disorder, and bulimia). The MAOIs commonly used in the United States at present are phenelzine (Nardil) and tranylcypromine sulfate (Parnate).

Common Adverse Reactions. Some common and troublesome long-term side effects of the MAOIs are orthostatic hypotension, weight gain, edema, change in cardiac rate and rhythm, constipation, urinary hesitancy, sexual dysfunction, vertigo, overactivity, muscle twitching, hypomanic and manic behavior, insomnia, weakness, and fatigue.

Potential Toxic Effects. The most serious reaction to the MAOIs is an increase in blood pressure, with the possible development of intracranial hemorrhage, hyperpyrexia, convulsions, coma, and death. Therefore, routine monitoring of blood pressure, especially during the first 6 weeks of treatment, is necessary.

Because so many other drugs, foods, and beverages can show adverse interactions with the MAOIs, increase in blood pressure is a constant concern. The beginning of a hypertensive crisis usually occurs within a few hours of ingestion of the contraindicated substance. The crisis may begin with headaches; stiff or sore neck; palpitations; increase or decrease in heart rate, often associated with chest pain; nausea; vomiting; or increase in temperature (pyrexia). When a hypertensive crisis is suspected, immediate medical attention is crucial. Antihypertensive medications, such as phentolamine (Regitine), are slowly administered intravenously. Pyrexia is treated with hypothermic blankets or ice packs. Table 18-15 identifies common side effects and toxic effects of the MAOIs. Box 18-7 can be used as a teaching guide for clients taking an MAOI and their families.

Contraindications. Use of MAOIs may be contraindicated when one of the following is present:

- Cerebrovascular disease
- Hypertension and congestive heart failure
- Liver disease
- Consumption of foods containing tyramine, tryptophan, and dopamine (see Table 18-14)
- Use of certain medications (see Box 18-6)
- Recurrent or severe headaches
- Surgery in the previous 10 to 14 days
- Age younger than 16 years

See Table 18-16 for an overview of side effects, MAOIs in current use, and dosage range.

Clients who do not improve with initial therapy often show improvement when switched to another class of antidepressants or when a drug from another class is added to the therapy.

TABLE 18-15

Common Adverse Reactions to and Toxic Effects of Monoamine Oxidase Inhibitors

Adverse Reactions	Comments
▪ Hypotension ▪ Sedation, weakness, fatigue ▪ Insomnia ▪ Changes in cardiac rhythm ▪ Muscle cramps ▪ Anorgasmia or sexual impotence ▪ Urinary hesitancy or constipation ▪ Weight gain	Hypotension is the most critical side effect (10%); the elderly, especially, may sustain injuries from it.

Toxic Effects	Comments

Hypertensive crisis*
▪ Severe headache
▪ Stiff, sore neck
▪ Flushing, cold, clammy skin
▪ Tachycardia
▪ Severe nosebleeds, dilated pupils
▪ Chest pains, stroke, coma, death
▪ Nausea and vomiting
	1. Client should go to local emergency department immediately—blood pressure should be checked.
	2. One of the following may be given to lower blood pressure:
	  ▪ 5 mg intravenous phentolamine (Regitine) or
	  ▪ Oral chlorpromazine or
	  ▪ Nifedipine (Procardia) (calcium channel blocker), 10 mg sublingually

*Related to interaction with foodstuffs and cold medication.

BOX 18-7

Client and Family Teaching About Monoamine Oxidase Inhibitors (MAOIs)

- Tell the client and the client's family to avoid certain foods and all medications (especially cold remedies) unless prescribed by and discussed with the client's physician (see Table 18-14 and Box 18-6 for specific food and drug restrictions).
- Give the client a wallet card describing the MAOI regimen.
- Instruct the client to avoid Chinese restaurants (sherry, brewer's yeast, and other contraindicated products may be used).
- Tell the client to go to the emergency department immediately if he or she has a severe headache.
- Ideally, monitor the client's blood pressure during the first 6 weeks of treatment (for both hypotensive and hypertensive effects).
- Instruct the client that, after the MAOI is stopped, dietary and drug restrictions should be maintained for 14 days.

TABLE 18-16

Monamine Oxidase Inhibitors (MAOIs): Overview of Adverse Reactions and Dosage Range

	Sedation	Weight Gain	Sexual Dysfunction	Other Key Adverse Reactions
MAOIs	Rare	Yes	Yes	■ Orthostatic hypotension ■ Insomnia ■ Peripheral edema (avoid use in patients with CHF) ■ Avoid phenelzine in patients with hepatitis ■ Potential life-threatening drug interactions ■ Strict dietary and medication restrictions (see Table 18-14 and Box 18-6)

Generic Name	Trade Name	Initial Dosage (mg/day)	Dosage After 4-8 Weeks (mg/day)	Maximum Dosage (mg/day)
Phenelzine	Nardil	45-75	45-75	75
Tranylcypromine	Parnate	20-30	20-60	30
Reversible Inhibitors of MAO Not Yet Available in United States				
Moclobemide	Manerix, Aurorix	300	300-600	900

Electroconvulsive Therapy

ECT remains one of the most effective yet most stigmatized treatments for depression (NIMH, 2000a). ECT can achieve a higher than 90% remission rate in depressed clients within 1 to 2 weeks. Because 20% to 30% of depressed individuals do not respond to antidepressants, ECT remains an effective treatment for depression (Mendelowitz, Dawkins, & Lieberman, 2000). According to Dubovsky and Buzan (1999), ECT is indicated when

- There is a need for a rapid, definitive response when a client is suicidal or homicidal.
- A client is in extreme agitation or stupor.
- The risks of other treatments outweigh the risks of ECT.
- The client has a history of poor drug response, a history of good ECT response, or both.
- The client prefers it.

ECT is useful in treating clients with major depressive and bipolar depressive disorders, especially when psychotic symptoms are present (delusions of guilt, somatic delusions, or delusions of infidelity). Clients who have depression with marked psychomotor retardation and stupor also respond well.

ECT is also indicated for manic clients whose conditions are resistant to treatment with lithium and antipsychotic drugs and for clients who are rapid cyclers. A **rapid cycler** is a client with bipolar disorder who has many episodes of mood swings close together (four or more in 1 year). People with schizophrenia (especially catatonia), those with schizoaffective syndromes, psychotic clients who are pregnant, and clients with Parkinson's disease can also benefit from ECT.

ECT is not necessarily effective, however, in clients with DD, those with atypical depression and personality disorders, those with drug dependence, or those with depression secondary to situational or social difficulties.

The usual course of ECT for a depressed client is two or three treatments per week to a total of 6 to 12 treatments. Although no absolute contraindications to ECT exist, several conditions pose particular risks, and special attention and skill are required in treating clients with these conditions. These conditions include recent myocardial infarction, cerebrovascular accident, and cerebrovascular malformation or intracranial mass lesion (Marangell et al., 2004). Clients with these high-risk conditions usually are not treated with ECT unless the need is compelling, and an additional special consent for this high-risk procedure is obtained.

Procedure. The procedure is explained to the client, and informed consent is obtained if the client is being treated voluntarily. For a client treated involuntarily, when informed consent cannot be obtained, permission may be obtained from the next of kin, although in some states treatment must be court ordered.

Use of a general anesthetic (e.g., a short-acting barbiturate such as methohexital sodium [Brevital]) and muscle-paralyzing agents (e.g., succinylcholine) have revolutionized the comfort and safety of ECT.

Potential Adverse Reactions. On awakening from ECT, the client may be confused and disoriented. The nurse and family may need to orient the client frequently during the course of treatment. Many clients state that they have memory deficits for the first few weeks after the course of treatment. Memory usually, although not always, recovers. ECT is not a permanent cure for depression, and maintenance treatment with TCAs or lithium decreases the relapse rate. Maintenance ECT (once a week to once a month) may also help to decrease relapse rates for clients with recurrent depression.

Integrative Approaches for Depression

Zahourek (2000) highlights an array of complementary, alternative, and integrative approaches in the treatment of depression that includes use of supplements, exercise, massage, light therapy, homeopathy, and rapid-rate transcranial magnetic stimulation (TMS). Many products are on the market over the counter for the treatment of dysphoric mood. Herbal products and supplements for depression have become a multimillion-dollar industry; however, the long-term effects of these products have not been studied nor are they presently known. Zahourek (2000) warns that, because many of these methods are not supported by research, they should be used with caution. It is important for psychiatric nurses to be knowledgeable about these alternatives so they can serve as a resource for clients. The approaches briefly discussed here are light therapy, use of St. John's wort, exercise, and TMS. Refer to Chapter 37 for more discussion of alternative and complementary approaches.

Light Therapy

Light therapy is the first-line treatment for SAD (see Table 18-3). People with SAD often live in climates in which there are marked seasonal differences in the amount of daylight. Seasonal variations in mood disorders in the southern hemisphere are the reverse of those in the northern hemisphere. Light therapy may also be useful as an adjunct in treating chronic MDD or dysthymia with seasonal exacerbations (APA, 2000b).

Light therapy is thought to be effective because of the influence of light on melatonin. Melatonin is secreted by the pineal gland and is necessary for maintaining and shifting biological rhythms. Exposure to light suppresses the nocturnal secretion of melatonin, which seems to have a therapeutic effect on people with SAD (Zahourek, 2000b). Treatments consist of exposure to light balanced to resemble sunlight; for example, a 10,000-lux light box is slanted toward the client's face to provide exposure for 30 minutes a day, either once or in two divided doses (APA, 2000b). Light treatment has been found to be as effective in reducing depressive symptoms as are medications in people with SAD (Zahourek, 2000).

St. John's Wort

St. John's wort (*Hypericum perforatum)* is a whole plant product with antidepressant properties that is not regulated by the U.S. FDA. In a recent review of 14 short-term double-blind studies in people with mild to moderate depression, St. John's wort demonstrated superior efficacy compared to placebo and was generally comparable in effect to low-dose TCAs (APA,

2000b). The herb is not to be taken in certain situations (e.g., major depression, pregnancy, age younger than 2 years) (Fuller & Sajatovic, 2000). Nor should St. John's wort be taken with certain substances, such as amphetamines or other stimulants, other antidepressants (MAOIs, SSRIs), levodopa, and 5-HT (Fuller & Sajatovic, 2000). When the herb is taken with other antidepressant medications, there is a potential for additive effects and central serotonin syndrome (Zahourek, 2000). A person taking this herb should also avoid tyramine-containing foods (see Table 18-14).

Research has shown that St. John's wort may also interact with certain drugs that control human immunodeficiency virus (HIV) infection, chemotherapeutic and other anticancer drugs, and drugs that help prevent the body from rejecting transplanted organs (National Center for Complementary and Alternative Medicine, 2004). Other adverse reactions include photosensitivity and hypersensitivity to sunlight, skin rash, gastrointestinal upset, sinus tachycardia, and abdominal pain. Nangia, Syed, and Doraiswamy (2000) have stressed the need for dose standardization and trials of adequate length before St. John's wort can be used as a first-line antidepressant.

Exercise

There is substantial evidence that exercise can enhance mood and reduce symptoms of depression (Mayo Foundation for Medical Education and Research, 2003). Andrew Weil's prescription is for 30 minutes of aerobic exercise at least five times per week (Zahourek, 2000).

Transcranial Magnetic Stimulation

Transcranial magnetic stimulation (TMS) is a newer technology that holds great promise, but clinical trials of TMS are in the early stages. TMS applies the principles of electromagnetism to deliver an electrical field to the cerebral cortices, but unlike in ECT, the waves do not result in generalized seizure activity (Rosenbaum, 2004). Early studies of this technique support further research into its use in the treatment of serious, relapsing medication-resistant depression. This is a potential treatment for the future, and some believe there is enough evidence to indicate that it will eventually become an accepted treatment for depression.

Future of Treatment

There is a great need for earlier detection, earlier interventions, achievement of remission, prevention of progression, and integration of neuroscience and behavioral science in the treatment of depression (Greden, 2004).

- There is a need to screen high-risk ages and groups:
  - Individuals in late adolescence and early adulthood
  - Women in reproductive years

– Adults and elderly with medical problems (e.g., pain)
– People with a family history of depression

■ There is a need for education, particularly about the linkage between physical symptoms and depression.

■ Psychopharmacological treatment should be augmented with cognitive-behavioral therapies.

■ There is need for more supplementary strategies, such as the following:

– Promotion of sleep hygiene
– Increase in exercise
– Better total health care

Greden (2004) speculates that the future will bring more genetic screening and pharmacogenetics and that the use of neuroimaging will become a diagnostic tool and will not be restricted to research. These advances are consistent with the goals of the President's New Freedom Commission on Mental Health (2003) for transforming mental health care in America (http://www.mentalhealthcommission.gov/reports/finalreport/toc.html).

■ EVALUATION

Short-term indicators and outcome criteria are frequently evaluated. For example, if the client comes into the unit with suicidal thoughts, the nurse evaluates whether suicidal thoughts are still present, whether the depressed person is able to state alternatives to suicidal impulses in the future, whether he or she is able to explore thoughts and feelings that precede suicidal impulses, and so forth. Outcomes relating to thought processes, self-esteem, and social interactions are frequently formulated because these areas are often problematic in people who are depressed. Physical needs warrant nursing or medical attention. If a person has lost weight because of anorexia, is the appetite returning? If a person was constipated, are the bowels now functioning normally? If the person was suffering from insomnia, is he or she now getting 6 to 8 hours of sleep per night?

If the indicators have not been met, an analysis of the data, nursing diagnoses, goals, and planned nursing interventions is made. The care plan is reassessed and reformulated when necessary.

CASE STUDY and NURSING CARE PLAN 18-1 Depression

Ms. Olston is a 35-year-old executive secretary. She has been divorced for 3 years and has two sons, 11 and 13 years of age. She is brought into the emergency department (ED) by her neighbor. She has some slashes on her wrists and is bleeding. The neighbor states that both of Ms. Olston's sons are visiting their father for the summer. Ms. Olston has become more and more despondent since terminating a 2-year relationship with a married man 4 weeks previously. According to the neighbor, for 3 years after her divorce, Ms. Olston talked constantly about not being pretty or good enough and doubted that anyone could really love her. The neighbor states that Ms. Olston has been withdrawn for at least 3 years. After the relationship with her boyfriend ended, she became even more withdrawn and sullen. Ms. Olston is about 20 lb overweight, and her neighbor states that Ms. Olston often stays awake late into the night, drinking by herself and watching television. She sleeps through most of the day on the weekends.

After receiving treatment in the ED, Ms. Olston is seen by a psychiatrist. The initial diagnosis is dysthymia with suicidal ideation. A decision is made to hospitalize her briefly for suicide observation and evaluation for appropriate treatment.

The nurse, Ms. Weston, admits Ms. Olston to the unit from the ED.

Nurse: Hello, Ms. Olston, I'm Marcia Weston. I will be your primary nurse.

Ms. Olston: Yeah . . . I don't need a nurse, a doctor, or anyone else. I just want to get away from this pain.

Nurse: You want to get away from your pain?

Ms. Olston: I just said that, didn't I? Oh, what's the use? No one understands.

Nurse: I would like to understand, Ms. Olston.

Ms. Olston: Look at me. I'm fat . . . ugly . . . and no good to anyone. No one wants me.

Nurse: Who doesn't want you?

Ms. Olston: My husband didn't want me . . . and now Jerry left me to go back to his wife.

Nurse: You think because Jerry went back to his wife that no one else could care for you?

Ms. Olston: Well . . . he doesn't anyway.

Nurse: Because he doesn't care, you believe that no one else cares about you?

Ms. Olston: Yes . . .

Nurse: Who do you care about?

Ms. Olston: No one . . . except my sons. . . . I do love my sons, even though I don't often show it.

Nurse: Tell me more about your sons.

Ms. Weston continues to speak with Ms. Olston. Ms. Olston talks about her sons with some affect and apparent affection; however, she continues to state that she does not think of herself as worthwhile.

Continued

Self-Assessment

Ms. Weston is aware that, when clients are depressed, they can be negative, think life is hopeless, and be hostile toward those who want to help. When Ms. Weston was new to the unit, she withdrew from depressed clients and sought out clients who appeared more hopeful and appreciative of her efforts. The unit coordinator was very supportive of Ms. Weston when she was first on the unit. Ms. Weston, along with other staff, was sent to in-service education sessions on working with depressed clients and was encouraged to speak up in staff meetings about the feelings that many of these depressed clients evoked in her. As a primary nurse, she was assigned a variety of clients. She found that as time went on, with the support of her peers and the opportunity to speak up at staff meetings, she was able to take what clients said less personally and not feel so responsible when clients did not respond as fast as she would like. After 2 years, she had had the experience of seeing many clients who seemed hopeless and despondent on admission respond well to nursing and medical interventions and go on to lead full and satisfying lives. This also made it easier for Ms. Weston to understand that, even though the client may think that life is hopeless and may believe that there is nothing in life to live for, change is always possible.

■ ASSESSMENT

Objective Data

- Slashed her wrists
- Recently broke off with boyfriend
- Has thought poorly of herself for 3 years, since divorce
- Has two sons she cares about
- Is 20 lb overweight
- Stays awake late at night, drinking by herself
- Has been withdrawn since divorce

Subjective Data

- "No one could ever love me."
- "I'm not good enough."
- "I just want to get rid of this pain."
- "I'm fat and ugly . . . no good to anyone."
- "I do love my sons, although I don't always show it."

■ NURSING DIAGNOSIS (NANDA)

The nurse evaluates Ms. Olston's strengths and weaknesses and decides to concentrate on two initial nursing diagnoses that seem to have the highest priority.

1. *Risk for suicide* related to separation from 2-year relationship, as evidenced by actual suicide attempt
   - Slashed her wrists
   - Recently broke off with boyfriend
   - Drinks at night by herself
   - Withdrawn for 3 years since divorce

2. *Situational low self-esteem* related to divorce and recent termination of love relationship, as evidenced by derogatory statements about self
   - "I'm not good enough."
   - "No one could ever love me."
   - "I'm fat and ugly . . . no good to anyone."
   - "I do love my sons, although I don't always show it."

■ OUTCOME CRITERIA (NOC)

Client refrains from attempting suicide.

■ PLANNING

Because Ms. Olston is discharged after 48 hours, the issue of disturbance in self-esteem continues to be addressed in her therapy after discharge. Ms. Weston later reviews the goals for her work with Ms. Olston in the community.

■ INTERVENTION (NIC)

Ms. Olston's plan of care is personalized as follows:

Short-Term Goal	Intervention	Rationale	Evaluation
1. Client expresses at least one reason to live, and this is apparent by the second day of hospitalization.	1a. Observe client every 15 minutes while she is suicidal. 1b. Remove all dangerous objects from client. 1c. Obtain a "no self-harm" contract with client for a specific period of time to be renegotiated. 1d. Spend regularly scheduled periods of time with client throughout the day. 1e. Assist client in evaluating positive as well as negative aspects of her life. 1f. Encourage appropriate expression of angry feelings. 1g. Accept client's negativism.	1a,b. Client safety is ensured. Impulsive self-harmful behavior is minimized. 1c. May help client gain a sense of control and a feeling of responsibility. 1d. This interaction reinforces that client is worthwhile, builds up experience to begin to relate better to nurse on one-to-one basis. 1e. A depressed person is often unable to acknowledge any positive aspects of her life unless they are pointed out by others. 1f. Providing for expression of pent-up hostility in a safe environment can reinforce more adaptive methods of releasing tension and may minimize need to act out self-directed anger. 1g. Acceptance enhances feelings of self-worth.	GOAL MET By the end of the second day, Ms. Olston states she really did not want to die, she just couldn't stand the loneliness in her life. She states that she loves her sons and would never want to hurt them.
2. Client will identify two outside supports she can call upon if she feels suicidal in the future.	2a. Explore usual coping behaviors. 2b. Assist client in identifying members of her support system. 2c. Suggest a number of community-based support groups she might wish to discuss or visit (e.g., hotlines, support groups, women's groups). 2d. Assist client in identifying realistic alternatives that she is willing to use.	2a. Behaviors that need reinforcing and new coping skills that need to be introduced can be identified. 2b. Strengths and weaknesses in support available can be evaluated. 2c. Client needs to be aware of community supports to use them. 2d. Unless client is in agreement with any plan, she will be unable or unwilling to follow through in a crisis.	GOAL MET By discharge, Ms. Olston states that she is definitely going to try cognitive-behavioral therapy. She also discusses joining a women's support group that meets once a week in a neighboring town.

■ EVALUATION

During the course of her work with Ms. Weston, Ms. Olston decides to go to some meetings of Parents Without Partners. She states that she is looking forward to getting back to work and feels much more hopeful about her life. She has also lost 3 lb while attending Weight Watchers. She states, "I need to get back into the world." Although Ms. Olston still has negative thoughts about herself, she admits to feeling more hopeful and better about herself, and she has learned important tools to deal with her negative thoughts.

evolve Visit the Evolve website at **http://evolve.elsevier.com/Varcarolis** for a full case study of this client and more case studies and nursing care plans.

■ ■ ■ KEY POINTS to REMEMBER

- Depression is probably the most commonly seen psychiatric disorder in the health care system.
- There are a number of subtypes of depression and depressive clinical phenomena. The two primary depressive disorders are MDD and DD.
- The symptoms in major depression are usually severe enough to interfere with a person's social or occupational functioning. A person with MDD may or may not have psychotic symptoms, and the symptoms a person usually exhibits during a major depression are different from the characteristics of the normal premorbid personality.
- In dysthymia, the symptoms are often chronic (lasting at least 2 years) and are considered mild to moderate. Usually, a person's social or occupational functioning is not greatly impaired. The symptoms in a dysthymic depression are often congruent with the person's usual pattern of functioning.
- Many theories exist about the cause of depression. The most accepted is psychophysiological theory; however, cognitive theory, learned helplessness theory, and psychodynamic and life events issues help explain triggers to depression and maintenance of depressive thoughts and feelings.
- Nursing assessment includes the evaluation of affect, thought processes (especially suicidal thoughts), feelings, physical behavior, and communication. The nurse also needs to be aware of the symptoms that mask depression.
- Nursing diagnoses can be numerous. Depressed individuals are always evaluated for *risk for suicide*. Some other common nursing diagnoses are *disturbed thought processes, chronic low self-esteem, imbalanced nutrition, constipation, disturbed sleep pattern, ineffective coping*, and *disabled family coping*.
- Working with people who are depressed can evoke intense feelings of hopelessness and frustration in health care workers. Initially, nurses need support and guidance to clarify realistic expectations of themselves and their clients and to sort out personal feelings from those communicated by the client via empathy. Peer supervision and individual supervision with an experienced nurse clinician or a psychiatric social worker or psychologist are useful in increasing therapeutic potential.
- Interventions with clients who are depressed involve several approaches. Basic level interventions include using specific principles of communication, planning activities of daily living, administering or participating in psychopharmacological therapy, maintaining a therapeutic environment, and teaching clients about the biochemical aspects of depression.
- Advanced practice interventions may include several short-term psychotherapies that are effective in the treatment of depression, including IPT, CBT, skills training (assertiveness and social skills), and some forms of group therapy.
- Evaluation is ongoing throughout the nursing process, and clients' outcomes are compared with the stated outcome criteria and short-term and intermediate indicators. The care plan is revised by use of the evaluation process when indicators are not being met.

■ ■ ■

Visit the Evolve website at **http://evolve.elsevier.com/Varcarolis** for a posttest on the content in this chapter. *evolve*

Critical Thinking and Chapter Review

Visit the Evolve website at **http://evolve.elsevier.com/Varcarolis/foundations** for additional self-study exercises.
evolve

■ ■ ■ CRITICAL THINKING

1. You are spending time with Mr. Plotsky, who is being given a workup for depression. He hardly makes eye contact, he slouches in his seat, and his expression appears blank, although sad. Mr. Plotsky has had numerous bouts of major depression in the past and says to you, "This will be my last depression. . . . I will never go through this again."

   A. If safety is the first concern, what are the appropriate questions to ask Mr. Plotsky at this time?
   B. Give an example of the kinds of signs and symptoms you might find when you assess a client with depression in terms of behaviors, thought processes, activities of daily living, and ability to function at work and at home?

   C. Mr. Plotsky tells you that he has been on every medication there is but that none have worked. He asks you about the herb St. John's wort. What is some information he should have about its effectiveness for severe depression, its interactions with other antidepressants, and its regulatory status?
   D. What might be some somatic options for a person who is resistant to antidepressant medications?
   E. Mr. Plotsky asks what causes depression. In simple terms, how might you respond to his query?
   F. Mr. Plotsky tells you that he has never tried therapy because he thinks it is for babies. What information could you give him about various therapeutic modalities that have proven effective for some other depressed clients?

Critical Thinking and Chapter Review—cont'd

Visit the Evolve website at **http://evolve.elsevier.com/Varcarolis/foundations** for additional self-study exercises.

2. When you are teaching Ms. Mac about her SSRI, sertraline (Zoloft), she asks you, "What makes this such a good drug?"

    A. What are some of the positive attributes of the SSRIs? What is one of the most serious, although rare, side effects of the SSRIs?

    B. Devise a teaching plan for Ms. Mac.

■ ■ ■ CHAPTER REVIEW

Choose the most appropriate answer.

1. Which statement, if made by a nurse, would indicate that the nurse subscribes to the theory that learned helplessness is a major factor in the development of depression?

    1. TCAs, MAOIs, and SSRIs are the most useful tools to combat depression.

    2. Depression develops when a person believes he or she is powerless to effect change in a situation.

    3. Depressive symptoms result from experiencing significant loss and turning aggression against the self.

    4. Psychosocial stressors and interpersonal events trigger neurophysical and neurochemical changes in the brain.

2. Which response by a nurse to a client experiencing depression would be helpful?

    1. "Don't worry, we all get down once in awhile."

    2. "Don't consider suicide. It's an unacceptable option."

    3. "Try to cheer up. Things always look darkest before the dawn."

    4. "I can see you're feeling down. I'll sit here with you for a while."

3. Which of the following is considered a vegetative symptom of depression?

    1. Sleep disturbance

    2. Trouble concentrating

    3. Neglected grooming and hygiene

    4. Negative expectations for the future

4. Which is true of the cognition of a person with severe depression?

    1. Reality testing remains intact.

    2. Concentration is unimpaired.

    3. Repetitive negative thinking is noted.

    4. Ability to make decisions is improved.

5. When the nurse is caring for a depressed client, the problem that should receive the highest nursing priority is

    1. powerlessness.

    2. suicidal ideation.

    3. inability to cope effectively.

    4. anorexia and weight loss.

■ STUDENT
■ STUDY
■ CD-ROM

Access the accompanying CD-ROM for animations, interactive exercises, review questions for the NCLEX examination, and an audio glossary.

■ NURSE,
■ CLIENT, AND
■ FAMILY RESOURCES

For suggested readings, information on related associations, and Internet resources, go to **http://evolve.elsevier.com/Varcarolis**.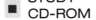

REFERENCES

Agency for Healthcare Research and Quality. (2004). *Improving depression care has long-lasting benefits for African Americans and Hispanics* [Press release]. Retrieved April 5, 2004, from http://www.ahrq.gov/news/press/pr2004/depminpr.htm.

Agras, W. S., & Berkowitz, R. I. (1999). Behavior therapies. In R. E. Hales, S. C. Yudofsky, & J. A. Talbott (Eds.), *Textbook of psychiatry*. Washington, DC: American Psychiatric Press.

American Psychiatric Association. (2000a). *Diagnostic and statistical manual of mental disorders (DSM-IV-TR)* (4th ed., text rev.). Washington, DC: Author.

American Psychiatric Association. (2000b). *Practice guidelines for the treatment of psychiatric disorders: Compendium 2000.* Washington, DC: Author.

Beck, A. T., & Rush, A. J. (1995). Cognitive therapy. In H. I. Kaplan & B. J. Sadock (Eds.), *Comprehensive textbook of psychiatry/VI* (6th ed., Vol. 2, pp. 1847-1856). Baltimore: Williams & Wilkins.

Bijl, D., et al. (2004). Effectiveness of disease management programmes for recognition, diagnosis and treatment of depression in primary care. *European Journal of General Practice, 10,* 6-12.

Culpepper, L., et al. (2003). *Spotlight on remission—achieving evidence-based goal in depression and anxiety.* Retrieved January 13, 2004, from Medscape website: http://www.medscape.com/viewprogram/2544.

Dochterman, J. M., & Bulechek, G. M. (2004). *Nursing interventions classification (NIC)* (4th ed.). St. Louis, MO: Mosby.

Dubovsky, S. L., & Buzan, R. (1999). Mood disorders. In R. E. Hales, S. C. Yudofsky, & J. A. Talbott (Eds.), *Textbook of psychiatry* (pp. 479-566). Washington, DC: American Psychiatric Publishing.

Dubovsky, S. L., Davies, R., & Dubovsky, A. N. (2004). Mood disorders. In R. E. Hales, & S. C. Yudofsky (Eds.), *Essentials of clinical psychiatry* (2nd ed., pp. 273-274). Washington, DC: American Psychiatric Publishing.

Fuller, M. A., & Sajatovic, M. (2000). *Drug information handbook* (2nd ed.). Cleveland, OH: Lexi-Comp.

Gitlin, M. (1999, November 11-14). *Psychopharmacology for psychotherapists* (Parts 1-3). Paper presented at 12th Annual U.S. Psychiatric and Mental Health Congress, New York.

Goldberg, R. J. (1998). *The care of the psychiatric patient*. St. Louis, MO: Mosby.

Golden, R. N., et al. (2004). Trazodone and other antidepressants. In A. F. Schatzberg & C. B. Nemeroff (Eds.), *The American Psychiatric Publishing textbook of psychopharmacology* (3rd ed., pp. 195-214). Washington, DC: American Psychiatric Publishing.

Greden, J. F. (2004, May 1-6). *Best practices for achieving remission in depression with physical symptoms: Current and future trends*. Paper presented in Symposium 10E conducted at the American Psychiatric Association Annual Meeting, New York.

Gruenberg, A. M., & Goldstein, R. D. (2003). Mood disorders: Depression. In A. Tasman, J. Kay, & J. A. Lieberman (Eds.), *Psychiatry* (2nd ed.). West Sussex, England: Wiley.

Guerrero-Berroa, E., & Phillips, R. S. C. (2001). Health care professionals' awareness of the symptoms of geriatric depression. *Journal of Psychosocial Nursing and Mental Health Services, 39*(11), 14-20.

Heim, C., & Nemeroff, C. B. (1999). The impact of early adverse experiences on brain systems involved in the pathophysiology of anxiety and affective disorders. *Social Biology and Psychiatry, 46*, 1-15.

Jain, R., & Russ, N. (2003). *Addressing both the emotional and physical symptoms in depression*. Retrieved March 21, 2003, from Medscape website: http://www.medscape.com/viewprogram/2240.

Kramer, T. A. M. (2004, May 1-6). *The relationship between depression and physical symptoms*. Paper presented at the American Psychiatric Association Annual Meeting, New York. Retrieved January 17, 2005, from http://www.medscape.com/viewarticle/480898.

Lenze, E. J. (2003). Comorbidity of depression and anxiety in the elderly. *Current Psychiatric Reports, 5*, 62-67.

Marangell, L. B., et al. (2004). Psychopharmacology and electroconvulsive therapy. In R. E. Hales, & S. C. Yudofsky (Eds.), *Essentials of clinical psychiatry* (4th ed.). Washington, DC: American Psychiatric Publishing.

Maxmen, J. S., & Ward, N. G. (2002). *Psychotropic drugs: Fast facts* (2nd ed.). New York: W. W. Norton.

Mayo Foundation for Medical Education and Research. (2003). *Exercise eases symptoms of anxiety and depression*. Retrieved February 28, 2005, from http://www.mayoclinic.com/invoke.cfm?objectid=8D173381-C07B-408F-88A4D285554134E5.

Mendelowitz, A. J., Dawkins, K., & Lieberman, J. A. (2000). Antidepressants. In J. A. Lieberman & A. Tasman (Eds.), *Psychiatric drugs*. Philadelphia: Saunders.

Montano, C. B. (2003). *New frontiers in the treatment of depression*. Retrieved September 30, 2003, from Medscape website: http://www.medscape.com/viewprogram/2689.

Moorhead, S., Johnson, M., & Maas, M. (2004). *Nursing outcomes classification (NOC)* (3rd ed.). St. Louis, MO: Mosby.

Nangia, M., Syed, W., & Doraiswamy, P. (2000). Efficacy and safety of St. John's wort for the treatment of major depression. *Public Health Nutrition, 3*(4A), 487-494.

National Center for Complementary and Alternative Medicine. (March 2004). *St. John's wort and the treatment of depression*. Retrieved February 28, 2005, from http://nccam.nih.gov/health/stjohnswort/.

National Institute of Mental Health. (2000a). *Depression: What every woman should know* (NIH Publication No. 004779). Washington, DC: Author. Retrieved February 28, 2005, from http://www.nimh.nih.gov/publicat/depwomenknows.cfm.

National Institute of Mental Health. (2000b). *Depression in children and adolescents: A fact sheet for physicians* (NIH Publication No. 004744). Washington, DC: Author. Retrieved March 7, 2005, from http://www.nimh.nih.gov/publicat/nimhdepchildresfact.pdf.

National Institute of Mental Health. (2001a). *The invisible disease: Depression* (NIH Publication No. 01-4591). Washington, DC: Author. Retrieved January 16, 2005, from http://www.nimh.nih.gov/publicat/invisible.cfm.

National Institute of Mental Health. (2001b). *The numbers count: Mental disorders in America* (NIH Publication No. 01-4584). Retrieved January 16, 2005, from http://www.nimh.nih.gov/publicat/numbers.cfm.

National Institute of Mental Health. (2002). *Depression research at the National Institute of Mental Health* (NIH Publication No. 004501). Bethesda, MD: National Institutes of Health.

National Institute of Mental Health. (2003a). *NIH News: Gene more than doubles risk of depression following life stresses*. Retrieved January 16, 2005, from http://www.nih.gov/news/pr/jul2003/nimh-17.htm.

National Institute of Mental Health. (2003b). *Older adults: Depression and suicide facts* (NIH publication No. 03-4593). Bethesda, MD: National Institutes of Health.

Rosenbaum, J. F. (2004, May 1-6). *New brain stimulation therapies for depression*. Paper presented at the American Psychiatric Association Annual Meeting, New York. Retrieved January 16, 2005, from http://www.medscape.com/viewarticle/480897.

Sadek, N., & Nemeroff, C. B. (2000). *Update on the neurobiology of depression*. Retrieved January 16, 2005, from Medscape website: http://www.medscape.com/viewprogram/142?src=search.

Seligman, M. E. (1973). Fall into hopelessness. *Psychology Today, 7*, 43.

Serby, M., & Yu, M. (2003, September 25). There is good news about depression in the elderly. *Clinical Advisor*, pp. 64-75.

Simon, N. M., & Rosenbaum, J. F. (2003, March 27). *Anxiety and depression comorbidity: Implications and intervention*. Retrieved January 16, 2005, from Medscape website: http://www.medscape.com/viewarticle/451325.

Stuart, D. E. (2003). Physical symptoms of depression: Emerging needs in special populations. *Journal of Clinical Psychiatry, 64*(7), 12-16.

Sutherland, J. E., Sutherland, S. J., & Hoehns, J. D. (2003). Achieving the best outcome in treatment of depression. *Journal of Family Practice, 52*(3), 201-209.

U.S. Food and Drug Administration, Center for Drug Evaluation and Research. (2004a). *Worsening depression and suicidality in patients being treated with antidepressant medications*. Retrieved January 16, 2005, from http://www.fda.gov/cder/drug/antidepressants/AntidepressanstPHA.htm.

U.S. Food and Drug Administration. (2004b). *FDA issues public health advisory on cautions for use of antidepressants in adults and children* (FDA Talk Paper T04-08). Retrieved January 16, 2005, from http://www.fda.gov/bbs/topics/ANSWERS/2004/ANS01283.html.

VanScoy, H. (2001). *Choosing the best SSRI*. Retrieved January 16, 2005, from Dr. John Grohol's Psych Central website: http://psychcentral.com/library/choosing_ssri.htm.

Young, J. E., Weinberger, A. D., & Beck, A. T. (2001). Cognitive therapy for depression. In D. H. Barlow (Ed.). *Clinical handbook of psychological disorders* (3rd ed.). New York: Guilford Press.

Zahourek, R. (2000). Alternative, complementary, or integrative approaches to treating depression. *Journal of the American Psychiatric Nurses Association, 6*(3), 77-86.

CHAPTER 19

Mood Disorders: Bipolar

ELIZABETH M. VARCAROLIS

 KEY TERMS and CONCEPTS

The key terms and concepts listed here appear in color where they are defined or first discussed in this chapter.

 OBJECTIVES

After studying this chapter, the reader will be able to

1. Assess a manic client's (a) mood, (b) behavior, and (c) thought processes and be alert to possible dysfunction.
2. Formulate three nursing diagnoses appropriate for a manic client and include supporting data.
3. Explain the rationale behind five methods of communication that may be used with a manic client.
4. Teach a classmate at least four expected side effects of lithium therapy.
5. Distinguish between signs of early and severe lithium toxicity.
6. Write a medication care plan specifying five areas of client teaching regarding lithium carbonate.
7. Contrast and compare basic clinical conditions that may respond better to anticonvulsant therapy with those that may respond better to lithium therapy.
8. Evaluate specific indications for the use of seclusion for a manic client.
9. Defend the use of electroconvulsive therapy for a client in specific situations.
10. Review with a bipolar client at least three of the items presented in the psychoeducation teaching plan (see Box 19-2).
11. Distinguish between the focus of treatment for a person in the acute manic phase and that for a person in the continuation or maintenance phase of a bipolar I disorder.

---

evolve Visit the Evolve website at **http://evolve.elsevier.com/Varcarolis** for a pretest on the content in this chapter.

Bipolar disorder is an illness that is biological in its origins, yet feels psychological in its experiences (Jamison, 1995b). Bipolar disorder is a chronic, recurrent illness that must be carefully managed throughout a person's life. Bipolar disorder frequently goes unrecognized, and people may suffer for years before receiving proper diagnosis and treatment. Bipolar disorder is marked by shifts in a person's mood, energy, and ability to function. Alternating mood episodes are characterized by mania, hypomania, depression, and concurrent mania and depression (mixed episodes in which depressive symptoms occur during a manic attack). Periods of normal functioning may alternate with periods of illness (highs, lows, or mixed highs and lows). However, some researchers suggest that 30% to 60% of individuals with bipolar disorder fail to regain full occupational and social functioning (MacQueen, Young, & Jaffe, 2001).

Indeed, many individuals with bipolar disorder experience chronic interpersonal or occupational difficulties during remission (Blairy et al., 2004). Not only is the morbidity rate high, but the mortality rate is equally severe: bipolar disorder is associated with the highest lifetime rate of suicide of any psychiatric illness (Jamison, 2000).

Bipolar disorders currently identified include the following:

Bipolar I disorder: At least one episode of mania alternating with major depression

Bipolar II disorder: Hypomanic episode(s) alternating with major depression

Cyclothymia: Hypomanic episodes alternating with minor depressive episodes (at least 2 years in duration)

The specifier rapid cycling (four or more mood episodes in a 12-month period) is used to indicate more severe symptoms such as poorer global functioning, high recurrence risk, and resistance to conventional somatic treatments (Schneck et al., 2003). The *Diagnostic and Statistical Manual of Mental Disorders,* fourth edition, text revision *(DSM-IV-TR)* (American Psychiatric Association [APA], 2000a) makes a distinction between mania and hypomania for diagnostic purposes, as shown in Figure 19-1.

DSM-IV-TR CRITERIA FOR BIPOLAR DISORDER

1. A distinct period of abnormality and persistently elevated, expansive, or irritable mood for at least:
   * 4 days for hypomania
   * 1 week for mania

2. During the period of mood disturbance, **three or more** of the following symptoms have persisted (four if the mood is only irritable) and have been present to a significant degree:
   * Inflated self-esteem or grandiosity
   * Decreased need for sleep (e.g., the person feels rested after only 3 hours of sleep)
   * More talkative than usual or pressure to keep talking
   * Flight of ideas or subjective experience that thoughts are racing
   * Distractibility (i.e., the person's attention is too easily drawn to unimportant or irrelevant external stimuli)
   * Increase in goal-directed activity (either socially, at work or school, or sexually) or psychomotor agitation
   * Excessive involvement in pleasurable activities that have a high potential for painful consequences (e.g., the person engages in unrestrained buying sprees, sexual indiscretions, or foolish business investments)

Hypomania

1. The episode is associated with an unequivocal change in functioning that is uncharacteristic of the person when not symptomatic.

2. The disturbance in mood and the change in functioning are observed by others.

3. Absence of marked impairment in social or occupational functioning.

4. Hospitalization is not indicated.

5. Symptoms are not due to direct physiological effects of substance (e.g., drug abuse, medication, or other medical conditions).

Mania

1. Severe enough to cause marked impairment in occupational activities, usual social activities, or relationships.

   or

2. Necessitate hospitalization to prevent harm to self or others, or there are psychotic features.

3. Symptoms are not due to direct physiological effects of substance (drug abuse, medication) or general medical condition (e.g., hyperthyroidism).

FIGURE 19-1 Diagnostic criteria for bipolar disorder. (Adapted from American Psychiatric Association. *Diagnostic and statistical manual of mental disorders* [4th ed., text rev.]. Washington, DC: Author.)

PREVALENCE

The lifetime prevalence of bipolar disorder in the U.S. population is estimated to range from 1.2% to 1.6% (APA, 2000a). Some put the prevalence of bipolar disorder as high as 3% (Bipolar Disorder Resource Center, 2004). Epidemiological surveys in general populations across different countries found a lifetime prevalence rate for bipolar I disorder of about 0.8% to 1.0%. Bipolar I disorder seems to be somewhat more common among males than among females (Wacker, 2000), but bipolar II disorder is more common among women (APA, 2000a). Whereas major depression usually starts between 25 and 30 years of age, bipolar disorders emerge between the ages of 18 and 30 (Wacker, 2000). Mean age of the first episode of the disorder appears lower for people with a family history of the disease (Dubovsky, Davies, & Dubovsky, 2004). A person 40 years or older who appears for treatment of a manic episode is more likely to have mania secondary to a general medical condition or substance abuse. The first episode in males is likely to be a manic episode, whereas in females the disease usually presents with a depressive episode. During the course of the illness, the episodes increase in number and severity as the person gets older.

Cyclothymia usually begins in adolescence or early adulthood. There is a 15% to 50% risk that an individual with cyclothymia will subsequently develop bipolar I or bipolar II disorder.

COMORBIDITY

Substance use disorders are exceptionally common in individuals with a bipolar disease. Substance-abusing clients seem to experience more rapid cycling and more mixed or dysphoric mania (Sonne & Brady, 1999). When this is the case, treatment for substance abuse and mood disorder should proceed at the same time whenever possible (APA, 2000a). Other associated disorders include personality disorders, anxiety disorders (panic disorder and social phobia), anorexia nervosa, bulimia nervosa, and attention deficit hyperactivity disorder (APA, 2000a). A study by Dunayevich and colleagues (2000) found that clients with bipolar disorders who had co-occurring personality disorders had poorer outcomes 12 months after hospitalization for mania than those who did not have personality disorders. A study by Colom and associates (2000) found that the client population with comorbid personality disorders also had a greater tendency toward medication nonadherence.

THEORY

Bipolar disorders (one or more episodes of both elated and depressed moods) are thought to be distinctly different from one another; for example, bipolar I disorder, bipolar II disorder, and cyclothymia have different characteristics. Other variants of bipolar disease are currently being evaluated.

Individuals with bipolar I disorder may become psychotic or display bizarre behavior and paranoia. Clients with bipolar II disorder are more likely to become depressed in winter than in summer (seasonal differences), make more suicide attempts, and display disorders in temperament (borderlinelike). A study by Judd and colleagues (2003) revealed that, compared with individuals with bipolar I disorder, people with bipolar II disorder have a higher lifetime prevalence of anxiety disorder and social and simple phobias, greater disease chronicity, and more subsequent depressions. These findings help highlight some of the less typical features of clients with bipolar II disorder (anxiety and characteristics of personality disorder) that may distract clinicians and impede recognition of bipolarity (Judd et al., 2003).

Bipolar depression is also different from unipolar depression. Bipolar depression affects younger people, produces more episodes of illness, and requires more frequent hospitalization. It is also characterized by higher rates of divorce and marital conflict.

Some theoretical conceptions pertaining specifically to the development of bipolar disorders are those focusing on biological, social, and psychosocial factors. Most likely, multiple independent variables contribute to the occurrence of bipolar disorder. For this reason, a biopsychosocial approach will likely be the most successful approach to treatment (Bauer, 2003).

Biological Theories

Genetic Factors

Significant evidence exists to support the view that bipolar disorders have a strong genetic component. For example, the rate of bipolar disorders in relatives of people with bipolar disorders can be as much as 5 to 10 times higher than the rates found in the general population (Bauer, 2003). A study conducted by the National Institute of Mental Health found that 25% of the relatives of clients with bipolar disorder had a bipolar or major depressive disorder. Some 20% of relatives of clients with a depressive disorder had a bipolar or major depressive disorder, compared with 7% of relatives of control clients (Nurnberger & Gershon, 1992). Twin studies confirm a genetic marker for both the bipolar disorders and the depressive disorders; however, the incidence of illness is significantly higher in those with the marker for bipolar disorder (Kelsoe, 1999). Identical twins are more concordant for bipolar disorder (78% to 80%) than fraternal twins (14% to 19%) (Merikangas & Kupfer, 1995; Nurnberger & Gershon, 1992). Twin, family, and adoption studies provide evidence for a partial genetic cause, but the modes of inheritance have not been identified (Ginns et al., 1996).

More recently, researchers have identified two genes (G72 and G30) located on the long arm of chromosome 13 that are associated with bipolar disorder as well as schizophrenia (Hattori et al., 2003).

Neurobiological Factors

Neurotransmitters (norepinephrine, dopamine, and serotonin) have been studied since the 1960s as causal factors in mania and depression. For example, during a manic episode, clients with bipolar disorder demonstrate significantly higher plasma levels of norepinephrine and epinephrine than they do when they are depressed or *euthymic* (have normal mood) (Freedman & McElroy, 1999; Nathan et al., 1995). Post, Rubinow, and Uhde (1989) found that acutely manic clients had higher cerebrospinal fluid levels of norepinephrine than depressed or euthymic persons. Among the manic clients, norepinephrine levels correlated with the degree of dysphoria, anger, and anxiety. Other research has found that the interrelationships in the neurotransmitter system are complex.

More elaborate theories have been developed since the amine hypotheses were originally proposed. Mood disorders are most likely a result of complex interactions among various chemicals, including neurotransmitters and hormones.

Neuroendocrine Factors

The hypothalamic-pituitary-thyroid-adrenal (HPTA) axis has been closely scrutinized in people with mood disorders. Hypothyroidism is known to be associated with depressed moods, and hypothyroidism is seen in some clients who are experiencing rapid cycling. Several studies have demonstrated that thyroid hormone administration may ameliorate mood disorders in some clients with bipolar disorder (Bauer, 2003).

Neuroanatomical Factors

Brain pathways implicated in the pathophysiology of bipolar disorder are in subregions of the prefrontal cortex (PFC) and medial temporal lobe (MTL). Dysregulation in the neurocircuits surrounding these areas have been viewed through functional imaging (e.g., positron emission tomography, magnetic resonance imaging) (Pollock & Kuo, 2004).

Sociological Findings

Some evidence suggests that the bipolar disorders may be more prevalent in the upper socioeconomic classes. The exact reason for this is unclear; however, people with bipolar disorders appear to achieve higher levels of education and higher occupational status than nonbipolar depressed individuals. The educational levels of individuals with nonbipolar depressive disorders, on the other hand, appear to be no different from those of nondepressed individuals within the same socioeconomic class. Also, the proportion of bipolar clients among creative writers, artists, highly educated men and women, and professional people is higher than in the general population.

Psychological Influences

Although there is increasing evidence for genetic and biological vulnerabilities in the etiology of the mood disorders, psychological factors may play a role in precipitating manic episodes for many individuals. Two studies of family atmosphere suggest an association between high expressed emotion and relapse. Another study of bipolar clients who suffered abuse as children revealed earlier onset of bipolar disorder, faster cycling frequencies, and an increase in comorbid disorders such as substance abuse (Leverich et al., 2002).

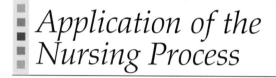

Application of the Nursing Process

■ ASSESSMENT

Individuals with bipolar disorder are often misdiagnosed or underdiagnosed. On average, people spend 8 years seeking treatment before receiving a correct diagnosis (Kahn et al., 2000). Early diagnosis and proper treatment can help people avoid the following (Goldberg & Ernst, 2002):

- Suicide (one out of five clients with bipolar disorder)
- Alcohol or substance abuse (50% abuse alcohol or drugs, which signals a worse outcome)
- Marital or work problems
- Development of medical comorbidity

Figure 19-2 presents the Mood Disorder Questionnaire (MDQ). This is *not* a diagnostic test; however, it is a helpful screening device.

Assessment of the Characteristics of Mania

The characteristics of mania discussed are (1) mood, (2) behavior, (3) thought processes, and (4) cognitive function.

Assessing Level of Mood

The euphoric mood associated with a bipolar illness is unstable. During euphoria, the client may state that he or she is experiencing an intense feeling of well-being, is "cheerful in a beautiful world," or is becoming "one with God." This mood may change to irritation and quick anger when the elated person is thwarted. The irritability and belligerence may be short-lived, or it may become

MOOD DISORDER QUESTIONNAIRE

Instructions: Please answer each question as best you can.

	Yes	No
1. **Has there ever been a period of time when you were not your usual self and....**		
you felt so good or so hyper that other people thought you were not your normal self or you were so hyper that you got into trouble?	○	○
you were so irritable that you shouted at people or started fights or arguments?	○	○
you felt much more self-confident than usual?	○	○
you got much less sleep than usual and found you didn't really miss it?	○	○
you were much more talkative or spoke much faster than usual?	○	○
thoughts raced through your head or you couldn't slow down your mind?	○	○
you were so easily distracted by things around you that you had trouble concentrating or staying on track?	○	○
you had much more energy than usual?	○	○
you were much more active or did many more things than usual?	○	○
you were much more social or outgoing than usual; for example, you telephoned friends in the middle of the night?	○	○
you were much more interested in sex than usual?	○	○
you did things that were unusual for you or that other people might have thought were excessive, foolish, or risky?	○	○
spending money got you or your family into trouble?	○	○
2. **If you answered "Yes" to more than one of the above, have several of these ever happened during the same period of time?**	○	○

3. **How much of a problem did any of these cause you — like being unable to work; having family, money, or legal troubles; or getting into arguments or fights? Please select one response only.**

    ○ No problem   ○ Minor problem   ○ Moderate problem   ○ Serious problem

	Yes	No
4. **Have any of your blood relatives (children, siblings, parents, grandparents, aunts, uncles) had manic-depressive illness or bipolar disorder?**	○	○
5. **Has a health care professional ever told you that you have manic-depressive illness or bipolar disorder?**	○	○

Criteria for Results: Answering "Yes" to 7 or more of the events in question 1, answering "Yes" to question 2, and answering "Moderate problem" or "Serious problem" to question 3 is considered a positive screen result for bipolar disorder.

FIGURE 19-2 The Mood Disorder Questionnaire. (From Hirschfeld, R. M. A., et al. [2000]. Development and validation of a screening instrument for bipolar spectrum disorder: The Mood Disorder Questionnaire, *American Journal of Psychiatry, 157*[11], 1873-1875. © 2004 Eli Lilly and Company.)

the prominent feature of a person's manic illness. When the person is elated, the overjoyous mood may seem out of proportion to what is going on, and a cheerful mood may be inappropriate to the circumstances.

People in a manic state may laugh, joke, and talk in a continuous stream, with uninhibited familiarity. Manic people demonstrate boundless enthusiasm, treat everyone with confidential friendliness, and incorporate everyone into their plans and activities. They know no strangers. Energy and self-confidence seem boundless.

Elaborate schemes to get rich and famous and acquire unlimited power may be frantically pursued, despite objections and realistic constraints. Excessive phone calls and e-mails are made, often to famous and influential people all over the world. People in the manic phase are busy all hours of the day and night furthering their grandiose plans and wild schemes. To the manic person, no aspirations are too high and no distances are too far. No boundaries exist in reality to curtail the elaborate schemes.

In the manic state, a person often gives away money, prized possessions, and expensive gifts. The manic person throws lavish parties, frequents expensive nightclubs and restaurants, and spends money freely on friends and strangers alike. This spending, excessive use of credit cards, and high living continue even in the face of bankruptcy. Intervention is often needed to prevent financial ruin.

Hypomania to Mania. As the clinical course progresses, sociability and euphoria are replaced by a stage of hostility, irritability, and paranoia. The following is a client's description of the painful transition from hypomania to mania (Jamison, 1995b):

> At first when I'm high, it's tremendous. . . . ideas are fast . . . like shooting stars you follow until brighter ones appear. . . . all shyness disappears, the right words and gestures are suddenly there. . . . uninteresting people, things become intensely interesting. Sensuality is pervasive; the desire to seduce and be seduced is irresistible. Your marrow is infused with unbelievable feelings of ease, power, well-being, omnipotence, euphoria. . . . you can do anything. . . . but somewhere this changes. . . .
>
> The fast ideas become too fast and there are far too many. . . . overwhelming confusion replaces clarity. . . . you stop keeping up with it—memory goes. Infectious humor ceases to amuse—your friends become frightened. . . . everything now is against the grain. . . . you are irritable, angry, frightened, uncontrollable, and trapped in the blackest caves of the mind—caves you never knew were there. It will never end. Madness carves its own reality.

Refer to Table 19-1 for further description of hypomania, acute mania, and delirious mania.

Assessing Behavior

During Mania. When in full-blown mania, a person constantly goes from one activity to another, one place to another, and one project to another. Many projects may be started, but few, if any, are completed. Inactivity is impossible, even for the shortest period of time. Hyperactivity may range from mild, constant motion to frenetic, wild activity. The writing of flowery and lengthy letters and the making of excessive long-distance telephone calls are accentuated. Individuals become involved in pleasurable activities that can have painful consequences. For example, spending large sums of money on frivolous items, giving money away indiscriminately, or making foolish business investments can leave a family penniless.

Sexual indiscretion can dissolve relationships and marriages.

Bipolar individuals can be manipulative, profane, fault finding, and adept at exploiting others' vulnerabilities. They constantly push limits. These behaviors often alienate family, friends, employers, health care providers, and others.

When people are hypomanic, they have voracious appetites for food as well as for indiscriminate sex. Although the constant activity of the hypomanic prevents proper sleep, short periods of sleep are possible. However, a reduced need for sleep is experienced by all manic clients, and some clients may not sleep for several days in a row. The manic person is too busy to eat, sleep, or engage in sexual activity. **This nonstop physical activity and the lack of sleep and food can lead to physical exhaustion and even death if not treated and therefore constitutes an emergency.**

Modes of dress often reflect the person's grandiose yet tenuous grasp of reality. Dress may be described as outlandish, bizarre, colorful, and noticeably inappropriate. Makeup may be garish or overdone. Manic people are highly distractible. Concentration is poor, and manic individuals go from one activity to another without completing anything. Judgment is poor. Impulsive marriages and divorces take place.

After Mania. People often emerge from a manic state startled and confused by the shambles of their lives. The following description conveys one client's experience (Jamison, 1995b):

> Now there are only others' recollections of your behavior— your bizarre, frenetic, aimless behavior—at least mania has the grace to dim memories of itself. . . . now it's over, but is it? . . . Incredible feelings to sort through. . . . Who is being too polite? Who knows what? What did I do? Why? And most hauntingly, will it, when will it, happen again? Medication to take, to resist, to resent, to forget . . . but always to take. Credit cards revoked . . . explanations at work . . . bad checks and apologies overdue . . . memory flashes of vague men (what did I do?) . . . friendships gone, a marriage ruined.

Assessing Thought Processes

Flight of ideas is a nearly continuous flow of accelerated speech with abrupt changes from topic to topic that are usually based on understandable associations or plays on words. At times, the attentive listener can keep up with the changes, even though direction changes from moment to moment. Speech is rapid, verbose, and circumstantial (including minute and unnecessary details). When the condition is severe, speech may be disorganized and incoherent. The incessant talking often includes joking, puns, and teasing:

> How are you doing, kid, no kidding around, I'm going home . . . home sweet home . . . home is where the heart is, the heart of the matter is I want out and that ain't hay, . . . hey, Doc . . . get me out of this place.

TABLE 19-1

Mania on a Continuum

Hypomania	Acute Mania	Delirious Mania
Communication		
1. Talks and jokes incessantly, is the "life of the party," gets irritated when not center of attention.	1. May go suddenly from laughing to anger or depression. *Mood is labile.*	1. Totally out of touch with reality.
2. Treats everyone with familiarity and confidentiality; often borders on crude.	2. Becomes inappropriately demanding of people's attention, and intrusive nature repels others.	—
3. Talk is often sexual—can reach obscene, inappropriate propositions to total strangers.	3. Speech may be marked by profanities and crude sexual remarks to everyone (nursing staff in particular).	—
4. Talk is fresh; flits from one topic to the next. Marked by *pressure of speech.*	4. Speech marked by *flight of ideas,* in which thoughts race and fly from topic to topic. May have *clang associations.*	4. Most likely has *clang associations.*
Affect and Thinking		
1. Full of pep and good humor, feelings of euphoria and sociability; may show inappropriate intimacy with strangers.	1. Good humor gives way to increased irritability and hostility, short-lived period of rage, especially when not getting his or her way or when controls are set on behavior. May have quick shifts of mood from hostility to docility.	1. May become destructive or aggressive—totally out of control.
2. Feels boundless self-confidence and enthusiasm. Has elaborate schemes for becoming rich and famous. Initially, schemes may seem plausible.	2. Grandiose plans are totally out of contact with reality. Thinks he or she is a musician, prominent businessman, great politician, or religious figure, without any basis in fact.	2. May experience undefined hallucinations and delirium.
3. Judgment often poor. Gets involved with schemes in which job, marriage, or financial status may be destroyed.	3. Judgment is extremely poor.	—
4. May write large quantities of letters to rich and famous people regarding schemes or may make numerous world-wide telephone calls.	—	—
5. Decreased attention span to both internal and external cues.	5. Decreased attention span and distractibility are intensified.	
Physical Behavior		
1. Overactive, distractible, buoyant, and busily occupied with grandiose plans (not delusions); goes from one action to the next.	1. Extremely restless, disorganized, and chaotic. Physical behavior may be difficult to control. May have outbursts, such as throwing things or becoming briefly assaultive when crossed.	1. *Dangerous state.* Incoherent, extremely restless, disoriented, and agitated. Hyperactive. Motor activity is totally aimless (must have physical or chemical restraints to prevent exhaustion and death).
2. Increased sexual appetite; sexually irresponsible and indiscreet. Illegitimate pregnancies in hypomanic women and venereal disease in both men and women are common. Sex used for escape, not for relating to another human being.	2. No time for sex—too busy. Poor concentration, distractibility, and restlessness are severe.	2. Same as in acute mania but in the extreme.
3. May have voracious appetite, eat on the run, or gobble food during brief periods.	3. No time to eat—too distracted and disorganized.	3. Same as acute mania but in the extreme.
4. May go without sleeping; unaware of fatigue. However, may be able to take short naps.	4. No time for sleep—psychomotor activity too high; if unchecked, can lead to exhaustion and death.	—
5. Financially extravagant, goes on buying sprees, gives money and gifts away freely, can easily go into debt.	5. Same as in hypomania but in the extreme.	5. Too disorganized to do anything.

The content of speech is often sexually explicit and ranges from grossly inappropriate to vulgar. Themes in the communication of the manic individual may revolve around extraordinary sexual prowess, brilliant business ability, or unparalleled artistic talents (e.g., writing, painting, and dancing). The person may actually have only average ability in these areas.

Speech is not only profuse but also loud, bellowing, or even screaming. One can hear the force and energy behind the rapid words. As mania escalates, flight of ideas may give way to clang associations. Clang associations are the stringing together of words because of their rhyming sounds, without regard to their meaning (Schiller & Bennett, 1994):

> Cinema I and II, last row. Row, row, row your boat. Don't be a cutthroat. Cut your throat. Get your goat. Go out and vote. And so I wrote.

Grandiosity (inflated self-regard) is apparent in both the ideas expressed and the person's behavior. Manic people may exaggerate their achievements or importance, state that they know famous people, or believe that they have great powers (Silverstone & Hunt, 1992). The boast of exceptional powers and status can take delusional proportions in mania. Grandiose persecutory delusions are common. For example, manic people may think that God is speaking to them or that the Federal Bureau of Investigation is out to stop them from saving the world. Sensory perceptions may become altered as the mania escalates, and hallucinations may occur. However, in hypomania, no evidence of delusions or hallucinations is present.

Assessing Cognitive Function

The onset of bipolar disease is often preceded by comparatively high cognitive function. However, there is growing evidence that about one third of bipolar clients display significant and persistent cognitive problems and difficulties in psychosocial areas (Martinez-Aran et al., 2000). Cognitive impairment appears to be a core feature of bipolar disorder.

The potential cognitive dysfunction among a large subgroup of bipolar clients has specific clinical implications (Spollen, 2003):

- Cognitive function greatly affects overall function.
- Cognitive deficits correlate with greater number of manic episodes, history of psychosis, chronicity of illness, and poor functional outcome.
- Early diagnosis and treatment are crucial to prevent illness progression, cognitive deficits, and poor outcome.
- Medication selection should consider not only the efficacy of the drug in reducing mood symptoms but also the cognitive impact of the drug on the client.

Self-Assessment

The manic client can elicit numerous intense emotions in the nurse. A manic client is out of control and resists being controlled. The client may use humor, manipulation, power struggles, or demanding behavior to prevent or minimize the staff's ability to set limits on and control dangerous behavior.

The behavior of a manic client is often aimed at decreasing the effectiveness of staff control. He or she might accomplish this by getting involved in power plays. For example, the client might taunt the staff by pointing out faults or oversights and drawing negative attention to one or more staff members. Usually, this is done in a loud and disruptive manner, which provokes staff to become defensive and thereby escalates the environmental tension and the client's degree of mania.

Another unconscious tactic is to divide staff as a ploy to keep the environment unsettled. The manic client is sensitive to the vulnerabilities and conflicts within a group. Often, a manic client manipulates staff by turning one group of staff members against another in an unconscious attempt to discourage outside controls. For example, a client might tell the day shift nurse, "You are the only nurse who listens. On evenings, they hardly look at you. You could drop dead, and the nurses wouldn't even know it." To the evening shift nurse the client might say, "Thank God you're here. At last, someone who cares. All the day people do is push pills and drink coffee." This manipulative tactic is a form of **splitting,** in which the client pits one person or group against another. Splitting is also seen with other client groups (e.g., clients with borderline and antisocial personality disorder, substance abusers).

The client can become aggressively demanding. This behavior often triggers frustration and exasperation in health care professionals. The manic individual is adept at distracting staff into defensive positions and setting up an environment that allows the manic defense to go unchecked. Setting limits is an important skill for staff to develop. Adequate administration of medications (anxiolytics, antipsychotics) is essential, particularly in the acute phase of mania.

When staff members start to feel confused and angry with each other, it is often an indication that a client is successfully splitting the staff. Frequent staff meetings dealing with the behaviors of the client and the nurses' responses to these behaviors can help minimize staff splitting and feelings of anger and isolation by the staff. The consistent setting of limits is the main theme in treating a person in mania.

Consistency among staff is imperative if the limit setting is to be carried out effectively.

Assessment Guidelines Bipolar Disorder

1. Assess whether the client is a danger to self and others:
   - Manic clients can exhaust themselves to the point of death.
   - Clients may not eat or sleep, often for days at a time.
   - Poor impulse control may result in harm to others or self.
   - Uncontrolled spending may occur.
2. Assess for need for controls. Controls may be needed to protect client from bankruptcy because manic clients may give away all of their money or possessions.
3. Assess for need for hospitalization to safeguard and stabilize the client.
4. Assess medical status. A thorough medical examination helps to determine whether mania is primary (a mood disorder—bipolar disorder or cyclothymia) or secondary to another condition.
   - Mania can be secondary to a general medical condition
   - Mania can be substance induced (caused by use or abuse of a drug or substance, or by toxin exposure)
5. Assess for any coexisting medical or other condition that warrants special intervention (e.g., substance abuse, anxiety disorder, legal or financial crises).
6. Assess the client's and family's understanding of bipolar disorder, knowledge of medications, and knowledge of support groups and organizations that provide information on bipolar disorder.

■ NURSING DIAGNOSIS

Nursing diagnoses vary for the manic client. A primary consideration for a client in acute mania is the prevention of exhaustion and death from cardiac collapse. Because of the client's poor judgment, excessive and constant motor activity, probable dehydration, and difficulty evaluating reality, *risk for injury* is a likely and appropriate diagnosis if the client's activity level is dangerous to his or her health. Refer to Table 19-2 for a list of potential nursing diagnoses for bipolar disorders.

■ OUTCOME CRITERIA

Outcome criteria will be based on which phase of the illness the client is experiencing. The Nursing Outcomes Classification (NOC) (Moorhead, Johnson, & Maas, 2004) provides useful outcomes.

Phase I: Acute Phase (Acute Mania)

The overall goal during the acute phase is to prevent injury. Outcomes in phase I reflect physiological as well as psychiatric issues. For example, the client will
- Be well hydrated.
- Maintain stable cardiac status.
- Maintain/obtain tissue integrity.
- Get sufficient sleep and rest.
- Demonstrate thought self-control.
- Make no attempt at self-harm.

Relevant NOC outcomes for this phase include the following: Hydration, Cardiac Pump Effectiveness, Tissue Integrity: Skin and Mucous Membrane, Sleep, Distorted Thought Self-Control, and Suicide Self-Restraint.

Phase II: Continuation of Treatment Phase

The continuation phase lasts for 4 to 9 months. Although the overall outcome of this phase is relapse prevention, many other outcomes must be accomplished to achieve relapse prevention. These outcomes include
- Psychoeducational classes for client and family related to
  - Knowledge of disease process
  - Knowledge of medication
  - Consequences of substance addictions for predicting future relapse
  - Knowledge of early signs and symptoms of relapse
- Support groups or therapy (cognitive-behavioral, interpersonal)
- Communication and problem-solving skills training

Relevant NOC outcomes for thise phase include the following: Compliance Behavior, Knowledge: Disease Process, Social Support, and Substance Addiction Consequences.

Phase III: Maintenance Treatment Phase

The overall outcomes for the maintenance phase continue to focus on prevention of relapse and to limit the severity and duration of future episodes. Relevant NOC outcomes include Knowledge: Disease Process, Compliance Behavior, and Family Support During Treatment. Additional outcomes include the following:
- Participation in learning interpersonal strategies related to work, interpersonal, and family problems
- Participation in psychotherapy, group, or other ongoing supportive therapy modality

TABLE 19-2

Potential Nursing Diagnoses for Bipolar Disorders

Signs and Symptoms	Nursing Diagnoses
Excessive and constant motor activity Poor judgment Lack of rest and sleep Poor nutritional intake (excessive or relentless mix of above behaviors can lead to cardiac collapse)	**Risk for injury**
Loud, profane, hostile, combative, aggressive, demanding behaviors	**Risk for other-directed violence** **Risk for self-directed violence** **Risk for suicide**
Intrusive and taunting behaviors Inability to control behavior Rage reaction	**Ineffective coping**
Manipulative, angry, or hostile verbal and physical behaviors Impulsive speech and actions Property destruction or lashing out at others in a rage reaction	**Defensive coping** **Ineffective coping**
Racing thoughts, grandiosity, poor judgment	**Disturbed thought processes** **Ineffective coping**
Giving away of valuables, neglect of family, impulsive major life changes (divorce, career changes)	**Interrupted family processes** **Caregiver role strain**
Continuous pressured speech jumping from topic to topic *(flights of ideas)*	**Impaired verbal communication**
Constant motor activity, going from one person or event to another Annoyance or taunting of others; loud and crass speech Provocative behaviors	**Impaired social interaction**
Failure to eat, groom, bathe, dress self because client is too distracted, agitated, and disorganized	**Imbalanced nutrition: less than body requirements** **Deficient fluid volume** **Self-care deficit (bathing/hygiene, dressing/grooming)**
Inability to sleep because client is too frantic and hyperactive (sleep deprivation can lead to exhaustion and death)	**Disturbed sleep pattern**

■ PLANNING

The planning of care for a bipolar individual usually is geared toward the particular phase of mania (acute mania, continuation of treatment, or maintenance treatment) as well as any other co-occurring issues identified in the assessment (e.g., risk of suicide, risk of violence to person or property, family crisis, legal crises, substance abuse, risk-taking behaviors).

Acute Phase

During the acute phase, planning focuses on medically stabilizing the client while maintaining safety. When mania is acute, hospitalization is usually the safest place for a client. Nursing care is often geared toward decreasing physical activity, increasing food and fluid intake, ensuring at least 4 to 6 hours of sleep per night, alleviating any bowel or bladder problems,

and intervening to see that self-care needs are met. Some clients may require seclusion or even electroconvulsive therapy and certainly need careful medication management.

Refer to Case Study and Nursing Care Plan 19-1 at the end of the chapter.

Continuation Phase

During the continuation phase (lasts 4 to 9 months), planning focuses on maintaining compliance with the medication regimen and preventing relapse. Interventions are planned in accordance with the assessment data regarding the client's interpersonal and stress reduction skills, cognitive functioning, employment status, substance-related problems, social support systems, and such. During this time psychoeducational teaching is a must for client and family. The need for referrals to community programs, groups, and support for any co-occurring disorders or problems (e.g., substance abuse, family problems, legal issues, and financial crises) is evaluated. Evaluation of the need for communication skills training and problem-solving skills training is an important consideration. People with bipolar disorders often have interpersonal problems that affect their work, family, and social lives, as well as other emotional problems. Residual problems resulting from reckless, violent, withdrawn, or bizarre behavior that may have occurred during a manic episode often leave lives shattered and family and friends hurt and distant. For some clients, specific psychotherapy (in addition to medication management) is needed to address these issues, although the focus of psychotherapeutic treatment will vary over time for each individual (Hirschfeld et al., 2000).

Maintenance Phase

During the maintenance phase, planning focuses on preventing relapse and limiting the severity and duration of future episodes. Clients with bipolar disorders require medications over long periods of time, if not a lifetime. Psychotherapy, support/psychoeducational groups, and periodic evaluations all help clients to maintain their family and social lives and to continue employment, if they are employed.

■ INTERVENTION

Clients with bipolar disorders are often ambivalent about treatment. Clients may minimize the destructive consequences of their behaviors or deny the seriousness of the disease. Some clients are reluctant to give up the increased energy, euphoria, and heightened sense of self-esteem of hypomania, before the devastating features of full-blown mania commence (Hirschfeld et al., 2000). Unfortunately, nonadherence to the regimen of mood-stabilizing medication is a major cause of relapse. Therefore, the establishment of a therapeutic alliance with the bipolar individual is crucial.

Acute Phase

Hospitalization provides safety for a client in acute mania (bipolar I disorder), imposes external controls on destructive behaviors, and provides medical stabilization. There are unique approaches to communicating with and maintaining the safety of the client during the hospitalization period. Table 19-3 presents these unique strategies. During this time, the staff members continuously set limits in a firm, nonthreatening, and neutral manner to prevent further escalation of mania and to provide safe boundaries for the client and others.

TABLE 19-3

Care of the Client in Acute Mania

Intervention	Rationale
Communication	
1. Use firm and calm approach: "John, come with me. Eat this sandwich."	1. Structure and control are provided for client who is out of control. Feelings of security can result: "Someone is in control."
2. Use short and concise explanations or statements.	2. Short attention span limits comprehension to small bits of information.
3. Remain neutral; avoid power struggles and value judgments.	3. Client can use inconsistencies and value judgments as justification for arguing and escalating mania.
4. Be consistent in approach and expectations.	4. Consistent limits and expectations minimize potential for client's manipulation of staff.
5. Have frequent staff meetings to plan consistent approaches and to set agreed-on limits.	5. Consistency of all staff is needed to maintain controls and minimize manipulation by client.
6. With other staff, decide on limits, tell client in simple, concrete terms with consequences; for example, "John, do not yell at or hit Peter. If you cannot control yourself, we will help you" or "The seclusion room will help you feel less out of control and prevent harm to yourself and others."	6. Clear expectations help client experience outside controls as well as understand reasons for medication, seclusion, or restraints (if he or she is not able to control behaviors).
7. Hear and act on legitimate complaints.	7. Underlying feelings of helplessness are reduced and acting-out behaviors are minimized.
8. Firmly redirect energy into more appropriate and constructive channels.	8. Distractibility is the nurse's most effective tool with the manic client.

Continued

TABLE 19-3

Care of the Client in Acute Mania—cont'd

Intervention	Rationale
Structure in a Safe Milieu	
1. Maintain low level of stimuli in client's environment (e.g., away from bright lights, loud noises, and people).	1. Escalation of anxiety can be decreased.
2. Provide structured solitary activities with nurse or aide.	2. Structure provides security and focus.
3. Provide frequent high-calorie fluids.	3. Serious dehydration is prevented.
4. Provide frequent rest periods.	4. Exhaustion is prevented.
5. Redirect violent behavior.	5. Physical exercise can decrease tension and provide focus.
6. When warranted in acute mania, use phenothiazines and seclusion to minimize physical harm.	6. Exhaustion and death can result from dehydration, lack of sleep, and constant physical activity.
7. Observe for signs of lithium toxicity.	7. There is a small margin of safety between therapeutic and toxic doses.
8. Protect client from giving away money and possessions. Hold valuables in hospital safe until rational judgment returns.	8. Client's "generosity" is a manic defense that is consistent with irrational, grandiose thinking.
Physiological Safety: Self-Care Needs	
Nutrition	
1. Monitor intake, output, and vital signs.	1. Adequate fluid and caloric intake are ensured; development of dehydration and cardiac collapse is minimized.
2. Offer frequent high-calorie protein drinks and finger foods (e.g., sandwiches, fruit, milkshakes).	2. Constant fluid and calorie replacement are needed. Client may be too active to sit at meals. Finger foods allow "eating on the run."
3. Frequently remind client to eat. "Tom, finish your milkshake." "Sally, eat this banana."	3. The manic client is unaware of bodily needs and is easily distracted. Needs supervision to eat.
Sleep	
1. Encourage frequent rest periods during the day.	1. Lack of sleep can lead to exhaustion and death.
2. Keep client in areas of low stimulation.	2. Relaxation is promoted and manic behavior is minimized.
3. At night, provide warm baths, soothing music, and medication when indicated. Avoid giving client caffeine.	3. Relaxation, rest, and sleep are promoted.
Hygiene	
1. Supervise choice of clothes; minimize flamboyant and bizarre dress (e.g., garish stripes or plaids and loud, unmatching colors).	1. The potential is decreased for ridicule, which lowers self-esteem and increases the need for manic defense. The client is helped to maintain dignity.
2. Give simple step-by-step reminders for hygiene and dress. "Here is your razor. Shave the left side . . . now the right side. Here is your toothbrush. Put the toothpaste on the brush."	2. Distractibility and poor concentration are countered through simple, concrete instructions.
Elimination	
1. Monitor bowel habits; offer fluids and foods that are high in fiber. Evaluate need for laxative. Encourage client to go to the bathroom.	1. Fecal impaction resulting from dehydration and decreased peristalsis is prevented.

Psychopharmacology: Mood Stabilizers

Individuals with bipolar disorder often require multiple medications. There may be times when an antianxiety agent can help reduce agitation or anxiety and/or an antipsychotic agent can reduce psychomotor activity and delusions or hallucinations. Antidepressants may be used periodically to help reduce bipolar depression. Antianxiolytics, antipsychotics, or antidepressants may be used for a limited time, but mood stabilizers are considered lifetime maintenance therapy for bipolar clients (Preston, O'Neal, & Talaga, 2005). Most treatment guidelines advocate lithium and divalproex (Depakote) as first-line agents (Preston et al., 2005).

Lithium Carbonate. Lithium carbonate ($LiCO_3$) is effective in the acute treatment of mania and depressive episodes and the prevention of recurrent mania and depressive episodes. Once primary acute mania has been diagnosed, lithium is most often the first choice of treatment.

Lithium aborts 60% to 80% of acute manic and hypomanic episodes within 10 to 21 days; in these 60% to 80% of cases, 65% to 70% of clients experience a full initial response, 20% experience a partial initial response, and 10% have no initial response (Maxmen & Ward, 2002). Lithium is less effective in people with mixed mania (elation and depression), those with rapid cycling, and those with atypical features.

Lithium is particularly effective in reducing the following (Maxmen & Ward, 2002):
- Elation, grandiosity, and expansiveness
- Flights of ideas
- Irritability and manipulativeness
- Anxiety

To a lesser extent, lithium controls
- Insomnia
- Psychomotor agitation
- Threatening or assaultive behavior
- Distractibility
- Hypersexuality
- Paranoia

Initially in the treatment of acute mania an antipsychotic or benzodiazepine can help calm manic symptoms. Antipsychotics act promptly to slow speech, inhibit aggression, and decrease psychomotor activity. The immediate action of the antipsychotic or benzodiazepine medication serves to prevent exhaustion, coronary collapse, and death until lithium reaches therapeutic levels.

Lithium must reach therapeutic levels in the client's blood to be effective. This usually takes from 7 to 14 days, or longer for some clients. As lithium become effective in reducing manic behavior, the antipsychotic drugs are usually discontinued. Although lithium is an effective intervention for treating the manic phase of a bipolar disorder, it is not a cure. Many clients receive lithium for maintenance indefinitely and experience manic and depressive episodes if the drug is discontinued.

Trade names for lithium carbonate include Lithane, Eskalith, and Lithonate. During the *active phase*, 300 to 600 mg by mouth is given two or three times a day, to reach a clear therapeutic result or a lithium level of 0.8 to 1.4 mEq/L. **The actual maintenance blood levels should range between 0.4 and 1.3 mEq/L.** However, levels of 0.6 to 0.8 mEq/L may be effective for many. To avoid serious toxicity, lithium levels should *not* exceed 1.5 mEq/L (Hopkins & Gelenberg, 2000). At serum levels above 1.5 mEq/L, early signs of toxicity can occur; at 1.5 to 2.0 mEq/L, advanced signs of toxicity may be seen; and at 2.0 to 2.5 mEq/L or above, severe toxicity can occur and emergency measures should be taken immediately.

Cases of severe lithium toxicity with levels of 2.0 mEq/L or above constitute a life-threatening emergency. In such cases, gastric lavage and treatment with urea, mannitol, and aminophylline can hasten lithium excretion. Hemodialysis may also be used in extreme cases.

Adverse Reactions. A small increment exists between the therapeutic dosage and the toxic dosage of lithium. Initially, blood levels are measured weekly or biweekly until the therapeutic level has been reached. After therapeutic levels have been reached, blood levels are determined every month. After 6 months to a year of stability, measurement of blood levels every 3 months may suffice (Freeman, Wiegand, & Gelenberg, 2004). Blood should be drawn 8 to 12 hours after the last dose of lithium is taken. Refer to Table 19-4 for side effects, signs of lithium toxicity, and interventions.

In elderly clients, the principle of **"start low and go slow"** still applies. Levels are often monitored every 3 or 4 days. Some elderly clients may respond to a dose as low as 0.3 to 0.4 mEq/L (Maxman & Ward, 2002). As mentioned earlier, toxic effects are usually associated with lithium levels of 2.0 mEq/L or higher, although they can occur at much lower levels (even within a therapeutic range).

Maintenance Therapy. Some clinicians suggest that clients with bipolar disorder need to be given lithium for 9 to 12 months, and some clients may need lifelong lithium maintenance to prevent further relapses. Many clients respond well to lower dosages during maintenance or prophylactic lithium therapy.

Lithium is unquestionably effective in preventing both manic and depressive episodes in clients with bipolar disorder. However, complete suppression occurs in only 50% of clients or fewer, even with compliance with the maintenance therapy regimen. Therefore, both the person with a bipolar disorder and his or her significant other should be given careful instructions about (1) the purpose and requirements of lithium therapy, (2) its adverse effects, (3) its toxic effects and complications, and (4) situations in which the physician should be contacted. The client and family should also be advised that suddenly stopping lithium can lead to relapse and recurrence of mania. Box 19-1 outlines client and family teaching regarding lithium therapy.

Clients need to know that **two major long-term risks of lithium therapy are hypothyroidism and impairment of the kidney's ability to concentrate urine.** Therefore, a person receiving lithium therapy must have periodic follow-ups to assess thyroid and renal function. Health care providers need to stress to bipolar clients and their families the importance of discontinuing maintenance therapy gradually.

Contraindications. Before lithium is administered, a medical evaluation is performed to assess the client's ability to tolerate the drug. In particular, baseline physical and laboratory examinations should include assessment of renal function; determination of thyroid status, including levels of thyroxine and thyroid-stimulating hormone; and evaluation for dementia or neurological disorders, which presage a poor response to lithium.

Other clinical and laboratory assessments, including an electrocardiogram, are performed as needed, depending on the individual's physical condition.

TABLE 19-4

Lithium Side Effects and Signs of Lithium Toxicity

Level	Signs	Interventions
Expected Side Effects		
<0.4-1.0 mEq/L (therapeutic level)	Fine hand tremor, polyuria, and mild thirst Mild nausea and general discomfort Weight gain	Symptoms may persist throughout therapy. Symptoms often subside during treatment. Weight gain may be helped with diet, exercise, and nutritional management.
Early Signs of Toxicity		
<1.5 mEq/L	Nausea, vomiting, diarrhea, thirst, polyuria, slurred speech, muscle weakness	Medication should be withheld, blood lithium levels measured, and dosage reevaluated.
Advanced Signs of Toxicity		
1.5-2.0 mEq/L	Coarse hand tremor, persistent gastrointestinal upset, mental confusion, muscle hyperirritability, electroencephalographic changes, incoordination	Interventions outlined above or below should be used, depending on severity of circumstances.
Severe Toxicity		
2.0-2.5 mEq/L	Ataxia, serious electroencephalographic changes, blurred vision, clonic movements, large output of dilute urine, seizures, stupor, severe hypotension, coma. Death is usually secondary to pulmonary complications.	There is no known antidote for lithium poisoning. The drug is stopped, and excretion is hastened. If client is alert, an emetic is administered. Otherwise, gastric lavage and treatment with urea, mannitol, and aminophylline are used to hasten lithium excretion.
>2.5 mEq/L	Confusion, incontinence of urine or feces, coma, cardiac arrhythmia, peripheral circulatory collapse, abdominal pain, proteinuria, oliguria, and death	In addition to the interventions above, hemodialysis may be used in severe cases.

Data from Lehne, R. A., et al. (2001). *Pharmacology for nursing care* (4th ed., p. 334). Philadelphia: Saunders; and Lieberman, J. A., & Tasman, A. (2000). *Psychiatric drugs.* Philadelphia: Saunders.

Lithium therapy is generally contraindicated in persons with cardiovascular disease and in people who have brain damage, renal disease, thyroid disease, or myasthenia gravis. Lithium may also harm the fetus and whenever possible is not given to women who are pregnant. Both the fear of pregnancy and the wish to become pregnant are major concerns for many bipolar women taking lithium. Lithium use is also contraindicated in mothers who are breast-feeding and in children younger than 12 years of age.

Antiepileptic Drugs. As many as 20% to 40% of bipolar clients may not respond or respond sufficiently to lithium, or they may not tolerate it. Some subgroups of bipolar clients may not respond well to lithium but may do well when treated with antiepileptic drugs (AEDs). These include clients with the following (Hopkins & Gelenberg, 2000):

- Dysphoric mania (depressive thoughts and feelings during manic episodes)
- Rapid cycling (four or more episodes a year)
- Electroencephalographic abnormalities
- Substance abuse not associated with mood episodes
- Progression in the frequency and severity of symptoms

- No family history of bipolar disorder among first-degree relations

Three AEDs have demonstrated efficacy for the treatment of mood disorders: carbamazepine (Tegretol), divalproex (Depakote), and lamotrigine (Lamictal). Newer anticonvulsants seem to be effective in some cases of refractory bipolar disease (those cases not responding to traditional approaches). AEDs are thought to be

- Superior for continuously cycling clients.
- More effective when there is no family history of bipolar disease.
- Effective at dampening affective swings in schizoaffective clients.
- Effective at diminishing impulsive and aggressive behavior in some nonpsychotic clients.
- Helpful in cases of alcohol and benzodiazepine withdrawal.
- Beneficial in controlling mania (within 2 weeks) and depression (within 3 weeks or longer).

Divalproex (Depakote). Valproic acid is useful in treating lithium nonresponders who are in acute mania, who experience rapid cycles, who are in dysphoric mania, or who have not responded to carbamazepine. It is also helpful in preventing future manic episodes. As with carbamazepine, it is important to

Client and Family Teaching About Lithium Therapy

The client and the client's family should receive the following teaching, should be encouraged to ask questions, and should be given the material in written form as well.

1. Lithium can treat your current emotional problem and also helps prevent relapse. Therefore, it is important to continue taking the drug after the current episode is over.
2. Because therapeutic and toxic dosage ranges are so close, it is important to monitor lithium blood levels very closely—more frequently at first, then once every several months after that.
3. Lithium is not addictive.
4. It is important to eat a normal diet with normal salt and fluid intake (1500-3000 mL/day or six 12-oz glasses of fluid). Lithium decreases sodium reabsorption in the kidneys; this could lead to a deficiency of sodium. A low sodium intake leads to a relative increase in lithium retention, which could produce toxicity.
5. You should stop taking lithium if you have excessive diarrhea, vomiting, or sweating. All of these symptoms can lead to dehydration. Dehydration can raise lithium levels in the blood to toxic levels. **Inform your physician if you have any of these problems.**
6. Do not take diuretics (water pills) while you are taking lithium.
7. Lithium is irritating to the lining in your stomach. It helps to take lithium with meals.
8. **It is important to have your kidneys and thyroid checked periodically, especially if you are taking lithium over a long period.** Talk to your doctor about this follow-up.
9. Don't take any over-the-counter medicines without checking first with your doctor.
10. If you find that you are gaining a lot of weight, you may need to talk this over with your physician or nutritionist.
11. Many self-help groups are available to provide support for people with bipolar disorder and their families. The local self-help group is (give name and telephone number).
12. You can find out more information by calling (give name and telephone number).
13. Keep a list of side effects and toxic effects handy along with the name and number of a contact person (see Table 19-4).
14. **If lithium is to be discontinued, your dosage will be tapered gradually to minimize risk of early relapse.**

monitor liver function and platelet count periodically, although serious complications are rare.

Lamotrigine (Lamictal). Lamotrigine is a first-line treatment for bipolar depression and is approved for acute and maintenance therapy. Lamotrigine is generally well tolerated, but there is one serious but rare dermatological reaction: a potentially life-threatening rash. Clients should be instructed to seek immediate medical attention if a rash appears, although most are likely benign (Preston et al., 2005).

Carbamazepine (Tegretol). Some clients with treatment-resistant bipolar disorder improve after taking carbamazepine and lithium or carbamazepine and an antipsychotic. Carbamazepine seems to work better in clients with rapid cycling and in severely paranoid, angry, manic clients than in euphoric, overactive, overfriendly manic clients. It is also thought to be more effective in dysphoric manic clients.

Blood levels of carbamazepine should be monitored at least weekly for the first 8 weeks of treatment, because the drug can increase the levels of liver enzymes that can speed its own metabolism. In some instances this can cause bone marrow suppression and liver inflammation.

Newer Antiepileptic Drugs. Other popular AEDs being used in the treatment of refractory bipolar disorder are gabapentin (Neurontin) and topiramate (Topamax). Gabapentin is effective in targeting anxiety and is unlikely to interact with other medications. Topiramate is helpful in mania and does not appear to cause weight gain.

See Table 19-5 for dosage range for and concerns regarding the AEDs.

Anxiolytics

Clonazepam (Klonopin) and Lorazepam (Ativan). Clonazepam and lorazepam are useful in the treatment of acute mania in some clients with treatment-resistant mania. These drugs are also effective in managing the psychomotor agitation seen in mania. They should be avoided, however, in clients with a history of substance abuse.

Antipsychotics. In addition to showing sedative properties during the early phase of treatment (help with insomnia, anxiety, agitation), the newer atypical antipsychotics seem to have mood-stabilizing properties. For example, an initial study showed that olanzapine (Zyprexa) is better tolerated and prevents mania relapse more effectively than lithium (Tohen, 2003). Quetiapine (Seroquel) is also effective in treating the anxiety symptoms in bipolar depression (Moyer, 2004).

Electroconvulsive Therapy

Electroconvulsive therapy (ECT) is also used to subdue severe manic behavior, especially in clients with treatment-resistant mania and clients with rapid cycling (i.e., those who experience four or more episodes of illness a year). ECT is effective in bipolar clients with rapid cycling and in those with paranoid-destructive features, who often respond poorly to lithium therapy (and in acutely suicidal clients). Refer to Chapter 18 for more on ECT.

TABLE 19-5

Antiepileptic Drugs (AEDs)

Drug	Dosage Range	Major Adverse Effects
Carbamazepine (Tegretol)	800-1200 mg/day	**Agranulocytosis** and **aplastic anemia** are most serious side effects. Blood levels should be monitored throughout first 8 weeks because drug induces liver enzymes that speed its own metabolism. Dosage may need to be adjusted to maintain serum level of 6-8 mg/L. Sedation is most common problem; tolerance usually develops. Diplopia, incoordination, and sedation can signal excessive levels.
Valproate (Depakene)	750-1000 mg/day	**Baseline liver function tests should be performed and results monitored** at regular intervals. Hepatitis, although rare, has been reported, with fatalities in children. Signs and symptoms to watch for include fever, chills, right upper quadrant pain, dark-colored urine, malaise, and jaundice. Common side effects include tremors, gastrointestinal upset, weight gain, and, rarely, alopecia.
Lamotrigine (Lamictal)	100-200 mg/day	**Life-threatening rash** reported in 3 out of every 1000 individuals. Use caution when renal, hepatic, or cardiac function is impaired. Dizziness, diplopia, headache, ataxia, and somnolence are among frequent side effects.
Gabapentin (Neurontin)	900-2000 mg/day	Most serious adverse effects are difficulty in breathing, swelling of the lips, rash, slurred speech, drowsiness, and diarrhea. Fatigue, somnolence, dizziness, ataxia, diplopia, hypertension are the more frequent side effects.
Topiramate (Topomax)	200-600 mg/day	Used in acute mania or in combination with other drugs. Adverse effects include weight loss, cognitive side effects, fatigue, dizziness, and paresthesia.

Milieu Therapy: Seclusion

Control during the acute phase of hyperactive behavior almost always includes immediate treatment with an antipsychotic. However, when a client is dangerously out of control, use of the seclusion room or restraints may also be indicated. The seclusion room provides comfort and relief to many clients who can no longer control their own behavior.

Seclusion serves the following purposes:

- Reduces overwhelming environmental stimuli
- Protects a client from injuring self, others, or staff
- Prevents destruction of personal property or property of others

Seclusion is warranted when documented data collected by the nursing and medical staff reflect the following points:

- Substantial risk of harm to others or self is clear.
- The client is unable to control his or her actions.
- Problematic behavior has been sustained (continues or escalates despite other measures).
- Other measures have failed (e.g., setting limits beginning with verbal deescalation, or using chemical restraints).

The use of seclusion or restraints is associated with complex therapeutic, ethical, and legal issues. Most state laws prohibit the use of unnecessary physical restraint or isolation. Barring an emergency, the use of seclusion and restraints warrants the client's consent. Therefore, most hospitals have well-defined protocols for treatment with seclusion. Seclusion protocol includes a proper reporting procedure through the chain of command when a client is to be secluded. For example, the use of seclusion and restraint is permitted only on the written order of a physician, which must be reviewed and rewritten every 24 hours. The order must include the type of restraint to be used. As-necessary (prn) orders are updated.

Only in an emergency may the charge nurse place a client in seclusion or restraint; under these circumstances, a written physician's order must be obtained within a specified period of time (15 to 30 minutes).

Seclusion protocols also identify specific nursing responsibilities, such as how often the client's behavior is to be observed and documented (e.g., every 15 minutes), how often the client is to be offered food and fluids (e.g., every 30 to 60 minutes), and how often the client is to be toileted (e.g., every 1 to 2 hours). Because phenothiazines are often administered to clients in seclusion, vital signs should be measured frequently (e.g., every 1 to 2 hours).

Careful and precise documentation is a legal necessity. The nurse documents the following:

- The behavior leading up to the seclusion or restraint

- The actions taken to provide the least restrictive alternative
- The time the client was placed in seclusion
- Every 15 minutes, the client's behavior, needs, nursing care, and vital signs
- The time and type of medications given and their effects on the client

When a client requires seclusion to prevent self-harm or violence toward others, it is ideal to have one nurse on each shift work with the client on a continuous basis. Communication with a client in seclusion is concrete and direct but also kind and limited to brief instructions. Clients need reassurance that seclusion is only a temporary measure and that they will be returned to the unit when their behavior is safer and quieter.

Frequent staff meetings regarding personal feelings about seclusion are necessary to prevent possible dangers. Dangers include using seclusion as a form of punishment and leaving a client in seclusion for long periods of time without proper supervision. **Restraints and seclusion are never to be used as punishment or for the convenience of the staff.** Chapter 8 discusses the legal implications of seclusion and restraints, and Chapter 24 provides more discussion and guidelines.

Continuation Phase

The treatment continuation phase is a crucial one for clients and their families. The outcome for this phase is to prevent relapse. Community resources are chosen based on the needs of the client, the appropriateness of the referral, and the availability of resources. Frequently, it is a case manager who evaluates appropriate follow-up care for clients and their families. Medication compliance during this phase is perhaps the most important treatment outcome. This follow-up is frequently handled in a mental health center. However, adherence to the medication regimen is also addressed in day hospitals and in psychiatric home care visits. Some clients may attend day hospitals if they are not too excitable and are able to tolerate a certain level of stimuli. In addition to medication oversight, day hospitals offer structure, decrease social isolation, and help clients channel their time and energy. If a client is homebound and unable to get to a mental health center or day hospital, then psychiatric home care is the appropriate modality for follow-up care.

Health Teaching

Clients and families need information about bipolar illness with particular emphasis on the chronic and highly recurrent nature of the illness. In addition, clients and families need to be taught the symptoms of impending episodes. For example, changes in sleep patterns are especially important, because they usually precede, accompany, or precipitate mania. Even a single night of unexplainable sleep loss can be taken as an early warning of impending mania. Health teaching stresses the importance of establishing regularity in sleep patterns, meals, exercise, and other activities. See Box 19-2 for guidelines for health teaching for clients with bipolar disorder and their families.

The role of psychoeducation in the prevention of relapse cannot be overstressed (see the Evidence-Based Practice box).

BOX 19-2

Health Teaching: Psychoeducation for Clients with Bipolar Disorder and Their Families

1. Clients with bipolar disorder and their families need to know the following:
   a. The chronic and episodic nature of bipolar disorder
   b. The fact that bipolar disorder is long term and that maintenance treatment therefore will require that one or more mood-stabilizing agents be taken for a long time
   c. The expected side effects and toxic effects of the prescribed medication, as well as whom to call and where to go in case of a toxic reaction
   d. The signs and symptoms of relapse that may "come out of the blue"
   e. The role of family members and others in preventing a full relapse
   f. The phone numbers of emergency contact people, which should be kept in an easily accessed place
2. The use of alcohol, drugs of abuse, even small amounts of caffeine, and over-the-counter medications can produce a relapse.
3. Good sleep hygiene is critical to stability. Frequently, the prodrome of a manic episode is lack of sleep. In some cases, mania may be averted by the use of sleep medications (e.g., temazepam [Restoril]).
4. Psychosocial strategies are important for dealing with work, interpersonal, and family problems; for lowering stress; for enhancing a sense of personal control; and for increasing community functioning.
5. Group and individual psychotherapy are invaluable for gaining insight as well as skills in relapse prevention, providing social support, increasing coping skills in interpersonal relations, improving compliance with the medication regimen, reducing functional morbidity, and decreasing rehospitalizations.

Health care workers need to remember the following:

1. Minimization and denial are common defenses that require gradual introduction of facts.
2. Anger and abusive remarks, although aimed at the health care provider, are symptoms of the disease and are not personal.

Adapted from Zerbe, K. J. (1999). *Women's mental health in primary care.* Philadelphia: Saunders; and Milkowitz, D. J. (2003). Bipolar disorder. In D. H. Barlow (Ed.), *Clinical handbook of psychological disorders* (pp. 523-560). New York: Guilford Press.

EVIDENCE-BASED PRACTICE

Use of Psychoeducation in Preventing Recurrences in Bipolar Clients Whose Disease Is in Remission

Background
Numerous studies have been published on the efficacy of individual therapies (especially cognitive-behavioral therapy) in the treatment of medicated clients with bipolar disorder. The study reported here was a well-designed, blinded, controlled study of the efficacy of group psychoeducation in the prevention of recurrences of bipolar episodes in individuals with bipolar I and bipolar II disorder.

Study
One hundred and twenty-one clients with bipolar I and bipolar II disorder in remission for at least 6 months who were receiving pharmacological treatment attended 21 sessions of group psychoeducation or 21 sessions of nonstructured group meetings. Subjects were assessed monthly during the 21-week treatment period and throughout the 2-year follow-up period.

Results of Study
Participation in group psychoeducation significantly reduced the number of relapses and the number of recurrences per client, while increasing the time to depressive, hypomanic, or mixed recurrences. The number and length of hospitalizations per client were also lower among clients who received psychoeducation.

Implications for Nursing Practice
Group psychoeducation (of families as well as clients) is an effective intervention to help pharmacologically treated clients with bipolar disorder prevent recurrences of the disorder. When a group format is used, many more clients and families can be educated at one time. Psychoeducation is within the purview of all nurses, because it includes medication instruction, information about the symptoms and course of the disorder as well as symptoms of potential relapse, information about useful therapies, and so on. Refer to Box 19-2 for psychoeducational guidance for nurses and others.

Colom, F., et al. (2003). Randomized trial on the efficacy of group psychoeducation in the prophylaxis of recurrences in bipolar patients whose disease is in remission. *Archives of General Psychiatry, 60*(4), 402-407.

Maintenance Phase

Maintenance therapy is aimed at preventing the recurrence of an episode of bipolar illness. Not only are some of the community resources cited earlier helpful, but clients and their families often greatly benefit from mutual support and self-help groups as mentioned later in this chapter.

Psychotherapeutic Approaches

Pharmacotherapy and psychiatric management are essential in the treatment of acute manic attacks. Individuals with bipolar disorder suffer from the psychosocial consequences of their past episodes and their vulnerability to experiencing future episodes. People who have bipolar disease also have to face the burden of long-term treatments that may involve some unpleasant side effects (APA, 2000b). During the course of their illness many clients have sustained strained interpersonal relationships, marriage and family problems, academic and occupational problems, and legal or other social difficulties. Psychotherapy can help people work through these difficulties and decrease some of the psychic distress and increase self-esteem. Psychotherapeutic treatments can also help clients improve their functioning between episodes and attempt to decrease the frequency of future episodes (APA, 2000b).

Cognitive-behavioral therapy (CBT) is typically used as an adjunct to pharmacotherapy and involves identifying maladaptive cognitions and behaviors that may be barriers to a person's recovery and ongoing mood stability (Fredman & Rosenbaum, 2004). It is also being used for bipolar disorder in children (Barclay, 2003). CBT in bipolar disorder focuses on adherence to the medication regimen, early detection and intervention, stress and lifestyle management, and the treatment of depression and comorbid conditions (Lam et al., 2003; Otto, Reilly-Harrington, & Sachs, 2003).

Behavioral family management, family therapy, and psychoeducation help families to stay together, lead to lower rates of rehospitalization, and improve family functioning (APA, 2000b; Miklowitz et al., 2000). Currently a formalized psychotherapy called *interpersonal and social rhythm therapy* is being tested in combination with pharmacotherapy in randomized clinical trials as treatment for clients during the maintenance phase of bipolar illness (APA, 2000b).

Psychotherapy is an important treatment in bipolar illness; it results in greater compliance with the lithium regimen (Jamison, 1995a). Often, the clients receiving medication and therapy place more value on psychotherapy than do clinicians. Moreover, clients treated with cognitive therapy are more likely to take their medications as prescribed than are clients who do not participate in therapy (Jamison, 1995a; Lam et al., 2003).

A client describes her feelings about drug therapy and psychotherapy as follows (Jamison, 1995b):

I cannot imagine leading a normal life without lithium. From startings and stoppings of it, I now know it is an essential part of my sanity. Lithium prevents my seductive but disastrous highs, diminishes my depressions, clears out the weaving of my disordered thinking, slows me, gentles me out, keeps me in my relationships, in my career, out of a hospital, and in psychotherapy. It keeps me alive, too. But psychotherapy heals, it makes some sense of the confusion, it reins in the terrifying thoughts and feelings, it brings back hope and the possibility of learning from it all. Pills cannot, do not, ease one back into reality. They bring you back headlong, careening, and faster than can be endured at times. Psychotherapy is a sanctuary, it is a battleground, and it is where I have come to believe that someday I may be able to contend with all of this. No pill can help me deal with the problem of not wanting to take pills, but no amount of therapy alone can prevent my manias and depressions. I need both.

Support Groups

Clients with bipolar disorder, as well as their friends and families, benefit from forming mutual support groups, such as those sponsored by the Depression and Bipolar Support Alliance (DBSA), the National Alliance for the Mentally Ill (NAMI), the National Mental Health Association, and the Manic-Depressive Association.

■ EVALUATION

Outcome criteria often dictate the frequency of evaluation of short-term and intermediate indicators. For example, are the client's vital signs stable and is he or she well hydrated? Is the client able to control own behavior or respond to external controls? Is the client able to sleep for 4 or 5 hours per night or take frequent short rest periods during the day? Does the family have a clear understanding of the client's disease and need for medication? Do the client and family know which community agencies may help them?

If outcomes or related indicators are not achieved satisfactorily, the preventing factors are analyzed. Were the data incorrect or insufficient? Were nursing diagnoses inappropriate or outcomes unrealistic? Was intervention poorly planned? After the outcomes and care plan are reassessed, the plan is revised, if indicated. Longer-term outcomes include compliance with the medication regimen; resumption of functioning in the community; achievement of stability in family, work, and social relationships and in mood; and improved coping skills for reducing stress.

CASE STUDY and NURSING CARE PLAN 19-1   Mania

Ms. Horowitz is brought into the emergency department after being found on the highway shortly after her car breaks down. When the police come to her aid, she tells them that she is "driving myself to fame and fortune." She appears overly cheerful, constantly talking, laughing, and making jokes. At the same time, she walks up and down beside the car, sometimes tweaking the cheek of one of the policemen. She is coy and flirtatious with the police officers, saying at one point, "Boys in blue are fun to do."

She is dressed in a long red dress, a blue and orange scarf, many long chains, and a yellow and green turban. When she reaches into the car and starts drinking from an open bottle of bourbon, the police decide that her behavior and general condition might result in harm to herself or others. When they explain to Ms. Horowitz that they want to take her to the hospital for a general checkup, her jovial mood

turns to anger and rage, yet 2 minutes after getting into the police car, she is singing Carry Me Back to Old Virginny.

On admission to the emergency department, she is seen by a psychiatrist, and her sister is called. The sister states that Ms. Horowitz stopped taking her lithium about 5 weeks ago and is becoming more and more agitated and out of control. She reports that Ms. Horowitz has not eaten in 2 days, has stayed up all night calling friends and strangers all over the country, and finally fled the house when the sister called an ambulance to take her to the hospital. The psychiatrist contacts Ms. Horowitz's physician, and her previous history and medical management are discussed. It is decided to hospitalize her during the acute manic phase and restart her lithium therapy. It is hoped that medications and a controlled environment will prevent further escalation of the manic state and prevent possible exhaustion and cardiac collapse.

Self-Assessment

Mr. Atkins has worked on the psychiatric unit for 2 years. He has learned to deal with many of the challenging behaviors associated with the manic defense. For example, he no longer takes most of the verbal insults personally, even when the remarks are cutting and hit close to home. He is also better able to recognize and set limits on some

of the tactics used by the manic client to split the staff. The staff on this unit work closely with each other, making the atmosphere positive and supportive; therefore, communication is good among staff. Frequent and effective communication is needed to prevent staff splitting, to maximize external controls, and to maintain consistency in nursing care.

Continued

The only aspect of Ms. Horowitz's behavior that Mr. Atkins thinks he may have difficulty with is the sexual advances and loud sexual comments she might make toward him. He knows that this could make him anxious, and his concern is that his anxiety might be picked up by the client.

When he discusses this with the unit coordinator, they both decide that two nurses should provide care for Ms. Horowitz. A female nurse will spend time with her in her room, and Mr. Atkins will spend time with her in quiet areas on the unit. It is decided that neither Mr. Atkins nor any male staff member will be alone with Ms. Horowitz in her room at any time. Mr. Atkins will ask for relief if Ms. Horowitz's sexual remarks and acting-out behaviors make him anxious.

◾ ASSESSMENT

Objective Data

- Little if anything to eat for days
- Little if any sleep for days
- History of mania
- History of lithium maintenance
- Constant physical activity: unable to sit
- Very loud and distracting to others
- Anger when wishes are curtailed
- Flight of ideas
- Dress loud and inappropriate
- Remarks suggestive of sexual themes: calls nurse "lover"
- Behavior that some clients find amusing
- Remarks that suggest grandiose thinking
- Poor judgment

Subjective Data

- "Driving myself to fame and fortune."
- "I'm untouchable . . . I'll get the FBI to set me free."
- "Let me be . . . set me free, lover."

◾ NURSING DIAGNOSIS (NANDA)

1. *Risk for injury* related to dehydration and faulty judgment, as evidenced by inability to meet own physiological needs and set limits on own behavior
   - Has not slept for days
   - Has not consumed food or fluids for days
   - Engages in constant physical activity, unable to sit

2. *Defensive coping* related to biochemical changes, as evidenced by change in usual communication patterns
   - Very loud and distracting to others
   - Remarks suggest sexual themes
   - Behavior some clients find amusing
   - Remarks suggesting grandiose thinking
   - Flight of ideas
   - Loud, hostile, and sexual remarks to other clients

◾ OUTCOME CRITERIA

Physical status will remain stable during manic phase.

◾ PLANNING

The nurse plans interventions that will help deescalate Ms. Horowitz's activity to minimize potential physical injury (dehydration, cardiac instability) through the use of medication and provision of a nonstimulating environment.

◾ INTERVENTION (NIC)

Mr. Atkins makes the following nursing care plan.

Short-Term Goal	Intervention	Rationale	Evaluation
1. Client will be well hydrated, as evidenced by good skin turgor and normal urinary output and specific gravity, within 24 hours.	1a. Give haloperidol (Haldol) intramuscularly immediately and as ordered.	1a. Continuous physical activity and lack of fluids can eventually lead to cardiac collapse and death.	GOAL MET After 3 hours, client takes small amounts of fluid (2-4 oz per hour). After 5 hours, client starts taking 8 oz per hour with a lot of reminding and encouragement. After 24 hours, urine specific gravity is within normal limits.
	1b. Check vital signs frequently (every 1-2 hours).	1b. Cardiac status is monitored.	
	1c. Place client in private or quiet room (whenever possible).	1c. Environmental stimuli are reduced—escalation of mania and distractibility is minimized.	
	1d. Stay with client and divert client away from stimulating situations.	1d. Nurse's presence provides support. Ability to interact with others is temporarily impaired.	
	1e. Offer high-calorie, high-protein drink (8 oz) every hour in quiet area.	1e. Proper hydration is mandatory for maintenance of cardiac status.	
	1f. Frequently remind client to drink: "Take two more sips."	1f. Client's concentration is poor; she is easily distracted.	
	1g. Offer finger food frequently in quiet area.	1g. Client is unable to sit; snacks she can eat while pacing are more likely to be consumed.	
	1h. Maintain record of intake and output.	1h. Such a record allows staff to make accurate nutritional assessment for client's safety.	
	1i. Weigh client daily.	1i. Monitoring of nutritional status is necessary.	
2. Client will sleep or rest 3 hours during the first night in the hospital with aid of medication and nursing interventions.	2a. Continue to direct client to areas of minimal activity.	2a. Lower levels of stimulation can decrease excitability.	Client is awake most of the first night. Sleeps for 2 hours from 4 to 6 AM. Client is able to rest on the second day for short periods and engage in quiet activities for short periods (5-10 minutes).
	2b. When possible, try to direct energy into productive and calming activities (e.g., pacing to slow, soft music; slow exercise; drawing alone; or writing in quiet area).	2b. Directing client to paced, nonstimulating activities can help minimize excitability.	
	2c. Encourage short rest periods throughout the day (e.g., 3-5 minutes every hour) when possible.	2c. Client may be unaware of feelings of fatigue. Can collapse from exhaustion if hyperactivity continues without periods of rest.	
	2d. Client should drink decaffeinated drinks only—decaffeinated coffee, tea, or colas.	2d. Caffeine is a central nervous system stimulant that inhibits needed rest or sleep.	
	2e. Provide nursing measures at bedtime that promote sleep—warm milk, soft music.	2e. Such measures promote nonstimulating and relaxing mood.	

Continued

Short-Term Goal	Intervention	Rationale	Evaluation
3. Client's blood pressure (BP) and pulse (P) will be within normal limits within 24 hours with the aid of medication and nursing interventions.	3a. Continue to monitor BP and P frequently throughout the day (every 30 minutes). 3b. Keep staff informed by verbal and written reports of baseline vital signs and client progress.	3a. Physical condition is presently a great strain on client's heart. 3b. Alerting all staff regarding client's status can increase medical intervention if a change in status occurs.	GOAL MET Baseline measures on unit are not obtained because of hyperactive behavior. Information from family physician states that baseline BP is 130/90 mm Hg and baseline P is 88 beats per minute. BP at end of 24 hours is 130/70 mm Hg; P is 80 beats per minute.

■ EVALUATION

After 2 days, the medical staff think that Ms. Horowitz's physical status is stable. Her vital signs are within normal limits, she is consuming sufficient fluids, and her urinary output is normal. Although her hyperactivity persists, it does so to a lesser degree, and she is able to get periods of rest during the day and is sleeping 3 to 4 hours during the night.

Ms. Horowitz's hyperactivity continues to be a challenge to the nurses; however, she is able to participate in some activities that require gross motor movement. These activities are useful in channeling some of her aggressive energy. Shortly after her arrival on the unit, Ms. Horowitz starts a fight with another client, but seclusion is avoided because she is able to refrain from further violent episodes as a result of medication and nursing interventions. She can be directed toward solitary activities, which channel some of her energies, at least for short periods.

As the effect of the drugs progresses, Ms. Horowitz's activity level decreases, and by discharge, she is able to discuss issues of concern with the nurse and make some useful decisions about her future. She is to come for follow-up at the community center and agrees to join a family psychoeducational group for clients with bipolar disorder and their families, which she will attend with her sister.

evolve Visit the Evolve website at **http://evolve.elsevier.com/Varcarolis** for a full case study of this client and more case studies and nursing care plans.

■■■ KEY POINTS to REMEMBER

- Biological factors appear to play a role in the etiology of the bipolar disorders. Strong genetic correlates have been revealed especially through twin studies. In addition, little doubt exists that an excess of, and imbalance in, neurotransmitters are also related to bipolar mood swings, which supports the existence of neurobiological influences. Neuroendocrine and neuroanatomical findings provide strong evidence for biological influences.

- Bipolar disorder often goes unrecognized, and early detection can help diminish comorbid substance abuse, suicide, and decline in social and personal relationships, and may help promote more positive outcomes.

- The nurse assesses the client's level of mood (hypomania, acute mania, delirious mania), behavior, and thought processes, and is alert to cognitive dysfunction.

- Analyzing the objective and subjective data helps the nurse to formulate appropriate nursing diagnoses. Some of the nursing diagnoses appropriate for a client who is manic are *risk for violence, defensive coping, ineffective coping, disturbed thought processes*, and *situational low self-esteem*.

- During the acute phase of mania, physical needs often take priority and demand nursing interventions. Therefore, deficient fluid volume and imbalanced nutrition or elimination, as well as disturbed sleep pattern, are usually addressed in the nursing plan.

- The diagnosis *interrupted family processes* is vital. Support groups, psychoeducation, and guidance for the family can greatly affect the client's compliance with the medication regimen.

- Planning nursing care involves identifying the specific needs of the client and family during the three phases of mania. Can the client benefit from communication skills training, improvement in coping skills, legal or financial counseling, or further psychoeducation? What community resources does the client need at this time?

- Manic clients can be very demanding and manipulative. Examples of manipulative behavior include pitting members of the staff against each other, loudly and persistently pointing to faults and shortcomings in staff, constantly demanding attention and favors from the staff, and provoking clients as well as staff with profane and lewd remarks. The manic client constantly interrupts activities and distracts groups with his or her continuous physical motion and incessant joking and talking. The nurse sets limits in a firm, neutral manner and tailors communication techniques as well as interventions to maintain the client's safety.

- Health care workers, family, and friends often feel angry and frustrated by the client's disruptive behaviors. When these feelings are not examined and shared with others, the therapeutic potential of the staff is reduced, and feelings of confusion and helplessness remain.
- Antimanic medications are available. Lithium has a narrow therapeutic index, which necessitates thorough client and family teaching and regular follow-up. AEDs such as carbamazepine and valproic acid are useful, especially in treating people with disease refractory to lithium therapy; newer AEDs are also useful in treating clients who need rapid deescalation and do not respond to other treatment approaches.
- Antipsychotic agents may be needed because of their sedating and mood-stabilizing properties, especially during initial treatment.

- For some clients ECT may be the most appropriate medical treatment.
- Client and family teaching takes many forms and is most important in encouraging compliance with the medication regimen and reducing the risk of relapse.
- Evaluation includes examining the effectiveness of the nursing interventions, changing the outcomes as needed, and reassessing the nursing diagnoses. Evaluation is an ongoing process and is part of each of the other steps in the nursing process.

Visit the Evolve website at **http://evolve.elsevier.com/Varcarolis** for a posttest on the content in this chapter. **evolve**

Critical Thinking and Chapter Review

Visit the Evolve website at **http://evolve.elsevier.com/Varcarolis** for additional self-study exercises. **evolve**

CRITICAL THINKING

1. Donald has a history of bipolar disorder and has been taking lithium for 4 months. During his clinic visit, he tells you, his caseworker, that he does not think he will be taking his lithium anymore because he feels great and he is able to function well at his job and at home with his family. He tells you his wife agrees that he "has this thing licked."
   A. What are Donald's needs in terms of teaching?
   B. What are the needs of the family?
   C. Write out a teaching plan, or use an already constructed plan. Include the following issues with sound rationales for these teaching topics:
      - Use of alcohol, drugs, caffeine, over-the-counter medications
      - Need for sleep, hygiene
      - Types of community resources available
      - Signs and symptoms of relapse
   D. Role-play with a classmate how you can teach this family about bipolar illness and approach effective medication teaching, stressing the need for compliance and emphasizing those things that may threaten compliance.
   E. What referral information (websites, associations) can you give Donald and his family if they ask where they can access further information regarding this disease?

CHAPTER REVIEW

Choose the most appropriate answer.

1. A major principle that should be observed when a nurse communicates with a client experiencing elated mood is to
   1. use a calm, firm approach.
   2. give expanded explanations.
   3. make use of abstract concepts.
   4. encourage lightheartedness and joking.
2. Which of the following is an outcome for a person in the continuation of treatment phase of bipolar disorder?
   1. Client will avoid involvement in self-help groups.
   2. Client will adhere to medication regimen.
   3. Client will demonstrate euphoric mood.
   4. Client will maintain normal weight.
3. A medication teaching plan for a client receiving lithium should include
   1. periodic monitoring of renal and thyroid function.
   2. dietary teaching to restrict daily sodium intake.
   3. the importance of blood draws to monitor serum potassium level.
   4. discontinuing the drug if weight gain and fine hand tremors are noticed.
4. Which symptom related to communication is likely to be present in a manic client?
   1. Mutism
   2. Verbosity
   3. Poverty of ideas
   4. Confabulation

Continued

Critical Thinking and Chapter Review—cont'd

Visit the Evolve website at **http://evolve.elsevier.com/Varcarolis** for additional self-study exercises.

5. For assessment purposes, the nurse should identify the body system most at risk for decompensation during a severe manic episode as

    1. renal.

    2. cardiac.

    3. endocrine.

    4. pulmonary.

■ **STUDENT**
■ **STUDY**
■ **CD-ROM**

Access the accompanying CD-ROM for animations, interactive exercises, review questions for the NCLEX examination, and an audio glossary.

■ **NURSE,**
■ **CLIENT, AND**
■ **FAMILY RESOURCES**

For suggested readings, information on related associations, and Internet resources, go to **http://evolve.elsevier.com/Varcarolis**.

REFERENCES

American Psychiatric Association. (2000a). *Diagnostic and statistical manual of mental disorders (DSM-IV-TR)* (4th ed., text rev.). Washington, DC: Author.

American Psychiatric Association. (2000b). *Practice guidelines for the treatment of psychiatric disorders: Compendium 2000.* Washington, DC: Author.

Barclay, L. (2003, October 20). *Cognitive behavioral therapy useful for bipolar disorder in children* [Abstract C6]. Paper presented at the 50th Annual Meeting of the American Academy of Child and Adolescent Psychiatry, Miami, FL.

Bauer, M. S. (2003). Mood disorders: Bipolar (manic depression) disorders. In A. Tasman, J. Kay, & J. A. Lieberman (Eds.), *Psychiatry* (2nd ed.). West Sussex, England: Wiley.

Bipolar Disorder Resource Center. (2004). Retrieved from http://www.medscape.com/pages/editorial/resourcescienters/public/bipolardisorder/rcbipolar.

Blairy, S., et al. (2004). Social adjustment and self-esteem of bipolar patients: A multicentric study. *Journal of Affective Disorders, 79,* 97-103.

Colom, F., et al. (2000). Clinical factors associated with treatment noncompliance in euthymic bipolar patients. *Journal of Clinical Psychiatry, 61*(8), 549-555.

Dubovsky, S. L., Davies, R., & Dubovsky, A. N. (2004). Mood disorders. In R. E. Hales & S. C. Yudofsky (Eds.), *Essentials of clinical psychiatry* (2nd ed.). Washington, DC: American Psychiatric Publishing.

Dunayevich, E., et al. (2000). Twelve month outcome in bipolar patients with and without personality disorders. *Journal of Clinical Psychiatry, 61*(2), 134-139.

Fredman, S. J., & Rosenbaum, J. F. (2004, May). *Psychosocial intervention for bipolar disorder.* Paper presented at the 157th Annual Meeting of the American Psychiatric Association, New York.

Freedman, M. P., & McElroy, S. L. (1999). Clinical picture and etiologic models of mixed states. *Psychiatric Clinics of North America, 22*(3), 535-546.

Freeman, M. P., Wiegand, C., & Gelenberg, A. J. (2004). Lithium. In A. F. Schatzberg & C. B. Nemeroff (Eds.), *The American Psychiatric Publishing textbook of psychopharmacology* (3rd ed., pp. 547-568). Washington, DC: American Psychiatric Publishing.

Ginns, E. I., et al. (1996). A genome-wide search for chromosomal loci linked to bipolar affective disorder in the Old Order Amish. *National Genetics, 12*(4), 431.

Goldberg, J. F., & Ernst, G. L. (2002). Features associated with delayed initiation of mood stabilizers at the onset of bipolar disorder. *Journal of Clinical Psychiatry, 63*(11), 985-991.

Hattori, E., et al. (2003). Polymorphisms at the G72/G30 gene locus, on L13q33, are associated with bipolar disorder in two independent pedigree series. *American Journal of Human Genetics, 72*(5), 1131-1140.

Hirschfeld, R. M. A., et al. (2000). Practice guidelines for the treatment of patients with bipolar disorder. In American Psychiatric Association, *Practice guidelines for the treatment of psychiatric disorders: Compendium 2000.* Washington, DC: Author.

Hopkins, H. S., & Gelenberg, A. J. (2000). Mood stabilizers. In J. A. Lieberman & A. Tasman (Eds.), *Psychiatric drugs.* Philadelphia: Saunders.

Jamison, K. R. (1995a, November 18). *Psychotherapy of bipolar patients.* Paper presented at the U.S. Psychiatric and Mental Health Congress, New York.

Jamison, K. R. (1995b). *An unquiet mind.* New York: Knopf.

Jamison, K. R. (2000). Suicide and bipolar disorder [Abstract]. *Journal of Clinical Psychiatry, 61*(Suppl. 19), 47-51.

Judd, L. L., et al. (2003). The comparative clinical phenotype and long term longitudinal episode course of bipolar I and II: A clinical spectrum or distinct disorders [Abstract]. *Journal of Affective Disorders, 73*(1), 19-32.

Kahn, D. A., et al. (2000). *Treatment of bipolar illness: A guide for patients and families.* Postgraduate Medicine, Special Report, April 2000. Retrieved February, 14, 2005, from http://www.psychguides.com/bipolar_2000_guide.pdf.

Kelsoe, J. R. (1999). Mood disorders: Genetics. In B. J. Sadock & V. A. Sadock (Eds.), *Kaplan and Sadock's comprehensive textbook of psychiatry* (7th ed., Vol. 2, pp. 1308-1317). Philadelphia: Lippincott Williams & Wilkins.

Lam, D. H., et al. (2003). A randomized controlled study of cognitive therapy for relapse prevention for bipolar affective disorder: Outcome of the first year. *Archives of General Psychiatry, 60,* 145-152.

Leverich, G. S., et al. (2002). Early physical and sexual abuse associated with an adverse course of bipolar illness. *Biological Psychiatry, 51*(4), 288-297.

MacQueen, G. M., Young, L T., & Jaffe, R. T. (2001). A review of psychosocial outcomes in patients with bipolar disorder [Abstract]. *Acta Psychiatrica Scandinavica, 103,* 163-170.

Martinez-Aran, A., et al. (2000). Cognitive dysfunction in bipolar disorder: Evidence of neuro-psychological disturbances [Abstract]. *Psychotherapy and Psychosomatics, 69*(2), 2-18.

Maxmen, J. S., & Ward, N. G. (2002). *Psychotropic drugs: Fast facts* (3rd ed.). New York: W. W. Norton.

Merikangas, K. R., & Kupfer, D. J. (1995). Mood disorders: Genetic aspects. In H. I. Kaplan & B. J. Sadock (Eds.), *Comprehensive textbook of psychiatry/VI* (6th ed., Vol. 1, pp. 1102-1115). Baltimore: Williams & Wilkins.

Miklowitz, D. J., et al. (2000). Family-focused treatment of bipolar disorder: 1-year effects of a psychoeducational program in conjunction with pharmacotherapy. *Biological Psychiatry, 48*(6), 582-592.

Moorhead, S., Johnson, M., & Maas, M. (2004). *Nursing outcomes classification (NOC)* (3rd ed.). St. Louis, MO: Mosby.

Moyer, P. (2004, May 5). *Quetiapine effective against anxiety in bipolar depression* [Abstract NR743]. Paper presented at the 157th Annual Meeting of the American Psychiatric Association, New York.

Nathan, K. I., et al. (1995). Biology of mood disorders. In A. F. Schatzberg & C. B. Nemeroff (Eds.), *The American Psychiatric Press textbook of psychopharmacology* (pp. 439-477). Washington, DC: American Psychiatric Press.

Nurnberger, J. I., Jr., & Gershon, E. S. (1992). Genetics. In E. S. Paykel (Ed.), *Handbook of affective disorders* (2nd ed., pp. 131-148). New York: Guilford Press.

Otto, M. W., Reilly-Harrington, N., & Sachs, G. S. (2003). Psychoeducational and cognitive-behavioral strategies in the management of bipolar disorder [Abstract]. *Journal of Affective Disorders, 73,* 171-181.

Pollock, R., & Kuo, I. (2004, February 9-13). *Neuroimaging in bipolar disorder.* Paper presented at the 5th Invitational Congress of Biological Psychiatry, Sydney, Australia.

Post, R. M., Rubinow, D. R., & Uhde, T. W. (1989). Dysphoric mania: Clinical and biological correlates. *Archives of General Psychiatry, 46,* 353-358.

Preston, J. D., O'Neal, J. H., & Talaga, M. C. (2005). *Handbook of clinical psychopharmacology for therapists* (4th ed.). Oakland, CA: New Harbinger Publications.

Schiller, L., & Bennett, A. (1994). *The quiet room.* New York: Warner Books.

Schneck, C. D., et al. (2003). Current concepts in rapid cycling-bipolar disorder [Abstract]. *Current Psychosis and Therapeutics Reports, 1,* 72-78.

Silverstone, T., & Hunt, N. (1992). Symptoms and assessment of mania. In E. S. Paykel (Ed.), *Handbook of affective disorders* (2nd ed., pp. 15-24). New York: Guilford Press.

Sonne, S. C., & Brady, K. T. (1999). Substance abuse and bipolar comorbidity. *Psychiatric Clinics of North America, 22*(3), 609-628.

Spollen, J. (2003, May 17-22). Impaired cognition in bipolar disorder: Something to think about. Paper presented at the American Psychiatric Association 156th Annual Meeting, San Francisco, CA.

Tohen, M. (2003, June 18). *Olanzapine more effective for preventing mania relapse.* Paper presented at the 5th Invitational Congress of Bipolar Disorders, Pittsburgh, PA.

Wacker, H. R. (2000). Epidemiology and comorbidity of depressive disorders. *Therapeutische Umschau, 57*(2), 53-58.

Zerbe, K. J. (1999). *Women's mental health in primary care.* Philadelphia: Saunders.

CHAPTER **20**

The Schizophrenias

ELIZABETH M. VARCAROLIS

■ KEY TERMS and CONCEPTS

The key terms and concepts listed here appear in color where they are defined or first discussed in this chapter.

acute dystonia, 408

affect, 388

akathisia, 408

ambivalence, 388

associative looseness, 388

atypical (novel) antipsychotics, 404

autism, 388

automatic obedience, 394

blocking, 415

clang association, 393

cognitive symptoms, 395

concrete thinking, 392

conventional (traditional) antipsychotics, 404

delusion of being controlled, 392

delusions, 391

depersonalization, 394

derealization, 394

echolalia, 393

echopraxia, 393

extrapyramidal side effects (EPSs), 405

hallucinations, 393

ideas of reference, 413

illusions, 393

negative symptoms, 394

negativism, 394

neologisms, 393

neuroleptic malignant syndrome (NMS), 410

paranoia, 412

positive symptoms, 391

pseudoparkinsonism, 408

stereotyped behaviors, 394

stupor, 394

tardive dyskinesia (TD), 410

thought broadcasting, 392

thought insertion, 392

thought withdrawal, 392

waxy flexibility, 394

word salad, 393

■ OBJECTIVES

After studying this chapter, the reader will be able to

1. Describe the progression of symptoms from the prepsychotic phase (prodromal symptoms) to the acute phase of schizophrenia.

2. Discuss at least three of the neurobiological-anatomical-nongenetic findings that indicate that schizophrenia is a neurological disease.

3. Differentiate between the positive and negative symptoms of schizophrenia with regard to (a) their response to traditional and atypical antipsychotic medications, (b) their effect on quality of life, and (c) their significance for the prognosis of the disease.

4. Formulate three nursing diagnoses that are appropriate for a person with schizophrenia.

5. Discuss how to deal with common reactions a nurse may experience while working with a schizophrenic client.

6. Role-play with a classmate interventions for a client who is hallucinating, delusional, and exhibiting looseness of associations.

7. Develop a teaching plan for a client with schizophrenia who is taking a traditional antipsychotic drug, such as haloperidol (Haldol).

8. Compare and contrast the properties of the conventional (traditional) with the newer atypical antipsychotic drugs in the following areas: (a) target symptoms, (b) indications for use, (c) adverse effects and toxic effects, (d) need for client and family teaching and follow-up, and (e) cost.

Continued

evolve Visit the Evolve website at **http://evolve.elsevier.com/Varcarolis** for a pretest on the content in this chapter.

9. Identify the effective strategies of individual, group, and family therapies that are most useful for clients with schizophrenia and their families.
10. Differentiate among the three phases of schizophrenia in terms of symptoms, focus of care, and intervention needs.
11. Apply the key elements of a teaching plan for a client with schizophrenia and a family member to the nursing care of one client with schizophrenia.
12. Analyze the different approaches to the care of a client with paranoid schizophrenia and a client with disorganized schizophrenia.

Schizophrenia is a devastating brain disease that affects a person's thinking, language, emotions, social behavior, and ability to perceive reality accurately. Unfortunately, people with this disease are often misunderstood and stigmatized not only by the general population but even by the medical community (Moller & Murphy, 2002). Schizophrenia is described as a psychotic disorder. The term **psychotic** refers to "delusions, any prominent hallucinations, disorganized speech, or disorganized catatonic behavior" (American Psychiatric Association [APA], 2000a, p. 297). Other psychotic disorders include schizophreniform disorder, brief psychotic disorder, schizoaffective disorder, delusional disorder, shared psychotic disorder, and psychosis related to substance abuse or a medical condition (see Box 20-1 for a description of each). Because schizophrenia is one of the most severe of the mental health disorders, it is placed under psychosis on the mental health continuum (Figure 20-1).

EPIDEMIOLOGY

The lifetime prevalence of schizophrenia is 1% worldwide with no differences related to race, social status, culture, or environment (Mariani, 2004).

The most typical age for onset of schizophrenia is during the late teens and early twenties, although cases of onset at age 5 or 6 have been reported (APA, 2000a). Men and women are equally represented in the population of individuals with this disease; however, there are some differences. Individuals with an early age of onset (18 to 25 years) are more often male and have poorer premorbid adjustment, more evidence of structural brain abnormalities, and more prominent negative symptoms (APA, 2000a). Individuals with a later onset (25 to 35 years) are more likely to be female, have less evidence of structural brain abnormalities, and have better outcomes (APA, 2000a). Childhood schizophrenia, although rare, does exist; schizophrenia occurs in 1 of 40,000 children compared to 1 of 100 adults (National Institute of Mental Health, 2003).

COMORBIDITY

Substance abuse disorders occur in approximately 40% to 50% of individuals with schizophrenia (Blanchard et al., 2000), and the lifetime incidence is

---

BOX 20-1

Psychotic Disorders Other Than Schizophrenia

Schizophreniform Disorder
The essential features of schizophreniform disorder are exactly those of schizophrenia except that
- The total duration of the illness is at least 1 month but less than 6 months.
- Impaired social or occupational functioning during some part of the illness may not be apparent (although it may appear).

This disorder may or may not have a good prognosis.

Brief Psychotic Disorder
Brief psychotic disorder is characterized by a sudden onset of psychotic symptoms (delusions, hallucinations, disorganized speech) or grossly disorganized or catatonic behavior. The episode lasts at least 1 day but less than 1 month, following which the individual returns to his or her premorbid level of functioning. Brief psychotic disorders are often precipitated by extremely stressful life events.

Schizoaffective Disorder
Schizoaffective disorder is characterized by an uninterrupted period of illness during which time there is a major depressive, manic, or mixed episode, concurrent with symptoms that meet the criteria for schizophrenia. The symptoms must not be due to any substance use or abuse or to a general medical condition.

Delusional Disorder
Delusional disorder involves nonbizarre delusions (situations that occur in real life, such as being followed, infected, loved at a distance, deceived by a spouse, or having a disease) of at least 1 month's duration. The person's ability to function is not markedly impaired nor is the person's behavior obviously odd or bizarre. Common types of delusions seen in this disorder are delusions of grandeur, persecution, or jealousy, somatic delusions, and mixed delusions.

Shared Psychotic Disorder (Folie à Deux)
A shared psychotic disorder is a condition in which one individual who is in a close relationship with another individual who has a psychotic disorder with a delusion eventually comes to share the delusional beliefs either in total or in part. Apart from the shared delusion, the behavior of the person who takes on the other's delusional behavior is not odd or unusual. Impairment of the person who shares the delusion is usually much less than that of the person who has the psychotic disorder with the delusion. The cult phenomenon is an example, as was demonstrated at Waco and Jonestown.

Induced or Secondary Psychosis
Psychosis may be induced by substances (drugs of abuse, alcohol, medications, or toxins) or caused by the physiological consequences of a general medical condition (delirium, neurological conditions, metabolic conditions, hepatic or renal diseases, and many others). Medical conditions and substances of abuse must always be ruled out before a primary diagnosis of schizophrenia or other psychotic disorder can be made.

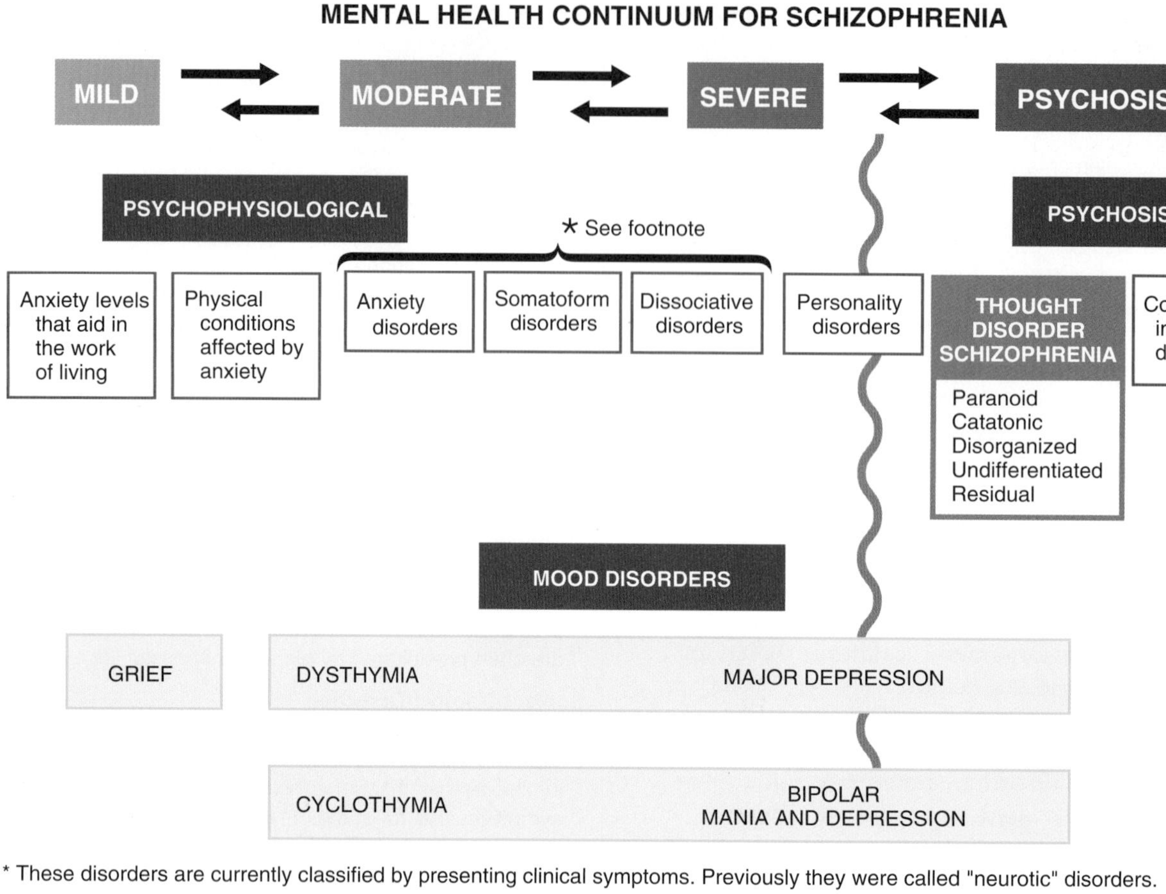

MENTAL HEALTH CONTINUUM FOR SCHIZOPHRENIA

* These disorders are currently classified by presenting clinical symptoms. Previously they were called "neurotic" disorders.

FIGURE 20-1 Mental health continuum for schizophrenia.

even higher at 60% (APA, 2000a). Substance abuse is associated with a variety of negative outcomes: incarceration, homelessness, violence, suicide, and infection with human immunodeficiency virus (HIV). Substance abuse in schizophrenia is also linked with male gender, more pronounced psychotic symptoms, nonadherence with medication regimen, and poor prognosis (Soyka, 2000).

Nicotine dependence is very common in schizophrenia and may be as high as 80% to 90% (APA, 2000a). Nicotine-addicted schizophrenic individuals have a high rate of emphysema and other pulmonary and cardiac problems (APA, 2000a).

Depressive symptoms occur frequently in schizophrenia. Suicide is the leading cause of premature death in this population, and occurs in 10% or perhaps more (Andreasen, 2000); 20% to 40% of individuals make at least one attempt over the course of the illness. A significant percentage of suicides in individuals with schizophrenia occur during periods of remission after 5 to 10 years of illness (APA, 2000a).

The rate of comorbid **anxiety disorders** in individuals with schizophrenia has also been found to be higher than the rate of anxiety disorders in the general population. **Psychosis-induced polydipsia** occurs in 6% to 20% of people with chronic mental illness. This

phenomenon is the compulsive drinking of 4 to 10 L of water a day.

THEORY

The cause of the group of disorders we call schizophrenia is clearly a complicated matter. What is known is that brain chemistry and brain activity are different in a person with schizophrenia than in a person without schizophrenia (Beng-Choon, Black, & Andreasen, 2004; Korn & Saito, 2000).

Schizophrenia most likely occurs as a result of a combination of inherited genetic factors and extreme nongenetic factors (e.g., virus infection, birth injuries, nutritional factors), which can affect the genes governing the brain or injure the brain directly (Andreasen, 2000). These factors may alter the structures of the brain, affect the brain's neurotransmitter system, and disrupt the neural circuits, resulting in impairment in cognition.

Once again, schizophrenia is not a single disease but a syndrome that involves neurobiochemical and neuroanatomical abnormalities with strong genetic links. It strikes early and relentlessly with a high heritability rate of about 80% (Bramon & Sham, 2001). Multiple nongenetic factors may also be present and may play a role in the development of schizophrenia.

Neurobiological Findings

Dopamine Hypothesis

For many years the most widely accepted explanation for the biochemical pathophysiology in schizophrenia was the dopamine hypothesis.

The dopamine theory of schizophrenia is derived from the study of the action of the antipsychotic drugs that block the activity of dopamine (D_2). These antipsychotics block some of the dopamine (D_2) receptors in the brain, thereby limiting the activity of dopamine and reducing some of the symptoms of schizophrenia. Amphetamines, cocaine, methylphenidate (Ritalin), and levodopa are drugs that increase the activity of dopamine in the brain. These drugs can exacerbate the symptoms of schizophrenia in psychotic clients. Amphetamines, cocaine, and other drugs can even simulate symptoms of paranoid schizophrenia in a person without schizophrenia.

Because the dopamine-blocking agents do not ameliorate all the symptoms of schizophrenia, the dopamine hypothesis is no longer considered conclusive. However, five subtypes of dopamine receptor have been discovered (D_1, D_2, D_3, D_4, D_5), and interest in dopamine receptors other than D_2 is rising (Patel, Pinals, & Breier, 2003).

Alternative Biochemical Hypotheses

More recent hypotheses postulate a role for other neurotransmitter systems (e.g., norepinephrine, serotonin, glutamate, γ-aminobutyric acid [GABA], neuropeptides, and neuromodulatory substances) in the pathophysiology of schizophrenia (Beng-Choon et al., 2004).

The development of the atypical antipsychotic drugs that block serotonin as well as dopamine suggests that **serotonin** may play a role in causing the symptoms of schizophrenia. If we can better understand how atypical antipsychotic agents modulate the expression and targeting of 5-hydroxytryptamine 2_A (5-HT$_{2A}$) receptors, we may gain unique insights into schizophrenia.

For quite some time researchers have been aware that phencyclidine piperidine (PCP) induces a state that closely resembles schizophrenia. This observation led to sustained interest in the N-methyl-D-aspartate (NMDA) receptor complex and the possible role of **glutamate** in the pathophysiology of schizophrenia. Glutamate is a crucial neurotransmitter during periods of neural maturation; abnormal maturation of the central nervous system (CNS) is considered to be a central factor in the development of schizophrenia (Korn & Saito, 2000).

Genetic Findings

Schizophrenia and schizophrenia-like symptoms occur at an increased rate in relatives of individuals with schizophrenia. For example (Beng-Choon et al., 2004; Mariani, 2004):

- If one parent has schizophrenia, about 12% of his or her children develop the disease.
- If both parents have schizophrenia, up to 46% of their children will get the disease.
- Among identical twins (from the same egg), the likelihood is 40% to 50% that the second twin will develop schizophrenia if one twin does.
- Among fraternal twins (from two eggs), the likelihood is 15% to 17% that the second twin will develop schizophrenia if one twin does.
- Children of nonschizophrenic parents who are placed in foster homes in which a foster parent later develops schizophrenia do not show an increased rate of schizophrenia.

Evidence suggests that several genes on different chromosomes interact with environmental factors to cause schizophrenia. The list of genes and loci potentially linked to schizophrenia continues to grow rapidly, which contributes to an overall picture of high complexity (Jones, 2003).

Neuroanatomical Findings

Disruptions in the connections and communication within neural circuitry (communication pathways) are thought to be severe in schizophrenia. Therefore, it is conceivable that structural cerebral abnormalities cause disruption to the entire circuitry of the brain.

Brain-imaging techniques, such as computed tomography (CT), magnetic resonance imaging (MRI), and positron emission tomography (PET), provide substantial evidence that some people with schizophrenia have structural brain abnormalities, including the following:

- Enlargement of the lateral cerebral ventricles, third ventricle dilation, and/or ventricular asymmetry
- Cortical atrophy
- Cerebellar atrophy
- Atrophy of the frontal lobe
- Increased size of the sulci (fissures) on the surface of the brain

In addition, MRI and CT scans demonstrate lower brain volume and more cerebrospinal fluid in people with schizophrenia than in healthy people.

During neurological testing, PET scans also show a low rate of blood flow and glucose metabolism in the frontal lobes of the cerebral cortex, which govern planning, abstract thinking, social adjustment, and decision making. Refer to Figure 3-5 for a PET scan that demonstrates reduced brain activity in the frontal lobe of a person with schizophrenia.

Postmortem studies performed on the brains of individuals who had schizophrenia revealed reduced volume of gray matter, especially in the temporal and frontal lobes. As expected, those with the most tissue loss had the worst symptoms (hallucinations, delusions, bizarre thoughts, and depression).

Nongenetic Risk Factors

Birth and Pregnancy Complications

Theories focusing on pregnancy- and birth-related factors arise from the fact that infants for whom there is a history of pregnancy or birth complications are at increased risk for developing schizophrenia as adults. Prenatal risk factors include viral infection, poor nutrition or starvation, or exposure to toxins. Lack of oxygen during birth is also considered a risk factor for the development of schizophrenia. Any of these factors can damage neurons or affect neurotransmitter systems in the fetus. Recently, a Swedish study indicated that individuals born to fathers aged 55 years or older were 1.84 times more likely to develop schizophrenia than those born to fathers aged 20 to 24 years (Byrne et al., 2003).

Stress

Although there is no evidence that stress causes schizophrenia, stress may precipitate the illness in a vulnerable individual. Developmental and family stress as well as social, psychological, and physical stress are all identified as playing a significant role in the severity and course of the disease, and in the person's quality of life.

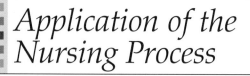

Application of the Nursing Process

ASSESSMENT

DSM-IV-TR Criteria for Schizophrenia

Eugen Bleuler (1857-1939), adding to the observations of Emil Kraepelin (1856-1926), coined the term *schizophrenia*. He first proposed that schizophrenia was not one illness but a heterogeneous group of illnesses with different characteristics and clinical courses. Bleuler's fundamental signs of schizophrenia are referred to as the four *A*'s. The four *A*'s are

1. Affect—refers to the outward manifestation of a person's feelings and emotions. In schizophrenia, clients may display flat, blunted, inappropriate, or bizarre affect.
2. Associative looseness—refers to haphazard and confused thinking that is manifested in jumbled and illogical speech and reasoning. The term *looseness of association* is also used.
3. Autism—refers to thinking that is not bound to reality but reflects the private perceptual world of the individual. Delusions, hallucinations, and neologisms are examples of autistic thinking in a person with schizophrenia.
4. Ambivalence—refers to simultaneously holding two opposing emotions, attitudes, ideas, or

wishes toward the same person, situation, or object. Ambivalence normally occurs in all relationships. Pathological ambivalence is paralyzing because the person continuously vacillates between opposing positions.

■ ■ ■ *VIGNETTE*

Sam, a 25-year-old man soon to be discharged from the hospital, constantly tells the social worker he wants his own apartment. When Sam is told that an apartment has been found for him, he states, "But who will take care of me?" Sam is acting out his ambivalence regarding his desire to be independent and his desire to be taken care of.

■ ■ ■

Kurt Schneider (1887-1957) developed a diagnostic system for schizophrenia in which ongoing symptoms are classified as first rank and second rank. In 1975, the World Health Organization (WHO) identified a standard set of symptoms specific to the diagnosis of schizophrenia; these symptoms are common to people with schizophrenia in numerous countries. Today clinicians in the United States use the criteria of the *Diagnostic and Statistical Manual of Mental Disorders,* fourth edition, text revision *(DSM-IV-TR)* for the diagnosis of schizophrenia (APA, 2000a). Subtypes of schizophrenia include paranoid, catatonic, disorganized, undifferentiated, and residual. Refer to Figure 20-2 for overall criteria for schizophrenia. Criteria and nursing guidelines for the subtypes of schizophrenia are presented in detail later.

Many symptoms are seen in schizophrenia, and not all people with schizophrenia have the same symptoms, even those with a specific subtype of the disease. Figure 20-3 organizes the signs and symptoms of schizophrenia into four main symptom groups or dimensions: positive symptoms, negative symptoms, cognitive symptoms, and depressive and other mood symptoms. These dimensions of schizophrenia appear to have different underlying mechanisms and show different patterns of response to various treatments (Tandon et al., 2003).

Course of the Disease

The course of the disease usually includes recurrent acute exacerbations of psychosis. Prevention of relapse can be more important than the risk of side effects from medications because most side effects are reversible, whereas the consequences of relapse may be irreversible. *With each relapse of psychosis, there is an increase in residual dysfunction and deterioration.* The phases in the course of the disease are the following:

Acute phase: periods of florid positive symptoms (e.g., hallucinations, delusions) as well as negative symptoms (e.g., apathy, withdrawal, lack of motivation)

Maintenance phase: period when acute symptoms decrease in severity

DSM-IV-TR Criteria for Schizophrenia

A. Characteristic Symptoms
Two or more of the following during a 1-month period (or less if successfully treated)
1. Delusions
2. Hallucinations
3. Disorganized speech (e.g., LOA)
4. Grossly disorganized or catatonic behavior
5. Negative symptoms (e.g., affective flattening, avolition, alogia)

If delusions bizarre or auditory hallucinations and
a. voices keep a running commentary about person's thoughts/behaviors **or**
b. two or more voices converse with each other
Then only one criterion is needed.

B. Social/Occupational Dysfunction
If one or more major areas of the person's life are markedly below premorbid functioning (work, interpersonal relationships, or self-care) **or**
If childhood or adolescence failure to achieve expected level of interpersonal, academic, or occupational achievement
Then meets criteria of **B**.

C. Duration
Continuous signs persist for at least 6 months with at least 1 month that meets criteria of **A** (active phase) and may include prodromal or residual symptoms.

D. 1. **All other mental diseases** (e.g., schizoaffective/ mood disorder) have been ruled out.
2. **All other medical conditions** (substance use/ medications or general medical conditions) have been ruled out.
3. **If history of pervasive developmental disorders**, then prominent hallucinations or delusions for 1 month are needed to make the diagnosis of schizophrenia.

FIGURE 20-2 Diagnostic criteria for schizophrenia. *LOA*, Looseness of association. (Adapted from American Psychiatric Association. [2000]. *Diagnostic and statistical manual of mental disorders* [4th ed., text rev.]. Washington, DC: Author.)

Stabilization phase: period in which symptoms are in remission, although there might be milder persistent symptoms

Prepsychotic Early Symptoms

Experts believe that adolescents who are premorbid for schizophrenia probably go through a prepsychotic phase in which the disorder is undiagnosed and untreated. This delay in diagnosis and treatment allows the psychotic process to become more entrenched.

Prodromal symptoms may appear a month to a year before the first psychotic break. These symptoms represent a clear deterioration in previous functioning. Frequently the history of a person with schizophrenia reveals that, during adolescence, the person was withdrawn from others, lonely, and perhaps depressed, and expressed vague or unrealistic plans regarding the future.

In the early phase complaints about acute or chronic anxiety, phobias, obsessions, and compulsions are common. The person may exhibit dissociative features. As anxiety mounts, indications of a thought disorder become evident. An adolescent experiences difficulty concentrating and completing school- or job-related work. Eventually, severe deterioration of work and the ability to cope with the environment occur. "Mind wandering" and the need to devote more time to maintaining one's thoughts are reported. It becomes impossible to control unwanted intrusions into one's thoughts. Eventually, the person finds that his or her mind becomes so distracted that the ability to have ordinary conversations with others is lost (Kolb & Brodie, 1982).

At first, an individual may feel that something "strange" or "wrong" is happening. The person misinterprets things occurring in the environment and may give mystical or symbolic meanings to ordinary events. For example, the individual may think that certain colors have special powers or that a thunderstorm is a message from God. Other people's actions or words may be mistaken for signs of hostility or evidence of harmful intent (Kolb & Brodie, 1982).

As the disease develops, strong feelings of rejection, lack of self-respect, loneliness, and hopelessness begin to emerge. Emotional and physical withdrawal increase feelings of isolation, as does an inability to trust or relate to others. Difficulty in reality testing is manifested in hallucinations, delusions, and odd mannerisms. Some individuals think that their thoughts are being controlled by others or that their thoughts are being broadcast to the world. Others may think that people are out to harm them or are spreading rumors about them. Voices are sometimes heard in the form of commands or derogatory statements about the person's character. The voices may seem to come from outside the room, from electrical appliances, or from other sources (auditory hallucinations).

Early in the disease a person may be preoccupied with religion, matters of mysticism, or metaphysical causes of creation. Speech may be characterized by obscure symbolism.

Later, words and phases may become indecipherable, and these can be understood only as part of the person's private world. Sometimes, the person makes up words (neologisms). People who have been ill with schizophrenia for a long time often have speech patterns that are incoherent, rambling, and devoid of meaning to the casual observer (looseness of association).

Sexual activity is frequently altered in mental disorders. Preoccupation with homosexual themes may be associated with all psychoses but is most prominent in people with paranoid schizophrenia. Doubts regard-

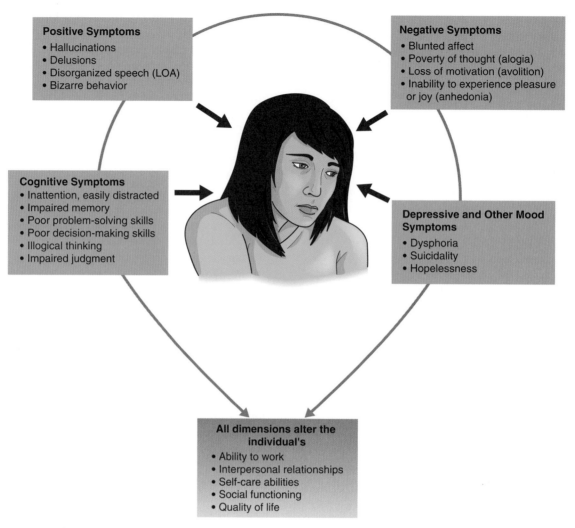

Positive Symptoms
• Hallucinations
• Delusions
• Disorganized speech (LOA)
• Bizarre behavior

Negative Symptoms
• Blunted affect
• Poverty of thought (alogia)
• Loss of motivation (avolition)
• Inability to experience pleasure or joy (anhedonia)

Cognitive Symptoms
• Inattention, easily distracted
• Impaired memory
• Poor problem-solving skills
• Poor decision-making skills
• Illogical thinking
• Impaired judgment

Depressive and Other Mood Symptoms
• Dysphoria
• Suicidality
• Hopelessness

All dimensions alter the individual's
• Ability to work
• Interpersonal relationships
• Self-care abilities
• Social functioning
• Quality of life

FIGURE 20-3 Treatment-relevant dimensions of schizophrenia. *LOA*, Looseness of association.

ing sexual identity, exaggerated sexual needs, altered sexual performance, and fears of intimacy are prominent in schizophrenia. As regression into the disease continues, the person becomes increasingly isolated and preoccupied with self, and engages in masturbatory behavior.

Treatment-Relevant Dimensions of Schizophrenia

No single symptom is always present in all cases of schizophrenia. An abrupt onset of symptoms with good premorbid functioning is usually a favorable prognostic sign. A slow, insidious onset over a period of 2 or 3 years is more ominous. Those whose prepsychotic personalities show good social, sexual, and occupational functioning have a greater chance for a good remission or a complete recovery. A childhood history of withdrawn, reclusive, eccentric, and tense behavior is an unfavorable diagnostic sign. The

younger the client is at the onset of schizophrenia, the more discouraging the prognosis.

The major symptoms of schizophrenia can be grouped into the positive, negative, cognitive, and depressive and other mood symptom dimensions. Tandon and colleagues (2003) and others refer to these four symptom groups as the *treatment-relevant dimensions of schizophrenia*. See Figure 20-3 for an overview of these dimensions and the way in which they can affect an individual's life.

The positive symptoms (e.g., hallucinations, delusions, bizarre behavior, and paranoia) are referred to as *florid psychotic symptoms*; they are the ones that capture our attention. Three decades of analysis of treatment and study findings indicate that perhaps these florid psychotic symptoms may not be the core deficiency after all. Actually, the crippling negative symptoms (e.g., apathy, lack of motivation, anhedonia, and poor thought processes) persist and seem the most destructive because they render the person inert and unmotivated (Beng-Choon et al., 2004). Refer to Box 20-2 for a listing of positive and negative symptoms and use it to follow the discussion of these symptoms.

Positive Symptoms

Positive symptoms, such as hallucinations, delusions, bizarre behavior, and paranoia, are associated with the following:

- Acute onset
- Normal premorbid functioning
- Normal social functioning during remissions
- Normal CT findings
- Normal neuropsychological test results
- Favorable response to antipsychotic medication

The positive symptoms appear early in the first phase of the illness and often precipitate hospitalization. They are, however, the least important prognostically and usually respond to antipsychotic medication. The positive symptoms are presented here in terms of alterations in thinking, speech, perception, and behavior.

Alterations in Thinking

Delusions. Alterations in thinking can take many forms. Delusions are most often defined as false fixed beliefs that cannot be corrected by reasoning. They may be simple beliefs or part of a complex delusional system. In schizophrenia, delusions are often loosely organized and may be bizarre. Most commonly, delusional thinking involves the following themes:

- Ideas of reference
- Persecution
- Grandiosity
- Somatic sensations
- Jealousy
- Control

Table 20-1 provides definitions and examples of delusions.

About 75% of schizophrenic people experience delusions at some time during their illness. In schizophrenia, the most common delusions are persecutory and grandiose, as well as those involving religious or hypochondriacal ideas.

In the acute phase of schizophrenia, the person is overwhelmed by anxiety and is not able to distinguish internal thoughts from external reality. Therefore, a delusion may stimulate behavior for dealing with confusion and the resulting anxiety. A person experiencing delusions is convinced that what he or she believes to be real *is* real. The person's thinking often reflects feelings of great fear and isolation: "I know the doctor talks to the FBI about getting rid of me" or "Everyone wants me dead." Delusions may reflect the person's feelings of low self-worth through the use of reaction formation (observed as grandiosity). "I'm the only one who can save the world, but they won't let me."

At times, delusions hold a kernel of truth. One client came into the hospital acutely psychotic. He repeatedly

---

BOX 20-2

Positive and Negative Symptoms of Schizophrenia

Positive Symptoms

Hallucinations
Auditory
- Voices commenting
- Voices conversing
Somatic-tactile
Olfactory
Visual

Delusions
Persecutory delusions
Jealous delusions
Grandiose delusions
Religious delusions
Somatic delusions
Delusions of reference
Delusions of being controlled
Delusions of mind reading
Thought broadcasting, insertion, withdrawal

Bizarre Behavior
Clothing, appearance
Social and sexual behavior
Aggressive, agitated behavior
Repetitive, stereotyped behavior

Positive Formal Thought Disorder and Speech Patterns
Derailment
Tangentiality
Incoherence
Illogicality
Circumstantiality
Pressure of speech
Distractible speech
Clang associations

Negative Symptoms

Affective Flattening
Unchanging facial expression
Decreased spontaneous movements
Paucity of expressive gestures
Poor eye contact
Inappropriate affect
Lack of vocal inflections

Alogia
Poverty of speech
Poverty of content of speech
Blocking

Avolition, Apathy
Impaired grooming and hygiene
Lack of persistence at work or school
Physical anergia

Anhedonia, Asociality
Few recreational interests or activities
Little sexual interest or activity
Impaired intimacy and closeness
Few relationships with friends or peers

Attention Deficits
Social inattentiveness

TABLE 20-1

Summary of Delusions*

Definition	Example
Ideas of Reference	
Misconstruing trivial events and remarks and giving them personal significance	When Maria saw the doctor and nurse talking together, she believed they were plotting against her. When she heard on the radio that a hurricane was coming, she believed this was really a message that harm was going to befall her.
Persecution	
The false belief that one is being singled out for harm by others; this belief often takes the form of a plot by people in power against the person	Sam believed that the Secret Service was planning to kill him. He believed that the Secret Service was poisoning his food. Therefore he would only eat food that he was certain was safe.
Grandeur	
The false belief that one is a very powerful and important person	Sally believed that she was Mary Magdalene and that Jesus controlled her thoughts and was telling her how to save the world.
Somatic Delusions	
The false belief that the body is changing in an unusual way (e.g., rotting inside)	David told the doctor that his brain was rotting away.
Jealousy	
The false belief that one's mate is unfaithful; may have so-called proof	Harry accused his girlfriend of going out with other men, even though this was not the case. His "proof" was that she came home from work late twice that week. He persisted in his belief, even when the girlfriend's boss explained that everyone had worked late.

*A false belief held and maintained as true, even with evidence to the contrary. This does not include unusual beliefs maintained by one's culture or subculture.

told the staff that the Mafia was out to kill him. Later, the staff learned that he had been selling drugs, that he had not paid his contacts, and that gang members were trying to find him to hurt or even kill him.

Other common delusions observed in schizophrenia are the following:

- **Thought broadcasting**—the belief that one's thoughts can be heard by others (e.g., "My brain is connected to the world mind. I can control all heads of state through my thoughts.")
- **Thought insertion**—the belief that thoughts of others are being inserted into one's mind (e.g., "They make me think bad thoughts.")
- **Thought withdrawal**—the belief that thoughts have been removed from one's mind by an outside agency (e.g., "The devil takes my thoughts away and leaves me empty.")
- **Delusion of being controlled**—belief that one's body or mind is controlled by an outside agency (e.g., "There is a man from darkness who controls my thoughts with electrical waves.")

Concrete Thinking. Concrete thinking refers to an overemphasis on specific details and impairment in the ability to use abstract concepts. For example, during an assessment, the nurse might ask what brought the client to the hospital. The client might answer "a cab" rather than explaining the reason for seeking medical or psychiatric aid. When asked to give the meaning of the proverb "People in glass houses shouldn't throw stones," the person with schizophrenia might answer, "Don't throw stones or the windows will break." The answer is literal; the ability to use abstract reasoning is absent.

Alterations in Speech

Associative Looseness. Zelda Fitzgerald wrote her husband, the writer F. Scott Fitzgerald, an account of going mad:

Then the world became embryonic in Africa—and there was no need for communication. . . . I have been living in vaporous places peopled with one-dimensional figures and tremulous buildings until I can no longer tell an optical illusion from a reality. . . . head and ears incessantly throb and roads disappear. (Vidal, 1982)

Associations are the threads that tie one thought to another and one concept to another. In schizophrenia, these threads are missing, and connections are interrupted. In looseness of association, thinking becomes haphazard, illogical, and confused:

Nurse: Are you going to the picnic today?

Client: I'm not an elephant hunter, no tiger teeth for me.

At times, the nurse may be able to decipher or decode the client's messages and begin to understand the client's feelings and needs. Any exchange in which a person feels understood is useful. Therefore, the nurse might respond to the client in this way:

Nurse: Are you saying, Tony, that you don't feel secure enough to go out with the others today?

Client: Yeah . . . no tiger getting me today.

Very often it is not possible to understand what the client may mean because the client's verbalizations are too fragmented. For example:

Client: I sang out for my mother . . . for this to hell I went. How long is road? These little said three hills hop aboard, share the appetite of the Christmas mice spread . . . within three round moons the devil will be washed away.

If the nurse does not understand what the client is saying, it is important to let the client know this. Clear messages and complete honesty are an important part of working effectively with a person with schizophrenia. An honest response lets the client know that the nurse does not understand, would like to understand, and will try to understand.

Neologisms. Neologisms are words a person makes up that have special meaning for the person. ("I was going to tell him the *mannerologies* of his hospitality won't do." "I want all the *vetchkisses* to leave the room and leave me be.")

Children and creative writers often make up their own words. Their creation of neologisms is imaginative, constructive, and adaptive. Neologisms in people with schizophrenia represent a disruption in thought processes.

Echolalia. Echolalia is the pathological repeating of another's word by imitation and is often seen in people with catatonia.

Nurse: Mary, come for your medication.

Mary: Mary, come for your medication.

Echolalia is the counterpart of echopraxia, mimicking of the *movements* of another, which is also seen in catatonia.

Clang Association. Clang association is the meaningless rhyming of words, often in a forceful manner ("On the track . . . have a Big Mac . . . or get the sack"), in which the rhyming is often more important than the context of the word. This form of speech pattern may be seen in individuals with schizophrenia; however, it may also be seen in persons in the manic phase of a bipolar disorder or in individuals with a cognitive disorder such as Alzheimer's disease or HIV-related dementia.

Word Salad. Word salad is a term used to identify a jumble of words that is meaningless to the listener and perhaps to the speaker as well. It may include a string of neologisms, as in the following example: "Frame woes oblivious waylaid cactus . . . mud and stars and thump-bump going" or "birdisms over squirrel gardening lexapedia listening."

Alterations in Perception. Hallucinations, especially auditory hallucinations, are the major example of an alteration in perception in schizophrenia. The perceptual alterations of hallucinations and loss of ego boundaries (depersonalization and derealization) are discussed in the following subsections.

Hallucinations. Hallucinations can be defined as sensory perceptions for which no external stimulus exists. The most common types of hallucination are the following:

- Auditory—hearing voices or sounds
- Visual—seeing persons or things
- Olfactory—smelling odors
- Gustatory—experiencing tastes
- Tactile—feeling bodily sensations

Table 20-2 provides examples of common hallucinations and also describes the difference between hallucinations and illusions.

It is estimated that up to 90% of people with schizophrenia experience hallucinations at some time during their illness. Although manifestations of hallucination are varied, auditory hallucinations are most common in schizophrenia. Voices may seem to come from outside or inside the person's head. The voices may be familiar or strange, single or multiple. Voices speaking directly to the person or commenting on the person's behavior are most common. A person may believe that the voices are from God, the devil, deceased relatives, or strangers. The auditory hallucinations may occasionally take the form of sounds rather than voices. **Command hallucinations** must be assessed carefully, because the voices may command the person to hurt self or others. For example, a client might state that "the voices" are telling him to "jump out the window" or "take a knife and kill my child." Command hallucinations are often terrifying for the individual. Command hallucinations may signal a psychiatric emergency. Clients who can give an identity to the hallucinated voice are at somewhat greater risk of compliance with the hallucinated command than are those who cannot (Junginger, 1995).

Evidence of possible auditory hallucinatory behavior is turning or tilting of the head, as if the client is talking to someone, or frequent blinking of the eyes and grimacing. Sometimes, clients verbally respond to "unseen others."

Visual hallucinations occur less frequently in people with schizophrenia and are more likely to occur in organic disorders. Olfactory, tactile, or gustatory hallucinations account for about 10% of hallucinations in people with schizophrenia (Moller & Murphy, 2002).

Personal Boundary Difficulties. People with schizophrenia often lack a sense of where their bodies end in relationship to where others begin. Clients might say that they are merging with others or are part of inanimate objects.

TABLE 20-2

Summary of Hallucinations*

Definition	Example
Auditory	
Hearing voices or sounds that do not exist in the environment but are projections of inner thoughts or feelings	Anna "hears" the voice of her dead mother call her a whore and a tramp.
Visual	
Seeing a person, object, or animal that does not exist in the environment	Charles, who is experiencing alcohol withdrawal delirium, "sees" hungry rats coming toward him.
Olfactory	
Smelling odors that are not present in the environment	Theresa "smells" her insides rotting.
Gustatory	
Tasting sensations that have no stimulus in reality	Sam will not eat his food because he "tastes" the poison the FBI is putting in his food.
Tactile	
Feeling strange sensations where no external objects stimulate such feelings; common in delirium tremens	Jack suffers from paranoid schizophrenia. He "feels" electrical impulses controlling his mind.

FBI, Federal Bureau of Investigation.

*A hallucination is a false sensory perception for which no external stimulus exists. Hallucinations are different from illusions in that illusions are misperceptions or misinterpretations of a real experience. For example, a man sees his coat hanging on a coat rack and believes it to be a bear about to attack him. He does see something real but misinterprets what it is.

Depersonalization is a nonspecific feeling that a person has lost his or her identity, that the self is different or unreal. People may be concerned that body parts do not belong to them. People may have an acute sensation that the body has drastically changed. For example, a woman may see her fingers as snakes or her arms as rotting wood. A man may look in a mirror and state that his face is that of an animal.

Derealization is the false perception by a person that the environment has changed. For example, everything seems bigger or smaller, or familiar surroundings have become somehow strange and unfamiliar.

Both depersonalization and derealization can be interpreted as **loss of ego boundaries,** sometimes referred to as *loose ego boundaries.*

Alterations in Behavior. Bizarre and agitated behaviors are associated with schizophrenia and may have a variety of manifestations. **Bizarre behavior** may take the form of a stilted rigid demeanor, eccentric dress or grooming, and rituals. The following behaviors are often seen:

- **Extreme motor agitation** is excited physical behavior, such as running about, in response to inner and outer stimuli. This behavior poses a risk to others as well as to the client, who is at risk for exhaustion, collapse, and even death.
- Stereotyped behaviors are motor patterns that originally had meaning to the person (e.g., sweeping the floor, washing windows) but are now mechanical and lack purpose.

- Automatic obedience is the performance by a catatonic client of all simple commands in a robotlike fashion.
- Waxy flexibility, seen in catatonia, is evidenced by excessive maintenance of posture. For example, the nurse raises the client's arm to bathe the client, and the client continues to hold this position until the nurse lowers the client's arm. Clients can hold unusual postures for long periods.
- Stupor refers to a state in which the catatonic client is motionless for long periods and may even appear to be in a coma.
- Negativism is equivalent to resistance. In *active negativism,* the client does the opposite of what he or she is told to do. When a person does not perform activities that are normal expectations, such as getting out of bed, dressing, and eating, the behavior is termed *passive negativism (catatonia).*

Slowness of movement, stupor, and negativism are considered negative symptoms.

When clients with schizophrenia are acutely ill, impulse control is lacking. Frequently the lack of impulse control is expressed in socially inappropriate **agitated behaviors** such as grabbing another's cigarette, throwing food on the floor, and obtaining the television remote control and changing channels abruptly.

Negative Symptoms

Negative symptoms, such as apathy, anhedonia, poor social functioning, and poverty of thought, are associated with the following:

- Insidious onset
- Premorbid history of emotional problems
- Chronic deterioration
- Demonstration of atrophy on CT scans
- Abnormal results on neuropsychological tests
- Poor response to antipsychotic therapy

The negative symptoms of schizophrenia develop over a long time. These are the symptoms that most interfere with the individual's adjustment and ability to survive. The presence of negative symptoms impedes the person's ability to

- Initiate and maintain relationships.
- Initiate and maintain conversations.
- Hold a job.
- Make decisions.
- Maintain adequate hygiene and grooming.

The presence of negative symptoms contributes to the person's poor social functioning and social withdrawal. During an acute psychotic episode, negative symptoms are difficult to assess because the positive and more florid symptoms, such as delusions and hallucinations, dominate. Some of the negative phenomena are outlined in Table 20-3.

Affect is the observable behavior that expresses a person's emotions. In schizophrenia, people's affect may not coincide with their inner emotions. The affect of a schizophrenic person can usually be categorized in one of three ways: flat or blunted, inappropriate, or bizarre.

A **flat affect** (immobile facial expression or a blank look) or **blunted affect** (minimal emotional response) is commonly seen in schizophrenia.

Inappropriate affect refers to an emotional response to a situation that is not congruent with the tone of the situation. For example, a young man breaks into laughter when told that his father has died.

Bizarre affect is especially prominent in the disorganized form of schizophrenia and includes grimacing, giggling, and mumbling to oneself. Bizarre affect is marked when the client is unable to relate logically to the environment.

Cognitive Symptoms

Cognitive symptoms represent the third dimension and affect at least 40% to 60% of people with schizophrenia. Cognitive impairment involves difficulty with attention, memory, and executive functions (e.g., decision making and problem solving) and is evident when the client is unable to manage his or her own health care, to hold a job, to initiate or maintain a social support system, or to live alone. The degree of cognitive deficit is associated with the severity of negative symptoms; the degree of **disorganized thinking** reflects the degree to which disorganized speech, disorganized behavior, or inappropriate affect is present (APA, 2000a).

Good verbal memory is one cognitive indicator that the individual eventually can function within the community, because it helps with acquisition of psychosocial skills, learning, and retention of skills. These are all necessary for eventual rehabilitation (Beng-Choon et al., 2004).

Depressive and Other Mood Symptoms

Depressive symptoms, the fourth dimension, increase the suffering of clients with schizophrenia and are common in schizophrenia. Recognition of depression

TABLE 20-3

Negative Phenomena

Phenomenon	Explanation
Affective blunting	In *affective blunting*, severe reduction in the expression and range and intensity of affect occurs; in *flat affect* no facial expression of emotion is present.
Anergia	Lack of energy: passivity, lack of persistence at work or school.
Anhedonia	Inability to experience any pleasure in activities that usually produce pleasurable feelings; result of profound emotional barrenness.
Avolition	Lack of motivation: inability to initiate tasks, such as social contacts, grooming, and other aspects of activities of daily living.
Poverty of content of speech	Speech that is adequate in amount but conveys little information because of vagueness, empty repetitions, or use of stereotypes or obscure phrases.
Poverty of speech	Restriction in the amount of speech—answers range from brief to monosyllabic one-word answers.
Thought blocking	May be signaled when a client stops talking in the middle of a sentence and remains silent. After a client stops abruptly: **Nurse:** What just happened now? **Client:** I forgot what I was saying. Something took my thoughts away.

during assessment is crucial for the following reasons (Tandon et al., 2003):

- Depression affects a majority of people with schizophrenia.
- Depression may herald a psychotic relapse and rehospitalization.
- Depression increases the likelihood of substance abuse.
- Depression increases the likelihood of suicide.
- Depression is associated with impaired functioning.

Self-Assessment

Working with individuals diagnosed with schizophrenia produces strong emotional reactions in most health care workers, including nurses. The psychotic client is intensely anxious, lonely, dependent, and distrustful. The intensity of these emotions evokes similarly intense, uncomfortable, and frightening emotions in others. It is important for the nurse to identify personal feelings and responses to clients with schizophrenia; otherwise, the nurse may experience helplessness and increased anxiety. Without support and the opportunity and willingness to explore these reactions with more experienced nursing staff, the nurse may adopt defensive behaviors such as denial, withdrawal, and avoidance. These behaviors not only thwart the client's progress but also undermine the nurse's self-esteem. Statements such as "These clients are hopeless," "You can't understand these people," and "You waste your time with them" are examples of unexamined or unrecognized emotional reactions to clients' behaviors or feelings.

For nurses new to the psychiatric setting, especially for student nurses, supportive supervision must be available if learning is to take place. The student's part in the supervisory process is a willingness to discuss and identify personal feelings and problem behaviors. This can be, and often is, accomplished in group supervision. Experienced psychiatric nurses call this process **peer group supervision.**

Years ago Menninger (1984) noted that staff experience extreme frustration because of the slow progress of clients with schizophrenia. This sense of frustration and accompanying feelings of helplessness are precursors to burnout. The antidote to this downward spiral is a team approach involving periodic reassessment of treatment outcomes with a willingness to scale down unrealistic expectations as well as periodic reassessment of clients who cause frustration to better understand each client's strengths and weaknesses. A team approach to reevaluating and establishing realistic, obtainable outcomes can increase nurses' skills and confidence and improve the quality of interpersonal relationships with clients, as well as relationships with others.

Assessment Guidelines Schizophrenia and Other Psychotic Disorders

1. Assess whether the client has had a medical workup; if so, was medical or substance-induced psychosis ruled out?
2. Assess whether the client is dependent on alcohol or drugs.
3. Assess for command hallucinations (e.g., voices telling the person to harm self or another). If present, ask the client:
   - Do you plan to follow the command?
   - Do you believe the voices are real?
   - Do you recognize the voices?
4. Assess the client's belief system. Is it fragmented, poorly or well organized? Is it systematized? Is the system of beliefs unsupported by reality (delusion)? If yes, then
   - Assess whether delusions focus on someone trying to harm the client; assess whether the client is planning to retaliate against a person or organization.
   - Assess whether precautions need to be taken.
5. Assess for co-occurring disorders:
   - Depression (suicidality)
   - Anxiety
   - Substance dependency
   - History of violence
6. Assess which medications the client is taking. Assess whether the client is adhering to the medication regimen.
7. Assess the family's response to increased symptoms. Are they overprotective? Hostile? Suspicious?
8. Assess the manner in which family members and the client relate.
9. Assess the support system. Is the family well informed about the disease? Does the family understand the need for medication adherence? Is the family familiar with what family support groups are available in the community or where to go for respite and family support? Have family members received or been referred for psychoeducation?
10. Assess the client's global functioning (using the Global Assessment of Functioning [GAF] Scale in Box 1-2).

■ NURSING DIAGNOSIS

People with schizophrenia have multiple disturbing and disabling symptoms that invite a multifaceted approach to care and treatment of the client as well as the client's family. See Table 20-4 for potential nursing diagnoses for a person with schizophrenia.

TABLE 20-4

Potential Nursing Diagnoses for Schizophrenia

Symptom	Nursing Diagnoses
Positive Symptoms	
Hallucinations	
Hears voices that others do not	**Disturbed sensory perception: auditory/visual**
Hears voices telling him or her to hurt self or others *(command hallucinations)*	**Risk for self-directed/other-directed violence**
Distorted Thinking Not Based on Reality	
Persecution: Thinks that others are trying to harm self	**Disturbed thought processes**
Jealousy: Thinks that spouse or lover is being unfaithful, or thinks others are jealous of self when they are not	**Defensive coping**
Grandeur: Thinks he or she has powers and talents that are not possessed or is someone powerful or famous	
Reference: Believes that all events within the environment are directed at or hold special meaning for self	
Looseness of association: Shows loose association of ideas	**Impaired verbal communication**
Clang association: Uses words that rhyme in a nonsensical fashion	**Disturbed thought processes**
Echolalia: Repeats words that are heard	
Mutism: Does not speak	
Circumstantiality: Delays getting to the point of communication because of unnecessary and tedious details	
Concrete thinking: Unable to abstract; uses literal translations concerning aspects of the environment	
Negative Symptoms	
Uncommunicative, withdrawn, makes no eye contact	**Social isolation**
Preoccupied with own thoughts	**Impaired social interaction**
Expresses feelings of rejection or aloneness (lies in bed all day, positions back to door)	**Risk for loneliness**
Talks about self as "bad" or "no good"	**Chronic low self-esteem**
Feels guilty because of "bad thoughts"; extremely sensitive to real or perceived slights	**Risk for self-directed violence**
Shows lack of energy **(anergia)**	**Ineffective coping**
Shows lack of motivation **(avolition)**, unable to initiate tasks (social contact, grooming, and other aspects of daily living)	**Self-care deficit (bathing/hygiene, dressing/grooming)**
	Constipation
Other	
Families and significant others become confused or overwhelmed, have lack of knowledge about disease or treatment, feel powerless in coping with client at home.	**Compromised family coping** **Impaired parenting** **Caregiver role strain** **Deficient knowledge**
Nonadherence to medication and treatment. Client stops taking medication (often from side effects), stops going to therapy groups, family and significant others not aware of need for medications and treatments.	**Nonadherence**

▪ OUTCOME CRITERIA

The desired outcome criteria may vary with the phase of the illness the client is experiencing. Nursing Outcomes Classification (NOC) (Moorhead, Johnson, & Maas, 2004) is a useful guide. Ideally, outcomes should focus on enhancing the person's strengths and minimizing effects of the client's deficits.

Phase I (Acute)

For the acute phase of the illness the overall goal is **client safety and medical stabilization.** Therefore, if the client is at risk for violence to self or others, initial outcome criteria address safety issues (e.g., *client consistently refrains from inflicting serious injury to self and/or others*). Another outcome might be *client consistently re-*

frains from acting upon delusions or hallucinations. Refer to Table 20-5 for selected short-term and intermediate indicators for the outcome *Distorted Thought Self-Control.*

Phase II (Maintenance) and Phase III (Stabilization)

Outcome criteria during phases II and III focus on helping the client to adhere to medication regimens, to understand schizophrenia, and to participate in available psychoeducational activities for both the client and the client's family.

During phase III the outcomes target the negative symptoms and may include ability to participate in social, vocational, or self-care skills training and involvement in socializing groups at various levels. It is also important to include outcomes that address anxiety control and relapse prevention. Mills (2000) identifies desired outcomes to reduce the client's vulnerability to psychosis:

- Maintain a regular sleep pattern.
- Reduce alcohol, drug, and caffeine intake.
- Keep in touch with supportive friends and family.
- Stay active (engage in exercise, hobbies, employment).
- Have a routine daily and weekly schedule including enjoyable activities.
- Take medication regularly.

■ PLANNING

The planning of appropriate interventions is guided by the phase of the illness.

Acute Phase

During the acute phase of schizophrenia, brief hospitalization is frequently indicated if the client is considered a danger to self or others, is refusing to eat or drink, or is too disorganized to provide self-care. Another indication for hospitalization is the need for specific observation, neurological workup, or other medically related tests or treatment. The planning process focuses on the best strategies to ensure client safety and to provide symptom stabilization.

At this time the treatment team identifies aftercare needs for follow-up and support as well as the appropriate referrals that will benefit the client and family. Discharge planning considers not only external factors such as the client's living arrangement, economic resources, social supports, and family relationships, but also the internal factor of the client's vulnerability to stress. Because relapse can be devastating to the client's long-term functioning, vigorous efforts are made to connect the client with community agencies that provide social supports and programs designed to help the client remain well.

Maintenance and Stabilization Phases

Planning during the maintenance and stabilization phases of treatment focuses on strategies to provide client and family education and skills training (psychosocial education). **Relapse prevention skills are vital.** Planning identifies what social, interpersonal, coping, and vocational skills are needed as well as how and where these needs can best be met within the community.

Refer to Table 20-6 for the treatment focus during the different phases of schizophrenia.

■ INTERVENTION

As with outcome criteria and planning, interventions are geared toward the phase of schizophrenia. For example, during phase I, the acute phase, the clinical focus is on crisis intervention, acute symptom stabilization (medication), and safety. Interventions are often hospital based; however, increasingly community-

---

TABLE 20-5

NOC Outcome: Distorted Thought Self-Control

Nursing Outcome and Definition	Intermediate Indicators	Short-Term Indicators
Distorted Thought Self-Control: Self-restraint of disruptions in perception, thought processes, and thought content*	Maintains affect consistent with mood Interacts with others appropriately Perceives environment accurately Exhibits logical thought flow patterns Exhibits reality-based thinking Exhibits appropriate thought content Exhibits ability to grasp ideas of others	Recognizes that hallucinations or delusions are occurring Refrains from attending to hallucinations or delusions Refrains from responding to hallucinations or delusions Describes content of hallucinations or delusions Reports decrease in hallucinations or delusions Asks for validation of reality

From Moorehead, S., Johnson, H., & Maas, M. (2004). *Nursing outcomes classification* (3rd ed.). St. Louis, MO: Mosby.
*Indicators measured on a five-point Likert scale ranging from 1 (never demonstrated) to 5 (consistently demonstrated).

TABLE 20-6

Treatment Focus at Different Phases of Schizophrenia

Phase I		Phase II	Phase III
Acute: Onset, Exacerbation, or Relapse	**Subacute or Convalescent**	**Maintenance Adaptive Plateau**	**Stable Plateau**
Clinical Focus			
Crisis intervention Safety Acute symptom stabilization	Social supports Stress and vulnerability assessment Living arrangements Daily activities Economic resources	Understanding and acceptance of illness	Social, vocational, and self-care skills Learning or relearning Identification of realistic expectations · Adaptation to deficits
Intervention			
Acute psychopharmacological treatment Limit setting Supportive and directive care Psychiatric, medical, neurological evaluation Meeting with family	Psychosocial evaluation Linkage with —Social services —Human services —Community treatment agencies Psychoeducational interventions with families	Support and teaching Medication teaching and side-effect management Direct assistance with situational problems Identification of prodromal and acute symptoms and signs of relapse Continued psychoeducational work with families as needed	Attention to details of self-care, social, and work functioning Direct intervention with family and/or employers Cognitive and social skills enhancement Medication maintenance Continued psychoeducational intervention with families as needed
Professional Collaboration			
Inpatient treatment team Residential alternative to hospitalization Community crisis intervention Internist Neurologist	Social work department Health and human services Day treatment or community support	Community support staff Family support groups Group therapists and self-help groups Practitioners of behavioral therapies using educational models	Group therapists Social, vocational, and self-care providers Family, employer, community support staff

Adapted from Gabard, G. O. (2001). *Treatment of psychiatric disorders* (3rd ed.). Washington, DC: American Psychiatric Publishing.

based providers and home care agencies are treating clients with acute schizophrenia in the community.

Basic Level Interventions

Basic level interventions are provided across the three phases of schizophrenia, take place in the hospital as well as in community-based facilities, and involve every intervention identified in the *Scope and Standards of Psychiatric-Mental Health Nursing Practice* (American Nurses Association, 2000). These interventions include milieu management, counseling, promotion of self-care activities, psychobiological interventions, health teaching, health promotion and health maintenance, and case management.

A number of factors affect the choice of treatment setting and include the following (APA, 2000b):
- Need to protect the person from harm to self or others
- Client's needs for external structure and support
- Client's ability to cooperate with treatment

- Client's need for a particular treatment that may be available only in one setting
- Client's need for treatment of a comorbid general, medical, or psychiatric condition
- Availability of psychosocial support to facilitate receipt of treatment and give critical information to staff about clinical status and response to treatment

Acute phase interventions include the following:
- Acute psychopharmacological treatment (psychobiological intervention)
- Supportive and directive communications (counseling)
- Limit setting (milieu management and counseling)
- Psychiatric, medical, and neurological evaluation

As a result of the recent trend toward decreasing the length of hospital stays, alternatives such as partial hospitalization, halfway houses, and day treatment centers are frequently used as cost-effective alternatives to hospitalization (Beng-Choon et al., 2004).

When clients are hospitalized during the acute phase, the length of hospitalization is often short (days). As soon as the acute symptoms are somewhat stabilized, the client is discharged to the community, where appropriate treatment can be carried out during the maintenance phase (phase II) and the stabilization phase (phase III) of the disease. Effective long-term care of an individual with schizophrenia relies on a three-pronged approach: medications, nursing interventions, and community support. **Family psychoeducation, which is a part of nursing interventions as well as community support, is a key component of effective treatment.**

Phase II and III interventions include the following:

Health teaching:
- Teaching the client and family about the disease
- Teaching the client and family about medication management
- Instructing in cognitive and social skills enhancement
- Teaching strategies to minimize stress and to control anxiety levels

Health promotion and maintenance:
- Teaching to identify signs of relapse and take preventive steps
- Improving deficits in self-care, social, and work functioning
- Encouraging participation in nonthreatening activities
- Encouraging social relationships
- Encouraging family interaction

Interventions are always geared to the client's strengths and healthy functioning as well as to areas of deficiency.

Milieu Therapy

Effective hospital care involves more than protection of the client from family, social, or work environments that are stressful or disruptive. Many clients need the structure provided by hospitalization. In fact, clients in the acute phase of schizophrenia improve more on a unit with a structured milieu than on an open unit that allows greater freedom. Partial hospitalization programs, halfway houses, and day treatment centers are other treatment options that provide a structured milieu. A therapeutic milieu provides safety, useful activities, resources for resolving conflicts, and opportunities for learning social and vocational skills.

Activities. Useful activities are often initiated in group settings that are oriented toward providing support and structure, as well as encouraging the development of social skills and friendships. Structured group therapy also targets the negative symptoms of schizophrenia, as well as some positive symptoms. For example, participation in activity groups appropriate to the client's level of functioning may decrease with-

drawal, promote motivation, modify unacceptable aggression, and increase social competence. Clients who respond to group therapy during hospitalization are likely to benefit from group therapy on an outpatient basis, and group therapy can then provide necessary structure within the client's community milieu.

Participation in group work carries additional benefits. Activities such as drawing pictures, reading poetry, and listening to music are used to focus conversation, which results in reduced anxiety and increased socialization. Self-esteem is enhanced as clients experience success at task completion. Group functions such as picnics facilitate growth in social concern as well as the ability to set limits on self and others. Furthermore, activity group therapy lends itself to many different settings.

Safety. A schizophrenic client, especially in the acute phase, is prone to physical violence, often in response to hallucinations or delusions. During this time, measures need to be taken to protect the client as well as others. If verbal deescalation efforts and chemical restraints (antipsychotic medication) fail to lessen the person's aggression, measures such as physical restraints and seclusion may be indicated. (Refer to Chapters 8, 19, and 24 for care of a client in seclusion or restraints.)

Counseling: Communication Guidelines

Therapeutic strategies for communicating with clients with schizophrenia address lowering the client's anxiety, decreasing defensive patterns, encouraging participation in the milieu, and raising the level of self-worth. Refer to the appropriate sections for specific counseling techniques to deal with paranoia, withdrawal, excitability, and regression.

Familiarity with the principles used for dealing with phenomena such as hallucinations, delusions, and looseness of association is vital for every nurse.

Hallucinations. As previously stated, hearing voices is the most common hallucinatory experience reported by clients. Initially the nurse tries to understand what the voices are saying or telling the person to do. Suicidal or homicidal messages necessitate initiation of safety measures for all members of the health care team.

Hallucinations are real to the person who is experiencing them. Nurses approach clients who are hallucinating in a nonthreatening and nonjudgmental manner (Moller & Murphy, 2002). Moller (1989) emphasizes that, often when a person is hallucinating, the individual is experiencing anxiety, fear, loneliness, and low self-esteem, and the brain is not processing stimuli accurately.

During the acute phase of the illness, the nurse maintains eye contact, calls the client by name, and speaks simply but in a louder voice than usual. Box 20-3 identifies basic communication strategies for use with a client who is hallucinating or delusional.

Delusions. Delusions reflect the misperception of cognitive stimuli. When the nurse attempts to see the world as it appears through the eyes of the client, it is easier to understand the client's delusional experience. For example:

> *Client:* You people are all alike . . . all in on the FBI plot to destroy me.

BOX 20-3

Techniques for Communicating with Clients with Thought Disorders

If the Client Is Hallucinating:

- Ask client directly about his or her hallucinations. For instance, you may say, "Are you hearing voices? What are they saying to you?"
- Watch client for cues that he or she is hallucinating, such as eyes darting to one side, muttering, or watching a vacant area of the room.
- Avoid reacting to hallucinations as if they are real. Do not argue back to the voices.
- Do not negate the client's experience but offer your own perceptions. For instance, you may say, "I don't see the devil standing over you, but I do understand how upsetting that must be for you."
- Focus on reality-based diversions and topics such as conversations or simple projects. Tell the client, "Try not to listen to the voices right now. I have to talk with you."
- Be alert to signs of anxiety in the client, which may indicate that hallucinations are increasing.

If the Client Is Experiencing Delusions:

- Be open, honest, and reliable in interactions to reduce suspiciousness.
- Respond to suspicions in a matter-of-fact and calm manner.
- Ask the client to describe the delusions, for instance, "Who is trying to hurt you?"
- Avoid arguing about the content but interject doubt where appropriate, for instance, "I don't think it would be possible for that petite girl to hurt you."
- Focus on the feelings the delusions generate, for example, "It must feel frightening to think there is a conspiracy against you."
- Once a client describes a delusion, do not dwell on it. Rather, focus conversation on more reality-based topics. If the client obsesses about delusions, set firm limits on the amount of time you will devote to talking about them.
- Observe for events that trigger delusions. If possible, discuss these with the client.
- Validate if part of the delusion is real, for instance, "Yes, there was a man at the nurse's station, but I did not hear him talk about you."

Data from Gorman, L. M., Sultan, D. F., & Raines, M. L. (1996). *Davis's manual of psychosocial nursing for general patient care.* Philadelphia: F. A. Davis.

> *Nurse:* I don't want to hurt you, Tom. Thinking that people are out to destroy you must be very frightening.

In this example, the nurse clarifies the reality of the client's experience and empathizes with the client's apparent experience and feelings of fear. The nurse avoids being drawn into the conversation regarding the content of the delusion (FBI and plot to destroy) but attempts to identify the feelings that the client is experiencing. Talking about the person's feelings is helpful; talking about delusional material is not.

It is *never* useful to argue with the client regarding the content of the delusion. Doing so can intensify the client's retention of irrational beliefs. However, it is helpful for the nurse to clarify misinterpretations of the environment. For example:

> *Client:* I see the doctor is here, and he is out to get me and destroy me.
>
> *Nurse:* It is true the doctor wants to see you, but he wants to talk to you about your treatment. Would you feel more comfortable talking to him in the day room?

Interacting with the client about concrete realities in the environment helps to minimize the time available for the client to focus on delusional thoughts. Performance of specific manual tasks within the scope of the client's abilities is also useful in distracting the client from delusional thinking. The more time the client spends engaged in reality-based activities or with people, the more opportunity the client has to become comfortable with reality.

Mills (2000) identifies useful coping strategies to help the client minimize the disturbing effect of voices and "worrying" thoughts. The counselor or nurse works with the client to find out which coping strategies work and how the client can make the best use of them (Box 20-4).

Associative Looseness. The symptom of associative looseness often mirrors the client's autistic thoughts and reflects the person's poorly organized thinking. An increase in this type of communication is often indicative that the client is feeling increased anxiety and an inability to respond to internal and external stimuli. The client's ramblings may also produce confusion and frustration in the nurse.

The following guidelines are useful for dealing with a client whose speech is confused and disorganized:

- Do not pretend that you understand the client's communications when you are confused by the client's words or meanings.
- Tell the client that you are having difficulty understanding the communications.
- Place the difficulty in understanding on yourself, *not* on the client. For example, say, "I am having trouble following what you are saying," *not* "You are not making any sense."

BOX 20-4

Ways of Coping with Voices and Worrying Thoughts

Distraction

Voices and strange, worrying thoughts:
- Listening to music
- Reading aloud
- Counting backwards from 100
- Describing an object in detail
- Watching television

Interaction

Voices:
- Telling the voices to go away
- Talking to the voices while pretending to use a mobile phone
- Agreeing to listen to the voices at particular times

Activity

Voices and strange, worrying thoughts:
- Walking
- Tidying the house
- Having a relaxing bath
- Playing the guitar
- Singing
- Going to the gym

Social Action

Voices and strange, worrying thoughts:
- Talking to a trusted friend or member of the family
- Phoning a help line
- Avoiding people
- Going to a drop-in center
- Visiting a favorite place

Physical Action

Voices and strange, worrying thoughts:
- Taking extra medication—call your doctor
- Using earplugs (voices)
- Doing breathing exercises
- Using relaxation methods

From Mills, J. (2000). Dealing with voices and strange thoughts. In C. Gamble & G. Brennan (Eds.), *Working with serious mental illness: A manual for clinical practice.* London: Baillière Tindall.

- Look for recurring topics and themes in the client's communications. For example, "You've mentioned trouble with your brother several times. Tell me about your brother and your relationship with him."
- Emphasize what is going on in the client's immediate environment (here and now) and involve the client in simple reality-based activities. These measures can help the client better focus thoughts.
- Tell the client what you do understand and reinforce clear communication and accurate expression of needs, feelings, and thoughts.

Client and Family Health Teaching

The family needs to be included in any psychological strategies aimed at reducing exacerbation of psychotic symptoms. Education is an essential strategy and includes teaching the client and family about the illness (causes, medications and side effects, prevention of relapse); helping the client and family to recognize the impact of stress; ensuring an understanding of the importance of medication to a good outcome; encouraging involvement in psychosocial activities; and identifying sources for ongoing support in dealing with the illness.

Some hospitals and clinics offer medication groups for clients (and sometimes family members as well). Medication groups can

- Help clients to deal more effectively with troubling side effects.
- Alert the nurse to potential adverse side effects or toxic effects.
- Minimize isolation among clients receiving antipsychotics.
- Increase adherence to the medication regimen.

Studies indicate that the family environment plays an important role in the stability of the client. When a client returns to an environment that is warm, concerned, and supportive, the client is less likely to experience relapse. An environment in which people are highly critical of the client's behavior or there is intrusive involvement into the client's life is highly correlated with recurrent episodes of schizophrenia.

Lack of understanding of the disease and its symptoms can lead family members to misinterpret the client's apathy and lack of drive as laziness. This erroneous assumption can foster hostility on the part of family members, caregivers, or people in the community. Thus, further teaching about the negative and positive symptoms of schizophrenia can reduce tensions in families as well as communities. The most effective education is that which occurs over time. Box 20-5 offers a guide for client and family teaching.

Case Management

Discharge planning is a vital aspect of the management of schizophrenia. With the shifting of care for the seriously mentally ill from inpatient to community-based treatment centers, the need for transitional care, with case management provided by nurses and other health care professionals, is heightened. Alternatives to hospitalization that work for many include partial hospitalization, halfway houses, and day treatment programs:

Partial hospitalization: Clients sleep at home and attend treatment sessions during the day or evening.

Halfway houses: Clients live in the community with a group of other clients, sharing expenses

BOX 20-5

Client and Family Teaching for Schizophrenia

1. **Learn all you can about the illness.**
   - Attend psychoeducational groups.
   - Attend support groups.
   - Join the National Alliance for the Mentally Ill (NAMI).
   - Contact the National Institute of Mental Health (NIMH).
2. **Develop a relapse prevention plan.**
   - Know the early warning signs of relapse (e.g., social withdrawal, trouble sleeping, increased bizarre or magical thinking).
   - Know whom to call and where to go when early signs of relapse appear.
   - **Relapse is part of the illness, not a sign of failure.**
3. **Take advantage of all psychoeducational tools.**
   - Participate in family, group, individual therapy.
   - Learn new behaviors and cognitive coping skills to help handle interfamily stress and interpersonal, social, and vocational difficulties. Get information from health care workers (nurse, case manager, physician), NAMI, community mental health groups, or a hospital.
   - **Everyone needs a place to address their fears and losses, and to learn new ways of coping.**
4. **Comply with treatment.**
   - Research has determined that people who do the best in coping with the disease comply with treatment that works for them.
   - Tell your health care worker (nurse, caseworker, physician, social worker) about troubling side effects (e.g., sexual problems, weight gain, "feeling funny"). Most side effects can be treated.
   - Keeping side effects a secret or stopping medication can prevent you from having the best quality of life. Share your concerns.
5. **Avoid alcohol and/or drugs; they can act on the brain and precipitate a relapse.**
6. **Keep in touch with supportive people.**
7. **Keep healthy—stay in balance.**
   - Self-care deficit is reflected in high rates of medical comorbidity.
   - Maintain a regular sleep pattern.
   - Maintain self-care (e.g., diet and hygiene).
   - Keep active (hobbies, friends, groups, sports, job, special interests).
   - Learn ways to reduce stress.

"I am always humbled by people's ability to bear the adversity associated with psychotic symptoms. Often people have adapted their lifestyle so much that the small sense of well-being they do have feels precariously balanced." (Mills, 2000)

Data from Zerbe, K. J. (1999). *Women's mental health in primary care.* Philadelphia: Saunders; Mills, J. (2000). Dealing with voices and strange thoughts. In C. Gamble & G. Brennan (Eds.), *Working with serious mental illness: A manual for clinical practice.* London: Baillière Tindall; and Tandon, R., et al. (2003, October 31). *Beyond symptoms control: Moving towards positive patient outcomes.* Paper presented at the American Psychiatric Association 55th Institute on Psychiatric Services, Boston, MA. Retrieved January 21, 2005, from http://www.medscape.com/viewprogram/2835_pnt.

and responsibilities. Staff are present in the house 24 hours a day, 7 days a week.

Day treatment programs: Clients live in a halfway house or on their own, sometimes with home visits, or in residential programs. Clients attend a structured program during the day.

Programs may include the following:
- Group therapy
- Supervised activities
- Individual counseling
- Specialized training and rehabilitation

It is vital that nurses, physicians, and social workers be aware of the community resources that provide support and make this information available to discharged clients as well as to their families. Examples of such resources include community mental health services, home health services, work support programs, day hospitals, social skills and support groups, family educational skills groups, and respite care.

Clients, siblings, or other family members should be given telephone numbers and addresses of local support groups that are affiliated with the National Alliance for the Mentally Ill (NAMI) (http://www.nami.org).

Advanced Practice Interventions

Psychotherapy

Medication maintenance is the single most important factor in the prevention of relapse in a person suffering from schizophrenia. However, adding psychosocial interventions to drug therapy results in an even lower rate of relapse than does drug therapy alone (Beng-Choon et al., 2004; Patel et al., 2003). Psychosocial therapies such as social skills training, cognitive remediation, cognitive adaptation training, and cognitive-behavioral therapies, considered advanced practice interventions, are particularly helpful in managing chronic schizophrenia in which there is cognitive impairment (Hirayasu, 2000).

Individual Therapy. Social skills training (SST) can improve the level of social activity, foster new social contacts, improve quality of life, and help lower anxiety (Patel et al., 2003).

Cognitive remediation through practice appears to improve cognitive dysfunction, helping individuals better cope with symptoms, the disorder itself, and everyday problems.

Cognitive adaptation training (CAT) is a novel technique aimed at improving adaptive functioning and compensating for the cognitive impairment associated with schizophrenia (Patel et al., 2003).

Cognitive-behavioral therapy (CBT) aims to change abnormal thoughts or responses to hallucinations through coping strategies such as listening to music (see Box 20-4).

Clients and their families benefit from individual therapy, ideally combined with group therapy, provided on an outpatient basis as well as during inpatient treatment.

Group Therapy. Group therapy is particularly useful for clients who have had one or more psychotic episodes. Groups help the client
- Develop interpersonal skills.
- Resolve family problems.
- Make effective use of community supports.

Clients with schizophrenia benefit the most from groups that are available on a continuing outpatient basis and that help develop abilities to solve day-to-day problems, to share relevant experiences, to listen, to ask questions, and to keep topics in focus.

Family Therapy. Families with members who are struggling with schizophrenia often endure considerable hardships while coping with the psychotic and residual symptoms of the illness. Often, these families become isolated from their relatives and communities. To make matters worse, until recently, families were often blamed for causing or triggering episodes of schizophrenia in their family member. NAMI and the National Alliance for Research in Schizophrenia and Depression are actively involved in efforts to develop new and effective treatment strategies that involve families, making them full partners in the treatment process.

Families are perhaps the most consistent factor in clients' lives. Over 60% of clients discharged from a psychiatric facility return to their family of origin (Bustillo, Keith, & Lauriello, 1999). Family education and family therapy improve the quality of family life for the client with schizophrenia. The combination of family therapy and pharmacological therapy is a particularly potent intervention, resulting in a 50% reduction in the relapse rate over the first year (Leff, 2000).

The following example shows how a family came to distinguish between "Martha's problem" and "the problem caused by schizophrenia":

It was a good idea, us all meeting in the comfort of our own home to discuss my sister's illness. We were all able to say how it felt and for the first time I realized that I knew very little about what she was suffering from or how much— the word *schizophrenia* meant nothing to me before but it's much clearer now. I used to think she was just being lazy until she told me in the meeting what it was really like. (Gamble & Brennan, 2000, p. 192)

Programs that provide support, education, coping skills training, and social network development are extremely effective. This approach is called **psychoeducational,** and it brings educational and behavioral approaches into family treatment. The psychoeducational approach does not blame families for their loved one's schizophrenia, but in fact recognizes that families are secondary victims of a biological illness. In family therapy sessions, fears, faulty communication patterns, and distortions are identified. Improved problem-solving skills can be taught, and healthier alternatives to situations of conflict can be explored. Family guilt and anxiety can be lessened, which facilitates change.

Families who receive psychoeducational treatment in multiple-family groups do even better than those treated in single-family groups. Although both single- and multiple-family treatments are cost effective, multiple-family groups are even more so and are the most beneficial to families as well as to the family members with schizophrenia. Improvement seems to stem from an expansion of the social network available to the family and client as well as an expansion in problem-solving capacity afforded by a group. Multiple-family groups also decrease emotional over-involvement while increasing the overall positive tone, which is characteristic of such groups.

Psychopharmacology

Until the 1960s, clients who had even one schizophrenic episode would have spent months to years in a state or private psychiatric hospital. Psychotic episodes, bizarre behavior, depression, and isolation resulted in great emotional and financial burdens to families as well as to individual clients. Refer to "A Nurse Speaks" at the beginning of Unit One. Only with the advent of antipsychotic drugs could symptoms be controlled and clients managed in the community. Although these drugs alleviate many of the symptoms of schizophrenia, they cannot cure the underlying psychotic processes. Therefore, when clients stop taking their medications, psychotic symptoms usually return. An additional concern is that, with each relapse following medication discontinuation, it takes longer to achieve remission after restarting medications. This leads to the possibility that the client will eventually become unresponsive to treatment (Tsung-Ung et al., 2004).

Drugs used to treat psychotic disorders are called *antipsychotic medications*. Two groups of antipsychotic drugs exist: conventional (traditional dopamine antagonists [D_2 receptor antagonists]) and atypical (serotonin-dopamine antagonists [$5\text{-}HT_{2A}$ receptor antagonists]). In addition, some drugs are used to augment the antipsychotic agents for treatment-resistant clients; they are discussed later in this chapter.

All antipsychotic drugs are effective for most acute exacerbations of schizophrenia and for prevention or mitigation of relapse. The conventional (traditional) antipsychotics target the positive symptoms of schizophrenia (e.g., hallucinations, delusions, disordered thinking, and paranoia). The newer atypical (novel) antipsychotics (e.g., clozapine, risperidone, olanzapine, quetiapine, ziprasidone, and aripiprazole) can diminish the negative symptoms as well (deficits in social interaction, blunted or inappropriate emotional expression, and lack of motivation). The atypical agents have fewer side effects and thus are better tolerated. The newer atypical agents also help with symptoms of anxiety and depression, decrease suicidal behavior, and increase neurocognitive functioning (Kuo, 2004).

Antipsychotic agents usually take effect 3 to 6 weeks after the regimen is started. Only about 10% of schizophrenic clients fail to respond to antipsychotic drug therapy. These clients should not continue to take medication that, for them, holds only risks and no benefit.

Because the newer atypical agents (except for clozapine) are generally the treatment of choice for clients experiencing their first episode of schizophrenia, these drugs are discussed first.

Atypical Antipsychotics

The atypical antipsychotics (AAPs) are a new generation of antipsychotics that first emerged in the early 1990s with clozapine (Clozaril). Clozapine unfortunately produces agranulocytosis in 0.8% to 1.0% of the people who take it; the drug also increases the risk for seizures. Fortunately, the AAPs developed after clozapine do not share these same disadvantages.

These newer atypical medications permit more than just control of the most alarming symptoms of this disease (e.g., hallucinations, delusions); they also allow for improvement in the quality of life of people with schizophrenia. **These drugs are often chosen as first-line antipsychotics** because they have the following characteristics (Kuo, 2004):

- Produce minimal to no extrapyramidal side effects (EPSs) or tardive dyskinesia
- Treat both the distressing positive symptoms as well as the disabling negative symptoms of schizophrenia (e.g., social withdrawal, cognitive dysfunction, inattention)
- May improve the neurocognitive defects associated with schizophrenia
- May decrease affective symptoms (anxiety and depression)
- Decrease suicidal behavior
- Target the neurocognitive symptoms
- Are associated with lower relapse rates

As noted earlier, the first of these newer drugs was clozapine, which produced dramatic changes in some clients whose disease had been resistant to the standard antipsychotics. Because of the risk for agranulocytosis and seizures, clients taking clozapine are required to have weekly white blood cell counts for the first 6 months, then frequent monitoring thereafter. The use of clozapine is declining because of the need for these precautions. After clozapine, risperidone (Risperdal) was the next AAP developed; it also improves the functioning of people with schizophrenia and it is used as a first-line drug without the hemato-

logical concerns of clozapine. Newer AAPs include olanzapine (Zyprexa), quetiapine (Seroquel), ziprasidone (Geodon), and, most recently, aripiprazole (Abilify). Each of these drugs is free of the potential hematological side effects of clozapine, and they are all good choices for first-line agents because of their lower side effect profile. One significant disadvantage of the AAPs is that they all (with the exception of ziprasidone and aripiprazole) have a tendency to cause significant weight gain in clients. Weight gain is a serious metabolic side effect of the AAPs and is associated with a cascade of additional side effects, including the following:

- Glucose dysregulation, which increases the propensity for diabetes
- Hypercholesterolemia, which increases the propensity for cardiovascular disease
- Hypertension
- Diminished self-esteem related to weight, which leads to problems with following the medication regimen

An additional disadvantage of the AAPs is that they are more expensive than the traditional antipsychotics. Refer to Table 20-7 for a list of the AAPs, their dosage ranges, some properties of these drugs, and comments.

Conventional (Traditional) Antipsychotics

The conventional antipsychotic agents are becoming obsolete in the treatment of schizophrenia because of their troubling side effects. These side effects lead to a decrease in medication compliance and therefore to an increase in relapse rates. Two of their distinct advantages, however, are that they are much less expensive than the atypical agents and they come in depot form. However, in 2003, risperidone, which is an AAP, was released in a depot form under the name of Risperdal Consta.

Dopamine neurotransmission plays a role in psychosis. The conventional antipsychotics are antagonists at the D_2 receptor site in both the limbic and motor centers. This blockage of D_2 receptor sites in the motor areas is responsible for some of the most troubling side effects of the conventional antipsychotics, namely, the extrapyramidal side effects (EPSs) (akathisia, dystonia, parkinsonism, and tardive dyskinesia). Other adverse reactions include anticholinergic effects, orthostasis, and lowered seizure threshold. When these agents are used, the specific drug is often chosen for its side effects profile. For example, chlorpromazine (Thorazine) is the most sedating agent and has fewer EPSs than do other antipsychotic agents, but it causes hypotension at large dosages. Haloperidol (Haldol) is the least sedating and is often used in large dosages to reduce assaultive behavior but has a high incidence of EPSs. The value of haloperidol for treating violent behaviors is its effectiveness in controlling hallucinatory phenomena with a low incidence of hypotension. People who are functioning at work or at

TABLE 20-7

Atypical Antipsychotic Agents (AAPs)

Pros
• Both atypical and conventional antipsychotic agents relieve the positive symptoms (e.g., hallucinations, delusions). The **atypical agents** target negative symptoms (e.g., cognitive dysfunction, social withdrawal, inattention) and have a lower risk for extrapyramidal symptoms.
• The more favorable side effects profile of the AAPs encourages medication compliance and can reduce the rate of relapse.
• AAPs help improve symptoms of depression and anxiety and decrease suicidal behavior.

Cons
With the exception of ziprasidone and aripiprazole, the AAPs can cause
• Weight gain
• Metabolic abnormalities (glucose dysregulation and hypercholesterolemia) that can increase the likelihood of cardiac conditions and diabetes

Drug	Route(s)	Maintenance Dosage Range (mg/day)	EPSs	ACh	OH	Sed	Comments/Notable Adverse Reactions
Clozapine (Clozaril)	*Oral* PO ODT†: FazaClo	300-900	No	High	High	High	■ **Not first line;** refractory cases only ■ Agranulocytosis in 0.8%-1.0%; scheduled WBC required* ■ High seizure rate ■ Significant weight gain (67%) ■ Excessive salivation ■ Tachycardia
Risperidone (Risperdal)	*Oral* ODT†: Risperdal M-TAB *Consta* Injectable (long-acting): Risperdal Consta	4-16	Mild	Very low	Moderate	Low	■ Hypotension ■ Insomnia ■ Sedation ■ Rarely NMS, TD ■ Sexual dysfunction ■ Weight gain (18%)
Olanzapine (Zyprexa)	*Oral* ODT†: Zyprexa *Injectable* (short-acting)	5-20‡	Low	Moderate	Moderate	Low	■ Significant weight gain (34%) ■ Drowsiness ■ Insomnia ■ Agitation and restlessness ■ Possibly akathisia or parkinsonism
Quetiapine (Seroquel)	Oral	300-800‡	Low	Mild	Moderate	Moderate	■ Weight gain (23%) ■ Headache ■ Drowsiness ■ Orthostasis
Ziprasidone (Geodon)	Oral Injectable (short-acting)	40-160	Low	Mild	Mild	Low	■ ECG changes§ ■ QT prolongation, not to be used with other drugs known to prolong QT interval ■ Low propensity for weight gain ■ Targets depressive symptoms
Aripiprazole (Abilify)	Oral/liquid	10-30	Low	Low-mild	Low-mild	Low	■ New class of AAP ■ Little or no weight gain or increase in glucose, HDL, LDL, or triglyceride levels

Drug dosages from Kane, J. M., et al. (2003). The expert consensus guidelines series: Optimizing pharmacological treatment of psychotic disorders. *Journal of Clinical Psychiatry, 64*(Suppl. 12), 21-51; and Preston, J. D., O'Neal, J. H., & Talaga, M. C. (2005). *Handbook of clinical psychopharmacology for therapists* (4th ed.). Oakland, CA: New Harbinger Publications.

ACh, Anticholinergic side effects (dry mouth, blurred vision, urinary retention, constipation, agitation); *ECG,* electrocardiogram; *EPSs,* extrapyramidal side effects; *HDL,* high-density lipoprotein; *LDL,* low-density lipoprotein; *NMS,* neuroleptic malignant syndrome; *ODT,* orally disintegrating tablet; *OH,* orthostatic hypotension; *Sed,* sedation; *TD,* tardive dyskinesia; *WBC,* white blood cell count.

*See Table 20-9 for more on agranulocytosis.

†An orally disintegrating tablet (ODT) is a fast-disintegrating tablet or wafer that dissolves on the tongue.

‡The safety of olanzapine at dosages of >20 mg/day and quetiapine at dosages of >800 mg/day has not been evaluated in clinical trials.

§Ziprasidone use may carry a risk for QT prolongation in clients with preexisting cardiac disease, low electrolyte levels, or family history of QTc syndrome or in clients taking other drugs that cause long QTc profiles.

home may prefer less sedating drugs; clients who are agitated or excitable may do better with a more sedating medication.

The conventional antipsychotics are often divided into low-potency and high-potency drugs on the basis of their anticholinergic side effects (ACh), EPSs, and sedative properties:

Low potency = high sedation + high ACh + low EPSs
High potency = low sedation + low ACh + high EPSs

All the traditional antipsychotic drugs can cause tardive dyskinesia, however. These drugs are used with caution in people who have seizure disorders because they can lower the seizure threshold. Table 20-8

TABLE 20-8

Typical (Traditional) Antipsychotics

Drug	Route(s) of Administration	Acute Dosage (mg/day)*	Maintenance Dosage (mg/day)*	Special Considerations
High Potency				
Haloperidol (Haldol)	PO, IM	3.0-18.5	1.5-13.5	Has low sedative properties; is used in large doses for assaultive clients to avoid the severe side effect of hypotension Appropriate for the elderly for the same reason as above; lessens the chance of falls from dizziness or hypotension High incidence of extrapyramidal side effects
Trifluoperazine (Stelazine)	PO, IM	5-35	5-30	Low sedative effect—good for symptoms of withdrawal or paranoia High incidence of extrapyramidal side effects Neuroleptic malignant syndrome may occur
Fluphenazine (Prolixin)	PO, IM, SC	2.5-20.0	2.5-15.0	Among the least sedating
Thiothixene (Navane)	PO, IM	6-30	5-40	High incidence of akathisia
Medium Potency				
Loxapine (Loxitane)	PO, IM	60-100	20-200	Possibly associated with weight reduction
Molindone (Moban)	PO	50-100	20-200	Possibly associated with weight reduction
Perphenazine (Trilafon)	PO, IM, IV	8-48	6-42	Can help control severe vomiting
Low Potency				
Chlorpromazine (Thorazine)	PO, IM, R	200-800	150-750	Increases sensitivity to sun (as do other phenothiazines) Highest sedative and hypotensive effects; least potent May cause irreversible retinitis pigmentosa at 800 mg/day
Chlorprothixene (Taractan)	PO, IM	50-600	75-600	Weight gain common
Thioridazine (Mellaril)	PO	225-650	150-550	**Not recommended as first-line antipsychotic** Dose-related severe ECG changes (prolonged QTc intervals), may cause sudden death
Mesoridazine (Serentil)	PO, IM	75-300	100-400	Among the most sedating; may cause severe nausea and vomiting in adults
Decanoate: Long-Acting				
Haloperidol decanoate (Haldol)	IM	0	50-250	Given deep muscle Z-track IM **Given every 3-4 weeks**
Fluphenazine decanoate (Prolixin)	IM	0	6.25-50.0	Given deep muscle Z-track IM **Effective when given every 2-4 weeks**

Drug dosages from Fuller, M. A., & Sajatovic, M. (2000). *Drug information handbook for psychiatry.* Hudson, OH: Lexi-Comp; and Kane, J. M., et al. (2003). The expert consensus guidelines series: Optimizing pharmacological treatment of psychotic disorders. *Journal of Clinical Psychiatry, 64*(Suppl. 12), 21-51.
*Dosages vary with individual response to the antipsychotic agent used.

identifies which drugs are low, medium, and high potency; gives dosages for treatment of acute symptoms and usual maintenance dosages; and lists other considerations.

Three of the more common EPSs are acute dystonia (muscle cramps of the head and neck), akathisia (internal restlessness and external restless pacing or fidgeting), and pseudoparkinsonism (stiffening of muscular activity in the face, body, arms, and legs). These side effects often appear early in therapy and can be minimized with treatment. Treatment usually consists of lowering the dosage or prescribing antiparkinsonian drugs, especially centrally acting anti-cholinergic drugs. Commonly used drugs include trihexyphenidyl (Artane) and benztropine mesylate (Cogentin). Diphenhydramine hydrochloride (Benadryl) and amantadine hydrochloride (Symmetrel) are also useful. Treatment with antiparkinsonian drugs is not completely benign, because the anticholinergic side effects of the antipsychotics may be intensified (e.g., urinary retention, constipation, failure of visual accommodation [blurred vision], cognitive impairment, and delirium).

Table 20-9 identifies common side effects of these antipsychotic medications as well as nursing and medical interventions for clients taking them.

TABLE 20-9

Nursing Measures for Side Effects of Traditional (Standard) Antipsychotics

Side Effect	Onset	Nursing Measures
Anticholinergic Symptoms (ACh)		
1. **Dry mouth**		1. Provide frequent sips of water and sugarless candy or gum. If severe, provide Xero-Lube, a saliva substitute.
2. **Urinary retention and hesitancy**		2. Check voiding; try warm towel on abdomen; consider catheterization if this doesn't work.
3. **Constipation**		3. Usually short term. May use stool softener. Assess for adequate water intake.
4. **Blurred vision**		4. Usually abates in 1 to 2 weeks. If client is taking thioridazine, do not give it, and check with physician.
5. **Photosensitivity**		5. Encourage client to wear sunglasses.
6. **Dry eyes**		6. Use artificial tears.
7. **Inhibition of ejaculation or impotence in men**		7. Alert physician; client may need alternative medication.
Extrapyramidal Side Effects (EPSs)		
1. **Pseudoparkinsonism:** masklike facies, stiff and stooped posture, shuffling gait, drooling, tremor, "pill-rolling" phenomenon	5 hours-30 days	1. Alert medical staff. An anticholinergic agent (e.g., trihexyphenidyl [Artane] or benztropine [Cogentin]) may be used.
2. **Acute dystonic reactions:** acute contractions of tongue, face, neck, and back (tongue and jaw first) ▪ **Opisthotonos:** tetanic heightening of entire body, head and belly up ▪ **Oculogyric crisis:** eyes locked upward	1-5 days	2. **First choice:** diphenhydramine hydrochloride (Benadryl) 25-50 mg IM/IV. Relief occurs in minutes. **Second choice:** benztropine, 1-2 mg IM/IV. **Prevent further dystonias** with any anticholinergic agent (see Table 20-10). Experience is very frightening. Take client to quiet area and stay with him or her until medicated.
3. **Akathisia:** motor inner-driven restlessness (e.g., tapping foot incessantly, rocking forward and backward in chair, shifting weight from side to side)	2 hours-60 days	3. Physician may change antipsychotic agent or give antiparkinsonian agent. Tolerance does not develop to akathisia, but akathisia disappears when neuroleptic is discontinued. Propranolol (Inderal), lorazepam (Ativan), or diazepam (Valium) may be used.
4. **Tardive dyskinesia:** ▪ **Facial:** protruding and rolling tongue, blowing, smacking, licking, spastic facial distortion, smacking movements	Months to years	4. **No known treatment.** Discontinuing the drug does not always relieve symptoms. Possibly 20% of clients taking these drugs for >2 years may develop tardive dyskinesia. Nurses and doctors should encourage clients to be screened for tardive dyskinesia at least every 3 months.

TABLE 20-9

Nursing Measures for Side Effects of Traditional (Standard) Antipsychotics—cont'd

Side Effect	Onset	Nursing Measures
Extrapyramidal Side Effects (EPSs)		
■ **Limbs:** —**Choreic:** rapid, purposeless, and irregular movements —**Athetoid:** slow, complex, and serpentine movements ■ **Trunk:** neck and shoulder movements, dramatic hip jerks and rocking, twisting pelvic thrusts		
α₂ Block: Cardiovascular Effects		
1. **Hypotension and postural hypotension**		1. Check blood pressure before giving agent; advise client to dangle feet before getting out of bed to prevent dizziness and subsequent falls. A systolic pressure of 80 mm Hg when standing is indication not to give the current dose. This effect usually subsides when drug is stabilized in 1 to 2 weeks. Elastic bandages may prevent pooling. If condition is serious, physician orders volume expanders or pressure agents.
2. **Tachycardia**		2. *Always* evaluate clients with existing cardiac problems before antipsychotic drugs are administered. Haloperidol (Haldol) is usually the preferred drug because of its low ACh effects.
Rare and Toxic Effects		
1. **Agranulocytosis:** symptoms include sore throat, fever, malaise, and mouth sores. It is a rare occurrence, but a possibility the nurse should be aware of; any flulike symptoms should be carefully evaluated.	Usually occurs suddenly and becomes evident in the first 12 weeks	1. Blood work usually done every week for 6 months, then every 2 months. Physician may order blood work to determine presence of leukopenia or agranulocytosis. If test results are positive, the drug is discontinued, and reverse isolation may be initiated. Mortality is high if the drug is not ceased and if treatment is not initiated.
2. **Cholestatic jaundice:** rare, reversible, and usually benign if caught in time; prodromal symptoms are fever, malaise, nausea, and abdominal pain; jaundice appears 1 week later.		2. Discontinue drug; give bed rest and high-protein, high-carbohydrate diet. Liver function tests should be performed every 6 months.
3. **Neuroleptic malignant syndrome (NMS):** somewhat rare, potentially fatal. ■ **Severe extrapyramidal:** severe muscle rigidity, oculogyric crisis, dysphasia, flexor-extensor posturing, cogwheeling ■ **Hyperpyrexia:** elevated temperature (over 103° F or 39° C) ■ **Autonomic dysfunction:** hypertension, tachycardia, diaphoresis, incontinence	Can occur in the first week of drug therapy but often occurs later. Rapidly progresses over 2 to 3 days after initial manifestation **Risk Factors:** ■ Concomitant use of psychotropics ■ Older age ■ Female gender (3:2) ■ Presence of a mood disorder (40%) ■ Rapid dose titration	3. ■ Stop neuroleptic. ■ Transfer STAT to medical unit. ■ Bromocriptine (Parlodel) can relieve muscle rigidity and reduce fever. ■ Dantrolene (Dantrium) may reduce muscle spasms. ■ Cool body to reduce fever. ■ Maintain hydration with oral and IV fluids. ■ Correct electrolyte imbalance. ■ Arrhythmias should be treated. ■ Small doses of heparin may decrease possibility of pulmonary emboli. ■ Early detection increases client's chance of survival.

STAT, Immediately.

Most clients develop tolerance to EPSs after a few months. Effective nursing and medical management is important to encourage compliance with the medication regimen until the disturbing and frightening side effects have been properly managed. Table 20-10 identifies some of the drugs most commonly used for the treatment of EPSs.

Perhaps the most troubling side effects for outpatients taking antipsychotic drugs are weight gain, impotence, and tardive dyskinesia. Weight gain is most frequently a problem for women, and as much as a 100-lb gain may occur in some clients. Discontinuation of the antipsychotic medication may be necessary, along with the use of an alternative drug. Impotence is occasionally reported (but frequently experienced) by men and may also necessitate switching to alternative drugs. Sexual dysfunctions are perhaps the most common reasons for male nonadherence to the medication regimen.

Tardive dyskinesia (TD), an EPS that usually appears after prolonged treatment, is more serious and is not always reversible. Tardive dyskinesia consists of involuntary tonic muscular spasms that typically involve the tongue, fingers, toes, neck, trunk, or pelvis. This potentially serious EPS is most frequently seen in women and older clients, and affects up to 50% of individuals receiving long-term high-dose therapy. Tardive dyskinesia varies from mild to moderate and

TABLE 20-10

Treatment of Acute Extrapyramidal Side Effects

Drug	Oral Dose (mg)	Intramuscular or Intravenous Dose (mg)	Chemical Type
Trihexyphenidyl* (Artane)	2-5 tid	—	ACA
Benztropine mesylate* (Cogentin)	1-3 bid	1-2	ACA
Biperiden* (Akineton)	2 bid or qid	2	ACA
Diphenhydramine hydrochloride (Benadryl)	25-50 tid or qid	25-50	Antihistamine
Procyclidine hydrochloride (Kemadrin)	2.5-5 tid	—	ACA
Bromocriptine mesylate (Parlodel)		1.25-2.0	

From Maxmen, J. S., & Ward, N. G. (2002). *Psychotropic drugs: Fast facts* (3rd ed.). New York: W. W. Norton.
ACA, Anticholinergic agent (after 1 to 6 months of long-term maintenance antipsychotic therapy, most ACAs can be withdrawn)
*Antiparkinsonian drug.

can be disfiguring or incapacitating. Early symptoms of tardive dyskinesia are fasciculations of the tongue or constant smacking of the lips. These early oral movements can develop into uncontrollable biting, chewing, or sucking motions, an open mouth, and lateral movements of the jaw. In many cases, the early symptoms of tardive dyskinesia disappear when the antipsychotic medication is discontinued. In other cases, however, early symptoms are not reversible and may progress. No proven cure for advanced tardive dyskinesia exists.

The National Institute of Mental Health developed a brief test for the detection of tardive dyskinesia. The test is referred to as the Abnormal Involuntary Movement Scale (AIMS) (Figure 20-4). The three areas of examination are facial and oral movements, extremity movements, and trunk movement.

Nurses need to know about some rare—but serious and potentially fatal—toxic effects of the antipsychotic drugs. Toxic effects include neuroleptic malignant syndrome, agranulocytosis, and liver involvement.

Neuroleptic malignant syndrome (NMS) occurs in about 0.2% to 1.0% of clients who have taken antipsychotic agents. It is believed that the acute reduction in brain dopamine activity plays a role in the development of neuroleptic malignant syndrome. Neuroleptic malignant syndrome is fatal in about 10% of cases. It usually occurs early in the course of therapy but has been reported in people after 20 years of treatment.

Neuroleptic malignant syndrome is characterized by decreased level of consciousness, greatly increased muscle tone, and autonomic dysfunction, including hyperpyrexia, labile hypertension, tachycardia, tachypnea, diaphoresis, and drooling. Treatment consists of early detection, discontinuation of the antipsychotic agent, management of fluid balance, reduction of temperature, and monitoring for complications. Mild cases of neuroleptic malignant syndrome are treated with bromocriptine (Parlodel), whereas more severe cases are treated with intravenous dantrolene (Dantrium) and even with electroconvulsive therapy in some cases (Wilkaitis, Mulvihill, & Nasrallah, 2004).

Agranulocytosis is also a serious side effect and can be fatal. Liver involvement may also occur. Nurses need to be aware of the prodromal signs and symptoms of these side effects and teach them to their clients and clients' families (see Table 20-9).

Adjuncts to Antipsychotic Drug Therapy

Antidepressants. Antidepressants are recommended along with antipsychotic agents for the treatment of depression, which is very common among individuals with schizophrenia. Refer to Chapter 18.

Antimanic Agents. Lithium has been helpful in suppressing episodic violence in schizophrenia as well

ABNORMAL INVOLUNTARY MOVEMENT SCALE (AIMS)

Public Health Service
Alcohol, Drug Abuse, and Mental Health Administration
National Institute of Mental Health

Name: _____

Date: _____

Prescribing Practitioner: _____

Code: 0 = None
1 = Minimal, may be extreme normal
2 = Mild
3 = Moderate
4 = Severe

Instructions: Complete Examination Procedure before making ratings.

Movement ratings: Rate highest severity observed. Rate movements that occur upon activation one *less* than those observed spontaneously. Circle movement as well as code number that applies.		Rater Date	Rater Date	Rater Date	Rater Date
Facial and Oral Movements	**1. Muscles of facial expression** (e.g., movements of forehead, eyebrows, periorbital area, cheeks, including frowning, blinking, smiling, grimacing)	0 1 2 3 4	0 1 2 3 4	0 1 2 3 4	0 1 2 3 4
	2. Lips and perioral area (e.g., puckering, pouting, smacking)	0 1 2 3 4	0 1 2 3 4	0 1 2 3 4	0 1 2 3 4
	3. Jaw (e.g., biting, clenching, chewing, mouth opening, lateral movement)	0 1 2 3 4	0 1 2 3 4	0 1 2 3 4	0 1 2 3 4
	4. Tongue: Rate only increases in movement both in and out of mouth — *not* inability to sustain movement. Darting in and out of mouth.	0 1 2 3 4	0 1 2 3 4	0 1 2 3 4	0 1 2 3 4
Extremity Movements	**5. Upper (arms, wrists, hands, fingers):** Include choreic movements (i.e., rapid, objectively purposeless, irregular, spontaneous) and athetoid movements (i.e., slow, irregular, complex, serpentine) *Do not include tremor* (i.e., repetitive, regular, rhythmic).	0 1 2 3 4	0 1 2 3 4	0 1 2 3 4	0 1 2 3 4
	6. Lower (legs, knees, ankles, toes) (e.g., lateral knee movement, foot tapping, heel dropping, foot squirming, inversion and eversion of foot)	0 1 2 3 4	0 1 2 3 4	0 1 2 3 4	0 1 2 3 4
Trunk Movements	**7. Neck, shoulder, hips** (e.g., rocking, twisting, squirming, pelvic gyrations)	0 1 2 3 4	0 1 2 3 4	0 1 2 3 4	0 1 2 3 4
Global Judgments	**8. Severity of abnormal movements overall**	0 1 2 3 4	0 1 2 3 4	0 1 2 3 4	0 1 2 3 4
	9. Incapacitation due to abnormal movements	0 1 2 3 4	0 1 2 3 4	0 1 2 3 4	0 1 2 3 4
	10. Patient's awareness of abnormal movements: Rate only patient's report. No awareness 0 Aware, no distress 1 Aware, mild distress 2 Aware, moderate distress 3 Aware, severe distress 4	0 1 2 3 4	0 1 2 3 4	0 1 2 3 4	0 1 2 3 4
Dental Status	**11. Current problems with teeth and/or dentures**	No Yes	No Yes	No Yes	No Yes
	12. Are dentures usually worn?	No Yes	No Yes	No Yes	No Yes
	13. Edentia	No Yes	No Yes	No Yes	No Yes
	14. Do movements disappear in sleep?	No Yes	No Yes	No Yes	No Yes

FIGURE 20-4 Abnormal Involuntary Movement Scale (AIMS). *Continued*

as in targeting many of the more disturbing symptoms when the agent is administered along with an antipsychotic, although data regarding the usefulness of lithium are mixed (Citrome, 2002). The addition of valproate can significantly enhance antipsychotic efficacy in some clients with schizophrenia that is nonresponsive to antipsychotic agents (Bowden, 2004; Citrome, 2002).

Benzodiazepines. Benzodiazepine augmentation can improve positive and negative symptoms by about 50% (Maxmen & Ward, 2002). Use of clonazepam as an

---

AIMS Examination Procedure

Either before or after completing the Examination Procedure, observe the patient unobtrusively, at rest (e.g., in waiting room).

The chair to be used in this examination should be a hard, firm one without arms.

1. Ask patient to remove shoes and socks.
2. Ask patient whether there is anything in his or her mouth (e.g., gum, candy) and, if there is, to remove it.
3. Ask patient about the *current* condition of his or her teeth. Ask patient if he or she wears dentures. Do teeth or dentures bother the patient *now?*
4. Ask patient whether he or she notices any movements in mouth, face, hands, or feet. If yes, ask to describe and to what extent they *currently* bother patient of interfere with his or her activities.
5. Have patient sit in chair with hands on knees, legs slightly apart, and feet flat on floor. Look at entire body movements while in this position.
6. Ask patient to sit with hands hanging unsupported: if male, between legs; if female and wearing a dress, hanging over knees. Observe hands and other body areas.
7. Ask patient to open mouth. Observe tongue at rest within mouth. Do this twice.
8. Ask patient to protrude tongue. Observe abnormalities of tongue movement. Do this twice.
9. Ask patient to tap thumb, with each finger, as rapidly as possible for 10 to 15 seconds, separately with right hand, then with left hand. Observe each facial and leg movement.
10. Flex and extend patient's left and right arms (one at a time). Note any rigidity.
11. Ask patient to stand up. Observe in profile. Observe all body areas again, hips included.
12. Ask patient to extend both arms outstretched in front with palms down. Observe trunk, legs, and mouth.
13. Have patient walk a few paces, turn, and walk back to chair. Observe hands and gait. Do this twice.

FIGURE 20-4, cont'd Abnormal Involuntary Movement Scale (AIMS).

---

adjunct to antipsychotics may diminish anxiety, agitation, and possibly psychosis (Maxmen & Ward, 2002).

When to Change an Antipsychotic Regimen

The following circumstances suggest the need to use a different antipsychotic agent:

- Clear lack of efficacy of the current drug regimen
- Need for supplemental medications (lithium, carbamazepine, valproate)
- Occurrence of intolerable or persistent side effects

Specific Nursing Interventions for Paranoid, Catatonic, and Disorganized Schizophrenia

The subtypes of schizophrenia defined by the *DSM-IV-TR* are found in Figure 20-5. In the following sections you are introduced to the paranoid, catatonic (excited and withdrawn phases), and disorganized subtypes. Each section identifies communication guidelines, self-care needs, and milieu needs. Descriptive vignettes are provided at the ends of some sections. Case Study and Nursing Care Plan 20-1 for a client with paranoid schizophrenia is found at the end of this chapter. Full nursing care plans for the other subtypes are found on the Evolve website.

Paranoia

Any intense and strongly defended irrational suspicion can be regarded as paranoia. Paranoid ideas cannot be corrected by experiences and cannot be modi-fied by facts or reality. **Projection** is the most common defense mechanism used by people who are paranoid. For example, when paranoid individuals feel self-critical, they experience others as being harshly critical toward them. When they feel angry, they experience others as being unjustly angry at them, as if to say, "I'm not angry, you are!"

Paranoid states may occur in numerous mental or organic disorders. For example, a person experiencing a psychotic depression or manic episode may display paranoid thinking. Paranoid symptoms can be secondary to physical illness, organic brain disease, or drug intoxication.

Paranoid schizophrenia is one of the **primary paranoid disorders** (i.e., those in which the primary symptom is paranoid thinking). The others are paranoid delusional disorder and paranoid personality disorder. Chapter 16 addresses paranoid personality disorder.

People with paranoid schizophrenia usually have a later age of onset of the disease (late twenties to thirties). Paranoid schizophrenia develops rapidly in individuals with good premorbid functioning and tends to be intermittent during the first 5 years of the illness. In some cases, the presence of paranoid schizophrenia is associated with a good outcome or with recovery. People with a paranoid disorder are usually frightened. Although not always consciously aware of their feelings, paranoid people have deep feelings of loneliness, despair, helplessness, and fear of abandonment. The paranoid facade is a defense against painful feelings. Useful nursing strategies are outlined in the following sections.

DSM-IV-TR CRITERIA FOR SCHIZOPHRENIA SUBTYPES

SCHIZOPHRENIC DISORDERS

Paranoid (Positive)

1. Dominant: hallucinations and delusions.

2. No disorganized speech, disorganized behavior, catatonia, or inappropriate affect present.

Disorganized

1. Dominant: disorganized speech and disorganized behavior and inappropriate affect.

2. Delusions and hallucinations, if present, are not prominent or fragmented.

3. Associated features include grimacing, mannerisms, and other oddities of behavior.

Catatonic

1. Motor immobility (waxy flexibility or stupor).

2. Excessive purposeless motor activity (agitation).

3. Extreme negativism or mutism.

4. Peculiar voluntary movement:
   • Posturing
   • Stereotyped movements
   • Prominent mannerisms
   • Prominent grimaces

5. Echolalia or echopraxis.

Residual

1. No longer has active-phase symptoms (e.g., delusions, hallucinations, or disorganized speech and behaviors).

2. However, persistence of some symptoms is noted, e.g.:
   • Marked social isolation or withdrawal
   • Marked impairment in role function (wage earner, student, or homemaker)
   • Markedly eccentric behavior or odd beliefs
   • Marked impairment in personal hygiene
   • Marked lack of initiative, interest, or energy
   • Blunted or inappropriate affect

Undifferentiated (Mixed Type)

1. Has active-phase symptoms (does have hallucinations, delusions, and bizarre behaviors).

2. No one clinical presentation dominates, e.g.:
   • Paranoid
   • Disorganized
   • Catatonic

FIGURE 20-5 Diagnostic criteria for schizophrenia subtypes. (Adapted from American Psychiatric Association. [2000]. *Diagnostic and statistical manual of mental disorders* [4th ed., text rev.]. Washington, DC: Author.)

Counseling: Communication Guidelines. Because persons who are paranoid are unable to trust the actions of those around them, they are usually guarded, tense, and reserved. Although clients may keep themselves aloof from interpersonal contacts, impairment in actual functioning may be minimal. To ensure interpersonal distance, they may adopt a superior, hostile, and sarcastic attitude. A common defense used by paranoid individuals to maintain self-esteem is to disparage others and dwell on the shortcomings of others. The client frequently misinterprets the messages of others or gives private meaning to the communications of others (ideas of reference). For example, a client might see his primary nurse talking to the physician and believe that they are planning to harm him in some manner. Minor oversights are often interpreted as personal rejection.

During hospitalization, a paranoid client may make offensive yet accurate criticisms of staff and of unit policies. It is important that staff not react to these criticisms with anxiety or rejection of the client. Staff conferences and peer group as well as clinical supervision are effective ways of looking behind the behaviors to the motivations of the client. This provides the opportunity to reduce the client's anxiety and increase staff effectiveness.

Self-Care Needs. People with paranoid schizophrenic disorder usually have stronger ego resources than do individuals with other schizophrenic disorders, particularly with regard to occupational functioning and capacity for independent living. Grooming, dress, and self-care may not be a problem. In fact, in some cases, grooming may be meticulous. Nutrition, however, may pose a difficulty. A common distortion or delusion is that the food is poisoned. In such a case, special foods should be provided in commercially sealed packaging—for example, peanut butter and crackers or nutritional drinks—to minimize the suspicion of tampering. If clients think that others will harm them when they are sleeping, they may be fearful of going to sleep. Therefore, adequate rest may become a problem that warrants nursing interventions.

Milieu Needs. A paranoid person may become physically aggressive in response to hallucinations or delusions. The client projects hostile drives onto others and then acts on these drives. Homosexual urges are projected onto the environment as well, and fear of sexual advances from others may stimulate aggression.

An environment that provides the client with a sense of security and safety minimizes anxiety and environmental distortions. Activities that distract the client from ruminating on hallucinations and delusions also help decrease anxiety.

Catatonia: Withdrawn Phase

The essential feature of catatonia is abnormal motor behavior. Clients show either extreme motor agitation or extreme psychomotor retardation (with mutism, even stupor). Other behaviors identified with catatonia include posturing, waxy flexibility, stereotyped behavior, extreme negativism or automatic obedience, echolalia, and echopraxia. The onset of catatonia is usually abrupt and the prognosis favorable. With pharmacotherapy and improved individual management, severe catatonic symptoms are rarely seen today. Useful nursing strategies are discussed in the following sections.

Counseling: Communication Guidelines. Clients in the withdrawn phase of catatonia can be so withdrawn that they appear comatose. They can be mute and may remain so for hours, days, or even weeks or months if they are not treated with antipsychotic medication. Although such clients may not appear to pay attention to events going on around them, clients are acutely aware of the environment and may accurately remember events at a later date. Withdrawn clients have special needs, and the nurse can use the guidelines in the following subsections. Developing skill and confidence in working with withdrawn clients takes practice.

Self-Care Needs. When a client is extremely withdrawn, physical needs take priority. A client may need to be hand fed or tube fed to maintain adequate nutritional status. Because normal control over bladder and bowel functions may be interrupted, an assessment of urinary or bowel retention is essential, and the appropriate interventions must be applied. Incontinence of urine and feces may cause skin breakdown and infection. In clients in whom physical movements are minimal or absent, range-of-motion exercises are necessary to prevent muscular atrophy, calcium depletion, and contractures. Dressing and grooming usually require direct nursing interventions.

The catatonic client's refusal to cooperate or to participate in activities frequently triggers staff resistance and frustration.

Milieu Needs. During the withdrawn state, the catatonic person may be on a continuum from decreased spontaneous movements to complete stupor. Waxy flexibility, or the ability to hold distorted postures for extensive periods, is often seen. The term *waxy* refers to the holding of any posture into which the staff may place the person. For example, if someone raises the client's arms over his head, the client may maintain that position for hours or longer. This phenomenon is often used as a diagnostic sign. When less withdrawn, a client may demonstrate stereotyped behavior, echopraxia, echolalia, or automatic obedience.

Caution is advised, because even after holding a single posture for long periods, the client may suddenly and without provocation show brief outbursts of gross motor activity in response to inner hallucinations, delusions, and change in neurotransmitter levels.

The following vignette applies to the client who is withdrawn.

■ ■ ■ *VIGNETTE*

Mrs. Chou is a 25-year-old woman. She left China for the United States 6 months ago to join her husband. Before she came to the United States, she lived with her parents and worked in a button factory. In China, Mrs. Chou had been educated to speak and understand English. She had always been shy and looked to her parents and then to her husband for guidance and support. Shortly after she arrived in the United States, her mother developed pneumonia and died, and Mrs. Chou was not able to go back to China for the funeral. Mr. Chou states that his wife thought that if she had stayed in China, her mother would not have become ill. She told him recently that evil would come to their 1-year-old child because she had been unable to take proper care of her mother. Three days before admission, Mrs. Chou became lethargic and spent most of the day staring into space and mumbling to herself. When Mr. Chou asked who she was talking to, she answered, "My mother." She has not eaten for 2 days; at the time of admission, Mrs. Chou sits motionless and mute and appears stuporous.

The physician notices that when he takes Mrs. Chou's pulse, her arm remains in midair until he replaces it by her side. Mr. Chou says that once his wife became extremely agitated and started to scream and cry while tearing the curtains and knocking over objects. Shortly afterward, she returned to a withdrawn, mute state. Mr. Chou is extremely distraught and confused, and he fears for the safety of their child. Mr. Nolan is assigned to Mrs. Chou as her primary nurse.

Mrs. Chou is sloppily dressed, and her hair and nails are dirty. She is pale, and her skin turgor is poor. She sits motionless and appears to be unaware of anything going on around her. Mr. Nolan introduces himself and explains what he will be doing before he does it—for example, that he will be taking her blood pressure and pulse and offering her fluids.

■ ■ ■

Refer to the Evolve website for a complete nursing care plan for Mrs. Chou.

Catatonia: Excited Phase

Counseling: Communication Guidelines. During the excited, or acute, stage of catatonia the person talks or shouts continually, and verbalizations may be incoherent. The nurse's communication needs to be clear and direct and to reflect concern for the safety of the client and others.

Self-Care Needs. A person who is constantly and intensely hyperactive can become completely exhausted and can even die if medical attention is not available. Most often, a standard antipsychotic agent is administered intramuscularly. The client may continue to be agitated, but within limits that are not potentially harmful. During this time of heightened physical activity, the client requires additional fluids, calories, and rest. It is not unusual for the client to be destructive and aggressive to others in response to hallucinations or delusions. Many of the concerns and interventions are the same as those for a bipolar client in a manic phase.

Disorganized Schizophrenia

Disorganized schizophrenia represents the most regressed and socially impaired of all the schizophrenias. A person diagnosed with disorganized schizophrenia (formally called *hebephrenia*) may have marked looseness of associations, grossly inappropriate affect, bizarre mannerisms, and incoherence of speech and may display extreme social withdrawal. Although delusions and hallucinations are present, they are fragmentary and poorly organized. Behavior may be considered odd, and giggling or grimacing in response to internal stimuli is common. Disorganized schizophrenia has an earlier age of onset (early to middle teens) and often develops insidiously. It is associated with poor premorbid functioning, a significant family history of psychopathological disorders, and a poor prognosis. Often, these clients are in state hospitals and can live in the community safely only in a structured and well-supervised setting. Unfortunately, a good portion of the homeless population consists of these clients. More fortunate clients may live at home. In such cases, their families need significant community support, respite care, and day hospital affiliations.

Counseling: Communication Guidelines. People with disorganized schizophrenia experience persistent and severe perceptual problems. Verbal responses are usually marked by looseness of associations or incoherence. Clang associations or word salad may be present. Blocking, a sudden cessation in the train of thought, is frequently observed.

Self-Care Needs. Grooming is neglected. Usually, hair is dirty and matted, and clothes are inappropriate and stained. The client has no awareness of social expectations. The client is frequently too disorganized to carry out simple activities of daily living.

Basic outcomes for nursing intervention include encouraging optimal level of functioning, preventing further regression, and offering alternatives for inappropriate behaviors whenever possible.

Milieu Needs. Behavior is often described as bizarre. A client may twirl around the room or make strange gestures with the hands and face. Social behavior is often primitive or regressed. For example, the client may eat with the hands, pick the nose, or masturbate in public. Typical behaviors include posturing, grimacing or giggling, and mirror gazing.

A vignette of a person with disorganized schizophrenia follows.

■ ■ ■ *VIGNETTE*

Martin Taylor, a 36-year-old unemployed man, has been referred to the mental health center. He is accompanied by his mother and sister. He had been hospitalized for 3 years in a state hospital with the diagnosis of chronic schizophrenia and was doing well at home until 2 months ago. His only employment was for 5 months as a janitor after high school graduation. Other significant family history includes a twin brother who died of a cerebral aneurysm in his teens. Martin tells the nurse he has used every street drug available, including LSD (lysergic acid diethylamide) and intravenous heroin. His mother states that when he was a teenager, before his substance abuse, he was an excellent athlete who received average grades. At the age of 17 years, he had his first psychotic break when taking a variety of street drugs. His behavior became markedly bizarre (e.g., eating cat food, swallowing a rubber-soled heel, which required an emergency laparotomy).

Ms. Lamb, a clinical nurse specialist, meets with Martin after speaking with his mother and sister. Martin is unshaven, and his appearance is disheveled. He is wearing a red headband in which he has placed Popsicle sticks and scraps of paper. He chain smokes during the interview and frequently gets up and paces back and forth. He tells the nurse that he is Alice from Alice in the Underground and that people from space hurt him with needles. His speech pattern is marked by associative looseness and occasional blocking. For example, he often stops in the middle of a phrase and giggles to himself. At one point, when he starts to giggle, Ms. Lamb asks him what he is thinking about. He states, "You interrupted me." At that point, he begins to shake his head while repeating in a sing-song voice, "Shake them tigers . . . shake them tigers . . . shake them tigers." He denies suicidal or homicidal ideation. Ms. Lamb notes that Martin has a great deal of difficulty accurately perceiving what is going on around him. He has markedly regressed social behaviors. For example, he eats with his hands and picks his nose in public. He has no apparent insight into his problems; he tells Ms. Lamb that his biggest problem is the people in space.

Undifferentiated Schizophrenia

In the undifferentiated type of schizophrenia, *active signs of the disorder* (positive or negative symptoms) are present, but the individual does not meet the criteria for paranoia, catatonia, or disorganized type (Beng-Choon et al., 2004). As does disorganized schizophrenia, undifferentiated schizophrenia begins early and has an insidious onset (early to middle teens). However, the premorbid state is less predictable, and the disability remains fairly stable, although persistent, over time.

Residual Type of Schizophrenia

In the residual type of schizophrenia, active-phase symptoms are no longer present, but evidence of two or more residual symptoms persists. Residual symptoms include the following:
- Lack of initiative, interests, or energy
- Marked social withdrawal
- Impairment in role function (wage earner, student, homemaker)
- Marked speech deficits (circumstantial, vague speech and poverty of speech or content of speech)
- Odd beliefs, magical thinking, and unusual perceptual experiences

Principles of care similar to those that pertain to withdrawn, paranoid, and disorganized schizophrenia apply to undifferentiated and residual schizophrenia, as dictated by the client's behavior.

■ EVALUATION

Evaluation is always an important step in the planning of care. Evaluation is especially important for people who have chronic psychotic disorders. Frequently outcomes are established that are too ambitious and serve only to discourage client and staff alike. It is critical for staff to remember that change is a process that occurs over time; for a person diagnosed with schizophrenia, the time period may be prolonged.

It is important to schedule regular evaluations for chronically ill clients so that new data can be considered and the client's problems can be reassessed. Questions to be asked include the following: Is the client not progressing because a more important need is not being met? Is the staff using the client's strengths and interests to achieve the outcomes? Are more appropriate interventions available for this client to facilitate progress? If a newer antipsychotic agent is being tried, is there evidence of improvement or a regression in functioning? Is the family involved, are family members supportive, and do they understand the client's disease and treatment issues?

Active staff involvement and interest in the client's progress communicates concern, helps the client to sustain interest, and prevents feelings of helplessness and burnout. Input from the client can offer valuable information about why a certain desired behavior or situation has not occurred.

■ ■ ■ KEY POINTS to REMEMBER

- Schizophrenia is a biologically based disease of the brain. It is not one disorder but a group of disorders. Psychotic symptoms in schizophrenia are more pronounced and disruptive than are symptoms found in other disorders. The basic differences are in the degree of severity, withdrawal, alteration in affect, impairment of intellect, and regression.
- Neurochemical (catecholamines and serotonin), genetic, and neuroanatomical findings help explain the symptoms of schizophrenia. However, at present no one theory accounts for all phenomena found in schizophrenic disorders.
- When the nurse works with clients with schizophrenia, four specific groups of symptoms may be evident. No one symptom is found in all cases. The positive and negative symptoms of schizophrenia are two of the major categories of symptoms.
- The positive symptoms are more florid (hallucinations, delusions, looseness of associations) and respond to antipsychotic drug therapy.
- The negative symptoms of schizophrenia (poor social adjustment, lack of motivation, withdrawal) are more debilitating and do not respond as well to antipsychotic therapy.
- The cognitive degree of impairment warrants careful assessment and interventions to increase the person's quality of life and ability to function in the community.

Continued, p. 419

CASE STUDY and NURSING CARE PLAN 20-1 Paranoid Schizophrenia

Tom is a 32-year-old man who is currently an inpatient at a Veterans Administration hospital. He has been separated from his wife and four children for 3 years. His medical records state that, because of his illness (which Tom describes as "hearing voices a lot"), he has been in and out of hospitals for 13 years. Tom is an ex-Marine who first "heard voices" at the age of 19, while he was serving in the first Gulf War. He subsequently received a medical discharge.

The hospitalization was precipitated by an exacerbation of auditory hallucinations. "I thought people were following me. I hear voices, usually a woman's voice, and she's tormenting me. People say that it happens because I don't take my medications. The medications make me tired and I can't have sex." Tom also admits to using cocaine and marijuana. He is aware that marijuana and cocaine increase his paranoia and that taking drugs usually precedes hospitalization but says that "they make me feel good." Tom finished 11 years of school but did not graduate from high school. He says that he has no close friends. He was in prison for 5 years for manslaughter and tells the nurse, "I was in prison because I did something bad." He was abusing alcohol and drugs at the time, and drug abuse has been related to each subsequent hospitalization.

Ms. Lally is Tom's primary nurse. When Tom meets the nurse, he is dressed in pajamas and bathrobe. His hygiene is good and he is well nourished. He tells the nurse that he does not sleep much because "the voices get worse at night." Ms. Lally notes in Tom's medical record that he has had two episodes of suicidal ideation. During those times, the voices were telling him to jump "off rooftops" and "in front of trains."

During the first interview, Tom only occasionally makes eye contact and speaks in a low monotone. At times, he glances about the room as if distracted, mumbles to himself, and appears upset.

Nurse: Tom, my name is Ms. Lally. I will be your nurse while you're in the hospital. We will meet every day for 30 minutes at 10 AM. During that time, we can discuss areas of concern to you.

Tom: Well . . . don't believe what they say about me. I want to start a new . . . Are you married?

Nurse: This time is for you to talk about your concerns.

Tom: Oh . . . (Looks furtively around the room, then lowers his eyes.) Someone is trying to kill me, I think. . . .

Nurse: You appear to be focusing on something other than our conversation.

Tom: The voices tell me things . . . I can't say . . .

Nurse: I don't hear any voices except yours and mine. I am going to stay with you. Tell me what is happening and I will try to help you.

Tom: The voices tell me bad things.

Ms. Lally stays with Tom and encourages him to communicate with her. As Tom focuses more on the nurse, his anxiety appears to lessen. His thoughts become more connected, he is able to concentrate more on what the nurse is saying, and he mumbles less to himself.

Self-Assessment

On the first day of admission, Tom assaults another male client, stating that the other client accused him of being a homosexual and touched him on the buttocks. After assessing the incident, the staff agrees that Tom's provocation came more from his own projections (Tom's sexual attraction to the other client) than from anything the other client did or said.

Tom's difficulty with impulse control frightens Ms. Lally. She has concerns regarding Tom's ability to curb his impulses and the possibility of Tom's striking out at her, especially when Tom is hallucinating and highly delusional. Ms. Lally mentions her concerns to the nursing coordinator, who suggests that Ms. Lally meet with Tom in the day room until he demonstrates more control and less suspicion of others. After 5 days, Tom is less excitable, and the sessions are held in a room set aside for client interviews. Ms. Lally also speaks with a senior staff nurse regarding her fear. By talking to the senior nurse and understanding more clearly her own fear, Ms. Lally is able to identify interventions to help Tom regain a better sense of control.

■ ASSESSMENT

Objective Data

- Speaks in low monotone
- Makes poor eye contact
- Appears well nourished, with adequate hygiene
- States that he has auditory hallucinations
- Has a history of drug abuse (cocaine and marijuana)
- Has no close friends
- Was first hospitalized at age 19 and has not worked since that time
- Has had suicidal impulses twice
- Was imprisoned for 5 years for violent acting out (manslaughter)
- Thoughts scattered when anxious

Subjective Data

- "Someone is trying to kill me, I think."
- "I don't take my medications. The medications make me tired and I can't have sex."
- "The voices get worse at night, and I can't sleep."
- Voices have told him to "jump off rooftops" and "in front of trains."

Continued

■ NURSING DIAGNOSIS (NANDA)

1. *Disturbed thought processes* related to alteration in biochemical compounds, as evidenced by persecutory hallucinations and intense suspiciousness
   - Voices have told him to "jump off rooftops" and "in front of trains."
   - "Someone is trying to kill me, I think."
   - Abuses cocaine and marijuana, although these increase paranoia, because "they make me feel good."

2. *Nonadherence* to medication regimen related to side effects of therapy, as evidenced by verbalization of noncompliance and persistence of symptoms
   - Failure to take prescribed medications because they "make me tired and I can't have sex"
   - Chronic history of relapse of symptoms when client is out of hospital

■ OUTCOME CRITERIA (NOC)

1. Tom consistently refrains from acting upon his "voices" and suspicions when they occur.
2. Tom consistently adheres to medication regimen.

■ PLANNING

The nurse plans intervention that will (1) help Tom deal with his disturbing thoughts and (2) minimize the adverse effects of medication to increase compliance and decrease the potential for relapse.

■ INTERVENTION (NIC)

Tom's plan of care was personalized as follows:

Nursing diagnosis: *Disturbed thought processes*
Outcome: Tom consistently refrains from acting upon his "voices" and suspicions when they occur.

Short-Term Goal	Intervention	Rationale	Evaluation
1. By the end of the first week, Tom will consistently recognize that hallucinations are occurring, as evidenced by Tom's telling his nurse when he is experiencing hallucinations.	1a. Meet with Tom each day for 30 minutes. 1b. Use clear, unambiguous statements. 1c. Provide activities that require concentration and are noncompetitive.	1a. Short, consistent meetings help establish contact and decrease anxiety. 1b. Minimizes potential for misconstruing messages. 1c. Increases time spent in reality-based activities and decreases delusional and hallucinatory experiences.	GOAL MET By the end of the first week, Tom tells the nurse that he is experiencing hallucinations.
2. By the end of the first week, Tom will consistently describe the content of the hallucinations to his nurse.	2a. Investigate content of hallucinations with Tom. 2b. Explore those times that voices are the most threatening and disturbing.	2a. Identifies suicidal or aggressive themes. 2b. Identifies events that increase anxiety.	GOAL MET Tom identifies that the voices tell him he is a loser and he needs to be careful "because someone is after me." He identifies that the voices are worse at nighttime. He also states that smoking marijuana and taking cocaine produce very threatening voices.
3. By discharge, Tom will consistently report a decrease in hallucinations.	3. Explore with Tom possible actions that can minimize anxiety.	3. Offers alternatives while anxiety level is relatively low.	GOAL MET Tom states that he is hearing voices less and they are less threatening to him. Tom identifies that if he whistles or sings he stays calm and can control the voices.

Nursing diagnosis: *Nonadherence*
Outcome: Tom consistently adheres to medication regimen.

Short-Term Goal	Intervention	Rationale	Evaluation
1. By discharge, Tom will consistently discuss his medication regimen with the nurse.	**1a.** Evaluate medication response with the physician in the hospital. **1b.** Initiate medication changed to olanzapine (Zyprexa). **1c.** Educate Tom regarding side effects—how long they last and what actions can be taken.	**1a.** Identifies drugs and dosages that have increased therapeutic value and decreased side effects. **1b.** Olanzapine causes no known sexual difficulties. **1c.** Can give increased sense of control over symptoms.	GOAL MET Tom is able to identify the reasons for not taking his medication as ordered; he expresses a willingness to try olanzapine because the physician assures him that the side effects will be less than those of his current medications. A large dose is taken at bedtime to increase sleep and a small dose is taken during the day to decrease fatigue. Tom states that he sleeps better at night but is still tired during the day.
2. By discharge, Tom will state that he will consistently attend the weekly support group for people with schizophrenia.	**2.** Encourage Tom to join support group for people with schizophrenia.	**2.** Provides peer support for drug therapy maintenance as well as suggestions for dealing with loneliness and other problems frequently encountered by clients with schizophrenia.	GOAL MET Week 1: Tom attends meeting. Week 2: He speaks in the group about "not feeling good." Several group members tell Tom that they understand and try to help him figure out why he is not feeling good. He is also encouraged by his peers to take his medication as a way of feeling better.

■ EVALUATION

When Tom is discharged home, he says he has a better understanding of his medications and what to do. He knows that marijuana and cocaine increase his symptoms, but he explains that when he gets lonely, he uses drugs to "feel good." Tom continues with the support group and outpatient counseling. Tom states that he decided to attend outpatient therapy because Ms. Lally really cared about him; this made him want to get better. He reports sleeping much better and says that he has more energy during the day.

evolve Visit the Evolve website at **http://evolve.elsevier.com/Varcarolis** for a full case study of this client and more case studies and nursing care plans.

■■■ KEY POINTS to REMEMBER—cont'd

- Comorbid depression needs to be identified and treated to lower the potential for suicide, substance abuse, and relapse.
- Some nursing diagnoses discussed include *disturbed sensory perception, disturbed thought processes, impaired verbal communication, ineffective coping, risk for self-directed or other-directed violence,* and *compromised or disabled family coping*.
- Planning of outcomes proceeds by identifying the phase of schizophrenia and assessing the client's individual needs based on functional ability, and involves identifying short-term and intermediate indicators.

- Interventions for people with schizophrenia include the use of special communication and counseling techniques, self-care strategies, and milieu intervention.
- Because antipsychotic medication is essential, the nurse must understand the properties, adverse effects, toxic effects, and dosages of the traditional, atypical, and other medications used to treat schizophrenia. This information must be shared with the client and family.
- Basic characteristics of paranoid schizophrenia, catatonia (withdrawn and excited phases), and disorganized schizophrenia are presented in this chapter. Specific nursing interventions are outlined in case studies found on the Evolve website.

Critical Thinking and Chapter Review

Visit the Evolve website at **http://evolve.elsevier.com/Varcarolis** for additional self-study exercises.

evolve

■ ■ ■ CRITICAL THINKING

1. Using Table 20-6, teach a group (study group, co-workers) about the acute and long-term needs of people with schizophrenia. Identify the basic focus and interventions for the different phases.

2. Jamie, a 29-year-old woman, is being discharged in 2 days from the hospital after her first psychotic break (paranoid schizophrenia). Jamie is recently divorced and has been working as a legal secretary, although her work had become erratic, and her suspicious behavior was calling attention to herself at work. Jamie will be discharged in her mother's care until she is able to resume working. Jamie's mother is overwhelmed and asks the nurse how she is going to cope. "Jamie has become so distant, and she always takes things the wrong way. I can hardly say anything to her without her misconstruing everything. She is very mad at me because I called 911 and had her admitted after she told me she was going to get justice back in the world by blowing up evil forces that have been haunting her life and then proceeded to try to run over her ex-husband, thinking he was the devil. She told me there is nothing wrong with her, and I am concerned she won't take her medication once she is discharged. What am I going to do?"

   Answer the following questions related to the case study just given. It is best if you can discuss and analyze responses to such situations with your classmates or instructor.

   A. What are some of the priority concerns that the nurse could address in the hospital setting before Jamie's discharge?

   B. How would you explain to Jamie's mother some of the symptoms that Jamie is experiencing? What suggestions could you give her to handle some of her immediate concerns?

   C. What issues could you bring up to the staff about Jamie's medication compliance? What would be some ways to deal with this issue?

   D. What are some of the community resources that the case manager could contact to help support this family and increase the chances of continuity of care? Identify some useful community referrals that would be supportive for Jamie and her mother. Choose at least three and describe how they could be supportive to this family.

   E. What do you think of the prognosis for Jamie? Support your hypothesis with data regarding influences on the course of schizophrenia.

■ ■ ■ CHAPTER REVIEW

Choose the most appropriate answer.

1. In which of the following situations can the nurse make the assessment that the client is experiencing auditory hallucinations?
   1. Mrs. D tells the nurse, "There are worms crawling on my arms and legs."
   2. Ms. E states, "I have seen the vorels who are planning to abduct me."
   3. Miss F mentions, "The food on my plate is poisoned. Take it away immediately."
   4. Mr. G, who is seated by himself, pleads, "I am a good person. Stop shouting those bad things about me."

2. To plan appropriate interventions the nurse must know that depersonalization and derealization are examples of
   1. delusions.
   2. hallucinations.
   3. automatic obedience.
   4. personal boundary difficulties.

3. Which symptoms of schizophrenia are most amenable to treatment with both low- and high-potency antipsychotic medications?
   1. Hallucinations, delusions
   2. Ambivalence, avolition
   3. Inadequate hygiene, grooming
   4. Poor social functioning, withdrawal

4. A nursing strategy that usually proves helpful when caring for a person with schizophrenia is
   1. asking directly about hallucinations or asking the client to describe a delusion he or she is experiencing.
   2. focusing on what is happening in the here and now.
   3. limiting contact to one or two short interactions daily.
   4. assuming knowledge of what is meant when the client talks about "they."

5. A nursing diagnosis that is universally applicable to clients with schizophrenia during the prodromal and acute phases is
   1. noncompliance.
   2. disturbed body image.
   3. disturbed thought processes.
   4. risk for other-directed violence.

Visit the Evolve website at **http://evolve.elsevier.com/Varcarolis** for a posttest on the content in this chapter.

evolve

■ STUDENT
■ STUDY
■ CD-ROM

Access the accompanying CD-ROM for animations, interactive exercises, review questions for the NCLEX examination, and an audio glossary.

■ NURSE,
■ CLIENT, AND
■ FAMILY RESOURCES

For suggested readings, information on related associations, and Internet resources, go to **http://evolve.elsevier.com/Varcarolis.** *evolve*

REFERENCES

American Nurses Association. (2000). *Statement on the scope and standards of psychiatric-mental health nursing practice.* Washington, DC: American Nurses Publishing.

American Psychiatric Association. (2000a). *Diagnostic and statistical manual of mental disorders (DSM-IV-TR)* (4th ed., text rev.). Washington, DC: Author.

American Psychiatric Association. (2000b). *Practice guidelines for the treatment of psychiatric disorders: Compendium 2000.* Washington, DC: Author.

Andreasen, N. C. (2000). Schizophrenia: The fundamental question. *Brain Research Review, 31*(2-3), 106-112.

Beng-Choon, H., Black, D. W., & Andreasen, N. C. (2004). Schizophrenia and other psychotic disorders. In R. E. Hales & S. C. Yudofsky (Eds.), *Essentials of clinical psychiatry* (2nd ed., p. 200). Washington, DC: American Psychiatric Publishing.

Blanchard, J. J., et al. (2000). Substance use disorders in schizophrenia: Review, integration, and a proposed model. *Clinical Psychological Review, 220*(2), 207-234.

Bowden, C. L. (2004). Valproate. In A. F. Schatzberg & C. B. Nemeroff (Eds.), *The American Psychiatric Publishing textbook of psychopharmacology* (3rd ed., pp. 572-573). Washington, DC: American Psychiatric Publishing.

Bramon, E., & Sham, P. C. (2001). The common liability link between schizophrenia and bipolar disorder: A review. *Current Psychiatric Reports, 3,* 332.

Bustillo, J., Keith, S. J., & Lauriello, J. (1999). Schizophrenia: Psychosocial treatment. In B. J. Sadock & V. A. Kaplan (Eds.), *Kaplan and Sadock's comprehensive textbook of psychiatry* (7th ed.). Philadelphia: Lippincott Williams & Wilkins.

Byrne, M. M., et al. (2003). Parental age and risk of schizophrenia: A case-control study. *Archives of General Psychiatry, 60*(7), 673-678.

Citrome, L. (2002, May 28). *Current treatments in agitation and aggression: CME. Medscape clinical update.* Retrieved February 14, 2005, from http://www.medscape.com/viewprogram/1866?src=search.

Gamble, C., & Brennan, G. (2000). Working with families and informed careers. In C. Gamble & G. Brennan (Eds.), *Working with serious mental illness: A manual for clinical practice.* London: Baillière Tindall.

Hirayasu, Y. (2000, May 17). *Management of schizophrenia with comorbid conditions.* Paper presented at the 153rd Annual Meeting of the American Psychiatric Association, Chicago, IL.

Jones, E. G. (2003, November 8-12). *Pathology of schizophrenia.* Paper presented at the 33rd Annual Meeting of the American Society of Neuroscience, New Orleans, LA.

Junginger, J. (1995). Common hallucinations and predictions of dangerousness. *Psychiatric Services, 46*(9), 911.

Kolb, L. C., & Brodie, H. K. H. (1982). *Modern clinical psychiatry* (10th ed.). Philadelphia: WB Saunders.

Korn, M. L., & Saito, T. (2000, July 9-13). *Glutamatergic and GABAergic based issues in schizophrenia.* Paper presented at the 22nd Congress of the Collegium International Neuro-Psychopharmacologicum, Brussels, Belgium.

Kuo, I. (2004, February 9-13). *Acute and long-term biological treatment of schizophrenia.* Paper presented at the International Congress of Biological Psychiatry, Sidney, Australia.

Leff, J. (2000). Family work for schizophrenia: Practical application. *Acta Psychiatrica Scandinavica, 102*(Suppl. 407), 78-82.

Mariani, S. (2004). Origin and neuropathology of schizophrenia. *Medscape Molecular Medicine, 6*(1). Retrieved January 21, 2005, from http://www.medscape.com/viewarticle/465642.

Maxmen, J. S., & Ward, N. G. (2002). *Psychotropic drugs: Fast facts* (2nd ed.). New York: W. W. Norton.

Menninger, W. W. (1984). Dealing with staff reactions to perceived lack of progress by chronic mental patients. *Hospital and Community Psychiatry, 35*(8), 805.

Mills, J. (2000). Dealing with voices and strange thoughts. In C. Gamble & G. Brennan (Eds.), *Working with serious mental illness: A manual for clinical practice.* London: Baillière Tindall.

Moller, M. D. (1989). *Understanding and communicating with an individual who is hallucinating* [Videotape]. Omaha, NE: NurScience.

Moller, M. D., & Murphy, M. F. (2002). *Recovering from psychosis: A wellness approach* (15th ed.). Nine Mile Falls, WA: Psychiatric Resource Network.

Moorhead, S., Johnson, M., & Maas, M. (2004). *Nursing outcomes classification (NOC)* (3rd ed.). St. Louis, MO: Mosby.

National Institute of Mental Health. (2003). *Childhood-onset schizophrenia: An update from the National Institute of Mental Health: A fact sheet that describes the symptoms, treatment, and causes of schizophrenia in children.* Retrieved January 21, 2005, from http://www.nimh.nih.gov/publicat/schizkids.cfm.

Patel, J. K., Pinals, D. A., & Breier, A. (2003). Schizophrenia and other psychoses. In A. Tasman, J. Kay, & J. A. Lieberman (Eds.), *Psychiatry* (2nd ed.). West Sussex, England: Wiley.

Soyka, Z. (2000). Substance misuse, psychiatric disorder and violent and disturbed behavior. *British Journal of Psychiatry, 176,* 345-350.

Tandon, R., et al. (2003, October 31). *Beyond symptoms control: Moving towards positive patient outcomes.* Paper presented at the American Psychiatric Association 55th Institute on Psychiatric Services, Boston, MA. Retrieved January 21, 2005, from http://www.medscape.com/viewprogram/2835_pnt.

Tsung-Ung, W. W., et al. (2004). Treatment of schizophrenia. In A. F. Schatzberg & C. B. Nemeroff (Eds.), *The American Psychiatric Publishing textbook of psychopharmacology* (3rd ed., pp. 885-912). Washington, DC: American Psychiatric Publishing.

Vidal, G. (1982). *The second American revolution and other essays (1976-1982).* New York: Random House.

Wilkaitis, J., Mulvihill, T., & Nasrallah, H. A. (2004). In A. F. Schatzberg & C. B. Nemeroff (Eds.), *The American Psychiatric Publishing textbook of psychopharmacology* (3rd ed., pp. 437-438). Washington, DC: American Psychiatric Publishing.

CHAPTER 21

Cognitive Disorders

CHARLOTTE ELIOPOULOS ▪ VERNA BENNER CARSON ▪ ELIZABETH M. VARCAROLIS

KEY TERMS and CONCEPTS

The key terms and concepts listed here appear in color where they are defined or first discussed in this chapter.

agnosia, 433

agraphia, 436

Alzheimer's disease, 431

amnestic disorder, 424

aphasia, 433

apraxia, 433

cognitive disorders, 423

confabulation, 433

delirium, 423

dementia, 424

hallucinations, 426

hypermetamorphosis, 436

hyperorality, 436

hypervigilance, 427

illusions, 426

perseveration, 433

primary dementia, 431

pseudodementia, 433

secondary dementia, 431

sundowning, 425

OBJECTIVES

After studying this chapter, the reader will be able to

1. Compare and contrast the clinical picture of delirium with the clinical picture of dementia.
2. Discuss three critical needs of a person with delirium, stated in terms of nursing diagnoses.
3. Identify three outcomes for clients with delirium.
4. Summarize the essential somatic and psychotherapeutic interventions for a client with delirium.
5. Compare and contrast the signs and symptoms occurring in the four stages of Alzheimer's disease.
6. Give an example of the following symptoms assessed during the progression of Alzheimer's disease: (a) amnesia (b) apraxia, (c) agnosia, and (d) aphasia.
7. Formulate at least three nursing diagnoses suitable for a client with Alzheimer's disease and define two outcomes for each.
8. Formulate a teaching plan for a caregiver of a client with Alzheimer's disease, including interventions for (a) communication, (b) health maintenance, and (c) safe environment.
9. Compose a list of appropriate referrals in the community for persons with Alzheimer's and their families. Include telephone numbers for at least one support group, hotline, source of further information, and caregiver respite service.

evolve Visit the Evolve website at **http://evolve.elsevier.com/Varcarolis** for a pretest on the content in this chapter.

The clarity and purpose of an individual's personal journey depend on the ability to reflect on its meaning. Cognition represents a fundamental human feature that distinguishes living from existing. This mental capacity has a distinctive, personalized impact on the individual's physical, psychological, social, and spiritual conduct of life. For example, the ability to "remember" the connections between related actions and how to initiate them depends on cognitive processing.

Moreover, this cognitive processing has a direct relationship to activities of daily living. Although primarily an intellectual and perceptual process, cognition is closely integrated with an individual's emotional and spiritual values. When human beings can no longer understand facts or connect the appropriate feelings to events, they have trouble responding to the complexity of life's challenges. Emotions take a back seat to profound disturbances in cognitive processing that either cloud or destroy the meaning of the journey. The labyrinth of current knowledge about cognitive disorders requires a compassionate understanding of the client and family. Nursing interventions are focused on protecting patient dignity, preserving functional status, and promoting quality of life for cognitively impaired clients.

There are three main cognitive disorders: delirium, dementia, and amnestic disorder. *Cognitive disorder not otherwise specified* is a category defined by the *Diagnostic and Statistical Manual of Mental Disorders,* fourth edition, text revision *(DSM-IV-TR)* that allows for the diagnosis of cognitive disorders that do not meet the criteria for delirium, dementia, or amnestic disorders (American Psychiatric Association [APA], 2000). Cognitive disorders not otherwise specified are presumed to be caused by a specific medical condition, a pharmacologically active agent, or possibly both (Sadock & Sadock, 2004). See Figure 21-1 for the location of these disorders on the mental health continuum.

Figure 21-2 identifies the three main cognitive disorders and gives the *DSM-IV-TR* criteria for each. This chapter addresses the broad categories of delirium and dementia because these are by far the most common conditions that nurses encounter.

PREVALENCE

Delirium "is characterized by a disturbance of consciousness and a change in cognition such as impaired attention span and disturbances of consciousness, that develop over a short period" (APA, 2000, p. 135; Sadock & Sadock, 2004, p. 46). Delirium is always secondary to another condition, such as a general medical condition or substance use (drugs of abuse, a medication, or toxin exposure), or it may have multiple causes. When the cause cannot be determined, delirium is classified as **delirium not otherwise specified.** Delirium is a transient disorder, and if the underlying medical cause is corrected, complete recovery should occur. Delirium secondary to substance abuse is discussed in Chapter 27. This chapter highlights delirium secondary to medical conditions, because delirium is one of the most commonly encountered mental disorders in medical practice; it is often overlooked or misdiagnosed.

Delirium is a significant risk for all hospitalized and elderly medically ill people. As many as 60% of nursing home residents 75 years of age or older may be delirious at any one time and up to 80% of those with

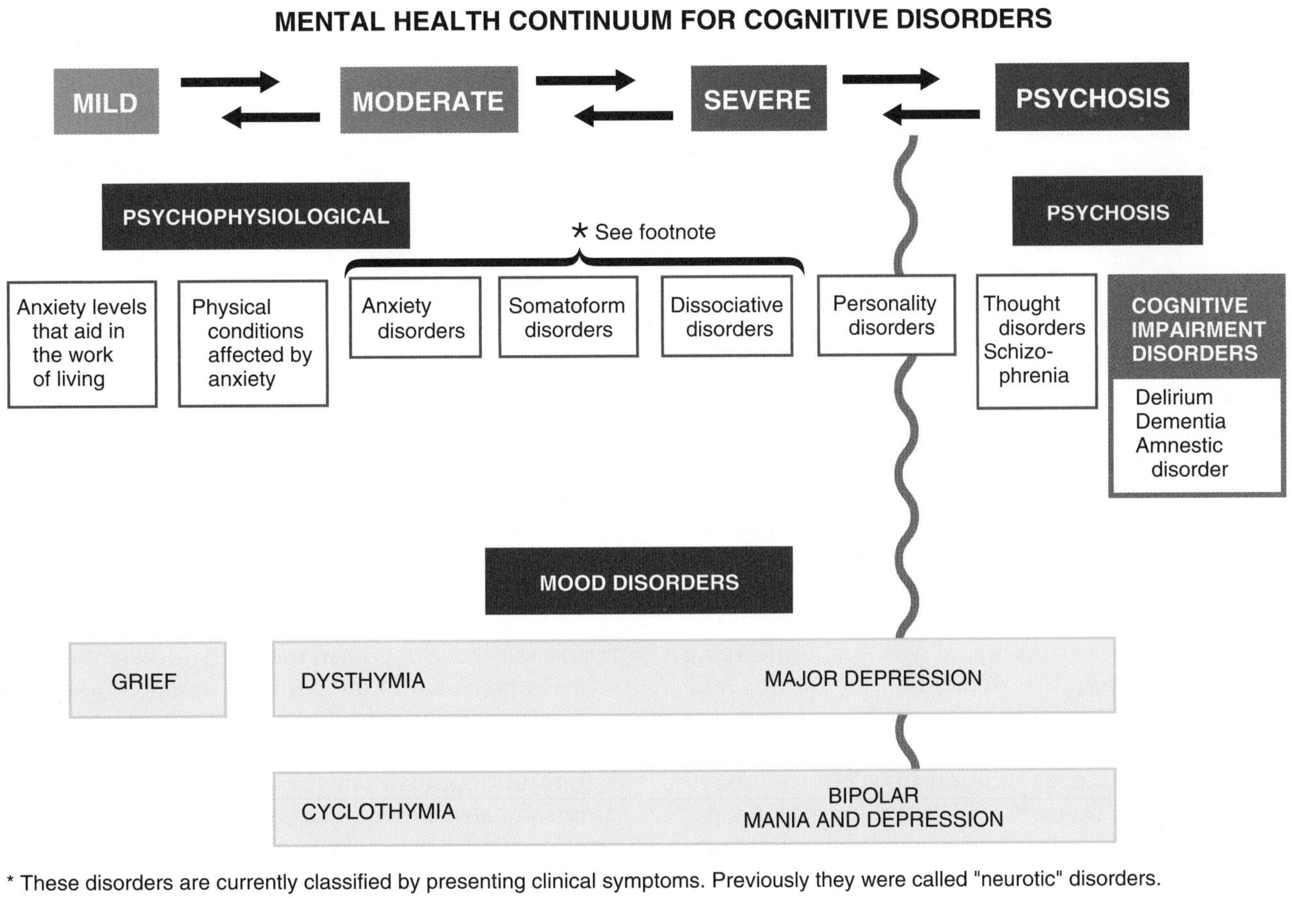

MENTAL HEALTH CONTINUUM FOR COGNITIVE DISORDERS

* These disorders are currently classified by presenting clinical symptoms. Previously they were called "neurotic" disorders.

FIGURE 21-1 Mental health continuum for cognitive disorders.

DSM-IV-TR CRITERIA FOR COGNITIVE DISORDERS

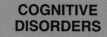

COGNITIVE DISORDERS

Delirium

A. Disturbance of consciousness (i.e., reduced clarity of awareness of the environment with reduced ability to focus, sustain, or shift attention).

B. A change in cognition (memory deficit, disorientation, language disturbance) or the development of a perceptual disturbance that is not better accounted for by a preexisting, established, or evolving dementia.

C. The disturbance develops over a short period of time (usually hours to days) and tends to fluctuate during the course of the day.

Due to:

1. A general medical condition
   or
2. Substance-induced (intoxication or withdrawal)
   or
3. Multiple etiologies (both 1 and 2 above)
   or
4. Not known (not otherwise specified)

Amnestic Disorder

A. The development of memory impairment as manifested by impairment in the ability to learn new information or the ability to recall previously learned information.

B. The memory disturbance causes significant impairment in social or occupational functioning and represents a significant decline from a previous level of functioning.

C. The memory disturbance does not occur exclusively during the course of a delirium or a dementia.

Dementia

A. The development of multiple cognitive deficits manifested by both:

1. **Memory impairment** (impaired ability to learn new information or to recall previously learned information).

2. One (or more) of the following cognitive disturbances:
   (a) **Aphasia** (language disturbance)
   (b) **Apraxia** (impaired ability to carry out motor activities despite intact motor function)
   (c) **Agnosia** (failure to recognize or identify objects despite intact sensory function)
   (d) Disturbance in executive functioning (i.e., planning, organizing, sequencing, abstracting)

B. The cognitive deficits in criteria A1 and A2 each cause significant impairment in social or occupational functioning and represent a significant decline from a previous level of functioning.

FIGURE 21-2 Diagnostic criteria for delirium, dementia, and amnestic disorder. (Adapted from American Psychiatric Association. [2000]. *Diagnostic and statistical manual of mental disorders* [4th ed., text rev.]. Washington, DC: Author.)

terminal illness develop delirium near death (APA, 2000).

Dementia usually develops more slowly and is characterized by multiple cognitive deficits that include impairment in memory without impairment in consciousness (Sadock & Sadock, 2004). The majority of dementias are irreversible; those dementias that have a reversible component are **secondary** to other pathological processes (e.g., neoplasms, trauma, infections, and toxin exposure). When the underlying causes are treated, the dementia often improves. However, most dementias, such as dementias of the Alzheimer type, are related to a **primary** encephalopathy. Alzheimer's disease accounts for 60% to 80% of all dementias in the United States. Vascular dementia, dementia with Lewy bodies, and frontotemporal dementia together account for 15% to 20% of dementias; other disorders (normal-pressure hydrocephalus, vita-

min B_{12} deficiency) account for 5% (Morris, 2000). The average lifetime prevalence of Alzheimer's disease is about 5% by age 65, 10% to 15% by age 75, and 20% to 40% by age 85 (Alzheimer's Disease and Related Disorders Association [ADRDA], 2004). Primary dementias have no known cause or cure; thus, they are progressive and irreversible.

Amnestic disorder is characterized by loss in both short-term memory (including the inability to learn information) and long-term memory, sufficient to cause some impairment in the person's functioning (Kaplan & Kaplan, 2004; Kochanek, Smith, & Andersen, 2001). This memory impairment exists in the absence of other significant cognitive impairments. These amnestic disorders are always **secondary** to underlying causes and are classified, for example, as general medical condition, substance induced; persistent amnestic disorder; and amnestic disorder not otherwise specified.

Delirium

Nurses frequently encounter delirium on medical and surgical units in the general hospital setting. During certain phases of a hospital stay, confusion may be noted (e.g., after surgery or after the introduction of a new drug). The second or third hospital day may herald the onset of confusion for older people and difficulty adjusting to an unfamiliar environment.

Delirium occurs more frequently in elderly than in younger clients. Surgery, drugs, urinary tract infections, pneumonia, cerebrovascular disease, and congestive heart failure are some of the most common causes. Delirium is also commonly seen in children with fever. Delirium often occurs in terminally ill clients.

A delayed or missed diagnosis can have serious implications, because the longer a condition goes untreated, the greater the risk that the condition can cause permanent damage. Table 21-1 offers some guidelines for distinguishing between delirium, depression, and dementia.

The essential feature of delirium is a disturbance in consciousness coupled with cognitive difficulties. Thinking, memory, attention, and perception are typically disturbed. The clinical manifestations of delirium develop over a short period (hours to days) and tend to fluctuate during the course of the day. Sundowning, in which symptoms and problem behaviors become more pronounced in the evening, may occur in both delirium and dementia.

Because delirium increases psychological stress, supportive interventions that lower anxiety and promote calm and security can foster a sense of control. Clients with delirium may appear withdrawn, agitated, or psychotic. Also, underlying personality traits often become exaggerated.

The priorities of treatment are to identify the cause and make an appropriate medical or surgical intervention. If the underlying disorder is corrected, complete recovery is possible. If, however, the underlying disorder is not corrected and persists, sustained neuronal damage can lead to irreversible changes. Box 21-1 lists common causes of delirium. Nursing concerns therefore center on the following:

- Performing a comprehensive nursing assessment to aid in identifying the cause
- Assisting with proper health management to eradicate the underlying cause

TABLE 21-1

Comparison of Delirium, Dementia, and Depression

	Delirium	Dementia	Depression
Onset	Sudden, over hours to days	Slowly, over months	May have been gradual with exacerbation during crisis or stress
Cause or contributing factors	Hypoglycemia, fever, dehydration, hypotension; infection, other conditions that disrupt body's homeostasis; adverse drug reaction; head injury; change in environment (e.g., hospitalization); pain; emotional stress	Alzheimer's disease, vascular disease, human immunodeficiency virus infection, neurological disease, chronic alcoholism, head trauma	Lifelong history, losses, loneliness, crises, declining health, medical conditions
Cognition	Impaired memory, judgment, calculations, attention span; can fluctuate through the day	Impaired memory, judgment, calculations, attention span, abstract thinking; agnosia	Difficulty concentrating, forgetfulness, inattention
Level of consciousness	Altered	Not altered	Not altered
Activity level	Can be increased or reduced; restlessness, behaviors may worsen in evening (sundowning); sleep-wake cycle may be reversed	Not altered; behaviors may worsen in evening (sundowning)	Usually decreased; lethargy, fatigue, lack of motivation; may sleep poorly and awaken in early morning
Emotional state	Rapid swings; can be fearful, anxious, suspicious, aggressive, have hallucinations and/or delusions	Flat; delusions	Extreme sadness, apathy, irritability, anxiety, paranoid ideation
Speech and language	Rapid, inappropriate, incoherent, rambling	Incoherent, slow (sometimes due to effort to find the right word), inappropriate, rambling, repetitious	Slow, flat, low
Prognosis	Reversible with proper and timely treatment	Not reversible; progressive	Reversible with proper and timely treatment

Common Causes of Delirium

Postoperative states
Drug intoxications and withdrawals
- Alcohol, anxiolytics, opioids, and central nervous system stimulants (e.g., cocaine and crack cocaine)

Infections
- Systemic: pneumonia, typhoid fever, malaria, urinary tract infection, and septicemia
- Intracranial: meningitis and encephalitis

Metabolic disorders
- Dehydration
- Hypoxia (pulmonary disease, heart disease, and anemia)
- Hypoglycemia
- Sodium, potassium, calcium, magnesium, and acid-base imbalances
- Hepatic encephalopathy or uremic encephalopathy
- Thiamine (vitamin B_1) deficiency (Wernicke's encephalopathy)
- Endocrine disorders (e.g., thyroidism or parathyroidism)
- Hypothermia or hyperthermia
- Diabetic acidosis

Drugs
- Digitalis, steroids, lithium, levodopa, anticholinergics, benzodiazepines, central nervous system depressants, tricyclic antidepressants
- Central anticholinergic syndrome due to use of multiple drugs with anticholinergic side effects

Neurological diseases
- Seizures
- Head trauma
- Hypertensive encephalopathy

Tumor
- Primary cerebral

Psychosocial stressors
- Relocation or other sudden changes
- Sensory deprivation or overload
- Sleep deprivation
- Immobilization
- Pain

- Preventing physical harm due to confusion, aggression, or electrolyte and fluid imbalance
- Using supportive measures to relieve distress

Application of the Nursing Process

ASSESSMENT

Overall Assessment

Generally, the nurse suspects the presence of delirium when a client abruptly develops a disturbance in consciousness that is manifested in reduced clarity of awareness of the environment. The person may have difficulty with orientation, first to time, then to place, and last to person. For example, a man with delirium may think that the year is 1972 instead of the correct year, that the hospital is home, and that the nurse is his wife. Orientation to person is usually intact to the extent that the person is aware of the self's identity. The ability to focus, sustain, or shift attention is impaired. Questions need to be repeated because the individual's attention wanders, and the person might easily get off track and need to be refocused. Conversation is made more difficult because the person may be easily distracted by irrelevant stimuli.

Fluctuating levels of consciousness are unpredictable. Disorientation and confusion are usually markedly worse at night and during the early morning. In fact, some clients may be confused or delirious only at night and may remain lucid during the day. Some clinicians use the Mini-Mental State Examination to screen or follow the progress of an individual with delirium.

Nursing assessment includes (1) cognitive and perceptual disturbances, (2) physical needs, and (3) mood and behavior.

Cognitive and Perceptual Disturbances

It may be difficult to engage delirious persons in conversation because they are easily distracted and display marked attention deficits. Memory is impaired. In mild delirium, memory deficits are noted on careful questioning. In more severe delirium, memory problems usually take the form of obvious difficulty in processing and remembering recent events. For example, the person might ask when a son is coming to visit, even though the son left only an hour earlier.

Perceptual disturbances are also common. Perception is the processing of information about one's internal and external environment. Various misinterpretations of reality may take the form of illusions or hallucinations.

Illusions are errors in perception of sensory stimuli. For example, a person may mistake folds in the bedclothes for white rats or the cord of a window blind for a snake. The stimulus is a real object in the environment; however, it is misinterpreted and often becomes the object of the client's projected fear. Illusions, unlike delusions or hallucinations, can be explained and clarified for the individual.

Hallucinations are false sensory stimuli (see Chapter 20). Visual hallucinations are common in delirium. Tactile hallucinations may also be present. For example, delirious individuals may become terrified when they "see" giant spiders crawling over the bedclothes or "feel" bugs crawling on or under their bodies. Auditory hallucinations occur more often in other psychiatric disorders, such as schizophrenia and depression.

The delirious individual generally possesses an awareness that something is very wrong. For example, the delirious person may state, "My thoughts are all jumbled." When perceptual disturbances are present, the emotional response is one of fear and anxiety. Verbal and psychomotor signs of agitation should be noted.

Physical Needs

Physical Safety. A person with delirium becomes disoriented and may try to "go home." Alternatively, a person may think that he or she *is* home and may jump out of a window in an attempt to get away from "invaders." Wandering, pulling out intravenous lines and Foley catheters, and falling out of bed are common dangers that require nursing intervention.

An individual experiencing delirium has difficulty processing stimuli in the environment. Confusion magnifies the inability to recognize reality. The physical environment should be made as simple and as clear as possible. Objects such as clocks and calendars can maximize orientation to time. Eyeglasses, hearing aids, and adequate lighting without glare can maximize the person's ability to interpret more accurately what is going on in the environment. The nurse should interact with the client whenever the client is awake. Short periods of social interaction help reduce anxiety and misperceptions.

Bacteriological Safety. Self-care deficits, injury, or hyperactivity or hypoactivity may lead to skin breakdown and may leave a person prone to infection. Often, this condition is compounded by poor nutrition, forced bed rest, and possible incontinence. These areas require nursing assessment and intervention.

Biophysical Safety. Autonomic signs, such as tachycardia, sweating, flushed face, dilated pupils, and elevated blood pressure, are often present. These changes must be monitored and documented carefully and may require immediate medical attention.

Changes in the sleep-wake cycle usually are noted, and in some cases, a complete reversal of the night-day sleep-wake cycle can occur. The client's level of consciousness may range from lethargy to stupor or from semicoma to hypervigilance. In hypervigilance clients are extraordinarily alert and their eyes constantly scan the room; they may have difficulty falling asleep or may be actively disoriented and agitated throughout the night.

It is also important that the nurse assess all medications, because the nurse is in a position to recognize drug reactions or potential interactions before delirium actually occurs.

Moods and Physical Behaviors

The delirious individual's behavior and mood may change dramatically within a short period. Moods may swing back and forth from fear, anger, and anxiety to euphoria, depression, and apathy. These labile moods are often accompanied by physical behaviors

associated with feeling states. A person may strike out from fear or anger or may cry, call for help, curse, moan, and tear off clothing one minute and become apathetic or laugh uncontrollably the next. In short, behavior and emotions are erratic and fluctuating. Lack of concentration and disorientation complicate interventions. The following vignette illustrates the fear and confusion a client may experience when admitted to an intensive care unit (ICU).

■ ■ ■ *VIGNETTE*

A 55-year-old married man, Mr. Arnold, is admitted to the ICU after having a three-vessel coronary artery bypass. Mr. Arnold's surgery has taken longer than usual and has necessitated his remaining on a cardiac pump for 3 hours. He arrives in the ICU without further complications. On awakening from the anesthesia, he hears the nurse exclaim, "I need to get a gas." Another nurse answers in a loud voice, "Can you take a large needle for the injection?" During this period, Mr. Arnold experiences the need to urinate and asks the nurse very calmly if he can go to the bathroom. Her reply is, "You don't need to go; you have a tube in." He again complains about his discomfort and assures the nurse that if she will let him go to the bathroom, he will be fine. The nurse informs Mr. Arnold that he cannot urinate and that he has to keep the "mask" on so that she can get the "gas" and check his "blood levels." On hearing this, Mr. Arnold begins to implore more loudly and states that he sees the bathroom sign. He assures the nurse that he will only take a minute. In reality, the sign is an exit sign.

To prove to him that a bathroom does not exist in the ICU and that the sign does not indicate a bathroom, the nurse takes off the restraints so that his head can be raised to see the sign. He abruptly breaks away from the nurse's grasp and runs toward the entrance to the ICU. He discovers a door, which is the entrance to the nurses' lounge, barricades himself in the room, and pulls out his chest tube, Foley catheter, and intravenous lines. He finds the bathroom that is connected to the lounge. Ten minutes later, the nurses and security personnel break through the barricade and escort Mr. Arnold back to bed.

When he becomes fully alert and oriented a day later, Mr. Arnold tells the nurses his perception of the previous day's events. Initially, he had thought he had been kidnapped and was being held against his will (the restraints had been tight). When the nurse yelled out about blood gas, he had thought she was going to kill him with noxious gas through his face mask (the reason he did not want to wear the face mask). All he could think about was escaping his tormentor and executioner. In this case, the nurse had not assessed the alteration in Mr. Arnold's mental status and allowed him to get out of bed. The medical jargon and loud voices had perpetuated his confusion and distortion of reality.

■ ■ ■

What are some more helpful interventions the nurses could have used? What could the nurses have done differently? What would you have done? What initial nursing actions would you have taken to assess his bladder?

For example, the nurses could have told Mr. Arnold where he was and that the nursing staff were caring for him; they could have better explained the function of his Foley catheter.

Self-Assessment

In many cases, delirium is easily associated with a medical disease. First, delirium is usually encountered on a medical or surgical unit; and second, delirium usually responds to specific medical or surgical interventions, depending on the underlying cause. Frequently, this syndrome reverses within a few days or less when the underlying cause is identified and treated. Because the behaviors exhibited by the client can be directly attributed to temporary medical conditions, intense personal reactions are less likely to arise. In fact, intense conflicting emotions are less likely to occur in nurses working with a client with delirium than in nurses working with a client with dementia, which is discussed later in this chapter.

Assessment Guidelines Delirium

1. Assess for fluctuating levels of consciousness, which is key in delirium.
2. Interview family or other caregivers to establish the client's normal level of consciousness and cognition.
3. Assess for past confusional states (e.g., prior dementia diagnosis).
4. Identify other disturbances in medical status (e.g., infection, dyspnea, edema, presence of jaundice).
5. Identify any electroencephalographic, neuroimaging, or laboratory abnormalities documented in the client's record.
6. Assess vital signs, level of consciousness, and neurological signs.
7. Assess potential for injury (is the client safe from falls, wandering?).
8. Assess the need for comfort measures (e.g., to address pain or cold, improve positioning).
9. Monitor factors that worsen or improve symptoms.
10. Assess for availability of immediate medical interventions to help prevent irreversible brain damage.
11. Remain nonjudgmental. Confer with other staff readily when questions arise.

■ NURSING DIAGNOSIS

Safety needs play a substantial role in nursing care. Clients with delirium often perceive the environment in a distorted way. Objects in the environment are often misperceived (illusions and/or hallucinations).

People and objects may be misinterpreted as threatening or harmful. Clients often act on these misinterpretations. For example, if feeling threatened or thinking that common medical equipment is harmful, the client may pull off an oxygen mask, pull out an intravenous or nasogastric tube, or try to flee. In such a case, the person demonstrates a *risk for injury* related to confusion, as evidenced by sensory deficits or perceptual deficits.

If fever and dehydration are present, fluid and electrolyte balance will need to be managed. If the underlying cause of the client's delirium results in fever, decreased skin turgor, decreased urinary output or fluid intake, and dry skin or mucous membranes, then the nursing diagnosis of *deficient fluid volume* is appropriate. Fluid volume deficit may be related to fever, electrolyte imbalance, reduced intake, or infection.

Perceptions are disturbed during delirium. Hallucinations, distractibility, illusions, disorientation, agitation, restlessness, and/or misperception are major aspects of the clinical picture. When some of these symptoms are present, *acute confusion* is an appropriate nursing diagnosis.

Because disruption in the sleep-wake cycle may be present, the client may be less responsive during the day and may become disruptively wakeful during the night. Restful sleep is not achieved, day or night; therefore, *disturbed sleep pattern* related to impaired cerebral oxygenation or disruption in consciousness is a likely diagnosis.

Sustaining communication with a delirious client is difficult. *Impaired verbal communication* related to cerebral hypoxia or decreased cerebral blood flow, as evidenced by confusion or clouding of consciousness, may be diagnosed.

Fear is one of the most common of all nursing diagnoses and may be related to illusions, delusions, or hallucinations, as evidenced by verbal and nonverbal expressions of fearfulness.

Other nursing concerns include *self-care deficit, disturbed thought processes,* and *impaired social interaction.*

Table 21-2 identifies nursing diagnoses for any confused client (with delirium or dementia).

■ OUTCOME CRITERIA

The overall outcome is that the delirious client will return to the premorbid level of functioning. Table 21-3 includes outcomes for acute confusion from the Nursing Outcomes Classification (NOC) (Moorhead, Johnson, & Maas, 2004). However, for many of the diagnoses that we would use for the delirious client, NOC is not specific enough. Although the client can demonstrate a wide variety of needs, *risk for injury* is always present. Appropriate outcomes are as follows:

- Client will remain safe and free from injury while in the hospital.

TABLE 21-2

Potential Nursing Diagnoses for the Confused Client

Symptoms	Nursing Diagnoses
Wanders, has unsteady gait, acts out fear from hallucinations or illusions, forgets things (leaves stove on, doors open)	**Risk for injury**
Awake and disoriented during the night (sundowning), frightened at night	**Disturbed sleep pattern** **Fear** **Acute confusion**
Too confused to take care of basic needs	**Self-care deficit (specify)** **Ineffective coping** **Functional urinary incontinence** **Imbalanced nutrition: less than body requirements** **Deficient fluid volume**
Sees frightening things that are not there (hallucinations), mistakes every-day objects for something sinister and frightening (illusions), may become paranoid and think that others are doing things to confuse him or her (delusions)	**Disturbed sensory perception** **Impaired environmental interpretation syndrome** **Disturbed thought processes**
Does not recognize familiar people or places, has difficulty with short- and/or long-term memory, forgetful and confused	**Impaired memory** **Impaired environmental interpretation syndrome** **Acute/chronic confusion**
Has difficulty with communication, cannot find words, has difficulty in recognizing objects and/or people, incoherent	**Impaired verbal communication**
Devastated over losing place in life as known (during lucid moments), fearful and overwhelmed by what is happening to him or her	**Spiritual distress** **Hopelessness** **Situational low self-esteem** **Grieving**
Family and loved ones overburdened and overwhelmed, unable to care for client's needs	**Disabled family coping** **Interrupted family processes** **Impaired home maintenance** **Caregiver role strain**

TABLE 21-3

NOC Outcomes Related to Acute Confusion

Acute confusion: Abrupt onset of a cluster of global, transient changes and disturbances in attention, cognition, psychomotor activity, level of consciousness, and/or sleep-wake cycle

Nursing Outcome and Definition	Intermediate Indicators	Short-Term Indicators
Cognitive Orientation: Ability to identify person, place and time accurately*	Identifies correct day Identifies correct month Identifies correct year Identifies correct season Identifies current place Identifies significant current events	Identifies self Identifies significant other
Neurological Status: Consciousness: Arousal, orientation, and attention to the environment*	Shows cognitive orientation Communicates appropriately for situation	Opens eyes to external stimuli Obeys commands Makes motor responses to noxious stimuli

From Moorhead, S., Johnson, M., & Maas, M. (2004). *Nursing outcomes classification (NOC)* (3rd ed.). St. Louis, MO: Mosby.

- During periods of lucidity, client will be oriented to time, place, and person with the aid of nursing interventions, such as the provision of clocks, calendars, maps, and other types of orienting information.

- Client will remain free from falls and injury while confused, with the aid of nursing safety measures. Because level of consciousness can change throughout the day, the client needs to be checked for orientation frequently.

INTERVENTION

The Nursing Interventions Classification (NIC) (Dochterman & Bulechek, 2004) can be used as a guide to develop interventions for a client with delirium (Box 21-2). Medical management of delirium involves treating the underlying organic causes. If the underlying cause of delirium is not treated, permanent brain damage may ensue. Judicious use of antipsychotic or antianxiety agents may also be useful in controlling behavioral symptoms.

A client in acute delirium should never be left alone. Because most hospitals and health facilities are unable to provide one-to-one supervision of the client, family members can be encouraged to stay with the client.

EVALUATION

Long-term outcome criteria for a delirious person include the following:

- Client will remain safe.
- Client will be oriented to time, place, and person by discharge.
- Underlying cause will be treated and ameliorated.

Dementia: Alzheimer's Disease

There are over 4 million people diagnosed with Alzheimer's disease. Over 19 million Americans are affected by the disease, including family members and other caretakers of individuals with Alzheimer's disease. The prediction is that 14 million Americans will be diagnosed with this disease by 2059 (ADRDA, 2004). It is the third most costly disease after heart disease and cancer, with the bulk of the financial burden carried by families. Although many of you reading this textbook will not choose to be psychiatric-mental health nurses, all of you will be confronted with the care of the client with Alzheimer's disease. You must be prepared to respond. It is a devastating disease.

BOX 21-2

Delirium Management (NIC)

Definition: Provision of a safe and therapeutic environment for the patient who is experiencing an acute confusional state

Activities:

- Identify etiological factors causing delirium.
- Initiate therapies to reduce or eliminate factors causing delirium.
- Monitor neurological status on an ongoing basis.
- Provide unconditional positive regard.
- Verbally acknowledge patient's fears and feelings.
- Provide optimistic but realistic reassurance.
- Allow patient to maintain rituals that limit anxiety.
- Provide patient with information about what is happening and what can be expected to occur in the future.
- Avoid demands for abstract thinking, if patient can only think in concrete terms.
- Limit need for decision making, if frustrating or confusing to patient.
- Administer prn (as needed) medications for anxiety or agitation.
- Encourage visitation by significant others, as appropriate.
- Recognize and accept patient's perceptions or interpretation of reality (hallucinations or delusions).
- State your perception in a calm, reassuring, and nonargumentative manner.
- Respond to the theme or feeling tone, rather than the content, of the hallucination or delusion.
- When possible, remove stimuli that create misperception in a particular patient (e.g., pictures on the wall or television).
- Maintain a well-lit environment that reduces sharp contrasts and shadows.

- Assist with needs related to nutrition, elimination, hydration, and personal hygiene.
- Maintain a hazard-free environment.
- Place identification bracelet on patient.
- Provide appropriate level of supervision and surveillance to monitor patient and to allow for therapeutic actions as needed.
- Use physical restraints, as needed.
- Avoid frustrating patient by quizzing with orientation questions that cannot be answered.
- Inform patient of person, place, and time, as needed.
- Provide a consistent physical environment and daily routine.
- Provide caregivers who are familiar to the patient.
- Use environmental cues (e.g., signs, pictures, clocks, calendars, and color coding of environment) to stimulate memory, reorient, and promote appropriate behavior.
- Provide a low-stimulation environment for patient in whom disorientation is increased by overstimulation.
- Encourage use of aids that increase sensory input (e.g., eyeglasses, hearing aids, and dentures).
- Approach patient slowly and from the front.
- Address patient by name when initiating interaction.
- Reorient patient to health care provider with each contact.
- Communicate with simple, direct, descriptive statements.
- Prepare patient for upcoming changes in usual routine and environment before their occurrence.
- Provide new information slowly and in small doses, with frequent rest periods.
- Focus interpersonal interactions on what is familiar and meaningful to patient.

From Dochterman, J. M., & Bulechek, G. M. (2004). *Nursing interventions classification (NIC)* (4th ed., pp. 275-276). St. Louis, MO: Mosby.

It is important to distinguish between normal forgetfulness and the memory deficit of Alzheimer's disease. Severe memory loss is *not* a normal part of growing older. Slight forgetfulness is a common phenomenon of the aging process (age-associated memory loss), but not memory loss that interferes with one's activities of daily living. Table 21-4 outlines memory changes in normal aging and memory changes seen in dementia.

Most people who live to a very old age never experience a significant memory loss or any other symptom of dementia. Most of us know of people in their eighties and nineties who lead active lives, with the intellect intact. Margaret Mead, Pablo Picasso, Duke Ellington, Count Basie, Ansel Adams, Sonny Coles, and George Burns are all examples of people who were still active in their careers when they died; all were older than 75 years of age (Picasso was 91 years; George Burns was 100 years). The slow, mild cognitive changes associated with aging should not impede social or occupational functioning.

Dementia, on the other hand, is marked by progressive deterioration in intellectual functioning, memory, and the ability to solve problems and learn new skills; a decline in the ability to perform activities of daily living; and a progressive deterioration of personality accompanied by impairment in judgment. A person's declining intellect often leads to emotional changes such as mood lability, depression, and aggressive acting out as well as to neurological changes that produce hallucinations and delusions. There are several types of dementia, including dementia of the Alzheimer's type, vascular dementia, Lewy body disease, Pick's disease, Huntington's chorea, alcohol-related dementias (including Korsakoff's syndrome), Creutzfeldt-Jakob disease, and the dementias associated with Parkinson's disease, acquired immunodeficiency syndrome (AIDS), and head trauma.

Dementias can be classified as primary or secondary. Primary dementia is not reversible, is progressive, and is not secondary to any other disorder. As mentioned, Alzheimer's disease accounts for about 70% of all dementias, and vascular dementia accounts for about 20% of all dementias (Kochanek et al., 2001). Both Alzheimer's and vascular dementias are primary, progressive, and irreversible.

Secondary dementia occurs as a result of some other pathological process (e.g., vascular, metabolic, nutritional, or neurological). AIDS-related dementia is an example of a secondary dementia that is increasingly seen in health care settings. The exact prevalence of AIDS-related dementia is not known, although it is estimated to occur in as many as 40% of individuals with human immunodeficiency virus (HIV) infection and in up to 90% of clients dying of AIDS (Ress, 2003). This phenomenon is now commonly referred to as HIV encephalopathy. Other secondary dementias can result from viral encephalitis, pernicious anemia, folic acid deficiency, and hypothyroidism.

Korsakoff's syndrome is an example of a secondary dementia and is caused by thiamine (vitamin B_1) deficiency, which may be associated with prolonged, heavy alcohol ingestion. Along with progressive mental deterioration, Korsakoff's syndrome is marked by peripheral neuropathy, cerebellar ataxia, confabulation, and myopathy (APA, 2000).

Alzheimer's disease attacks indiscriminately, striking men and women, black and white, rich and poor, and individuals with varying degrees of intelligence. Although the disease can occur at a younger age (early onset), most of those with the disease are 65 years of age or older (late onset).

THEORY

Although the cause of Alzheimer's disease is not known, numerous hypotheses have been put forward regarding its cause.

Pathological Findings

Alzheimer's Tangles

Alzheimer's disease results in cerebral atrophy with neuritic plaques and neurofibrillary tangles, which are microscopic abnormalities in brain tissue. β-amyloid

TABLE 21-4

Memory Deficit: Normal Aging Versus Dementia

Parameter	Normal Aging	Dementia
Degree of change	Slowing	More severe and increasing
	Cautiousness	Variable
	Reduced ability to solve new problems	More severe and increasing
	Mildly impaired memory	More severe and increasing
	Mild decline in fluid intelligence	More severe and increasing intellectual impairment
Extent of damage	Difficulty in word finding, but no dysphasia, dyspraxia, agnosia	Dysphasia, dyspraxia, agnosia often found
Rate of change	Very slow change over many years	More rapid though gradual changes

protein is the main component of neuritic plaques, one of the abnormal structures found in the brains of Alzheimer's clients. These abnormalities can be described as follows:

Neurofibrillary tangles are mainly composed of hyperphosphorylated tau protein and initially form in the neurons in the hippocampus, the part of the brain responsible for recent (short-term) memory. Therefore, memory is negatively affected.

Neuritic plaques are cores of degenerated neuron material that lie free of the cell bodies on the ground substances of the brain. The quantity of plaques has been correlated with the degree of mental deterioration.

Granulovascular degeneration is the filling of brain cells with fluid and granular material. Increased degeneration accounts for increased loss of mental function.

Brain atrophy is observable, with wider cortical sulci and enlarged cerebral ventricles, as demonstrated by computed tomography (CT) and magnetic resonance imaging (MRI) (APA, 2000).

Genetic Findings

Family members of people with Alzheimer's dementia are at greater risk for developing the disease than are those in the general population (Prasher et al., 2003).

Recent developments have helped in the understanding of Alzheimer's disease. A study of sibling pairs ($N = 292$) who showed evidence of late-onset Alzheimer's disease were studied. The genes that seemed to show the highest hereditary link were on chromosomes 1, 9, 10, and 19 (Alzheimer's Disease Education and Referral [ADEAR] Center, 2004; Korn, 2000). Although each of these chromosomes is suspected of carrying genetic risk factors for late-onset Alzheimer's disease, chromosome 19 has received the greatest attention.

The apolipoprotein E (APOE) gene on chromosome 19, which occurs in several different forms, or alleles, has been implicated in late-onset Alzheimer's disease. The alleles that occur most frequently are the following:

- APOE ε4
- APOE ε2
- APOE ε3

People inherit one APOE allele from each parent. Having one or two copies of the ε4 allele increases a person's risk of getting Alzheimer's disease. However, it is important to note that the presence of two copies of the ε4 allele does not guarantee that the person will develop the disease. Some people with two copies of the ε4 allele do not develop clinical signs of Alzheimer's disease, whereas others with no ε4 alleles do. The ε3 allele is the most common form found in the general population and may play a neutral role in the development of Alzheimer's disease. The rarer ε2 form appears to be associated with lower risk for the disease (ADEAR Center, 2004).

Herpes simplex virus type 1 (HSV-1) has been found on autopsy in the brains of many elderly people who died with dementia. Researchers believe that HSV-1 in the nervous systems of ε4 allele carriers is a risk factor for Alzheimer's disease (Strandberg et al., 2003).

Nongenetic Findings

Until recently, the only risk factors that seemed to play a role in noninherited cases of Alzheimer's disease were increasing age, Down syndrome, and, most likely, head injury.

An interesting research discovery, however, is the finding of inflammation and high cholesterol levels in the brains of clients who died with Alzheimer's disease. These findings suggest that antiinflammatory agents and the statins (cholesterol-lowering drugs) may help to prevent Alzheimer's disease. The Framingham study confirms that elevated homocysteine levels and folic acid deficiency may also be risk factors for Alzheimer's disease (ADEAR Center, 2002).

Neurochemical Changes

Some studies have indicated that people with Alzheimer's dementia have drastically reduced levels of the enzyme acetyltransferase, which is needed to synthesize the neurotransmitter acetylcholine. Some theorists propose that the cognitive defects that occur in Alzheimer's disease, especially memory loss, are a direct result of the reduction in the amount of acetylcholine available to the brain.

There is also ongoing investigation as to the role of estrogen in the development of Alzheimer's disease. Prior to the release of findings from the Women's Health Initiative Memory Study, researchers believed that estrogen was protective against Alzheimer's disease. However, this study demonstrated an increased risk for dementia in postmenopausal women taking estrogen with progestin (Shumaker et al., 2003).

Application of the Nursing Process

■ ASSESSMENT
Overall Assessment

Alzheimer's disease is commonly characterized by progressive deterioration of cognitive functioning. Initially, deterioration may be so subtle and insidious that others may not notice. In the early stages of the disease, the affected person may be able to compensate for loss of memory. Some people may have superior social graces and charm that give them the ability to hide severe deficits in memory, even from experienced health care professionals. This hiding is actually a form of **denial**, which is an unconscious protective defense against the terrifying reality of losing one's place in the world. Family members may also unconsciously deny that anything is wrong as a defense against the painful awareness that a loved one is deteriorating. As time goes on, symptoms become more obvious, and other defensive maneuvers become evident. Confabulation (making up stories or answers to maintain self-esteem when the person does not remember) is noticed. For example, the nurse addresses a client who has remained in a hospital bed all weekend:

> *Nurse:* Good morning, Ms. Jones. How was your weekend?
>
> *Client:* Wonderful. I discussed politics with the President, and he took me out to dinner.
>
> *or*
>
> I spent the weekend with my daughter and her family.

Confabulation is not the same as lying. When people are lying, they are aware of making up an answer; confabulation is an **unconscious** attempt to maintain self-esteem.

Perseveration (the repetition of phrases or behavior) is eventually seen and is often intensified under stress. The avoidance of answering questions is another mechanism by which the client is able to maintain self-esteem unconsciously in the face of severe memory deficits.

Therefore, (1) denial, (2) confabulation, (3) perseveration, and (4) avoidance of questions are four defensive behaviors the nurse might notice during assessment.

Cardinal symptoms observed in Alzheimer's disease are the following (APA, 2000):

- **Amnesia or memory impairment.** Initially, the person has difficulty remembering recent events. Gradually, deterioration progresses to include both recent and remote memory.
- Aphasia (loss of language ability), which progresses with the disease. Initially, the person has difficulty finding the correct word, then is reduced to a few words, and finally is reduced to babbling or mutism.
- Apraxia (loss of purposeful movement in the absence of motor or sensory impairment). The person is unable to perform once-familiar and purposeful tasks. For example, in apraxia of gait, the person loses the ability to walk. In apraxia of dressing, the person is unable to put clothes on properly (may put arms in trousers or put a jacket on upside down).
- Agnosia (loss of sensory ability to recognize objects). For example, the person may lose the ability to recognize familiar sounds (auditory agnosia), such as the ring of the telephone, a car horn, or the doorbell. Loss of this ability extends to the inability to recognize familiar objects (visual or tactile agnosia), such as a glass, magazine, pencil, or toothbrush. Eventually, people are unable to recognize loved ones or even parts of their own bodies.
- **Disturbances in executive functioning** (planning, organizing, abstract thinking). The degeneration of neurons in the brain results in the wasting away of working components in the brain. These cells contain memories, receive sights and sounds, cause hormones to secrete, produce emotions, and command muscles into motion.

A person with Alzheimer's disease loses a personal history, a place in the world, and the ability to recognize the environment and, eventually, loved ones. Alzheimer's disease robs family and friends, husbands and wives, and sons and daughters of valuable human relatedness and companionship, which results in a profound sense of grief. Alzheimer's disease robs society of productive and active participants. Because of these devastating effects, it challenges mental health professionals and social agencies, the medical and nursing professions, and researchers looking for possible solutions.

Diagnostic Tests for Dementia

A wide range of problems may masquerade as dementia and may be mistaken for Alzheimer's disease. For example, in the elderly depression and dementia present with similar symptoms. It is important that nurses and other health care professionals be able to assess some of the important differences among depression, dementia, and delirium. See Table 21-1 for important differences among these three phenomena.

Other disorders that often mimic dementia include drug toxicity, metabolic disorders, infections, and nutritional deficiencies. A disorder that mimics dementia is sometimes referred to as a pseudodementia. That is, although the symptoms may suggest dementia, a careful examination may reveal another diagnosis altogether. This reinforces the importance of performing a comprehensive assessment when symptoms of dementia are present to identify nondementia causes.

Making a diagnosis of Alzheimer's disease includes ruling out all other pathophysiological conditions through the history and through physical and laboratory tests, many of which are identified in Box 21-3.

CT, positron emission tomography, and other developing scanning technologies have diagnostic capabilities because they reveal brain atrophy and rule out other conditions, such as neoplasms. The use of mental status questionnaires such as the Mini-Mental State Examination and various other tests to identify deterioration in mental status and brain damage are important parts of the assessment.

BOX 21-3

Basic Workup for Dementia

- Chest and skull radiographic studies
- Electroencephalography
- Electrocardiography
- Urinalysis
- Sequential multiple analyzer 12-test serum profile
- Thyroid function tests
- Folate level
- Venereal Disease Research Laboratories (VDRL), human immunodeficiency virus tests
- Serum creatinine assay
- Electrolyte assessment
- Vitamin B_{12} level
- Liver function tests
- Vision and hearing evaluation
- Neuroimaging (when diagnostic issues are not clear)

In addition to performing a complete physical and neurological examination, it is important to obtain a complete medical and psychiatric history, description of recent symptoms, review of medications used, and nutritional evaluation. The observations and history provided by family members are invaluable to the assessment process.

As already mentioned, depression in the elderly is the disorder frequently confused with dementia. Medical and nursing personnel should be cautioned, however, that dementia and depression or dementia and delirium *can* coexist in the same person. In fact, studies indicate that many people diagnosed with Alzheimer's dementia also meet the *DSM-IV-TR* criteria for a depressive disorder.

Assessment for Stage of the Disease

Alzheimer's disease is classified according to the stage of the degenerative process. The number of stages defined ranges from three to seven, depending on the source. However, four stages, as discussed subsequently, are commonly used to categorize the progressive deterioration seen in those diagnosed with Alzheimer's disease. Table 21-5 can be used as a guide as we review the four stages of Alzheimer's disease and highlight the deficits associated with each stage.

Stage 1: Mild Alzheimer's Disease. The loss of intellectual ability is insidious. The person with mild Alzheimer's disease loses energy, drive, and initiative and has difficulty learning new things. Because personality and social behavior remain intact, others tend to minimize and underestimate the loss of the individual's abilities. The individual may still continue to work, but the extent of the dementia becomes evident

in new or demanding situations. Depression may occur early in the disease but usually lessens as the disease progresses. Activities such as doing the marketing or managing finances are noticeably impaired during this phase.

■ ■ ■ ■ *VIGNETTE*

Mr. Collins, 56 years of age, is a lineman for a telephone company. He feels that he is getting old. He keeps forgetting things and writes notes to himself on scraps of paper. One day on the job, he forgets momentarily which wires to connect and connects all the wrong ones, causing mass confusion for a few hours. At home, Mr. Collins flies off the handle when his wife suggests that they invite the new neighbors for dinner. It is hard for him to admit that anything new confuses him, and he often forgets names (aphasia) and sometimes loses the thread of conversations. Once, he even forgot his address when his car broke down on the highway. He is moody and depressed and becomes indignant when his wife finds 3 months' worth of unpaid bills stashed in his sock drawer. Mrs. Collins is bewildered, upset, and fearful that something is terribly wrong.

■ ■ ■

The rate of progression varies from person to person. Some individuals in stage 1 Alzheimer's disease decline quickly and may die within 3 years. Others, although their condition worsens, may still function in the community with support. Still others may remain at this level for 3 years or more. The duration of the disease from onset of symptoms to death averages 8 to 10 years but can range from 3 to 20 years (APA, 2000). Stage 2: Moderate Alzheimer's Disease. Deterioration becomes evident during the moderate phase. Often, the person with moderate Alzheimer's disease cannot remember his or her address or the date. There are memory gaps in the person's history that may fluctuate from one moment to the next. Hygiene suffers, and the ability to dress appropriately is markedly affected. The person may put on clothes backward, button the buttons incorrectly, or not fasten zippers (apraxia). Often, the person has to be coaxed to bathe.

Mood becomes labile, and the individual may have bursts of paranoia, anger, jealousy, and apathy. Activities such as driving are hazardous; families are faced with the difficulty of taking away the car keys from their loved one. Care and supervision become a full-time job for family members. Denial mercifully takes over and protects people from the realization that they are losing control, not only of their minds but also of their live. Along with denial, people begin to withdraw from activities and from others, because they often feel overwhelmed and frustrated when they try to do things that once were easy. They may also have moments of becoming tearful and sad.

As important as it is to recognize all of the deficits of stage 2 disease, it is helpful for caretakers to realize that the client still retains abilities that influence care.

TABLE 21-5

Stages of Alzheimer's Disease

Stage	Hallmarks
Stage 1 (Mild) *Forgetfulness*	Shows short-term memory losses; loses things, forgets Memory aids compensate: lists, routine, organization Aware of the problem; concerned about lost abilities Depression common—worsens symptoms Not diagnosable at this time

Stage 2 (Moderate)
 Confusion
	Shows progressive memory loss; short-term memory impaired; memory difficulties interfere with
	     all abilities
	 Withdrawn from social activities
	 Shows declines in instrumental activities of daily living (ADLs), such as money management,
	     legal affairs, transportation, cooking, housekeeping
	 Denial common; fears "losing his or her mind"
	 Depression increasingly common; frightened because aware of deficits; covers up for memory
	     loss through confabulation
	 Problems intensified when stressed, fatigued, out of own environment, ill
	 Commonly needs day care or in-home assistance

Stage 3 (Moderate to Severe)
  Ambulatory dementia
	Shows ADL losses (in order): willingness and ability to bathe, grooming, choosing clothing,
	     dressing, gait and mobility, toileting, communication, reading, and writing skills
	 Shows loss of reasoning ability, safety planning, and verbal communication
	 Frustration common; becomes more withdrawn and self-absorbed
	 Depression resolves as awareness of losses diminishes
	 Has difficulty communicating; shows increasing loss of language skills
	 Shows evidence of reduced stress threshold; institutional care usually needed

Stage 4 (Late) *End stage*	Family recognition disappears; does not recognize self in mirror Nonambulatory; shows little purposeful activity; often mute; may scream spontaneously Forgets how to eat, swallow, chew; commonly loses weight; emaciation common Has problems associated with immobility (e.g., pneumonia, pressure ulcers, contractures) Incontinence common; seizures may develop Most certainly institutionalized at this point Return of primitive (infantile) reflexes

From Hall, G. R. (1994). Caring for people with Alzheimer's disease using the conceptual model of progressively lowered stress threshold in the clinical setting. *Nursing Clinics of North America, 29*(1), 129-141.

BOX 21-4

Abilities of the Client in Stage 2 Alzheimer's Disease

- Able to initiate familiar activity if supplies are available and within reach
- Able to perform steps of self-care with verbal and tactile cues
- Able to tell stories from past
- Able to read words slowly out loud
- Able to follow simple instructions
- Able to speak in short sentences or phrases; able to make needs known
- Able to sort, stack objects, count
- Able to ambulate if no physical disability is present
- Able to feel and name objects

Box 21-4 describes the abilities of clients in the second stage of Alzheimer's disease.

■ ■ ■ *VIGNETTE*

For a short period, Mr. Collins is transferred to a less complicated work position after his inability to function is recognized. His wife drives him to work and picks him up. Mr. Collins often forgets what he is doing and stares blankly. He accuses the supervisor of spying on him. Sometimes, he disappears at lunch and is unable to find his way back to work. The transfer lasts only a few months, and Mr. Collins is forced to take an early retirement. At home, Mr. Collins sleeps in his clothes. He loses interest in reading and watching sports on television and often breaks into angry outbursts, seemingly over nothing. Often, he becomes extremely restless and irritable and wanders around the house aimlessly.

■ ■ ■

Stage 3: Moderate to Severe Alzheimer's Disease. At the moderate to severe stage, the person is often unable to identify familiar objects or people, even a spouse (severe agnosia). The person needs repeated instructions and directions to perform the simplest tasks (advanced apraxia): "Here is the face cloth, pick up the soap. Now, put water on the face cloth and rub the face cloth with soap." Often, the individual cannot remember where the toilet is and becomes incontinent. Total care is necessary at this point, and the burden on the family can be emotionally, financially, and physically devastating. The world is very frightening to the person with Alzheimer's disease because nothing makes sense any longer. Agitation, violence, paranoia, and delusions are commonly seen. Another problem that is frightening to family members and caregivers is wandering behavior. An estimated 60% of people with Alzheimer's disease wander and are at risk for becoming lost (ADRDA, 2004).

Institutionalization may be the most appropriate recourse at this time, because the level of care is so demanding, and violent outbursts and incontinence may be burdens that the family can no longer handle. The following are some criteria that indicate the need for placement in a skilled nursing facility:

- The person wanders.
- The person is a danger to self and others.
- The person is incontinent.
- The person's behavior affects the sleep and general health of others.
- The person is totally dependent on others for physical care.

■ ■ ■ *VIGNETTE*

Mr. Collins is terrified. Memories come and then slip away. People come and go, but they are strangers. Someone is masquerading as his wife, and it is hard to tell what is real. Things never stay in the same place. Sometimes, people hide the bathroom where he cannot find it. He in turn hides things to keep them safe, but he forgets where he hides them. Buttons and belts are confusing, and he does not know what they are doing there, anyway. Sometimes, he tries to walk away from the terrifying feelings and the strangers. He tries to find something he has lost long ago . . . if he could only remember what it is.

■ ■ ■

Stage 4: Late Alzheimer's Disease. Late in Alzheimer's disease the following symptoms may occur: agraphia (inability to read or write), hyperorality (the need to taste, chew, and put everything in one's mouth), blunting of emotions, visual agnosia (loss of ability to recognize familiar objects), and hypermetamorphosis (manifested by touching of everything in sight).

At this stage, the ability to talk, and eventually the ability to walk, is lost. The end stage of Alzheimer's disease is characterized by stupor and coma. Death frequently is secondary to infection or choking.

■ ■ ■ *VIGNETTE*

Mrs. Collins and the children keep Mr. Collins at home until his outbursts become frightening. Once, he is lost for 2 days after he somehow unlocks the front door. Finally, Mrs. Collins has her husband placed in a Veterans Administration (VA) hospital. When his wife comes to visit, Mr. Collins sometimes cries. He never talks and is always tied into his chair when she comes to see him. The staff explain to her that, although Mr. Collins can still walk, he keeps getting into other people's beds and scaring them. They explain that perhaps he wants comfort and misses human touch. They encourage her visits, even though Mr. Collins does not seem to recognize her. He does respond to music. His wife brings a radio, and when she plays the country and western music he has always loved, Mr. Collins nods and claps his hands.

Mrs. Collins is torn between guilt and love, anger and despair. She is confused and depressed. She is going through the painful process of mourning the loss of the man she has loved and shared a life with for 34 years.

Three months after his admission to the VA hospital, and 8 years after the incident of the crossed wires at the telephone company, Mr. Collins chokes on some food, develops pneumonia, and dies.

■ ■ ■

Self-Assessment

Nurses working in any setting with cognitively impaired clients are aware of the tremendous responsibility placed on the caregivers. The behavioral problems that these clients display can cause tremendous stress for professional and family caregivers. Taking care of clients who are unable to communicate and who have lost the ability to relate and respond to others is extremely difficult, especially for student nurses or nurses who do not understand dementia or Alzheimer's disease.

Nurses working in facilities for clients who are cognitively impaired (e.g., nursing homes and extended care facilities) need special education and skills. Education must include information about the process of the disease and effective interventions, as well as knowledge regarding antipsychotic drugs. Support and educational opportunities should be readily available, not just to nurses but also to nurse's aides, who are often directly responsible for administering basic care.

Because stress is a common occurrence when working with persons with cognitive impairments, staff need to be proactive in minimizing its effects; this can be facilitated by:

- Having a realistic understanding of the disease so that expectations for the client are realistic.
- Establishing realistic outcomes for the client and recognizing when they are achieved. These out-

comes may be as minor as *client feeds self with spoon*, yet it must be remembered that even the smallest achievement can be a significant accomplishment for the impaired individual.

■ Maintaining good self-care. Nurses need to protect themselves from the negative effects of stress by obtaining adequate sleep and rest, eating a nutritious diet, exercising, engaging in relaxing activities, and addressing their own spiritual needs.

Assessment Guidelines Dementia

1. Assess to help identify the underlying cause.
2. Explore how well the family is prepared for and informed about the progress of the client's dementia (e.g., the phases and course of Alzheimer's disease, vascular dementia, AIDS-related dementia, or dementia associated with multiple sclerosis, lupus erythematosus, or brain injury).
3. Review the medications (herbs, complementary agents) the client is currently taking.
4. Evaluate the client's current level of cognitive functioning.
5. Discuss with the family members how they are coping with the client and their main issues at this time.
6. Review the resources available to the family. Ask the family members to describe the help they receive from other family members, friends, and community resources. Determine if caregivers are aware of community support groups and resources.
7. Determine the appropriate safety measures needed by the client and arrange for them to be implemented.
8. Evaluate the safety of the client's home environment (e.g., with regard to wandering, eating inedible objects, falling, engaging in provocative behaviors toward others).
9. Identify the needs of the family for teaching and guidance (e.g., how to manage catastrophic reactions; lability of mood; aggressive behaviors; and nocturnal delirium and increased confusion and agitation at night, or sundowning).

■ NURSING DIAGNOSIS

Caring for a client with dementia requires a great deal of patience, creativity, and maturity. The needs of such a client can be enormous for nursing staff and for families who care for their loved ones in the home. As the disease progresses, so do the needs of the client and the demands on the caregivers, staff, and family.

One of the most important areas of concern identified by both staff and families is the client's safety. Many people with Alzheimer's disease wander and

may be lost for hours or days. Wandering, along with behaviors such as rummaging, may be perceived as purposeful to the person with Alzheimer's disease. Wandering may result from changes in the physical environment, fear caused by hallucinations or delusions, or lack of exercise. Refer to the Evidence-Based Practice box for protocol for responding to wandering behaviors.

Seizures are common in the later stages of this disease. Injuries from falls and accidents can occur during any stage as confusion and disorientation progress. The potential for burns exists if the client is a smoker or is unattended when using the stove. Prescription drugs can be taken incorrectly, or bottles of noxious fluids can be mistakenly ingested, which results in a medical crisis. Therefore, *risk for injury* is always present.

As the person's ability to recognize or name objects is decreased, *impaired verbal communication* becomes a problem. As memory diminishes and disorientation increases, *impaired environmental interpretation syndrome, impaired memory,* and *confusion* occur.

During the course of the disease, people show personality changes, increased vulnerability, and often inappropriate behaviors. Common behaviors include hoarding, regression, and being overly demanding. Therefore, nurses and family members often intervene in behaviors that signal *ineffective coping*. Family caregivers may experience compromised or even disabling family coping.

Additional family issues may emerge. Perhaps some of the most crucial aspects of the client's care are support, education, and referrals for the family. The family loses an integral part of its unit. Family members lose the love, the function, the support, the companionship, and the warmth that this person once provided. *Caregiver role strain* is always present, and planning with the family and offering community support is an integral part of appropriate care. *Anticipatory grieving* is also an important phenomenon to assess and may be an important target for intervention. Helping the family grieve can make the task ahead somewhat clearer and, at times, less painful. Refer back to Table 21-2 for potential nursing diagnoses for confused and demented clients.

■ OUTCOME CRITERIA

Families who have a member with dementia are faced with an exhaustive list of issues that need addressing. Table 21-6 provides a checklist that may help the nurse and families identify areas for intervention. Self-care needs, impaired environmental interpretation, chronic confusion, ineffective individual coping, and caregiver role strain are just a few of the areas nurses and other health care members will need to target. See Box 21-5 for some suggestions.

EVIDENCE-BASED PRACTICE

Wandering

Background
Clinically, the causes of wandering behavior in individuals with Alzheimer's disease remain unidentified, and the behavior poses considerable management problems for both professional and lay caregivers.

Study
This review examined available research that met the study criteria, which included the following: the study had to be written in English or have available English transcripts; wandering had to be operationally defined as a physical activity versus a cognitive distraction; the studies had to be either qualitative or quantitative in data generation. A sample of 31 articles was selected from 278 articles. Articles were reviewed for the following:
- Goal or purpose of the study
- Use of a theoretical framework
- Definition and operationalization of wandering
- Specific research questions or hypotheses
- Sample size and type
- Findings or outcomes

Results of Study
From this review, the researchers were able to define a protocol for responding to wandering behaviors. This protocol specifies the following:
- Assessment criteria, which should incorporate evaluation for cognitive decline and for depression, anxiety, and agitation; determination of the frequency with which

behavior problems including wandering occur; identification of what environmental strategies are currently used by formal and informal caregivers; identification of wandering pattern; and assessment of premorbid lifestyle to identify individuals likely to wander.
- Environmental modifications such as providing a safe place to wander; enhancing the visual appeal of the environment; placing grid lines in front of doors to decrease exit seeking; making exits less accessible by covering panic bar with cloth and allowing walking where doors are not in the path; installing safety locks; using less accessible door latches; decreasing clutter; and providing environmental stimulation.
- Technology and safety devices, including such additions as a verbal alarm system and the use of mobile locator devices for quickly locating wanderers.
- Physical and psychological interventions such as assessing and treating depression; increasing structured activities; using music sessions; allowing walking in safe places; and providing regular exercise.
- Caregiving support and education to assist caregivers in their ability to care for the wanderer.

Implications for Nursing Practice
This protocol identifies specific assessment and intervention strategies for nurses involved in the care of the Alzheimer's client regardless of where the nurse-client encounter occurs. The nurse may encounter this client in an inpatient medical unit, a geriatric psychiatric unit, a skilled nursing facility, an assisted living facility, an adult day treatment program, or the client's home.

Futrell, M., & Melillo, K. D. (2002, March). *Evidence-based protocol: Wandering.* Iowa City: University of Iowa Gerontological Nursing Interventions Research Center, Research Dissemination Core. Retrieved February 1, 2005, from http://www.guideline.gov.

TABLE 21-6

Problems That May Affect Dementia Sufferers and Their Families

Problem	Examples
Memory impairment	Forgets appointments, visits, etc.
	Forgets to change cloths, wash, go to the toilet
	Forgets to eat, take medications
	Loses things
Disorientation	Time: mixes night and day, mixes days of appointments, wears summer clothes in winter, forgets age
	Place: loses way around house
	Person: has difficulty recognizing visitors, family, spouse
Need for physical help	Dressing
	Washing, bathing
	Toileting
	Eating
	Performing housework
	Maintaining mobility
Risks in the home	Falls
	Fire from cigarettes, cooking, heating
	Flooding
	Admission of strangers to home
	Wandering out

TABLE 21-6

Problems That May Affect Dementia Sufferers and Their Families—cont'd

Problem	Examples
Risks outside the home	Competence, judgment, and risks at work
	Driving, road sense
	Getting lost
Apathy	Little conversation
	Lack of interest
	Poor self-care
Poor communication	Dysphasia
Repetitiveness	Repetition of questions or stories
	Repetition of actions
Uncontrolled emotion	Distress
	Anger or aggression
	Demands for attention
Uncontrolled behavior	Restlessness day or night
	Vulgar table or toilet habits
	Undressing
	Sexual disinhibition
	Shoplifting
Incontinence	Urine
	Feces
	Urination or defecation in the wrong place
Emotional reactions	Depression
	Anxiety
	Frustration and anger
	Embarrassment and withdrawal
Other reactions	Suspiciousness
	Hoarding and hiding
Mistaken beliefs	Still at work
	Parents or spouse still alive
	Hallucinations
Decision making	Indecisive
	Easily influenced
	Refuses help
	Makes unwise decisions
Burden on family	Disruption of social life
	Distress, guilt, rejection
	Family discord

■ PLANNING

The planning of care for a client with dementia is geared toward the client's immediate needs. Refer to Table 21-6 for help in identifying areas of care needed. See Figure 21-3 for the Functional Dementia Scale, which can be used by nurses and families to plan strategies for addressing immediate needs and to track progression of the dementia.

Identifying level of functioning and assessing caregivers' needs help the nurse identify appropriate community resources. Does the client or family need the following?

- Transportation services
- Supervision and care when primary caregiver is out of the home
- Referrals to day care centers
- Information on support groups within the community
- Meals on Wheels
- Information on respite and residential services
- Telephone numbers for help lines
- Home health aides
- Home health services
- Additional psychopharmaceuticals to manage distressing or harmful behaviors

■ INTERVENTION

The nurse's attitude of unconditional positive regard is the single most effective tool in caring for demented clients. It induces clients to cooperate with care, reduces catastrophic outbreaks, and increases

Suggested Outcome Criteria for Dementia*

Injury

- Client will remain safe in the hospital or at home.
- With the aid of an identification bracelet and neighborhood or hospital alert, client will be returned within 1 hour of wandering.
- Client will remain free of danger during seizures.
- With the aid of interventions, client will remain burn free.
- With the aid of guidance and environmental manipulation, client will not hurt himself or herself if a fall occurs.
- Client will ingest only correct doses of prescribed medications and appropriate food and fluids.

Communication

- Client will communicate needs.
- Client will answer yes or no appropriately to questions.
- Client will state needs in alternative modes when he or she is aphasic (e.g., will signal correct word on hearing it or will refer to picture or label).
- Client will wear prescribed glasses or hearing aid each day.

Caregiver Role Strain

- Family members will have the opportunity to express "unacceptable" feelings in a supportive environment.
- Family members will have access to professional counseling.
- Family members will name two organizations within their geographical area that can offer support.
- Family members will participate in ill member's plan of care, with encouragement from staff.
- Family members will state that they have outside help that allows them to take personal time for themselves each week or month.
- Family members will have the names of three resources that can help with financial burdens and legal considerations.

Impaired Environmental Interpretation: Chronic Confusion

- Client will acknowledge the reality of an object or a sound that was misinterpreted (illusion), after it is pointed out.
- Client will state that he or she feels safe after experiencing delusions or illusions.
- Client will remain nonaggressive when experiencing paranoid ideation.

Self-Care Needs

- Client will participate in self-care at optimal level.
- Client will be able to follow step-by-step instructions for dressing, bathing, and grooming.
- Client will put on own clothes appropriately, with aid of fastening tape (Velcro) and nursing supervision.
- Client's skin will remain intact and free from signs of pressure.

*Based on the Nursing Outcomes Classification; not an exhaustive list.

FUNCTIONAL DEMENTIA SCALE

Circle one rating for each item:
1. None or little of the time
2. Some of the time
3. Good part of the time
4. Most or all of the time

Client: _____
Observer: _____
Position or relation to patient: _____
Facility: _____
Date: _____

1	2	3	4	1. Has difficulty in completing simple tasks on own (e.g., dressing, bathing, doing arithmetic).
1	2	3	4	2. Spends time either sitting or in apparently purposeless activity.
1	2	3	4	3. Wanders at night or needs to be restrained to prevent wandering.
1	2	3	4	4. Hears things that are not there.
1	2	3	4	5. Requires supervision or assistance in eating.
1	2	3	4	6. Loses things.
1	2	3	4	7. Appearance is disorderly if left to own devices.
1	2	3	4	8. Moans.
1	2	3	4	9. Cannot control bowel function.
1	2	3	4	10. Threatens to harm others.
1	2	3	4	11. Cannot control bladder function.
1	2	3	4	12. Needs to be watched so doesn't injure self (e.g., by careless smoking, leaving the stove on, falling).
1	2	3	4	13. Destructive of materials around him/her (e.g., breaks furniture, throws food trays, tears up magazines).
1	2	3	4	14. Shouts or yells.
1	2	3	4	15. Accuses others of doing bodily harm or stealing his or her possessions — when you are sure the accusations are not true.
1	2	3	4	16. Is unaware of limitations imposed by illness.
1	2	3	4	17. Becomes confused and does not know where he or she is.
1	2	3	4	18. Has trouble remembering.
1	2	3	4	19. Has sudden changes of mood (e.g., gets upset, angered, or cries easily).
1	2	3	4	20. If left alone, wanders aimlessly during the day or needs to be restrained to prevent wandering.

FIGURE 21-3 Functional Dementia Scale. (From Moore, J. T., et al. [1983]. A functional dementia scale. *Journal of Family Practice, 16,* 498.)

family members' satisfaction with care. Refer to Box 21-6 for NIC interventions related to the management of dementia.

A considerable number of individuals with dementia have secondary behavioral disturbances, including depression, hallucinations and delusions, agitation, insomnia, and wandering. Because these symptoms impair the person's ability to function, increase the need for supervision, and influence the need for institutionalization, the control of these symptoms is a priority in managing Alzheimer's disease. Helping the individual achieve the highest possible level of independence and function is the foundation of care.

Intervention with family members is critical. The effects of losing a family member to dementia—that is, watching the deterioration of a person who has had an important role within the family unit and who is loved and is a vital part of his or her family's history—can be devastating. The interventions discussed subsequently are useful.

BOX 21-6

Dementia Management (NIC)

Definition: Provision of a modified environment for the patient who is experiencing a chronic confusional state

Activities:

- Include family members in planning, providing, and evaluating care, to the extent desired.
- Identify usual patterns of behavior for such activities as sleep, medication use, elimination, food intake, and self-care.
- Determine physical, social, and psychological history of patient, usual habits, and routines.
- Determine type and extent of cognitive deficit(s), using standardized assessment tool.
- Monitor cognitive functioning, using standardized assessment tool.
- Determine behavioral expectations appropriate for patient's cognitive status.
- Provide a low-stimulation environment (e.g., quiet, soothing music; nonvivid and simple, familiar patterns in décor; performance expectations that do not exceed cognitive processing ability; and dining in small groups).
- Provide adequate but nonglare lighting.
- Identify and remove potential dangers in environment for patient.
- Place identification bracelet on patient.
- Provide a consistent physical environment and daily routine.
- Prepare for interaction with eye contact and touch, as appropriate.
- Introduce self when initiating contact.
- Address patient distinctly by name when initiating interaction and speak slowly.
- Give one simple direction at a time.
- Speak in a clear, low, warm, respectful tone of voice.
- Use distraction, rather than confrontation, to manage behavior.
- Provide unconditional positive regard.
- Avoid touch and proximity, if this causes stress or anxiety.
- Provide caregivers that are familiar to the patient (e.g., avoid frequent rotations of staff assignments).
- Avoid unfamiliar situations, when possible (e.g., room changes and appointments without familiar people present).
- Provide rest periods to prevent fatigue and reduce stress.
- Monitor nutrition and weight.
- Provide space for safe pacing and wandering.

- Avoid frustrating patient by quizzing with orientation questions that cannot be answered.
- Provide cues—such as current events, seasons, location, and names—to assist orientation.
- Seat patient at small table in groups of three to five for meals, as appropriate.
- Allow patient to eat alone, if appropriate.
- Provide finger foods to maintain nutrition for patient who will not sit and eat.
- Provide patient a general orientation to the season of the year by using appropriate cues (e.g., holiday decorations, seasonal decorations and activities, and access to contained, out-of-doors area).
- Decrease noise levels by avoiding paging systems and call lights that ring or buzz.
- Select television or radio programs based on cognitive processing abilities and interests.
- Select one-to-one and group activities geared to patient's cognitive abilities and interests.
- Label familiar photos with names of the individuals in the photos.
- Select artwork for patient's rooms featuring landscapes, scenery, or other familiar images.
- Ask family members and friends to see patient one or two at a time, if needed, to reduce stimulation.
- Discuss with family members and friends how best to interact with patient.
- Assist family to understand that it may be impossible for patient to learn new material.
- Limit number of choices patient has to make, so as not to cause anxiety.
- Provide boundaries, such as red or yellow tape on the floor, when low-stimulus units are not available.
- Place patient's name in large block letters in room and on clothing, as needed.
- Use symbols, rather than written signs, to assist patient in locating room, bathroom, or other area.
- Monitor carefully for physiological causes of increased confusion that may be acute and reversible.
- Remove or cover mirrors, if patient is frightened or agitated by them.
- Discuss home safety issues and interventions.

From Dochterman, J. M., & Bulechek, G. M. (2004). *Nursing interventions classification (NIC)* (4th ed.). St. Louis, MO: Mosby.

Counseling: Communication Guidelines

How nurses choose to communicate with clients with dementia affects the client's maintenance of self-esteem and ability to participate in care. People with dementia often find it difficult to express themselves. They

- Have difficulty finding the right words.
- Use familiar words repeatedly.
- Invent new words to describe things.
- Frequently lose their train of thought.
- Rely on nonverbal gestures.

Table 21-7 provides special guidelines for nurses and family members to use in communicating with a cognitively impaired person.

Health Teaching

Educating families who have a cognitively impaired member is one of the most important areas for nurses. Families who are caring for a member in the home need to know about strategies for communicating and for structuring self-care activities (Table 21-8). Visit the Evolve website for additional family teaching tools regarding the management of challenging behaviors.

Most important, families need to know where to get help. Help includes professional counseling and education regarding the process and the progression of the disease. Families especially need to know about, and be referred to, community-based groups that can help shoulder this tremendous burden (e.g., day care cen-

TABLE 21-7

Guidelines for Communicating with Clients with Dementia

Intervention	Rationale
Chronic Confusion	
1. Always identify yourself and call the person by name at each meeting.	1. Client's short term memory is impaired—requires frequent orientation to time and environment.
2. Speak slowly.	2. Client needs time to process information.
3. Use short, simple words and phrases.	3. Client may not be able to understand complex statements or abstract ideas.
4. Maintain face-to-face contact.	4. Verbal and nonverbal clues are maximized.
5. Be near client when talking, one or two arm-lengths away.	5. This distance can help client focus on speaker as well as maintain personal space.
6. Focus on one piece of information at a time.	6. Attention span of client is poor and client is easily distracted—helps client focus. Too much data can be overwhelming and can increase anxiety.
7. Talk with client about familiar and meaningful things.	7. Self-expression is promoted and reality is reinforced.
8. Encourage reminiscing about happy times in life.	8. Remembering accomplishments and shared joys helps distract client from deficit and gives meaning to existence.
9. When client is delusional, acknowledge client's feelings and reinforce reality. Do not argue or refute delusions.	9. Acknowledging feelings helps client feel understood. Pointing out realities may help client focus on realities. Arguing can enhance adherence to false beliefs.
10. If a client gets into an argument with another client, stop the argument and get individuals out of each other's way. After a short while (5 minutes), explain to each client matter-of-factly why you had to intervene.	10. Escalation to physical acting out is prevented. Client's right to know is respected. Explaining in an adult manner helps maintain self-esteem.
11. When client becomes verbally aggressive, acknowledge client's feelings and shift topic to more familiar ground (e.g., "I know this is upsetting for you, because you always cared for others. Tell me about your children.")	11. Confusion and disorientation easily increase anxiety. Acknowledging feelings makes client feel more understood and less alone. Topics client has mastery over can remind him or her of areas of competent functioning and can increase self-esteem.
12. Have client wear prescription eyeglasses or hearing aid.	12. Environmental awareness, orientation, and comprehension are increased, which in turn increases awareness of personal needs and the presence of others.
13. Keep client's room well lit.	13. Environmental clues are maximized.
14. Have clocks, calendars, and personal items (e.g., family pictures or Bible) in clear view of client while he or she is in bed.	14. These objects assist in maintaining personal identity.
15. Reinforce client's pictures, nonverbal gestures, Xs on calendars, and other methods used to anchor client in reality.	15. When aphasia starts to hinder communication, alternate methods of communication need to be instituted.

*Based on the Nursing Interventions Classification.

TABLE 21-8

Family and Health Care Guidelines for Client Self-Care

Intervention	Rationale
Dressing and Bathing	
1. Always have client perform all tasks within his or her present capacity.	1. Maintains client's self-esteem and uses muscle groups; impedes staff burnout; minimizes further regression.
2. Always have client wear own clothes, even if in the hospital.	2. Helps maintain client's identity and dignity.
3. Use clothing with elastic, and substitute fastening tape (Velcro) for buttons and zippers.	3. Minimizes client's confusion and eases independence of functioning.
4. Label clothing items with client's name and name of item.	4. Helps identify client if he or she wanders and gives client additional clues when aphasia or agnosia occurs.
5. Give step-by-step instructions whenever necessary (e.g., "Take this blouse. . . . Put in one arm . . . now the next arm. . . . Pull it together in the front. . . . Now . . . ")	5. Client can focus on small pieces of information more easily; allows client to perform at optimal level.
6. Make sure that water in faucets is not too hot.	6. Judgment is lacking in client; client is unaware of many safety hazards.
7. If client is resistant to performing self-care, come back later and ask again.	7. Moods may be labile, and client may forget but often complies after short interval.
Nutrition	
1. Monitor food and fluid intake.	1. Client may have anorexia or be too confused to eat.
2. Offer finger food that client can take away from the dinner table.	2. Increases input throughout the day; client may eat only small amounts at meals.
3. Weigh client regularly (once a week).	3. Monitors fluid and nutritional status.
4. During periods of hyperorality, watch that client does not eat nonfood items (e.g., ceramic fruit or food-shaped soaps).	4. Client puts everything into mouth; may be unable to differentiate inedible objects made in the shape and color of food.
Bowel and Bladder Function	
1. Begin bowel and bladder program early; start with bladder control.	1. Establishing same time of day for bowel movements and toileting—in early morning, after meals and snacks, and before bedtime—can help prevent incontinence.
2. Evaluate use of disposable diapers.	2. Prevents embarrassment.
3. Label bathroom door as well as doors to other rooms.	3. Additional environmental clues can maximize independent toileting.
Sleep	
1. Because client may awaken, be frightened, or cry out at night, keep area well lighted.	1. Reinforces orientation, minimizes possible illusions.
2. Maintain a calm atmosphere during the day.	2. Encourages a calming night's sleep.
3. Order nonbarbiturates (e.g., chloral hydrate) if necessary.	3. Barbiturates can have a paradoxical reaction, causing agitation.
4. If medications are indicated, consider neuroleptics with sedative properties, which may be the most helpful (e.g., haloperidol [Haldol]).	4. Helps clear thinking and sedates.
5. Avoid the use of restraints.	5. Can cause client to become more terrified and fight against restraints until exhausted to a dangerous degree.

ters, senior citizen groups, organizations providing home visits and respite care, and family support groups). A list with definitions of some of the types of services available in the client's community, as well as the names and telephone numbers of the providers of these services, should be given to the family.

Support

The Alzheimer's Disease and Related Disorders Association (ADRDA), or simply Alzheimer's Association, is a national umbrella agency that provides various forms of assistance to persons with the disease and their families. The Alzheimer's Association has launched Safe Return, the first nationwide program to help locate and return missing people with Alzheimer's disease and other memory impairments. Wandering is a common behavior during the second and third stages of Alzheimer's disease, and the Safe Return program offers peace of mind to families. Information regarding housekeeping, home health aides, and companions is also available through this organization. Such outside resources can help prevent the total emotional and physical fatigue of family members. Family members can call 800-272-3900 to locate the Alzheimer's Association chapter nearest them. Types of resources that might be available in some communities are found in Table 21-9.

Although many families manage the care of their loved one until death, other families eventually find that they can no longer deal with their loved ones' labile and aggressive behavior, incontinence, wandering, unsafe habits, or disruptive nocturnal activity. Family members need to know where and how to place their loved one for care if this becomes necessary. Families need information, support, and legal and financial guidance at this time. When the nurse is unable to provide the relevant information, proper referrals by the social worker are needed. Information regarding advance directives, durable power of attorney, guardianship, and conservatorship should be included in the communication with the family. Useful guidelines for families in structuring a safe environment and planning appropriate activities are found in Table 21-10.

Psychopharmacology

Cognitive Impairment

There is as yet no cure for Alzheimer's disease. There are, however, five Alzheimer's disease drugs approved by the Food and Drug Administration (FDA) that demonstrate positive effects not only on cognition but also on behavior and function in activities of daily living. These drugs include tacrine (Cognex), donepezil (Aricept), rivastigmine (Exelon), galantamine (Reminyl), and memantine (Namenda). All these drugs except memantine work to increase the brain's supply of acetylcholine, a nerve communicator that is deficient in people with Alzheimer's disease. Memantine blocks overstimulation by glutamate, which contributes to neurodegenerative disease (O'Boyle, 2003; U.S. FDA, 2003).

Tacrine (THA, Cognex) was the first cholinesterase inhibitor to be approved by the U.S. FDA for the treatment of mild to moderate symptoms of Alzheimer's disease. It improves functioning and slows the

---

TABLE 21-9

Types of Services That May Be Available to People with Dementia

Type of Service	Services Provided
Family/caregiver Some clients may live by themselves in the community; active case management is vital when this is the case.	Caregivers have a right to: ▪ Easy access to services ▪ Respite care ▪ Full involvement in decision making ▪ Assessment of the needs of the caregiver as well as those of the client ▪ Information and referral ▪ Case management: coordination of community resources and follow-up
Community services	▪ Adult day care: provides activities, socialization, supervision ▪ Physician services ▪ Protective services: prevent, eliminate, and/or remedy effects of abuse or neglect ▪ Recreational services ▪ Transportation ▪ Mental health services ▪ Legal services
Home care	▪ Meals on Wheels ▪ Home health aide services ▪ Homemaker services ▪ Hospice services ▪ Occupational therapy ▪ Paid companion or sitter services ▪ Physical therapy ▪ Skilled nursing ▪ Personal care services: assistance in basic self-care activities ▪ Social work services ▪ Telephone reassurance: regular telephone calls to individuals who are isolated and homebound* ▪ Personal emergency response systems: telephone-based systems to alert others that a person who is alone is in need of emergency assistance*

*Vital for those living alone.

TABLE 21-10

Guidelines for Family Care at Home

Intervention	Rationale
Safe Environment	
1. Gradually restrict use of the car.	1. As judgment becomes impaired, client may be dangerous to self and others.
2. Remove throw rugs and other objects in person's path.	2. Minimizes tripping and falling.
If client is in hospital or living with family:	
3. Minimize sensory stimulation.	3. Decreases sensory overload, which can increase anxiety and confusion.
4. If client becomes verbally upset, listen briefly, give support, then change the topic.	4. Goal is to prevent escalation of anger. When attention span is short, client can be distracted to more productive topics and activities.
5. Label all rooms and drawers. Label often-used objects (e.g., hairbrushes and toothbrushes).	5. May keep client from wandering into other client's rooms. Increases environmental clues to familiar objects.
6. Install safety bars in bathroom.	6. Prevents falls.
7. Supervise client when he or she smokes.	7. Danger of burns is always present.
8. If client has history of seizures, keep padded tongue blades at beside. Educate family on how to deal with seizures.	8. Seizure activity is common in advanced Alzheimer's disease.
Wandering	
1. If client wanders during the night, put mattress on the floor.	1. Prevents falls when client is confused.
2. Have client wear medical alert bracelet that cannot be removed (with name, address, and telephone number). Provide police department with recent pictures.	2. Client can easily be identified by police, neighbors, or hospital personnel.
3. Alert local police and neighbors about wanderer.	3. May reduce time necessary to return client to home or hospital.
4. If client is in hospital, have him or her wear brightly colored vest with name, unit, and phone number printed on back.	4. Makes client easily identifiable.
5. Put complex locks on door.	5. Reduces opportunity to wander.
6. Place locks at top of door.	6. In moderate and late Alzheimer's-type dementia, ability to look up and reach upward is lost.
7. Encourage physical activity during the day.	7. Physical activity may decrease wandering at night.
8. Explore the feasibility of installing sensor devices.	8. Provides warning if client wanders.
Useful Activities	
1. Provide picture magazines and children's books when client's reading ability diminishes.	1. Allows continuation of usual activities that client can still enjoy; provides focus.
2. Provide simple activities that allow exercise of large muscles.	2. Exercise groups, dance groups, and walking provide socialization as well as increased circulation and maintenance of muscle tone.
3. Encourage group activities that are familiar and simple to perform.	3. Activities such as group singing, dancing, reminiscing, and working with clay and paint all help to increase socialization and minimize feelings of alienation.

progress of the disease, particularly in the areas of cognition and memory, in about 20% to 50% of clients with Alzheimer's disease. Unfortunately, tacrine is associated with a high frequency of side effects, including elevated liver transaminase levels, gastrointestinal effects, and liver toxicity. The hepatic effects, along with the inconvenience of multiple dosing, have drastically reduced the use of this drug (Keltner, Zielinshi, & Hardin, 2001).

Donepezil (Aricept) inhibits acetylcholine breakdown and was approved by the FDA in December 1996. It is the most prescribed of the Alzheimer's

drugs, with 1.7 million people currently taking the drug (ADRDA, 2004). It also appears to slow down deterioration in cognitive functions but without the potentially serious liver toxicity attributed to tacrine. In studies of donepezil, some individuals with Alzheimer's disease did experience diarrhea and nausea when taking the drug. Donepezil has been shown to slow down cognitive deterioration by about 2 years (Alzheimer's Association, 2004).

Rivastigmine (Exelon), a brain selective acetylcholinesterase inhibitor, was approved in 2000. In clinical trials rivastigmine helped slightly more than half of the people who took it. The most common side effects are nausea, vomiting, loss of appetite, and weight loss. In most cases these side effects are temporary (ADRDA, 2004).

Galantamine (Reminyl) is a reversible cholinesterase inhibitor approved for use in the United States in February 2001 (CenterWatch, 2001). Galantamine also works to increase the concentration of acetylcholine by blocking the action of acetylcholinesterase, the enzyme that breaks down acetylcholine. Galantamine is prescribed in the first and second stages of Alzheimer's disease.

Other cholinesterase inhibitors are being developed in other countries and are being studied in clinical trials.

Memantine (Namenda) is a drug that was developed in Germany and marketed there under the name of Axura. It was approved for use in the United States in October 2003 and became available to physicians, patients, and pharmacies in January 2004 (FDA News, 2003). Memantine is the first drug to target symptoms of Alzheimer's disease during the moderate to severe stages of the disorder. In one study memantine was added to the daily drug regimen of clients already taking donepezil and produced significant additional benefits (O'Boyle, 2003). This drug works by affecting the N-methyl-D-aspartate (NMDA) receptors, another chemical and structural system involved in memory (ADRDA, 2004).

Alzheimer's Therapy: Future. Perhaps the most exciting development is the start of clinical trials of an amyloid **vaccine (AN-1792),** which it is hoped will clear the brain of β-amyloid plaques. Scientists have hypothesized that these plaques, found in the brains of people with Alzheimer's disease, impede nerve cell function and cause nerve cell death (ADRDA, 2004). In a phase I safety study, AN-1792 was administered in multiple dosage regimens to more than 100 clients with mild to moderate Alzheimer's disease. It appeared to be safe and well tolerated. A phase IIa clinical trial was halted because 15 cases of encephalitis, paralysis, or death occurred in the United States, United Kingdom, and France. Passive immunization is currently being investigated (Sabbagh, 2003).

Additional research is ongoing, with focuses on:
- The development of other cholinesterase inhibitors.
- The use of cholesterol-lowering agents, which is being investigated through multicenter trials.
- The use of antiinflammatory agents as a preventive measure. The Alzheimer's Disease Anti-Inflammatory Prevention Trial (ADRDA, 2004) is a multicenter trial funded by the National Institutes of Health to determine whether the use of antiinflammatory agents can prevent Alz-

heimer's disease in people at risk (70 years of age and older with a first-degree relative with Alzheimer's disease, senility, dementia, or memory loss).
- The use of neurotrophic agents with the potential to regenerate brain cells.
- The use of diabetic treatments that might decrease blood vessel inflammation in the brain.

Behavioral Symptoms

Other medications are often useful in managing the behavioral symptoms of individuals with dementia, but these need to be used with extreme caution. The rule of thumb for elderly clients is **"start low and go slow."** Some of the troubling behaviors exhibited by Alzheimer's clients with which their caregivers must cope are (1) psychotic symptoms (hallucinations, paranoia), (2) severe mood swings (depression is very common), (3) anxiety (agitation), and (4) verbal or physical aggression (combativeness). Table 21-11 lists acceptable medications for management of these behavioral symptoms.

Alternative and Complementary Treatments

A number of **herbal or all-natural drugs** are currently under investigation. However, there is not yet enough scientific evidence concerning their effectiveness or harmfulness. Keep in mind that the designation *all-natural* or *herbal* does not mean that a substance is safe. Some alternative treatments being investigated are *Ginkgo biloba,* dong quai, and vitamins B_6, B_{12}, C, and E (Howes, Perry, & Houghton, 2003) (see the Integrative Therapy box). Refer to the Evolve website as well as the website of the national Alzheimer's Association (http://www.alz.org) for more on these substances.

■ EVALUATION

The outcome criteria set for clients with cognitive impairment need to be measurable, be within the capabilities of the client, and be evaluated frequently. As the person's condition continues to deteriorate, outcomes need to be altered to reflect the person's diminished functioning. Frequent evaluation and reformulation of outcome criteria and short-term indicators also help diminish staff and family frustration, as well as minimize the client's anxiety by ensuring that tasks are not more complicated than the person can accomplish. The overall outcomes for treatment are to promote the client's optimal level of functioning and to retard further regression, whenever possible. Working closely with family members and providing them with the names of available resources and support sources may help increase the quality of life for both the family and the client (see Case Study and Nursing Care Plan 21-1).

TABLE 21-11

Acceptable Medications to Target Specific Problems in Dementia

Symptom or Behavior	Comments and Cautions
Psychotic Symptoms (Delusions and Hallucinations)	
Antipsychotics ■ Haloperidol (Haldol) ■ Olanzapine (Zyprexa) ■ Quetiapine (Seroquel) ■ Risperidone (Risperdal)	The traditional antipsychotic drugs can produce akathisia, with increased restlessness and agitation. Clients can become more incapacitated by the parkinsonian and anticholinergic side effects.
Affective Symptoms (Depression)	
Antidepressants ■ Bupropion (Wellbutrin) ■ Fluoxetine (Prozac) ■ Nefazodone (Serzone) ■ Paroxetine (Paxil) ■ Sertraline (Zoloft) ■ Trazodone (Desyrel)	Agents with high anticholinergic activity should be avoided. The selective serotonin reuptake inhibitors appear to be well tolerated and effective in geriatric clients.
Anxiety	
Buspirone (BuSpar)	Has no serious side effects for the elderly and should be considered.
Benzodiazepines ■ Alprazolam (Xanax) ■ Diazepam (Valium) ■ Lorazepam (Ativan)	Have side effects. Produce psychomotor impairment, drowsiness, or cognitive impairment. Shorter-acting agents should be used at dosages as low as possible.
Agitated or Combative Behavior	
Antipsychotics	Used when the behavior is a consequence of underlying psychotic process only.
Buspirone	Can decrease episodic agitation in dementia clients (5 mg tid).
Trazodone	Appears to decrease aggressive behavior in agitated demented clients over 3-4 weeks.
Benzodiazepines	May nonspecifically sedate agitated clients; however, oversedation impairs function and can increase cognitive disability and psychomotor impairment.

Data from Goldberg, R. J. (1998). *Practical guide to the care of the psychiatric patient* (2nd ed.). St. Louis, MO: Mosby; and Skidmore-Roth, L. (2005). Mosby's nursing drug reference. St. Louis, MO: Mosby.

 INTEGRATIVE THERAPY

Ginkgo Biloba

As many as 11 million Americans take *Ginkgo biloba* to improve memory and increase blood circulation. Because *Ginkgo biloba* is an herbal product, people may assume that it is harmless and completely safe. This attitude prevents disclosure of herbal use to health care providers. However, ginkgo may reduce the level of platelets, which are needed for blood to clot. Use of ginkgo could pose a serious risk for consumers who are taking warfarin, heparin, aspirin, or other anticoagulants, and the use of this herbal product should be shared with health professionals.

Data from American Society of Anesthesiologists. (1999, March 24). *Anesthesiologists warn: If you're taking herbal products, tell your doctor before surgery.* Retrieved February 1, 2005, from http://medicalreporter.health.org/tmr0799/herbs&anesthesia.htm; RainforestTreasure.com. (n.d.). *Herbs with drug interactions—a partial list.* Retrieved February 1, 2005, from http://rainforesttreasure.com/drug_interact.asp.

■ ■ ■ KEY POINTS to REMEMBER

■ *Cognitive disorder* is a term that refers to disorders marked by disturbances in orientation, memory, intellect, judgment, and affect resulting from changes in the brain.

■ Delirium and dementia are discussed in this chapter because they are the cognitive disorders most frequently seen by health care workers.

■ Delirium is marked by acute onset, disturbance in consciousness, and symptoms of disorientation and confusion that fluctuate by the minute, hour, or time of day.

■ Delirium is always secondary to an underlying condition; therefore, it is temporary, transient, and may last from hours to days once the underlying cause is treated. If the cause is not treated, permanent damage to neurons can result.

■ Dementia usually has a more insidious onset than delirium. Global deterioration of cognitive functioning (e.g., memory, judgment, ability to think abstractly, and orientation) is often progressive and irreversible, depending on the underlying cause.

Continued, p. 452

CASE STUDY and NURSING CARE PLAN 21-1 Cognitive Impairment

During the past 4 years, Mr. Ludwik has demonstrated rapidly progressive memory impairment, disorientation, and deterioration in his ability to function, related to Alzheimer's disease. He is a 67-year-old man who retired at age 62 to spend some of his remaining "youth" with his wife and to travel, garden, visit family, and finally implement the plans they made over the previous 40 years. He was diagnosed with Alzheimer's disease at age 63.

Mr. Ludwik has been taken care of at home by his wife and his daughter Daisy. Daisy is divorced and has returned home with her two young daughters.

The family members find themselves progressively closer to physical and mental exhaustion. Mr. Ludwik has become increasingly incontinent when he cannot find the bathroom. He wanders away from home constantly, despite close supervision. The police and neighbors bring him back home an average of four times a week. Once, he was lost for 5 days after he had somehow boarded a bus for Pittsburgh, 1000 miles from home. He was robbed and beaten before being found by the police and returned home.

He frequently wanders into his granddaughters' rooms at night while they are sleeping and tries to get into bed with them. Too young to understand that their grandfather is lonely and confused, they fear that he is going to hurt them. Four times in the past 2 weeks, he has fallen while getting out of bed at night, thinking he is in a sleeping bag camping out in the mountains. After a conflicted and painful 2 months, the family places him in a special hospital for people with Alzheimer's disease.

Mrs. Ludwik tells the admitting nurse, Mr. Jackson, that her husband wanders almost all the time. He has difficulty finding the right words for things (aphasia) and becomes frustrated and angry when that happens. Sometimes, he does not seem to recognize the family (agnosia). Once, he thought that Daisy was a thief breaking into the house and attacked her with a broom handle. Telling this story causes Daisy to break down into heavy sobs: "What's happened to my father? He was so kind and gentle. Oh, God . . . I've lost my father."

Mrs. Ludwik tells Mr. Jackson that her husband can sometimes participate in dressing himself; at other times, when he appears confused over what goes where, he needs total assistance. At this point, Mrs. Ludwik begins to cry uncontrollably, saying "I can't bear to part with him . . . but I can't do it anymore. I feel as if I've betrayed him."

Mr. Jackson then focuses his attention on Mrs. Ludwik and her experience. He states, "This a difficult decision for you." He says that he supports their decision to move Mr. Ludwik to the Alzheimer's unit. However, he is also aware that families usually have conflicting and intense emotional reactions of guilt, depression, loss, anger, and other painful feelings. Mr. Jackson suggests that Mrs. Ludwik talk to other families with a cognitively impaired member. "It might help you to know that you are not alone, and having contact with others to share your grief can be healing." One of the groups he suggests is the Alzheimer's Association, a well-known self-help group.

Self-Assessment

Mr. Jackson has worked on his particular unit for 4 years. It is a unit especially designed for cognitively impaired individuals, which makes nursing care easier than on a regular unit. However, Mr. Jackson would be the first to admit that he has come a long way during the time he has worked on the unit.

Four years ago, he found himself getting constantly frustrated and angry. He had entered this special unit enthusiastically and had worked hard setting goals and trying to implement them. However, he thought that no one, especially the clients, cared about what he was doing for them. When the nursing coordinator asked him what made him come to that conclusion, he burst out, "Nothing I do seems to make any difference. . . . No one listens to me."

Mr. Jackson had a lot to learn about Alzheimer's disease, and he found that the more he learned, the more he understood why change took so long or, in some cases, could not take place. He, like everyone before him, learned

to become more realistic in formulating goals, which lessened his frustration.

From his co-workers, he also learned many nursing care strategies that increased competent care and decreased frustration. For example, he learned that he could distract certain clients from inappropriate behaviors (e.g., arguing with others or taking things out of other people's rooms) by engaging them in another, enjoyable activity, such as talking about something they were interested in. This reduced Mr. Jackson's initial response of scolding the client, which had usually resulted in escalating the client's anxiety, confusion, and sometimes aggression, and left Mr. Jackson annoyed and upset.

As time progressed, Mr. Jackson found that he was well suited to this kind of nursing. He has an enthusiastic manner, and his patience, wit, and genuine liking of his clients make him an ideal role model for staff new to the unit. He does a lot of teaching on the unit, both formal and informal. He is compiling a workbook for caregivers of the cognitively impaired.

■ ASSESSMENT

Objective Data

- Wanders away from home about four times a week
- Was lost for 5 days and was robbed and beaten
- Often incontinent when he cannot find the bathroom
- Has difficulty finding words
- Has difficulty identifying members of the family at times
- Has difficulty dressing himself at times
- Falls out of bed at night
- Has memory impairment
- Is disoriented much of the time
- Gets into bed with granddaughters at night when wandering
- Family undergoing intense feelings of loss and guilt

Subjective Data

- "I can't bear to part with him."
- "I feel as if I've betrayed him."
- "I've lost my father."

■ NURSING DIAGNOSIS (NANDA)

1. *Risk for injury* related to confusion, as evidenced by wandering
   - Wanders away from home about four times a week
   - Wanders despite supervision
   - Falls out of bed at night
   - Gets into other people's beds
   - Wanders at night

2. *Functional urinary incontinence* related to disturbed cognition, as evidenced by inability to find the toilet
   - Incontinent when he cannot find the bathroom

3. *Self-care deficit* (self-dressing deficits) related to impaired cognitive functioning, as evidenced by impaired ability to put on and take off clothing
   - Sometimes is able to dress with help of wife
   - At other times is too confused to dress self at all

4. *Anticipatory grieving* related to loss and deterioration of family member
   - "I can't bear to part with him."
   - "I feel as if I've betrayed him."
   - "I've lost my father."
   - Family undergoing intense feelings of loss and guilt

■ PLANNING

Mr. Jackson plans care to ensure Mr. Ludwik's safety, to provide for the maintenance of his hygiene needs and incontinence, and to assist Mrs. Ludwik as she deals with her husband's deterioration.

■ OUTCOME CRITERIA (NOC)

Although Mr. Ludwik has many unmet needs that require nursing interventions, Mr. Jackson decides to focus on the four initial nursing diagnoses. As other problems arise, they will be addressed.

Continued

Nursing Diagnosis	Long-Term Goals	Short-Term Goals
1. *Risk for injury* related to confusion, as evidenced by wandering	1. Client will remain safe in nursing home.	1a. Throughout nursing home stay, client will not fall out of bed. 1b. Throughout nursing home stay, client will wander only in protected area. 1c. Client will be returned within 2 hours if he succeeds in escaping from the unit.
2. *Functional urinary incontinence* related to disturbed cognition, as evidenced by inability to find the toilet	2. Client will experience less incontinence (fewer episodes) by fourth week of hospitalization.	2a. By the end of 4 weeks, client will participate in toilet training. 2b. By the end of 4 weeks, client will find the toilet most of the time.
3. *Self-care deficit* (self-dressing) related to impaired cognitive functioning, as evidenced by impaired ability to put on and take off clothes	3. Client will participate in dressing himself 80% of the time.	3a. By the end of 4 weeks, client will follow step-by-step instructions for dressing most of the time. 3b. By the end of 4 weeks, client will dress in own clothes with aid of fastening tape.
4. *Anticipatory grieving* related to loss and deterioration of family member	4. All family members will state, in 3 months' time, that they feel they have more support and are able to talk about their grieving.	4a. After 3 months, family members will state that they have opportunity to express "unacceptable" feelings in supportive environment. 4b. After 3 months, family members will state that they have found support from others who have a family member with Alzheimer's disease.

■ INTERVENTION (NIC)

Nursing diagnosis: *Risk for injury* related to confusion, as evidenced by wandering
Supporting Data
- Wanders away from home about four times a week
- Wanders despite supervision
- Falls out of bed at night
- Gets into other people's beds
- Wanders at night

Outcome criteria: Client will remain safe in nursing home.

Short-Term Goal	Intervention	Rationale	Evaluation
1. Throughout nursing home stay, client will not fall out of bed.	**1a.** Spend time with client on admission.	**1a.** Lowers anxiety, provides orientation to time and place. Client's confusion is increased by change.	GOAL MET Mattress on floor prevents falls out of bed.
	1b. Label client's room in big, colorful letters.	**1b.** Offers clues in new surroundings.	
	1c. Remove mattress from bed and place on floor.	**1c.** Prevents falling out of bed.	
	1d. Keep room well lit at all times.	**1d.** Provides important environmental clues; helps lower possibility of illusions.	
	1e. Show client clock and calendar in room.	**1e.** Fosters orientation to time.	
	1f. Keep window shade up.	**1f.** Allows day-night variations.	
2. Throughout nursing home stay, client will wander only in protected area.	**2a.** At night, take client to large, protected, well-lit room.	**2a.** Client is able to wander safely in protected environment.	GOAL MET Client continues to wander at night; with supervision, keeps out of other clients' rooms most of the time. By fourth week, client starts to nap on couch in large room after snacks during the night.
	2b. Alert physician to check client for cardiac decompensation.	**2b.** Addresses possible underlying cause of nocturnal wakefulness and wandering.	
	2c. Offer snacks when client is up—milk, decaffeinated tea, sandwich.	**2c.** Helps replace fluid and caloric expenditure.	
	2d. Allow soft music on radio.	**2d.** Helps induce relaxation.	
	2e. Spend short, frequent intervals with client.	**2e.** Decreases client's feelings of isolation and increases orientation.	
	2f. Take client to bathroom after snacks.	**2f.** Helps prevent incontinence.	
	2g. During day, offer activities that include use of large muscle groups.	**2g.** For some clients, helps decrease wandering.	
3. Client will be returned within 2 hours if he succeeds in escaping from the unit.	**3a.** Order medical alert bracelet for client (with name, unit, or hospital, phone number).	**3a.** If client gets out of hospital, he can be identified.	GOAL MET By fourth week, client wanders off unit only once; is found in lobby and returned by security guard within 45 minutes.
	3b. Place brightly colored vest on client with name, unit, and phone number taped on back.	**3b.** If client wanders in hospital, he can be identified and returned.	
	3c. Check client's whereabouts periodically during the day and especially at night.	**3c.** Helps monitor client's activities.	

■ EVALUATION

Although Mr. Ludwik continues to display wandering behaviors, his wandering is contained to safe areas of the unit except for one instance when he wanders to the lobby. He is stopped by security and safely returned to the unit within 45 minutes. He has not fallen out of bed. Nursing interventions such as placing his mattress on the floor as well as ensuring adequate lighting increase his safety while at the same time acknowledging that he continues to exhibit wandering behaviors.

■■■ KEY POINTS to REMEMBER—cont'd

■ Dementia may be primary (e.g., Alzheimer's disease, vascular dementia, Pick's disease, Lewy body disease). In this case, the disease is irreversible.

■ Alzheimer's disease accounts for up to 70% of all cases of dementia, and vascular dementia accounts for about 20%.

■ There are various theories regarding the cause of Alzheimer's disease; none is definitive.

■ Signs and symptoms change according to the four stages of Alzheimer's disease: stage 1 (mild), stage 2 (moderate), stage 3 (moderate to severe), and stage 4 (late).

■ The behavioral manifestations of Alzheimer's disease include confabulation, perseveration, aphasia, apraxia, agnosia, and hyperorality.

■ No known cause or cure exists for Alzheimer's disease, although a number of drugs that increase the brain's supply of acetylcholine (a nerve communication chemical) are helpful in slowing the progress of the disease.

■ People with Alzheimer's disease have many unmet needs and present many management challenges to their families as well as to health care workers.

■ Specific nursing interventions for cognitively impaired individuals can increase communication, safety, and self-care and are described in the chapter. The need for family teaching and support is strong.

■■■

Visit the Evolve website at **http://evolve.elsevier.com/Varcarolis** for a posttest on the content in this chapter. *evolve*

Critical Thinking and Chapter Review

Visit the Evolve website at **http://evolve.elsevier.com/Varcarolis** for additional self-study exercises.
evolve

■■■ CRITICAL THINKING

1. Mrs. Kendel is an 82-year-old woman who has progressive Alzheimer's disease. She lives with her husband, who has been trying to care for her in their home. Mrs. Kendel often wears evening gowns in the morning, puts her blouse on backwards, and sometimes puts her bra on backwards outside her blouse. She often forgets where things are. She makes an effort to cook but often confuses frying pans and pots and sometimes has trouble turning on the stove. Once in a while, she cannot find the bathroom in time, often mistaking it for a broom closet. She becomes frightened of noises and is terrified when the telephone or doorbell rings. At times, she cries because she is aware that she is losing her sense of her place in the world. She and her husband have always been close, loving companions, and he wants to keep her at home as long as possible.

   A. Help Mr. Kendel by writing out a list of suggestions that he can try at home that might help facilitate (a) communication, (b) activities of daily living, and (c) maintenance of a safe home environment.

   B. Identify at least seven interventions that are appropriate to this situation for each of the areas cited above.

   C. Identify possible types of resources available for maintaining Mrs. Kendel in her home for as long as possible. Provide the name of one self-help group that you would urge Mr. Kendel to join.

   D. Share with your clinical group the name and function of at least three community agencies in your area that could be an appropriate referral for a family in your neighborhood with a member with dementia. (For one, you can call the Alzheimer's Association at 800-272-3900 to find a local chapter that might help you with this information. Another resource is the ADEAR Center at 800-438-4380; website: http://www.alzheimers.org.)

■■■ CHAPTER REVIEW

Choose the most appropriate answer.

1. The nurse assessing a client with suspected delirium will expect to find that the client's symptoms developed
   1. over a period of hours to days.
   2. over a period of weeks to months.
   3. with no relationship to another condition.
   4. during the years of life after middle age.

2. An outcome that would be appropriate for a client with cognitive impairment related to delirium would be
   1. Client will participate fully in self-care from admission on.
   2. Client will have stable vital signs 6 hours after admission.
   3. Client will participate in simple activities that bring enjoyment.
   4. Client will return to the premorbid level of functioning.

3. The nursing diagnosis of highest priority for clients with late Alzheimer's disease is
   1. risk for injury.
   2. self-care deficit.
   3. chronic low self-esteem.
   4. impaired verbal communication.

Critical Thinking and Chapter Review—cont'd

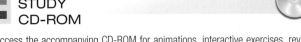

4. Strategies to help staff caring for cognitively impaired clients avoid developing burnout include
   1. setting realistic client goals.
   2. insulating self from emotional involvement with clients.
   3. sedating clients to promote rest and minimize catastrophic episodes.
   4. encouraging the family to permit the use of restraint to promote client safety.

5. Psychobiological agents showing promise for the treatment of cognitive impairment associated with Alzheimer's disease include
   1. cholinesterase inhibitors.
   2. herbals, including *Ginkgo biloba*.
   3. selective serotonin reuptake inhibitors and trazodone.
   4. benzodiazepines and buspirone.

STUDENT
STUDY
CD-ROM

Access the accompanying CD-ROM for animations, interactive exercises, review questions for the NCLEX examination, and an audio glossary.

NURSE,
CLIENT, AND
FAMILY RESOURCES

For suggested readings, information on related associations, and Internet resources, go to **http://evolve.elsevier.com/Varcarolis**. *evolve*

REFERENCES

Alzheimer's Association. (2004, June 24). Alzheimer's Association statement on research published in *The Lancet* regarding cost effectiveness of a current Alzheimer treatment. Retrieved March 7, 2005, from http://www.alz.org/Media/newsreleases/2004/062404aricept.asp.

Alzheimer's Disease Education and Referral Center. (2002, February). *High homocysteine levels may double risk of dementia, Alzheimer's disease, new report suggests.* Retrieved February 1, 2005, from http://www.alzheimers.org/nianews/nianews44.html.

Alzheimer's Disease Education and Referral Center. (2004, August). *Alzheimer's disease genetics fact sheet.* Retrieved September 13, 2004, from http://www.alzheimers.org/pubs/genefact.html.

Alzheimer's Disease and Related Disorders Association. (2004, February 1). *Statistics.* Retrieved March 7, 2005, from http://www.alz.org/Resources/FactSheets/FSAlzheimerStats.pdf.

American Psychiatric Association. (2000). *Diagnostic and statistical manual of mental disorders (DSM-IV-TR)* (4th ed., text rev.). Washington, DC: Author.

CenterWatch. (2001). *Drugs approved by the FDA: Drug name: Reminyl (galantamine hydrobromide).* Retrieved February 1, 2005, from http://www.centerwatch.com/patient/drugs/dru666.html.

Dochterman, J. M., & Bulechek, G. M. (2004). *Nursing interventions classification (NIC)* (4th ed.). St. Louis, MO: Mosby.

Howes, M. J., Perry, N. S., & Houghton, P. J. (2003, January). Plants with traditional uses and activities, relevant to the management of Alzheimer's disease and other cognitive disorders. *Phytotherapy Research, 17*(1), 1-18.

Kaplan, B. J., & Kaplan, V. A. (2004). *Kaplan & Sadock's concise textbook of clinical psychiatry* (2nd ed.). Philadelphia: Lippincott Williams & Wilkins.

Keltner, N. L, Zielinshi, A. L., & Hardin, M. S. (2001). Drugs used for the cognitive symptoms of Alzheimer's disease. *Perspectives in Psychiatric Care, 37*(1), 31-34.

Kochanek, K. D., Smith, B. L., & Andersen, R. N. (2001). Deaths: Preliminary data for 1999. *National Vital Statistics Reports, 49*(3).

Korn, M. (2000, April 29-May 6). *Dementia from many perspectives.* Paper presented at the 22nd Congress of the Collegium Internationale Neuro-Psycopharmacologicum, San Diego, CA.

Moorhead, S., Johnson, M., & Maas, M. (2004). *Nursing outcomes classification (NOC)* (3rd ed.). St. Louis, MO: Mosby.

Morris, J. C. (2000, April 29-May 6). Alzheimer's disease: Unique, differentiable and treatable. Paper presented at the 22nd Congress of the Collegium Internationale Neuro-Psycopharmacologicum, San Diego, CA.

O'Boyle, R. (2003, October 17). *Memantine officially approved for use in U.S.* Retrieved February 1, 2005, from http://www.ec-online.net/knowledge/Articles/memantine.html.

Prasher, V., et al. (2003). Magnetic resonance imaging, Down's syndrome and Alzheimer's disease: Research and clinical implications. *Journal of Intellectual Disabilities Research, 47*(Pt 2), 90-100.

Ress, B. (2003). HIV disease and aging: The hidden epidemic. *Critical Care Nursing, 5,* 38-42.

Sabbagh, M. N. (2003, March 21). *Alzheimer's disease diagnosis and treatment: Past, present and future.* Paper presented at the 12th Annual Caregiver Conference, "Visions of Hope: Living Today, Planning Tomorrow," Alzheimer's Association Desert Southwest Chapter, Central Arizona Region, Phoenix, AZ.

Sadock, B. J., & Sadock, V. A. (2004). *Concise textbook of clinical psychiatry* (2nd ed.). Philadelphia: Lippincott Williams & Wilkins.

Shumaker, S. A., et al. (2003). Estrogen plus progestin and the incidence of dementia and mild cognitive impairment in postmenopausal women. The Women's Health Initiative Memory Study: A randomized controlled trial. *Journal of the American Medical Association, 289*(20), 2651.

Strandberg, T. E., et al. (2003). Impact of viral and bacterial burden on cognitive impairment in elderly persons with cardiovascular diseases. *Stroke, 34*(9), 2126-2131.

U.S. Food and Drug Administration. (2003, October 17). *FDA News: FDA approves memantine (Namenda) for Alzheimer's disease.* Retrieved February 1, 2005, from http://www.fda.gov/bbs/topics/NEWS/2003/NEW00961.html.

A CLIENT SPEAKS

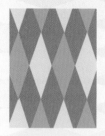

Hello, my name is Patty, and I am an alcoholic. When I was 16 years of age, my friends and I started skipping school on a regular basis to buy alcohol and drugs. At first it was just for kicks. Eventually I ended up drinking on almost a daily basis and stole from parents to buy drugs and alcohol. The more I drank, the worse things got at home. My whole existence revolved around drugs and alcohol. In the process I was losing everything. My poor parents had no idea what to do. I lied, stole, and hurt everyone who ever really cared for me.

Around this time I was diagnosed with bipolar disorder. Unfortunately, I was allergic to the only medication they had for bipolar disease at that time. I was left untreated for the next 16 years.

I married, but my drinking escalated, and my marriage deteriorated and ended. I was able to care for my son, Teddy, only with my parents help. I started nursing school, and things were finally looking up. I graduated and became an LPN. For the first time ever I was proud of myself and had accomplished something great. It wasn't long before I fell off the wagon again. My parents took care of my son.

One day I went to New York City to get some dope and never came home. I was living on the streets. All I cared about was the next high. I quickly became one of those homeless people you step over on the street . . . selling aluminum cans for a quarter just to buy one cigarette. All that mattered was staying high.

The day I went home, I was emaciated and was virtually on my death bed. My parents took me to a hospital, and I was in life-threatening withdrawal from drugs and alcohol. I almost died.

Later, looking at pictures of my son, I knew I had missed so many precious times with him that I will never get back. Hurting people you love is one of the things you can't take back or make up for. Now, even after 10 years of being clean and sober, I doubt my sister will ever forgive me. I love my sister. When I was pregnant with my first son, she helped me and stepped in for me when I was gone. I will never forget that. Thank you, Lisa.

I was unaware that addiction was disease until I went to Alcoholics Anonymous (AA). I stopped feeling helpless, and I saw that other people who had similar problems were alive and well and able to stay sober. I owe my sobriety to the people in those rooms of AA over the years.

The important things to me now are family, religion, and my home. I have a terrific husband and another wonderful little boy, and my life is full. Staying sober is a daily struggle. Being bipolar and a recovering alcoholic and drug addict makes for a challenging existence. I have learned to stay around people that truly understand me and stay away from people who don't. If you don't, you set yourself up for a miserable life. I hope my story might help someone else struggling with this disease and help others know that when treated like a disease, alcoholism can be treated successfully.

PSYCHIATRIC EMERGENCIES

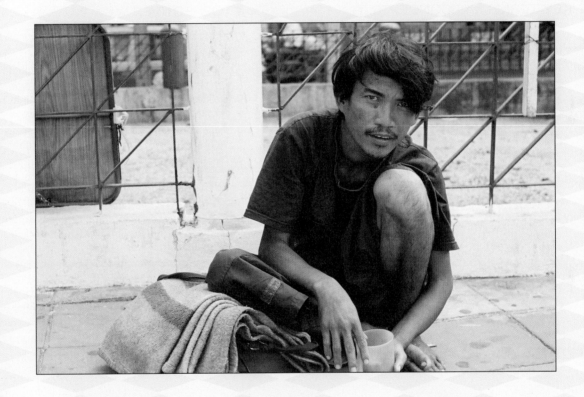

WHAT LIES BEHIND US AND WHAT LIES BEFORE US ARE SMALL MATTERS
COMPARED TO WHAT LIES WITHIN US.

Ralph Waldo Emerson

CHAPTER 22

Crisis

CAROLYN M. SCOTT ■ ELIZABETH M. VARCAROLIS

KEY TERMS and CONCEPTS

The key terms and concepts listed here appear in color where they are defined or first discussed in this chapter.

adventitious crisis, 459

crisis intervention, 457

critical incident stress debriefing (CISD), 465

maturational crisis, 458

phases of crisis, 459

primary care, 465

secondary care, 465

situational crisis, 458

tertiary care, 465

OBJECTIVES

After studying this chapter, the reader will be able to

1. Differentiate among the three types of crisis discussed in this chapter and give an example of each from the reader's own experience.
2. Delineate at least six aspects of crisis that have relevance for nurses involved in crisis intervention.
3. Develop a handout including areas to assess during crisis, with at least two sample questions for each area.
4. Discuss four common problems in the nurse-client relationship that are frequently encountered by beginning nurses when starting crisis intervention and discuss at least two interventions for each problem.
5. Compare and contrast the differences among primary, secondary, and tertiary intervention, including appropriate intervention strategies.
6. Explain to a classmate four potential crisis situations, common in the hospital setting, that a client may face and give concrete examples of how they can be minimized.
7. Make a list of at least five resources in the community that could be used as referrals for a person in crisis.

evolve Visit the Evolve website at **http://evolve.elsevier.com/Varcarolis** for a pretest on the content in this chapter.

The Homeland Security Department raises the terror alert to "high" and warns American citizens to be watchful for any suspicious behavior. A child is killed in a drive-by shooting—the bullet intended for a neighborhood drug dealer. A tornado touches down in a small Midwestern town leveling an entire neighborhood and leaving 10 residents dead and many more homeless. Hurricane Isabel tears through the mid-Atlantic and northeastern states leaving a wake of devastation in her path. A child is diagnosed with cancer. A 35-year employee in a manufacturing company is laid off. A teenaged boy armed with several guns enters his high school and randomly shoots everyone who crosses his path. A husband announces to his wife of 30 years that he no longer loves her and wants a divorce. A young nursing student discovers she is pregnant, and the father of the baby abandons her. What do these situations have in common? Each of these situations could be the precipitant of a crisis—leaving individuals, families, and whole communities struggling to cope with the impact of the event.

Everyone experiences crises. The experience itself is not pathological but rather represents a struggle for equilibrium and adjustment when problems seem unsolvable. A crisis presents both a danger to personality organization and a potential opportunity for personality growth. The outcome depends on how the individual, family, or community perceives and deals with the crisis and what outside supports are available at the time the crisis occurs.

Crises are acute, time-limited occurrences experienced as overwhelming emotional reactions to

- A stressful situational event,
- A developmental event,
- A societal event,
- A cultural event, or
- The perception of that event.

Crisis intervention is what nurses and other health professionals do to assist those in crisis to cope. Interventions are broad, creative, and flexible.

COMORBIDITY

Many factors may limit a person's ability to problem-solve or cope with stressful life events or situations, such as

- The number of other stressful life events with which the person is currently coping.
- The presence of other unresolved losses with which the person may be dealing.
- The presence of concurrent psychiatric disorders.
- The presence of concurrent medical problems.
- The presence of excessive fatigue or pain.
- The quality and quantity of a person's usual coping skills.

Coping skills are often acquired through a variety of sources, for example, cultural responses, the modeling behaviors of others, and life opportunities that broaden our experience and allow us to acquire new responses (Aguilera, 1998; Greenstone & Leviton, 2002).

Chapter 28 discusses the vulnerability of people with severe mental illness and their susceptibility to crisis as well as crisis interventions. Nurses, perhaps more than any other group, deal with people who are experiencing disruption in their lives. People often experience increased stress and anxiety in medical and surgical and psychiatric settings, as well as in community settings.

THEORY

An early crisis theorist, **Erich Lindemann,** conducted a classic study in the 1940s on the grief reactions of close relatives of victims who died in the Coconut Grove nightclub fire in Boston. This study formed the foundation of crisis theory and clinical intervention. Lindemann was convinced that, even though acute grief is a normal reaction to a distressing situation, preventive interventions could eliminate or decrease serious personality disorganization and devastating psychological consequences from the sustained effects of severe anxiety. He believed that the same interventions that were helpful in bereavement would prove just as helpful in dealing with other types of stressful events and proposed a crisis intervention model as a major element of preventive psychiatry in the community.

In the early 1960s, **Gerald Caplan** (1964) further elaborated crisis theory and outlined crisis intervention strategies. Since that time, our understanding of crisis and effective intervention has continued to be refined and enhanced by numerous contemporary clinicians and theorists (Behrman & Reid, 2002; Roberts, 2000).

In 1961, a report of the Joint Commission on Mental Illness and Mental Health addressed the need for community mental health centers throughout the country. This report stimulated the establishment of crisis services, which are now an important part of mental health programs in hospitals and communities.

Donna Aguilera and **Janice Mesnick** (1970) provided a framework for nurses for crisis assessment and intervention, which has grown in scope and practice. Aguilera (1998) continues to set a standard in the practice of crisis assessment and intervention.

Roberts' seven-stage model of crisis intervention (2000) is a more contemporary model that is useful in helping individuals who have suffered from an acute situational crisis as well as people who are diagnosed with acute stress disorder. See Figure 22-1 for a diagram of Roberts' model.

The devastating effects of the 9/11 World Trade Center terrorist attack emphasized the need for crisis assessment and intervention by community mental health providers throughout the country to deal with all types of crises experienced by people who had been traumatized—victims, families, rescue workers, and observers (Behrman, 2002; Everly, 2000; Howard & Goelitz, 2004; Lowry & Lating, 2002).

The ways of assessing crisis described in the following sections are derived from established crisis theory and constitute a sound knowledge base for the application of the nursing process to treatment of a client in crisis. An understanding of three areas of crisis theory enables application of the nursing process: (1) types of crisis, (2) phases of crisis, and (3) aspects of crisis that have relevance for nurses.

Types of Crisis

There are three basic types of crisis situation: (1) maturational, (2) situational, and (3) adventitious. People who have preexisting mental health problems are very vulnerable and are prone to crisis. Chapter 28 addresses crisis in and rehabilitation of the mentally ill. Psychiatric emergencies (suicide, family violence, sexual assault, uncontrollable anger) are covered in Unit Six. Drug overdoses and alcohol intoxication and withdrawal are discussed in Chapter 27.

Maturational Crisis

A process of maturation occurs throughout life. Erik Erikson (1902-1994) identified eight stages of growth and development in which specific maturational tasks must be mastered. The path (stages) to adulthood is

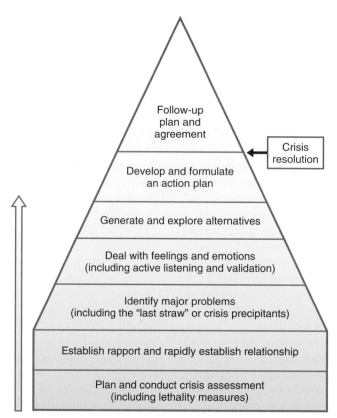

FIGURE 22-1 Roberts' seven-stage model of crisis intervention. (From Roberts, A. R. [Ed.]. [2000]. *Crisis intervention handbook* [3rd ed.]. New York: Oxford University Press.)

stressful and at times can be overwhelming. Erikson declared that each of these stages constitutes a crisis in personal growth and development.

Each developmental stage can thus be referred to as a maturational crisis. When a person arrives at a new stage, formerly used coping styles are no longer appropriate, and new coping mechanisms have yet to be developed. For a time, the person is without effective defenses. This often leads to increased anxiety, which may manifest as variations in the person's normal behavior. Marriage, the birth of a child, and retirement are all examples of maturational crises. Successful resolution of these maturational tasks leads to development of basic human qualities. Erikson believed that the way these crises are resolved at one stage affects the ability to pass through subsequent stages, because each crisis provides the starting point for moving to the next stage. If a person lacks support systems and adequate role models, successful resolution may be difficult or may not occur. Unresolved problems in the past and inadequate coping mechanisms can adversely affect what is learned in each developmental stage. When a person is experiencing severe difficulty during a maturational crisis, professional intervention may be indicated.

Alcohol and drug addiction interrupt an individual's progression through the maturational stages. This phenomenon is too often seen among teenagers today.

When the addictive behavior is controlled (by the late teens), the young person's growth and development will resume at the point at which it was interrupted. A young person whose addiction is arrested at 19 years of age may have the social and problem-solving skills of a 14-year-old. Often these teenagers do not receive treatment, and their adult coping skills are diminished or absent.

Situational Crisis

A situational crisis arises from an external rather than an internal source. Often the crisis is unanticipated. Examples of external situations that can precipitate a crisis include the loss of a job, the death of a loved one, an abortion, a change of job, a change in financial status, divorce, and severe physical or mental illness.

Situations such as these were referred to as life events by Holmes and Rahe (1967). Each life event is assigned stress points that, when totaled, may predict the risk for illness. A high point count can indicate a higher risk of physical or psychological illness.

Some authors refer to these events as critical life problems because these problems are encountered by most people during the course of their lives. Whether or not these events precipitate a crisis depends on such factors as the degree of support available from caring friends and family members, a person's general emotional and physical status, and a person's ability to understand and cope with the meaning of the stressful event.

As in all crises or potential crisis situations, the stressful event involves a loss or change that threatens a person's self-concept and self-esteem. To varying degrees, successful resolution of a crisis depends on resolution of the grief associated with the loss.

Adventitious Crisis

An **adventitious crisis**, or crisis of disaster, is not a part of everyday life; it is unplanned and accidental. Adventitious crises may result from (1) a natural disaster (e.g., flood, fire, earthquake), (2) a national disaster (e.g., acts of terrorism, war, riots, airplane crashes), or (3) a crime of violence (e.g., rape, assault or murder in the workplace or school, bombing in crowded areas, spousal or child abuse).

The recent literature includes numerous studies related to the psychological sequelae suffered by people after the 9/11 World Trade Center disaster (Behrman & Reid, 2002; Jordan, 2003; Regehr, 2001). Common phenomena experienced were acute stress disorder, posttraumatic stress disorder, and depression. **The need for psychological first aid (crisis intervention) and debriefing after any crisis situation for all age groups (children, adolescents, adults, and the elderly) cannot be overstressed.** *Critical incident debriefing* is discussed later in this chapter.

It is possible to experience two types of crisis situations simultaneously. For example, a 51-year-old woman may be going through a midlife crisis (maturational) when her husband dies suddenly of cancer (situational). The presence of more than one crisis further taxes the individual's coping skills.

Phases of Crisis

Caplan (1964) identified four distinct phases of crisis.

Phase 1

A person confronted by a conflict or problem that threatens the self-concept responds with increased feelings of anxiety. The increase in anxiety stimulates the use of problem-solving techniques and defense mechanisms in an effort to solve the problem and lower anxiety.

Phase 2

If the usual defensive response fails, and if the threat persists, anxiety continues to rise and produce feelings of extreme discomfort. Individual functioning becomes disorganized. Trial-and-error attempts at solving the problem and restoring a normal balance begin.

Phase 3

If the trial-and-error attempts fail, anxiety can escalate to severe and panic levels, and the person mobilizes automatic relief behaviors, such as withdrawal and

flight. Some form of resolution (e.g., compromising needs or redefining the situation to reach an acceptable solution) may be made in this stage.

Phase 4

If the problem is not solved and new coping skills are ineffective, anxiety can overwhelm the person and lead to serious personality disorganization, depression, confusion, violence against others, or suicidal behavior (Greenstone & Leviton, 2002; Jordan, 2003; Lowry & Lating, 2002).

Aspects of Crisis That Have Relevance for Nurses

Crisis theory defines specific aspects of crisis that are basic to crisis intervention. These are listed in Box 22-1.

BOX 22-1

Foundation for Crisis Intervention

1. A crisis is self-limiting and is usually resolved within 4 to 6 weeks.
2. The resolution of a crisis results in achievement of one of three different functional levels. The person will emerge at
   - a higher level of functioning.
   - the same level of functioning.
   - a lower level of functioning.
3. The goal of crisis intervention is to return the individual to the precrisis level of functioning.
4. The form of resolution of the crisis depends on the actions of the individual and the intervention of others.
5. During a crisis, people are often more open to outside intervention than they are at times of stable functioning. With intervention, the person can learn different adaptive means of problem solving to correct inadequate solutions.
6. The person in a crisis situation is assumed to be mentally healthy and to have functioned well in the past but is presently in a state of disequilibrium.
7. Crisis intervention deals with the person's present problem and resolution of the immediate crisis only. Dealing with material not directly related to the crisis can take place at a later time. Crisis intervention deals with the "here and now."
8. The nurse must be willing to take an active, even directive, role in intervention; this is in direct contrast to what occurs in conventional therapeutic intervention, which stresses a more passive and nondirective role for the practitioner.
9. Early intervention probably increases the chances for a good prognosis.
10. The client is encouraged to set realistic goals and plan an intervention with the nurse that is focused on the current situation.

Application of the Nursing Process

ASSESSMENT
Overall Assessment

A person's equilibrium may be adversely affected by one or more of the following: (1) an unrealistic perception of the precipitating event, (2) inadequate situational supports, and (3) inadequate coping mechanisms (Aguilera, 1998). It is crucial to assess these factors when a crisis situation is evaluated, because data gained from the assessment are used as guides for both the nurse and the client in setting realistic and meaningful goals as well as in planning possible solutions to the problem situation.

After determining whether there is a need for external controls because of suicidal or homicidal ideation or gestures, the nurse assesses three main areas: (1) the client's perception of the precipitating event, (2) the client's situational supports, and (3) the client's personal coping skills.

Assessing the Client's Perception of the Precipitating Event

The nurse's initial task is to assess the individual or family and the problem. The more clearly the problem can be defined, the better the chance that an effective solution will be found. Sample questions that may facilitate the assessment include the following:

- Has anything particularly upsetting happened to you within the past few days or weeks?
- What was happening in your life before you started to feel this way?
- What leads you to seek help now?
- Describe how you are feeling right now.
- How does this situation affect your life?
- How do you see this event as affecting your future?
- What would need to be done to resolve this situation?

■ ■ ■ VIGNETTE

Susan, a 25-year-old woman, is brought to the emergency department after being beaten by her husband. She was found bleeding from her head by her upstairs neighbor. Her neighbor called the police, and they rushed Susan to the hospital. After Susan is seen by the medical personnel, she is interviewed by the psychiatric nurse working in the emergency department. The nurse calmly introduces herself and tells Susan she would like to spend some time with her. The nurse says, "It looks as if things are pretty overwhelming. Is that how you're feeling?" The nurse makes the observation that things must be very bad if Susan stays with an abusive husband. Susan sits slumped in a chair with her hands in her lap and her head hanging down, tears in her eyes.

Example: Assessing Susan's Perception of the Precipitating Event

Nurse: Susan, tell me what has happened.
Susan: I can't . . . I can't go home. . . . No one cares. . . . No one believes me. . . . I can't go through it again.
Nurse: Tell me what you can't go through again, Susan. (Susan starts to cry, shaking with sobs. The nurse sits quietly for a while, offers her some tissues, then speaks.)
Nurse: Tell me what is so terrible. Let's look at it together.

After a while, Susan starts telling the nurse that her husband has been beating her on a regular basis, particularly after a night out drinking with his male friends. The beatings have gotten much worse over time. Susan states, "I'm afraid that eventually I will end up dead. He becomes so violent when he is drunk."

Assessing Situational Supports

The client's support systems are assessed to determine the resources available to the person. Does the stressful event involve important people in the support system? Is the client isolated from others, or are there family and friends who can provide the vital support? Family and friends may be called upon to aid the individual by offering material or emotional support, for example, lending money, offering services, or being available to give affection and understanding. If these resources are not available, the nurse or counselor acts as a temporary support system while relationships with individuals or groups in the community are established. The following are some sample questions to ask:

- With whom do you live?
- To whom do you talk when you feel overwhelmed?
- Whom can you trust?
- Who is available to help you?
- Where do you go to worship (or talk to God)? Where do you go to school or to other community-based activities?
- During difficult times in the past, who did you want most to help you?
- Who is the most helpful?

Example: Assessing Susan's Situational Supports

Nurse: Susan, who can you go to? Do you have any other family?
Susan: No. My family is in another state. We stay pretty much alone.
Nurse: Do you have anyone you can talk to?
Susan: No, I really don't have any friends. My husband's jealousy makes it a real problem for me to have friends. He doesn't like anyone that I would want as a friend.
Nurse: What about people at your place of worship, or co-workers?
Susan: My co-workers are nice, but I can't tell them things like this. Besides, they wouldn't believe me either.

Assessing Personal Coping Skills

In crisis situations, it is important to evaluate the person's level of anxiety. Common coping mechanisms may be overeating, drinking, smoking, withdrawing, seeking out someone to talk to, yelling, fighting, or engaging in other physical activity (Behrman & Reid, 2002). The potential for suicide or homicide must be assessed. If the client is suicidal, homicidal, or unable to take care of personal needs, hospitalization should be considered (Aguilera, 1998). Some sample questions to ask are the following:

- Have you thought of killing yourself or someone else? If yes, have you thought of how you would do this?
- What do you usually do to feel better?
- Did you try it this time? If so, what was different?
- What helped you through difficult times in the past?
- What do you think might happen now?

The nurse learns that Susan does very well at her job. Susan explains that when she is at work, she can forget her problems for a little while. Getting good job reviews also has another reward: it is the only time her husband says anything nice about her.

Example: Assessing Susan's Personal Coping Style

Nurse: What do you think would help your situation?
Susan: I don't want to be in an abusive marriage. I just don't know where to turn.

The nurse tells Susan that she wants to work with her to find a solution and that she is concerned for Susan's safety and well-being.

Self-Assessment

Nurses need to constantly monitor personal feelings and thoughts when dealing with a person in crisis. It is important to recognize one's own level of anxiety to prevent closing off the expression of painful feelings by the client. The nurse may respond with anxiety to the client's situation or anxiety level and try to repress such feelings to maintain personal comfort. When the nurse is not aware of personal feelings and reactions, she or he may unconsciously prevent the expression of the painful feelings in the client that are precipitating the nurse's own discomfort. Thus, closing off feelings in the client can render the nurse ineffective. There may be times when the nurse, perhaps for personal reasons, feels he or she cannot deal effectively with a client's situation at this time. Therefore, the nurse might ask another colleague to work with a particular client. This will give the nurse a chance to work through some uncomfortable or painful personal issues.

Beginning nurses in crisis intervention often face common problems that must be dealt with before the nurses become comfortable and competent in the role of a crisis counselor. Four of the more common problems are the following:

1. The nurse needs to be needed.
2. The nurse sets unrealistic goals for clients.
3. The nurse has difficulty dealing with the issue of suicide.
4. The nurse has difficulty terminating the nurse-client relationship.

Refer to Table 22-1 for examples and results of these problems, appropriate interventions, and desired outcomes. It is crucial in beginning crisis intervention that supervision be available as an integral part of the training process. The supervisor should be an experienced professional, such as a nurse counselor or a nursing supervisor.

Nurses working in disaster situations can become overwhelmed by witnessing catastrophic loss of human life (as in acts of terrorism, plane crashes, school shootings) and/or mass destruction of people's homes and belongings (as in floods, fires, tornadoes) that leave many families bereft of a sense of stability, well-being, and shelter. Disaster nurses need both supportive ties and access to debriefing.

Debriefing is an important step for staff in coming to terms with overwhelming violent or otherwise disastrous situations once they are over. It helps staff place the crisis in perspective and begin healing themselves. Debriefing is discussed in detail later in the chapter.

Assessment Guidelines **Crisis**

1. Identify whether the client's response to the crisis warrants psychiatric treatment or hospitalization to minimize decompensation (suicidal behavior, psychotic thinking, violent behavior).
2. Identify whether the client is able to identify the *precipitating event*.
3. Assess the client's understanding of his or her present *situational supports*.
4. Identify the client's usual *coping styles* and determine what coping mechanisms may help the present situation.
5. Determine whether there are certain religious or cultural beliefs that need to be considered in assessing and intervening in this person's crisis.
6. Assess whether this situation is one in which the client needs primary intervention (education, environmental manipulation, or new coping skills), secondary intervention (crisis intervention), or tertiary intervention (rehabilitation).

■ NURSING DIAGNOSIS

A person in crisis may exhibit various behaviors that indicate a number of human problems. For example, when a person is in crisis, the nursing diagnosis of

TABLE 22-1

Common Problems in the Nurse-Client Relationship Faced by Beginning Nurses

Examples	Results	Interventions	Outcome
Problem 1: *Nurse needs to feel needed.* Feels total responsibility to "care for" or "cure" client's problems.			
Nurse allows excessive phone calls between sessions. Nurse gives direct advice without sufficient knowledge of client's situation. Nurse attempts to influence lifestyle of client on a judgmental basis.	Client becomes more dependent on nurse and relies less on own abilities. Nurse reacts to client's not getting "cured" or taking advice by projecting feelings of frustration and anger onto client.	Nurse evaluates with an experienced professional nurse's needs versus client's needs. Nurse discourages dependency by client. Nurse encourages goal setting and problem solving by client. Nurse takes control only if suicide or homicide is a possibility.	Client is free to grow and problem-solve own life crises. Nurse's skills and effectiveness grow as comfort with role increases and own goals are clarified.
Problem 2: *Nurse sets unrealistic goals for clients.* Goals become nurse's goals and not mutually determined goals for the client.			
Nurse expects physically abused woman to leave battering partner. Nurse expects man who abuses alcohol to stop drinking when loss of family or job is imminent.	Nurse feels anxious and responsible when expectations are not met; anxiety resulting from feelings of inadequacy are projected onto the client in the form of frustration and anger.	Nurse examines with an experienced professional realistic expectations of self and client. Nurse reevaluates client's level of functioning and works with client on his level. Nurse encourages setting of goals by client.	Nurse's ability to assess and problem-solve increases as anger and frustration decrease. Client feels less alienated, and a working relationship can ensue.
Problem 3: *Nurse has difficulty dealing with a suicidal client.*			
Nurse selectively inattends by ■ Denying possible clues. ■ Neglecting to follow up on verbal suicide clues. ■ Changing topic to less threatening subject when self-destructive themes come up.	Client is robbed of opportunity to share feelings and find alternatives to intolerable situation. Client remains suicidal. Nurse's crisis intervention ceases to be effective.	Nurse assesses own feelings and anxieties with help of an experienced professional. Nurse evaluates all clues or slight suspicions and acts on them; for example, "Are you thinking of killing yourself?" If yes, nurse assesses ■ Suicide potential. ■ Need for hospitalization.	Client experiences relief in sharing feelings and evaluating alternatives. Suicide potential can be minimized. Nurse becomes more adept at picking up clues and minimizing suicide potential.
Problem 4: *Nurse has difficulty terminating* after crisis has resolved.			
Nurse is tempted to work on other problems in client's life to prolong contact with client.	Nurse steps into territory of traditional therapy without proper training or experience.	Nurse works with an experienced professional to ■ Explore own feelings regarding separations and termination. ■ Reinforce crisis model; crisis intervention is a preventative tool, not psychotherapy. Nurse becomes better able to help client with his or her feelings when nurse's own feelings are recognized.	Client is free to go back to his or her life situation or request appropriate referral to work on other issues of importance to client.

Data from Finkleman, A. W. (1977). The nurse therapist: Outpatient crisis intervention with the chronic psychiatric patient. *Journal of Psychosocial Nursing and Mental Health Services, 8,* 27; and Wallace, M. A., & Morley, W. E. (1970). Teaching crisis intervention. *American Journal of Nursing, 7,* 1484.

ineffective coping is often evident. Because anxiety may escalate to moderate or severe levels, the ability to solve problems is usually impaired, if it is present at all. Ineffective coping may be evidenced by inability to meet basic needs, inability to meet role expectations, alteration in social participation, use of inappropriate defense mechanisms, or impairment of usual patterns of communication. See Table 22-2 for some signs and symptoms of people in crisis that may be used as a guide for identifying potential nursing diagnoses.

For the example in the preceding vignette, the assessment of Susan's (1) perception of the precipitating event, (2) situational supports, and (3) personal coping skills provides the nurse enough data to formulate two diagnoses and to work with Susan in setting goals and planning interventions.

TABLE 22-2

Potential Nursing Diagnoses for Crisis Intervention

Symptoms	Nursing Diagnosis
Overwhelmed, depressed, states that has nothing in life worthwhile, self-hate and feelings of being in-effectual are assessed	**Risk for self-directed violence** **Chronic low self-esteem** **Spiritual distress** **Hopelessness** **Powerlessness**
Confused, highly anxious, incoherent, crying or sob-bing, shows extreme emotional pain	**Anxiety (moderate, severe, panic)** **Acute confusion** **Disturbed thought processes** **Sleep deprivation**
Has difficulty with interper-sonal relationships, iso-lated, has few or no social supports	**Social isolation** **Risk for loneliness** **Impaired social interaction**
Unable to function at work, school, and/or home at previous level, has diffi-culty concentrating or completing simple tasks	**Ineffective coping** **Interrupted family processes** **Caregiver role strain**
Has experienced traumatic, emotionally overwhelming event or loss; unable to work through overwhelm-ing loss or event	**Risk for posttrauma syndrome** **Rape-trauma syndrome** **Dysfunctional grieving** **Chronic sorrow**

Example: Nursing Diagnosis for Susan

The nurse formulates the following nursing diagnoses:

Anxiety (moderate/severe) related to mental and physical abuse, as evidenced by ineffectual problem solving and feelings of impending doom

Compromised family coping related to the constant threat of violence

■ OUTCOME CRITERIA

Relevant outcomes of the Nursing Outcomes Clas-sification (NOC) (Moorhead, Johnson, & Maas, 2004) for a person experiencing a crisis include *Coping, Decision Making, Role Performance,* and *Stress Level.* The planning of realistic client outcomes is done together with the client or family. Realistic outcomes are made to fit within the person's cultural and personal values. Without the client's involvement, the outcome criteria (goals at the end of 4 to 8 weeks) may be irrelevant or unacceptable solutions to that person's crisis.

For example, a nurse new to crisis intervention who suggests that a woman leave her husband because he beats her may be surprised to find that the woman has different thoughts on what she wants as a final solu-tion. Thus, outcomes are always established with the

client, and they have to be congruent with clients' needs, values, and (in some instances) cultural expec-tations. The nurse evaluates the outcome for safety as well as other factors and works on contingency plans when necessary.

Refer to Table 22-3 for selected NOC outcomes with supporting intermediate and short-term indicators for a client in crisis.

A social worker is called. Susan, the nurse, and the social worker meet together. All agree that Susan should not return to her home because of the husband's frequent abuse. The nurse then meets with Susan to establish goals and to plan interventions.

The nurse and Susan set four goals together:

Susan will return to her precrisis state within 2 weeks.
Susan, with the support of staff, will find a safe environment.
Susan, with the support of staff, will have at least two outside supports available within 24 hours.
Susan will receive continued evaluation and support until the immediate crisis is over (6 to 8 weeks).

■ PLANNING

Nurses are called upon to plan and intervene through a variety of crisis intervention modalities, such as dis-aster nursing, mobile crisis units, group work, health education and crisis prevention, victim outreach pro-grams, and telephone hotlines.

The nurse may be involved in planning and inter-vention for an individual (e.g., cases of physical abuse), for a group (e.g., students after a classmate's suicide event or shooting), or for a community (e.g., disaster nursing after tornadoes, shootings, and air-plane crashes).

The following questions are answered (Aguilera, 1998):

1. How much has this crisis affected the person's life? Can the client still go to work? Attend school? Care for family members?
2. How is the state of disequilibrium affecting sig-nificant people in the client's life (wife, husband, children, other family members, boss, boyfriend, girlfriend)?

Data from the answers to these two questions will guide the nurse in determining what kinds of immedi-ate action to take.

■ INTERVENTION

Crisis intervention is considered to be a function of the basic level nurse and has two basic initial goals:

1. **Client safety.** External controls may be applied for protection of the person in crisis if the person is suicidal or homicidal.

TABLE 22-3

NOC Outcomes for a Client in Crisis

Nursing Outcome and Definition	Intermediate Indicators	Short-Term Indicators
Coping: Personal actions to manage stressors that tax an individual's resources*	Modifies lifestyle as needed Uses effective coping strategies Reports decrease in negative feelings Reports decrease in physical symptoms of stress	Identifies effective coping patterns Identifies ineffective coping patterns Reports decrease in stress Uses available social support Verbalizes need for assistance
Decision-Making: Ability to make judgments and choose between two or more alternatives†	Chooses among alternatives	Identifies relevant information Identifies alternatives Weighs alternatives
Role Performance: Congruence of an individual's role behavior with role expectations‡	Able to meet role expectations	Performance of family role behaviors Description of role changes based on illness or disability Description of role changes with elderly dependents/with new family member/when family member leaves home Performance of family/parental/intimate/community/work/friendship role behaviors
Stress Level: Severity of manifested physical or mental tension resulting from factors that alter an existing equilibrium§		Elevated blood pressure Increased radial pulse rate Upset stomach Forgetfulness and blocking Compulsive behavior Restlessness Emotional outbursts

From Moorhead, S., Johnson, M., & Maas, M. (2004). *Nursing outcomes classification (NOC)* (3rd ed.). St. Louis, MO: Mosby.
*Evaluated on a five-point Likert scale ranging from 1 (never demonstrated) to 5 (consistently demonstrated).
†Evaluated on a five-point Likert scale ranging from 1 (severely compromised) to 5 (not compromised).
‡Evaluated on a five-point Likert scale ranging from 1 (not adequate) to 5 (totally adequate).
§Evaluated on a five-point Likert scale ranging from 1 (severe) to 5 (none).

2. **Anxiety reduction.** Anxiety reduction techniques are used, so that inner resources can be mobilized.

During the initial interview, the person in crisis first needs to gain a feeling of safety. Solutions to the crisis may be offered, so that the client is aware of other options. Feelings of support and hope will temporarily diminish anxiety. The nurse needs to play an active role by indicating that help is available. The availability of help is conveyed by the competent use of crisis intervention skills and genuine interest and support. It is not conveyed by the use of false reassurances and platitudes, such as "Everything will be all right." Crisis intervention requires a creative and flexible approach through the use of traditional and nontraditional therapeutic methods. The nurse may act as educator, advisor, and model, always keeping in mind that it is the client who solves the problem, not the nurse. The following are important assumptions when working with a client in crisis:

- The person is in charge of his or her own life.
- The person is able to make decisions.
- The crisis counseling relationship is one between partners.

The nurse helps the client refocus to gain new perspectives on the situation. The nurse supports the client during the process of finding constructive ways to solve or cope with the problem. It is important for the nurse to be mindful of how difficult it is for the client to change his or her behavior. See Table 22-4 for guidelines for nursing interventions and corresponding rationales.

After talking with the nurse and the social worker, Susan seems open to going to a safe house for battered women. She also agrees to talk to a counselor at a mental health facility. The nurse sets up an appointment at which she, Susan, and the counselor will meet. The nurse will continue to see Susan twice a week.

Counseling Strategies

There are three levels of nursing care in crisis intervention. These three levels are (1) primary, (2) secondary, and (3) tertiary. Psychotherapeutic nursing interventions in crisis are directed toward these three levels of care.

TABLE 22-4

Overall Guidelines for Nursing Intervention

Intervention	Rationale
1. Assess for any suicidal or homicidal thoughts or plans.	1. Safety is always the first consideration.
2. Take initial steps to make client feel safe and to lower anxiety.	2. When a person feels safe and anxiety decreases, the individual is able to problem-solve solutions with the nurse.
3. Listen carefully (e.g., make eye contact, give frequent feedback to make sure you understand, summarize what client says at the end).	3. When a person believes that someone is really listening, this can translate into the belief that someone cares about the person's situation and that help may be available. This offers hope.
4. Crisis intervention calls for directive and creative approaches. Initially, the nurse may make phone calls (arrange baby-sitters, schedule a visiting nurse, find shelter, contact a social worker).	4. Initially, a person may be so confused and frightened that performing usual tasks is not possible at this moment.
5. Identify needed social supports (with client's input) and mobilize the most needed first.	5. Client's needs for shelter, help with care for children or elders, medical workup, emergency medical attention, hospitalization, food, safe housing, and self-help group are determined.
6. Identify needed coping skills (problem solving, relaxation, assertiveness, job training, newborn care, self-esteem raising).	6. Increasing coping skills and learning new ones can help with current crisis and help minimize future crises.
7. Plan with client interventions acceptable to both counselor and client.	7. Client's sense of control, self-esteem, and compliance with plan are increased.
8. Plan regular follow-up to assess client's progress (e.g., phone calls, clinic visits, home visits as appropriate).	8. Plan is evaluated to see what works and what doesn't work.

Primary

Primary care promotes mental health and reduces mental illness to decrease the incidence of crisis. On this level the nurse can

- Work with an individual to recognize potential problems by evaluating the stressful life events the person is experiencing.
- Teach an individual specific coping skills, such as decision making, problem solving, assertiveness skills, meditation, and relaxation skills, to handle stressful events.
- Assist an individual in evaluating the timing or reduction of life changes to decrease the negative effects of stress as much as possible. This may involve working with a client to plan environmental changes, make important interpersonal decisions, and rethink changes in occupational roles.

Secondary

Secondary care establishes intervention during an acute crisis to *prevent* prolonged anxiety from diminishing personal effectiveness and personality organization. The nurse's primary focus is to ensure the safety of the client. After safety issues are dealt with, the nurse works with the client to assess the client's problem, support systems, and coping styles. Desired goals are explored and interventions planned. Secondary care lessens the time a person is mentally disabled during a crisis. Secondary-level care occurs in hospital units, emergency departments, clinics, or mental health centers, usually during daytime hours.

Tertiary

Tertiary care provides support for those who have experienced a severe crisis and are now recovering from a disabling mental state. Social and community facilities that offer tertiary intervention include rehabilitation centers, sheltered workshops, day hospitals, and outpatient clinics. Primary goals are to facilitate optimal levels of functioning and prevent further emotional disruptions. People with severe and persistent mental problems are often extremely susceptible to crisis, and community facilities provide the structured environment that can help prevent problem situations. Refer to Chapter 28 for strategies for crisis intervention and rehabilitation for people with severe and long-term mental illness. Box 22-2 lists Nursing Interventions Classification (NIC) interventions for responding to a crisis (Dochterman & Bulechek, 2004).

Critical Incident Stress Debriefing. Critical incident stress debriefing (CISD) is an example of a tertiary intervention directed toward a group that has experienced a crisis (Everly, Lating, & Mitchell, 2000). CISD consists of a seven-phase group meeting that offers individuals the opportunity to share their

BOX 22-2

Crisis Intervention (NIC)

Definition: Use of short-term counseling to help the patient cope with a crisis and resume a state of functioning comparable to or better than the precrisis state
Activities:

- Provide an atmosphere of support.
- Determine whether the patient presents a safety risk to self or others.
- Initiate necessary precautions to safeguard the patient or others at risk for physical harm.
- Encourage expression of feelings in a nondestructive manner.
- Assist in identification of the precipitants and dynamics of the crisis.
- Assist in identification of past and present coping skills and their effectiveness.
- Assist in identification of personal strengths and abilities that can be used in resolving the crisis.
- Assist in development of new coping and problem-solving skills, as needed.
- Assist in identification of available support systems.
- Provide guidance about how to develop and maintain support system(s).
- Introduce the patient to persons (or groups) who have successfully undergone the same experience.
- Assist in identification of alternative courses of action to resolve the crisis.
- Assist in evaluation of the possible consequences of the various courses of action.
- Assist the patient to decide on a particular course of action.
- Assist in formulating a time frame for implementation of the chosen course of action.
- Evaluate with the patient whether the crisis has been resolved by the chosen course of action.
- Plan with the patient how adaptive coping skills can be used to deal with crises in the future.

From Dochterman, J. M., & Bulechek, G. M. (2004). *Nursing interventions classification (NIC)* (4th ed.). St. Louis, MO: Mosby.

thoughts and feelings in a safe and controlled environment. CISD is used to debrief staff on an inpatient unit following the suicide of a client; to debrief staff following incidents of client violence; to debrief crisis hotline volunteers; to debrief schoolchildren and school personnel after multiple shootings have occurred in a school; and to debrief rescue and health care workers who have responded to a natural disaster or a terrorist attack such as that on the World Trade Center (Hammond & Brooks, 2001).

The phases of CISD are the following (Everly et al., 2000):

- *Introductory phase*—The purpose of the meeting is explained; an overview of the debriefing process is provided; participants are motivated; confiden-

tiality is assured; guidelines are explained; team members are identified; and questions are answered.
- *Fact phase*—Participants are assisted in discussing the facts of the incident; participants are asked to introduce themselves and tell how they were involved in the incident and what happened from their perspective.
- *Thought phase*—Every participant is asked to discuss his or her first thoughts of the incident.
- *Reaction phase*—Participants engage in freewheeling discussion and talk about the worst thing about the incident—what they would like to forget and what was most painful.
- *Symptom phase*—Participants describe cognitive, physical, emotional, or behavioral experiences that they had at the scene of the incident and describe any symptoms they felt following the initial experience.
- *Teaching phase*—The normality of the symptoms that have been expressed is acknowledged and affirmed; anticipatory guidance is offered regarding future symptoms that may be experienced by participants; the group is involved in stress management techniques.
- *Reentry phase*—Participants review old material discussed; introduce new topics they want to discuss; ask questions; and discuss how they would like to bring closure to the debriefing. Debriefing team members answer questions, inform, and reassure; provide handouts and other written material; provide information on referral sources for additional help; and summarize the debriefing experience with encouragement, support, and appreciation.

The nurse performs secondary crisis intervention and meets with Susan twice weekly during the next 4 weeks. Susan is motivated to work with the social worker and the nurse to find another place to live. The nurse suggests several times that Susan start to see a counselor in the outpatient clinic after the crisis is over, so that she can talk about some of her pain. Susan is ambivalent and is already thinking she will return to her husband.

Three weeks after the battering episode, Susan has returned to her husband; she has convinced herself that he has changed his behavior despite the fact that he has not sought any help to control his anger.

■ EVALUATION

NOC includes a built-in measurement for each outcome and for the indicators that support the outcome. Each outcome is measured on a five-point Likert scale. This measurement allows the nurse to evaluate the effectiveness of the crisis intervention.

This evaluation is usually performed 4 to 8 weeks after the initial interview, although it can be done earlier (e.g., by the end of the visit the anxiety level will decrease from 1 = severe to 3 = moderate). If the intervention has been successful, the person's level of anxiety and ability to function should be at precrisis levels. Often, a person chooses to follow up on additional areas of concern and is referred to other agencies for more long-term work. Crisis intervention often serves to prepare a person for further treatment.

After 6 weeks, Susan and the nurse decide that the crisis is over. Susan remains aloof and distant. The nurse evaluates Susan as being in a moderate amount of emotional pain, but Susan feels she is doing well. The nurse's assessment indicates that Susan has other serious issues (e.g., low self-esteem, childhood abuse), and the nurse strongly suggests that she could benefit from further counseling. The decision, however, is up to Susan, who says she is satisfied with the way things are and again states that if she has any future problems she will return to the safe house counselor.

CASE STUDY and NURSING CARE PLAN 22-1   Crisis

Ms. Greg, the psychiatric nurse consultant, is called to the neurological unit. She is told that Mr. Raymond, a 43-year-old man with Guillain-Barré syndrome, is presenting a serious nursing problem and the staff has requested a consult. The disease has caused severe muscle weakness to the point that he is essentially paralyzed; however, he is able to breathe on his own.

The head nurse says that Mr. Raymond is hostile and sexually abusive to the nursing staff. His abusive language, demeaning attitude, and angry outbursts are having an adverse effect on the unit as a whole. The other nurses state that they feel ineffective and angry and that they have tried

to be patient and understanding; however, nothing seems to get through to him. The situation has affected the morale of the staff and, the nurses believe, the quality of their care.

Mr. Raymond, an American Indian, was employed as a taxicab driver. Six months before his admission to the hospital, he had given up drinking after years of episodic alcohol abuse. He is engaged to a woman who visits him every day.

He needs a great deal of assistance with every aspect of his activities of daily living. Because his muscle weakness is so severe, he has to be turned and positioned every 2 hours. He is fed through a gastrostomy tube.

■ ASSESSMENT

Ms. Greg gathers data from Mr. Raymond and the nursing staff and speaks with Mr. Raymond's fiancée.

Mr. Raymond's Perception of the Precipitating Event
During the initial interview, Mr. Raymond speaks to Ms. Greg angrily, using profanity and making lewd sexual suggestions. He also expresses anger about needing a nurse to "scratch my head and help me blow my nose." He still cannot figure out how his illness suddenly developed. He says the doctors told him that it was too early to know for sure if he would recover completely, but that the prognosis was good.

Mr. Raymond's Support System
Ms. Greg speaks with Mr. Raymond's fiancée. Mr. Raymond's relationships with his fiancée and with his American Indian cultural group are strong. With minimal ties outside their reservation, neither Mr. Raymond nor his fiancée have much knowledge of outside supportive agencies.

Mr. Raymond's Personal Coping Skills
Mr. Raymond comes from a strongly male-dominated subculture in which the man is expected to be a strong leader. His ability to be an independent person with the power to affect the direction of his life is central to his perception of being acceptable as a man.

Mr. Raymond feels powerless, out of control, and enraged. He is handling his anxiety by displacing these feelings onto the environment, namely, the staff and his fiancée. This redirection of anger temporarily lowers his anxiety and distracts him from painful feelings. When he intimidates others through sexual profanity and hostility, he feels temporarily in control and experiences an illusion of power. He uses displacement to relieve his painful levels of anxiety when he feels threatened.

Mr. Raymond's use of displacement is not adaptive, because the issues causing his distress are not being resolved. His anxiety continues to escalate. The effect his behavior is having on others causes them to move away from him. This withdrawal further increases his sense of isolation and helplessness.

Self-Assessment
Ms. Greg meets with the staff twice. The staff discuss their feelings of helplessness and lack of control stemming from their feelings of rejection by Mr. Raymond. They talk of their anger about Mr. Raymond's demeaning behavior and frustration about the situation. Ms. Greg points out to the staff that Mr. Raymond's feelings of helplessness, lack of control, and anger at his situation are the same feelings the staff are experiencing. Displacement of his feelings of helplessness and frustration by intimidating the staff gives

Continued

Mr. Raymond a brief feeling of control. It also distracts him from his own feelings of helplessness.

The nurses become more understanding of the motivation for the behavior Mr. Raymond employs to cope with moderate to severe levels of anxiety. The staff begins to focus more on the client and less on personal reactions, and decide together on two approaches they can try as a group. First, they will not take Mr. Raymond's behavior personally. Second, Mr. Raymond's feelings that are displaced will be refocused back to him.

■ NURSING DIAGNOSIS (NANDA)

On the basis of her assessment, Ms. Greg identifies three main problem areas in order of importance and formulates the following nursing diagnoses:

1. *Ineffective coping* related to inadequate coping methods, as evidenced by inappropriate use of defense mechanisms (displacement)
   - Anger directed toward staff and fiancée
   - Profanity and crude sexual remarks aimed at staff
   - Isolation related to staff withdrawal
   - Continued escalation of anxiety

2. *Powerlessness* related to lack of control over his health care environment, as evidenced by frustration over inability to perform previously uncomplicated tasks
   - Anger over nurses' having to "scratch my head and blow my nose"
   - Minimal awareness of available supports in larger community

3. *Ineffective coping* related to exhaustion of staff supportive capacity toward client, as evidenced by staff withdrawal and limited personal communication with client
   - Staff feels ineffective.
   - Morale of staff is poor.
   - Nurses believe that the quality of their care has been adversely affected.

■ OUTCOME CRITERIA (NOC)

Ms. Greg speaks to Mr. Raymond and tells him she would like to spend time with him for 15 minutes every morning and talk about his concerns. She suggests that there might be alternative ways he can handle his feelings, and community resources can be explored. Mr. Raymond gruffly agrees, saying, "You can visit me, if it will make you feel better." They make arrangements to meet at 7:30 AM for 15 minutes each morning.

For each nursing diagnosis the following outcomes are set:

Nursing Diagnosis	Short-Term Goal
1. *Ineffective coping* related to inadequate coping methods, as evidenced by inappropriate use of defense mechanisms (displacement)	1. Mr. Raymond will be able to name and discuss at least two feelings about his illness and lack of mobility by the end of the week.
2. *Powerlessness* related to lack of control over health care environment, as evidenced by frustration over inability to perform previously uncomplicated tasks	2. Mr. Raymond will be able to name two community organizations that can offer him information and support by the end of 2 weeks.
3. *Ineffective coping* related to exhaustion of staff supportive capacity toward client, as evidenced by staff withdrawal and limited personal communication with client	3. Staff and nurse consultant will discuss reactions and alternative nursing responses to Mr. Raymond's behavior twice within the next 7 days.

■ PLANNING

Ms. Greg creates a nursing care plan and shares it with the staff.

Nursing diagnosis: *Ineffective coping* related to inadequate coping methods, as evidenced by inappropriate use of defense mechanisms (displacement)

Supporting data

- Anger directed toward staff and fiancée
- Profanity and crude sexual remarks aimed at staff
- Isolation related to staff withdrawal
- Continued escalation of anxiety

Outcome criteria: By discharge, Mr. Raymond will state that he feels more comfortable discussing difficult feelings.

Short-Term Goal	Intervention	Rationale	Evaluation
1. By the end of the week, Mr. Raymond will be able to name and discuss at least two feelings about his illness and lack of mobility.	**1a.** Nurse will meet with client for 15 minutes at 7:30 AM each day for a week.	**1a.** Night is usually the most frightening for client; in early morning, feelings are closer to surface.	GOAL MET Within 7 days, Mr. Raymond is able to speak to nurse more openly about feelings of anger and frustration.
	1b. When client lashes out with verbal abuse, nurse will remain calm.	**1b.** Client perceives that nurse is in control of her feelings. This can be reassuring to client and can increase client's sense of security.	
	1c. Nurse will consistently redirect and refocus anger from environment back to client (e.g., "It must be difficult to be in this situation.").	**1c.** Refocusing feelings offers client opportunity to cope effectively with his anxiety and decreases need to act out toward staff and fiancée.	
	1d. Nurse will come on time each day and stay for allotted time.	**1d.** Consistency sets stage for trust and reinforces that client's anger will not drive nurse away.	

Nursing diagnosis: *Powerlessness* related to lack of control over health care environment, as evidenced by frustration over inability to perform previously uncomplicated tasks

Supporting data

- Anger over nurses' having to "scratch my head and help me blow my nose"
- Minimal awareness of available supports in larger community

Outcome criteria: By discharge, Mr. Raymond will have contacted at least one outside community support source.

Short-Term Goal	Intervention	Rationale	Evaluation
1. By the end of the 2 weeks, Mr. Raymond will be able to name and discuss at least two community organizations that can offer information and support.	**1a.** Nurse will spend time with client and his fiancée. Role of specific agencies and how they may be of use will be discussed.	**1a.** Both client and fiancée will have opportunity to ask questions with nurse present.	GOAL MET By the end of 10 days, Mr. Raymond and his fiancée can name two community resources they are interested in.
	1b. Nurse will introduce one agency at a time.	**1b.** Gradual introduction allows time for information to sink in and minimizes feeling of being pressured or overwhelmed.	At the end of 6 weeks, Mr. Raymond has contacted the Guillain-Barré Society.
	1c. Nurse will follow up but not push or persuade client to contact any of the agencies.	**1c.** Client is able to make own decisions once he has appropriate information.	

■ **INTERVENTION (NIC)**

The following morning, Ms. Greg goes into Mr. Raymond's room at 7:30 AM and sits by his bedside. At first, Mr. Raymond's comments are hostile.

Continued

Dialogue	Therapeutic Tool/Comment
Nurse: Mr. Raymond, I'm here as we discussed. I'll be spending 15 minutes with you every morning. We could use this time to talk about some of your concerns.	Nurse offers herself as a resource, gives information, and clarifies her role and client expectations. Night is the most difficult time for Mr. Raymond. In the early morning he will be the most vulnerable and open for therapeutic intervention and support.
Mr. R: Listen, sweetheart, my only concern is how to get a little sexual relief, get it?	
Nurse: Being hospitalized and partially paralyzed can be overwhelming for anyone. Perhaps you wish you could find some relief from your situation.	Nurse focuses on the process "need for relief" and not the sexual content. Encourages discussion of feelings. Sexual issues are often challenging to new nurses, and discussing their feelings and appropriate interventions with an experienced professional is important for their own growth and to the quality of the care they give.
Mr. R: What do you know, Ms. Know-it-all? I can't even scratch my nose without getting one of those fools to do it for me . . . and half the time those bitches aren't even around.	
Nurse: It must be difficult to have to ask people to do everything for you.	Nurse restates what the client says in terms of his feelings. Continues to refocus away from the environment back to the client.
Mr. R: Yeah. . . . The other night a fly got into the room and kept landing on my face. I had to shout for 5 minutes before one of those bitches came in, just to take the fly out of the room.	
Nurse: Having to rely on others for everything can be a terrifying experience for anyone. It sounds extremely frustrating for you.	Nurse acknowledges that frustration and anger would be a normal and healthy response for anyone in this situation. This encourages the client to talk about these feelings instead of acting them out.
Mr. R: Yeah. . . . It's a bitch . . . like a living hell.	

Ms. Greg continues to spend time with Mr. Raymond in the mornings. He is gradually able to talk more about his feelings of anger and frustration and is less apt to act with hostility toward the staff. As he begins to feel more in control, he becomes less defensive about others' caring for him.

After 2 weeks, Ms. Greg cuts her visits down to twice a week. Mr. Raymond is beginning to get back gross motor movements but is not walking yet. He still displaces much of his frustration and lack of control onto the environment, but he is better able to acknowledge the reality of his situation. He can identify what he is feeling and talk about those feelings briefly.

Dialogue	Therapeutic Tool/Comment
Nurse: What's happening? Your face looks tense this morning, Mr. Raymond.	Nurse observes the client's clenched fists, rigid posture, and tense facial expression.
Mr. R: I had to wait 10 minutes for a bedpan last night.	
Nurse: And you're angry about that.	Nurse verbalizes the implied.
Mr. R: Well, there were only two nurses on duty for 30 people, and the aide was on her break. . . . You can't expect them to be everywhere . . . but still. . . .	
Nurse: It may be hard to accept that people can't be there all the time for you.	Nurse validates the difficulty of accepting situations one does not like when one is powerless to make changes.
Mr. R: Well . . . that's the way it is in this place.	

■ EVALUATION

After 6 weeks, Mr. Raymond is able to get around with assistance, and his ability to perform his activities of daily living is increasing. Although Mr. Raymond is still angry and still feels overwhelmed at times, he is able to identify more of his feelings. He does not need to act them out so often. He is able to talk to his fiancée about his feelings, and he lashes out at her less. He is looking forward to going home, and his boss is holding his old job.

Mr. Raymond contacts the Guillain-Barré Society, which makes arrangements for a meeting with him. He is still thinking about Alcoholics Anonymous but believes he can handle this problem himself.

The staff feel more comfortable and competent in their relationships with Mr. Raymond. The goals have been met. Mr. Raymond and Ms. Greg both believe that the crisis is over, and their visits are terminated. Mr. Raymond is given the number of the crisis unit and encouraged to call if he has questions or feels the need to talk.

evolve Visit the Evolve website at http://evolve.elsevier.com/Varcarolis for a full case study for this client and more case studies and nursing care plans.

▪▪▪ KEY POINTS to REMEMBER

- A crisis is not a pathological state but a struggle for emotional balance.
- Crises offer opportunities for emotional growth but can also lead to personality disorganization.
- There are three types of crisis: maturational, situational, and adventitious.
- Crises are usually resolved within 4 to 6 weeks.
- Crisis intervention therapy is short term, from 1 to 6 weeks, and focuses on the present problem only.
- Resolution of a crisis takes three forms: a person emerges at a higher level, at the precrisis level, or at a lower level of functioning.
- Social support and intervention can promote successful resolution.
- Crisis therapists take an active and directive approach with the client in crisis.
- The client is an active participant in setting goals and planning possible solutions.

- Crisis intervention is usually aimed at the mentally healthy person who generally is functioning well but is temporarily overwhelmed and unable to function.
- The crisis model can be adapted to meet the needs of people in crisis who have long-term and persistent mental problems.
- The steps in crisis intervention are consistent with the steps of the nursing process.
- Specific qualities in the nurse that can facilitate effective intervention are a caring attitude, flexibility in planning care, an ability to listen, and an active approach.
- The basic goals of crisis intervention are to reduce the individual's anxiety level and to support the effort to return to the person's precrisis level of functioning.
- Critical incident stress debriefing is a group approach that helps groups of people who have been exposed to a crisis situation.

Visit the Evolve website at **http://evolve.elsevier.com/Varcarolis** for a posttest on the content in this chapter. *evolve*

Critical Thinking and Chapter Review

Visit the Evolve website at **http://evolve.elsevier.com/Varcarolis** for additional self-study exercises.
evolve

▪▪▪ CRITICAL THINKING

Write a short paragraph in response to each of the following questions.

1. List the three important areas of the crisis assessment once safety concerns have been identified. Give examples of two questions in each area that need to be answered before planning can take place.

2. Barbara, 21 years old and a junior in nursing school, tells her nursing instructor that her father (age 45 years) has just lost his job. Her father has been drinking heavily for years, and Barbara is having difficulty coping. Because of her father's alcoholism and the increased stress in her family, Barbara wants to leave school. Her mother has multiple sclerosis and thinks Barbara should quit school to take care of her.

   A. How many different types of crisis are going on in this family? Discuss the crises from the viewpoint of each individual family member.

   B. If this family came for crisis counseling, what areas would you assess and what kinds of questions would you ask to evaluate each member's individual needs and the needs of the family as a unit (perception of events, coping styles, social supports)?

   C. Formulate some tentative goals you might set in conjunction with the family.

   D. Identify by name appropriate referral agencies in your area that would be helpful if members of this

family were willing to expand their use of outside resources and stabilize the situation.

   E. How would you set up follow-up visits for this family? Would you see the family members together, alone, or in a combination during the crisis period (4 to 6 weeks)? How would you decide whether follow-up counseling was indicated?

▪▪▪ CHAPTER REVIEW

Choose the most appropriate answer.

1. Which statement about crisis theory will provide a basis for nursing intervention?

   1. A crisis is an acute, time-limited phenomenon experienced as an overwhelming emotional reaction to a problem perceived as unsolvable.

   2. A person in crisis has always had adjustment problems and has coped inadequately in his or her usual life situations.

   3. Crisis is precipitated by an event that enhances the person's self-concept and self-esteem.

   4. Nursing intervention in crisis situations rarely has the effect of ameliorating the crisis.

Continued

Critical Thinking and Chapter Review—cont'd

Visit the Evolve website at **http://evolve.elsevier.com/Varcarolis** for additional self-study exercises.

evolve

2. Ms. T, a single mother of four, comes to the crisis center 24 hours after an apartment fire in which all the family's household goods and clothing were lost. Ms. T. has no family in the area. Her efforts to mobilize assistance have been disorganized, and she is still without shelter. She is distraught and confused. The nurse assesses the situation as
   1. a maturational crisis.
   2. a situational crisis.
   3. an adventitious crisis.
   4. evidence of an inadequate personality.

3. As the nurse responds to the client in Question 2, the intervention that takes priority is to
   1. reduce anxiety.
   2. arrange shelter.
   3. contact out-of-area family.
   4. hospitalize and place on suicide precautions.

4. Which belief would be least helpful for a nurse working in crisis intervention to hold?
   1. A person in crisis is incapable of making decisions.
   2. The crisis counseling relationship is one between partners.
   3. Crisis counseling helps the client refocus to gain new perspectives on the situation.
   4. Anxiety reduction techniques are used so the client's inner resources can be accessed.

5. The highest-priority goal of crisis intervention is
   1. client safety.
   2. anxiety reduction.
   3. identification of situational supports.
   4. teaching of specific coping skills that are lacking.

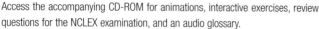

■ **STUDENT**
■ **STUDY**
■ **CD-ROM**

Access the accompanying CD-ROM for animations, interactive exercises, review questions for the NCLEX examination, and an audio glossary.

■ **NURSE,**
■ **CLIENT, AND**
■ **FAMILY RESOURCES**

For suggested readings, information on related associations, and Internet resources, go to **http://evolve.elsevier.com/Varcarolis**.   **evolve**

REFERENCES

Aguilera, D. C. (1998). *Crisis intervention: Theory and methodology* (8th ed.). St. Louis, MO: Mosby.

Aguilera, D. C., & Mesnick, J. (1970). *Crisis intervention: Theory and methodology.* St. Louis, MO: Mosby.

Behrman, G., & Reid, W. J. (2002). Post-trauma intervention: Basic tasks. *Brief Treatment and Crisis Intervention, 2,* 39-48.

Caplan, G. (1964). *Symptoms of preventive psychiatry.* New York: Basic Books.

Dochterman, J. M., & Bulechek, G. M. (2004). *Nursing interventions classification (NIC)* (4th ed.). St. Louis, MO: Mosby.

Everly, G. S., Jr. (2000). Crisis management briefings (CMB): Large group crisis intervention in response to terrorism, disasters and violence. *International Journal of Emergency Mental Health, 2,* 53-57.

Everly, G. S., Jr., Lating, J. M., & Mitchell, J. T. (2000). Innovations in group crisis intervention: Critical incident debriefing (CISD) and critical incident stress management (CISM). In A. R. Roberts, *Crisis interventions handbook: Assessment, treatment, and research* (2nd ed., pp. 77-100). New York: Oxford University Press.

Greenstone, J. L., & Leviton, S. C. (2002). *Elements of crisis intervention: Crises and how to respond to them* (2nd ed.). Pacific Grove, CA: Brooks/Cole.

Hammond, J., & Brooks, J. (2001). The world trade center attack. Helping the helpers: The role of critical incident stress management. *Critical Care, 5*(6), 315-317.

Holmes, T. H., & Rahe, R. H. (1967). The social readjustment rating scale. *Journal of Psychosomatic Research, 11*(2), 213-218.

Howard, J. M., & Goelitz, A. (2004). Psychoeducation as a response to community disaster. *Brief Treatment and Crisis Intervention, 4,* 1-10.

Joint Commission on Mental Illness and Health. (1961). *Action for mental health: Final report, 1961.* New York: Basic Books.

Jordan, K. (2003). A trauma and recovery model for victims and their families after a catastrophic school shooting: Focusing on behavioral, cognitive, and psychological effects and needs. *Brief Treatment and Crisis Intervention, 3,* 397-411.

Lowry, J. L., & Lating, J. M. (2002). Reflections on the response to mass terrorist attacks: An elaboration on Everly and Mitchell's 10 commandments. *Brief Treatment and Crisis Intervention, 2,* 95-104.

Moorhead, S., Johnson, M., & Maas, M. (2004). *Nursing outcomes classification (NOC)* (3rd ed.). St. Louis, MO: Mosby.

Regehr, C. (2001). Crisis debriefing groups for emergency responders: Reviewing the evidence. *Brief Treatment and Crisis Intervention, 1,* 87-100.

Roberts, A. R. (Ed.). (2000). *Crisis intervention handbook: Assessment, treatment, and research* (2nd ed., pp. 77-100). New York: Oxford University Press.

CHAPTER 23

Suicide

NANCY CHRISTINE SHOEMAKER ■ ELIZABETH M. VARCAROLIS

KEY TERMS and CONCEPTS

The key terms and concepts listed here appear in color where they are defined or first discussed in this chapter.

completed suicides, 473

copycat suicide, 475

lethality, 477

no-suicide contract, 481

parasuicide, 476

postvention, 480

primary intervention, 480

psychological autopsies, 475

SAD PERSONS scale, 478

secondary intervention, 480

suicidal ideation, 476

suicide, 475

suicide attempt, 476

tertiary intervention, 480

OBJECTIVES

After studying this chapter, the reader will be able to

1. Describe the profile of suicide in the United States, noting psychosocial and cultural factors that affect risk.
2. Identify three common precipitating events.
3. Name the most frequent coexisting psychiatric disorders.
4. Using the SAD PERSONS scale, explain ten risk factors to consider when assessing for suicide.
5. Describe three expected reactions a nurse may have when beginning work with suicidal clients.
6. Give examples of primary, secondary, and tertiary (postvention) interventions.
7. Describe basic level interventions that take place in the hospital or in the community.
8. Identify key elements of suicide precautions and environmental safety factors in the hospital.

evolve Visit the Evolve website at **http://evolve.elsevier.com/Varcarolis** for a pretest on the content in this chapter.

Suicide is a significant public health problem, and nurses frequently encounter clients at risk for suicide in inpatient settings, in outpatient treatment settings, and in the community. No age group, gender, or ethnic group is protected from this phenomenon, and each suicide traumatizes multiple suicide "survivors" (family and friends of a person who has committed suicide). However, suicide is largely preventable. The majority of people with suicidal ideation have a treatable psychiatric disorder and give clues about their suffering. It is estimated that only 1% of the people with suicidal ideation actually follow through and commit suicide (Shea, 1999, p. 19). This chapter reviews the facts about suicide and discusses approaches for assessment and care of suicidal clients and their loved ones.

PREVALENCE

In the United States, approximately 75 people commit suicide every day (Roy, 2000). In 2001, suicide was the eleventh leading cause of death, with 30,622 completed suicides or an age-adjusted rate of 10.7 per 100,000 (National Institute of Mental Health [NIMH], 2003). Suicide is the third leading cause of death among 14- to 25-year-olds, and the rate is 13 per 100,000 in this age group (American Psychiatric Association [APA], 2003). The elderly, defined as those aged 65 years and older, have the highest risk, with a rate of 15.3 per 100,000 (APA, 2003). It is estimated that at least 4.4 million Americans are suicide survivors, facing emotional distress and an increased risk of suicide themselves (American Association of Suicidology [AAS], 2004). Box 23-1 provides some facts about suicide, including data for specific age groups.

COMORBIDITY

Suicide is not a disorder per se, but studies show that more than 90% of suicide victims meet criteria for at least one psychiatric disorder at the time of death (APA, 2003, p. 11). Suicide occurs more frequently among those with the following disorders (Roy, 2000):

- Major depression and bipolar disorder
- Schizophrenia
- Alcohol and substance use disorders
- Borderline and antisocial personality disorders
- Panic disorder

It is estimated that two thirds of people who commit suicide are depressed at the time. One in 16 clients diagnosed with depression will commit suicide (AAS, 2000). Bipolar disorder is also a risk factor: 18.9% of deaths among bipolar clients are due to suicide (Russ, 2003). Loss of relationships, financial difficulty, and impulsivity are factors in this population (Roy, 2000).

Suicide risk is high among schizophrenic clients, especially during the first few years of the illness. Up to 10% of these clients die from suicide, which is usually related to depressive symptoms rather than to command hallucinations or delusions (Roy, 2000).

Clients with alcohol or substance use disorders also have a higher suicide risk. Years of abuse and comorbidity with depression or antisocial personality disorder are also factors associated with increased risk (Roy, 2000).

BOX 23-1

Suicide Facts

Overall

- Suicide is the eleventh leading cause of death in the United States, occurring at a rate of 10.7 per 100,000 persons (based on 2001 mortality data as coded according to the *International Statistical Classification of Diseases and Related Health Problems,* 10th revision)
- It is the eighth leading cause of death for males and the nineteenth leading cause of death for females.
- Suicides outnumber homicides by 3:2.
- More men than women die by suicide, with a gender ratio of 4:1.
- Suicide by firearm is the most common method for both men and women.
- The highest suicide rate is in white men older than 85 years, among whom the rate is 54 per 100,000.
- Suicide rates are highest in the mountain states, in which the rates of firearms ownership are also the highest (APA, 2003).
- Occupations with the highest risk of suicide are physician and dentist; nursing and social work also have elevated risk compared to other occupations (APA, 2003).

Suicide in the Elderly

- The elderly (over 65 years of age) make up 12.6% of the population but account for 18.1% of suicides.
- For persons aged 65 to 74 years, the rate is 12.6 per 100,000; for persons 75 to 84 years, the rate is 17.7 per 100,000.
- Eighty-four percent of elderly suicide victims are men, five times the number of elderly women dying by suicide.
- The elderly attempt suicide less often but have a higher completion rate because their methods are more lethal.
- Two thirds of adults in their sixties, seventies, and eighties were in relatively good health when they died by suicide.
- Seventy-five percent of elderly victims over the age of 75 years were seen by a primary care physician within a month of their suicide.

- Some 66% to 90% of elderly suicide victims had at least one psychiatric diagnosis; two thirds of these diagnoses were late-onset, single-episode depression.

Suicide in Youth

- Suicide is the third leading cause of death for youth 14 to 24 years of age, after accidents and homicides.
- In 2000, 13.6% of all suicides in the United States were committed by persons under the age of 25 years.
- The suicide rate for adolescents 14 to 19 years of age is 7.9 per 100,000, and the rate for young adults 20 to 24 years of age is 12 per 100,000.
- Suicide rates for 14- to 24-year-olds doubled from the 1950s to the 1970s, were stable at this high level up to the mid-1990s, and showed a slight decline by 2000.
- Firearms are the most commonly used suicide method, accounting for almost three of five completed suicides.
- Male to female ratios are 3:1 for 10- to 14-year-olds; 5:1 for 15- to 19-year-olds; and 7:1 for 20- to 24-year-olds.
- The largest increase in suicide rates since 1980 has been among black male youth (10 to 19 years).
- Self-report surveys show that, nationwide, one in five high school students has seriously considered attempting suicide in the preceding 12 months.

Attempted Suicide

- There are an estimated 8 to 25 attempted suicides for each suicide death.
- Women report more history of attempted suicide than men, with a gender ratio of 3:1.
- Most adolescent suicide attempts are precipitated by interpersonal conflicts.
- As many as 75% of depressed older Americans are not receiving treatment, which places them at increased risk for suicide.

Data from American Association of Suicidology. (2002, October 4). *Elderly suicide fact sheet.* Retrieved February 8, 2005, from http://www.suicidology.org; and National Institute of Mental Health (2004, April 19). *Suicide facts and statistics.* Retrieved April 13, 2005, from http://www.nimh.nih.gov/suicideprevention/suifact.cfm.

Clients with borderline and antisocial personality disorder are at risk, and comorbid substance use or depression is frequent (Roy, 2000). Among clients with borderline personality disorder, the suicide rate is 10%; such suicides often occur in females later in their course of treatment when they perceive that treatment is unsuccessful (Paris, 2002).

The NIMH Epidemiologic Catchment Area Study found that 20% of people with panic disorder had made a suicide attempt (Roy, 2000). This rate is similar to that of clients with major depression. Among adolescents, in particular, one study noted that a history of panic attacks is associated with a three times greater likelihood of suicidal ideation and two times greater likelihood of suicide attempts (Brown, 2003).

It is important to keep in mind, however, that suicide is not necessarily synonymous with a mental disorder. The act of purposeful self-destruction represented by taking one's own life is usually accompanied by intense feelings of pain and hopelessness, coupled with the belief that there are no solutions.

THEORY
Biological Factors

Twin studies and adoption studies suggest the presence of genetic factors in suicide (Roy, 2000). For example, suicide rates in twins are higher among monozygotic twins than among dizygotic twins. Studies found a significantly higher incidence of suicide among biological relatives of adoptees who committed suicide than among the biological relatives of control subjects.

Low levels of the neurotransmitter serotonin are thought to play a part in the decision to commit suicide (Roy, 2000). Low serotonin levels are related to depressed mood. Studies have found low levels of serotonin or its metabolites in the cerebrospinal fluid of suicidal clients. Postmortem studies of suicide victims also reveal a low level in the brainstem or the frontal cortex.

Suicidal behavior seems to run in families. For example, Margaux Hemingway's death in 1996 was the fifth suicide among four generations of Ernest Hemingway's family. However, it is difficult to distinguish biochemical or genetic predisposition to suicide from predisposition to depression or alcoholism.

A final point related to biological risk factors is the role of physical disorders in suicide. Physical illness is considered an important factor in 11% to 51% of suicides, and the percentage increases with age (Roy, 2000). Refer to Box 23-2 for a list of diagnoses associated with increased risk. It is notable that depression often accompanies these conditions and may be the causative factor.

BOX 23-2

Somatic Conditions Associated with Increased Suicide Risk

- Acquired immunodeficiency syndrome (AIDS)
- Cancer
- Cardiovascular disease
- Cerebrovascular disease
- Chronic renal failure with hemodialysis
- Cirrhosis
- Cushing's disease
- Dementia
- Epilepsy
- Head injury
- Huntington's disease
- Multiple sclerosis
- Peptic ulcer
- Prostatic hypertrophy

Psychosocial Factors

Freud originally theorized that suicide resulted from aggression turned inward toward an internalized love object (i.e., a repressed desire to kill someone). Karl Menninger added to Freud's thought by describing three parts of suicidal hostility: the wish to kill, the wish to be killed, and the wish to die (Roy, 2000). Aaron Beck identified a central emotional factor underlying suicide intent as hopelessness. The suicidal persons most likely to act out suicidal fantasies are those who have experienced the following (Roy, 2000):

- A loss of love
- A narcissistic injury (humiliation, loss of job, threat of incarceration)
- Overwhelming moods such as rage or guilt
- Identification with a suicide victim (copycat suicide)

Other motivations include revenge, reunion with a loved one, or rebirth. Adolescents have a special risk of impulsive suicide known as copycat suicide. A copycat suicide follows a highly publicized suicide of a public figure, an idol, or a peer in the community (Pataki, 2000). Certain cognitive styles also contribute to higher risk: rigid all-or-nothing thinking, inability to see different options, and perfectionism (APA, 2003). The suicidal client is often ambivalent about death and therein lies the key to helping the individual examine alternative actions to reduce the pain. Extensive data are available about risk factors for suicide, based on epidemiological studies and psychological autopsies (i.e., retrospective reviews of the deceased person's life within several months of death to establish likely diagnoses at the time of death) (APA, 2003). There is also evidence concerning protective factors (those that tend to reduce risk). Refer to Box 23-3

BOX 23-3

Suicide Risk Factors and Protective Factors

Risk Factors
- Suicidal ideation with intent
- Lethal suicide plan
- History of suicide attempt
- Co-occurring psychiatric illness (see text)
- Co-occurring medical illness (see Box 23-2)
- History of childhood abuse
- Family history of suicide
- Recent lack of social support (isolation)
- Unemployment
- Recent stressful life event (e.g., death, other loss)
- Hopelessness
- Panic attacks
- Feeling of shame or humiliation
- Impulsivity
- Aggressiveness
- Loss of cognitive function (e.g., loss of impulse control)
- Access to firearms
- Substance abuse (without formal disorder)

Protective Factors
- Sense of responsibility to family (spouse, children)
- Pregnancy
- Religious beliefs
- Satisfaction with life
- Positive social support
- Effective coping skills
- Effective problem-solving skills
- Intact reality testing

Data from American Psychiatric Association. (2003). Practice guidelines for the assessment and treatment of patients with suicidal behaviors. *American Journal of Psychiatry, 160*(11 Suppl.), 12.

for a description of significant psychosocial risk and protective factors for suicide.

Cultural Factors

Cultural factors, including religious beliefs, family values, and attitude toward death, have an impact on suicide rates. Generally, in the United States, European Americans have twice the suicide rate of minority groups (Hispanic Americans, African Americans, and Asian Americans) (APA, 2003). The exception is Native Americans, among whom the suicide rate is equal to that of European Americans. Refer to the Culturally Speaking box for a description of factors related to suicide among Native Americans.

Among African Americans, men commit suicide more often than women and the peak rate occurs in adolescence and young adulthood. Protective factors for this group as a whole include religion and the role of the extended family, both of which provide a strong social support system. Similarly, among Hispanic

■ ■ ■ CULTURALLY SPEAKING

The suicide rate among Native Americans—13.6 per 100,000—is higher than the overall United States rate and twice as high as the rate for other minority groups (APA, 2003). The male to female ratio is 12:1 and the median age of the Native American victim is 25 years. Although the rates are different in various tribes, the factors that seem to contribute to the higher risk include frequent alcohol or substance abuse; high unemployment; loss of tribal identity and cohesion with westernization; poor living conditions on the reservation; and a more accepting view toward death, including beliefs about the close contact between the human and spirit worlds and belief in reincarnation.

Data from Range, L. M., et al. (1999). Multicultural perspectives on suicide. *Aggression and Violent Behavior, 4*(4), 413-430; and American Psychiatric Association. (2003). Practice guideline for the assessment and treatment of patients with suicidal behaviors. *American Journal of Psychiatry, 160*(11 Suppl.), 1-60.

Americans, Roman Catholic religion (in which suicide is a sin) and the importance given to the extended family decrease the risk for suicide. There is also the philosophy of *fatalismo,* a belief that divine providence regulates the world, so that the individual is deemed unable to control adverse events and is more likely to accept misfortune instead of blaming the self.

Among Asian Americans, suicide rates are noted to increase with age. Beliefs that reduce suicide include adherence to religions that tend to emphasize interdependence between the individual and society (i.e., self-destruction is seen as disrespectful to the group or selfish). However, the high value given to the reputation of the family may lead at times to the conclusion that suicide is preferable if it prevents shame to the family. Also, the Japanese Shinto religion includes a belief in reincarnation, so that death may be seen as a potential honorable solution to life problems (Range et al., 1999).

■ *Application of the Nursing Process*

The process of suicide risk assessment is comprehensive and is based on identifying specific risk factors, taking a psychosocial and medical history, and interacting with the client during the interview. The nurse usually completes this assessment in conjunction with a physician or other clinician. In fact, comparison of data from two interviewers is often a significant element of the evaluation. Not all clients who show suicidal ideation or who make a suicide attempt truly want to die. Parasuicide (i.e., nonfatal self-injury with a clear intent to cause bodily harm or death) is a common event (Comtois, 2002). Parasuicide is a clear risk factor for suicide—about half of all people who kill themselves have a history of parasuicide. Parasuicide with a lethal intent requires emergency hospitalization just as does any other behavior carrying serious risk.

If there is not a clear desire to die, however, suicidal or self-destructive feelings can be treated in the outpatient setting. Follow-up studies of suicidal clients who came to the emergency department sometimes show that hospitalization was not necessary. Clients may report suicidal ideation when they are desperate about social problems such as homelessness or legal charges. One study evaluated 137 hospital admissions and coined the term *contingent suicidality* (i.e., clients told emergency staff that they would kill themselves if they were not admitted or, after admission, confessed that they had exaggerated their symptoms to get into the hospital) (Lambert, 2002, p. 12). Over the following 7 years, none of the contingently suicidal clients committed suicide, but 10 of 92 noncontingently suicidal clients did kill themselves. Alternate services that could be offered to contingently suicidal clients include crisis intervention, addiction treatment, social services, and legal assistance. In another study in Canada, treatment of suicidal adolescents by a rapid-response outpatient team immediately after emergency evaluation produced improved functioning without subsequent hospitalizations or suicide attempts (Greenfield et al., 2002).

■ ASSESSMENT
Verbal and Nonverbal Clues

Almost all people considering suicide send out clues, especially to people they think of as supportive. Nurses often fit into this category. There may be overt or covert verbal clues and nonverbal signals. Examples include the following:

Overt statements
- "I can't take it anymore."
- "Life isn't worth living anymore."
- "I wish I were dead."
- "Everyone would be better off if I died."

Covert statements
- "It's OK now. Soon everything will be fine."
- "Things will never work out."
- "I won't be a problem much longer."
- "Nothing feels good to me anymore, and probably never will."
- "How can I give my body to medical science?"

Most often it is a relief for people contemplating suicide finally to talk to someone about their despair and loneliness. **Asking someone if he or she is thinking of suicide does not "give a person ideas."** Self-destructive ideas are a personal decision. Talking openly about suicide leads to a decrease in isolation and can increase problem-solving alternatives for living. People who attempt suicide, even those who re-gret the failure of their attempt, are often extremely receptive to talking about their suicide crisis. Specific questions to ask about suicidal ideation include the following (APA, 2003):

- Have you ever felt that life was not worth living?
- Have you been thinking about death recently?
- Did you ever think about suicide?
- Have you ever attempted suicide?
- Do you have a plan for committing suicide?
- If so, what is your plan for suicide?

The following dialogue illustrates how the nurse can make covert messages more open:

Nurse: You haven't eaten or slept well for the past few days, Mary.

Mary: No, I feel pretty low lately.

Nurse: How low are you feeling?

Mary: Oh, I don't know. Nothing seems to matter to me anymore. It's all so meaningless. . . .

Nurse: What is meaningless, Mary?

Mary: Life . . . the whole thing . . . nothingness. Life is a bad joke.

Nurse: Are you saying that you don't think life is worth living?

Mary: Well . . . yes. It's all so hopeless anyway.

Nurse: Are you thinking of killing yourself, Mary?

Mary: Oh, I don't know. Well, sometimes I think about it. I probably would never go through with it.

Nurse: Let's talk more about what you are thinking and feeling. Since this is important, Mary, I will need to share your thoughts with other members of the staff.

The nurse should also be alert for nonverbal behavioral clues, including showing a sudden brightening of mood with more energy, giving away possessions, or organizing financial affairs.

Lethality of Suicide Plan

The evaluation of a suicide plan is extremely important in determining the degree of suicidal risk. Three main elements must be considered when evaluating lethality (APA, 2003): (1) Is there a specific plan with details? (2) How lethal is the proposed method? (3) Is there access to the planned method? People who have definite plans for the time, place, and means are at high risk.

Based on the lethality of a method, which indicates how quickly a person would die by that mode, a method can be classified as higher or lower risk. Higher-risk methods, also referred to as "hard" methods, include
- Using a gun.
- Jumping off a high place.
- Hanging oneself.
- Poisoning with carbon monoxide.
- Staging a car crash.

Examples of lower-risk methods, also referred to as "soft" methods, are

- Slashing one's wrists.
- Inhaling natural gas.
- Ingesting pills.

When the proposed method is available, the situation is more serious. For example, a man who has access to a high building and states that he will jump from it, or a woman who has a gun and says that she will shoot herself, is at serious risk for suicide. When people are psychotic, they are at high risk regardless of the specificity of details, because impulse control and judgment are grossly impaired. A psychotic person is particularly vulnerable if depressed or experiencing command hallucinations.

Assessment Tools

Many tools have been developed to aid a health care worker in assessing suicidal potential. Patterson and co-workers (1983) devised an assessment aid with the acronym *SAD PERSONS* to evaluate 10 major risk factors for suicide (Box 23-4). The SAD PERSONS scale is a simple, clearcut, and practical guide for gauging suicide potential. Ten categories are described in the assessment tool, and the person being evaluated is assigned one point for each applicable characteristic. The total points for the individual are compared with a

BOX 23-4

SAD PERSONS Scale

S	Sex	1 if male
A	Age	1 if 25 to 44 years or 65+ years
D	Depression	1 if present
P	Previous attempt	1 if present
E	Ethanol use	1 if present
R	Rational thinking loss	1 if psychotic for any reason
S	Social supports lacking	1 if lacking, especially recent loss
O	Organized plan	1 if plan with lethal method
N	No spouse	1 if divorced, widowed, separated, or single male
S	Sickness	1 if severe or chronic

Guidelines for Action

Points	Clinical Action
0-2	Send home with follow-up
3-4	Closely follow up; consider hospitalization
5-6	Strongly consider hospitalization
7-10	Hospitalize or commit

From Patterson, W. M., et al. (1983). Evaluation of suicidal patients: The SAD PERSONS scale. *Psychosomatics, 24*(4), 343.

scale, which assists health care workers in determining whether hospital admission is advisable.

Self-Assessment

People who are suicidal demonstrate behavior that is difficult for nurses to manage effectively. *All* health care professionals who work with suicidal people need supervision and guidance by a more experienced clinician. Most people who are suicidal experience extreme feelings: hopelessness, helplessness, ambivalence, and anger. Affects such as these can stir up strong negative reactions in others. Staff often respond with fear, grief, anger, puzzlement, or condemnation (Shea, 1999). If these intense emotional responses are not acknowledged, the countertransference will limit effective intervention, because suicidal clients are especially sensitive to rejection.

The following are universal reactions toward suicidal clients in any health care setting.

Anxiety. Anxiety may have numerous sources: concern about professional consequences if the client is injured; response to the suicidal ideation as a personal rejection; thoughts about one's own death. Nurses must become aware of their own anxiety and attempt to identify the unmet need or expectation. Personal anxiety can then be reduced and not transferred to the client.

Irritation. People who make repeated suicide attempts are often accused by family as well as health care workers of just "trying to get attention" or "looking for sympathy." It is common to hear frustrated friends or family members telling a suicidal person to "go ahead and get it over with." Such remarks by family and health providers strip the suicidal person of all hope and serve as an encouragement to act. No matter how trivial the suicide attempt may appear, it must be taken seriously. It is a genuine communication that the person is unable to find a way out of a desperate situation or state of mind.

Avoidance. People who are suicidal are frequently kept at a distance when they do not show improvement. Staff avoid situations or people that stimulate feelings of helplessness and incompetence. Clinical supervision can help the nurse reduce the need to feel "in control" or to feel responsible for client decisions. Then the nurse can refocus energy back to the client.

Denial. Denying or minimizing suicidal ideation or gestures is a defense against experiencing the feelings aroused by a suicidal person. Denial can be seen in statements such as "I can't understand why anyone would want to take his own life." Often, family members and health care professionals are unable to acknowledge suicidal tendencies in someone close to them. Denial also occurs when identification with a suicidal person is strong, such as when a colleague commits suicide. As noted in Box 23-1, health care professionals are at higher risk for suicide. It has been suggested that the topic should be openly discussed with physicians, starting in medical school and continuing through all work sites (Myers & Fine, 2003). This same advice can be applied to nursing professionals. If you ever feel suicidal, remember the following:

- Do not remain alone.
- Call 911 or the emergency telephone number listed in the front of the telephone book or on-line.
- If you cannot talk to a stranger, contact a relative, friend, or another health care professional.
- There is always another point of view for your situation, no matter how desperate you feel. The immediate crisis will pass if you seek help (Mayo clinic.com, 2004).

Assessment Guidelines Suicide

1. Assess risk factors, including history of suicide (in family, friends), degree of hopelessness and helplessness, and lethality of plan.
2. If there is a history of suicide attempt, assess
   - Intent: Was there a high probability of being discovered?
   - Lethality: Was the method used highly lethal or less lethal?
   - Injury: Did the client suffer physical harm (e.g., was client admitted to intensive care unit)?
3. Determine whether the client's age, medical condition, or psychiatric diagnosis put the client at higher risk.
4. Consider a red flag to be raised if the client suddenly goes from sad or depressed to happy and peaceful. Often a decision to commit suicide gives a feeling of relief and calm.
5. If the client is to be managed on an outpatient basis, also assess
   - Social supports.
   - Significant others' knowledge of the signs of potential suicidal ideation (e.g., increasing withdrawal, preoccupation, silence, and remorse).

■ NURSING DIAGNOSIS

The nursing diagnoses for a person who is suicidal may address many areas. However, the nursing diagnosis with the highest priority is *risk for suicide* related to various emotional states. As noted earlier, feelings of hopelessness, anger, frustration, abandonment, and rejection are common among people who are suicidal. Table 23-1 identifies a number of nursing diagnoses that may apply.

TABLE 23-1

Potential Nursing Diagnoses for the Suicidal Client

Signs and Symptoms	Potential Nursing Diagnoses
Gives overt or covert clues (e.g., "I can't stand the pain"), has a plan (gun), is in high-risk category on assessment (elderly or teenager, isolated, depressed, has had a recent loss), has a psychiatric diagnosis (substance abuse, depression, borderline personality disorder, psychosis)	**Risk for suicide**
Overwhelmed with situational crises, relies heavily on drugs or alcohol, has few supportive systems, shows poor problem-solving skills, has "tunnel vision"; no family available, or crisis in the family, poor family communication	**Ineffective coping** **Disabled family coping**
Lacks hope for the future; believes that nothing can change intolerable situation; has intense feelings of isolation, deprivation, lack of love, having nowhere to turn; believes that he or she has no control over the future	**Hopelessness** **Powerlessness** **Social isolation** **Spiritual distress** **Loneliness**
Believes that he or she is no good, worthless, ineffective, a burden to others, can't do anything right	**Situational low self-esteem** **Chronic low self-esteem**
Does not understand age-related crises; does not know of available resources	**Deficient knowledge**

■ OUTCOME CRITERIA

Relevant Nursing Outcomes Classification (NOC) outcomes include *Suicide Self-Restraint, Coping, Hope, Social Support, Spiritual Health,* and *Self-Esteem* (Moorhead, Johnson, & Maas, 2004). Refer to Table 23-2 for examples of short-term and intermediate indicators for suicidal clients.

■ PLANNING

The plan of care for the suicidal client is based on the assessment of risk factors. When a psychiatric disorder is present, the treatment plan includes appropriate

TABLE 23-2

NOC Outcomes for Suicidal Clients

Nursing Outcome and Definition	Intermediate Indicators	Short-Term Indicators
Suicide Self-Restraint: Personal actions to refrain from gestures and attempts at killing self*	Maintains self-control without supervision	Discloses plan for suicide if present Refrains from attempting suicide
Coping: Personal actions to manage stressors that tax an individual's resources*	Reports decrease in stress	Verbalizes need for assistance
Hope: Optimism that is personally satisfying and life-supporting*	Sets goals	Expresses will to live
Self-Esteem: Personal judgment of self-worth†	Verbalizations of self-acceptance	Feelings about self-worth
Social Support: Perceived availability and actual provision of reliable assistance from others‡	Emotional assistance provided by others	Willingness to call on others for help
Spiritual Health: Connectedness with self, others, higher power, all life, nature, and the universe that transcends and empowers the self§	Connectedness with others	Interaction with others to share thoughts, feelings, and beliefs

From Moorhead, S., Johnson, M., & Maas, M. (2004). *Nursing outcomes classification (NOC)* (3rd ed.). St. Louis, MO: Mosby.
*Evaluated on a five-point Likert scale from 1 (never demonstrated) to 5 (consistently demonstrated).
†Evaluated on a five-point Likert scale from 1 (never positive) to 5 (consistently positive).
‡Evaluated on a five-point Likert scale from 1 (not adequate) to 5 (totally adequate).
§Evaluated on a five-point Likert scale from 1 (severely compromised) to 5 (not compromised).

nursing approaches (e.g., care for depressed or schizophrenic clients). The client's significant others need to be involved in the plan, because the client's perception of total isolation is a significant cause of hopelessness. Refer to Case Study and Nursing Care Plan 23-1 at the end of the chapter.

■ INTERVENTION

The Surgeon General's *Call to Action* (U.S. Public Health Service, 1999) emphasizes the following factors regarding suicide prevention:

- Interventions are more likely to be successful if they involve a variety of services and providers.
- Interventions must be developed and tested to provide a "fit." Factors such as age, gender, and ethnic and cultural group are considerations in formulating effective interventions.
- Suicide prevention must recognize and affirm the value, dignity, and importance of each person.

Levels of Intervention

Nursing interventions for suicide take place at three different levels: primary, secondary, and tertiary.

1. Primary intervention includes activities that provide support, information, and education to prevent suicide. Primary intervention can be practiced in schools, homes, hospitals, and work settings. See Box 23-5 for methods of developing effective suicide prevention strategies.

BOX 23-5

Methodology to Advance the Science of Suicide Prevention

- Enhance research to understand risk factors and protective factors related to suicide, their interaction, and their effects on suicide and suicidal behaviors. In addition, increase research on effective suicide prevention programs, clinical treatments for suicidal individuals, and culture-specific interventions.
- Develop additional scientific strategies for evaluating suicide prevention interventions and ensure that evaluation components are included in all suicide prevention programs.
- Establish mechanisms for federal, regional, and state interagency public health collaboration toward improving monitoring systems for suicide and suicidal behaviors and develop and promote standard terminology in these systems.
- Encourage the development and evaluation of new prevention technologies, including firearm safety measures, to reduce easy access to lethal means of suicide.

U.S. Public Health Service. (1999). *The Surgeon General's call to action to prevent suicide.* Washington, DC: Author.

2. Secondary intervention is treatment of the actual suicidal crisis. It is practiced in clinics, in hospitals, and on telephone hotlines.
3. Tertiary intervention (or postvention) refers to interventions with the family and friends of a person who has committed suicide to reduce the traumatic aftereffects.

Basic Level Interventions

The Nursing Interventions Classification (NIC) offers the following topics pertinent to the care of the suicidal client: *Suicide Prevention, Hope Instillation, Coping Enhancement, Self-Esteem Enhancement, Family Mobilization,* and *Support System Enhancement* (Dochterman & Bulechek, 2004).

In the hospital or community setting, the basic level registered nurse (RN) utilizes counseling, health teaching, case management, and psychobiological interventions. During the acute suicidal crisis on the inpatient unit, suicide precautions are carried out as a specialized form of milieu therapy.

Milieu Therapy with Suicide Precautions

Implementing suicide precautions for the acutely suicidal client is one of the most challenging roles for the inpatient nurse. In accordance with unit policies and procedures, the client is observed continuously by nursing staff. Refer to Table 23-3 for a general description of suicide precautions. This intense attention from the nurse provides for safety and also allows for constant reassessment of risk. Monitoring flow sheets for suicide precautions are more clinically useful if they include a description of affect as well as behavior. For example, instead of noting "Client watching television," the nurse can describe the client's affect at each observation interval (hostile, fearful, calm, etc.). Flow sheets should also indicate clear accountability for staff starting and ending their periods of observation

(Temkin & Crotty, 2004). In addition to observing the client, the nurse is responsible for monitoring the environment for safety hazards. Review Box 23-6 for guidelines on how to minimize physical risks in the milieu.

Studies show that acute care of suicidal clients is usually effective. Only 15% of psychiatric clients who commit suicide do so as inpatients (Roy, 2000). Even in these cases, the suicide usually does not happen on the unit but in stairwells, in other hospital buildings, or on the grounds. Suicide risk is highest in the first few days of admission and during times of staff rotation, particularly rotation of psychiatric residents. Assessment of suicidal risk must be an ongoing process; assessment should be performed particularly before a change in level of observation or upon sudden improvement or worsening of symptoms.

Counseling

Counseling skills, including interviewing, crisis care, and problem-solving techniques, are used in both the inpatient and outpatient settings. The key element is establishing a working alliance to encourage the client to engage in more realistic problem solving. Helpful staff characteristics include warmth, sensitivity, interest, and consistency. After hospitalization, the nurse may see these clients in the clinic, in a partial hospital program, or in home care. One particular aspect of counseling is the use of a no-suicide contract (also called a *no-harm contract*). This is a written contract in which the client agrees not to harm himself or herself but to take an alternative action if feeling suicidal (e.g.,

TABLE 23-3

Suicide Precautions with Constant One-to-One Observation

Staff Assessment	Possible Client Symptoms	Nursing Responsibilities
Client with suicidal ideation or delusions of self-mutilation who, according to assessment by unit staff, presents clinical symptoms that suggest a clear intent to follow through with the plan or delusion	1. Client is currently verbalizing a clear intent to harm self. 2. Client is unwilling to make a no-suicide contract. 3. Client shows no insight into existing problems. 4. Client has poor impulse control. 5. Client has already attempted suicide in the recent past by a particularly lethal method (e.g., hanging, gun, carbon monoxide poisoning).	1. Conduct one-to-one nursing observation and interaction 24 hours a day (never let client out of staff's sight). 2. Maintain arm's length at all times. 3. Chart client's whereabouts and record mood, verbatim statements, and behavior every 15 to 30 minutes per protocol. 4. Ensure that meal trays contain no glass or metal silverware. 5. During observation when client is sleeping, **hands should always be in view,** not under the bedcovers. 6. Carefully observe client swallow each dose of medication. 7. The nurse and physician should explain to the client what they will be doing and why; both document this in the chart.

BOX 23-6

Environmental Guidelines for Minimizing Suicidal Behavior on the Psychiatric Unit

1. Use plastic eating utensils.
2. Do not assign client to a private room.
3. Jump-proof and hang-proof the bathrooms by installing break-away shower rods and recessed shower nozzles.
4. Keep electrical cords to a minimal length.
5. Install unbreakable glass in windows. Install tamper-proof screens or partitions too small to pass through. Keep all windows locked.
6. Lock all utility rooms, kitchens, adjacent stairwells, and offices. All nonclinical staff (e.g., housekeepers, maintenance workers) should receive instructions to keep doors locked.
7. Take all potentially harmful gifts (e.g., flowers in glass vases) from visitors before allowing them to see clients.
8. Go through client's belongings with client and remove all potentially harmful objects (e.g., belts, shoelaces, metal nail files, tweezers, matches, razors, perfume, and shampoo).
9. Ensure that visitors do not leave potentially harmful objects in client's room (e.g., matches, nail files).
10. Search client for harmful objects (e.g., drugs, sharp objects, cords) on return from pass.

talk with staff, call a crisis line). Refer to the Evidence-Based Practice box for an evaluation of the use of no-suicide contracts.

Health Teaching

The nurse teaches the client about any psychiatric diagnosis present and about medications, age-related crises, community resources, coping skills, and communication skills, especially the expression of anger. When possible, the family or significant others are included to strengthen the client's support system.

Case Management

Case management is an important aspect of nursing care for the suicidal client. The client's perception of being alone without supports often blinds the person to the real support figures who are present. Reconnecting the client with family and friends is a major focus, whether in the hospital or in the community. Referrals to community services are also essential. In addition to the aftercare referral, information on the following resources may be given: substance treatment centers, crisis hotlines, support groups for clients or families, and recreational activities to enhance socialization and self-esteem. Encouraging the client to get reacquainted with a previous spiritual support system can also be beneficial.

EVIDENCE-BASED PRACTICE

Suicide Prevention Contracts

Background
Suicide prevention contracts or no-suicide (no-harm) contracts have been used by clinicians to work with suicidal clients in inpatient and outpatient settings. The contract is verbal or written, and the client agrees to take an alternate action rather than harming self if feeling suicidal (e.g., call a crisis line or 911, go to the emergency department). In the era of managed care the use of such contracts has increased, and clinicians may believe that they can gauge suicidal intent by the client's willingness to enter into a contract.

Study
In 2003, the American Psychiatric Association published guidelines for the assessment and treatment of suicidal clients. An expert work group conducted an exhaustive review of the literature and research related to suicide published from 1966 to 2002, including 17,589 articles in English.

Results of Study
No studies have demonstrated the effectiveness of suicide contracts in reducing suicide. Some studies noted that a significant number of suicide attempts and suicides occurred despite the presence of a contract. The contract is only as reliable as the therapeutic alliance between the client and the clinician. In situations in which the client is unknown (e.g., in the emergency department or with clients newly admitted to the inpatient unit), use of a contract is not recommended. The use of contracts is also discouraged with clients who are in crisis, intoxicated, psychotic, agitated, or impulsive.

Implications for Nursing Practice
The nurse should follow agency policy regarding the use of suicide prevention contracts. It is important to know that willingness to enter into a contract does not objectively measure the client's suicidal intention, and the contract has no legal authority. With new clients, the use of a contract does not lessen the need for suicide observation. With clients in an ongoing relationship, the contract may serve as a behavioral tool to reinforce teaching and remind the client of available resources to contact outside of scheduled appointments with the nurse.

American Psychiatric Association. (2003). Practice guidelines for the assessment and treatment of patients with suicidal behaviors. *American Journal of Psychiatry, 160*(11 Suppl.), 1-60.

Psychobiological Interventions

A significant nursing intervention to assist the suicidal client in regaining self-control is the careful administration of medication. All medications given to high-risk clients are monitored carefully. Nevertheless, lethal overdose is nearly impossible with selective serotonin reuptake inhibitors (SSRIs), unlike with the previously used tricyclic antidepressants and monoamine oxidase inhibitors, which did present such a risk. Mouth checks may be used in the hospital, whereas in the community, provision of a limited-day supply or family supervision is required. The following recommendations for somatic treatment were included in the APA's guidelines for treatment of the suicidal client (2003).

Antidepressants are ordered for clients who have depressive or anxiety disorders, with an emphasis on administering an adequate dosage and providing appropriate clinical evaluation during the use of SSRIs. Some case reports have suggested that SSRIs increase aggressive or impulsive behavior, but review of the evidence does not show increased suicidal behavior. Rather, the illness being treated carries the risk of agitation and suicide.

There is clear evidence that long-term lithium treatment for bipolar disorder and major depression significantly reduces suicide and suicide attempts. Because lithium does frequently cause side effects and periodic blood work is required to test for therapeutic level, client and family education is important to support compliance.

For psychotic or bipolar manic clients, antipsychotic medication is usually ordered. Second-generation antipsychotics are usually preferable to the traditional ones because they have fewer adverse effects. Some studies have shown a reduced suicide rate among schizophrenic clients receiving clozapine. Its use must be monitored closely, however, because of the risk of severe medical side effects (e.g., agranulocytosis, myocarditis, and altered glucose metabolism).

Finally, antianxiety medication may help to treat panic and insomnia. As of this writing, no clinical studies have examined the effect of antianxiety treatment on suicide risk. But short-term use of long-acting benzodiazepines may be helpful for management of panic symptoms. For insomnia, second-generation antipsychotics or the anticonvulsants divalproex (Depakote) or gabapentin (Neurontin) may be used.

An alternative somatic treatment for acute suicidal risk is electroconvulsive therapy (ECT). Evidence suggests that ECT decreases acute suicidal ideation. This treatment is useful for certain types of clients: severely depressed or psychotic clients whose behavior is considered life threatening and for whom waiting for medication to take effect is not feasible; pregnant clients; clients with certain medical conditions who cannot tolerate medication; and clients who do not respond to multiple trials of medication. Refer to Chapter 18 for further discussion of ECT.

Advanced Practice Interventions

The psychiatric advanced practice RN (APRN) may treat suicidal clients directly with several types of psychotherapy, provide clinical supervision for direct care staff, or provide consultation in nonpsychiatric settings (e.g., medical unit, nursing home, or forensic site). Following acute hospitalization, the APRN provides aftercare for the client with coexisting psychiatric disorders, including individual therapy and family therapy. The APA review of the literature found a consensus that various forms of therapy are effective in treating depression and borderline personality disorder. These include cognitive-behavioral therapy, psychodynamic therapy, and interpersonal therapy. In particular, for clients with borderline personality disorder, dialectical behavior therapy has been helpful, because it focuses on improving specific skills such as impulse control, anger management, and assertiveness.

In nonpsychiatric settings, the APRN may function as a consultant to assess suicidal risk or to recommend treatment. As noted earlier in this chapter, some clients who receive news of a devastating medical illness or who are suffering from a difficult chronic condition may become suicidal. Studies report that 15% to 50% of nursing home clients are depressed and may show indirect self-destructive behavior (e.g., not eating, not taking prescribed medication) (APA, 2003, p. 28). The APRN may be called to perform a suicide assessment or to give a recommendation to the medical team regarding an appropriate level of care. Likewise, APRNs may perform suicide screening in emergency departments or in forensic settings. One study noted suicidal behavior in 38% of the clients seeking psychiatric evaluation in the emergency department (Dhossche, 2000). Emergency care nurses note that all psychiatric clients need to be screened for suicide risk, not just those who offer suicidal ideation as a chief complaint (Rose & Jagim, 2003). The high rate of suicide in jails and prisons has led many facilities to institute admission screening for suicide risk. Refer to the Forensic Highlights box for a review of data for this population. With increased public awareness of the prevalence of suicide in the elderly, research is focused on finding innovative ways to screen for risk. An NIMH study conducted at 20 primary care sites in three major cities showed a significant reduction in suicidal ideation and depression in clients 60 years of age and older treated under a protocol of SSRI therapy and care by a master's level clinician (Barclay, 2004).

FORENSICS HIGHLIGHTS

Rates of suicide are higher among those in jails and prisons than in the general population. The U.S. Department of Justice Bureau of Justice Statistics estimated that, in 1999, the suicide rate among prison inmates was 14 per 100,000 and the rate among jail inmates was 55 per 100,000 (jails are short-term local facilities, whereas prisons are facilities where longer-term sentences are carried out). Most suicides occur in the first 24 hours of incarceration in a jail. Other risk factors include learning of new legal complications, receiving bad news from home, and experiencing sexual assault. The typical person who commits suicide is young, white, male, single, intoxicated, and has a history of substance abuse. The most common method is hanging. Suicide prevention programs have been shown to be effective in reducing suicide rates. The National Commission on Correctional Health Care had adopted standards for assessment and intervention. Nurses in the forensic setting may play a key role in admission screening and ongoing monitoring of suicidal inmates.

Data from American Psychiatric Association. (2003). Practice guidelines for the assessment and treatment of patients with suicidal behaviors. *American Journal of Psychiatry*, *160*(11 Suppl.) 1-60.

Survivors of Completed Suicide: Postvention

A discussion of suicidal clients is incomplete without noting the issues surrounding a completed suicide. Surviving family and friends experience overwhelming guilt and shame, compounded by the difficulty of discussing the taboo subject of suicide (Fine & Myers, 2003). The usual social supports of neighbors and church are sometimes lacking for these mourners. Within 6 months of a suicide, 45% of bereaved adults report mental deterioration, with symptoms of depression or posttraumatic stress disorder. Adolescent siblings of youth suicide victims have a seven times higher risk of developing major depressive disorder over the 6-month period. Adolescent friends who suffer traumatic grief are more likely to report suicidal ideation within 6 years of the suicide (APA, 2003). Family members of a suicide victim develop a higher risk of suicide, 4.5 times greater than the risk in families in which no suicide occurred.

One survivor wrote a personal account 25 years after the suicide of her brother:

> The first year after was a blur. . . . I became so severely depressed that I had to withdraw from school. . . . I am still plagued by what I call the 'if onlys'—if only I could have switched places with him, if only he had been in restraints. . . . despite the progress I have made, the death of anyone close to me rips open the wound. Even fictional suicides on television lead to uncontrollable crying. (Simon, 2003, p. 1597)

Despite their suffering, only approximately 25% of survivors seek treatment (APA, 2003).

Survivors give the following suggestions to health care professionals:

- If being a survivor is the main reason treatment has been sought, remember that the survivor is the client and not the deceased. Focus on the client's thoughts and feelings and do a thorough assessment as you usually would.
- If the deceased was your client, clarify why the relative is coming to you—for more information, for consolation, or for treatment.
- If being a survivor comes out as an incidental finding during an assessment, ask open-ended questions and evaluate how much the loss has been resolved.
- Do not say "successful suicide." More acceptable phrases are "died by suicide" or "killed himself or herself."
- Do recommend community resources and survivor support groups and show empathy about the loss of someone to suicide.
- Do examine you own feelings and countertransference if you treat a suicide survivor. Use clinical supervision or a mentor or therapy to help yourself.

Staff members who have cared for a suicide victim are similarly traumatized by suicide. Staff may also experience symptoms of posttraumatic stress disorder with guilt, shock, anger, shame, and decreased self-esteem (APA, 2003). Group support is essential as the treatment team conducts a thorough psychological postmortem assessment. The event is carefully reviewed to identify the potential overlooked clues, faulty judgments, or changes that are needed in agency protocols. Most facilities have a clear policy about communication with families after suicide. Although some lawyers advise having no contact except through them, others recommend designating a spokesperson who can address the feelings of the family without discussing the details of the client's care. In fact, referrals should be given to family members to try to assist them in dealing with their grief and to address any emotional problems that develop, especially in adolescents. The team needs to discuss any clinician's plan to attend the funeral. As for documentation, all staff need to ensure that the record is complete and that any late entries are identified as such. Legal cases have shown that the courts require that the client be periodically evaluated for suicidal risk, that the treatment plan provide for high-level security, and that staff members follow the individual treatment plan (Roy, 2000).

EVALUATION

Evaluation of a suicidal client is an ongoing part of the assessment. The nurse must be constantly alert to changes in the suicidal person's mood, thinking, and behavior. As mentioned earlier, sudden behavioral changes can signal suicidal intent, especially when the client's depression is lifting and more energy is available to carry out a preconceived plan. A person with a diagnosis of schizophrenia is also at risk when recov-

ering from a psychotic episode. Anniversaries of losses and holidays may have special significance for the suicidal person.

In evaluation, the nurse also looks for indications that the client is communicating thoughts and feelings more readily and that the client's social network is widening. For example, if the person is able to talk about his or her feelings and engage in problem solving with the nurse, this is a positive sign. Is the client increasing his or her social activities and expanding his or her interests? Essentially, the nurse evaluates each short-term goal and establishes new ones as the client progresses toward the long-term goal of resolving suicidal ideation.

CASE STUDY and NURSING CARE PLAN 23-1 A Suicidal Client in the Outpatient Setting

Mr. Martin is a 46-year-old divorced social worker who is brought to the emergency department by ambulance after a suicide attempt. He had taken a bottle of sleeping pills and consumed half of a bottle of scotch whiskey at home. He was found by his landlady after a co-worker called about his absence. His stomach is lavaged and he remains under observation for 16 hours. When he is no longer groggy, he is interviewed by the psychiatric nurse and psychiatrist on call. He states that he has been divorced for 2 years but has seen his 8-year-old son weekly. Three days before his suicide attempt, his ex-wife informed him that she was moving out of state. Because Mr. Martin continues to state that he wants to kill himself, because he lives alone without any apparent support system, and because his score on the SAD PERSONS scale is 5, the decision is made to hospitalize him. After 3 days on suicide precautions, he is no longer acutely suicidal and agrees to continue treatment in the outpatient division of the hospital. In this system, outpatient nurses rotate through the emergency department. Mr. Martin requests assignment to the nurse who has seen him initially.

Self-Assessment

Mrs. Ruiz is an RN with a bachelor's degree and 5 years of experience. She remembers Mr. Martin from the emergency evaluation and immediately wants to refuse the assignment. She seeks out the APRN clinical supervisor to discuss the case. In talking about her feelings, she realizes that she wants to avoid this client for two reasons. He makes her feel anxious and inadequate, showing a sarcastic, angry attitude belittling all women but nurses in particular. Also, she feels disapproving of his attempt to end his life because of his profession—"He's a social worker, he should know better." Once she recognizes her own feelings, Mrs. Ruiz can focus on Mr. Martin's issues: he feels angry and helpless about his son's leaving; his isolation seems self-imposed because he pushes people away, probably due to low self-esteem. After consultation, Mrs. Ruiz agrees with her supervisor that she can work with Mr. Martin.

ASSESSMENT

Objective Data
- First suicide attempt in a 46-year-old divorced male
- High-risk profession
- Isolated without social support system
- Impending separation from son
- No history of psychiatric disorder or substance abuse

Subjective Data
- "My son is the only thing that matters to me."
- "All my family died when I was a kid."
- "I don't need other people."
- "People don't seem to like me much."

NURSING DIAGNOSIS (NANDA)

1. *Risk for suicide* related to loss of son, as evidenced by suicide attempt
   Supporting Data
   - Suicide attempt with lethal intent
   - "I don't want to live if I can't see my son."
   - "I don't need other people."
   - Impending loss of son

Continued

2. *Impaired social interaction* related to social isolation, as evidenced by lack of support system
   Supporting Data
   - "He (son) is all I have left."
   - "All my family died when I was a kid."
   - "I don't go out to drink with co-workers."
   - "People don't seem to like me much."

■ OUTCOME CRITERIA (NOC)

1. Client will consistently use suicide prevention resources and social support groups within the community (long-term outcome).

2. Client will have adequate supportive social contacts (long-term outcome).

■ PLANNING

The initial plan is to establish a working relationship with Mr. Martin, involving him in planning his own treatment and identifying alternative actions for suicidal ideation in the future.

■ INTERVENTION (NIC)

Mr. Martin's plan of care is personalized as follows.

Nursing diagnosis: *Risk for suicide* related to loss of son, as evidenced by suicide attempt
Outcome criteria: Client will consistently use suicide prevention resources and social support groups within the community.

Short-Term Goal	Intervention	Rationale	Evaluation
1. Mr. Martin will immediately seek help when feeling self-destructive.	1a. Assess suicide status. 1b. Even if Mr. Martin denies suicidal ideas, make a future plan.	1a. Ongoing periodic check of suicidal status. Higher rate of suicide for those who have attempted suicide. 1b. Demonstrates concern and offers alternatives if suicidal thoughts return.	GOAL MET Mr. Martin agrees to talk to the nurse about suicidal feelings. If clinic is closed, he will call the crisis hotline (first session).
2. Mr. Martin will talk about painful feelings by the fourth week.	2a. Remain neutral in face of hostility and put-downs. 2b. Refocus attention back to Mr. Martin. 2c. Give frequent opportunities for discussion of feelings through verbal invitation and stated concern.	2a. Diminishes power struggles and discourages continuing acting-out behaviors. 2b. Arguments and power struggles keep attention away from important issues. 2c. Aggressive, hostile communications are cover for painful feelings. When client can express feelings in words, there is less need for client to act them out.	GOAL MET During the first to third weeks, hostile and sarcastic communication is constant. By the fourth week, Mr. Martin states, "You really want to know." Mr. Martin talks of feeling like a failure as a husband and father.
3. Mr. Martin will look at alternative ways he can keep in touch with his son by the fifth week.	3. Alternative solutions can be problem-solved once feelings and problems are identified.	3. Acceptable alternatives increase a future orientation and decrease hopelessness. Client can experience feelings of control over situation.	GOAL MET By the fifth week, Mr. Martin talks about taking his son on a camping trip during summer recess.

Nursing diagnosis: *Impaired social interaction* related to social isolation, as evidenced by lack of support system
Outcome criteria: Client will have adequate supportive social contacts.

Short-Term Goal	Intervention	Rationale	Evaluation
1. Mr. Martin will discuss feelings of isolation and loneliness by the fourth week.	1. Provide opportunities for Mr. Martin to express feelings and thoughts regarding his self-imposed isolation.	1. Before change can take place, clarification of personal feelings and thoughts is necessary.	GOAL MET By the fourth week, Mr. Martin speaks of feeling alone—son is only contact to life.
2. Mr. Martin will identify three positive aspects of self and job by the fifth week.	2a. Validate Mr. Martin's strengths.	2a. Positive as well as negative feedback aids in more realistic perception of self.	GOAL MET By the fifth week, Mr. Martin states that he thinks he is a good worker and is respected (if not liked) by his peers.
	2b. Encourage self-evaluation of positive as well as negative aspects of Mr. Martin's life.	2b. Client can begin to see himself more clearly, with increase in self-esteem.	
3. Mr. Martin will state that he enjoys one new weekly activity with at least one other person by the seventh week.	3a. Review previous activities that Mr. Martin enjoyed before his marriage ended.	3a. Change focus from negative present to positive aspects of client's past. Can help increase hope and self-esteem.	GOAL MET By the seventh week, Mr. Martin states that he has started bowling again and is surprised that he has a good time.
	3b. Have Mr. Martin choose an activity that he is willing to participate in.	3b. Participating in own problem solving and decision making offers client a sense of control and an increase in self-esteem.	

■ EVALUATION

See individual outcomes and evaluation within the care plan.

evolve Visit the Evolve website at **http://evolve.elsevier.com/Varcarolis** for a full case study of this client and more case studies and nursing care plans.

■ ■ ■ KEY POINTS to REMEMBER

- Suicide is a significant public health problem in the United States.
- Specific biological, psychosocial, and cultural factors are known to increase the risk of suicide.
- Most suicidal clients can be helped by treatment of a coexisting psychiatric disorder.
- Certain medical conditions and psychiatric diagnoses are associated with increased risk for suicide.
- Every suicide attempt must be taken seriously, even if the person has a history of multiple attempts.
- The nurse can have a real impact on suicide prevention through primary, secondary, and tertiary interventions.

- Nursing care of the suicidal client is challenging but rewarding: clients evoke intense reactions in staff due to their desperate feelings, but most people with suicidal ideation respond to treatment and do not complete suicide.
- If a client completes suicide, family, friends, and health care workers are traumatized and need support, including possibly referrals for psychiatric treatment.

■ ■ ■

Visit the Evolve website at **http://evolve.elsevier.com/Varcarolis** for a posttest on the content in this chapter. *evolve*

Critical Thinking and Chapter Review

Visit the Evolve website at **http://evolve.elsevier.com/Varcarolis** for additional self-study exercises.

■ ■ ■ CRITICAL THINKING

1. Read the suicide protocol at your hospital unit or community center. Are there any steps you anticipate having difficulty carrying out? Discuss these difficulties with your peers or clinical group.

2. How would you respond to a staff person who expresses guilt over the completed suicide of a client on your unit?

3. Identify three common and expected emotional reactions that a nurse might have when initially working with people who are suicidal. How do you think you might react? What actions could you take to deal with the event and obtain support?

■ ■ ■ CHAPTER REVIEW

Choose the most appropriate answer.

1. Charles Brown, age 52, lost his wife in an automobile accident 4 months earlier. Since that time he has been severely depressed, has withdrawn from contacts with family and friends, and has taken to drinking to "numb the pain." On the SAD PERSONS assessment scale, how many points does Mr. Brown have?
    1. Three
    2. Four
    3. Five
    4. Six

2. Which of the following cannot be relied upon to provide a basis for nursing intervention with a suicidal client?
    1. Most people who are planning suicide give clues.
    2. The nurse should not bring up the subject of suicide with a client.
    3. When depression is lifting there is more energy to carry out a suicide plan.
    4. Most people who contemplate suicide are highly ambivalent about dying.

3. Select the example of primary intervention in suicide.
    1. Working with the family of a recent suicide victim.
    2. Placing a hospitalized client on suicide precautions.
    3. Keeping the caller to a crisis hotline on the phone and working out alternatives to suicide.
    4. Providing a seminar for the elderly focusing on coping with loneliness and physical changes.

4. Miss B. has a concrete plan to commit suicide by hanging. She refuses to make a no-suicide contract because she believes there is no hope for a better life now that her fiancé has left her and God has abandoned her. She believes the breakup with her fiancé was because he found out "how worthless I am." Which of Miss B.'s nursing diagnoses is of highest priority?
    1. Hopelessness
    2. Spiritual distress
    3. Low self-esteem
    4. Risk for suicide

5. Which of the following cultural groups is known to have the highest suicide rate?
    1. Asian Americans
    2. African Americans
    3. Native Americans
    4. Hispanic Americans

■ **STUDENT**
■ **STUDY**
■ **CD-ROM**

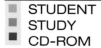

Access the accompanying CD-ROM for animations, interactive exercises, review questions for the NCLEX examination, and an audio glossary.

■ **NURSE,**
■ **CLIENT, AND**
■ **FAMILY RESOURCES**

For suggested readings, information on related associations, and Internet resources, go to **http://evolve.elsevier.com/Varcarolis.**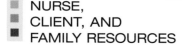

REFERENCES

American Association of Suicidology. (2000). *Some facts about suicide and depression.* Retrieved February 8, 2005, from http://www.suicidology.org.

American Association of Suicidology. (2004, March 20). *Some facts about suicide in the U.S.A.* Retrieved February 8, 2005, from http://www.suicidology.org.

American Psychiatric Association. (2003). Practice guideline for the assessment and treatment of patients with suicidal behaviors. *American Journal of Psychiatry, 160*(11 Suppl.), 1-60.

Barclay, L. (2004). Primary care intervention reduces suicidal ideation in older patients with depression. *Journal of the American Medical Association, 291,* 1081-1091.

Brown, A. B. (2003). Panic disorder: Highly disabling, yet treatable. *NARSAD Research Newsletter, 15*(3), 24-28.

Comtois, K. A. (2002). A review of interventions to reduce the prevalence of parasuicide. *Psychiatric Services, 53*(9), 1138-1144.

Dhossche, D. M. (2000). Suicidal behavior in psychiatric emergency room patients. *Southern Medical Journal, 93*(3), 310-314.

Dochterman, J. M., & Bulechek, G. M. (2004). *Nursing interventions classification (NIC)* (4th ed.). St. Louis, MO: Mosby.

Fine, C., & Myers, M. (2003, September 17). Suicide survivors: Tips for health professionals. *Medscape General Medicine, 5*(3). Retrieved February 8, 2005, from http://www.medscape.com/viewarticle/460958?src=search.

Greenfield, B., et al. (2002). A rapid-response outpatient model for reducing hospitalization rates among suicidal adolescents. *Psychiatric Services, 53*(12), 1574-1579.

Lambert, M. T. (2002). Seven-year outcomes of patients evaluated for suicidality. *Psychiatric Services, 53*(1), 92-94.

Mayo Clinic.com. (2004). *Considering suicide: Don't let despair obscure other options.* Retrieved March 12, 2005, from http://www.mayoclinic.com/invoke.cfm?id=mH00054.

Moorhead, S., Johnson, M., & Maas, M. (2004). *Nursing outcomes classification (NOC)* (3rd ed.). St. Louis, MO: Mosby.

Myers, M., & Fine, C. (2003, October 21). Suicide in physicians: Toward prevention. *Medscape General Medicine, 5*(4). Retrieved February 8, 2005, http://www.medscape.com/viewarticle/462619?src=search.

National Institute of Mental Health. (2004, April 9). *Suicide facts and statistics.* Retrieved April 13, 2005, from http://www.nimh.nih.gov/suicideprevention/suifact.cfm.

Paris, J. (2002). Chronic suicidality among patients with borderline personality disorder. *Psychiatric Services, 53*(6), 738-742.

Pataki, C. S. (2000). Mood disorders and suicide in children and adolescents. In B. J. Sadock & V. A. Sadock (Eds.), *Comprehensive textbook of psychiatry* (7th ed., Vol. II, pp. 2740-2757). Philadelphia: Lippincott Williams & Wilkins.

Patterson, W., et al. (1983). Evaluation of suicidal patients: The SAD PERSONS scale. *Psychosomatics, 24*(4), 343-345, 348, 349.

Range, L. M., et al. (1999). Multicultural perspectives on suicide. *Aggression and Violent Behavior, 4*(4), 413-430.

Rose, C., & Jagim, M. (2003). Psychiatric triage RNs in the ED. *American Journal of Nursing, 103*(9), 101-105.

Roy, A. (2000). Psychiatric emergencies: Suicide. In B. J. Sadock & V. A. Sadock (Eds.), *Comprehensive textbook of psychiatry* (7th ed., Vol. II, pp. 2031-2040). Philadelphia: Lippincott Williams & Wilkins.

Russ, N. (2003, May 20). Current topic review: The role of comorbid substance abuse in suicide risk for bipolar patients. *Medscape Psychiatry & Mental Health, 8*(1). Retrieved February 8, 2005, from http://www.medscape.com/viewarticle/455675?src=search.

Shea, S. C. (1999). *The practical art of suicide assessment.* New York: Wiley.

Simon, L. (2003). Surviving suicide: The ones left behind. *Psychiatric Services, 54*(12), 1596-1597.

Temkin, R. M., & Crotty, M. (2004). Suicide and other risk monitoring in inpatient psychiatry. *Journal of American Psychiatric Nurses Association, 10*(2), 73-80.

U.S. Public Health Service. (1999). *The Surgeon General's call to action to prevent suicide.* Washington, DC: Author.

CHAPTER 24

Anger and Aggression

VERNA BENNER CARSON ▪ CARROL ALVAREZ

■ KEY TERMS and CONCEPTS

The key terms and concepts listed here appear in color where they are defined or first discussed in this chapter.

aggression, 490

anger, 490

deescalation techniques, 496

restraint, 496

seclusion, 496

■ OBJECTIVES

After studying this chapter, the reader will be able to

1. Compare and contrast three theories that explore the nature of aggression.
2. Compare and contrast interventions for a client with healthy coping skills with those for a client with marginal coping behaviors.
3. Explain why behavioral and cognitive-behavioral techniques are useful modalities for anger management.
4. Apply at least four principles of deescalation with a moderately angry client.
5. Describe four criteria for the use of seclusion or restraint over verbal intervention.
6. Role-play with classmates by using understandable but unhelpful responses to anger and aggression in clients; discuss how these responses can affect nursing interventions.

evolve Visit the Evolve website at **http://evolve.elsevier.com/Varcarolis** for a pretest on the content in this chapter.

It is impossible to pick up a newspaper, watch a news broadcast on television, or tune in to a radio program and not be assailed by some story of out-of-control anger that has escalated into violence. Anger is expressed in many ways, from episodes of "road rage" that often end in tragedy to bursts of profanity in the workplace. The media have coined new terms such as *desk rage* and *air rage* to describe the increasing tendency of Americans to erupt and lash out (Thomas, 2003). Nurse researcher Linda Aiken used the phrase *ward rage* to describe the epidemic of anger and frustration in hospitals (Bergstrom, 2001). Clients and families get angry at hospital personnel, nurses get angry at each other, and physicians get angry at nurses. It seems that there is an epidemic of anger!

Anger and aggression are difficult targets for nursing intervention, particularly if their focus is the nurse, because they imply threat and generate feelings of fear, hurt, and helplessness. Anger is an emotional response to the perception of frustration of desires, threat to one's needs (emotional or physical), or challenge, and as such anger is a normal response. Aggression is harsh physical or verbal action that reflects rage, hostility, and potential for physical or verbal destructiveness. Anger and aggression are the last two stages of a response that begins with feelings of vulnerability and then uneasiness. Clients often communicate their anxiety before escalating to anger. Nursing interventions for anger and aggression begin at these early stages, with accurate assessment of clients' behaviors, appropriate intervention, and care to reassess that the intervention was effective. See Chapters 13 and 14 for interventions that can be used when anxiety is escalating.

PREVALENCE

As a nurse you can be assured that you will deal with anger and aggression, because these are universal emotions. Anger is included in all descriptions of primary emotions and is one of six emotions that can generally be identified across cultures via facial expression (Ekman, 2003).

The Centers for Disease Control and Prevention (CDC) (2003) reported more than 50,000 deaths from suicide and homicide in 2001. Homicide is the leading cause of death overall for persons 15 to 34 years of age; it is also the leading cause of death for African Americans in this age group and the second leading cause of death for Hispanic youth (CDC, 2003). In 2001 more than 2 million people were victims of nonfatal violence. The CDC suggests that the widespread incidence of aggression and violence indicates that these are common parts of social interactions in many environments, including hospitals. The National Institute for Occupational Safety and Health reports that in 1999 the rate of assaults on hospital workers was 8.3 assaults per 10,000 workers, which contrasts with a much lower rate of 2 per 10,000 workers in private-sector industries (CDC, 2002). Although anyone working in a hospital may become a victim of violence, nurses and aides who have the most contact with clients are at higher risk. Violence can occur anywhere in the hospital, but it is most frequent in the following areas:

- Psychiatric units
- Emergency departments
- Waiting rooms
- Geriatric units

Refer to Chapter 25 for statistics on family violence and to Chapter 26 for statistics on sexual assault.

COMORBIDITY

Although anger is a universal emotion experienced by everyone, not everyone responds to the anger with aggression and violence. There is evidence that anger coexists with attention deficit hyperactivity disorder, oppositional defiant disorder, and impulsivity in children, especially male children. In addition, anger frequently co-occurs with depression, suicide, posttraumatic stress disorder, mania, psychotic disorders with paranoid delusions, Alzheimer's disease, personality disorders, and Tourette's disease (Sadock & Sadock, 2004).

Anger and hostility are also risk factors for hypertension and cardiovascular disease, including ischemic heart disease and cerebral vascular attacks. Hostility has been shown to increase adrenocorticotropin and cardiovascular responses to stress and, in longitudinal studies, to increase illness (Davis, Matthews, & McGrath, 2000; Suinn, 2001; Williams, et al., 2000).

THEORY

Another Look at an Old Theory

In 1982 a psychologist, Carol Tavris, wrote a popular book entitled *Anger: The Misunderstood Emotion*. At that time Ms. Tavris sought to dispel a number of misconceptions regarding anger, including the widespread but erroneous belief that "getting anger off your chest" is a good thing to do. Research has since shown that the expression of anger is not always beneficial to clients; moreover, it can lead to escalation of anger with negative physiological changes. In addition, venting of anger in close relationships actually blocks the development of healthier interaction patterns. However, it is worth restating that anger is a normal emotion, experienced by everyone. The *experience* of anger should not make us feel guilty; it is *how we respond* to anger that may be a problem.

The physiological changes associated with anger expression are significant because they reflect a cardiac reactivity in men that is associated with coronary heart disease. In other research, the opposite approach to anger—repression—has been associated with essential hypertension and cardiac reactivity in women (Siegman et al., 2000). These changes are strongest in African Americans, who show longer-lasting cardiac reactivity to anger than white research subjects (Fredrickson et al., 2000).

Clearly, the venting of anger is not always useful. However, other anger management techniques can be taught, and these techniques are beneficial to many who struggle with anger control. These techniques are derived from two theoretical bases.

Behavioral Theory Base

Early behaviorists held that emotions, including anger, were learned responses to environmental stimuli (Skinner, 1953). Social learning theorists adapted this theory through research which showed that children learn aggression by imitating others and that people repeat behavior that is rewarded (Bandura, 1973). Thus, children who watch television violence learn violent ways of resolving problems. Not only is television violence portrayed as an option for resolving conflict, but 73% of violent acts are also shown without negative consequences (Fenichel, 2005; National Television Violence Study Council, 1996). When parents are not present or are too preoccupied to teach their children alternative ways of dealing with problems, the range of skills learned by the children for managing frustration remains limited. Similarly, children who grow up in angry families learn to respond to frustration with anger and violence (Partenheimer, 2003). In addition, children and young adults with mental problems are particularly vulnerable to experiencing explosive anger because they may be unable to incorporate anger management skills taught by parents and schools.

Cognitive Theory Base

Individuals appraise events as threatening, and this cognition leads to the emotional and physiological arousal necessary to take action. Although threat is usually understood as an alert to physical danger, Beck (1976) noted that perceived assault on areas of personal domain, such as values, moral code, and protective rules, can also lead to anger. For example, clinic clients kept waiting for long periods of time without explanation may interpret this as neglect and a lack of respect. Anger may escalate when the initial appraisal is followed by cognitions such as "They have no right to treat me this way. I am a person too." These additional cognitions lead to escalating behavior that can erupt into violence unless the situation is defused through successful interventions. In some individuals, the period of escalation can be rapid. In contrast, clients less predisposed to anger might interpret the wait as a sign that the clinic is busy. These clients might be frustrated by the situation, but in the absence of anger they might access and utilize skills such as asking how much longer the wait is likely to be, finding distractions in the environment, or rescheduling the appointment.

As nurses, of course, we are not immune to anger. A client who is shouting angrily may reasonably be apprised as a potential threat. This appraisal may lead to anger on the nurse's part, as well as an impulse for self-protection (Thomas, 2003). One study found that the nurse's response to anger in a client varied according to the interpretation given to the client's anger and to the nurse's self-appraised ability to manage the situation. Only when self-efficacy was perceived as adequate did the nurse move to help the client. When self-efficacy was not seen as adequate, the nurse showed a decreased ability to process the client's message and a decreased ability to problem solve (Smith & Hart, 1994).

Neurobiology of Anger and Aggression

Brain Abnormalities

Many neurological conditions are associated with anger and aggression. For example, certain brain tumors, Alzheimer's disease, temporal lobe epilepsy, and traumatic injury to certain parts of the brain result in changes to personality that includes increased violence. Many clients with brain injury have severe behavior disorders, including aggressiveness, that disrupts their lives.

One site known to be associated with aggression is the limbic system, which mediates primitive emotion and behaviors that are necessary for survival. The limbic system contains several structures that appear to have a role in the production of aggression. The area of the brain called the *amygdala* mediates anger experiences, judging events as either aversive or rewarding. For example, in animal studies, stimulation of the amygdala produces rage responses, whereas lesions in the same structure produce docility.

The temporal lobe of the brain shares some structures with the limbic system. Here, in the temporal lobe, memory is thought to be integrated; memory of previous insult is important in the cognitive appraisal of threat in the face of new stimuli. This lobe is also the source of complex partial seizures, which may give rise to aggressive behavior. Interestingly, high violence scores correlate with computed tomographic and electroencephalographic abnormalities in the temporal lobes of clients in maximum security (Kavoussi, Armstead, & Coccaro, 1997).

Serotonin

Studies have shown a relationship between impulsive aggression and low levels of the neurotransmitter serotonin (Kavoussi et al., 1997). There is also preliminary evidence for a genetic disturbance in serotonergic function that may predispose individuals to impulsive aggressive behaviors (Kavoussi et al., 1997).

Genetic and Environmental Factors

Finally, research findings indicate that violence is a function of both genetics and childhood environment. For example, researchers have noted that family dynamics affect the dispositions of infant members; disorganized, unpredictable families, or those high in conflict, tend to have more irritable infants than families that are stable (Brackbill et al., 1990; Eisenberg et al., 1997). Similarly, anger in toddlers has been seen to be related to child-rearing variables in their mothers; nonconflictual parent-child relationships are most highly correlated with low toddler anger (Brook, Whiteman, & Brook, 1999). Of course, family dynamics may themselves reflect genetic variables.

Clearly, some individuals are biologically more predisposed than others to respond to life events with irritability, easy frustration, and anger. This predisposition may be a function of genetics or of neurological development that occurs in the context of certain infant and childhood environments. These two risk factors appear to combine in an exponential way. Nevertheless, if all the dimensions of anger are centrally mediated, then successful interventions can be designed to target any of its manifestations. This is likely the reason biological, pharmacological, behavioral, and cognitive strategies are all useful in the management of anger and aggression.

Application of the Nursing Process

◾ ASSESSMENT

Overall Assessment

Accurate and early assessment can many times identify client anxiety before it escalates to anger and aggression. Such assessment also leads directly to the appropriate nursing diagnosis and intervention. Client expressions of anxiety and of anger generally look similar. Both may involve increased demands, irritability, frowning, redness of the face, pacing, and twisting of the hands or clenching and unclenching of the fists. Speech either may be increased in rate and volume or may be slowed, pointed, and quiet. Box 24-1 identifies signs and symptoms that indicate the risk of escalating anger leading to aggressive behavior. Simple observation of these signs, however, does not provide the information necessary to drive the appropriate intervention. Taking an accurate history of the client's background and usual coping skills, as well as determining the client's perception of the issue (if possible), are required.

The importance of history in predicting violence was highlighted in a violence reporting program established at the Veterans Administration Medical Center in Portland, Oregon. Clients with a history of violence were identified in a computerized database. This program helped reduce the number of violent attacks by 91.6% by alerting staff to take additional safety measures when serving these clients (CDC, 2002).

Self-Assessment

The nurse's ability to intervene safely in situations of anger and potential violence depends on the nurse's self-awareness. Without this awareness, nursing interventions are marked by impulsive or emotion-based responses, which are generally nontherapeutic and may be harmful. Self-awareness includes knowledge of personal responses to anger and aggression, including choice of words and tone of voice, as well as nonverbal communication via body posture and facial expressions. Awareness of the norms brought from the nurse's own family and of norms brought from the larger society is also essential. In addition, staff must be aware of personal dynamics that may trigger emotions and reactions that are not therapeutic with specific clients. Finally, the nurse must assess situational factors (e.g., fatigue, insufficient staff) that may decrease normal competence in the management of complex client problems.

BOX 24-1

Some Predictive Factors of Violence

1. Signs and symptoms that usually *(but not always)* precede violence*:
   a. Hyperactivity: most important predictor of imminent violence (e.g., pacing, restlessness)
   b. Increasing anxiety and tension: clenched jaw or fist, rigid posture, fixed or tense facial expression, mumbling to self (client may have shortness of breath, sweating, and rapid pulse)
   c. Verbal abuse: profanity, argumentativeness
   d. Loud voice, change of pitch, or very soft voice forcing others to strain to hear
   e. Intense eye contact or avoidance of eye contact
2. Recent acts of violence, including property violence
3. Stone silence
4. Alcohol or drug intoxication
5. Possession of a weapon or object that may be used as a weapon (e.g., fork, knife, rock)
6. Milieu characteristics conducive to violence:
   a. Overcrowding
   b. Staff inexperience
   c. Provocative or controlling staff
   d. Poor limit setting
   e. Arbitrary revocation of privileges

*Sometimes violence may be perceived to come from "out of the blue."

Self-assessment promotes calm responses to client anger and potential aggression. These responses are further supported by use of the following techniques:
- Deep breathing
- Relaxation of muscles that are not in use
- Empathetic interpretation of the client's distress
- Review of intervention strategies
- Review of prevention strategies

In settings in which staff can reasonably expect episodes of client anger and aggression, regular teaching and practice of verbal and nonverbal interventions are essential. This fosters nurses' increased confidence in their own abilities and those of co-workers.

Assessment Guidelines   Anger and Aggression

1. A history of violence is the single best predictor of future violence.
2. Clients who are hyperactive, impulsive, or predisposed to irritability are at higher risk for violence.
3. Assess client risk for violence:
   - Does the client have a wish or intent to harm?
   - Does the client have a plan?
   - Does the client have means available to carry out the plan?

- Does the client have demographic risk factors: male gender, age 14 to 24 years, low socioeconomic status, low support system?

4. Aggression by clients occurs most often in the context of limit setting by the nurse.

5. Clients with a history of limited coping skills, including lack of assertiveness or use of intimidation, are at higher risk of using violence.

6. Assess self for personal triggers and responses likely to escalate client violence, including client characteristics or situations that trigger impatience, irritation, or defensiveness.

7. Assess personal sense of competence when in any situation of potential conflict; consider asking for the assistance of another staff member.

NURSING DIAGNOSIS

When potential aggression is identified, *ineffective coping* (overwhelmed or maladaptive), *risk for self-directed violence,* and *risk for other-directed violence* are important nursing diagnoses.

Clients may have coping skills that are adequate for day-to-day events in their lives but are overwhelmed by the stresses of illness or hospitalization. Other clients may have a pattern of maladaptive coping that is marginally effective and consists of a set of coping strategies that have been developed to meet unusual or extraordinary situations (e.g., abusive families).

Ideally, intervention occurs at the point of ineffective coping. Nurses work with clients to support or teach ways of coping that will decrease anxiety and distress. However, client behavior may escalate quickly, or the client may mask early signs of distress. Nurses may be distracted and may miss those early signs, even when they are visible. Other clients may be acutely intoxicated and not amenable to early nursing interventions. In these situations, the problem with anger may not be resolved before the risk for violence arises. When this diagnosis is used, deescalation of anger is the primary nursing intervention. Seclusion, restraint, or psychopharmacological means may be necessary to ensure the safety of clients and staff.

OUTCOME CRITERIA

Having clearly defined outcome criteria when interventions are planned for angry and aggressive clients is important for identifying the behaviors that staff can encourage if their interventions have been successful. The Nursing Outcomes Classification outlines specific outcome criteria for use with angry and aggressive clients (Moorhead, Johnson, & Maas, 2004). See Table 24-1 for selected potential outcomes for aggressive behaviors.

PLANNING

Planning interventions necessitates having a sound assessment; for example, past history (previous acts of violence, comorbid disorders), present coping skills, and willingness and capacity of the client to learn alternative and nonviolent ways of handling angry feelings.

Does the client have
- Good coping skills but is presently overwhelmed?
- Marginal coping skills and uses anger or violence as a way to cover other feelings and gain a sense of mastery or control?
- A neuropsychotic or chronic psychotic disorder and is prone to violence?
- Cognitive deficits that predispose to anger in the form of misinterpretation of environmental stimuli?

Does the situation call for
- Psychotherapeutic approaches to teach the client new skills for handling anger?

TABLE 24-1

Aggression Self-Control (NOC)

Nursing Outcome and Definition	Intermediate Indicators	Short-Term Indicators
Aggression Self-Control: Self-restraint of assaultive, combative, or destructive behaviors toward others*	Maintains self-control without supervision Upholds contract to restrain aggressive behaviors	Identifies when angry Identifies when frustrated Communicates needs appropriately Vents negative feelings appropriately Refrains from striking others Refrains from destroying property Uses specific techniques to control anger

From Moorhead, S., Johnson, M., & Maas, M. (2004). *Nursing outcomes classification (NOC)* (3rd ed., pp. 142-143). St. Louis, MO: Mosby.
*Evaluated on a five-point Likert scale from 1 (never demonstrated) to 5 (consistently demonstrated).

■ Immediate intervention to prevent overt violence (deescalation techniques, restraints or seclusion, and/or medications)?

Does the environment provide

■ Privacy for the client?

■ Enough space for clients or is there overcrowding?

■ A healthy balance between structured time and quite time?

Do the skills of the staff call for

■ Additional education for staff in verbal deescalation techniques?

■ Counseling of staff regarding use of punitive and arbitrary approaches to clients?

■ Additional training in restraint techniques?

Planning also involves attention to the numbers of personnel who are available to respond to a potentially violent situation.

■ INTERVENTION

Basing Interventions on Stages of the Violence Cycle

When interventions to prevent or deal with client violence are considered, it is important to take into account the stages of the violence cycle. These stages include the preassaultive stage, the assaultive stage, and the postassaultive stage when the client returns to baseline. Let's take a look at each of these stages and the appropriate interventions for each. Interventions presented here reflect a nursing diagnosis of *risk for other-directed (or self-directed) violence.*

Preassaultive Stage: Deescalation Approaches

During the preassaultive stage the client is increasingly agitated. Staff require training in both verbal techniques of deescalation and physical techniques to restrain without harm. The better trained the staff, the less chance that either staff or client will be injured. Frequently verbal interventions are sufficient during this stage. Interventions at this stage include the following:

Analyze the client and situation. As you try to determine what the client is feeling, you have already begun to intervene. During this process you are attempting to hear the client's feelings and concerns. If you already know the client well, this time initially spent listening and attending to the client's concerns may allow you to determine the problem as well as an acceptable solution. If you do not know the client well, your role is primarily as an observer, gathering sufficient information with which to plan an intervention. Encouraging the client to move to a place that is quiet and safe is a good first sugges-

tion. Frequently this can be accomplished by telling the client that you are concerned and want to listen. The client needs reassurance that people are interested and willing to help. It is essential during this stage to acknowledge the client's needs regardless of whether the expressed needs are rational or irrational, possible or impossible to meet. It is important to clearly and simply state your expectations for the client's behavior: "I expect that you will stay in control." Offer prn (as needed) medication if it is available and appropriate.

Use verbal techniques of deescalation. You need to be an excellent listener and be able to respond to the client in a therapeutic manner. You want to convey that you are calm, controlled, open, nonthreatening, and caring. You want to maintain a relaxed posture. If you are feeling fear, you may find that this is quite challenging. Maintaining a calm exterior while your interior is in an upheaval requires considerable self-discipline.

Demonstrate respect for the client's personal space. If the client is sitting, you should sit. Your eyes should be on the same level as the client's eyes to decrease a sense of intimidation and to communicate to the client that you are speaking as equals. Allow the client enough personal space so that the client does not perceive you as intrusive but not so much space that the client cannot speak in a normal voice. Clients who are poised for violence need much more space than clients who are not. While you are giving the client space, the client may be invading your space with verbal abuse and the use of profanity. This may be the only way the client can express feelings. As uncomfortable as this may be for you, you cannot take the client's words personally or respond in kind. It is also important not to end the conversation because of the client's verbal abusiveness or to forbid the client from communicating in this way.

Interact with the client. Speak to the client in a low and calm voice. Never yell, but continue to model controlled behavior. Use open-ended statements such as "You think people are always unkind to you?" rather than challenging statements such as "What is wrong with you?" Avoid ending statements with "okay?" because it may create ambivalence in the client and give the erroneous impression that choices exist. It is important to avoid punitive, threatening, accusatory, or challenging statements to the client; rather, find out what is behind the client's feelings and behaviors. Honestly verbalize the client's options and encourage the client to assume responsibility for choices made. This approach decreases the sense of powerlessness that often precipitates violence. Do not, however, offer options that are not possible; this will only increase the client's anger. If the client is unable to make a choice, acknowledge the client's decision-making difficulty: "You seem too upset to make a decision right now. I will make the decision for you now."

Invest time in the process. It is important when you begin a verbal intervention to have a time frame in mind. The amount of time needed varies with the client and the particular situation. Depressed, suicidal, or frightened clients may require more time; manipulative clients should be given less time. You may decide initially that you will spend 8 to 10 minutes, and if progress is being made, you can extend the time. It is important to gently but firmly set limits regarding time. When the time limit is reached, you inform the client that you will not discuss the matter further. Once these limits have been set, they must be consistently enforced.

Pay attention to the environment. The environment is critical. Choose a quiet place, but one that is visible to staff. This is most beneficial in helping a client regain control. Staff should know who is working with the client and for how long, so that uninterrupted time is allowed.

Assure your safety. You must feel safe to be able to communicate in a calm manner. There are six basic considerations for ensuring your safety. First, avoid wearing dangling earrings or necklaces. The client may become focused on these and grab at them, causing serious injury. If you are wearing such jewelry, it is important to remove it before dealing with an agitated client. Second, having enough staff for backup is essential. Only one person should talk to the client, but staff need to maintain an unobtrusive presence in case the situation escalates. Third, always know the layout of the area. Correct placement of furniture and elimination of obstacles or hazards are important to prevent injury if the client requires physical interventions. Fourth, do not stand directly in front of the client or in front of the doorway; this position could be interpreted as confrontational. It is better to stand off to the side and encourage the client to have a seat. Fifth, if you are interviewing a client whose behavior begins to escalate, provide feedback about what you observe: "You seem to be very upset." Such an observation allows exploration of the client's feelings and may lead to deescalation of the situation. If the client's behavior continues to escalate, end the interview and assure the client that the staff will provide for the client's as well as everyone else's safety. Sixth, avoid confrontation with the client either through verbal means or

through a "show of force" with security guards. Verbal confrontation and discussion of the incident must occur when the client is calm. A show of force by security guards may serve to escalate the client's behavior; therefore, security personnel are better kept in the background until they are needed to assist).

Refer to Box 24-2 for some principles underlying deescalation techniques.

Assaultive Stage: Restraint, Medication, Seclusion

If the client progresses to the assaultive stage, the staff must respond quickly. Generally, a team approach with about five staff members is advisable, but the team may be larger if the client requires it. One leader speaks to the client and instructs members of the team. The interventions include the use of physical restraints and seclusion of the client.

Use of Physical Restraints and Seclusion. Seclusion refers to "the involuntary confinement of a client alone in a room, which the client is prevented from leaving" (Health Care Financing Administration [HCFA], 1999, p. 27). The goal of seclusion is never punitive. Rather, *the goal is safety of the client and others.* Restraint refers to "any manual method, or mechanical device, material or equipment attached or adjacent

---

BOX 24-2

Deescalation Techniques: Practice Principles

1. Maintain the client's self-esteem and dignity.
2. Maintain calmness (your own and the client's).
3. Assess the client and the situation.
4. Identify stressors and stress indicators.
5. Respond as early as possible.
6. Use a calm, clear tone of voice.
7. Invest time.
8. Remain honest.
9. Establish what the client considers to be his or her need.
10. Be goal oriented.
11. Maintain a large personal space.
12. Avoid verbal struggles.
13. Give several options.
14. Make clear the options.
15. Utilize a nonaggressive posture.
16. Use genuineness and empathy.
17. Attempt to be confidently aware.
18. Use verbal, nonverbal, and communication skills.
19. Be assertive (not aggressive).
20. Assess for personal safety.

From Mason, T., & Chandley, M. (1999). *Management of violence and aggression* (p. 73). Philadelphia: Churchill Livingstone.

to the client's body that he or she cannot easily remove that restricts freedom of movement or normal access to one's body" (HCFA, 1999, p. 41). Seclusion or physical restraint is used only after alternative interventions have been tried, including verbal intervention, behavioral care plan, medication, decrease in sensory stimulation, removal of a particular problematic stimulus, presence of a significant other, frequent observation, and use of a sitter who provides 24-hour one-on-one observation of the client. Seclusion or restraint is used in the following circumstances (American Psychiatric Nurses Association, 2000):

- The client presents a clear and present danger to self.
- The client presents a clear and present danger to others.
- The client has been legally detained for involuntary treatment and is thought to pose an escape risk.
- The client requests to be secluded or restrained.

A client may not be held in seclusion or restraint without a physician's order. Once in restraint, a client must be directly observed and formally assessed at frequent, regular intervals for level of awareness, level of activity, safety within the restraints, hydration, toileting needs, nutrition, and comfort. The frequency of observation is mandated by licensing and accreditation agencies. Refer to Chapter 8 for more on the legalities of the use of seclusion and restraints.

Each team member is trained in the correct use of physical restraining maneuvers as well as the use of physical restraints. The team is organized before approaching the client so that each team member knows his or her individual responsibility regarding limb securing. Before approaching the client, the team is prepared with the correct number and size of restraints and with medication, if ordered. The team leader explains to the client in a matter-of-fact manner exactly what the team is about to do and why. If restraints are to be used, the client is informed at this point of the team's intent and the reason for the team's actions. Sometimes, the client is ready to cooperate and moves to the seclusion room, where he or she is restrained with either four-point or two-point restraints. The team remains calm and acts as quickly as possible. Guidelines for the use of mechanical restraints are given in Box 24-3.

Once the client is restrained, the nurse might administer an intramuscular injection of a benzodiazepine, a major tranquilizer, or an antihistamine, depending on the physician's order. The nurse's role is to provide an explanation to the client for the medication and to make sure that the client is properly restrained so that the medication can be safely administered. Throughout this time, the team leader continues to relate to the client in a calm, steady voice, communicating decisiveness, consistency, and control.

BOX 24-3

Some Guidelines for Use of Mechanical Restraint

Indications for Use
- To protect the client from self-harm
- To prevent the client from assaulting others

Legal Requirements
- Multidisciplinary involvement
- Physician's signature
- Client advocate or relative notification
- Client agreement

Clinical Assessments
- Client's mental state
- Risks to the client
- Need for restraints

Observation
- Have nurse in constant attendance
- Complete written record every 15 minutes
- Release limb from restraint every 2 hours
- Stretch limb through range of movement
- Monitor vital signs
- Observe blood flow
- Observe that restraint is not rubbing
- Provide for nutrition, hydration, and elimination

Release Procedure
- Limit on time in restraint
- Behaviors required before release
- Release protocol—graduated versus complete
- Termination of restraints

Documentation
- Restraint documentation
- Client's record
- Day report

Adapted from Mason, T., & Chandley, M. (2000). *Management of violence and aggression* (p. 179). Philadelphia: Churchill Livingstone.

While the client is restrained and in seclusion, staff closely monitor the client to determine the client's ability to reintegrate into the unit activities. Reintegration is gradual and is geared to the client's ability to handle increasing amounts of stimulation. If the reintegration proves to be too much for the client and results in increased agitation, the client is returned to the room or another quiet area.

Generally a structured reintegration is the best approach. For instance, reintegration can begin by reducing four-point restraints to two-point restraints. Once the client no longer requires the locked seclusion room, the client may be given specified time-out periods to leave the room and move slowly into the milieu of the unit. The time-out periods are gradually lengthened until the client is able to maintain control within the unit.

Postassaultive Stage

Once the client no longer requires seclusion and restraints, the staff should review the incident with the client as well as among themselves. Discussion with the client is an important part of the therapeutic process. Going over what has occurred allows the client to learn from the situation, to identify the stressors that precipitated the out-of-control behavior, and to plan alternative ways of responding to these stressors in the future.

Return to Baseline: Critical Incident Debriefing

Staff analysis of the episode of violence, referred to as critical incident debriefing, is crucial for a number of reasons. First, a review is necessary to ensure that quality care was provided to the client. Staff members need to critically examine their response to the client. Questions to be answered include the following:

- Could we have done anything that would have prevented the violence?
- If the answer is yes, then what could have been done, and why wasn't it done in this situation?
- Did the team respond as a team? Were team members acting according to the policies and procedures of the unit? If not, why not?
- How do staff members feel about this client? About this situation? Feelings of fear and anger must be discussed and handled. Otherwise the client may be dealt with in a punitive and nontherapeutic manner. Employee morale, productivity, use of sick leave time, transfer requests, and absenteeism are all affected by client violence, especially if a staff member has been injured. Staff members must feel supported by their peers as well as by the organizational policies and procedures established to maintain a safe environment.
- Is there a need for additional staff education regarding how to respond to violent clients?

Refer to Chapter 22 for additional information on critical incident debriefing.

Documentation of a Violent Episode

There are a number of areas in which the nurse must provide documentation in situations in which violence was either averted or actually occurred:

- Assessment of behaviors that occurred during the preassaultive stage
- Nursing interventions and the client's responses
- Evaluation of the interventions used
- Detailed description of the client's behaviors during the assaultive stage
- All nursing interventions used to defuse the crisis
- Client's response to those interventions
- Observations of and interventions performed while the client was in restraints and/or seclusion

- The way in which the client was reintegrated into the unit milieu

Box 24-4 lists selected potential interventions for *Anger Control Assistance* (Dochterman & Bulechek, 2004).

Let's take a closer look at intervening in different settings with clients who are exhibiting ineffective coping skills.

General Hospital Settings

Angry Clients with Healthy Coping Who Are Overwhelmed

A careful assessment, with history and information from family members, determines whether a client's anger is a usual or an unusual way of managing stress. Interventions for clients whose usual coping strategies are healthy involve finding ways to reestablish or substitute similar means of dealing with the hospitalization. This problem solving occurs in collaboration with the client, in interactions in which the nurse acknowledges the client's distress, validates it as understandable under the circumstances, and indicates a willingness to search for solutions. Validation includes making an apology to the client when appropriate, such as when a promised intervention (e.g., changing a dressing by a certain time) has not been delivered.

BOX 24-4

NIC Interventions for Anger Control Assistance

Definition: Facilitation of the express of anger in an adaptive, nonviolent manner

Activities*:

- Establish basic trust and rapport with patient.
- Use calm, reassuring approach.
- Determine appropriate behavioral expectations for expression of anger, given patient's level of cognitive and physical functioning.
- Limit access to frustrating situations until patient is able to express anger in an adaptive manner.
- Encourage patient to seek assistance from nursing staff or responsible others during periods of increasing tension.
- Monitor potential for inappropriate aggression and intervene before its expression.
- Prevent physical harm if anger is directed at self or others (e.g., restrain and remove potential weapons).
- Provide reassurance to patient that nursing staff will intervene to prevent patient from losing control.
- Use external controls (e.g., physical or manual restraint, time-outs, and seclusion) as needed to calm patient who is expressing anger in a maladaptive manner.

From Dochterman, J. M., & Bulechek, G. M. (2004). *Nursing interventions classification (NIC)* (4th ed., p. 166). St. Louis, MO: Mosby.
*Partial list.

Finally, clients who have become angry may be unable to moderate this emotion enough to problem solve with their nurses; others may be unable to communicate the source of their anger. Often, the nurse, knowing the client and the context of the anger, can make an accurate guess at what feeling is behind the anger. Naming this feeling can lead to a dissipation of the anger, can help the client to feel understood, and can lead to a calmer discussion of the distress. Some of the feelings that can precipitate anger are listed in Box 24-5. The following vignette provides an example of nursing interventions that are helpful in dissipating anger in a hospital situation.

▪ ▪ ▪ VIGNETTE

A 41-year-old woman with a long history of peripheral vascular disease and of surgeries for vascular grafts and repair of graft occlusions is admitted to the hospital with severe pain in her left foot. Tests reveal that vessels to the foot are occluded. Additional surgery is ruled out, and medication is prescribed. Unfortunately, the medication is ineffective, and the foot begins to become necrotic. Physicians then discuss amputation with the client. The client refuses the surgery, demands a series of unproven alternative therapies, and is extremely angry with all members of the hospital staff. The treatment team becomes increasingly impatient to schedule further surgery before the necrosis worsens and the client begins to experience signs of systemic infection. This impatience aggravates the client's feelings of being out of control and erodes her belief that she is a competent partner in her treatment.

Intervention. The nurse is aware that before the client became disabled by progressive vascular disease, she had been employed for many years as a buyer at a local department store. The nurse knows, too, that the client's family lives some distance from the hospital and is unable to visit regularly. The nurse recognizes that the client is in the preassaultive stage of the violence cycle and may respond to verbal interventions. Finally, the nurse understands that, when the client was admitted, she had expected medical intervention once more to save her leg. Nursing intervention is twofold. First, the client's anger and unwillingness to discuss her condition end when the nurse names her feelings of fear and being out of control. Once the client's anger is reduced, the nurse is able to help her negotiate more time for the final decision; this allows the client to complete her anticipatory grieving (including stages of denial, anger, and bargaining). In this interval, the client's wish to explore alternative therapies is addressed via second and third medical opinions; she is also able to consult further with her family.

▪ ▪ ▪

Angry Clients with Marginal Coping Skills

Clients whose coping skills were marginal before hospitalization need a different set of interventions than those with basically healthy ways of coping. Clients with maladaptive coping are poorly equipped to use alternatives when their initial attempts to cope are unsuccessful or are found to be inappropriate. Such clients frequently manifest anger that moves quickly from the preassaultive stage to the assaultive stage of the violence cycle. For some, anger and intimidation are primary strategies used to obtain their short-term goals of feelings of control or mastery. For others, the anger occurs when limited or primitive attempts at coping are unsuccessful and alternatives are unknown. For these clients, anger and violence are particular risks in inpatient settings.

This is especially true for hospitalized clients with chemical dependence who may be anxious about being cut off from their substance of choice; they may have well-founded concerns that any physical pain will be inadequately addressed. Many clients with marginal coping also have personality styles that externalize blame. That is, they see the source of their discomfort and anxiety as being outside themselves; relief must therefore also come from an outside source (e.g., the nurse, medication).

Interventions begin with attempts to understand and meet the client's needs. For instance, baseline anxiety can be moderated by the provision of comfort items before they are requested (e.g., decaffeinated coffee, deck of cards); this can build rapport and acts symbolically to reassure. Anxiety can also be minimized by reducing ambiguity. This strategy includes clear and concrete communication. An interaction providing clarity about what the nurse can and cannot do is most usefully ended by offering something within the nurse's power to provide (i.e., leaving the client with a "yes").

Interventions for anxiety might also include the use of distractions, such as magazines, action comics, and video games. Generally, distractions that are colorful and do not require sustained attention work best, al-

BOX 24-5

Feelings That May Underlie Anger

- Discounted
- Embarrassed
- Frightened
- Found out
- Guilty
- Humiliated
- Hurt
- Ignored
- Inadequate
- Insecure
- Not heard
- Out of control of the situation
- Rejected
- Threatened
- Tired
- Vulnerable

though this varies according to the client's interests and abilities. Finally, clients with a high level of baseline anxiety and limited coping skills are helped when their interactions with the treatment team are predictable; this might include speaking with the physician at a specific time each day or having the client see a single spokesperson from the treatment team each day.

Because these clients have limited coping skills, once anxiety is moderated, nursing interventions include teaching alternative behaviors and strategies. For clients who externalize blame, such teaching may best be preceded by a gentle challenge. The challenge serves to engage the client's interest in teaching that might otherwise be seen as irrelevant.

■ ■ ■ *VIGNETTE*

A 21-year-old man who was in an automobile accident is bedridden with a pelvic fracture. During his first day of admission, he yells at each nurse who walks by his room, using expletives in his demands that the nurse enter the room.

Intervention. The nurse who is assigned to the client for the evening stops in his doorway after he yells at her and asks in mild disbelief, "Is this working for you? Do nurses really come in here when you yell at them that way?" The client responds sullenly, justifying his behavior by complaining about his care. However, the nurse's challenge has caught his attention, and she goes on to suggest (i.e., teach) alternative strategies for contacting her and other nurses. The strategies are immediately put into use by the client.

■ ■ ■

This intervention is also important in that the nurse has (1) avoided a punitive or demeaning response that might have fueled escalation of the client's anger, (2) taught a couple of strategies, and (3) provided the client with choices and thus with more control.

Often, anger may be communicated via long-term verbal abuse. If attempts to teach alternatives have not been successful, three interventions can be used:

1. The first is to leave the room as soon as the abuse begins; the client can be informed that the nurse will return in a specific amount of time (e.g., 20 minutes) when the situation is calmer. A matter-of-fact, neutral manner is important because fear, indignation, and arguing are gratifying to many verbally abusive clients. Alternatively, if the nurse is in the midst of a procedure and cannot leave immediately, the nurse can break off conversation and eye contact, completing the procedure quickly and matter-of-factly before leaving the room. Note that the nurse avoids chastising, threatening, or responding punitively to the client.
2. Withdrawal of attention to the abuse is successful only if a second intervention is also used. This step requires attending positively to, and thus reinforcing, nonabusive communication by the client. Interventions can include discussing

non–illness-related topics, responding to requests, and providing emotional support.

3. Clients who are regularly verbally abusive may respond best to the predictability of routine, such as scheduled contacts with the nurse (e.g., every 30 minutes or every 60 minutes). Use of such contacts provides nursing attention that is not contingent on the client's behavior and therefore does not reinforce the abuse. This intervention works only to the extent that the nurse maintains the scheduled contacts as agreed on. In addition, other staff members must be informed of the care plan so that they do not inadvertently sabotage it by responding to incidental requests by the client. Of course, the client's illness or injury may sometimes require nursing visits for assessment or intervention outside the scheduled contact times. These visits can be carried out in a calm, brief, matter-of-fact manner. This care plan is best negotiated with the client and can be presented as supportive in that it attempts to address client anxiety about getting needs met (anxiety that is reflected in the verbal abuse and also manifested by frequent angry demands) through the predictability of the nurse's contacts.

Implementing appropriate interventions can be difficult when the nurse is feeling threatened. Remaining matter-of-fact with clients who habitually use anger and intimidation can be difficult, because these people are often skillful at making personal and pointed statements. It is important for the nurse to remember that clients do not know their nurses personally and thus have no basis on which they can make accurate judgments. Nurses can also vent their own responses elsewhere, with other staff or family members or via critical incident debriefing.

Inpatient Psychiatric Settings

It is important to know that not all psychiatric clients are potentially violent, and aggression appears to be correlated less with certain illnesses than with certain client characteristics. For example, the two most significant predictors of violence are a history of violence and impulsivity.

Situational factors contribute to client anger and aggression. For instance, feelings of vulnerability and powerlessness resulting from trying to come to grips with depersonalized hospital routines, intrusive procedures, and restrictions on freedom lead to anger and possibly aggression (Thomas, 2003). Additional causes of clients' anger include (1) unrealistic expectations that their nurses will be angels of mercy, (2) the feeling that their physical and psychological needs are being ignored (Shattell, 2002), and (3) the feeling that health care providers fail to recognize the uniqueness and wholeness of the client (Plaas, 2002).

If staff can identify clients who have a potential for violence, early intervention becomes possible. Nurses can work with the clients to recognize their early signs of anger and can teach them strategies to manage the anger and to prevent aggression.

▪ ▪ ▪ *VIGNETTE*

A 19-year-old man has a 2-year history of quadriplegia. This client also has a history of drug abuse that began in grade school, an inability to set or work toward long-term goals, and a primary coping style of anger and intimidation. The client is admitted to an inpatient psychiatric unit because of increasing suicidal ideation. He clearly communicates to staff that his preferred means of coping with anger is to "cuss people out" and run into them with his wheelchair. However, in the hospital, the consequence of wheelchair assaults is that the client is secluded in his room, which he finds intolerable. The client asks the staff to help him manage his anger.

Intervention. The nurse assigned to this young man sets aside time to interview him regarding the triggers for his anger. He identifies several issues that "make him angry." These typically relate to feeling unheard and controlled by the staff. Together the nurse and client examine alternative ways for him to deal with these situations, such as telling the staff that he doesn't feel that they are listening to him and letting them know that he needs to be involved in the planning of his care to increase his own sense of control. The client and nurse role-play a situation in which the client is told by a staff member that he must attend a group session. Such a situation would usually result in the client's becoming angry and aggressive, but in the role play he is willing to "try out" alternative communication techniques to communicate his feelings to the staff member and thus to handle his anger. In addition, the client is willing to enter into a behavioral contract with the nurse which states that he will not curse at staff nor assault anyone with his wheelchair. Instead, he will let the staff know when he is feeling angry and what the triggering issue is so that a nonaggressive resolution can be found.

Response. Because this client is intelligent and motivated to gain increased personal control, he responds positively to these suggestions. In addition, once it becomes clear that issues of feeling unheard and out of control underlie most episodes of anger, the client is able to target these issues for problem solving. He rapidly develops effective and appropriate ways to make himself heard and understood. He also becomes adept at communicating when he feels out of control and at finding ingenious ways of negotiating control on issues that are particularly important to him. The client's suicidal impulses, which occur when he is frustrated, also diminish.

▪ ▪ ▪

Clients with Cognitive Deficits

Clients with cognitive deficits are particularly at risk for acting aggressively. Such deficits may result from delirium, dementias (e.g., Alzheimer's disease, multi-infarct dementia), or brain injury (see Chapter 21).

Traditional approaches to disorientation and to the agitation that it can cause have relied heavily on reality orientation and medication. Reality orientation consists of providing the correct information to the client about place, date, and current life circumstances. For many clients, this is comforting because it reminds them of pertinent information and helps them feel grounded. For others, reality orientation does not work; because of their cognitive disorder they can no longer "enter into our reality"; they become frightened and more agitated, and may become aggressive.

Sedating medication may calm agitation, but the risks often outweigh the benefits. Sedation only further clouds a client's sensorium, which makes disorientation worse and increases the risks of falls and injuries. It is better to examine alternative interventions.

Orientation aids, such as a calendar and a clock, can provide easy reference and increased autonomy. Such aids must be prominent and easily read by clients with diminished eyesight. Because such clients have difficulty interpreting environmental stimuli, another set of interventions involves making the environment as simple, predictable, and comfortable as possible. Simplicity includes decreasing sensory stimuli. In the hospital, this might include placing the client's bed away from doorways that enter onto the hall and choosing not to turn on the television. Establishing a routine of activities for each day and displaying the day's schedule prominently in the client's room can provide predictability. The comfort of the client is enhanced by provision of familiar photographs and objects from home. The availability of a rocking chair can provide a rhythmic source of self-soothing.

Sometimes the client with a cognitive disorder experiences such severe agitation and aggression that it is referred to as a catastrophic reaction. The client may scream, strike out, or cry because of overwhelming fear. Adopting a calm and unhurried manner is the best response to such a client. The steps for making contact with a client experiencing a catastrophic reaction are listed in Box 24-6.

To respond effectively to episodes of agitation, it is crucial to identify the antecedents, or what preceded the episode, and the consequences of such episodes. Once antecedents are understood, interventions are often obvious.

▪ ▪ ▪ *VIGNETTE*

An 81-year-old woman with Alzheimer's disease always becomes agitated during her morning care; this comes to be a time dreaded by her caregivers. Careful observation of the antecedents to episodes of agitation reveals a natural course to the morning problems. The client is initially calm when care begins. However, one staff person gives morning care to the client and her roommate at the same time, moving between the two. Observation of the process reveals that the client becomes distracted by cues being given to her roommate and often startles when the caregiver returns

BOX 24-6

Cognitive Deficits

The Catastrophic Reaction: Making Contact
Cognitive deficits result in
- A decreased ability to interpret sensory stimuli.
- A decreased ability to tolerate sensory stimuli.

Striking out represents fear or the feeling that the environment is out of control.
Presence of a second agitated person (e.g., staff member) leads to increased agitation.
Therefore:
1. Face the client from within 2 feet, remaining as calm and unhurried as possible.
2. Say the client's name.
3. Gain eye contact.
4. Smile.
5. Repeat (2) through (4) several times if necessary, to gain and maintain contact.
6. Use gentle touch, keep voice soft (the person often matches this tone and lowers his or her voice also).
7. Ask the client if he or she needs the bathroom.
8. Help the client regain a sense of control—ask what he or she needs.
9. Validate the client's feelings: "You look upset. This can be a confusing place."
10. Use short, simple sentences; complex explanations just represent more noise.
11. Decrease sensory stimulation.
12. Get the client to use rhythmic sources of self-stimulation (e.g., humming, a rocking chair).

Adapted from Rader, J., Doan, J., & Schwab, M. (1985). How to decrease wandering, a form of agenda behavior. *Geriatric Nursing, 6*(4), 196-199.

to her. As this process continues over several minutes, the client becomes increasingly distressed and then agitated. When a change is made so that the client's care is provided by one person who remains with her throughout the process, the client's morning agitation ends.

Consequences of agitation may also be a factor if they serve to reinforce the behaviors. For example, an elderly man who loves ice cream and who becomes calm when it is given to him becomes agitated more often when ice cream is routinely used to stop his angry behaviors.

Finally, clients who misperceive their setting or life situation may be calmed by **validation therapy** (Feil, 1992). Some disoriented clients believe that they are young and feel the need to return to important tasks that were a significant part of those earlier years. For example, an elderly woman may insist that she must go home to take care of her babies. Telling the client that her babies have grown up and there is no home to return to is not only cruel but nontherapeutic and will result in increased agitation. It is often more helpful to reflect back to the client the feelings behind her de-

mand and to show understanding and concern for her worry.

Rather than attempting to reorient the client, the nurse asks him or her to further describe the setting or situation that the client has reported to be a problem (e.g., the need to return home). During the conversation, the nurse can comment on what appears to be underlying the client's distress, thus validating it. For example, the elderly woman who believes that she needs to return home to care for her children is asked to tell the nurse more about her children. The nurse may note that the client misses her children and that the current setting gets lonely at times. For example:

Nurse: Mrs. Green, you miss your children, and this can be a lonely place.

As the nurse shows interest in aspects of the client's life, the nurse establishes himself or herself as a safe, understanding person. In turn, the client often becomes calmer and more open to redirection. As clients reminisce in this fashion, they often bring themselves into the present: "Of course, they're all grown and doing well on their own now." Refer to Chapter 21 for more on interventions for people with cognitive impairments. Box 24-7 provides a framework for validation therapy. Refer to Chapter 34 for more on the use of validation and reminiscent therapeutic modalities for the elderly.

BOX 24-7

Validation Therapy for Clients with Cognitive Deficits

Validation therapy lets you begin emotionally where the client is.
Validation therapy "grounds" the client where he or she feels most secure.
Reality orientation is the first intervention. Resistance to this intervention may represent an increased feeling by the client that the environment makes no sense.
Therefore:
1. Make a connection with the person as outlined in Box 24-6.
2. Repeat some part of what the client has said: "You need to go home to fix dinner for your children?"
3. Reflect what seems to be the underlying feeling (usually related to a lack of connectedness or security): "You miss your children. And this can be a lonely place."
4. Continue to talk with the client about the topic (e.g., the children); this establishes you as a safe, understanding person.
5. As the client becomes calmer and more secure, redirect him or her (e.g., back to the client's room).
6. Provide a parting reinforcer (e.g., food, rocking chair), an esteem-enhancing comment, or a reassuring comment.
7. Provide orienting information again only if the person requests it.

Adapted from Rader, J., Doan, J., & Schwab, M. (1985). How to decrease wandering, a form of agenda behavior. *Geriatric Nursing, 6*(4), 196-199.

EVALUATION

Evaluation of the care plan is essential for clients who are potentially angry and aggressive. A well-considered plan has specific outcome criteria (see Table 24-1). Evaluation provides information about the extent to which the interventions have achieved the outcomes. If the outcomes have not been achieved to at least a level of 3 on the five-point Likert scale, the plan must be revised. Revision focuses on all aspects of the nursing process:

- Was the assessment accurate and thorough?
- Were the nursing diagnoses applicable to the assessment data? Did the nursing diagnoses accurately drive nursing interventions?
- Was the plan comprehensive and individualized?

For instance, the initial plan may have included assessment of the environmental stimuli that precede a client's agitation. Once these are identified, the plan provides interventions that are specific to those stimuli. However, the plan can work only if staff members evaluate the effectiveness of the approach by noting the extent to which agitation is decreased. Evaluation may reveal that the client's agitation has decreased except in specific situations. The plan is then revised to include these situations.

▪▪▪ KEY POINTS to REMEMBER

- Angry emotions and aggressive actions are difficult targets for nursing intervention.
- Nurses benefit from an understanding of how the angry and aggressive client should be handled.
- Understanding client cues to escalating aggression, appropriate goals for intervention for individuals in a variety of situations, and helpful nursing interventions is important for nurses in any setting.
- The expression of anger can lead to increased anger and to negative physiological changes.
- Behavioral, cognitive, and biological theories provide explanations for anger and aggression.
- It is helpful for providers of care to know what cues should be looked for and what should be assessed when a client's anger is escalating (verbal cues, nonverbal cues that include facial expression, breathing, body language, and posture).
- A client's past aggressive behavior is the most important indicator of future aggressive episodes.
- Working with angry and aggressive clients is a challenge for all nurses, and a careful understanding and recognition of one's personal responses to angry or threatening clients can be crucial.
- Many approaches are effective in helping clients deescalate and maintain control.
- Different interventions are used depending on the client's coping abilities, cognitive status, and potential for violence.
- Guidelines for deescalation of client behavior are given.
- Specific medications such as antipsychotics, lithium, and antianxiety medications may be useful.
- Restraints may be needed to ensure the safety of the client as well as the safety of other clients and the staff.
- Each unit has a clear protocol for the safe use of restraints and for the humane management of care during the time the client is restrained, as well as clear guidelines for understanding and protecting the client's legal rights.

▪ ▪ ▪

Visit the Evolve website at **http://evolve.elsevier.com/Varcarolis** for a posttest on the content in this chapter. **evolve**

Critical Thinking and Chapter Review

Visit the Evolve website at **http://evolve.elsevier.com/Varcarolis** for additional self-study exercises.
evolve

▪▪▪ CRITICAL THINKING

1. A 24-year-old man with mania is admitted to an inpatient unit. Staff note that the client is irritable and has a history of assault. What interventions should be built into the care plan?
    A. Identify appropriate responses the nurse can make to the client.
    B. Identify at least three long-term outcomes to consider when planning care.

2. Identify some assessment data that can be used as predictors of potential violence.

3. What are the four indicators for the use of seclusion and restraint rather than verbal interventions?

Critical Thinking and Chapter Review—cont'd

Visit the Evolve website at **http://evolve.elsevier.com/Varcarolis** for additional self-study exercises.

evolve

■ ■ ■ CHAPTER REVIEW

Choose the most appropriate answer.

1. Which is a clinical example of the use of predictability when caring for an anxious, angry client who possesses limited coping skills?
   1. The nurse refocuses conversation to minimize client tangentiality.
   2. The nurse empathizes with the client's underlying fear and anxiety.
   3. The nurse agrees to meet with the client for 10 minutes every 2 hours.
   4. The nurse teaches the client techniques to manage auditory hallucinations.

2. In planning intervention for an angry client, the nurse must understand that withdrawal of attention to verbally abusive behaviors works only if the strategy is accompanied by
   1. attending positively to nonabusive communication.
   2. requiring the client to wait before granting requests.
   3. giving large doses of antipsychotic medication.
   4. using empathetic communication.

3. To act to prevent displays of anger and aggression, the nurse must understand that anger and aggression are preceded by feelings of
   1. vulnerability.
   2. depression.
   3. elation.
   4. isolation.

4. Which information is most useful to the nurse planning intervention for an angry client?
   1. Client facial expression
   2. Client body language
   3. Client medical diagnosis
   4. Client perception of the situation

5. The nurse should understand that encouraging a client to vent anger
   1. is a strategic nursing intervention.
   2. should always be taught as a beneficial anger management technique.
   3. is not always useful.
   4. is useful only in a well-controlled inpatient setting.

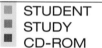

■ STUDENT
■ STUDY
■ CD-ROM

Access the accompanying CD-ROM for animations, interactive exercises, review questions for the NCLEX examination, and an audio glossary.

■ NURSE,
■ CLIENT, AND
■ FAMILY RESOURCES

For suggested readings, information on related associations, and Internet resources, go to **http://evolve.elsevier.com/Varcarolis.**

REFERENCES

American Psychiatric Nurses Association. (2000). *Position statement on the use of seclusion and restraint.* Retrieved March 7, 2005, from http://www.apna.org.

Bandura, A. (1973). *Aggression: A social learning analysis.* New York: Prentice Hall.

Beck, A. (1976). *Cognitive therapy and the emotional disorders.* New York: International Universities Press.

Bergstrom, B. (2001, May 7). One out of 3 nurses under 30 plans to quit in next year, study finds. *Knoxville News-Sentinel,* p. A-13.

Brackbill, W., et al. (1990). Family dynamics as predictors of infant disposition. *Infant Mental Health Journal, 11,* 113-126.

Brook, J., Whiteman, M., & Brook, D. (1999). Transmission of risk factors across three generations. *Psychological Reports, 85*(1), 227-241.

Centers for Disease Control and Prevention, National Center for Injury Prevention and Control. (2003). Web-based Injury Statistics Query and Reporting System [Interactive database system]. Retrieved from http://www.cdc.gov/ncipc/wisqars.

Centers for Disease Control and Prevention, National Institute for Occupational Safety and Health. (2002, April). *Violence: Occupational hazards in hospitals* (DHHS [NIOSH] Publication 2002-101). Retrieved March 7, 2005, from http://www.cdc.gov/niosh/2002-101.html.

Davis, M., Matthews, K., & McGrath, C. (2000). Hostile attitudes predict elevated vascular resistance during interpersonal stress in men and women. *Psychosomatic Medicine, 62*(1), 17-25.

Dochterman, J. M., & Bulechek, G. M. (2004). *Nursing interventions classification (NIC)* (4th ed.). St. Louis, MO: Mosby.

Eisenberg, N., et al. (1997). Contemporaneous and longitudinal prediction of children's social functioning from regulation and emotionality. *Child Development, 68,* 642-664.

Ekman, P. (2003). *Emotions revealed: Understanding faces and feelings.* London: Weidenfeld & Nicolson.

Feil, N. (1992). *V/F validation: The Feil method.* Cleveland, OH: Edward Feil Productions.

Fenichel, M. (2005). *Children and violence.* Retrieved March 7, 2005, from http://www.fenichel.com/violence.shtml.

Fredrickson, B., et al. (2000). Hostility predicts magnitude and duration of blood pressure responses to anger. *Journal of Behavioral Medicine, 23*(3), 229-243.

Health Care Financing Administration, Medicare and Medicaid Programs. (1999). *Hospital conditions of patient's rights: Interim final rule.* Washington, DC: Author.

Kavoussi, R., Armstead, P., & Coccaro, E. (1997). The neurobiology of impulsive aggression. *Psychiatric Clinics of North America, 20*(2), 395-401.

Moorhead, S., Johnson, M., & Maas, M. (2004). *Nursing outcomes classification (NOC)* (3rd ed.). St. Louis, MO: Mosby.

National Television Violence Study Council. (1996). *National violence study: Council statement.* Studio City, CA: MediaScope.

Partenheimer, D. (July 24, 2003). *Exposure to violence between parents and harsh punishment during childhood significantly increases risk for adult partner violence.* Retrieved February 11, 2005, from http://www.apa.org/releases/partnerviolence.html.

Plaas, K. (2002). Like a bunch of cattle: The patient's experience of the outpatient health care environment. In S. B. Thomas & H. R. Pollio (Eds.), *Listening to patients: A phenomenological approach to nursing research and practice* (pp. 237-251). New York: Springer Publishing.

Sadock, B. J., & Sadock, V. A. (2004). *Kaplan & Sadock's concise textbook of clinical psychiatry* (2nd ed.). Philadelphia: Lippincott Williams & Wilkins.

Shattell, M. (2002). Eventually it'll be over: The dialectic between confinement and freedom in the world of the hospitalized patient. In S. P. Thomas & H. R. Pollio (Eds.), *Listening to patients: A phenomenological approach to nursing research and practice* (pp. 214-236). New York: Springer Publishing.

Siegman, A., et al. (2000). Antagonistic behavior, dominance, hostility, and coronary heart disease. *Psychosomatic Medicine, 62*(2), 248-257.

Skinner, B. (1953). *Science and human behavior.* New York: Macmillan.

Smith, M., & Hart, G. (1994). Nurses' responses to patient anger: From disconnecting to connecting. *Journal of Advanced Nursing, 20*(4), 643-651.

Suinn, R. (2001). The terrible twos—anger and anxiety: Hazardous to your health. *American Psychologist, 56,* 27-36.

Tavris, C. (1982). *Anger: The misunderstood emotion.* New York: Simon & Shuster.

Thomas, S. P. (2003). Anger: The mismanaged emotion. *Dermatologic Nursing, 15*(4), 351-357.

Williams, J. E., et al. (2000). Anger proneness predicts coronary heart disease risk: Prospective analysis from the Atherosclerosis Risk in Communities (ARIC) Study. *Circulation, 101,* 2034-2039.

CHAPTER 25

Family Violence

VERNA BENNER CARSON ■ KATHLEEN SMITH-DIJULIO

■ KEY TERMS and CONCEPTS

The key terms and concepts listed here appear in color where they are defined or first discussed in this chapter.

acute battering stage, 510

crisis situation, 510

economic maltreatment, 511

emotional violence, 511

escalation-deescalation, 510

family violence, 508

health care record, 517

honeymoon stage, 510

neglect, 511

perpetrators, 508

physical violence, 510

primary prevention, 520

safety plan, 521

secondary prevention, 520

sexual violence, 510

shelters or safe houses, 521

tension-building stage, 510

tertiary prevention, 521

vulnerable person, 509

■ OBJECTIVES

After studying this chapter, the reader will be able to

1. Discuss the epidemiological theory of violence in terms of stresses on the perpetrator, vulnerable person, and environment that could escalate anxiety to the point at which violence becomes the relief behavior.
2. Contrast and compare three characteristics of perpetrators with three characteristics of a vulnerable person.
3. Name three indicators of (a) physical violence, (b) sexual violence, (c) neglect, and (d) emotional violence.
4. Describe four areas to assess when interviewing a person who has experienced family violence.
5. Formulate four nursing diagnoses for the survivor of violence and list supporting data from the assessment.
6. Write out a safety plan, including the essential elements, for an abused spouse.
7. Compare and contrast primary, secondary, and tertiary levels of intervention, giving two examples of intervention for each level.
8. Identify two common emotional responses the nurse might experience when faced with a person subjected to family violence.
9. Describe at least three possible referrals for a violent family (child, adult, elder abuse) and write down the telephone numbers of the corresponding agencies in the community.
10. Name and discuss three psychotherapeutic modalities that are useful in working with violent families.

evolve Visit the Evolve website at **http://evolve.elsevier.com/Varcarolis** for a pretest on the content in this chapter.

PREVALENCE

Violence is among America's most important public health issues. A violent family is one in which at least one family member is using physical or sexual force against another that results in physically or emotionally destructive injury, or both. The true prevalence of child, spouse-partner, and elder abuse is not known because of underreporting and variability in reporting methods, instruments, sites, and reporters.

In a 2003 survey conducted by the Center for the Advancement of Women, led by former Planned Parenthood president Faye Wattleton, the chief concern voiced by American women was the reduction of domestic violence and sexual assault. Of over 3300 women surveyed by Princeton Survey Research Associates from 2001 to 2003, 92% cited reducing violence as their top priority, whereas only 41% of women surveyed identified keeping abortion legal as a top priority (Center for the Advancement of Women, 2003). Approximately 20% to 30% of the women in this country will experience domestic violence during their lives (Mayes, 2003). Estimates are that 2% to 4% of all women seen in hospital emergency departments have acute trauma associated with domestic violence and another 10% to 12% have a recent history of domestic violence. In addition, an estimated 73,000 hospitalizations and 1500 deaths among women are attributed to domestic violence each year (Agency for Healthcare Research and Quality, 2002).

Estimates are that half of all Americans have experienced violence in their families. A substantial percentage of childhood injuries are due to abuse (DiScala, 2000; Reece & Sege, 2000). Every year more than 2 million older Americans are victims of physical, psychological, or other forms of abuse and neglect, and experts estimate that for every case of elder abuse and neglect that is reported to the authorities, there may be as many as five cases that are not reported (American Psychological Association, 2003). The occurrence of one type of violence is a fairly strong predictor of the occurrence of another type. This connection calls for more coordinated efforts at prevention and intervention. To this end, the President's Family Justice Center Initiative was passed in 2004 to provide for planning and development of a comprehensive domestic violence victim service and support centers (U.S. Department of Justice, 2004).

Violence can also occur in gay and lesbian relationships. Domestic violence is the third largest health problem for gay men, following substance abuse and acquired immunodeficiency syndrome (Seelau, Seelau, & Poorman, 2003). Violence between siblings is one of the most common and unrecognized forms of domestic violence. Another alarming and often unreported form of domestic violence is that of children against parents. Although it is often not reported or even discussed, violence toward men by women also occurs and goes unrecognized as a problem.

COMORBIDITY

The secondary effects of violence, such as anxiety, depression, and suicidal ideation, are health care issues that can last a lifetime. Family violence is common in the childhood histories of juvenile delinquents, runaways, violent criminals, prostitutes, and those who in turn are violent toward others. Exposure to violence can adversely affect children's development, because the energy needed to accomplish developmental tasks successfully goes to coping with violence (Bensley, Van Eenwyk, & Wynkoop Simmons, 2003; Desai, 2002). Abused adolescents report more psychopathological changes, poorer coping and social skills, a

higher incidence of dissociative identity disorder, and poorer impulse control than do other adolescents. Women who are victims of prolonged childhood sexual abuse are more likely to develop major psychiatric distress. When health care providers do not routinely assess for history of sexual abuse, symptoms arising in times of crisis may be labeled as adult psychopathological disorders and not understood as possible post-trauma response (Stevens, 2003). Box 25-1 identifies some of the long-term effects of family violence.

Social factors that reinforce violence include the wide acceptance of the hitting of children (corporal punishment); the celebration of increasingly violent movies, video games, Internet sites, and comic books;

BOX 25-1

Long-Term Effects of Family Violence

People involved in family violence are found to have a higher incidence of
- Depression.
- Suicidal feelings.
- Self-contempt.
- Inability to trust.
- Inability to develop intimate relationships in later life.

Victims of severe violence are also at higher risk for experiencing recurring symptoms of posttraumatic stress disorder:
- Flashbacks
- Dissociation—out-of-body experiences
- Poor self-esteem
- Compulsive or impulsive behaviors (e.g., substance abuse, excessive spending, gambling, and promiscuity)
- Multiple somatic complaints

Children who witness violence in their homes
- After the age of 5 or 6 years show an indication of identifying with the aggressor and losing respect for the victim.
- Are at greater risk for developing behavioral and emotional problems throughout their lives.

Some mental and behavioral disorders are associated with violence in childhood:
- Depressive disorders
- Posttraumatic stress disorder
- Somatic complaints
- Low self-esteem
- Phobias (agoraphobia, social and specific phobias)
- Antisocial behaviors
- Child or spouse abuse

Adolescents are more likely to have behavioral symptoms such as
- Failing grades.
- Difficulty forming relationships.
- Increased incidence of theft, police arrest, and violent behaviors.
- Seductive or promiscuous behaviors.
- Running away from home.

the violent themes in rap music; and the increase in the total volume of pornography (which is strongly associated with physical abuse of women).

THEORY

Family violence refers to physical injury or mental anguish (e.g., putdowns, demeaning actions toward partners, controlling behavior) inflicted by one family member upon another and the omission or deprivation of essential services by a caregiver. To be more effective in working with victims, the nurse needs an understanding of the conditions for violence and the types of maltreatment. Fundamental to this entire discussion is self-understanding, which is addressed in the Self-Assessment section.

Conditions for Violence

Abuse occurs across all segments of American society and is reinforced by the society and the culture. The actual occurrence of violence requires (1) a perpetrator; (2) someone who by age or situation is vulnerable (i.e., children, women, the elderly, and the mentally ill or physically challenged person); and (3) a crisis situation.

Perpetrator

The propensity for violence is rooted in childhood and manifested by a general lack of self-regard, dissatisfaction with life, and inability to assume adult roles. Often the abuser lacked good role models and was deprived of the opportunity to develop learning and problem-solving skills. Witnessing family violence, experiencing family violence, and experiencing neglectful or abusive parenting are contributing factors.

Perpetrators, those who initiate violence, often consider their own needs to be more important than anyone else's and look toward others to meet their needs. Specific characteristics of violent parents and of those who maltreat elders are listed in Boxes 25-2 and 25-3, respectively.

Even though the majority of victims are women, men are also abused. The principles discussed in this chapter apply to any member of a household who is violent toward another member (e.g., siblings, same-sex partners, extended family members).

■ ■ ■ ■ **VIGNETTE**

A 53-year-old man came to the ambulatory care clinic looking very fatigued and complaining of pain in his left shoulder "since last night." Holding his left arm close to his side,

---

BOX 25-2

Characteristics of Violent Parents

- A history of violence, neglect, or emotional deprivation as a child
- Family authoritarianism: raise children as they were raised by their own parents
- Low self-esteem, feelings of worthlessness, depression
- Poor coping skills
- Social isolation (may be suspicious of others): few or no friends, little or no involvement in social or community activities
- Involvement in a crisis situation: unemployment, divorce, financial difficulties
- Rigid, unrealistic expectations of child's behavior
- Frequent use of harsh punishment
- History of severe mental illness, such as schizophrenia
- Violent temper outbursts
- Looking to child for satisfaction of needs for love, support, and reassurance (often unmet because of parenting deficits in family of origin)
- Projection of blame onto the child for parents' "troubles" (e.g., stepparent may project hostility toward new mate onto a child)
- Lack of effective parenting skills
- Inability to seek help from others
- Perception of the child as bad or evil
- History of drug or alcohol abuse
- Feeling of little or no control over life
- Low tolerance for frustration
- Poor impulse control

Data from Warner, C. G. (Ed.). (1981). *Conflict intervention in social and domestic violence.* Bowie, MD: Robert J. Brady.

BOX 25-3

Characteristics of Elder Abusers

Physical and Psychological Violence
The perpetrator may have
- A history of mental illness.
- A recent decline in mental status.
- Recent medical problems.
- A financial dependence on the victim.
- Shared living arrangements with the victim.
- A history of alcohol or drug abuse.
- Pathological family dynamics.

Neglect
The perpetrator may
- Abuse alcohol or drugs.
- Not live with the victim.
- Not have a decline in mental status.
- Not have recent medical problems.
- Not experience the victim as a source of stress.

Financial Maltreatment
The perpetrator may
- Abuse alcohol or drugs.
- Be a distant relative.
- Be financially dependent on the victim.
- Be greedy.

Data from Wolf, R. S., & Pillemer, K. A. (1989). *Helping elderly victims: The reality of elder abuse.* New York: Columbia University Press; and Wolf, R. S. (1990). Elder abuse: Scope, characteristics, and treatment. *Nurse Practitioner Forum, 1*(2), 102.

he averted his eyes from those of the receptionist, nurse, and doctor. When asked if anything had occurred that might have caused the pain, he answered, "I fell." Asked why he had not sought care the previous night, he stated, "I . . . I . . . thought it would go away overnight."

Upon further examination and x-ray imaging, it was determined that the patient had sustained a fractured clavicle. Additional direct, supportive questioning elicited the information that the patient had been injured when pushed down the stairs by his 17-year-old stepson.

■ ■ ■

Men and women who are violent are found in all segments of society. Men who abuse believe in male supremacy, being in charge, and being dominant. "Acting out" physically makes them feel more in control, more masculine, and more powerful. Parent-child interactions, peer-group experiences, observations of the partner dyad, and the influence of the media (television, comics, video games, movies) all support the same message: males can expect to be in a position of power in relationships and may use physical aggression to maintain that position.

Extreme pathological jealousy is characteristic of an abuser. Many refuse to allow their partners to work outside the home; others demand that their partners work in the same place as they do so that they can monitor activities and friendships. Many accompany their partners to and from all activities and forbid them to have personal friends or to participate in recreational activities outside the home. When this is not possible, a man or woman may restrict mobility by monitoring the odometer and keeping clock watches. Even with such restrictions, abusers accuse their partners of infidelity. Many perpetrators maintain their possessiveness by controlling the family finances so tightly that there is barely enough money for daily living. These abusive men and women may appear to outsiders as ordinary doctors, nurses, machinists, lawyers, salesmen, executives, and plumbers—or even police officers, judges, and politicians. It is important to recognize that there are a wide variety of cultural norms dictating male-female relationships, some of which might appear to be abusive. Learning about the cultural backgrounds of clients can prevent mistaking

common cultural norms for abuse. Misunderstandings frequently exist regarding traditional culture-bound health practices and the knowledge level of health care providers caring for specific populations (Davis, 2000). The Culturally Speaking box describes Asha Family Services, which focuses on the needs of African Americans.

Individuals are more likely to engage in family violence when they use substances. Alcohol and other drugs (illicit or prescribed) tend to weaken inhibitions and lead to a disregard of social rules prohibiting violence against children, women, and the elderly, whom perpetrators view as weak and inferior. The consumption of alcohol and drugs is often used as a rationalization by the victim to excuse the behavior ("He was drunk, and he didn't know what he was doing"). In fact, when drug and alcohol use is reduced or eliminated, family violence still occurs.

Both male and female perpetrators perceive themselves as having poor social skills. They describe their relationships with their spouses as being the closest they have ever known, which is typical in enmeshed and codependent relationships. They lack supportive relationships outside the marriage.

Vulnerable Person

The **vulnerable person** is the one in the family unit on whom violence is perpetrated. In some situations, violence does not occur until after the legal marriage of couples who have lived together or dated for a long time.

Pregnancy often serves to increase violence even further (Gazmararian et al., 2000). An estimated 15% to 25% of women experience violence during pregnancy. One reason may be that the husband resents the added responsibility that a baby entails, or he may resent the relationship that the baby will have with his mate. Violence also escalates when the wife makes a move toward independence, such as visiting friends without permission, getting a job, or going back to school. Victims are at greatest risk for violence when they attempt to leave the relationship.

Children are most likely to be abused if they are younger than 3 years of age; are perceived as being dif-

---

■ ■ ■ **CULTURALLY SPEAKING**

Although violence against women is a worldwide phenomenon, the response of victims is influenced by cultural factors. Asha Family Services, based in Milwaukee, Wisconsin, is designed to meet the cultural needs of African American women. The center is committed to providing a spiritually based, holistic, and culturally responsive service designed to end violence against African American women and children specifically and

families of other communities of color and all families in general. The services are informed by the belief that, to adequately address family violence and promote healthy living, the abuser as well as the abused must be treated. The center recognizes the importance of shared cultural values, history, language, experience, traditions, and spirituality of people of color.

Vann, A. A. (2003). *Developing culturally-relevant responses to domestic abuse: Asha Family Services, Inc.* Harrisburg, PA: National Resource Center on Domestic Violence

ferent because of temperamental traits, congenital abnormalities, or chronic disease; remind the parents of someone they do not like (perhaps an ex-spouse); are different from the parents' fantasy of what the child should be like; or are a product of an unwanted pregnancy. Interference with emotional bonding between parents and child (e.g., because of a premature birth or prolonged illness requiring hospitalization) has also been found to increase the risk for future abuse. Adolescents are abused at least as frequently as younger children, yet such abuse is often overlooked.

Elderly adults may become vulnerable because they are in poor mental or physical health or are disruptive (e.g., a person with Alzheimer's disease). The dependency needs of elderly persons are usually what puts them at risk for abuse. The typical victim is female, over 75 years of age, white, living with a relative, and experiencing a physical and/or mental impairment. Dealing with the problems of the elderly can be stressful for adult caregivers in the best of cases, but in families in which violence was a coping strategy, the potential for abuse is great. Other scenarios include the elderly male cared for by a daughter whom he abused as a child and who now is abusive toward him, or the elderly woman abused by her husband as part of a longstanding abusive relationship. Many caregivers become angry because of the failing health of a loved one.

Crisis Situation

Anyone may be at risk for abuse in a crisis situation, one that puts stress on a family with a violent member. Stressful life events tax coping skills, leaving the perpetrator incapable of dealing with what is going on. A person with good impulse control who can solve problems and has a healthy support system is less likely to resort to violence. Social isolation caused by frequent moves or an inability to make friends contributes to ineffective coping during crisis situations. Refer to Chapter 22 for more on crisis and crisis intervention.

Cycle of Violence

Periods of intense violence alternate with periods of safety, hope, and trust. This pattern has been described as a process of escalation-deescalation.

The tension-building stage is characterized by minor incidents such as pushing, shoving, and verbal abuse. During this time the victim does not say that the abuse is unacceptable, for fear that more severe abuse will follow. Abusers then rationalize that their abusive behavior is acceptable.

As the tension escalates, both spouses may try to reduce it. The batterer may try to reduce the tension with the use of alcohol or drugs. The vulnerable person may try to reduce the tension by minimizing the importance of the incidents ("I should have had the house neater . . . dinner ready"). The abused person may also try to reduce the tension by somatizing, thus perpetuating the "poor-me" image.

During the acute battering stage, the perpetrator releases the built-up tension by brutal and uncontrollable beatings. The perpetrator is unable to control the amount of damage inflicted on the victim. Severe injuries can and do result. The perpetrator may have amnesia and may not remember what happened during the battering. The victim usually depersonalizes the incident and is able to remember the beatings in detail. After the beatings, both are in shock.

The honeymoon stage may be characterized by kindness and loving behaviors. The perpetrator, at least initially, feels remorseful and apologetic and may bring presents, make promises, and tell the victim how much she or he is loved and needed. The victim usually believes the promises, feels needed and loved, and drops any legal proceedings or plans to leave that may have been initiated during the acute battering stage. Unfortunately, without intervention the cycle will repeat itself. The honeymoon stage will fade away as tension starts to build.

When escalation-deescalation occurs, conditions of anger and fear escalate until an incident of violence takes place, after which there is a defusing of tension and a brief feeling of safety. Over time, the periods of calmness and safety become briefer and the periods of anger and fear are more intense. There are intervals of stability, but the violence increases over time. With each repeat of the pattern, the self-esteem of the person experiencing the violence becomes more and more eroded. The victim either believes that the violence was deserved or accepts the blame for it. This can lead to feelings of depression, hopelessness, immobilization, and self-deprecation. Figure 25-1 illustrates the cycle of violence.

Types of Maltreatment

Five specific types of maltreatment have been identified: (1) physical violence, (2) sexual violence, (3) emotional violence, (4) neglect, and (5) economic maltreatment.

1. Physical violence is the infliction of physical pain or bodily harm (e.g., slapping, punching, hitting, pushing, restraining, biting, throwing, burning).
2. Sexual violence is any form of sexual contact or exposure without consent, or in circumstances in which the victim is incapable of giving consent. Childhood sexual abuse destroys an individual's positive self-concept and can interfere with the learning of self-care skills. Sexual abuse of adults is usually referred to as sexual assault or rape, and is discussed in Chapter 26.

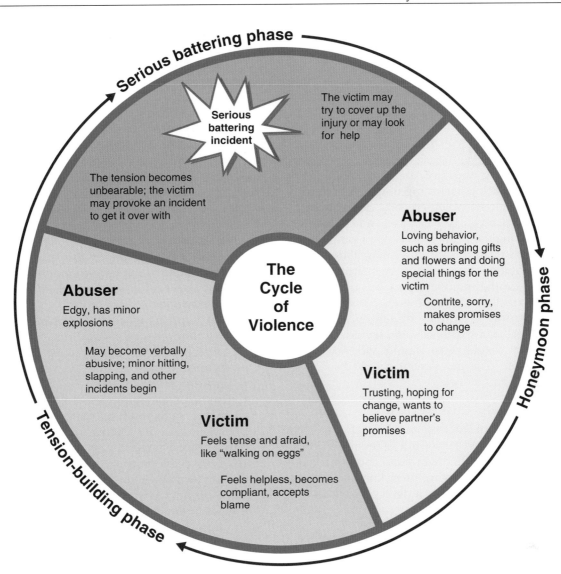

FIGURE 25-1 The cycle of violence. (Redrawn from YWCA of Annapolis and Anne Arundel County, 1517 Ritchie Highway, Arnold, MD 21012.)

3. **Emotional violence** is the infliction of mental anguish (e.g., threatening, humiliating, intimidating, and isolating). It can take the form of any of the following:
   - Terrorizing an individual through verbal threats
   - Demeaning an individual's worth or putting the person down
   - Directing blatant or subtle hostility and hatred toward an individual—or omitting positive behaviors
   - Persistently ignoring an individual and her or his needs
   - Consistently belittling and criticizing an individual
   - Withholding warmth and affection from an individual

   - Threatening an individual with abandonment or institutionalization (nursing home, psychiatric hospital)

4. **Neglect** can be physical, developmental, or educational. **Physical neglect** is failure to provide the medical, dental, or psychiatric care needed to prevent or treat physical or emotional illnesses. **Developmental neglect** is failure to provide emotional nurturing and the physical and cognitive stimulation needed to ensure freedom from developmental deficits. **Educational neglect** occurs when a child's caretakers deprive the child of the education available in accordance with the state's education laws.

5. **Economic maltreatment** is illegal or improper exploitation of funds or other resources for one's personal gain or withholding of support.

Application of the Nursing Process

■ ASSESSMENT
Overall Assessment

Persons experiencing violence are encountered in every health care setting, including outpatient clinics, community health centers, emergency departments, general hospitals, physicians' offices, and nursing homes, and during home health visits. Complaints may be vague and can include insomnia, abdominal pain, hyperventilation, headache, or menstrual problems. Attention to the interview process and setting are important to facilitate accurate assessment of physical and behavioral indicators of family violence (Stevens, 2003). All assessments should include identifying a history of sexual abuse, family violence, and drug use or abuse. The assessment should be completed with the victim alone.

Interview Process and Setting

Important and relevant information about the family situation can be gathered by routine assessment conducted with tact, understanding, and a calm, relaxed attitude. Important interviewing guidelines are listed in Box 25-4. A person who feels judged or accused of

---

<table>
<tr><td>

BOX 25-4

Interview Guidelines

Do
- Conduct the interview in private.
- Be direct, honest, and professional.
- Use language the client understands.
- Ask the client to clarify words not understood.
- Be understanding.
- Be attentive.
- Inform the client if you must make a referral to children's or adult protective services and explain the process.
- Assess safety and help reduce danger (at discharge).

Don't
- Do *not* try to "prove" abuse by accusations or demands.
- Do *not* display horror, anger, shock, or disapproval of the perpetrator or situation.
- Do *not* place blame or make judgments.
- Do *not* allow the client to feel "at fault" or "in trouble."
- Do *not* probe or press for answers the client is not willing to give.
- Do *not* conduct the interview with a group of interviewers.
- Do *not* force a child or anyone else to remove clothing.

</td></tr>
</table>

---

wrongdoing is likely to become defensive, and any attempts at changing coping strategies in the family are thwarted. It is better to ask about ways of solving disagreements or methods of disciplining children rather than to use the words *abuse* or *violence*.

When interviewing, sit near the abused client and spend some time establishing trust and rapport before focusing on the details of the violent experience. Reassure the client that he or she did nothing wrong. The interview should be nonthreatening and supportive. The person who experienced the violence should be allowed to tell the story and not be interrupted. Establishing trust is crucial if the client is to feel comfortable enough to self-disclose. Verbal approaches may include the following:
- Tell me about what happened to you.
- Who takes care of you? (for children and dependent elders)
- What happens when you do something wrong? (for children) *or* How do you and your partner/caregiver resolve disagreements? (for women and the elderly)
- What do you do for fun?
- Who helps you with your child(ren)/parent?
- What time do you have for yourself?

Questions that are open ended and require a descriptive response can be less threatening and elicit more relevant information than questions that are direct or can be answered with yes or no. Here are some examples of how to approach parents:
- What arrangements do you make when you have to leave your child alone?
- How do you discipline your child?
- When your infant cries for a long time, how do you get him or her to stop?
- What about your child's behavior bothers you the most?

When trust has been established, openness and directness about the situation can strengthen the relationship with those experiencing violence. The Nursing Research Consortium on Violence and Abuse (1989) has developed a five-question assessment tool that has been used extensively to assist in the routine identification of domestic violence (see Figure 25-2, p. 517). It can be used in clinical settings without requesting permission. The following vignette illustrates the key points in assessing a woman in crisis at the initial interview, as well as suggested follow-up.

■ ■ ■ VIGNETTE

Darnell Peters is a 42-year-old married woman in a relationship she describes as "bad for a long time. We don't communicate." She is brought to the emergency department by ambulance with lacerations to her face and swollen eyes, lips, and nose. She tells the nurse that her husband had been in bed asleep for hours before she joined him. On getting into bed, she attempted to redistribute the blankets.

Suddenly, he leaped from the bed, started punching her in the face, and began to throw her against the wall. She called out to her 11-year-old son to call the police. The police arrived, called an ambulance, and took Mr. Peters to jail.

The nurse takes Mrs. Peters to an individual examination room (to emphasize confidentiality) to assess the whole problem. Mrs. Peters states that her relationship with her husband is always stormy. "He is always putting me down and yelling at me." He started hitting her 5 years earlier when she became pregnant with her second and last child. The beatings have increased in intensity over the past year, and this emergency department visit is the fifth this year. Tonight is the first time she has ever called the police.

Mrs. Peters has visibly lost control. Periods of crying alternate with periods of silence. She appears apathetic and depressed. The nurse remains calm and objective. After Mrs. Peters has finished talking, the nurse explores alternatives designed to help her reduce the danger when she is discharged. "I'm concerned that you will be hurt again if you go home. What options do you have?" Acknowledging the escalating intensity of the violence, Mrs. Peters is able to make arrangements with a shelter to take in her and her two children until after she has secured a restraining order.

The nurse charts the abuse referrals. The keeping of careful and complete records helps ensure that Mrs. Peters will receive proper follow-up care and will assist Mrs. Peters when and if she pursues legal action.

Self-Assessment

In all areas of psychiatric nursing and counseling, the nurse should be aware of personal emotions and thoughts. Strong negative feelings can cloud one's judgment and interfere with assessment and intervention, no matter how well the nurse tries to cover or deny feelings. Intense and overwhelming feelings may be aroused by working with those experiencing violence. The nurse may also have come from a violent environment and thus identify too closely with the victim; old personal issues connected with the abuse may surface, further clouding judgment (Thomas, 2003). Many nurses do not believe that they are adequately prepared or have not had enough supervisory experience to intervene in cases of family violence. Supervision needs to be made available to nurses when working with victims of violence. These situations are often complex and entail multifaceted interventions and follow-up when possible.

Nurses with a personal history of abuse and those working with family violence need a source of psychological support. Interdisciplinary team conferences can be especially helpful in clarifying reactions and neutralizing intense emotions. Information from physicians, psychologists, nurses, and social workers can assist in refocusing efforts to work constructively with a family in crisis. Sharing perceptions and feelings with other professionals can help reduce feelings of isolation and discomfort for nurses.

Awareness of personal feelings in response to those experiencing violence stimulates an examination of personal views toward violence and the status of children, women, and elders. This is most effectively done through professional or peer supervision. Common responses of health care professionals to violence are listed in Table 25-1.

When determining the need for further help, it is also useful to assess (a) violence indicators, (b) levels of anxiety and coping responses, (c) family coping patterns, (d) support systems, (e) suicide potential, (f) homicide potential, and (g) drug and alcohol use.

TABLE 25-1

Common Responses of Health Care Professionals to Violence

Response	Source
Anger	Anger may be felt toward the person responsible for the violence, toward those who allowed it to happen, and toward society for condoning its occurrence through attitudes, traditions, and laws.
Embarrassment	The victim is a symbol of something close to home: the stress and strain of family life unleashed as uncontrollable anger.
Confusion	Our cherished view of the family as a haven of safety and privacy is challenged.
Fear	A small percentage of perpetrators are dangerous to others.
Anguish	The nurse may have experienced family violence.
Helplessness	The nurse may want to do more, to eliminate the problem, to cure the victim.
Discouragement	Discouragement may result if no long-term solution is achieved.
"Blame the victim" mentality	Lay people as well as health care workers can get caught up in "blaming the victim" for not having the house neat, serving food on time, keeping clothes neat. There is never an excuse for violence, and no one has the right to hurt another person. "Blaming the victim" can occur when health care professionals feel overwhelmed. Supervision is a must for therapeutic intervention.

Assessing Types of Maltreatment

Physical Violence. A series of minor complaints, such as headaches, "back trouble," dizziness, and "accidents," especially falls, may be covert indications of violence. Overt signs of battering include bruises, scars, burns, and other wounds in various stages of healing, particularly around the head, face, chest, arms, abdomen, back, buttocks, and genitalia. Injuries seen in emergency departments, clinics, and offices that should arouse the nurse's suspicion are listed in Box 25-5. If the explanation does not match the injury seen, or if the client minimizes the seriousness of the injury, violence may be suspected. The key to identification is a high index of suspicion.

Nonspecific bruising in older children is common. Any bruises on an infant younger than 6 months of age should be considered suspicious. **Shaken baby syndrome** is frequently overlooked, yet shaking is one of the most serious types of child abuse. A baby who has been shaken may often present with respiratory problems. If the pulmonary examination is not normal, the possibility of rigorous shaking must be considered. Full, bulging fontanelles and a head circumference greater than the 90th percentile are also suggestive. Shaking can cause intracranial hemorrhage leading to cerebral edema and death (Starling & Holden, 2000).

Ask clients directly, but in a nonthreatening manner, whether the injury has been caused by someone close to them. Observe the nonverbal response, such as hesitation or lack of eye contact, as well as the verbal response. Then ask specific questions, such as: When was the last time it happened? How often does it happen? In what ways are you hurt?

Nurses not only recognize the indicators of physical violence but also note the alleged method of injury. Inconsistent explanations serve as a warning that further investigation is necessary. Vague explanations such as "She fell from a chair (a lap, down the stairs)," "He was running away," or "The hot water was turned on by mistake" should alert the nurse to possible violence.

Sexual Violence. Patients with a history of sexual abuse often display various psychopathologies (Stevens, 2003). Childhood sexual violence is likely to be a significant factor in the development of depression in many women (Bensley et al., 2003). Sexual abuse of boys appears to be common, underreported, underrecognized, and untreated (Desai et al., 2002).

■ ■ ■ *VIGNETTE*

Ms. Randall, 83 years old, is admitted from an adult foster home for evaluation of deterioration in her mental status. She is confused and disoriented as to time and place and is unable to give a coherent history. Blood and urine are collected for diagnostic evaluation. The laboratory report notes semen in the urine. Adult Protective Services is called to begin an investigation into the adult family home.

■ ■ ■

Emotional Violence. Whenever physical or sexual violence is occurring, emotional violence also occurs. Emotional violence may also exist alone. When there is emotional violence, the victim experiences low self-esteem, anguish, and isolation instead of love and acceptance. Emotional violence is less obvious and more difficult to assess than physical violence.

Neglect. Neglected children and elders often appear undernourished, dirty, and poorly clothed. Neglect is also manifested by inadequate medical care, such as lack of immunizations or untreated medical conditions.

Economic Maltreatment. Failure to provide for the needs of the victim even when adequate funds are available is a sign of economic maltreatment.

BOX 25-5

Presenting Problems of Victims of Family Violence

Emergency Department

- Bleeding injuries, especially to head and face
- Internal injuries, concussions, perforated eardrum, abdominal injuries, severe bruising, eye injuries, strangulation marks on neck
- Back injuries
- Broken or fractured jaw, arms, pelvis, ribs, clavicle, legs
- Burns from cigarettes, appliances, scalding liquids, acids
- Psychological trauma, anxiety, attacks of hyperventilation, heart palpitations, severe crying spells, suicidal tendencies
- Miscarriage

Ambulatory Care Settings

- Perforated eardrum, twisted or stiff neck and shoulder muscles, headache
- Depression, stress-related conditions (e.g., insomnia, violent nightmares, anxiety, extreme fatigue, eczema, loss of hair)
- Talk of having "problems" with husband or son, describing person as very jealous, impulsive, or an alcohol or drug abuser
- Repeated visits with new complaints
- Bruises of various ages and specific shapes (fingers, belt)

Both Settings

- Signs of stress due to family violence: emotional, behavioral, school, or sleep problems and increase in aggressive behavior
- Injuries in a pregnant woman
- Recurrent visits for injuries attributed to being "accident prone"

Another sign is unpaid bills when another person is supposed to handle their payment, which may result in disconnection of the heat or electricity (Stevens, 2003).

Assessing Level of Anxiety and Coping Responses

Nonverbal responses to history taking can be indicative of the victim's anxiety level. The identification of anxiety level is described in Chapter 14. Hesitation, lack of eye contact, and use of vague statements such as "It's been rough lately" indicate that the situation is difficult to talk about.

Agitation and anxiety bordering on panic are often present in victims experiencing violence. Because they live in terror, battered individuals remain vigilant, unable to relax or sleep. Signs of the effects of living with chronic stress and severe levels of anxiety may be present (e.g., hypertension, irritability, gastrointestinal disturbances).

■ ■ ■ *VIGNETTE*

Bilateral corneal abrasions in a woman coming to the walk-in clinic raises the suspicion of an astute nurse, who notes the client's vague responses to history questions and her unrelenting checking of the clock followed by the urgent statement, "I've got to get home." On further questioning, the woman reveals that she is often quite fatigued because of caring for her five children, all younger than 7 years of age. Yet her husband, who works until 2 AM, expects her to be awake when he comes home from work and to have a warm meal ready in the oven. "He hits me if I'm asleep." She had taped her eyes open so that even if she were lying down when he came home she would look awake. "I didn't even think about taking my contacts out."

■ ■ ■

The coping mechanisms used by many battered individuals to endure living in violent and terrifying situations often prevent the dissolution of the marriage. These coping mechanisms take in the form of beliefs or

TABLE 25-2

Myth Versus Fact: Family Violence

Myth	Fact
Ninety-five percent of abuse victims are women.	Recent surveys report that from 30% to 40%, perhaps 50%, of abuse victims are men.
The victim's behavior often causes violence.	The victim's behavior is *not* the cause of the violence. Violence is the abuser's pattern of behavior, and the victim cannot learn how to control it.
Men have the right to keep their wives and/or children in line.	No person has the right to beat or hurt another person.
Spouse abuse is a minor problem.	There is a *real* danger that a woman may be killed by a violent partner.
Battered women are masochistic and like to be beaten. (The abuse cannot be that bad or they would leave.)	Women do not like, ask, or deserve to be abused. Economic considerations are usually the only reason they stay.
Family violence is most prevalent in those from poor working class backgrounds who are usually poorly educated.	Violence occurs in families of all socioeconomic, religious, cultural, and educational backgrounds.
The family is sacred and should be allowed to take care of its own problems.	Intervention in family violence is justified because such violence always escalates in frequency and intensity, can end in death, and is passed on to future generations.
Victims of abuse tacitly accept the abuse by trying to conceal it, by not reporting it, or by failing to seek help.	When attempting to disclose their situation, many women are met with disbelief. This discourages them from persevering.
Myths abused women believe: "I can't live without him." "If I hadn't done ____, it wouldn't have happened." "He will change." "I stay for the sake of the children." "His jealousy and possessiveness prove he really loves me."	These myths are coping mechanisms women use to allay panic in a situation of random and brutal violence. They give the illusion of control and rationality.
Alcohol and stress are the major causes of physical and verbal abuse.	This myth offers an explanation of and tolerance for verbal abuse and battering. There are no excuses and it is not acceptable behavior. Abuse is a learned behavior, not an uncontrollable reaction. People are abusive because they have acquired the belief that violence and aggression are acceptable and effective responses to read or imagined threats.
Violence occurs only between heterosexual partners.	Gay and lesbian partners experience violence for reasons similar to those in heterosexual relationships.
Pregnancy protects a woman from battering.	Battering frequently begins or escalates during pregnancy.

myths (Table 25-2). Because of feelings of confusion, shame, despair, and powerlessness, victims may withdraw from interaction with others.

Assessing Family Coping Patterns

When assessing family violence, the nurse should show a willingness to listen and avoid any judgmental tone. Questioning about memories of early family relationships can provide additional information about attitudes in the home and the way they might influence coping. Living with children and older adults in the same household can cause frustration, stress, and anger. Unless there are appropriate outlets for stress, violence can occur. Box 25-6 is a useful guide for assessing the risk of child and/or elder abuse in the home.

Assessing Support Systems

The person experiencing violence is usually in a dependent position, relying on the perpetrator (spouse, parent, other family member, or caregiver) for basic needs. Such situations foster isolation from others. Children's options are especially limited, as are those of the physically and mentally challenged. Assessing for support should focus on intrapersonal, interpersonal, and community resources (e.g., the school system for school-aged victims).

Assessing Suicide Potential

A person experiencing violence may feel so trapped in a detrimental relationship, yet so desperate to get out, that suicide may seem the only answer. The threat of suicide may also be used by an emotionally violent person in an attempt to manipulate the partner or spouse into caving in to demands ("Don't leave me or I'll kill myself" or "I took all my pills. . . . I said I would the next time you were late").

A suicide attempt may be the presenting symptom in the emergency department. It has been estimated that at least 10% of abused women attempt suicide. With sensitive questioning conducted in a caring manner, the nurse can elicit the history of violence. Often the means of attempted suicide is overdose with a combination of alcohol and other central nervous system depressants, tranquilizers, or sleeping medications that have been prescribed in previous visits to physicians' offices, clinics, or emergency departments.

When the crisis of the immediate suicide attempt has been resolved, careful questioning to determine lethality is in order. For example, if the client still feels that life is not worth living, has a suicide plan, and has the means to carry it out, admission to an inpatient psychiatric unit must be considered. On the other hand, if the client is talking about future plans and about hanging in there "for the sake of the children," outpatient referrals are appropriate.

BOX 25-6

Factors to Assess During a Home Visit

For Child
- Responsiveness to infant's crying
- Responsiveness to infant's signals related to feeding
- Caregiver's facial expressions in response to infant
- Holding of child
- Playfulness of caregiver with infant
- Type of physical contact during feeding
- Temperament of infant: average, quiet, or active
- Parental attitudes signaling possible warnings:
  —Complaints of inadequacy as a parent
  —Complaints of inadequacy of child
  —Fear of "doing something wrong"
  —Attribution of badness to newborn
  —History of a destructive childhood
  —Misdirected anger
  —Continued evidence of isolation, apathy, anger, frustration, projection
  —Adult conflict
- Environmental conditions:
  —Sleeping arrangements
  —Child management
  —Home management
  —Use of supports (formal and informal)
- Need for immediate services for situational (economics, child care), emotional, or educational information:
  —Information about hotlines, baby-sitters, homemakers, parent groups
  —Information about child development
  —Information about child care and home management services

For Elder
- Environmental conditions:
  —House in poor repair
  —Inadequate heat, lighting, furniture, cooking utensils
  —Presence of garbage or vermin
  —Old food in kitchen
  —Lack of assistive devices
  —Locks on refrigerator
  —Blocked stairways
  —Victim lying in urine, feces, or food
  —Unpleasant odors
- Medication:
  —Medication not being taken as prescribed (e.g., medication not available, elder confused about procedure, elder physically unable to take medication)

Data from Galbraith, M. (1986). *Elder abuse: Perspective on an emerging crisis.* Kansas City, KS: Mid-American Congress on Aging; and Unwin, B. K., & Jerant, A. F. (1999). The home visit. *American Family Physician, 60*(5), 1481-1488.

Assessing Homicide Potential

Inquire whether the client feels safe going home and, if so, whether a safety plan is in place for when the violence recurs. Certain factors place a vulnerable person at greater risk for homicide from continuing and escalating violence:

- The presence of a gun in the home
- Alcohol and drug abuse
- History of violence on the part of the perpetrator in other situations (harmed pets, beat spouse when she was pregnant, forced sex on spouse)
- Extreme jealousy and obsessiveness on the part of the perpetrator regarding the relationship with the victim and attempt to control all the victim's daily activities

Persons victimized by violence should be asked if they have ever felt like killing the perpetrator and, if so, whether they have the current desire and means to do so. If the answer is yes, intervention is required.

Assessing Drug and Alcohol Use

A person experiencing violence may self-medicate with alcohol or other drugs as a way of escaping a dreadful situation. The drugs are usually central nervous system depressants (e.g., benzodiazepines) prescribed by physicians in response to the battered person's presentation with vague complaints, which are often stress related (e.g., insomnia, gastrointestinal upsets, jittery feeling, difficulty concentrating).

The degree of intoxication can be determined by history, physical examination, and blood alcohol level. If a battered client is intoxicated on presentation, allow the client to sober up before initiating referral. Referral information will not be understood or assimilated if the client is intoxicated. The client should not be discharged to the client's spouse.

Assess for a chronic alcohol or drug problem (see Chapter 27) and provide appropriate treatment referrals. Treatment choices can include both inpatient and outpatient options.

Maintaining Accurate Records

Because of the possibility of legal action, it is essential that the health care record contain an accurate and detailed description of the victim's medical history, the psychosocial history of the family, and observations of

---

ABUSE ASSESSMENT SCREEN

1. Within the last year, have you been hit, slapped, kicked, or otherwise physically hurt by someone?

☐ Yes ☐ No

If yes, by whom? _____

Total number of times: _____

2. Since you've been pregnant, have you been hit, slapped, kicked, or otherwise physically hurt by someone?

☐ Yes ☐ No

If yes, by whom? _____

Total number of times: _____

Mark the area of injury on the body map below.

3. Within the last year, has anyone forced you to have sexual activities?

☐ Yes ☐ No

If yes, who? _____

Total number of times: _____

4. Have you ever been emotionally or physically abused by your partner or someone important to you?

☐ Yes ☐ No

If yes, by whom? _____

Total number of times: _____

5. Are you afraid of your partner or anyone listed above?

☐ Yes ☐ No

Score each incident according to the following scale:

1 = Threats of abuse including use of a weapon

2 = Slapping, pushing; no injuries and/or continuing pain

3 = Punching, kicking, bruises, cuts, and/or continuing pain

4 = Beating up, severe contusions, burns, broken bones

5 = Head injury, internal injury, permanent injury

6 = Use of weapon, wound from weapon

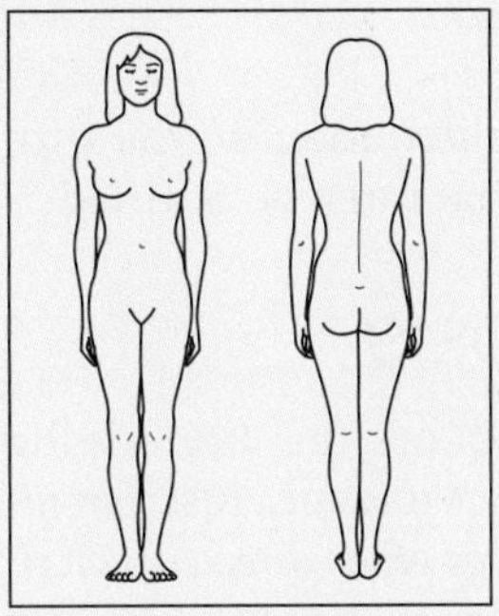

SCORE

_____

_____

_____

_____

FIGURE 25-2 Abuse assessment screen. (Developed by the Nursing Research Consortium on Violence and Abuse, 2004.)

the family interactions during the interviews. Especially important in documentation of findings from the initial assessment are (1) verbatim statements of who caused the injury and when it occurred; (2) a body map to indicate size, color, shape, areas, and types of injuries, with explanations (Figure 25-2); and (3) physical evidence of sexual abuse, when possible. Procedures for evidence collection must be followed carefully or legal action can be thwarted. If the beating has just occurred, ask the client to return in a day or two for more photographs; bruises may be more evident at that time. The client must be assured of the confidentiality of the record and of its power should legal action be initiated. Even if intervention does not occur at this time, the record is begun; the next provider will not have to stumble across the problem and will be in a better position to offer support.

Because many victims of violence are seen in emergency departments, the Emergency Nurses Association (ENA) issued a position statement urging "emergency nurses to take an active role in the development, implementation, and ongoing maintenance of hospital and community protective service teams to ensure consistent and accurate assessments and protection of all individuals and/or families at risk for domestic violence, maltreatment and neglect" (ENA, 2003, p. 2).

Assessment Guidelines Family Violence

During your assessment and counseling, maintain an interested and empathetic manner. Refrain from displaying horror, anger, shock, or disapproval of the perpetrator or the situation. Assess for

1. Presenting signs and symptoms of victims of family violence.
2. Potential problem in vulnerable families; for example, some indicators of vulnerable parents who might benefit from education and instruction in effective coping techniques.
3. Physical, sexual, and/or emotional abuse and neglect and economic maltreatment in elders.
4. Family coping patterns.
5. Client's support system.
6. Drug or alcohol use.
7. Suicidal or homicidal ideas.
8. Posttrauma syndrome.

If the client is a child or an elder, identify the protective agency in your state that must be notified.

■ NURSING DIAGNOSIS

Nursing diagnoses are focused on the underlying causes and symptoms of family violence. *Risk for injury, risk for violence (self-directed or other-directed), anxiety,* and *fear* are nursing diagnoses that apply. *Disabled family coping, powerlessness,* and *caregiver role strain* are others. Feelings of helplessness, hopelessness, and powerlessness contribute to the diagnoses of *disturbed*

body image and *chronic low self-esteem.* The crisis of family violence precipitates *interrupted family process* or *impaired parenting* as the family system becomes less able to meet the emotional, physical, and security needs of its members.

Pain related to physical injury or trauma would most certainly take high priority and need immediate attention. Table 25-3 lists potential nursing diagnoses for family violence.

The identification of desired outcomes and design of nursing interventions that facilitate achieving those outcomes should be developed as much as possible in collaboration with the survivor and primary support person. These outcomes should be continually reassessed and revised as new information about the survivor's needs emerges. A comprehensive plan can also be the coordinating framework for the work of an interdisciplinary team.

■ OUTCOME CRITERIA

The Nursing Outcomes Classification (NOC) (Moorhead, Johnson, & Maas, 2004) identifies the following indicators for the outcome of *Abuse Cessation,* which is defined as "evidence that the victim is no longer hurt or exploited":

- Physical abuse has ceased.
- Emotional abuse has ceased.
- Sexual abuse has ceased.
- Financial abuse has ceased.
- Financial exploitation has ceased.

TABLE 25-3

Potential Nursing Diagnoses for Family Violence

Signs and Symptoms	Potential Nursing Diagnoses
Bruises, cuts, broken bones, lacerations, scars, burns, wounds in various phases of healing, particularly when explanations do not match injury, or explanations are vague	**Risk for injury** **Pain** **Risk for infection** **Impaired skin integrity** **Risk for posttrauma syndrome**
Isolation, fear, feelings of shame and low self-esteem, feelings of worthlessness, depression, feelings of helplessness	**Powerlessness** **Ineffective coping** **Fear** **Risk for self-directed violence** **Chronic or situational low self-esteem** **Helplessness** **Spiritual distress**
Vaginal-anal bruises, sores, discharge, peritoneal pain, positive VDRL test results	**Rape-trauma syndrome** **Risk for infection**

VDRL, Venereal Disease Research Laboratories.

The outcome and indicators are evaluated on a scale from 1 (no evidence) to 5 (extensive evidence).

NOC offers other abuse-specific categories of outcome, including *Abuse Protection; Abuse Recovery Status; Abuse Recovery: Emotional; Abuse Recovery: Financial; Abuse Recovery: Physical;* and *Abuse Recovery: Sexual.* In addition, it is appropriate to include outcomes focusing on improved coping, self-esteem, social support, and pain control, to name just a few.

Table 25-4, building on the language of NOC, may be used as a guideline for specific outcome criteria, along with short-term and intermediate indicators, for child, spouse, and elder abuse clients and for the abuser.

■ PLANNING

Family violence is all too common, and nurses and other health care workers encounter it frequently in community health clinics, emergency departments, doctors' offices, obstetrical units, schools, and nursing homes; on home visits and in home health care; and in any other arena in which nurses meet the public. You may even find that your neighbor, a colleague, your best friend, your sister-in-law, or another member of your family is involved in abusive situations (either as the abused or the abuser).

Violence within families is seldom recognized by outsiders, including nurses. Yet the nurse is often the first point of contact for people experiencing family violence and thus is in an ideal position to contribute to prevention, detection, and effective intervention. The Joint Commission on Accreditation of Healthcare Organi-

zations requires staff education in family violence as well as the development of standards of care to guide clinical practice (Family Violence Prevention Fund, 2004a, 2004b). The Nursing Network on Violence Against Women encourages the development of a nursing practice that focuses on health issues relating to the effects of violence on women's lives. Altering the pattern of violence against women can also affect child abuse, because the main predictor of violence toward children is violence toward their mothers. Ultimately, the general tolerance of violence in the United States must be addressed if long-lasting changes are to be made.

Most hospitals and community centers provide protocols for dealing with child, spouse, or elder abuse that may or may not meet all the needs of a given client. Unless it is a case of child abuse in which the child has been removed from the home, most interventions performed after necessary emergency care will take place within the community. Plans should center around the client's safety first and, whenever it is possible or in the best interest of the client, should be discussed with the client (partner or spouse, parents, or elder). Planning also needs to take into consideration the needs of the abuser (e.g., parents, caretakers, spouse or partner), if the abuser seem willing to learn violent-free alternatives to frustration and aggression.

■ INTERVENTION

Nurses have a legal responsibility and are mandated to report suspected or actual cases of child and elder abuse. The appropriate agency may be the state or

---

TABLE 25-4

NOC Outcomes for Family Violence

Nursing Outcome and Definition	Short-Term and Intermediate Indicators
Child	
Abuse Cessation: Evidence that the victim is no longer hurt or exploited*	Evidence that physical abuse has ceased Evidence that emotional abuse has ceased Evidence that sexual abuse has ceased
Spouse Abuse Client	
Abuse Recovery: Physical: Extent of healing of physical injuries due to abuse*	Timely treatment of injuries Healing of physical injuries Resolution of physical health problems
Elder Abuse Client	
Abuse Recovery: Financial: Extent of control of monetary and legal matters following financial exploitation*	Control of Social Security and pension checks Protection of financial assets Control of withdrawal of money from account(s)
Abuser	
Abusive Behavior Self-Restraint: Self-restraint of abusive and neglectful behaviors toward others†	Seeks treatment as needed Controls impulses Discusses the abusive behavior

From Moorhead, S., Johnson, M., & Maas, M. (2004). *Nursing outcomes classification (NOC)* (3rd ed.). St. Louis, MO: Mosby.
*Evaluated on a five-point Likert scale from 1 (none) to 5 (extensive).
†Evaluated on a five-point Likert scale from 1 (never demonstrated) to 5 (consistently demonstrated).

county child welfare agency, law enforcement agency, juvenile court, or county health department. Each state has specific guidelines for reporting, including whether the report can be oral or written, or both, and within what time period the suspected abuse or neglect must be reported (immediately, within 24 hours, or within 48 hours). Every battered person is a crime victim, and assault with a weapon is reportable in most states. Also, all 50 states have marital rape statutes. The following vignette gives an example of a case to report.

■ ■ ■ VIGNETTE

Two nurses who work in a family practice clinic are suspicious of child abuse. A 12-year-old girl has recurrent urinary tract infections. She is always accompanied to clinic visits by her father, who even goes into the bathroom with her when she is producing urine samples. He answers all questions for the girl even when they are directed toward her. He has recently refused the next diagnostic test to attempt to ascertain the reason for the recurrent infections.

After pressure by the nurses, the physician agrees to ask the girl some questions in private. The nurses think the physician has discounted the problem, asked superficial questions, and dismissed their concerns. They attempt without success to get the girl alone for a discussion. After consultation with clinical resources, they decide to report their concerns to Children's Protective Services. They inform the father, who becomes outraged at their accusations and threatens to change doctors. The nurses try to reassure him about the nature of the referral, to no avail. Subsequent investigation confirms the likelihood of sexual abuse, and the child is placed in temporary foster care with follow-up counseling. The father refuses treatment and threatens to sue the nurses. Four months later the father leaves the family.

■ ■ ■

The case in the preceding vignette illustrates that a reasonable basis for suspecting maltreatment, not proof, is all that is required to report. Nurses must attempt to maintain both an appropriate level of suspicion and a neutral, objective attitude. One can be too concerned and jump to conclusions (which is what the physician in this case thought the nurses were doing) or not be concerned enough and rationalize an incomplete examination to avoid confrontation (which is what the nurses thought the physician was doing). Given these opposing stances, the case was reported, as required by law and ethical standards, and Children's Protective Services was given the opportunity to sort it out.

Competency may be a consideration in a situation of elder mistreatment. Unless the elderly person has been found legally incompetent, he or she has the right to self-determination. Some institutions and health care agencies have developed guidelines for dealing with actual or suspected situations of mistreatment. These protocols list possible behaviors or conditions of the elderly and the most appropriate intervention. The establishment of such protocols is highly recommended because it gives support to the nurse's actions.

Quality nursing care for those experiencing violence must be culturally sensitive. The nurse must be aware of the cultural issues that may affect response to violence and to intervention. For example, Cambodian women control their responses to stress and violence through nonconfrontation and withdrawal, which are designed to restore equilibrium. Culture is important because it is central to how people organize their experience. Even the most acculturated people have a tendency to revert to their cultural past in organizing coping strategies after a stressful event. If there is a language barrier, the nurse should speak slowly and clearly in English, without using jargon, and allow time for the response. If the client speaks no English, a trained medical interpreter should be provided. A family member should *not* be used as interpreter, to ensure confidentiality and to protect the person from future retaliation.

Primary prevention consists of measures taken to prevent the occurrence of family violence. Identifying people at high risk, providing health teaching, and coordinating supportive services to prevent crises are examples of primary prevention. Specific strategies include (1) reducing stress, (2) reducing the influence of risk factors, (3) increasing social support, (4) increasing coping skills, and (5) increasing self-esteem. Community health nurses are also in a position to assess family functioning in the home during visits for such matters as assisting children with chronic health problems. In addition, the community health nurse and clinic nurse maintain contact with the family over time, which allows for assessment of changes. They are also in an excellent position to connect parents to appropriate resources in the community that can meet their needs.

Secondary prevention involves early intervention in abusive situations to minimize their disabling or long-term effects. Nurses can establish screening programs for individuals at risk, participate in the medical treatment of injuries resulting from violent episodes, and coordinate community services to provide continuity of care. Stress and depression can be reduced by providing supportive psychotherapy, support groups, pharmacotherapy, and telephone numbers to safe houses. Social dysfunction or lack of information can be addressed by counseling and education. Caregiver burden can be reduced by arranging assistance in caregiving, nursing, or housekeeping or (in cases in which caregiving needs exceed even optimized caregiver capacity) by placing the patient in a more appropriate setting. The following vignette illustrates a successful secondary prevention effort.

Billy, age 4 years, is brought into the physician's office by 15-year-old Mary, the children's baby-sitter, with second-degree burns on his right hand. Mary frequently baby-sits for Billy and his younger brother Jimmy, age 2 years, and older brother Tom, age 6 years. Mary appears apprehensive and says she is very concerned. Mary tells the nurse that the children have told her in the past that their mother has threatened them with burning if they do not behave. Billy told her that his mother once held his hands on a cold stove and told him that, if he was bad, she would burn him. Mary is shocked that Billy's mother would do such a thing, but at the same time she mentions that she feels guilty for "telling on Ms. J."

Mary also states that the older brother told Mary what had happened but was afraid that, if his mother found out, she would burn him also. Mary says she is aware that the mother hits the children, but she did not believe that anyone would burn her own child.

The nurse reports what happened to the physician, and the mother is called and asked to come to the office.

Billy appears frightened and in pain. The nurse asks Mary to come with Billy while she examines him.

Nurse: Tell me about your hand, Billy. *(Billy looks down and starts to cry.)*

Nurse: It's OK if you don't want to talk about it, Billy.

Billy: *(Does not look at the nurse and speaks softly.)* My mommy burned my hand on the stove.

Nurse: Tell me what happened before that happened.

Billy: Mommy was mad because I didn't put my toys away.

Nurse: What does your mommy usually do when she gets mad?

Billy: She yells mostly. Sometimes she hits us. Mommy is going to be so mad at Tommy for telling.

Nurse: Tell me about the hitting.

Billy: Mommy hits us a lot since Daddy left us. *(Billy starts to cry to himself.)*

On examination, the nurse notices a ringed pattern of burns across Billy's right palm like the burner of an electric stove. There are blisters on the fingers. Billy appears well nourished and properly dressed. He is at his approximate developmental age except for some language delay.

Because of the physical evidence and history, there is strong suspicion of child abuse. Children's Protective Services is notified, and the family situation is evaluated for possible placement of Billy in protective custody. The initial evaluation concludes that there is no indication of serious potential harm to the child and that Billy should return home.

The mother, who is initially defensive, starts to cry and states, "I can't cope with being alone and I don't know where to turn." The intervention that the nurse facilitates centers around caring for Billy's immediate health needs; finding supports for the mother to help her cope with crises; providing a counseling referral for the mother to learn alternative ways of expressing anger and frustration; informing the mother of parents' groups; providing referrals to play groups or day care for the children to help increase their feelings of self-esteem and security; and providing a break, and perhaps some instruction in parenting, for the mother.

■ ■ ■

Tertiary prevention involves nurses' facilitating the healing and rehabilitative process by counseling individuals and families; providing support for groups of survivors; and assisting survivors of violence to achieve their optimal level of safety, health, and well-being. Tertiary interventions often occur in mental health settings.

Basic Level Interventions

The specific interventions performed by the basic level practitioner include counseling, case management, milieu therapy, self-care activities, and health teaching.

Counseling

Counseling includes crisis intervention measures. It is useful to emphasize that people have a right to live without fear of violence or physical harm and without fear of assault. The role of the nurse is to support the victim, counsel about safety, and facilitate access to other resources as appropriate. By listening, giving support, discussing options, and describing other ways of living, the nurse initiates an awareness of other possibilities.

All persons experiencing violence should be counseled about developing a safety plan, a plan for a fast escape when violence recurs. They should be asked to identify the signs of escalation of violence and to pick a particular sign that will tell them in the future that "now is the time to leave." If children are present, they can all agree on a code word that, when spoken by their parent, means "it is time to go." If the individual plans ahead, it may be possible to leave before the violence occurs. It is important that the plan include a destination and a way to get there. The nurse should suggest packing ahead of time with the items designated in Box 25-7. The packed bag should be kept in a place where the perpetrator will not find it.

If the battered person chooses to leave, shelters or safe houses (for both sexes) are available in many communities (although, sadly, at only half the rate of animal shelters—a reflection of our social values). They are open 24 hours a day and can be reached through hotline information numbers, hospital emergency departments, YWCAs, or the local office of the National Organization for Women. The address of the house is usually kept secret to protect battered persons from attack by their mates. Besides offering protection, many of these safe shelters serve important education and consciousness-raising functions. Clients should be given the number of the nearest available shelter, even if they decide for the present to stay with their partners. Referral phone numbers may be kept for years before the decision to call is made. Having the number and a contact person all that time contributes to thinking about options.

BOX 25-7

Personalized Safety Guide

Suggestions for Increasing Safety—in the Relationship

- I will have important phone numbers available to my children and myself.
- I can tell _____ and _____ about the violence and ask them to call the police if they hear suspicious noises coming from my home.
- If I leave my home, I can go to (list four places)
  _____ , _____ , _____ , or _____.
- I can leave extra money, car keys, clothes, and copies of documents with _____.
- If I leave, I will bring _____ (see checklist below).
- To ensure safety and independence, I can keep change for phone calls with me at all times; open my own savings account; rehearse my escape route with a support person; and review safety plan on _____ (date).

Suggestions for Increasing Safety—When the Relationship Is Over

- I can change the locks; install steel or metal doors, a security system, smoke detectors, and an outside lighting system.
- I will inform _____ and _____ that my partner no longer lives with me and ask them to call the police if he or she is observed near my home or my children.
- I will tell people who take care of my children the names of those who have permission to pick them up. The people who have permission are _____ , _____ and _____.
- I can tell _____ at work about my situation and ask _____ to screen my calls.
- I can avoid stores, banks, and _____ that I used when living with my battering partner.

- I can obtain a protective order from _____. I can keep it on or near me at all times as well as have a copy with _____.
- If I feel down and ready to return to a potentially abusive situation, I can call _____ for support or attend workshops and support groups to gain support and strengthen my relationships with other people.

Important Phone Numbers
Police _____
Hotline _____
Friends _____
Shelter _____

Checklist of Items to Take
- Identification
- Birth certificates for me and my children
- Social Security card
- School and medical records
- Money, bank books, credit cards
- Keys to house, car, office
- Driver's license and registration
- Medications
- Change of clothes
- Welfare identification
- Passport(s), green card, work permit
- Divorce papers
- Lease or rental agreement, house deed
- Mortgage payment book, current unpaid bills
- Insurance papers
- Address book
- Pictures, jewelry, items of sentimental value
- Children's favorite toys and/or blankets

Case Management

Community mental health centers are becoming increasingly involved in the delivery of services to victims and perpetrators of domestic violence. Nurses working in these settings have the opportunity to be case managers to coordinate community, medical, criminal justice, and social services to provide comprehensive assistance to violent families. Strategies must encompass needs for housing, child care, economic stability, physical and emotional safety, counseling, legal protection, career development or job training, education, ongoing support groups, and health care. The myriad of agencies and people that those seeking help must reach can be daunting and confusing. A nurse functioning in a case manager role can assist the client in choosing the best options and coordinating the interventions of several agencies. Box 25-8 lists selected abuse interventions according

to Nursing Interventions Classification (NIC) (Dochterman & Bulechek, 2004).

Milieu Therapy

Interventions are geared toward stabilizing the home situation and maintaining a violence-free environment. The interventions offered should leave options for growth, increase in self-esteem, and a higher quality of life for all family members (Lawson, 1998). Some mental health agencies have family-based units in which a caseworker or clinician comes to the home instead of the family going to the agency. Providing and maintaining a therapeutic environment in the home ideally involves three levels of help for violent families:

1. Provide the family with economic support, job opportunities, and social services, such as through family service agencies.
2. Arrange social support in the form of a public health nurse, lay home visitor, day care teacher,

BOX 25-8

NIC Interventions for Children, Domestic Partners, and the Elderly

Abuse Protection Support: Child

Definition: Identification of high-risk, dependent child relationships and actions to prevent possible or further infliction of physical, sexual, or emotional harm or neglect of basic necessities of life

Activities*:

- Identify mothers who have a history of late (4 months or later) or no prenatal care.
- Identify parents who have had another child removed from the home or have placed previous children with relatives for extended periods.
- Identify parents with a history of domestic violence or a mother who has a history of numerous "accidental" injuries.
- Determine whether a child demonstrates signs of physical abuse, including numerous injuries in various stages of healing; unexplained bruises and welts; unexplained pattern, immersion, and friction burns; facial, spiral, shaft, or multiple fractures; unexplained facial lacerations and abrasions; human bite marks; intracranial, subdural, intraventricular, and intraocular hemorrhaging; whiplash shaken infant syndrome; and diseases that are resistant to treatment and/or have changing signs and symptoms.
- Encourage admission of child for further observation and investigation as appropriate.
- Monitor parent-child interactions and record observations.
- Report suspected abuse or neglect to proper authorities.

Abuse Protection Support: Domestic Partner

Definition: Identification of high-risk, dependent domestic relationships and action to prevent possible or further infliction of physical, sexual, or emotional harm or exploitation of a domestic partner

Activities*:

- Screen for risk factors associated with domestic abuse (e.g., history of domestic violence, abuse, rejection, excessive criticism, or feelings of being worthless and unloved; difficulty trusting others or feeling disliked by others; feeling that asking for help is an indication of personal incompetence; high physical care needs; intense family care responsibilities; substance abuse; depression; major psychiatric illness; social isolation; poor relationships between domestic partners; multiple marriages; pregnancy; poverty; unemployment; financial dependence; homelessness; infidelity; divorce; or death of a loved one).
- Document evidence of physical or sexual abuse using standardized assessment tools and photographs.
- Listen attentively to individual who begins to talk about own problems.
- Encourage admission to a hospital for further observation and investigation, as appropriate.
- Provide positive affirmation of worth.
- Report any situations in which abuse is suspected in compliance with mandatory reporting laws.

Abuse Protection Support: Elder

Definition: Identification of high-risk, dependent elder relationships and actions to prevent possible or further infliction of physical, sexual, or emotional harm; neglect of basic necessities of life; or exploitation

Activities*:

- Identify elderly patients who perceive themselves to be dependent on caretakers due to impaired health status, functional impairment, limited economic resources, depression, substance abuse, or lack or knowledge of available resource and alternatives for care.
- Identify family caretakers who have a history of being abused or neglected in childhood.
- Monitor patient-caretaker interactions and record observations.
- Report suspected abuse or neglect to proper authorities.

From Dochterman, J. M., & Bulechek, G. M. (2004). *Nursing interventions classification (NIC)* (pp. 131-137). St. Louis, MO: Mosby.
*Partial list.

---

schoolteacher, social worker, respite worker, or any other potential contact person who has a good relationship with the family.

3. Encourage and provide family therapy.

Self-Care Activities

The primary goal of intervention is empowerment. Supporting the client to act on her or his own behalf can decrease feelings of helplessness and hopelessness. The initial phase of recovery begins when a client first makes steps to leave the abusive relationship. Giving referral numbers and providing an opportunity for the client to call from your office, or inquiring at the next visit whether the client was successful in reaching the appropriate agency, demonstrates confidence in the client's ability to take care of herself or himself.

Specific referrals regarding emergency monetary assistance and legal counseling should be made available to each client. Vocational counseling is another referral that may be appropriate. Battered clients should be given referrals to parenting resources that enable them to explore alternative approaches to discipline (i.e., no hitting, slapping, or other expressions of violence).

Health Teaching

In families at risk for violence, health teaching includes meeting with both the client and the family and discussing associated risk factors. The client, caregiver, and family need to learn to recognize behaviors and situations that might trigger violence.

Normal developmental and physiological changes should be explained to enable family members to gain a more positive view of the victim and the crisis situation. Gaining a more complete understanding can help family members broaden their insight and thus increase their compassion. They may then begin to anticipate new stress situations and be able to prepare for them before a crisis occurs.

Nurses who work on a maternity unit are often in a position to spot potential violence in new families and initiate appropriate interventions, including education about effective parenting as well as coping techniques. Information about these interventions should be shared with the client's ambulatory care nurse for appropriate monitoring and follow-up. Parents who are candidates for special attention include

- New parents whose behavior toward the infant is rejecting, hostile, or indifferent.
- Teenage parents, most of whom are children themselves and who require special help and guidance in handling the baby and discussing their expectations of the baby and their support systems.
- Retarded parents, for whom careful, explicit, and repeated instructions on caring for the child and recognizing the infant's needs are indicated.
- Parents who grew up watching their mothers being beaten. This is the biggest risk factor for perpetuation of family violence.

Nurses can also recognize the vulnerable child. When it is known that specific children are at risk, referrals to community resources are in order. These may include emergency child care facilities, emergency telephone numbers, numbers of 24-hour crisis centers or hotlines, and respite programs in which volunteers take the child for an occasional weekend so that parents can get some relief. Public health nurses can make home visits; such visits allow assessment of potential violence in the crucial first few months of life. This early period is when the style of parent-child interactions is set for later life. Important factors for the community health nurse to assess are noted in Box 25-7. Such observations made by nurses in clinic and public health settings are fundamental in case finding and evaluation.

Advanced Practice Interventions

Psychotherapy is carried out by a nurse who is educated at the master's level in psychiatric nursing and is certified or eligible for certification. Therapy is most effective after crisis intervention, when the situation is less chaotic and tumultuous. A variety of therapeutic modalities are available for treatment of violent families.

Individual Therapy

The goals of individual therapy for a survivor are empowerment and practice in recognizing and selecting productive life options and developing a solid sense of self. People who have either experienced violence as a child or have left a violent relationship may choose individual therapy to work out symptoms of depression, anxiety, somatization, or posttraumatic stress disorder. Many of the psychological symptoms shown by battered women can be understood as complex survival strategies and responses to violence. This constellation of symptoms has been referred to as the "battered woman syndrome," the posttraumatic stress disorder category in the *Diagnostic and Statistical Manual of Mental Disorders,* fourth edition, text revision *(DSM-IV-TR)* (American Psychiatric Association, 2000).

Individual therapy is often indicated for the perpetrator also, particularly when an individual psychopathological process is identified. Many perpetrators meet the *DSM-IV-TR* criteria for intermittent explosive disorder, which involves repeated episodes of assault or destruction of property out of proportion to precipitating stressors that cannot be accounted for by another mental disorder, the physiological effects of a substance, or a general medical condition. Therapy for the perpetrator is most effective when it is court mandated, because then the perpetrator is more likely to complete the course of treatment.

Family Therapy

Because family violence is a symptom of a family in crisis, each part of the family system needs attention. Also, because change in one member of the family system affects the whole system, support and understanding are needed by all members. Family interventions may maximize positive interactions among family members. Family therapy should take place *only* if the violence is recent and if *both* partners agree to be involved. The perpetrator should have taken steps to control violent behavior that are verified by the survivor.

Expected outcomes are that the perpetrator will recognize inner states of anger and learn alternative ways of dealing with anger. Intermediate goals are that members of the family will openly communicate and learn to listen to each other. Refer to Chapter 36 for more information on family therapy.

Group Therapy

Participation in therapy groups provides assurances that one is not alone and that positive change is possible. Because many survivors have been isolated over time, they have been deprived of validation and positive feedback from others. Working in a group can help diminish feelings of isolation, strengthen feelings of self-esteem and self-worth, and increase the potential for realistic problem solving in a supportive atmosphere.

Self-help groups serve a vital function for many people. Hotlines provide emergency resources and information on how to contact self-help groups within the community, such as Parents Anonymous.

The real problem in a violent relationship is the perpetrator. Nurses engaged in therapy with perpetrators have a duty to warn potential victims if they conclude that the perpetrator is a danger (see Chapter 8). In therapy groups for perpetrators, these individuals are taught to recognize signs of escalating anger and learn ways of channeling their anger nonviolently. Perpetrators who have never discussed problems with anyone before are encouraged to discuss their thoughts and feelings. Group therapy can help create a community of healing and restoration. Refer to Chapter 35 for more information on group therapy.

■ EVALUATION

Failures in interventions with abusive families often are due not to our lack or to theirs but to deficits in the social, economic, and political systems in which

we live. A very real problem is that of social exclusion by which multidimensionally disadvantaged individuals are prohibited from obtaining formal helping services (Hilbert & Krishnan, 2000). Nurses can direct their interventions to the social environment and can question, among other things, the acceptance of corporal punishment as a technique for guiding behavior in children, the unequal burden of caregiving responsibilities placed on women, the low priority given to education and preparation for parenthood, and the belief that one has little social value if one is elderly.

Evaluation of brief interventions can be based on whether the survivor acknowledges the violence, is willing to accept intervention, and/or is removed from the violent situation. With more long-term interventions, evaluation should be made by all members of the health care team on an ongoing basis. Because violence is a symptom of a family in distress, diagnosis, interventions, and evaluation should ideally be carried out by a multidisciplinary team that includes a physician, a nurse, a social worker, an attorney, and perhaps a psychiatrist. Follow-up is crucial in helping decrease the frequency of family violence.

CASE STUDY and NURSING CARE PLAN 25-1 Family Violence

Mrs. Rob, a recently widowed 84-year-old woman, moved to her son's apartment 3 months ago. She had been living in her third-floor walk-up in the city. Because of her declining health, crime in the neighborhood, and the need to climb three flights of stairs, and with her son John's encouragement, she went to live with him. He and his wife Judy, who have been married for almost 20 years, have five children 6 to 18 years of age, all living in a rather cramped three-bedroom apartment.

Mrs. Rob is being cared for by a visiting nurse, who monitors her blood pressure and adjusts her medication. Over a series of visits, the nurse, Ms. Green, notices that Mrs. Rob is looking unkempt, pale, and withdrawn. While taking her blood pressure, Ms. Green observes bruises on Mrs. Rob's arms and neck. When questioned about the bruises, Mrs. Rob appears anxious and nervous. She says

that she had slipped in the bathroom. Mrs. Rob becomes increasingly apprehensive and stiffens up in her chair when her daughter-in-law Judy comes into the room, asking when the next visit is. The nurse notices that Judy avoids eye contact with Mrs. Rob.

When the injuries are brought to Judy's attention, she responds by becoming angry and agitated, blaming Mrs. Rob for causing so many problems. She will not explain the reason for the change in Mrs. Rob's behavior or the origin of the bruises to the nurse. She merely comments, "I have had to give up my job since my mother-in-law came here. It's been difficult and crowded ever since she moved in. The kids are complaining. We are having trouble making ends meet since I gave up my job. And my husband is no help at all."

Self-Assessment

Ms. Green has worked in a number of situations with violent families, but this is the first time she has encountered elder maltreatment. She discusses her reactions with the other team members. She is especially angry at Judy, although she is able to understand the daughter-in-law's frustration. The team concurs with Ms. Green that there seems to be potential for positive change in this family. If abuse does not abate, more drastic measures will need to be taken and legal services contacted.

Continued

ASSESSMENT

Objective Data

- Physical symptoms of violence (bruises, unkempt appearance, withdrawn attitude)
- Stressful, crowded living conditions
- No eye contact between Mrs. Rob and her daughter-in-law
- Economic hardships leading to stress
- No support for the daughter-in-law from the rest of the family for care of Mrs. Rob

Subjective Data

- Mrs. Rob states she slipped in the bathroom, but physical findings do not support this explanation.
- Judy states, "It's been difficult and crowded ever since she moved in."
- Mrs. Rob exhibits withdrawn and apprehensive behavior.

NURSING DIAGNOSIS (NANDA)

On the basis of the data, the nurse formulates the following nursing diagnoses:

1. *Risk for injury* related to increase in family stress, as evidenced by signs of violence
   - Mrs. Rob states she slipped in the bathroom, but physical findings do not support this explanation.
   - Physical symptoms of violence (bruises, unkempt appearance, withdrawn attitude)
   - Stressful, crowded living conditions

2. *Ineffective coping* related to helplessness, as evidenced by inability to meet role expectations
   - Mrs. Rob appears unkempt, anxious, depressed.
   - Mrs. Rob exhibits withdrawn and apprehensive behavior.

3. *Risk for other-directed violence* related to increased stressors within a short period, as evidenced by probable elder abuse and feelings of helplessness verbalized by the primary caregiver
   - Judy states, "It's been difficult and crowded ever since she moved in."
   - No eye contact between Judy and Mrs. Rob
   - Signs and symptoms of physical abuse on Mrs. Rob
   - Judy says, "My husband is no help at all."

4. *Caregiver role strain* related to extreme feelings of being overwhelmed and of helplessness
   - Family not helping with care of mother-in-law; burden of care on Judy
   - Economic hardships leading to stress when Judy gave up her job to care for Mrs. Rob

OUTCOME CRITERIA (NOC)

Overall outcome: *Abuse Cessation:* Evidence that the victim is no longer hurt or exploited
Short-term indicators:
- Evidence that physical abuse has ceased
- Evidence that emotional abuse has ceased

Short-term indicators are evaluated on a five-point Likert scale from 1 (none) to 5 (extensive).

PLANNING

Ms. Green discusses several possible outcomes with members of her team, giving attention to the priority of outcomes and to whether they are realistic in this situation. She also plans to report the elder abuse to Adult Protective Services and to work with Mrs. Rob, Judy, and the rest of the family to improve this situation for everyone.

INTERVENTION (NIC)

Mrs. Rob's plan of care is personalized as follows:

Nursing diagnosis: *Risk for injury* related to increase in family stress, as evidenced by signs of violence
Outcome criteria: Abuse Cessation

Short-Term Goal	Interventions	Rationale	Evaluation
1. On each visit made by the nurse, the client will state that abuse has decreased using a scale from 1 to 5 (1 being the least abuse).	1a. Follow state laws and guidelines for reporting elder abuse.	1a. Provides maximum protection under the law. Provides data for future use.	GOAL MET Client states that after family talked to the nurse and planned strategies, physical abuse no longer occurs.
	1b. Assess severity of signs and symptoms of abuse.	1b. Accurate charting (body map, pictures with permission, verbatim statements) helps follow progress and provides legal data.	
	1c. Do a careful home assessment to identify other areas of abuse and neglect.	1c. Check for adequacy of food, presence of vermin, blocked stairways, medication safety, etc. All indicate abuse and neglect. Determine the kinds of problems in the home to plan intervention. Identify community resources that could help the elder and caregivers.	
	1d. Discuss with client factors leading to abuse and concern for safety.	1d. Allows family stressors and potential areas for intervention to be identified. Validates that situation is serious and increases client's knowledge base.	
2. Within 2 weeks client will be able to identify at least two supportive services to deal with emergency situations.	2. Discuss with client supportive services such as hotlines and crisis units to call in case of emergency situations.	2. Maximizes client's safety through use of support systems.	GOAL MET Client has been talking to two old friends who she had stopped talking to because of shame and depression. She has called the hotline once to get information on transportation to the senior center in town.
3. Within 3 weeks family members will be able to identify difficult issues that increase their stress levels.	3. Discuss with family members their feelings and identify at least four areas that are most difficult for the various family members.	3. Listening to each family member and identifying unmet needs helps family as well as nurse identify areas that require changing and interventions.	GOAL MET Family members identify areas such as overwork, lack of free time, lack of privacy, and financial difficulties, all of which increase their stress levels.
4. Within 3 weeks family will seek out community resources to help with anger management, need for homemaker support, and other needs.	4. Identify potential community supports, skills training, respite places, homemakers, financial aids, etc., that might help meet family's unmet needs.	4. When stressed, individuals solve problems poorly and do not know about or cannot manage to organize outside help. Finances are often a problem.	GOAL MET The daughter-in-law is glad to get out of the house for anger management classes, and the son states he will try to take on more responsibility, but he often feels guilty and angry, too. Reluctantly, he and his wife agree to try a support group with other caregivers in similar situations.

■ EVALUATION

Eight weeks after Ms. Green's initial visit, Mrs. Rob appears well groomed, friendly, and more spontaneous in her conversation. She comments, "Things are better with my daughter-in-law." No bruises or other signs of physical violence are noticeable. She is considerably more outgoing and has even taken the initiative to contact an old friend. Mrs. Rob has talked openly to her son and daughter-in-law about stress in the family. Mrs. Rob says that she went for a walk when her daughter-in-law Judy appeared tense and returned to find that the tension had lessened. Neither Mrs. Rob nor her family has initiated plans for alternative housing.

- Family violence occurs across all age groups and can be predicted with some accuracy by examining the characteristics of perpetrators, vulnerable people, and situations in which violence is likely.
- Maltreatment can be physical, sexual, emotional, or economic, or caused by neglect.
- Assessment includes identifying indicators of mistreatment, levels of anxiety, coping mechanisms, support systems, and suicide and homicide potential as well as alcohol and drug abuse.

■■■

Visit the Evolve website at **http://evolve.elsevier.com/Varcarolis** for a posttest on the content in this chapter.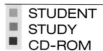

■ STUDENT
■ STUDY
■ CD-ROM

Access the accompanying CD-ROM for animations, interactive exercises, review questions for the NCLEX examination, and an audio glossary.

■ NURSE,
■ CLIENT, AND
■ FAMILY RESOURCES

For suggested readings, information on related associations, and Internet resources, go to **http://evolve.elsevier.com/Varcarolis**. *evolve*

Critical Thinking and Chapter Review

Visit the Evolve website at **http://evolve.elsevier.com/Varcarolis** for additional self-study exercises.
evolve

■■■ CRITICAL THINKING

1. How would you respond to a colleague who has witnessed a child being abused and stated, "I don't think it's any of our business what people do in the privacy of their own homes"? What would you do legally? Ethically?
2. Congratulations! You successfully convinced your colleagues to assess routinely for family violence. Now they want to know how to do it. How would you go about teaching them to assess for child abuse? Spouse abuse? Elder abuse?
3. Your health maintenance organization's routine health screening form for adolescents, adults, and elders has just been changed to include questions about family violence. How would you respond to patients who indicate on this form that family violence occurs in their home?
4. Write out a safety plan that could be adopted with other clients who are being abused.
5. Identify at least four referrals in your community for a battered person.
6. Identify two referrals in your community for a violent person, partner, or parent.

■■■ CHAPTER REVIEW

Choose the most appropriate answer.

1. Identifying people at high risk and providing health teaching about recognizing behaviors and situations that might trigger violence are examples of
    1. primary prevention.
    2. secondary prevention.
    3. tertiary prevention.
    4. nonintervention.

2. Which example of thinking is *not* a myth that would keep a woman locked in an abusive relationship?
    1. "If I'm patient, he'll change."
    2. "I deserved to be beaten."
    3. "I'll stay for the sake of the children."
    4. "No adult has the right to control or harm another."

3. When making assessments the nurse should bear in mind that a common characteristic of an abusing parent is
    1. being female.
    2. having poor coping skills.
    3. having realistic expectations of child behavior.
    4. abstaining from use of chemical substances of abuse.

4. Which of the following is a "red flag" for suspecting physical violence during assessment of a client?
    1. Client's explanation does not match the injury.
    2. Client has no history of stress-related physical problems.
    3. Client mentions having a concerned, supportive spouse.
    4. Client is anxious but open and direct in explaining the complaint or injury.

5. Which nursing diagnosis should be considered for the Jones family? The husband is disabled, unable to work, drinks episodically, and abuses the two preschool children when in this cycle. The wife works outside the home.
    1. Powerlessness
    2. Caregiver role strain
    3. Low self-esteem
    4. Disabled family coping

REFERENCES

Agency for Healthcare Research and Quality. (2002, October 9). *AHRQ unveils new web-based instrument to help hospitals assess domestic violence programs* [Press release]. Retrieved February 18, 2005, from http://www.ahrq.gov/news/press/pr2002/domvpr.htm.

American Psychiatric Association. (2000). *Diagnostic and statistical manual of mental disorders (DSM-IV-TR)* (4th ed., text rev.). Washington, DC: Author.

American Psychological Association. (2003). *Elder abuse and neglect: In search of solutions.* Retrieved February 18, 2005, from http://www.apa.org/pi/aging/eldabuse.html.

Bensley, L., Van Eenwyk, J., & Wynkoop Simmons, K. (2003). Childhood family violence history and women's risk for intimate partner violence and poor health. *American Journal of Preventive Medicine, 25,* 38-44.

Center for the Advancement of Women. (2003, June 24). *Is your mother's feminism dead? New agenda for women revealed in landmark two-year study* [Press release]. Retrieved February 17, 2004, from http://advancewomen.org/for_reporters/press_releases.php.

Davis, R. E. (2000). Cultural health care of child abuse: The Southeast Asian practice of cao gio. *Journal of American Academy of Nurse Practitioners, 12*(3), 89-95.

Desai, S., et al. (2002). Childhood victimization and subsequent adult revictimization assessed in a nationally representative sample of women and men. *Violence and Victims, 17,* 639-653.

DiScala, C. (2000). Child abuse and unintentional injuries: A 10-year retrospective. *Archives of Pediatric and Adolescent Medicine, 154*(1), 16.

Dochterman, J. M., & Bulechek, G. M. (2004). *Nursing interventions classification (NIC)* (4th ed.). St. Louis, MO: Mosby.

Emergency Nurses Association. (2003). *Emergency Nurses Association Position Statements: Domestic violence, maltreatment, and neglect* (pp. 1-6). Retrieved February 18, 2005, http://www.ena.org/about/position/domesticviolence.asp.

Family Violence Prevention Fund. (2004a). *Comply with JCAHO Standard PC.3.10 on victims of abuse.* Retrieved February 18, 2005, from http://endabuse.org/programs/display.php3?DocID=266.

Family Violence Prevention Fund. (2004b). *Staff education for elder abuse, neglect and exploitation.* Retrieved February 18, 2005, from http://endabuse.org/programs/display.php3?DocID=268.

Gazmararian, J. A., et al. (2000). Violence and reproductive health: Current knowledge and future research directions. *Maternal and Child Health Journal, 4*(2), 79-84. Retrieved February 18, 2005, from Centers for Disease Control and Prevention (CDC) website: http://www.cdc.gov/reproductivehealth/wh_viol_mchjv4n2.htm.

Hilbert, J. C., & Krishnan, S. P. (2000). Addressing barriers to community care of battered women in rural environments: Creating a policy of social inclusion. *Journal of Health and Social Policy, 12*(1), 41-52.

Lawson, L. (1998). Milieu management of traumatic youngsters. *Journal of Child and Adolescent Psychiatric Nursing, 11*(3), 99.

Mayes, G. (2003). Medical screening for domestic violence should be routine. *Medscape Ob/Gyn & Women's Health 8*(2), 1-2.

Moorhead, S., Johnson, M., & Maas, M. (2004). *Nursing outcomes classification (NOC)* (3rd ed.). St. Louis, MO: Mosby.

Nursing Research Consortium on Violence and Abuse. (1989). *Abuse assessment screen.* Baltimore, MD: University of Maryland.

Reece, R. M., & Sege, R. (2000). Childhood head injuries: Accidental or inflicted? *Archives of Pediatric and Adolescent Medicine, 154*(1), 11.

Seelau, E. P., Seelau, S. M., & Poorman, P. B. (2003). Gender and role-based perceptions of domestic abuse: Does sexual orientation matter? *Behavioral Sciences and the Law, 21,* 199-214.

Starling, S. P., & Holden, J. R. (2000). Perpetrators of abusive head trauma: A comparison of two geographic populations. *Southern Medical Journal, 93*(5), 463-465.

Stevens, L. (2003). *Clinical update: Improving screening of women for violence—basic guidelines for physicians.* Retrieved February 17, 2004, from http://www.medscape.com/viewprogram/2777.

Thomas, S. P. (2003). Anger: The mismanaged emotion. *Dermatologic Nursing, 15*(4), 351-357.

U.S. Department of Justice, Office on Violence Against Women. (2004). *President's Family Justice Center Initiative.* Retrieved February 22, 2004, from http://www.ojp.usdoj.gov/vawo/pfjci.htm.

CHAPTER 26

Sexual Assault

VERNA BENNER CARSON ▪ KATHLEEN SMITH-DIJULIO

KEY TERMS and CONCEPTS

The key terms and concepts listed here appear in color where they are defined or first discussed in this chapter.

acquaintance or date rape, 531

acute phase, 532

blame, 538

compound reaction, 536

controlled style of coping, 535

expressed style of coping, 534

long-term reorganization phase, 533

rape-trauma syndrome, 531

silent reaction, 537

spousal or marital rape, 531

OBJECTIVES

After studying this chapter, the reader will be able to

1. Define sexual assault (rape).
2. Discuss the reasons that rapes go unreported.

3. Distinguish between the acute and long-term phases of the rape-trauma syndrome and identify some common reactions during each phase.
4. Identify and give examples of five areas to assess when working with a person who has been sexually assaulted.
5. Formulate two long-term outcomes and two short-term goals for the nursing diagnosis *rape-trauma syndrome.*
6. Analyze one's own thoughts and feelings regarding the myths about rape and its impact on survivors.
7. Identify six overall guidelines for nursing interventions related to sexual assault.
8. Describe the role of the sexual assault nurse examiner to a colleague.
9. Discuss the responsibilities of the nurse when a rape survivor is discharged from the emergency department, citing specific referrals in the community.
10. Develop a handout delineating the nurse's role when staffing a rape-crisis hotline.
11. Discuss the long-term psychological effects of sexual assault that might lead to a survivor's seeking psychotherapy.
12. Identify three outcome criteria that would signify successful interventions for a person who has suffered a sexual assault.

evolve Visit the Evolve website at **http://evolve.elsevier.com/Varcarolis** for a pretest on the content in this chapter.

Imagine that a friend has been sexually assaulted. She comes to you crying and fearful. She tells you that she has been brutally raped. It terrifies you just as it has terrified her. You want to help her, but initially you are not sure what to do. She is paralyzed with fear, shame, and pain. As a nursing student or a nurse, as a friend, or as a parent, it is likely that you will encounter someone who has been raped. Or it could be you who is sexually assaulted, and you are feeling the pain, shame, and guilt. The whole notion of rape is horrifying. Rape is an act of violence, and sex is the weapon used by the perpetrator. Rape engulfs its victims in fear, resulting in

withdrawal for some and causing severe panic reactions in others. After being traumatized, the person raped often carries an additional burden of shame, guilt, fear, anger, distrust, and embarrassment. It is important that as a nurse you know how to respond to individuals undergoing the trauma of rape.

Sexual assault is any type of sexual activity that the victim does not want or agree to. It ranges from inappropriate touching to penetration, or intercourse. Sexual assault can occur verbally over the telephone or electronically over the Internet. Being forced into activities such as prostitution, posing for pornographic photographs, and appearing in pornographic videos are all examples of sexual assaults. Children and elders, women and men can all be victims of sexual assault.

Rape is one type of sexual assault. Rape is nonconsensual vaginal, anal, or oral penetration, obtained by force or by threat of bodily harm, or when a person is incapable of giving consent. It is usually men who rape, and most of those raped are women. However, about 12.8% (31,640) of all rape victims are male (Rape Abuse and Incest National Network [RAINN], 2002). When men are raped, the rape is generally perpetrated by a heterosexual male.

A male who is raped is more likely to experience physical trauma and to have been victimized by several assailants than is a female who is raped. Reported homosexual rape occurs primarily in closed institutions, such as prisons and maximum-security hospitals. The psychodynamics are the same as those of heterosexual rape, and males experience the same devastation and emotional consequences as do females (Porcerelli et al., 2003).

According to the National Crime Victimization Survey, in 2002 there were 216,090 female rape victims (1.8 per 1000 persons aged 12 years and older). This figure reflects an overall decline in rapes from 1993 through 2002. Rape is down by 60%; attempted rape is down by 57.1% (RAINN, 2002). Experts attribute this decline to two trends. The first trend reflects policies that are tough on crime, including imposition of longer sentences, "three-strike" laws, and mandatory minimum sentences, which mean that fewer criminals are on the street (RAINN, 2002). The second trend is generational. Eighty percent of rape victims are under 30 years of age. This current generation has grown up knowing that "no means no," and young women today are more willing to express their own desires assertively and to go to the authorities to report sexual abuse.

The remainder of this chapter focuses on rape as an example of sexual assault. Nurses are very involved in the assessment and treatment of those who have been sexually assaulted through rape. Therefore, it is essential that nurses be adequately informed about their roles and responsibilities with regard to these clients. Also, the female pronoun is used throughout the remainder of this chapter in recognition of the fact that women are more frequently assaulted sexually. However, the principles discussed apply to anyone who is raped.

THEORY

Stranger rape is what most people envisage when they think of sexual assault, yet this is the least common type. The 2002 National Crime Victimization Survey indicated that 69% of rapes were perpetrated by someone known to the victim (RAINN, 2003). The terms *spousal or marital rape* and *acquaintance or date rape* de-

scribe the nature of the relationship between victim and rapist. In recent years the courts have recognized spousal or marital rape, in which the perpetrator (nearly always the male) is married to the person raped. In acquaintance or date rape, the perpetrator is known to, and presumably trusted by, the person raped. The incidence of rape is four times higher among young women aged 16 to 24 years than among women in other age groups (Lynch, 2003). The psychological and emotional outcomes of rape seem to vary depending on the level of intimacy of the perpetrator. Sexual distress is more common among women who have been sexually assaulted by intimates; fear and anxiety are more common in those assaulted by strangers; depression occurs in both groups.

Date or acquaintance rape has increased in the United States in recent years, with drugs, often combined with alcohol, used to commit sexual assault. Alcohol is implicated in 69% of date rapes (King, 2003). Other drugs used as "knockout drugs" may render a woman incapable of resisting the rape attack and are purported to facilitate acquaintance rape (Lynch, 2003). Often these drugs are slipped unknowingly to the victim (e.g., "the new Mickey Finn"). Once they are ingested, victims lose their ability to ward off attackers, develop amnesia, and are unreliable witnesses. Because the symptoms mimic those of alcohol, victims are not always screened for these drugs. The increase in prevalence and incidence of drug-assisted rape led to the passage of the Drug-Induced Rape Prevention and Punishment Act in 1996. This law provides for up to 20 years' imprisonment and fines for anyone who intends to commit a violent crime by administering a controlled substance to an unknowing individual (U.S. Department of Justice, 1997). Table 26-1 provides information on date-rape drugs. Most people who are raped suffer severe and long-lasting emotional trauma. Long-term psychological effects of sexual assault may include depression, suicide, anxiety, and fear; difficulties with daily functioning; low self-esteem; sexual dysfunction; and somatic complaints. Incest victims may experience a negative self-image, depression, eating disorders, personality disorders, self-destructive behavior, and substance abuse. Timely intervention can greatly help to minimize the devastating aftermath of rape. A history of sexual abuse in psychiatric clients is associated with a characteristic pattern of symptoms that may include depression, anxiety disorders, chemical dependency, suicide attempts, self-mutilation, compulsive sexual behavior, and psychosis-like symptoms (Vaughn, Vaughn, & Wiemann, 2003).

The rape-trauma syndrome is a variant of posttraumatic stress disorder (PTSD) and consists of (1) an acute phase and (2) a long-term reorganization process that occurs after an actual or attempted sexual assault. Each phase has separate symptoms. Refer to Chapter 14 for more on PTSD.

TABLE 26-1

Currently Available Drugs Associated with Date Rape

Name of Drug	Street Name(s) of Drug	Mechanism of Action	Effect on Victim	Treatment of Overdose
GHB (γ-hydroxy-butyric acid)	Georgia home boy, liquid ecstasy, salty water, scoop	Central nervous system depressant	Onset is within 5-20 minutes; duration is dose related and is from 1 to 12 hours. Produces euphoria, amnesia, hypotonia, and depressed respiration. Can also cause seizures, unconsciousness, nausea, and vomiting.	Intubation for severe respiratory distress; atropine for bradycardia and benzodiazepines for seizure activity. Vomiting should always be induced whenever possible.
Rohypnol (flunitrazepam)	"Forget" drug; also roofies, club drug, roachies, and rophies	A potent benzodiazepine; 10 times stronger than diazepam	Impact is within 10-30 minutes and lasts 2-12 hours; becomes more potent when combined with alcohol; causes dizziness, amnesia, lack of motor coordination, confusion, nausea and vomiting, respiratory depression, and blackout episodes lasting 8-24 hours.	Airway protection and gastrointestinal decontamination.
Ketamine	Special K, K, vitamin K, bump, kitkat, purple, super C	An anesthetic frequently used in veterinary practice; also a hallucinogenic substance related to PCP (phencyclidine)	Onset is rapid, within 30 seconds intravenously and 20 minutes orally; duration is only 30-60 minutes; amnesia effects may last longer; usually administered as a powder that is snorted, smoked, injected, or dissolved in drinks. Causes dissociative reaction with a dreamlike state leading to deep amnesia and analgesia and complete compliance of the victim. Later, victim may be confused, paranoid, delirious, combative, with drooling and hallucinations.	Airway maintenance and use of anticholinergics such as atropine and benzodiazepines.
Burundanga or datura	Nightshade, angel trumpet, CIA drug, jimson weed	Datura is an anticholinergic and hallucinogenic substance consisting of refined scopolamine. Used for motion sickness and as an adjunct to anesthesia to produce sedation and amnesia.	Ingestion or inhalation of datura produces amnesia, submissive behavior, hypnosis, hallucinations, and confusion. An anticholinergic syndrome may occur, leading to coma, seizures, and death.	Airway maintenance and administration of physostigmine for severe anticholinergic symptoms.

Data from Lynch, J. S. (2003, October 15-18). *Date rape and drug-assisted rape: Clinical implications.* Paper presented at the National Association of Nurse Practitioners in Women's Health 6th Annual Conference, Savannah, GA.
CIA, Central Intelligence Agency.

Acute Phase of Rape-Trauma Syndrome

The acute phase of the rape-trauma syndrome occurs immediately after the assault and may last for a couple of weeks. This is the stage at which clients are seen by emergency department personnel. Nurses are the ones most involved in dealing with these initial reactions. During this phase, there is a great deal of disorganization in the person's lifestyle, and somatic symptoms are common. This disorganization can be described in terms of impact, somatic, and emotional reactions (Box 26-1).

Acute Phase of Rape-Trauma Syndrome

Impact Reaction

Expressed Style

Overt behaviors:

- Crying, sobbing
- Smiling, laughing, joking
- Restlessness, agitation, hysteria
- Volatility, anger
- Confusion, incoherence, disorientation
- Tenseness

Controlled Style

Ambiguous reactions:

- Confusion, incoherence, disorientation
- Masked facies
- Calm, subdued appearance
- Shock, numbness, confusion, disbelieving appearance
- Distractibility, difficulty making decisions

Somatic Reaction

Evidenced within first several weeks after a rape

Physical Trauma

- Bruises (breasts, throat, or back)
- Soreness

Skeletal Muscle Tension

- Headaches
- Sleep disturbances
- Grimaces, twitches

Gastrointestinal Symptoms

- Stomach pains
- Nausea
- Poor appetite
- Diarrhea

Genitourinary Symptoms

- Vaginal itching
- Vaginal discharge
- Pain or discomfort

Emotional Reaction

- Fear of physical violence and death
- Denial
- Anxiety
- Shock
- Humiliation
- Fatigue
- Embarrassment
- Desire for revenge
- Self-blame
- Lowered self-esteem
- Shame
- Guilt
- Anger

Data from Burgess A. W. (1995). Rape trauma syndrome: A nursing diagnosis. *Occupational Health Nursing, 33*(8), 405; and Burgess, A. W., & Holstrom, L. L. (1974). The rape victim in the ER. *American Journal of Nursing, 73*(10), 1740.

The most common initial reaction is shock, numbness, and disbelief. Outwardly, the person may appear self-contained and calm and may make remarks such as "It doesn't seem real" or "I don't believe this really happened to me." Sometimes, cognitive functions may be impaired, and the traumatized person may appear extremely confused and have difficulty concentrating and making decisions. Alternatively, the person may become hysterical or restless, or may cry or even smile. These reactions to crisis are typical and reflect cognitive, affective, and behavioral disruptions.

People who have experienced an emotionally overwhelming event may find it too painful to discuss. Examples of this response are found in statements such as "I don't want to talk about it" or "I just want to forget what happened." Behaviors that minimize the magnitude of the event include reluctance to seek medical attention and failure to follow up with legal counsel.

Long-Term Reorganization Phase of Rape-Trauma Syndrome

The long-term reorganization phase of rape-trauma syndrome occurs 2 or more weeks after the rape. Nurses who initially care for the survivors can help them anticipate and prepare for the reactions they are likely to experience. These include the following:

Intrusive thoughts of the rape break into the survivor's conscious mind during the day and during sleep. These thoughts commonly include anger and violence toward the assailant, flashbacks (reexperiencing of the traumatic event), dreams with violent content, and insomnia.

Increased motor activity follows, such as moving, taking trips, changing telephone numbers, and making frequent visits to old friends. This activity stems from the fear that the assailant will return.

Increased emotional lability occurs, including intense anxiety, mood swings, crying spells, and depression.

Fears and phobias develop as a defensive reaction to the rape. Typical phobias include

- Fear of the indoors (if the rape occurred indoors).
- Fear of the outdoors (if the rape occurred outdoors).
- Fear of being alone (common for most women after an assault).
- Fear of crowds. Women may believe that any person in the crowd might be a rapist.
- Fear of sexual encounters and activities. Many women experience acute disruption of their sex lives with their partners. Rape is especially disruptive for those with no previous sexual experience.

As mentioned, the consequences of sexual assault may be severe, debilitating, and long term. Intervention and support for the survivor can help prevent some of the complications mentioned: anxiety, depression, suicide, difficulties with daily functioning and interpersonal relationships, sexual dysfunction, and somatic complaints.

Application of the Nursing Process

■ ASSESSMENT

Once the rape survivor is in the emergency department, the attention received depends on the protocol of the particular hospital. The Emergency Nurses Association position statement on care of sexual assault victims (2001) suggests the following interventions:

- Use a nonjudgmental and empathetic approach.
- Provide rapid assessment of the needs and support required to prevent further trauma.
- Treat and document injuries.
- Provide a private environment and limit personnel to examining health care professionals, a translator if needed, and (with the consent of the client) a specially trained advocate if indicated.
- Assist with or conduct a physical examination.
- Obtain pertinent laboratory tests (e.g., human immunodeficiency virus [HIV] testing, hepatitis profiles).
- Assist with or perform collection of evidence with appropriate documentation and preservation of evidence.
- Evaluate for and treat sexually transmitted diseases.
- Conduct pregnancy risk evaluation and prevention.
- Provide crisis intervention and arrange follow-up counseling.

The nurse talks with the survivor, the family or friends who accompany the survivor, and the police to gather as much data as possible for assessing the crisis. The nurse then assesses the survivor's (1) level of anxiety, (2) coping mechanisms, (3) available support systems, (4) signs and symptoms of emotional trauma, and (5) signs and symptoms of physical trauma. Information obtained from the assessment is then analyzed, and nursing diagnoses are formulated.

Overall Assessment

Assessing the Level of Anxiety

A client who is experiencing severe to panic levels of anxiety will not be able to problem solve or process information. The nurse uses approaches that can lower the client's anxiety so that mutual goals can be set and information can be assimilated. Support, reassurance, and appropriate therapeutic techniques can help diminish anxiety. Refer to Chapters 12 and 13 for more detailed discussion of levels of anxiety and therapeutic interventions.

Assessing Coping Mechanisms Used

The same coping skills that have helped the survivor through other difficult problems will be used in adjusting to the rape. In addition, new ways of getting through the difficult times may be developed, for both the short- and long-term adjustment.

Behavioral responses include crying; withdrawing; smoking; abusing alcohol and drugs; wanting to talk about the event; acting hysterical, confused, disoriented, or incoherent; and even laughing or joking. These behaviors are examples of an **expressed style of coping** (see Box 26-1).

Cognitive coping mechanisms are the thoughts people have that help them deal with high anxiety levels. If thoughts are verbalized, the nurse will know what the survivor is thinking. If not, the nurse can ask questions such as, "What do you think might help?" or "What can I do to help you in this difficult situation?" or "What has helped in the past?"

Assessing Support Systems Available

The availability, size, and usefulness of a survivor's social support system must be assessed. Often partners or family members do not understand the survivor's feelings about the sexual assault, and they may not be the best supports available. Pay careful attention to verbal and nonverbal cues of the survivor that may communicate the strength of her social network.

■ ■ ■ *VIGNETTE*

Ms. Ruiz, age 18 years, is brought to the emergency department by a concerned neighbor. She was found wandering aimlessly outside her house, sobbing and muttering, "He had no right to do that to me." Because of Ms. Ruiz's distraught appearance and her statement, the triage nurse suspects sexual assault and brings Ms. Ruiz to the office of the psychiatric nurse, Ms. Wong. Ms. Wong introduces herself, explains her role, and states that she is there to help. Ms. Wong then asks Ms. Ruiz what happened. After careful, sensitive, nonthreatening questioning, Ms. Ruiz divulges that she had been out with her boyfriend, who took her to a "rave" party and then raped her. She got a ride back home but no one else was at home. She was so upset and afraid, she did not go inside, and the neighbor, Ms. Green, had seen her outside.

After the entire history and examination are completed, plans for discharge are discussed. Ms. Ruiz states that no one will be home until Sunday night, 2 days away, and that she does not feel comfortable calling any friends because she does not want them to know what happened. The neighbor, Ms. Green, has told the nurse earlier that Ms. Ruiz can stay with her family.

Nurse: Earlier, your neighbor, Ms. Green, told me that you are welcome to spend the weekend with her family.

Ms. Ruiz: (Loudly, sharply, with eyes wide) Oh, no, I couldn't do that.

Nurse: You don't seem to like that idea.

Ms. Ruiz: Oh, I just wouldn't want to bother them.

Nurse: Ms. Green seems quite concerned about your welfare.

Ms. Ruiz: Oh, yes, she's very nice. (Pause)

Nurse: But not someone you would want to spend the weekend with?

Ms. Ruiz: Her children are too noisy. I've got homework to do.

Nurse: You might not get the quiet you need to study. (Pause) Yet you also do not want to be alone?

Ms. Ruiz: (Wringing a tissue in her hands, head hanging, voice soft) I can't go in her house anymore.

Nurse: Something about being in that house disturbs you?

Ms. Ruiz: Mr. Green (deep sigh, pause) used to . . . uh . . . take advantage of me when I used to baby-sit his children.

Nurse: Take advantage?

Ms. Ruiz: Yes . . . (sobbing) he used to force me to have sex with him. He said he'd blame it on me if I told anyone.

Nurse: What a frightening experience that must have been for you.

Ms. Ruiz: Yes.

Nurse: I can see why you would not want to spend the night there. Let's continue to explore other options.

A suitable place to stay is finally arranged. Ms. Ruiz is given counseling referrals that will help her deal with the process of reorganization after this current rape experience. Her counselor will explore her feelings about past sexual abuse she has suffered at the hands of her neighbor when she is ready.

Assessing Signs and Symptoms of Emotional Trauma

Nurses work most frequently with sexual assault survivors in the emergency department soon after the rape has occurred. Rape is a psychological emergency and should receive immediate attention. Some emergency departments provide the services of sexual assault nurse examiners (SANEs) or clinicians who are specially trained to meet the myriad needs of the sexual assault survivor (Ledray, 1998, 2001).

The extent of the psychological and emotional trauma sustained may not be readily apparent from behavior, especially if the person uses the controlled style of coping during the acute phase of the rape trauma (see Box 26-1).

A nursing history is obtained and properly recorded. When taking a history, the nurse determines only the details of the assault that will be helpful in addressing the immediate physical and psychological needs of the survivor. The nurse allows the survivor to talk at a comfortable pace; poses questions in nonjudgmental, descriptive terms; and refrains from asking "why" questions. The survivor frequently finds that relating the events of the rape is traumatic and embarrassing.

If suicidal thoughts are expressed, the nurse assesses what precautions are needed by asking direct questions, such as "Are you thinking of harming yourself?" and "Have you ever tried to kill yourself before or after this attack occurred?" If the answer is yes, the nurse conducts a thorough suicide assessment (plan, means to carry it out) as described in Chapter 23.

Assessing Signs and Symptoms of Physical Trauma

It is essential that nurses provide psychological support while collecting and preserving potentially crucial legal evidence such as hair, skin, and semen samples. The most characteristic physical signs of sexual assault are injuries to the face, head, neck, and extremities. Any noted injuries should be carefully documented, preferably on a body map (Ledray, 2001).

The nurse takes a brief gynecological history, including date of last menstrual period, the likelihood of current pregnancy, and any history of a sexually transmitted disease. If the survivor has never undergone a pelvic examination, the steps of the examination will need to be explained. The nurse plays a crucial role in giving support and minimizing the trauma of the examination. The survivor may feel that it is another violation of her body. Recognizing this, the nurse can explain the examination procedure in a way that will be reassuring and supportive. Allowing the survivor to participate in all decisions affecting care helps her regain a sense of control over her life.

The survivor has the right to refuse either a legal or a medical examination. Consent forms must be signed to take photographs, perform a pelvic examination, and carry out whatever other procedures might be needed to collect evidence and provide treatment. The correct preservation of body fluids and swabs is essential, because DNA (genetic mapping) may identify the rapist. A shower and fresh clothing should be made available to the survivor immediately after the examination, if possible.

Providing prophylactic treatment for syphilis, chlamydiosis, and gonorrhea, according to guidelines of the Centers for Disease Control and Prevention, is common practice.

HIV exposure is an ever-growing concern of sexual assault survivors. This concern is always addressed, and the rape survivor is given the information needed to evaluate the likely risk. With this information, the person and her sexual partner(s) can make educated choices about HIV testing and safer sex practices until testing can be done.

About 3% to 5% of women who are raped become pregnant as a result. Pregnancy prophylaxis can be offered in the emergency department or at follow-up, after the results of the pregnancy test are obtained.

All data are carefully documented, including verbatim statements by the survivor, detailed observations of emotional and physical status, and all results of the physical examination. All laboratory tests performed are noted and findings recorded as soon as they are available. The Emergency Nurses Association position statement on forensic evidence collection (2003) spells out the role of the nurse in collecting medical and legal evidence.

Self-Assessment

Nurses' attitudes influence the physical and psychological care administered to rape survivors. Knowing the myths and facts surrounding sexual assault can increase nurses' awareness of their personal beliefs and feelings regarding rape. Nurses who examine their personal feelings and reactions before encountering a rape survivor are better prepared to give empathetic and effective care. Nurses must also examine their feelings about abortion, because a client might choose to abort a fetus produced as a result of rape. It is the patient's choice, and if an individual nurse is too conflicted to work with the patient, then the nurse should switch duties with another nurse. It is better to ask for help with a client than to make the client uncomfortable. The process is the same as that described for caring for survivors of other types of violence (see Chapter 25). Table 26-2 compares rape myths and facts.

Assessment Guidelines Sexual Assault

1. Assess psychological trauma. Write down verbatim statements of the client.
2. Assess level of anxiety. If the client is in a severe to panic level of anxiety, the client will not be able to problem solve or process information.
3. Assess physical trauma. Use a body map and ask permission to take photographs.
4. Assess available support system. Often partners or family members do not understand the trauma of rape, and they may not be the best supports to draw on at this time.
5. Identify community supports (e.g., attorneys, support groups, therapists) that work in the area of sexual assault.
6. Encourage the clients to tell his or her experience. Do not press the client to tell.

■ NURSING DIAGNOSIS

Rape-trauma syndrome is the nursing diagnosis that applies to the physical and psychological effects resulting from an episode of sexual assault. It includes an acute phase of disorganization of the survivor's lifestyle and a long-term phase of reorganization.

Rape-Trauma Syndrome: Compound Reaction. Compound reaction includes
- All symptoms listed under rape-trauma syndrome (see Box 26-1).
- Reliance on alcohol or other drugs.

TABLE 26-2

Myth Versus Fact: Rape

Myth	Fact
Many women really want to be raped.	Women do not ask to be raped—no matter how they are dressed, what their behavior is, or where they are at any given time. Studies show that violence toward women in the media leads to attitudes that foster tolerance of rape.
Most rapists are oversexed.	Sex is used as an instrument of violence in rape. Rape is an act of aggression, anger, or power.
Most women are raped by strangers.	The majority (69%) of rape victims are raped by someone they knew.
No healthy adult female who resists vigorously can be raped by an unarmed man.	Most men can overpower most women because of differences in body build. Also, the victim may panic, which makes her actions less effective than usual.
Most charges of rape are unfounded.	There is no evidence to show that there are more false reports for rape than for other crimes. Most rape victims do not even report the rape.
Rapes usually occur in dark alleys.	Over 50% of all rapes occur in the home.
Rape is usually an impulsive act.	Most rapes are planned; over 50% involve a weapon.
Nice girls don't get raped.	Any woman is a potential rape victim. Victims range in age from 6 months to 90 years.
There was not enough time for a rape to occur.	There is no minimal time limit that characterizes rape. It can happen very quickly.
Do not fight or try to get away because you will just get hurt.	There are no verifiable data to substantiate the theory that a victim will be injured if he or she tries to get away.
Only females are raped.	There are a growing number of male rape victims.
Rape is a sexual act.	Rape is a violent expression of aggression, anger, and need for power.

- Reactivated symptoms of previous conditions, such as physical or psychiatric illness.

Rape-Trauma Syndrome: Silent Reaction.
Silent reaction is a complex stress reaction to rape in which an individual is unable to describe or discuss the rape. Symptoms include
- Abrupt changes in relationships with sexual partners.
- Nightmares.
- Increasing anxiety during the interview, such as blocking of associations, long periods of silence, minor stuttering, or physical distress.
- Marked changes in sexual behavior.
- Sudden onset of phobic reactions.
- No verbalization of the occurrence of rape.

OUTCOME CRITERIA

The long-term outcome includes the absence of any residual symptoms after the trauma. The Nursing Outcomes Classification (NOC) (Moorhead, Johnson, & Maas, 2004) identifies additional outcomes that are appropriate for the rape survivor: *Abuse Protection; Abuse Recovery: Emotional; Abuse Recovery: Sexual; Coping; Sexual Functioning;* and *Stress Level.* Some of the suggested indicators for these outcomes include the following:
- Client will demonstrate positive interpersonal relationships.
- Client will demonstrate adequate social interactions.
- Client will demonstrate healing of physical injuries.
- Client will demonstrate evidence of appropriate same-sex relationships.
- Client will demonstrate evidence of appropriate opposite-sex relationships.
- Client will verbalize accurate information about sexual functioning.
- Client will express comfort with body.
- Client will express sexual interest.
- Client will express willingness to be sexual.
- Client will report increased psychological comfort.
- Client will report a decrease in physical symptoms of stress.

PLANNING

The majority of rape survivors are seen in the emergency department. Unless the survivor has sustained serious physical injury, treatment is offered and the client is released. However, because the ramifications of rape are experienced for an extended time after the acute phase, the plan of care must include information for follow-up care. The survivor needs information

about what community supports are available and how to access these supports. In addition, nurses may encounter rape survivors in many other settings when they are no longer in the acute phase but still are dealing with the aftermath of rape; such settings include inpatient facilities, community, and home. The plan of care needs to address the continuing needs of the rape survivor wherever the nurse encounters her.

INTERVENTION

The occurrence of rape can be the most devastating experience in a person's life and constitutes an acute adventitious crisis. Typical crisis reactions reflect cognitive, affective, and behavioral disruptions. For survivors to return to their previous level of functioning, it is necessary for them to fully mourn their losses, experience anger, and work through their terrifying fears. Box 26-2 provides Nursing Interventions Classification (NIC) interventions for rape-trauma treatment (Dochterman & Bulechek, 2004).

BOX 26-2

Rape-Trauma Treatment (NIC)

Definition: Provision of emotional and physical support immediately following a reported rape
Activities:
- Provide support person to stay with patient.
- Explain legal proceedings available to patient.
- Explain rape protocol and obtain consent to proceed through protocol.
- Document whether patient has showered, douched, or bathed since incident.
- Document mental state, physical state (clothing, dirt, and debris), history of incident, evidence of violence, and prior gynecological history.
- Determine presence of cuts, bruises, bleeding, lacerations, or other signs of physical injury.
- Implement rape protocol (e.g., label and save soiled clothing, vaginal secretions, and vaginal hair combings).
- Secure samples for legal evidence.
- Implement crisis intervention counseling.
- Offer medication to prevent pregnancy, as appropriate.
- Offer prophylactic antibiotic medication against sexually transmitted disease.
- Inform patient of availability of human immunodeficiency virus testing, as appropriate.
- Give clear, written instructions about medication use, crisis support services, and legal support.
- Refer patient to rape advocacy program.
- Document according to agency policy.

From Dochterman, J. M., & Bulechek, G. M. (2004). *Nursing interventions classification (NIC)* (4th ed., p. 593). St. Louis, MO: Mosby.

Basic Level Interventions

Basic level nursing interventions include counseling, promotion of self-care activities, and case management.

Counseling

The rape survivor may be too traumatized, ashamed, or afraid to come to the hospital. Cultural definitions of what constitutes rape may also affect the decision to seek treatment. For these reasons, most communities provide 24-hour telephone hotlines. The trained phone counselor talks briefly with the person to determine where she is, what has happened, and what kind of help she needs. The counselor provides empathetic listening and the survivor is further encouraged to go to the hospital. The main focus in the telephone contact is on the immediate steps the survivor may take. The counselor provides the necessary information for the woman to make decisions.

The most effective approach for counseling in the emergency department or crisis center is to provide nonjudgmental care as well as optimal emotional support. Displays of shock, horror, disgust, surprise, or disbelief are not appropriate. Confidentiality is crucial. The most helpful things the nurse can do are to listen and to let the survivor talk. A woman who feels understood is no longer alone; she then feels more in control of her situation.

It is especially important to help the survivor and her significant others separate issues of vulnerability from blame. Although the person may have made choices that made her more vulnerable, she is not to blame for the rape, no matter what she did. She may, however, decide to avoid some of those choices in the future (e.g., walking alone late at night or excessive use of alcohol). Focusing on one's behavior (which is controllable) allows the survivor to believe that similar experiences can be avoided in the future.

■ ■ ■ *VIGNETTE*

Mary comes to see that it was not her fault that she was raped. However, she is now adamant about not walking from the bus stop alone late at night, and from now on will take a cab, get a lift from a friend, or take a safer alternative route when she goes home.

■ ■ ■

If the survivor consents, involve her support system (e.g., family or friends) and discuss with them the nature and trauma of sexual assault and possible delayed reactions that may occur. One survivor expressed it this way:

It takes a few days to hit you. It was bad. It was really rough for my husband. I needed to be reassured. I needed to be told that there was nothing I could do to prevent it. Understanding helps.

Social support effectively moderates somatic symptoms and subjective health ratings. The survivor who is able to confide comfortably in one or two friends or family members, especially immediately after the assault, is likely to experience fewer somatic manifestations of stress. In many cases, family and friends need support and reassurance as much as the survivor does. This is especially true for those from traditional cultures. The long-standing cultural myth that women are the property of men still prevents some people from empathizing with the woman's severe psychic injury and from being supportive. Instead, in these cases, the woman is devalued.

Promotion of Self-Care Activities

When preparing the survivor to go home, the nurse provides all referral information and follow-up instructions in writing, detailing likely physical concerns and emotional reactions, legal matters, victim compensation, and ways that family and friends can help. This is important, because the amount of verbal information the client can retain will likely be limited owing to anxiety. Written material can be referred to repeatedly over time. Legal referrals (i.e., names of attorneys who specialize in rape cases and options for low-cost legal assistance) can also be given.

Case Management

Caring for the survivor is not completed in a single visit. Her emotional state and other psychological needs should be reassessed by telephone or personal contact within 24 to 48 hours after discharge from the hospital. Repeat referrals should be made for needed resources or support services at this time. Effective crisis intervention and continuity of care require outreach activities and services beyond the emergency medical setting.

Survivors may seek help from medical professionals rather than from mental health professionals because medical treatment is more socially sanctioned and they are likely to be experiencing the physical symptoms of stress. By being aware of this, the outpatient nurse can make a more focused assessment of stress-related symptoms and/or depression and ascertain the need for mental health referral. Reporting symptoms and seeking medical treatment are adaptive coping behaviors and can be reinforced as such.

Follow-up visits should occur at least 2, 4, and 6 weeks after the initial evaluation. At each visit, the survivor should be assessed for psychological progress, the presence of a sexually transmitted disease, and pregnancy.

Case Study and Nursing Care Plan 26-1 describes the care of a client who has been raped.

Advanced Practice Interventions

Psychotherapy

The advanced practice nurse may offer individual or group psychotherapy for either the rape survivor or the perpetrator.

Survivor. Most of those who have been raped are eventually able to resume their previous lives after supportive services and crisis counseling. However, many continue to experience emotional trauma: flashbacks, nightmares, fear, phobias, and other symptoms associated with PTSD (see Chapter 14). Some people who survive rape may be susceptible to a psychotic episode or an emotional disturbance so severe that hospitalization is required. Others whose emotional lives may be overburdened with multiple internal and external pressures may require individual psychotherapy.

Depression and suicidal ideation frequently follow rape. Depression is more common in those who do not disclose the assault to significant others because they have concerns about being stigmatized, have children living at home, or have a pending civil lawsuit. Any exposure to stimuli related to the traumatic event may activate a reliving of the traumatic state.

People who have been raped are likely to benefit from group therapy or support groups. These modalities may be particularly beneficial for survivors from cultures that are group oriented rather than individualistic, and for women who derive much of their self-definition from cultural norms. Group therapy can make the difference between a person's coming out of the crisis at a lower level of functioning or gradually adapting to the experience with an increase in coping skills.

Rapist. Psychotherapy is essential for rapists if behavioral change is to occur. Unfortunately, most rapists do not acknowledge the need for behavioral change, and no single method or program of treatment has been found to be totally effective. If a nurse is the counselor for the rapist, the nurse's awareness of his or her own feelings and reactions will be crucial so as to avoid interference with the therapeutic process.

■ EVALUATION

Rape survivors are recovered if they are relatively free of any signs or symptoms of PTSD; that is, if they are

- Sleeping well, with very few instances of episodic nightmares or broken sleep.
- Eating as was their pattern before the rape. (Clients may respond to the crisis of rape by undereating or overeating.)
- Calm and relaxed or only mildly suspicious, fearful, or restless.
- Getting support from family and friends. Some strain might still be present in relationships, but it should be minimal.
- Generally positive about themselves. On occasion, doubts about self-worth may occur.
- Free from somatic reactions. If mild symptoms persist and minor discomfort is reported, the survivor should be able to talk about it and feel in control of the symptoms.
- Showing a return to prerape sexual functioning and interest.

In general, the closer the survivor's lifestyle is to the pattern that was present before the rape, the more complete the recovery has been.

CASE STUDY and NURSING CARE PLAN 26-1 Rape

Latisha Smith, a 36-year-old single mother of two, goes out one evening with some friends. Her children are at a slumber party and she "needs to get away and have a little rest and relaxation." She and her friends go bowling. Later in the evening, Latisha is tired and ready to go home. A man who has joined the group offers to take her home. She has seen the man at the bowling alley before but does not know much about him. Not in the habit of going home alone with men she does not know, she hesitates. A friend whom she trusts encourages her to go with James because he is a nice man.

James drives Latisha home. He then asks if he can come into her house to use the bathroom before driving the long distance to his house. She reluctantly agrees and sits on the living room couch. After using the bathroom, James sits next to Latisha and begins to kiss her and fondle her breasts. As she protests, James becomes more forceful in his advances. Latisha is confused and frightened. She manages to get away from him briefly, but he begins grabbing, squeezing, and biting her. He tells her gruffly, "If you don't do what I say, I'll break your neck." She screams, but he proceeds to rape her. James becomes nervous that the noise will alert the neighbors and races out of the house. A neighbor does in fact arrive just after James flees. The neighbor calls the police and then brings Latisha to the local hospital emergency department for a physical examination, crisis intervention, and support.

In the emergency department, Latisha is visibly shaken. She keeps saying, over and over, "I shouldn't have let him take me home. I should have fought harder, I shouldn't have let him do this."

The nurse takes Latisha to a quiet cubicle. She doesn't want Latisha to stay alone and asks the neighbor to stay with her. The nurse then notifies the doctor and the rape-

Continued

victim advocate. When the nurse comes back, she tells Latisha that she would like to talk to her before the doctor comes. Latisha looks at her neighbor and then down. The nurse asks the neighbor to wait outside for a while and says she will call her later.

Latisha: It was horrible. I feel so dirty.

Nurse: You have had a traumatic experience. Do you want to talk about it?

Latisha: I feel so ashamed. I never should have let that man take me home.

Nurse: You think that if you hadn't gone home with a stranger this wouldn't have happened?

Latisha: Yes. . . . I shouldn't have let him do it to me anyway, I shouldn't have let him rape me.

Nurse: You mentioned that he said he would break your neck if you didn't do as he said.

Latisha: Yes, he said that . . . he was going to kill me, it was awful.

Nurse: It seems you did the right thing in order to stay alive.

As the nurse continues to talk with Latisha, Latisha's anxiety level seems to lessen. The nurse talks to Latisha about the kinds of experiences rape victims often have after the rape and explains that the reactions she might have 2 or 3 weeks from now are normal in these circumstances. The nurse continues to collect the necessary information. She says that the doctor will want to examine Latisha and explains the procedure to her. She then asks Latisha to sign a consent form. While preparing Latisha for examination, the nurse notices bite marks and bruises on both breasts. She also notes Latisha's lower lip, which is cut and bleeding. The nurse keeps detailed notes on her observations and draws a body map of the injuries. After the examination, Latisha is given clean clothes and a place to shower.

Self-Assessment

The nurse has worked with rape survivors before and has helped develop the hospital protocol. It took a while for her to be able to remain neutral as well as responsive, because her own anger at rapists had initially interfered. She also remembers a time when a woman came in stating that she was raped but was so calm, smiling, and polite that the nurse initially did not believe her story. She had not, at that point, examined her own feelings or dealt with the popular societal myths regarding rape. It was only later, when she had talked to more experienced health care personnel, that she learned that crisis reactions can seem bizarre, confusing, and contradictory.

The nurse learned that staying with the survivor, encouraging her to express her reactions and feelings, and listening are effective methods of reducing feelings of anxiety. Once the nurse learned through supervision and peer discussion to let go of her personal anger at the attacker and her ambivalence toward the survivor, her care and effectiveness improved greatly. All of this growth took time and support from more experienced nurses and other members of the health care team.

■ ASSESSMENT

The nurse organizes her data into subjective and objective components.

Objective Data

- Crying and sobbing
- Bruises and bite marks on each breast
- Lip cut and bleeding
- Rape reported to the police

Subjective Data

- "He was going to kill me."
- "It was horrible. I feel so dirty."
- "I shouldn't have let him rape me."

■ NURSING DIAGNOSIS (NANDA)

The nurse formulates the following diagnosis:

Rape-trauma syndrome

- "I shouldn't have let him rape me."
- "He was going to kill me."
- Crying and sobbing.
- Bruises and bite marks on both breasts.
- Rape reported to the police.
- "It was horrible. I feel so dirty."

■ OUTCOME CRITERIA (NOC)

Overall outcome: *Abuse Recovery: Emotional*
Short-term indicator: Latisha will demonstrate appropriate affect for the situation.
Intermediate indicator: Latisha will demonstrate confidence.
Short-term and intermediate outcome indicators are measured on a five-point Likert scale from 1 (none) to 5 (extensive).

■ PLANNING

The nurse plans to provide emotional and physical support to Latisha while she receives care in the emergency setting and to make sure that Latisha is aware of the importance of follow-up care.

■ INTERVENTION (NIC)

Latisha's plan of care is personalized as follows.

Short-Term Goal	Intervention	Rationale
1. Latisha will demonstrate appropriate affect by discharge from the emergency department.	**1a.** Remain neutral and nonjudgmental and assure survivor of confidentiality.	**1a.** Lessens feelings of shame and guilt and encourages sharing of painful feelings.
	1b. Do not leave survivor alone.	**1b.** Deters feelings of isolation and escalation of anxiety.
	1c. Allow client negative expressions and behavioral self-blame while using reflective techniques.	**1c.** Fosters feelings of control.
	1d. Assure survivor she did the right thing to save her life.	**1d.** Decreases burden of guilt and shame.
	1e. When anxiety level is down to moderate, encourage problem solving.	**1e.** Increases survivor's feeling of control in her own life. (When in severe anxiety, a person cannot problem-solve.)
	1f. Tell survivor of common reactions experienced by people in long-term reorganization phase (e.g., phobias, flashbacks, insomnia, increased motor activity).	**1f.** Helps survivor anticipate reactions and understand them as part of recovery process.
	1g. Explain emergency department procedure to survivor.	**1g.** Lowers anticipatory anxiety.
	1h. Explain physical examination.	**1h.** Allows for questions and concerns; victim may be too traumatized and may refuse.
	1i. Nurse/female rape advocate should stay with survivor during physical examination.	**1i.** Physical examination may be experienced as a second assault. Nurse provides comfort and support.

■ EVALUATION

Latisha is able to express her feelings in the emergency department as well as talk about the possible reactions she might experience as she moves through the reorganization phase. The indicator is achieved at a level of 3 (moderate).

evolve Visit the Evolve website at **http://evolve.elsevier.com/Varcarolis** for a full case study of this client and more case studies and nursing care plans.

■■■ KEY POINTS to REMEMBER

- A rape survivor experiences a wide range of feelings, which may or may not be exhibited to others.
- Feelings of fear, degradation, anger and rage, helplessness, and nervousness; sleep disturbances; disturbed relationships; flashbacks; depression; and somatic complaints are all common.
- The circumstances of the initial medical evaluation may be frightening and stressful. Police interrogation, repeated questioning by health professionals, and the physical examination itself all have the potential to add to the trauma of the sexual assault.

- Nurses, in their role as case managers, can serve to minimize repetition of questions and support the survivor as she goes through the entire ordeal.
- Survivors require long-term health care that can include counseling to minimize the long-term effects of the rape and to assist in an early return to a normal living pattern.
- Most metropolitan areas now have special programs to assist rape survivors.

■■■

Visit the Evolve website at **http://evolve.elsevier.com/Varcarolis** for a posttest on the content in this chapter. **evolve**

Critical Thinking and Chapter Review

Visit the Evolve website at **http://evolve.elsevier.com/Varcarolis/foundations** for additional self-study exercises.

evolve

■■■■ CRITICAL THINKING

Sal Petrillo, 18 years of age, is brutally beaten and sexually assaulted by an unidentified male as he makes his way home from a party in an unfamiliar part of town. He is found semiconscious by a passerby and taken to the emergency department. Sal has extensive bruises around his head, chest, and buttocks and has sustained a cracked rib and anal tears. Ms. Santinez, a nurse and rape counselor in the emergency department, works with Sal using the hospital's rape protocol. Sal appears stunned and confused, and has difficulty focusing on what the nurse says. He states repeatedly, "This is crazy, this can't be happening. . . . I can't believe this has happened to me. . . . Oh, my God, I can't believe this."

1. What areas will Ms. Santinez and her staff most likely assess while Sal is in the emergency department?

2. Chart signs and symptoms of Sal's physical and emotional trauma and verbatim statements in as much detail as you can. How else can his physical trauma be documented?

3. What are some of the pivotal issues that need to be addressed in terms of assessing Sal's signs and symptoms of physical trauma? Although the risk of pregnancy is not present, what other real physical risks need to be assessed?

4. What are some of the signs and symptoms of rape-trauma syndrome? Of rape-trauma silent reaction?

5. Identify the short-term outcome criteria for Sal Petrillo that ideally would be met before he leaves the emergency department.

6. What information does Sal need to have regarding potential signs and symptoms that may occur in the near future? Why is this important for him to understand at present?

7. Identify specific indicators that will be met if Sal recovers with minimal trauma from the event. How would you evaluate these criteria?

■■■■ CHAPTER REVIEW

Choose the most appropriate answer.

1. The rape-trauma syndrome is most similar to
    1. posttraumatic stress disorder.
    2. dissociative identity disorder.
    3. unresolved grief reaction.
    4. developmental crisis.

2. Data that are inappropriate to document in the medical record of a survivor of rape are
    1. observations of the client's physical trauma using a body map.
    2. assessment of signs and symptoms of emotional trauma.
    3. verbatim statements made by the client.
    4. details of the client's sexual history.

3. The most important element of care for an emergency department nurse to provide to a rape survivor is
    1. encouraging the client to give a complete report of the incident.
    2. helping the client to make a decision about where she will go after leaving the emergency department.
    3. providing the telephone number of a 24-hour hotline.
    4. assuring confidentiality.

4. An intervention that would be useful when working with a person in the emergency department who has been sexually assaulted is
    1. interacting in a cool and reserved fashion.
    2. helping the client separate issues of vulnerability from blame.
    3. structuring communication to minimize expression of strong feelings.
    4. expecting family and friends to provide the majority of emotional support for the client.

5. Identify the observation that, if found in the medical record of a sexual assault survivor, would indicate that reorganization after a rape crisis is not yet complete.
    1. Free from somatic reactions
    2. Generally positive about self
    3. Calm and relaxed during interactions
    4. Frequently experiences nightmares

▪ STUDENT
▪ STUDY
▪ CD-ROM

Access the accompanying CD-ROM for animations, interactive exercises, review questions for the NCLEX examination, and an audio glossary.

▪ NURSE,
▪ CLIENT, AND
▪ FAMILY RESOURCES

For suggested readings, information on related associations, and Internet resources, go to **http://evolve.elsevier.com/Varcarolis.** *evolve*

REFERENCES

Dochterman, J. M., & Bulechek, G. M. (2004). *Nursing interventions classification (NIC)* (4th ed.). St. Louis, MO: Mosby.

Drug-Induced Rape Prevention and Punishment Act, 21 U.S.C. § 841(b)(7) (1996).

Emergency Nurses Association. (2001). *Emergency Nurses Association position statements: Care of sexual assault victims.* Retrieved March 7, 2005, from http://www.ena.org/about/position/caresexualassault.asp.

Emergency Nurses Association. (2003). *Emergency Nurses Association position statements: Forensic evidence collection.* Retrieved February 20, 2005, from http://www.ena.org/about/position/forensicevidence.asp.

King, J. (2003, October 15-18). *Date rape: All rape is real rape.* Paper presented at the National Association of Nurse Practitioners in Women's Health 6th Annual Conference, Savannah, GA.

Ledray, L. E. (1998). SANE development and operation guide. *Journal of Emergency Nursing, 24*(2), 197-198.

Ledray, L. E. (2001). *Evidence collection and care of the sexual assault survivor: The SANE-SART response.* Retrieved February 20, 2005, from http://www.vaw.umn.edu/documents/commissioned/2forensicevidence/2forensicevidence.html.

Lynch, J. S. (2003, October 15-18). *Date rape and drug-assisted rape: Clinical implications.* Paper presented at the National Association of Nurse Practitioners in Women's Health 6th Annual Conference, Savannah, GA.

Porcerelli, J., et al. (2003). Violent victimization of women and men: Physical and psychiatric symptoms. *Journal of American Board of Family Practice, 16,* 32-39.

Rape Abuse and Incest National Network. (2002). *RAINN News: New report shows dramatic increase in willingness to report rape to police.* Retrieved February 20, 2005, from http://www.rainn.org/news/ncvs2002.html.

U.S. Department of Justice, Office of the Attorney General. (1997, September 23). *Memorandum for all United States attorneys.* Retrieved February 21, 2005, from http://www.usdoj.gov/ag/readingroom/drugcrime.htm.

Vaughn, I. R., Vaughn, R. D., & Wiemann, C. M. (2003). Violence against young women: Implications for clinicians. *Contemporary OB/GYN, 48*(2), 30-45.

A CLIENT SPEAKS

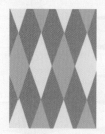

I am a 35-year-old female, and I was born in Tennessee. I grew up with my parents and my two younger sisters. My mother said that I was a jolly, friendly baby and that everyone was always holding and playing with me. Growing up, I was very quiet and shy and I did not make friends easily. I was an average student and I graduated from high school. I started working as a secretary and I also took some college courses. I have never married, although I have had a few male acquaintances.

When I was 26, I began to hear voices. I remember thinking that I was hearing people talking outside. And I was thinking, "Am I crazy? It sounds like they are talking about me." Except that the talking never stopped. No matter where I went, I kept hearing people talking. I had what I considered to be a weird life, so I just brushed it off as something else weird. Then one day it dawned on me that something was not right, and I sat down in a stupor and realized that I was hearing things. I was really scared. There were four different voices: a loud, shrill female voice that kept telling me to kill myself; another female voice that sounded like a nerd; a male voice that was kind of deep but sweet; and another male voice that had an "I don't care" attitude. They told me all sorts of things, like they did not know who they were, or I was going to die before the next day. They even told me a story about my childhood best friend and her family going to hell. They had a lot of personality and they often said things that sounded comical. They talked nonstop unless I fell asleep for a little while. My mother noticed me sitting around staring, and took me to a hospital.

I was diagnosed with schizophrenia and started on medication, which made me so tired that I thought that I was dying. I stayed in the hospital for 2 weeks and then I started seeing a community psychiatrist. I have taken several different medications, and the psychological change that took place is that the four voices decreased to two constant voices (although, under stress, I still hear four).

I never used alcohol or illegal drugs to cope with my illness.

With regard to the stigma of mental illness, I really do not talk much about my illness to anyone unless it is necessary. The times that I do talk, people may act a little hesitant. Currently, my social support system includes my family and several other groups. My relationship with my mother is good and we talk often. I have just completed an online nursing assistant course, although I am not sure if I want to go into that work right now. I enjoy working on the computer, exercising, and listening to music or news programs. I really like my living situation—I have my own apartment in a group of apartments supervised by a mental health case manager. I have not had an actual friend since high school because I feel tense around people. I am not working right now, but I hope to become self-supporting some day, by which I mean not having to depend on charity (Social Security). For now, I am continuing to learn how to be happy and strong.

INTERVENTIONS FOR SPECIAL POPULATIONS

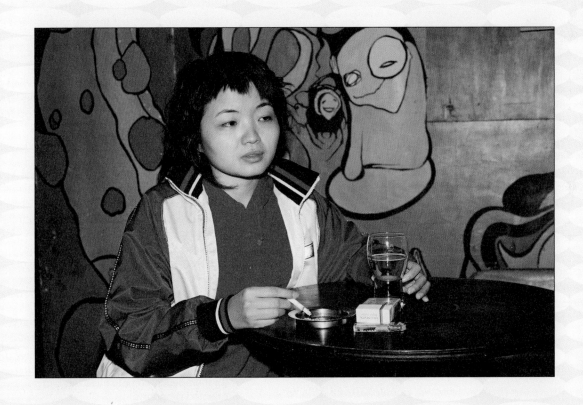

THE GREATEST DISCOVERY OF MY GENERATION IS THAT A HUMAN BEING CAN ALTER HIS LIFE BY ALTERING HIS ATTITUDES OF MIND.

William James

CHAPTER 27

Care of the Chemically Impaired

KATHLEEN SMITH-DIJULIO

KEY TERMS and CONCEPTS

The key terms and concepts listed here appear in color where they are defined or first discussed in this chapter.

addiction, 548

Al-Anon, 565

Alateen, 565

Alcoholics Anonymous (AA), 566

antagonistic effect, 549

blood alcohol level (BAL), 554

Cannabis sativa, 557

codependence, 551

dual diagnosis, 547

enabling, 560

flashbacks, 549

relapse prevention, 564

substance-abuse intervention, 563

synergistic effects, 549

tetrahydrocannabinol (THC), 557

therapeutic communities, 566

tolerance, 549

withdrawal, 549

OBJECTIVES

After studying this chapter, the reader will be able to

1. Compare and contrast the terms *substance abuse* and *substance dependence,* as defined by the *Diagnostic and Statistical Manual of Mental Disorders.*

2. Explain the difference between tolerance and withdrawal, and give a clinical definition of each.

3. Discuss four components of the assessment process to be used with a person who is chemically dependent.

4. Describe the difference between the behaviors of an alcoholic person and a nondrinker in relation to blood alcohol level.

5. Compare and contrast the symptoms seen in alcohol withdrawal and those seen in alcohol delirium.

6. List the appropriate steps to take if one observes an impaired co-worker.

7. Describe aspects of enabling behaviors and give examples.

8. Compare and contrast the signs and symptoms of intoxication, overdose, and withdrawal for cocaine and amphetamine.

9. Distinguish between the symptoms of narcotic intoxication and those of narcotic withdrawal.

10. Discuss the effects of the techno drugs ecstasy (MDMA), Rohypnol, γ-hydroxybutyric acid (GHB), and Eve (MDE).

11. Discuss treatment of a person who is withdrawing from alcohol delirium, including nursing care and pharmacological therapy.

12. Discuss the synergistic and antagonistic effects of drugs in polydrug abusers and give an example of each.

13. Formulate six nursing diagnoses that might apply to substance-abusing clients, including diagnoses in the physical, medical, and safety areas.

14. Develop three short-term outcomes relating to (a) withdrawal, (b) active treatment, and (c) health maintenance.

15. Analyze the pros and cons of the following treatments for narcotic addictions: (a) methadone or L-α-acetylmethadol, (b) therapeutic communities, and (c) self-help, abstinence-oriented programs.

16. Recognize the phenomenon of relapse as it affects substance abusers during different phases of treatment.

17. Plan steps in relapse prevention.

18. Evaluate four indications that a person is successfully recovering from substance abuse.

evolve Visit the Evolve website at **http://evolve.elsevier.com/Varcarolis** for a pretest on the content in this chapter.

PREVALENCE

The United States is a drug-oriented society. People use a host of drugs for various purposes: to restore health, reduce pain and anxiety, increase energy, create a feeling of euphoria, induce sleep, and enhance alertness. Two thirds of the nation's adult population consumes alcohol regularly. Studies indicate that 13.8% of American adults have had either an alcohol dependence or alcohol abuse problem at one point in their lives. Estimates suggest that about 2.7% (2.4 million) of the U.S. population over the age of 12 years needs treatment for drug use disorders. An additional 13 million people need treatment for alcohol use disorders (American Psychiatric Association [APA], 2000b).

COMORBIDITY
Psychiatric Comorbidity

Approximately 50% of people with a serious mental illness have a substance use disorder at some point in their lives (Mueser et al., 2001). Data from the Epidemiologic Catchment Area Study found that 55% of schizophrenic clients and 62% of bipolar clients had a comorbid substance use disorder (Minkoff, 2003). Other psychiatric disorders that may be seen concurrently in people addicted to substances include acute and chronic cognitive impairment disorders, attention deficit disorder, borderline and antisocial personality disorders, anxiety disorders, and depression. Substance abuse contributes to emotional problems in young and old alike. Eating disorders and compulsive behaviors (e.g., gambling) are also associated with substance use. **Suicide** is a high risk. The rate of suicide is three to four times higher in substance abusers than in the general population, with a lifetime mortality rate of 15% in this group (APA, 2000b).

Compared with people who have a mental health disorder or a substance abuse problem alone, clients with comorbid mental illness or dual diagnosis often experience more severe and chronic medical, social, and emotional problems. Because they have two or more disorders, they are vulnerable to both substance abuse relapse and worsening of the psychiatric disorder. In addition, substance abuse relapse often leads to psychiatric decompensation, and worsening of psychiatric problems often leads to substance abuse relapse. Compared with clients who have a single disorder, clients with dual disorders often require longer treatment, experience more crises, and progress more gradually in treatment (Compton et al., 2003; Cornelius et al., 2003; Judd et al., 2003). Common examples of dual disorders include the combination of major depression with cocaine addiction, alcohol addiction with generalized anxiety disorder, alcoholism and polydrug addiction with schizophrenia, and borderline personality disorder with episodic polydrug abuse (Farris et al., 2003; Frye et al., 2003; Negrete, 2003).

Medical Comorbidity

Alcohol abuse is the most prevalent of the substance abuse disorders. Therefore, alcohol-related medical problems are the comorbidities most commonly seen in medical settings. Alcohol can affect all organ systems, in particular the central nervous system (Wernicke's encephalopathy and Korsakoff's psychosis) and the gastrointestinal system (esophagitis, gastritis, pancreatitis, alcoholic hepatitis, and cirrhosis of the liver). Also commonly associated with long-term alcohol use or abuse are tuberculosis, all types of accidents, suicide, and homicide. Alcohol use during pregnancy can have negative consequences for the fetus and result in fetal alcohol syndrome.

Cocaine abusers may experience extreme weight loss and malnutrition, myocardial infarction, and stroke. The route of drug administration influences medical complications. **Intravenous drug users** have a higher incidence of infections and sclerosing of veins. **Intranasal users** may have sinusitis and a perforated nasal septum. **Smoking a substance** increases the likelihood of respiratory problems. Refer to Table 27-1 for a look at physical complications associated with various classes of drugs and their routes of administration.

TABLE 27-1

Drug Information: Physical Complications Related to Drug Abuse

Drug	Physical Complications
Route: Intravenous*	
Narcotics (e.g., heroin)	Acquired immunodeficiency
Phencyclidine	syndrome
piperidine (PCP)	Hepatitis
Cocaine or crack	Bacterial endocarditis
	Renal failure
	Cardiac arrest
	Coma
	Seizures
	Respiratory arrest
	Dermatitis
	Pulmonary emboli
	Tetanus
	Abscesses—osteomyelitis
	Septicemia
Route: Intravenous, Intranasal, Smoking	
Cocaine	Perforation of nasal septum (when taken intranasally)
	Respiratory paralysis
	Cardiovascular collapse
	Hyperpyrexia

**Note:* The complications listed can result from any drug taken intravenously.

Continued

TABLE 27-1

Drug Information: Physical Complications Related to Drug Abuse—cont'd

Drug	Physical Complications
Route: Ingestion	
Caffeine	Gastroesophageal reflux
	Peptic ulcer
	Increased intraocular pressure in unregulated glaucoma
	Tachycardia
	Increased plasma glucose and lipid levels
PCP	Respiratory arrest
Route: Smoking, Ingestion	
Marijuana	Impaired lung structure
	Chromosomal mutation— increased incidence of birth defects
	Micronucleic white blood cells— increased risk of disease due to decreased resistance to infection
	Possible long-term effects on short-term memory
Route: Smoking, Chewing	
Nicotine	Heavy chronic use associated with:
	Emphysema
	Cancer of the larynx and esophagus
	Lung cancer
	Peripheral vascular diseases
	Cancer of the mouth
	Cardiovascular disease
	Hypertension
Route: Intravenous,* Smoking	
Heroin	Constipation
	Dermatitis
	Malnutrition
	Hypoglycemia
	Dental caries
	Amenorrhea
Route: Sniffing, Snorting, Bagging (Inhalation of Fumes from a Plastic Bag), Huffing (Placement of Inhalant-Soaked Rag in the Mouth)	
Inhalants	Respiratory arrest
	Tachycardia
	Arrhythmias
	Nervous system damage

THEORY

Addiction is characterized by (1) loss of control of substance consumption, (2) substance use despite associated problems, and (3) tendency to relapse. The reason one person becomes addicted and another does not seems to relate to physical, developmental, psychosocial, and environmental factors as well as genetic predisposition (Lingford-Hughes et al., 2003; Sinha, Drummond, & Orford, 2001). The difficulty in determining cause and effect is that the diagnosis of addiction generally occurs many years after the onset of use. Various factors are involved over the course of those years. Biological, psychological, and sociocultural theories are examined here briefly.

Biological Theories

Interest in biological theories was augmented by the observation that substance use problems seem to run in families. If a person's ancestors had such problems, the likelihood is increased that the person will also be susceptible. Alcoholism is three to four times more likely to occur in children of alcoholic parents than in children of nonalcoholic parents (APA, 2000a).

It has been demonstrated more recently that alcohol and drug use has specific effects on selected neurotransmitter systems. The main systems that seem to be involved in substance abuse are the opioid, catecholamine (especially dopamine), and γ-aminobutyric acid (GABA) systems (Sadock & Sadock, 2003). Opioid drugs act on opioid receptors. Alcohol and other central nervous system (CNS) depressants act on GABA receptors. This finding helps explain the addictive and cross-tolerance effects that occur when the use of alcohol is combined with use of barbiturates and benzodiazepines. Cocaine and amphetamines act on the dopamine system. New studies demonstrate that inactivating both the dopamine and the serotonin transporters in the brains of mice drastically reduces their experience of cocaine's reward system National Institute on Drug Abuse, 2001).

Psychological Theories

Although no known addictive personality type exists, associated psychodynamic factors have been identified, including the following:

- Lack of tolerance for frustration and pain
- Lack of success in life
- Lack of affectionate and meaningful relationships
- Low self-esteem, lack of self-regard
- Risk-taking propensity

Psychodynamic theories view substance use as a defense against anxious impulses, a form of oral regression (dependency), or self-medication for depression (Sadock & Sadock, 2003). Persons who are polysubstance abusers are more likely to report an unstable childhood and self-medication than are persons who abuse alcohol. Multiple studies link personality disorders and substance abuse.

Behavioral theory focuses on the positive reinforcing effects of drug-seeking behavior.

Sociocultural Theories

Sociocultural theories attempt to explain differences in the incidence of substance use in various groups. Social and cultural norms influence when, what, and how a person uses substances. For example, in Asian cultures, the prevalence rate for alcohol abuse is relatively low. This is due in part to a deficiency in about 50% of the population of aldehyde dehydrogenase, the chemical that breaks down alcohol acetaldehyde. As the level of alcohol acetaldehyde increases in the blood, a severe flush and palpitations may occur (APA, 2000a). This reaction effectively keeps many Asians from drinking. In contrast, in Native Americans and Alaska Natives, the prevalence rate for alcohol dependence and/or abuse is quite high: 70% compared to 11% to 32% for their white, African American, and Japanese American counterparts (U.S. Department of Health and Human Services, 1999).

Another theory correlates substance use with the degree of socioeconomic stress people experience (Sinha et al., 2001). Being a drug addict can give a person a feeling of acceptance in his or her subculture. This is most true in economically deprived and unstable environments, where drugs may be taken to provide a person with a sense of belonging and identity.

Women in general are diagnosed with substance use at lower rates than men (Becker & Walton-Moss, 2001). Addicted women are viewed much more negatively than addicted men in many cultural groups. This negative attitude may lead to avoidance of the diagnosis and thus to a lack of treatment services.

In summary, there is no single cause of substance abuse. Multiple factors contribute to substance use, abuse, and addiction in any individual. For example, a child of an alcoholic parent may have a biochemical deficiency predisposing him or her to alcoholism and may grow up with low self-esteem in a society that has no rituals governing alcohol use. Because of complex biological, psychological, and sociocultural factors, this person is at risk for developing alcoholism.

DEFINITIONS

The diagnostic scheme in the *Diagnostic and Statistical Manual of Mental Disorders*, fourth edition, text revision *(DSM-IV-TR)* (APA, 2000a) focuses on the behavioral aspects and the pathological patterns of substance use, emphasizing the physical symptoms of tolerance and withdrawal. An overview of *DSM-IV-TR* diagnostic criteria for substance abuse and dependence is provided in Figure 27-1.

Tolerance and Withdrawal

The diagnosis of substance dependence involves the concepts of tolerance and withdrawal. Tolerance is a need for higher and higher doses to achieve the desired effect. Withdrawal occurs after a long period of continued use, so that stopping or reducing use results in specific physical and psychological signs and symptoms. Because alcohol is still the most common drug of abuse in the United States and poses the greatest withdrawal danger, *DSM-IV-TR* diagnostic criteria for alcohol intoxication, withdrawal, and delirium are highlighted in Figure 27-2. Information on signs and symptoms of intoxication and withdrawal from other substances of abuse is given later in this chapter.

Other phenomena frequently encountered in substance abuse are flashbacks, synergistic effects, and antagonistic effects. These are discussed briefly here, although they are seen in many situations, not just in substance abuse.

Flashbacks

Flashbacks are transitory recurrences of perceptual disturbance caused by a person's earlier hallucinogenic drug use when he or she is in a drug-free state (APA, 2000a). Experiences such as visual distortions, time expansion, loss of ego boundaries, and intense emotions are reported. Often flashbacks are mild and perhaps pleasant, but at other times, individuals experience repeated recurrences of frightening images or thoughts.

Synergistic Effects

When some drugs are taken together, the effect of either or both of the drugs is intensified or prolonged. For example, combinations of alcohol plus a benzodiazepine, alcohol plus an opiate, and alcohol plus a barbiturate all produce synergistic effects. All these drugs are CNS depressants. Taking two of these drugs together results in far greater CNS depression than the simple sum of the effects of each drug. Many unintentional deaths have resulted from lethal combinations of drugs.

Antagonistic Effects

Many people combine drugs to weaken or inhibit the effect of one of the drugs (i.e., for antagonistic effect). For example, cocaine is often mixed with heroin (speedball). The heroin (CNS depressant) is meant to soften the intense letdown of withdrawal from cocaine (CNS stimulant). **Naloxone (Narcan),** an opiate antagonist, is often given to people who have overdosed on an opiate (usually heroin) to reverse respiratory and CNS depression. Because the duration of action of naloxone may be less than that of the narcotic that was taken, further monitoring and possible additional doses of naloxone may be needed.

DSM-IV-TR CRITERIA FOR SUBSTANCE ABUSE AND DEPENDENCE

SUBSTANCE ABUSE AND DEPENDENCE

Substance Abuse

Maladaptive pattern of substance use leading to clinically significant impairment or distress, manifested by one or more of the following within a 12-month period:

1. Inability to fulfill major role obligations at work, school, and home

2. Participation in physically hazardous situations while impaired (driving a car, operating a machine, exacerbating existing problem [e.g., ulcer])

3. Recurrent legal or interpersonal problems

4. Continued use despite recurrent social and interpersonal problems

Substance Dependence

Maladaptive pattern of substance use leading to clinically significant impairment or distress, manifested by three or more of the following within a 12-month period:

1. Presence of tolerance to the drug

2. Presence of withdrawal syndrome

3. Substance is taken in larger amounts/for longer period than intended

4. Unsuccessful or persistent desire to cut down or control use

5. Increased time spent in getting, taking, and recovering from the substance; may withdraw from family or friends

6. Reduction or absence of important social, occupational, or recreational activities

7. Substance used despite knowledge of recurrent physical or psychological problems or that problems were caused or exacerbated by one substance

FIGURE 27-1 Diagnostic criteria for substance abuse and dependence. (Adapted from American Psychiatric Association. [2000]. *Diagnostic and statistical manual of mental disorders* [4th ed., text rev.]. Washington, DC: Author.)

DSM-IV-TR CRITERIA FOR ALCOHOL-RELATED DISORDERS

ALCOHOL-RELATED DISORDERS

Alcohol Intoxication

1. Recent ingestion

2. Clinically significant, maladaptive behavior or psychological changes (sexual, aggressive, mood, and judgment)

3. At least one of the following:
   - Slurred speech
   - Incoordination
   - Unsteady gait
   - Nystagmus
   - Impairment in attention or memory
   - Stupor or coma

4. Symptoms not due to another medical/mental condition

Alcohol Withdrawal

1. Cessation (reduction) of alcohol use that has been heavy or prolonged

2. Two (or more) of the following:
   - Nausea or vomiting
   - Anxiety
   - Transient visual, tactile, or auditory hallucinations or illusions
   - Autonomic hyperactivity (e.g., sweating, increased pulse over 100 beats/min)
   - Psychomotor agitation
   - Insomnia
   - Grand mal seizures
   - Increased hand tremor

Substance-Induced Delirium

1. Impaired consciousness (reduced awareness of environment)

2. Changes in cognition (memory impairment, disorientation, language impairment, visual or tactile hallucinations, illusions)

3. Develops over short period of time — hours to days — and fluctuates over a day

4. Evidence of substance use (history, physical, laboratory findings) and symptoms developed during withdrawal

FIGURE 27-2 Diagnostic criteria for alcohol-related disorders. (Adapted from American Psychiatric Association. [2000]. *Diagnostic and statistical manual of mental disorders* [4th ed., text rev.]. Washington, DC: Author.)

Codependence

Codependence is a cluster of behaviors originally identified through research involving the families of alcoholic clients. Living with a substance-abusing or alcoholic individual is a source of stress and requires family system adjustments. People who are codependent often exhibit overresponsible behavior—doing for others what others could just as well do for themselves. They have a constellation of maladaptive thoughts, feelings, behaviors, and attitudes that effectively prevent them from living full and satisfying lives. Symptomatic of codependence is valuing oneself by what one does, what one looks like, and what one has, rather than by who one is (Box 27-1).

Application of the Nursing Process

■ ASSESSMENT

Assessment of chemical impairment is becoming more complex because of the increase in the simultaneous use of many substances **(polydrug abuse),** the coexistence of psychiatric disease with substance abuse **(dual diagnosis),** and associated comorbid physical illnesses, including human immunodeficiency virus (HIV) infection, acquired immunodeficiency syndrome (AIDS), dementia, and encephalopathy.

Sensitivity to multicultural and racial issues is important in interpreting symptoms, making diagnoses, providing clinical care, and designing prevention strategies. Refer to Box 27-2 for areas to be covered in overall assessment for clients who use substances.

Interview Guidelines

Current alcohol and/or other drug problems can be detected by asking two questions that are easily integrated into a clinical interview (Brown et al., 2001). These two questions are: (1) In the last year, have you ever drunk or used drugs more than you meant to? (2) Have you felt you wanted or needed to cut down on your drinking or drug use in the last year? From that initial questioning the nurse can then pinpoint specific drugs depending on the particular clinical situation. The nurse should ask questions in a matter-of-fact, nonjudgmental fashion. Specific details include name(s) of drug(s) used, route, quantity, time of last use, and usual pattern of use.

Responses that serve as red flags indicating the need for further assessment are rationalizations ("You'd smoke dope, too, if . . ."); automatic responses, as if the question were predicted; and slow, prolonged

---

BOX 27-1

Overresponsible (Codependent) Behaviors

Codependent individuals find themselves
1. Attempting to control someone else's drug use.
2. Spending inordinate time thinking about the addicted person.
3. Finding excuses for the person's substance abuse.
4. Covering up the person's drinking/drug taking or lying.
5. Feeling responsible for the person's drinking/drug use.
6. Feeling guilty for the addicted person's behavior.
7. Avoiding family and social events because of concerns or shame about the addicted member's behavior.
8. Making threats regarding the consequences of the alcoholic's/drug abuser's behavior and failing to follow through.
9. Eliciting promises for change.
10. Feeling like they are "walking on eggshells" on a routine basis to avoid causing problems, especially in relation to alcohol or drug use.
11. Allowing moods to be influenced by those of the addicted person.
12. Searching for, hiding, and destroying the abuser's drug or alcohol supply.
13. Assuming the alcoholic's/substance abuser's duties and responsibilities.
14. Feeling forced to increase control over the family's finances.
15. Often bailing the addicted person out of financial or legal problems.

---

responses, as if the person were being careful about what to say. If the person is not able to provide a drug history, the nurse should assess for indications of substance abuse, such as dilated or constricted pupils, abnormal vital signs, needle marks, tremors, and alcohol on the breath, and obtain history information from family and friends. The clothing is checked for drug paraphernalia, such as used syringes, crack vials, white powder, razor blades, bent spoons, and pipes.

There is a consistent and significant association between alcohol and/or drug use and the occurrence of injury (Miller, Lestina, & Smith, 2001). Intracranial hematomas, subdural hematomas, and other conditions can go unnoticed if symptoms of acute alcohol intoxication and withdrawal are not distinguished from the symptoms of a brain injury. Therefore, neurological signs (pupil size, equality, and reaction to light) should be assessed, especially in comatose clients suspected of having traumatic injuries. In addition, questions about alcohol abuse should be asked as part of the assessment of any trauma. A urine **toxicology screen** and/or **blood alcohol level** can be useful for assessment purposes. See the Forensic Highlights box for guidance about preserving confidentiality while collecting necessary information for treatment.

BOX 27-2

Overall Assessment Guide

History of Client's Past Substance Use

1. What are the date of first use, number of substances being taken, pattern of use, amount, frequency, periods of sobriety, time last taken?
2. Was client treated previously for substance abuse? What was the outcome?
3. Is there a history of blackouts, delirium, or seizures?
4. Is there a history of withdrawal symptoms, overdoses, and complications from past substance use?
5. Is there a family history of drug or alcohol problems?

Medical History

1. Does the client have any coexisting physical conditions (e.g., human immunodeficiency virus infection)?
2. What medications does the client presently take?
3. What is the client's current medical status?
4. What is the client's present mental status?

Psychiatric History

1. Is there a history of comorbid psychiatric problems (dual diagnosis)? Depression? Personality disorder? Conduct disorder? Schizophrenia?
2. Has the client undergone treatment for a specific disorder? What medications were given and what was the outcome?
3. Is there a history of abuse (physical, sexual)? Family violence?
4. Is there a history of suicide? Violence toward others?
5. Is the client presently having suicidal thoughts?

Psychosocial Issues

1. Does the client have a poor work record related to substance use?
2. How has the client's substance use affected his or her relationships with others?
   - Family
   - Friends
   - Professional relationships
   - Community involvement
3. How has the substance use affected the client's ability to meet usual role expectations (e.g., parent, spouse, friend, employee)?
4. Is there a police or criminal record or legal problems related to substance use (e.g., vehicle accidents, driving while intoxicated, physical violence)?
5. Whom does the client identify as his or her support system? Whom does the client trust? Who cares for the client? Who will help the client if the client asks for help?
6. Does the client use coping styles that contribute to the maintenance of his or her drug/alcohol lifestyle?

FORENSICS HIGHLIGHTS

Impairment caused by alcohol is the leading risk factor for trauma. It is important to evaluate blood alcohol level to aid in decisions about treatment and to guide brief interventions designed to promote abstinence and treatment. However, screening for alcohol use is often not carried out in emergency departments or trauma units because of concerns about confidentiality and denial of insurance coverage. In fact, federal regulations protecting confidentiality of alcohol screening data depend on how such information is acquired and do not routinely cover trauma patients. Prudent measures for providers are to

1. Segregate information about alcohol use in the medical record.
2. Assign psychiatric nurses, chemical dependency counselors, or other professionals with expertise in the area to screen all trauma patients.

Implementing these two measures would ensure confidentiality of alcohol information under federal regulations and allow denial of release of information except under subpoena.

Rivara, F. P., et al. (2000). Screening trauma patients for alcohol problems: Are insurance companies barriers? *Journal of Trauma, 48*(1), 115-118.

out obvious reason, chronic noncompliance with treatment regimens, and self-medication or use of a substance in response to symptomatology secondary to psychiatric impairment or social stressors (Compton et al., 2003). Substance abuse can go undetected in those who are depressed, suicidal, or anxious unless a thorough history is taken. Similarly, the understanding and treatment of substance-dependent people are enhanced by inquiries about symptoms of depression and anxiety.

Once specific data are obtained, it is helpful to know if the person is abusing a substance or is actively dependent on the substance. Refer back to Figure 27-1 for guidance in making this distinction.

Assessing Psychological Changes

Certain psychological characteristics are associated with substance abuse, including denial, depression, anxiety, dependency, hopelessness, low self-esteem, and various psychiatric disorders. It is often difficult to determine which comes first, psychological changes or substance abuse. Some people self-medicate to cope with psychiatric symptoms. For these people, symptoms of psychological difficulty remain, even after months of sobriety.

Substance-abusing people are threatened on many levels in their interactions with nurses. First, they are concerned about being rejected. They are acutely aware that not all nurses are equally willing to care for addicted people, and in fact, many clients have experienced instances of rejection in past encounters with nursing personnel. Second, substance abusers may be

Assessment strategies must include collection of data pertaining to both substance dependence and psychiatric impairment. Individuals with previously established psychiatric impairment may be experiencing substance abuse or dependence if they exhibit increasing frequency of symptoms, exacerbation with-

anxious about recovering because to do so they must give up the substance they think they need to survive. Third, addicts are concerned about failing at recovering. Addiction is a chronic relapsing condition. In fact, relapse is one of the criteria for diagnosing addiction. Most addicts have tried recovery at least once before and have experienced relapse. As a result, many become discouraged about their chances of ever succeeding.

These concerns can threaten the addict's sense of security and sense of self, increasing anxiety levels. To protect against these feelings, the addict establishes a **predictable defensive style.** The elements of this style include various defense mechanisms (denial, projection, rationalization) as well as characteristic thought processes (all-or-none thinking, selective attention) and behaviors (conflict minimization and avoidance, passivity, and manipulation). The substance abuser is not able to give up these maladaptive coping styles until more positive and functional skills are learned.

Assessing Signs of Intoxication and Withdrawal

Central Nervous System Depressants

CNS depressant drugs include alcohol, benzodiazepines, and barbiturates. Symptoms of intoxication, overdose, and withdrawal, along with possible treatments, are presented in Table 27-2.

Withdrawal reactions to alcohol and other CNS depressants are associated with severe morbidity and mortality, unlike withdrawal from other drugs. The syndrome for alcohol withdrawal is the same as that for the entire class of CNS depressant drugs. Alcohol is used here as the prototype. The time intervals are delayed when other CNS depressants are the main drugs of choice or are used in combination with alcohol. In addition, as clients age, their symptoms of withdrawal continue for longer periods and are more severe than in younger clients.

TABLE 27-2

Central Nervous System Depressants

| Drug | Intoxication | Overdose | | Withdrawal | |
		Effects	Possible Treatments	Effects	Possible Treatments
Barbiturates **Benzodiazepines** **Chloral hydrate** **Glutethimide** **Meprobamate** **Alcohol (ETOH)**	*Physical:* Slurred speech Incoordination Unsteady gait Drowsiness Decreased blood pressure *Psychological-perceptual:* Disinhibition of sexual or aggressive drives Impaired judgment Impaired social or occupational function Impaired attention or memory Irritability	Cardiovascular or respiratory depression or arrest (mostly with barbiturates) Coma Shock Convulsions Death	*If awake:* Keep awake. Induce vomiting. Give activated charcoal to aid absorption of drug. Every 15 minutes check vital signs (VS). *Coma:* Clear airway; insert endotracheal tube. Give intravenous (IV) fluids. Perform gastric lavage with activated charcoal. Check VS frequently for shock and cardiac arrest after client is stable. Initiate seizure precautions. Possibly perform hemodialysis or peritoneal dialysis. Administer flumazenil (Romazicon) IV.	*Cessation of prolonged-heavy use:* Nausea and vomiting Tachycardia Diaphoresis Anxiety or irritability Tremors in hands, fingers, eyelids Marked insomnia Grand mal seizures *After 5-15 years of heavy use:* Delirium	Perform carefully titrated detoxification with similar drug. *Note:* Abrupt withdrawal can lead to death.

Data from American Psychiatric Association. (2000). *Diagnostic and statistical manual of mental disorders* (4th ed., text rev.). Washington, DC: Author; and Bohn, M. J. (2000). Alcoholism. *Psychiatric Clinics of North America, 16*(4), 679.

Multiple drug and alcohol dependencies can result in simultaneous withdrawal syndromes that present a bizarre clinical picture and may pose problems for safe withdrawal. Family and friends may help provide important information that can assist in care planning. The *DSM-IV-TR* identifies two alcohol withdrawal syndromes: (1) alcohol withdrawal and (2) the more severe alcohol withdrawal delirium (see Figure 27-2).

Alcohol Withdrawal. The early signs of withdrawal develop within a few hours after cessation or reduction of alcohol (ethanol) intake; they peak after 24 to 48 hours and then rapidly and dramatically disappear, unless the withdrawal progresses to alcohol withdrawal delirium. The person may appear hyperalert, manifest jerky movements and irritability, startle easily, and experience subjective distress often described as "shaking inside." Grand mal seizures may appear 7 to 48 hours after cessation of alcohol intake, particularly in people with a history of seizures. Careful assessment followed by appropriate medical and nursing interventions can prevent the more serious withdrawal reaction of delirium.

A kind, warm, and supportive manner on the part of the nurse can allay anxiety and provide a sense of security. Consistent and frequent orientation to time and place may be necessary. Encouraging the family or close friends (one at a time) to stay with the client in quiet surroundings can also help increase orientation and minimize confusion and anxiety. **Illusions** are usually terrifying for the client. Illusions are misinterpretations of objects in the environment, usually of a threatening nature. For example, a person may think that spots on the wallpaper are blood-sucking ants. However, illusions can be clarified; this reduces the client's terror: "See, they are not ants, they are just part of the wallpaper pattern." If a person experiencing withdrawal is argumentative, hostile, or demanding, it is often because of deep-seated anxiety and feelings of guilt and shame. The nurse can make relief and hope possible by demonstrating an accepting attitude and showing strong support for efforts at recovery.

Alcohol Withdrawal Delirium. Alcohol withdrawal delirium is considered a medical emergency and can result in death even if treated (Webb, Carlton, & Geehan, 2000). Death is usually due to sepsis, myocardial infarction, fat embolism, peripheral vascular collapse, electrolyte imbalance, aspiration pneumonia, or suicide. The state of delirium usually peaks 2 to 3 days (48 to 72 hours) after cessation or reduction of intake (although it can occur later) and lasts 2 to 3 days.

In addition to anxiety, insomnia, anorexia, and delirium, features include the following:

- Autonomic hyperactivity (e.g., tachycardia, diaphoresis, elevated blood pressure)
- Severe disturbance in sensorium (e.g., disorientation, clouding of consciousness)
- Perceptual disturbances (e.g., visual or tactile hallucinations)
- Fluctuating levels of consciousness (e.g., ranging from hyperexcitability to lethargy)
- Delusions (paranoid), agitated behaviors, and fever (100°F to 103°F).

Immediate medical attention is warranted (see the Psychopharmacology section for a full discussion of medical treatments).

Alcohol is the only drug for which objective measures of intoxication exist. The relationship between blood alcohol level (BAL) and behavior in a nontolerant individual is shown in Table 27-3. Knowledge of the BAL assists the nurse in determining the level of intoxication and the level of tolerance, and in ascertaining whether the person accurately reported recent drinking during the nursing history. These factors are also assessed by means of behavioral cues. As tolerance develops, a discrepancy is seen between BAL and expected behavior. A person with tolerance to alcohol may have a high BAL but minimal signs of impairment, as indicated in the following vignette.

■ ■ ■ *VIGNETTE*

Clarence comes to the emergency department with a BAL of 0.51 mg%. He is stuporous and ataxic, and has slurred speech. The fact that he is still alive indicates a high toler-

TABLE 27-3

Relationship Between Blood Alcohol Level and Effects in a Nontolerant Drinker

Blood Alcohol Level	Blood Alcohol Accumulation	Effects
0.05 mg%	1-2 drinks	Changes in mood and behavior; impaired judgment
0.10 mg%	5-6 drinks	Clumsiness in voluntary motor activity; **legal level of intoxication in most states**
0.20 mg%	10-12 drinks	Depressed function of entire motor area of the brain, causing staggering and ataxia; emotional lability
0.30 mg%	15-18 drinks	Confusion, stupor
0.40 mg%	20-24 drinks	Coma
0.50 mg%	25-30 drinks	Death due to respiratory depression

ance for alcohol. A nursing history conducted as the client sobers up reveals an extensive drinking history. When the blood alcohol level is this high, assessing for withdrawal symptoms is important.

■ ■ ■

The nursing history, physical examination, and laboratory tests are methods used to gather data about drug-related physical problems (Becker & Walton-Moss, 2001; Resnick et al., 2003; Sommers et al., 2003; Tuttle et al., 2002). The extent of impairment depends on individual susceptibility as well as the amount of drug used and the route of administration. Each class

of drugs has its own physiological signs and symptoms of intoxication, which are summarized in the tables for each substance class.

Central Nervous System Stimulants

Table 27-4 outlines the physical and psychological effects of intoxication from abuse of amphetamines and other psychostimulants, possible life-threatening results of overdose, and emergency measures for both overdose and withdrawal. All stimulants accelerate the normal functioning of the body and affect the CNS. Common signs of stimulant abuse include dilation of

TABLE 27-4

Central Nervous System Stimulants

| Drug | Intoxication | Overdose | | Withdrawal | |
		Effects	Possible Treatments	Effects	Possible Treatments
Cocaine, crack (short acting) *Note:* High obtained in: snorted, 3 minutes; injected, 30 seconds; smoked, 4-6 seconds (crack) Average high lasts 15-30 minutes for cocaine; 5-7 minutes for crack	*Physical:* Tachycardia Dilated pupils Elevated blood pressure Nausea and vomiting Insomnia *Psychological-perceptual:* Assaultiveness Grandiosity Impaired judgment Impaired social and occupational functioning Euphoria	Respiratory distress Ataxia Hyperpyrexia Convulsions Coma Stroke Myocardial infarction Death	Antipsychotics Medical and nursing management for: Hyperpyrexia (ambient cooling) Convulsions (diazepam) Respiratory distress Cardiovascular shock Acidification of urine (ammonium chloride for amphetamine)	Fatigue Depression Agitation Apathy Anxiety Sleepiness Disorientation Lethargy Craving	Antidepressants (desipramine) Dopamine agonist Bromocriptine
Amphetamines (long-acting) Dextroamphetamine Methamphetamine Ice (synthesized for street use)	Increased energy *Severe effects:* State resembling paranoid schizophrenia Paranoia with delusions Psychosis Visual, auditory, and tactile hallucinations Severe to panic levels of anxiety Potential for violence ***Note:* Paranoia and ideas of reference may persist for months afterward**	Same as above	Same as above	Same as above	Same as above

Data from American Psychiatric Association. (2000). *Diagnostic and statistical manual of mental disorders* (4th ed., text rev.). Washington, DC: Author; O'Connor, P. G., Samet, J. H., & Stein, M. D. (1994). Management of hospitalized drug users: Role of the internist. *American Journal of Medicine, 96,* 551; and Bell, K. (1992). Identifying the substance abuser in clinical practice. *Orthopedic Nursing, 11*(2), 29.

the pupils, dryness of the oronasal cavity, and excessive motor activity.

When a person who has ingested a stimulant experiences chest pain, has an irregular pulse, or has a history of heart trouble, the person should be taken to an emergency department immediately.

Cocaine and Crack. Cocaine is a naturally occurring stimulant extracted from the leaf of the coca bush. Crack is a cheap, widely available alkalinized form of cocaine. When crack is smoked, it takes effect in 4 to 6 seconds, producing a fleeting high (5 to 7 minutes) followed by a period of deep depression that reinforces addictive behavior patterns and guarantees continued use of the drug. Cocaine is classified as a schedule II substance—"high abuse potential with some recognized medical use." Cocaine exerts two main effects on the body: anesthetic and stimulant. As an anesthetic, it blocks the conduction of electrical impulses within the nerve cells that are involved in sensory transmission, primarily pain transmission. It also acts as a stimulant for both sexual arousal and violent behavior. Cocaine produces an imbalance of neurotransmitters (dopamine and norepinephrine) that may be responsible for many of the physical withdrawal symptoms reported by heavy chronic cocaine users: depression, paranoia, lethargy, anxiety, insomnia, nausea and vomiting, and sweating and chills—all signs of the body's struggling to regain its normal chemical balance.

Nicotine and Caffeine. Most people consume caffeine by way of coffee, tea, or cola drinks. People ingest coffee as a drug ("I've got to have two cups in the morning to function"), for social reasons ("Let's get together for coffee"), or as a reward ("After I finish this job, I'm going to take a coffee break").

About one out of four Americans is an active smoker, with 20% of the population meeting the criteria for nicotine dependence. A high proportion of psychiatric outpatients are nicotine dependent: 90% of clients with schizophrenia and 70% of clients with bipolar I disorder or another substance abuse disorder (Sadock & Sadock, 2003).

Nicotine can act as a stimulant, depressant, or tranquilizer. Nicotine can also be chewed (in smokeless tobacco), which adds mouth cancer to the list of dangers. Lung cancer is highly correlated with smoking tobacco. Wellbutrin (Zyban) and nicotine replacement therapy are successful treatments for many individuals during smoking cessation.

Opiates

The opiate drug class includes opium, morphine, heroin, codeine, fentanyl and its analogues, methadone, and meperidine. Use of heroin by American teenagers is increasing as it becomes cheaper and more potent (Hopfer et al., 2002). Novices are starting with nasal administration. Table 27-5 lists signs and symptoms of intoxication, overdose, and withdrawal, and possible treatments.

TABLE 27-5

Opiates

| Drug | Intoxication | Overdose | | Withdrawal | |
		Effects	Possible Treatments	Effects	Possible Treatments
Opium **(paregoric)** **Heroin** **Meperidine** **(Demerol)** **Morphine** **Codeine** **Methadone** **(Dolophine)** **Hydromorphone** **(Dilaudid)** **Fentanyl** **(Sublimaze)** **Fentanyl** **analogues**	*Physical:* Constricted pupils Decreased respiration Drowsiness Decreased blood pressure Slurred speech Psychomotor retardation *Psychological-perceptual:* Initial euphoria followed by dysphoria and impairment of attention, judgment, and memory	Possible dilation of pupils due to anoxia Respiratory depression or arrest Coma Shock Convulsions Death	Narcotic antagonist (e.g., naloxone [Narcan]) to quickly reverse central nervous system depression	Yawning Insomnia Irritability Runny nose (rhinorrhea) Panic Diaphoresis Cramps Nausea and vomiting Muscle aches ("bone pain") Chills Fever Lacrimation Diarrhea	Methadone tapering Clonidine-naltrexone detoxification Buprenorphine substitution

Data from American Psychiatric Association. (2000). *Diagnostic and statistical manual of mental disorders* (4th ed., text rev.). Washington, DC: Author; O'Connor, P. G., Samet, J. H., & Stein, M. D. (1994). Management of hospitalized drug users: Role of the internist. *American Journal of Medicine, 96,* 551; and Bell, K. (1992). Identifying the substance abuser in clinical practice. *Orthopedic Nursing, 11*(2), 29.

Note: An opiate is a derivative or synthetic that affects the central nervous system and the autonomic nervous system. Medically used primarily as an analgesic (pain killer). Consistent use causes tolerance and distressing withdrawal symptoms.

Marijuana *(Cannabis sativa)*

Cannabis sativa is an Indian hemp plant. **Tetrahydrocannabinol (THC)** is the active ingredient found in the resin secreted from the flowering tops and leaves of the cannabis plant. THC has mixed depressant and hallucinogenic properties. Marijuana, the leaves of the cannabis plant, is generally smoked (joint, reefer, roach), but it can be ingested. It is the most widely used illicit drug in the United States. Desired effects include euphoria, detachment, and relaxation. Other effects include talkativeness, slowed perception of time, inappropriate hilarity, heightened sensitivity to external stimuli, and anxiety or paranoia. Long-term dependence on cannabis can result in lethargy, anhedonia, difficulty concentrating, and loss of memory for some people.

Overdose and withdrawal (other than craving) rarely occur. Medical indications exist for the use of THC (e.g., control of chemotherapy-induced nausea, reduction of intraocular pressure in glaucoma, and appetite stimulation in AIDS wasting syndrome).

Hallucinogens

See Table 27-6 for signs and symptoms of hallucinogen intoxication and overdose.

TABLE 27-6

Hallucinogens

| Drug | Intoxication | | Overdose | |
	Physical Effects	Psychological-Perceptual Effects	Effects	Possible Treatments
Lysergic acid diethylamide (LSD) **Mescaline (peyote)** **Psilocybin**	Pupil dilation Tachycardia Diaphoresis Palpitations Tremors Incoordination Elevated temperature, pulse, respiration	Fear of going crazy Paranoid ideas Marked anxiety, depression Synesthesia (e.g., colors are heard; sounds are seen) Depersonalization Hallucinations, although sensorium is clear Grandiosity (e.g., thinking one can fly)	Psychosis Brain damage Death	Keep client in room with low stimuli—minimal light, sound, activity. Have one person stay with client; reassure client, "talk down" client. Speak slowly and clearly in low voice. Give diazepam or chloral hydrate for extreme anxiety or tension.
Phencyclidine piperidine (PCP)	Vertical or horizontal nystagmus Increased blood pressure, pulse, and temperature Ataxia Muscle rigidity Seizures Blank stare Chronic jerking Agitated, repetitive movements Belligerence, assaultiveness, impulsiveness Impaired judgment, impaired social and occupational functioning	*Severe effects:* Hallucinations, paranoia Bizarre behavior (e.g., barking like a dog, grimacing, repetitive chanting speech) Regressive behavior **Violent bizarre behaviors** Very labile behaviors	Psychosis Possible hypertensive crisis or cardiovascular accident Respiratory arrest Hyperthermia Seizures	*If alert:* *Caution:* Gastric lavage can lead to laryngeal spasms or aspiration. Acidify urine (cranberry juice, ascorbic acid); in acute stage, ammonium chloride acidifies urine to help excrete drug from body—may continue for 10-14 days. Put in room with minimal stimuli. Do not attempt to talk down! Speak slowly, clearly, and in a low voice. Administer diazepam. Haloperidol may be used for severe behavioral disturbance (*not* a phenothiazine). *Institute medical intervention for:* Hyperthermia High blood pressure Respiratory distress Hypertension

Data from American Psychiatric Association. (2000). *Diagnostic and statistical manual of mental disorders* (4th ed., text rev.). Washington, DC: Author; and Bell, K. (1992). Identifying the substance abuser in clinical practice. *Orthopedic Nursing, 11*(2), 29.

Note: A hallucinogen produces *abnormal mental phenomena* in the cognitive and perceptual spheres; for example, distortion in space and time, hallucinations, delusions (paranoid or grandiose), and synesthesia may occur.

Lysergic Acid Diethylamide (LSD) and LSD-Like Drugs. LSD (also known as "acid"), **mescaline** (peyote), and **psilocybin** (magic mushroom) are hallucinogens. Mescaline and the mushroom *Psilocybe mexicana* (from which psilocybin is isolated) have been used for centuries in religious rites by Native Americans living in the southwestern United States and northern Mexico. The hallucinogenic experience produced by LSD is called a trip.

Phencyclidine Piperidine (PCP). PCP is also known as angel dust, horse tranquilizer, and peace pill. When it is taken orally, the onset of symptoms occurs about 1 hour after ingestion. When the drug is taken intravenously, sniffed, or smoked, the onset of symptoms may occur within 5 minutes. The signs and symptoms of PCP intoxication range from acute anxiety to acute psychosis. The drug produces a generalized anesthesia that lessens the sensations of touch and pain and makes staff interventions difficult. Chronic use of PCP can result in long-term effects such as dulled thinking, lethargy, loss of impulse control, poor memory, and depression.

Suicidal risk is always assessed, especially in cases of toxicity or coma. If the client awakens and appears to be suicidal, the nurse should determine whether previous suicide attempts have occurred. Information regarding suicide history of family members is also elicited. Additional history may be obtained through family as well as a review of medical records. Refer to Chapter 23 for more information on suicide assessment.

Inhalants

About 19% of adolescents in the United States say that they have sniffed inhalants—usually volatile solvents such as spray paint, glue, cigarette lighter fluid, and propellant gases used in aerosols—at least once in their lives (Espeland, 2000). Types of inhalants, signs of intoxication, and side effects are given in Table 27-7. Inhalant use may be an early marker of substance abuse and should be the focus of increased preventive efforts and early diagnosis and treatment (Espeland, 2000).

Rave and Techno Drugs, Club Drugs, Date Rape Drugs

Raves or techno dances are all-night dance parties attended by large numbers of youth, sometimes in excess of 20,000 (Weir, 2000). Raves are known for their electric music and the liberal use of techno drugs such as ecstasy. **Ecstasy** (3,4-methylenedioxy-methamphetamine), also called MDMA, Adam, yaba, and XTC, is a prototype of a class of substituted amphetamines that

TABLE 27-7

Inhalants

Drug	Intoxication	Side Effects/Overdose	Treatment

Volatile solvents: gases or liquids that vaporize at room temperature:
   Butane
   Paint thinner
   Paint and wax removers
   Propellant gases used in aerosols (e.g., dispensers for whipped cream, hair spray)
   Airplane glue
   Nail polish remover
   Dry cleaning fluid
	Excitation followed by drowsiness, disinhibition, staggering, lightheadedness, and agitation	Damage to the nervous system
		 Death
			Support affected systems.

Nitrates: Room deodorizers (less common because products containing butyl and propyl were banned in 1991)	Enhancement of sexual pleasure		Neurological symptoms may respond to vitamin B_{12} and folate.

Anesthetics:
   Gas—especially nitrous oxide
   Liquid
   Local
	Giggling, laughter
	 Euphoria
		Possible polyneuropathy and myelopathy in chronic users	

From National Institute on Drug Abuse. (1998). *Research report series: Inhalant use* (NIH Publication No. 94-3818). Washington, DC: U.S. Department of Health and Human Services.

also includes MDA (methylenedioxy-amphetamine, or "love") and MDE (3,4-methylenedioxy-ethylamphetamine, or "Eve"). These recreational drugs produce subjective effects resembling those of stimulants and hallucinogens.

After the usual dose (100 to 150 mg) of MDMA is taken, subjective side effects include euphoria, increased energy, increased self-confidence, increased sociability, and a feeling of closeness to people (Leshner, 2000). Due to their psychostimulant and psychedelic effects, ecstasy and the other drugs listed are increasingly abused, especially within the rave subculture.

Adverse effects such as hyperthermia, heart failure, and kidney failure have occurred. Deaths from acute dehydration have been reported (Leshner, 2000). Morgan (2000) states that there is growing evidence that chronic heavy recreational use of ecstasy is associated with sleep disorders, depressed mood, persistent elevation of anxiety level, impulsiveness, and hostility as well as selective impairment of episodic memory and weakening of memory and attention.

The drugs most frequently used to facilitate a sexual assault (rape) are flunitrazepam (Rohypnol or "roofies"), which is a fast-acting benzodiazepine, and γ-hydroxybutyric acid (GHB) and its congeners (Schwartz, Milteer, & LeBeaur, 2000). They are odorless, tasteless, and colorless, mix easily with drinks, and can leave a person unconscious in a matter of minutes. Perpetrators use these drugs because they rapidly produce disinhibition and relaxation of voluntary muscles; they also cause the victim to have lasting anterograde amnesia for events that occur. Alcohol potentiates their effects. Refer to Chapter 26 for additional discussion of the use of these drugs in sexual assault.

Self-Assessment

Although you may identify with, and have empathy for, clients addicted to caffeine or tobacco, your responses to clients who abuse other substances may not be so empathetic. A client who has overdosed on heroin or cocaine, or who comes in with complications from use of ecstasy or other techno drugs, may be met with disapproval, intolerance, and condemnation or may be considered morally weak. Also, the manipulative behaviors often seen in these clients may lead you to feel angry and exploited. You may want to help but may perceive the client who abuses drugs to be willful, uncooperative, and impossible to work with.

In some areas of the United States, the recreational use of cocaine, marijuana, and amphetamine is so common that the nurse may not have much emotional reaction. This attitude is as detrimental as is strong emotional disapproval, because the nurse may underestimate the importance of supportive measures and client education and the need for follow-up psychotherapeutic intervention.

To come to a true personal understanding means that you must examine your own attitudes, feelings, and beliefs about addicts and addiction. It often means that you must examine your own substance use and that of others you know, and this is not always pleasant work.

A history of substance abuse in a nurse's own family can overshadow the nurse's interactions with addicts. The negative or positive experiences a nurse has had with addicted family members can influence interpersonal interactions with present or future clients.

Therefore, it is important that nurses attend to personal feelings that arise when they work with addicts. All health care professionals require supervision if they are not experienced in this area. Nurses who do not attend to, and work through, expected negative feelings that arise during treatment have power struggles with clients, and the therapeutic process is generally ineffective. These issues can become evident when it is a fellow nurse who has a substance abuse problem.

Chemically Impaired Nurse

Nurses have a 32% to 50% higher rate of chemical dependency than the general population. Estimates of the proportion of practicing nurses who are chemically dependent range from 10% to 20%. Helping the chemically impaired nurse is difficult but not impossible. The choices for action are varied, and the only choice that is clearly wrong is to do nothing. Without intervention or treatment, the problems associated with the chemical dependency escalate, and the potential for client harm increases.

Often, the impaired nurse volunteers to work additional shifts to be nearer to the source of the drug. The nurse may leave the unit frequently or spend a lot of time in the bathroom. When the impaired nurse is on duty, more clients may complain that their pain is unrelieved by their narcotic analgesic or that they are unable to sleep, despite receiving sedative medications. Increases in inaccurate drug counts and vial breakage may occur.

If indicators of impaired practice are observed, the observations need to be reported to the nurse manager. Intervention is the responsibility of the nurse manager and other nursing administrators. However, clear documentation by co-workers (specific dates, times, events, consequences) is crucial. The nurse manager's major concerns are with job performance and client safety. Once the nurse manager has been informed, the legal and ethical responsibilities for in-house reporting have been met. If the impaired nurse remains in the situation and no action is taken by the nurse manager, then the information must be taken to the next level in the chain of command. These measures can prevent harm to clients under the impaired nurse's care and can save a colleague's professional career or even life (Sloan & Vernarec, 2001).

Reporting an impaired colleague is not easy, even though it is our responsibility. In order not to see what is going on, nurses may deny or rationalize, thus *enabling* the impaired nurse to potentially endanger lives while becoming sicker and more isolated. Box 27-3 can be used as a check to discern enabling behaviors with regard to a nurse colleague.

Referral to a treatment program should always be an option. Programs for chemically dependent nurses have been developed in some states in response to a policy statement issued by the American Nurses Association. Some state boards of nursing allow impaired nurses to avoid disciplinary action if they seek treatment. The aim of these programs is to protect clients and to keep the nurse in active practice (perhaps with limitations) or to return the nurse to practice after suspension and professional help. Nurses who continue to show signs of impaired practice should not be returned to direct patient care.

Assessment Guidelines Chemically Impaired Clients

1. Assess for a severe or major withdrawal syndrome.
2. Assess for an overdose to a drug or alcohol that warrants immediate medical attention.

BOX 27-3

Have I Enabled?

Have I

Excused or ignored behaviors in a peer that may be suggestive of impairment and justified those behaviors as "just having a bad day" or "stress"?

Never told the supervisor about behaviors possibly indicative of impairment that I observed because I was afraid of being wrong and did not want anyone to get angry at me?

Accepted responsibility for my colleague's unfinished work and at times attempted to counsel and solve his or her problem?

Believed that nurses do not use drugs or alcohol to the point of practice impairment and that substance use can be stopped at any time unless the person is morally weak?

Liked to use drugs or alcohol myself to relax or enjoy with friends? I do not want anyone to look at me. In fact, I have used a few discontinued drugs from work myself. Doesn't everyone?

Exonerated a peer's irresponsible actions by covering for attendance or tardiness? Have I cosigned wastes I have not truly witnessed or corrected the narcotic count to account for a discrepancy?

Defended a colleague when it was suggested there may be a problem with impairment?

From Smith, L., Taylor, B. B., & Hughes, T. L. (1998). Effective peer response to impaired nursing practice. *Nursing Clinics of North America, 33*(1), 105-118.

---

3. Assess the client for suicidal thoughts or other self-destructive behaviors.
4. Evaluate the client for any physical complications related to drug abuse.
5. Explore the client's interests in doing something about his or her drug or alcohol problem.
6. Assess the client and family for knowledge of community resources for alcohol and drug treatment.

■ NURSING DIAGNOSIS

Formulation of appropriate nursing diagnoses depends on accurate assessment. Whereas the *DSM-IV-TR* criteria emphasize patterns of use and physical symptoms, nursing diagnoses identify how dependence on substances of abuse interferes with a person's ability to deal with the activities and demands of daily living.

Nursing diagnoses for clients with psychoactive substance use disorders are many and varied because of the large range of physical and psychological effects of drug abuse or dependence on the user and his or her family. Comorbid psychiatric problems also must be addressed. Potential nursing diagnoses for people with substance use disorders are listed in Table 27-8.

■ OUTCOME CRITERIA

Nursing Outcomes Classification (NOC) categories (Moorhead, Johnson, & Maas, 2004) for outcome criteria for clients with substance use disorders can be divided into three phases. When the client has a dual diagnosis, outcomes for the psychiatric disorder are also developed. NOC outcomes and examples of client goal statements follow.

Withdrawal

Fluid Balance: Client's blood pressure will not be compromised.
Neurological Status: Consciousness: Client will have no seizure activity.
Distorted Thought Self-Control: Client will consistently describe content of hallucinations.

Initial and Active Drug Treatment

Risk Control: Alcohol Use: Client will consistently demonstrate a commitment to alcohol use control strategies.
Risk Control: Drug Use: Client will consistently demonstrate acknowledgment of personal consequences associated with drug misuse.
Substance Addiction Consequences: Client will demonstrate no difficulty supporting self financially.

TABLE 27-8

Potential Nursing Diagnoses for Substance Abuse

Signs and Symptoms	Nursing Diagnoses
Vomiting, diarrhea, poor nutritional and fluid intake	**Imbalanced nutrition: less than body requirements** **Deficient fluid volume**
Audiovisual hallucinations, impaired judgment, memory deficits, cognitive impairments related to substance intoxication or withdrawal (deficits in problem solving, ability to attend to tasks and grasp ideas)	**Disturbed thought processes** **Disturbed sensory perception**
Changes in sleep-wake cycle, interference with stage 4 sleep, inability to sleep or long periods of sleeping related to effects of or withdrawal from substance	**Disturbed sleep pattern**
Lack of self-care (hygiene, grooming), failure to care for basic health needs	**Ineffective health maintenance** **Self-care deficit** **Nonadherence to health care regimen**
Feelings of hopelessness, inability to change, feelings of worthlessness, feeling that life has no meaning or future	**Hopelessness** **Spiritual distress** **Situational low self-esteem** **Chronic low self-esteem** **Risk for self-directed violence** **Risk for suicide**
Family crises and family pain, ineffective parenting, emotional neglect of others, increased incidence of physical and sexual abuse of others, increased self-hate projected to others	**Interrupted family processes** **Impaired parenting** **Risk for other-directed violence**
Excessive substance abuse affecting all areas of a person's life: loss of friends, poor job performance, increased illness rates, proneness to accidents and overdoses	**Ineffective coping** **Impaired verbal communication** **Social isolation** **Risk for loneliness** **Anxiety** **Risk for suicide**
Increased health problems related to substance used and route of use, as well as overdose	**Activity intolerance** **Ineffective airway clearance** **Ineffective breathing pattern** **Impaired oral mucous membrane** **Risk for infection** **Decreased cardiac output** **Sexual dysfunction**
Total preoccupation with and majority of time consumed by taking and withdrawing from drug	**Delayed growth and development** **Ineffective coping** **Impaired social interaction** **Dysfunctional family processes: substance dependence**

Health Maintenance

Knowledge: Substance Abuse Control: Client will describe actions to prevent and manage relapses in substance use.

Family Coping: Family will consistently demonstrate care for needs of all family members.

■ PLANNING

Planning care requires attention to the client's social status, income, ethnic background, sex, age, substance use history, and current condition. It is safest to propose abstinence as a treatment goal for all addicts. Abstinence is strongly related to good work adjustment, positive health status, comfortable interpersonal relationships, and general social stability. Planning must also address the client's major psychological, social, and medical problems as well as the substance-using behavior. Involvement of appropriate family members is essential.

Unfortunately, a person's social status and social relations often deteriorate as a result of addiction. Job demotion or loss of job, with resultant reduced or nonexistent income, may occur. Meeting basic needs for food, shelter, and clothing is thereby hampered. Marriage and other close relationships deteriorate and fail, and the person is often left alone and isolated. The lack of interpersonal and social supports is a complicating factor in treatment planning for the addict. Refer to Case Study and Nursing Care Plan 27-1 for a dual-diagnosis client at the end of the chapter.

■ INTERVENTION

The aim of treatment is self-responsibility, not compliance. A major challenge is improving treatment effectiveness by matching subtypes of clients to specific types of treatment. Although addicts share some characteristics and dynamics, significant differences exist within the addict population with regard to physiological, psychological, and sociocultural processes. These differences influence the recovery process either positively or negatively.

Often, the choice of inpatient or outpatient care depends on cost and the availability of insurance coverage. Outpatient programs work best for employed substance abusers who have an involved social support system. People who have no support and structure in their day often do better in inpatient programs when these programs are available.

In addition, neuropsychological deficits have been associated with long-term alcohol abuse. Impairment has been found in abstract reasoning ability, ability to use feedback in learning new concepts, attention and concentration spans, cognitive flexibility, and subtle memory functions. These deficits undoubtedly have an impact on the process of alcoholism treatment.

At all levels of practice, the nurse can play an important role in the intervention process by recognizing the signs of substance abuse in both the client and the family and by being familiar with the resources available to help with the problem.

Communication Guidelines

Communication strategies are designed to address behaviors that almost all substance abusers have in common, including dysfunctional anger, manipulation, impulsiveness, and grandiosity. The nurse's ability to develop a warm, accepting relationship with an addicted client can help the client feel safe enough to start looking at problems with some degree of openness and honesty. The following is an example of a portion of the intake interview with a client upon admission to a treatment program.

DIALOGUE	THERAPEUTIC TOOL/COMMENT
Nurse: Elyse, I get the impression that life must have been getting very difficult for you lately.	Validating and empathizing
Elyse: (Silence) I don't think you would understand.	
Nurse: I guess sometimes it feels as if no one understands, but I would like to try.	Reflecting and empathizing
Elyse: At times . . . I feel I can't go on any more . . . so many losses.	
Nurse: Loss is difficult. Elyse, tell me about your losses.	Encouraging the client to share her painful feelings
Elyse: My brother's sudden death. . . . We were so close. . . . I depended on him so much.	
Nurse: It must have been difficult for you to lose him so suddenly.	Empathizing
Elyse: (Silence) No one knows. . . . Then Harry, he left. . . . (Elyse starts to cry.)	
Nurse: Tell me what you are feeling right now.	Encouraging the expression of feelings while feelings are close to the surface
Elyse: I don't know . . . angry maybe. . . . Why does everyone leave me? . . . Oh, I hate them. . . . Oh, I wish I had a Valium now. . . .	
Nurse: And what does the Valium do to help you?	Beginning to explore the drug dependence in a gentle, nonthreatening manner

The following example demonstrates the use of therapeutic leverage (i.e., making abstinence and sobriety worthwhile for the substance abuser). It is presented as a dialogue between a nurse and a 17-year-old young man. His parents are divorced, and his father abuses him when drinking. He was picked up three times during the preceding 7 months for possession of cocaine.

DIALOGUE	THERAPEUTIC TOOL/COMMENT
Nurse: I understand you entered the treatment program yesterday afternoon following your court appearance.	Placing the event in time and sequence, validating the precipitating event
Frank: Yeah—it was my dad's idea.	
Nurse: Well, what do you think of the idea?	Encouraging evaluation (actions first, thoughts, then feelings)
Frank: I don't like it. I don't need this place. I'm not a junkie—I just use cocaine, that's all. I can handle it.	
Nurse: From what I've heard, your involvement with cocaine has gotten you into trouble.	Pointing out realities
Frank: Yeah, well, I guess I can't deny that . . . but I still don't think I need this place.	
Nurse: Are you saying that you don't think you need a treatment program?	Validating the client's perception
Frank: Well, I don't know, I guess maybe I am messed up a bit.	
Nurse: "Messed up."	Restating
Frank: Yeah.	
Nurse: What is one thing about you that's messed up?	Encouraging the client to be specific rather than global
Frank: (Silence) I guess I feel like I don't belong anywhere.	
Nurse: Talk more about that.	Clarifying

■■■ CULTURALLY SPEAKING

Little is known about designing culturally appropriate approaches for preventing alcohol and drug abuse. A study to develop such guidelines was conducted in Hawaii using the American Nurses Association's adaptation of *Put Prevention into Practice—Clinician's Handbook of Preventative Services*. The study groups were Hispanic, Japanese, Filipino, part-Hawaiian, and white women. The part-Hawaiian women were in alcohol or drug treatment at the time of the study. Using a focus group process, the women identified culturally appropriate material for inclusion into the guidelines. The identified content was then incorporated into the alcohol and drug abuse prevention protocol.

The groups consistently noted several characteristics that would discourage them from discussing alcohol or drug use, including the following:
- The counselor is of a different gender or ethnicity than the woman.
- The clinician speaks a language not familiar to the woman, including "scientific" or medical language.
- The clinician appears to be busy.
- The clinician tells the woman what to do.
- The clinician wears a suit or sits behind a desk.

Building a foundation for disclosure requires
- Connection to the community.
- Demonstrated concern for the woman and her children.
- Demonstrated willingness to build a relationship with the woman.
- Trusting relationship between the woman and the clinician.

Adapted protocols are needed to address cultural perceptions and preferences to increase the probability that strategies used for health promotion, disease prevention, and treatment are appropriate.

Shoultz, J., Tanner, B., & Harrigan, R. (2000). Culturally appropriate guidelines for alcohol and drug use prevention. *Nurse Practitioner, 25*(11), 50-56.

It is also important to communicate in culturally appropriate ways. The Culturally Speaking box provides guidelines for finding out what factors are important to enable clients from different cultural groups to open up and share information about their substance abuse problems.

A useful tool for helping the resistant addict develop a willingness to engage in treatment is known as substance-abuse intervention. The concept behind this approach is that addiction is a progressive illness and rarely goes into remission without outside help. Significant others arrange for a meeting with the addict to point out current problems and to offer treatment alternatives. The steps or elements are outlined in Box 27-4 and can be applied not only to alcohol but also to other substances.

Intervention Strategies

Primary Prevention

Primary prevention through health teaching can have an important impact on how youngsters and adolescents choose to solve problems and relate interpersonally. Young people who participate in groups such as scouting, 4-H clubs, school clubs, and organized church activities are at a lower risk for substance abuse. Activities such as these help develop self-confidence and self-esteem. Elderly individuals who are experiencing stressful life events are also at risk. This population may be reached through senior citizen centers and other community social or spiritual groups and organizations.

Primary prevention of HIV infection in the drug-using population is facilitated by needle exchange programs, in which addicts return their used needles for

BOX 27-4

Steps in Substance-Abuse Intervention (for the Resistant Addict)

1. All the people concerned about, and affected by, the person's substance abuse are gathered together to present their case. The intervention must be rehearsed before it is actually carried out, usually with the support and guidance of a counselor.
2. Specific evidence related to the substance abuse is presented by each person, and it is written down so that each person does not have to rely on memory in a tense situation.
3. Timing must be right:
   - There must be current evidence available.
   - The intervention must take place after a crisis is precipitated by substance use and *not* when the person is under the influence of the substance or in severe withdrawal.
4. The intervention requires privacy. It is held in a place where no interruptions can occur.
5. The use of defenses is anticipated. No reaction is made to them.
6. Genuine, but firm, concern is demonstrated.
7. Substance abuse is understood as a disease.
8. Treatment alternatives are presented.
9. Responses to possible outcomes are prepared. The goal is to get the affected person into treatment. If the substance abusing person agrees to accept treatment, then he or she is taken immediately to a detoxification unit, where arrangements have been made previously. If the person refuses, then family members state that his or her decision must force them to make decisions of their own because they are no longer willing to live with the addicted person's behavior.

Adapted from Johnson, V. E. (1986). *Intervention: How to help someone who doesn't want help.* Minneapolis, MN: Johnson Institute.

sterile ones. One in three people with AIDS in the United States is an intravenous drug user or the sexual partner of an intravenous drug user. Reducing needle sharing can decrease the spread of HIV.

Brief Interventions

Use of brief interventions to effect behavior change allows the nurse to take advantage of any interaction with a substance-abusing client and use it as an opportunity for managing associated behaviors. Key interventions can be remembered by using the acronym *FRAMES*. The elements are the following (Becker & Walton-Moss, 2001):

Feedback of personal risk
Responsibility of the patient (personal control)
Advice to change
Menu of ways to reduce substance use (options)
Empathetic counseling
Self-efficacy or optimism of the patient

A case manager focuses on these elements when conducting a comprehensive needs assessment to (1) identify presenting problems; (2) develop an individualized plan, including client goals and a plan to reach those goals; (3) link clients with various treatment providers; (4) monitor the treatment process and its progress; and (5) serve as the client's advocate when needed.

Nursing Interventions Classification (NIC) categories that are applicable to clients with substance use disorders include *Substance Use Treatment, Family Support, Health Education, Coping Enhancement,* and *Self-Esteem Enhancement* (Dochterman & Bulechek, 2004).

Dual-Diagnosis Principles

The nurse also needs to be aware of clinical practice guidelines that have been developed through research involving the dual-diagnosis population. The following six principles are applicable in both inpatient and outpatient settings (Minkoff, 2003):

1. Expect a client to have a dual diagnosis—it is not the exception.
2. Treatment success is increased when providers are empathetic and hopeful, and work together as a team.
3. Addiction programs and mental health programs both need a dual focus, which requires appropriate training for staff.
4. The substance use disorder and the psychiatric disorder are both considered primary and need simultaneous treatment.
5. Recovery occurs in stages, and treatment should be matched to the client's needs and level of motivation and engagement.
6. Outcomes must be individualized to support progress in small steps over a long period of time.

Psychotherapy

Nurses with advanced training may be involved in psychotherapy with substance-using clients. Psychotherapy assists clients in identifying and using alternative coping mechanisms to reduce reliance on substances. Eventually, psychotherapy can assist recovering addicts to become increasingly comfortable with sobriety.

Evidence-based practice and data indicate that cognitive-behavioral therapies, psychodynamic and interpersonal therapies, group therapy, and family therapy are all effective for selected substance use disorders (APA, 2000b). See Chapters 35 and 36 for discussion of group and family therapy.

Confidentiality must be maintained throughout therapy *except* when this conflicts with requirements for mandatory reporting in certain circumstances (e.g., child abuse, danger to self or others).

Many critical issues arise during the first 6 months of sobriety. These include the following:

- Physical changes take place as the body adapts to functioning without substances.
- Numerous signals occur in the client's internal and external world that previously were cues to drinking and drug use. Different responses to these cues need to be learned.
- Emotional responses (feelings that were formerly diluted by substance use) are now experienced full strength. Because they are so unfamiliar, they can produce anxiety.
- Responses of family and co-workers to the client's new behavior must be addressed. Sobriety disrupts a system, and everyone in that system needs to adjust to the change.
- New coping skills must be developed to prevent relapse and ensure prolonged sobriety.

Psychotherapy needs to be directive, open and honest, and caring. The therapeutic process involves teaching the client to identify the physical and emotional changes that are occurring in the here and now. The nurse therapist can then assist in the problem-solving process.

Relapse Prevention

Relapses are common during a person's recovery. The goal of relapse prevention is to help the person learn from these situations so that periods of sobriety can be lengthened over time and so that lapses and relapses are not viewed as total failure. Relapse can result in a renewed and refined effort toward change.

■ ■ ■ *VIGNETTE*

Bill, a 20-year-old single man, is brought to the emergency department in a coma. He is accompanied by his mother, with whom Bill lives in a small apartment. Bill had been in his room at home. When his mother was not able to rouse him, she dialed 911 for an ambulance. A syringe and some white powder were found next to Bill. Bill's breathing is labored, and his pupils are constricted. Vital signs are taken; his blood pressure is 60/40 mm Hg, and his pulse is 132 beats per minute. Bill's situation is determined to be life threatening. Bill's mother is extremely distressed, but she is able to report to the staff that Bill has a substance abuse problem and had been taking heroin for 6 months before entering a methadone maintenance program. It is decided at this point to administer a narcotic antagonist, and naloxone is given intramuscularly. After this, Bill's breathing improves, and he responds to verbal stimuli. Bill's mother later tells staff that Bill has been in the methadone maintenance program for the past year but has not attended the program or received his methadone for the past week. At their urging, she calls the program, which arranges to send an outreach worker, Mr. Rodriguez, to talk to her and Bill. Bill makes an appointment with Mr. Rodriguez for the following Monday. Mr. Rodriguez knows that Bill's future ultimately rests with Bill. On Monday, Mr. Rodriguez talks to Bill regarding how Bill perceives his situation, where Bill wants to go, and what Bill thinks he needs to get there.

DIALOGUE	THERAPEUTIC TOOL/COMMENT
Mr. Rodriguez: I was in the emergency department Friday afternoon when you were brought in by ambulance.	Placing the event in time and sequence, validating the precipitating event
Bill: Were you? I guess a lot of people thought it was over for me.	
Mr. Rodriguez: It certainly looked quite serious.	Emphasizing the reality—prevents minimizing the situation
Bill: Yeah. I should never have left the program. I was doing better, and I just didn't think I needed it anymore.	
Mr. Rodriguez: You said you were doing well.	Reflecting
Bill: Yeah. I had a job, and I was beginning to save some money. Wow! I can't believe I blew this whole thing.	
Mr. Rodriguez: I don't know that you really did. Your counselor for the program phoned your doctor this morning to find out how you were doing.	Pointing out reality
Bill: Do you think they will take me back?	
Mr. Rodriguez: Why don't we talk some more, and after we finish, I'll speak with the other staff about your situation. If you would like to get back into the program, you can call your counselor and we'll support your decision.	Gathering information

After reviewing Bill's history, the health care team decides that a self-help, abstinence-oriented recovery program might be the most helpful treatment. Bill has not been taking drugs a long time, he has a job, and he appears motivated. Naltrexone (Trexan) will be given in conjunction with relapse prevention training, and Bill will regularly attend Narcotics Anonymous meetings.

General strategies for relapse prevention are cognitive and behavioral: recognizing and learning how to avoid or cope with threats to recovery; changing lifestyle; learning how to participate fully in society without drugs; and securing help from other people, or social support. Box 27-5 and the Integrative Therapy box identify relapse prevention strategies.

Self-Help Groups for Client and Family

Counseling and support should be encouraged for all families with a drug-dependent member. **Al-Anon** and **Alateen** are self-help groups that offer support and guidance for adults and teenagers, respectively, in families with a chemically dependent member. Other such organizations include Adult Children of Alcoholics (ACA), Pills Anonymous (PA), and Narcotics Anonymous (NA), to name but a few.

BOX 27-5

Relapse Prevention Strategies

Basics
1. Keep the program simple at first; 40% to 50% of clients who abuse substances have mild to moderate cognitive problems while actively using.
2. Review instructions with health team members.
3. Use a notebook and write down important information and telephone numbers.

Skills
Take advantage of cognitive-behavioral therapy to increase your coping skills. Identify which important life skills are needed:
1. Which situations do you have difficulty handling?
2. Which situations are you managing more effectively?
3. For which situations would you like to develop more skills to act more effectively?

Relapse Prevention Groups
Become a member of a relapse prevention group. These groups work on
1. Rehearsing stressful situations using a variety of techniques.
2. Finding ways to deal with current problems or ones that are likely to arise as you become drug free.
3. Providing role models to help you make necessary life changes.

Enhancement of Personal Insight
Therapy—group, individual, or family—can help you gain insight and control over a variety of psychological concerns, for example:
1. What drives your addictions?
2. What constitutes a healthy supportive relationship?
3. How can you increase your sense of self and self-worth?
4. What does your addictive substance give you that you think you need and cannot find otherwise?

Adapted from Zerbe, K. J. (1999). *Women's mental health in primary care* (pp. 94-95). Philadelphia: Saunders.

INTEGRATIVE THERAPY

Therapeutic touch (TT) is an alternative, nontraditional health care practice used by some nurses in traditional health care settings. TT has been endorsed by the National League for Nursing. Nurses who practice TT use their hands to direct energy into the fields of the patient to redirect flow in areas of accumulated tension and transmit energy. Balance in the patient's energy field translates into a state of health. Fewer relapses occurred in a group of alcohol and drug abusers who received TT than in a group who did not. Perhaps this is because TT elevated the mood in the intervention group and improved family and social relationships.

Hagemaster, J. (2000). Use of therapeutic touch in treatment of drug addictions. *Holistic Nursing Practice, 14*(3), 14-20.

Self-help groups assist family members in dealing with many common issues. Their work is based on a combination of educational and operational principles centered around acceptance of the disease model of addiction, including pragmatic methods for avoiding enabling behaviors.

Twelve-Step Programs

The most effective treatment modality for all addictions has been the 12-step program. Alcoholics Anonymous (AA) is the prototype for all the 12-step programs that were subsequently developed for many types of addiction. These programs offer the behavioral, cognitive, and dynamic structure needed in recovery. Three basic concepts are fundamental to all 12-step programs:

1. Individuals with addictive disorders are powerless over their addiction, and their lives are unmanageable.
2. Although individuals with addictive disorders are not responsible for their disease, they are responsible for their recovery.
3. Individuals can no longer blame people, places, and things for their addiction; they must face their problems and their feelings.

Using the 12 steps is often referred to as "working the steps" and helps a person refrain from addictive behaviors as well as fostering individual change and growth. In addition to AA, other 12-step programs include PA, NA, Cocaine Anonymous (CA), and Valium Anonymous.

Residential Programs

Residential treatment programs are best suited for individuals who have a long history of antisocial behavior. The goal of treatment is to effect a change in lifestyle, including abstinence, development of social skills, and elimination of antisocial behavior. Follow-up studies suggest that clients who stay in such programs 90 days or longer exhibit a significant decrease in illicit drug use and recorded arrests and an increase in legitimate employment. Length of stay increases when treatment is family focused (McComish et al., 2000). Synanon, Phoenix House, and Odyssey House are three of the more familiar names among the 300-plus therapeutic communities in the United States.

Intensive Outpatient Programs

Most treatment for substance-abusing clients takes place in the community. Clinical Pathway 27-1 provides an example of the steps addicted people follow in an intensive outpatient program, which includes a variety of psychotherapeutic and pharmacological interventions along with behavioral monitoring.

Intensive outpatient treatment programs are becoming more popular because they are viewed as flexible, diverse, cost effective, and responsive to the specific needs of the individual. Reduction in program length can significantly increase the number of patients completing a program without affecting clinical effectiveness (Bamford et al., 2003).

Outpatient Drug-Free Programs and Employee Assistance Programs

Outpatient drug-free programs are better suited to the polydrug-abusing or alcoholic client than to the client who is heavily addicted to heroin. These centers may offer vocational education and placement, counseling, and individual or group psychotherapy. Employee assistance programs have been developed to provide the delivery of mental health services in occupational settings. Many hospitals and corporations offer their employees counseling and support as an alternative to job termination when the employee's work performance is negatively affected by his or her impairment.

Psychopharmacology

The predominant somatic therapies are intended to support detoxification (management of withdrawal) or to alter drug use (e.g., disulfiram [Antabuse], methadone, and naltrexone).

Alcohol Withdrawal Treatment

Not all people who stop drinking require management of withdrawal. This decision depends on the length of time and the amount the client has been drinking, the prior history of withdrawal complications, and overall health status. Medication should not be given until the symptoms of withdrawal are seen. Drugs that are useful in treating alcohol withdrawal delirium are listed in Table 27-9.

Treatment of Alcoholism

Naltrexone (Trexan, Revia). Naltrexone—an agent used for narcotic addiction—is sometimes used in the treatment of alcoholism, especially for those with high levels of craving and somatic symptoms.

Intensive Outpatient Program for Substance Abuse

First 4 Weeks	Next 6 Weeks	Next 2 Weeks
Assessment		
Evaluation (CAC) H&P (MDs, NPs, PAs)	Completion of initial treatment plan Completion of diagnostic summary First treatment plan review	Ongoing monitoring of abstinence Second treatment plan review
Diagnostic Studies		
Routine laboratory tests* Complete or partial physical examination	Review of laboratory results	Follow-up laboratory tests and workup as needed
Medications		
Written orders	Medication monitoring, prn Routine laboratory tests and measure- ment of medication levels*	
Treatment Activity		

Individual counseling, psychoeducational
    groups, random drug screens—
    monitoring of results; random alcohol
    saliva tests—monitoring of results;
    attendance at AA/NA meetings.
	→	→

Teaching		

Explanation of disease concept of
    alcoholism/addiction
Beginning of family education sessions;
    explanation of rules and regulations
	Education on feelings, 12 steps, relapse
	    prevention, post–acute withdrawal
	    symptoms, anger management,
	    spirituality of recovery
		→

Discharge Planning		
Initial assessment of discharge needs	Review of discharge status	Revision of discharge needs Transfer of client to aftercare phase
Consults		
Psychiatric specialists (for evaluations) Subspecialists or legal authorities*	→	→
Patient Outcomes		
Verbalizes understanding of concept	Verbalizes feeling states Verbalizes relapse triggers	Presents first step Receives peer evaluation
Attends 12-step AA meeting 3 times per week	→	Gives life story
Abstains from all mood-altering substances	→	Gives peer goals to complete Presents completed peer goals to peers
	Develops strategies to avoid relapse Prepares first step: relapse prevention	Graduates to aftercare phase of program

Modified from Mary T. Pfister, RN, MHA, Mountainside Hospital, Glen Ridge/Montclair, NJ.
AA, Alcoholics Anonymous; *CAC*, community alcohol center; *H&P*, history and physical; *NA*, Narcotics Anonymous; *MDs*, physicians; *NPs*, nurse practitioners; *PAs*, physician assistants.
*As indicated.

Naltrexone works by blocking opiate receptors, thereby interfering with the mechanism of reinforcement and reducing or eliminating the alcohol craving (Srisurapanont & Jarusuraisin, 2002) (see the Evidence-Based Practice box). As of 2004, clinical trials are showing promising results for a long-acting injectable form called Vivitrex.

Acamprosate (Campral). **Acamprosate** is a second medication used to treat alcoholism that was approved by the Food and Drug Administration in 2004. It has been widely used in Europe for 15 years, and studies show that it helps clients abstain from alcohol, although the mechanism of action is not understood (HealthDayNews, 2004).

TABLE 27-9

Treatment of Alcohol Withdrawal Delirium

Drug	Dosage	Purpose
Sedatives		
Benzodiazepines		
Chlordiazepoxide (Librium) (drug of choice)	25-100 mg PO q4h tapered to zero over 5-7 days	Chlordiazepoxide and diazepam are cross-addicting, provide *safe* withdrawal, and have *anticonvulsant* effects
Diazepam (Valium)	5-10 mg PO q2-4h in tapering doses	Has anticonvulsant qualities
Oxazepam (Serax) or lorazepam (Ativan)	30-90 mg PO qid and 45 mg at bedtime and tapered to zero over 5-7 days	Not metabolized in the liver
Thiamine (vitamin B$_1$) Given intramuscularly or intravenously before glucose loading	100 mg PO qd for 3 days	Prevents Wernicke's encephalopathy
Magnesium sulfate Especially if history of seizures	1 g IM q6h for 2 days	Increases effectiveness of vitamin B$_1$ Helps reduce postwithdrawal seizures
Anticonvulsant Phenobarbital		For seizure control
Folic acid	1 mg PO qid	Most effective in short time
Multivitamins	1 daily	Malabsorption due to heavy long-term alcohol abuse causes deficiencies in many vitamins

Data from Weinrieb, R. M., & O'Brien, C. P. (1997). Diagnosis and treatment of alcoholism. In D. L. Dunner (Ed.), *Current psychiatric therapy II* (pp. 153-156). Philadelphia: Saunders; Franklin, J. E., & Frances, R. F. (1999). Alcohol and other psychoactive substances use disorders. In R. E. Hales, S. C. Yudofsky, & J. A. Talbott (Eds.), *The American Psychiatric Press textbook of psychiatry* (3rd ed.). Washington, DC: American Psychiatric Press.

 EVIDENCE-BASED PRACTICE

Use of Opioid Antagonists for Alcohol Dependence

Background

Many clients recovering from alcohol dependence complain of alcohol cravings, and medication might be able to reduce this risk for relapse. The results of animal studies suggest that opioid antagonists may prevent the reinforcing effects of alcohol consumption. Naltrexone, an opioid antagonist, has been studied for its benefits in treating alcohol dependence.

Studies

Nineteen controlled studies have been completed to determine the effectiveness of opioid antagonists in relapse prevention, in comparison to placebo, other medications, and psychosocial treatments. Discontinuation rate, death, client satisfaction, functioning, health-related quality of life, and economic outcomes were evaluated.

Results of Studies

Clients who took naltrexone were significantly less likely to return to drinking and spent less time drinking than clients who took a placebo. However, treatment discontinuation rates were similar for both groups. The naltrexone-treated clients consumed smaller amounts of alcohol than placebo-treated clients for 6 months. It is concluded that 50 mg/day of naltrexone is effective for treatment of alcohol dependence in short-term therapy, perhaps no longer than 3 to 6 months. Naltrexone should be given concurrently with psychosocial intervention.

Implications for Nursing Practice

The nurse should encourage the client's consistent compliance with the daily medication regimen. Positive changes in drinking patterns such as lower consumption and fewer drinking episodes need to be reinforced. The nurse can also recommend that psychosocial intervention accompany any naltrexone treatment.

Srisurapanont, M., & Jarusuraisin, N. (2005). Opioid antagonists for alcohol dependence (Cochrane Review). *The Cochrane Library*, Issue 4, 1-2.

Disulfiram (Antabuse). **Disulfiram** is used with motivated clients who have shown the ability to stay sober. Disulfiram works on the classical conditioning principle of inhibiting impulsive drinking because the client tries to avoid the unpleasant physical effects caused by the alcohol-disulfiram reaction. These effects consist of facial flushing, sweating, throbbing headache, neck pain, tachycardia, respiratory distress, a potentially serious decrease in blood pressure, and nausea and vomiting. The adverse reaction usually begins within minutes to a half-hour after drinking and may last 30 to 120 minutes. These symptoms are usually followed by drowsiness and are gone after the person naps.

Disulfiram must be taken daily. The action of the drug can last from 5 days to 2 weeks after the last dose. It is most effectively used early in the recovery process while the individual is making the major life changes associated with long-term recovery from alcoholism. Disulfiram should always be prescribed with the full knowledge and consent of the client. The client needs to be told about the side effects and must be well aware that any substances that contain alcohol can trigger an adverse reaction. Three primary sources of hidden alcohol exist—food, medicines, and preparations that are applied to the skin. People also need to be careful to avoid inhaling fumes from substances that might contain alcohol, such as paints, wood stains, and stripping compounds. Voluntary compliance with the disulfiram regimen is often poor. Counseling is recommended as an adjunct to treatment (O'Farrell & Fals-Stewart, 2002). Court-ordered disulfiram treatment can also be helpful (Martin et al., 2003).

Treatment of Opioid Addiction

Methadone (Dolophine). **Methadone** is a synthetic opiate that blocks the craving for and effects of heroin. It has to be taken every day, is highly addicting, and when stopped produces withdrawal. For methadone to be effective, the client must take a dose that will prevent withdrawal symptoms, block drug craving, and block any effects of illicit use of short-acting narcotics.

A methadone maintenance program is not considered to be an effective treatment in itself. At times, it keeps the client out of the illegal drug subculture, but to be successful, programs must include counseling and job training (Sees et al., 2000). Methadone maintenance reduces heroin addicts' risk of infection with HIV by reducing the occurrence of drug injection.

Methadone is the only medication currently approved for the treatment of the pregnant opioid addict. The clinical studies available demonstrate that methadone maintenance at the appropriate dosage, when combined with prenatal care and a comprehensive program of support, can significantly improve fetal and neonatal outcome.

L-α-Acetylmethadol (LAAM). As an alternative to methadone, **LAAM** is effective for up to 3 days (72 to 96 hours), so clients need to come to an outpatient facility for their medication only three times a week. This regimen makes it easier for clients to keep jobs and gives them more freedom than is available with methadone maintenance. LAAM is also an addictive narcotic: its therapeutic effects and side effects are the same as those of morphine.

Naltrexone (Trexan, Revia). **Naltrexone** is a relatively pure antagonist that blocks the euphoric effects of opioids. It has low toxicity and few side effects. A single dose provides an effective opiate blockade for up to 72 hours. Taking naltrexone three times a week is sufficient to maintain a fairly high level of opiate blockade. For many clients, long-term use results in gradual extinction of drug-seeking behaviors. Naltrexone does not produce dependence. As previously mentioned, it has also been approved for the treatment of alcoholism because it decreases the pleasant, reinforcing effects of alcohol.

Clonidine (Catapres). **Clonidine** was initially marketed for high blood pressure, but it is also an effective somatic treatment for some chemically dependent individuals when combined with naltrexone. Clonidine is a nonopioid suppresser of opioid withdrawal symptoms. It is also nonaddicting.

Buprenorphine (Subutex). **Buprenorphine** is a partial opioid agonist. At low doses (2 to 4 mg/day sublingually), the drug blocks signs and symptoms of opioid withdrawal. In experimental studies, buprenorphine has been shown to suppress heroin use in both inpatient and outpatient settings (APA, 2000b).

Treatment of Nicotine Addiction

Transdermal administration of nicotine doubles long-term tobacco abstinence rates. The nicotine patch is preferred over nicotine gum because compliance with the treatment regimen is better, blood levels are steadier, little long-term dependence occurs, and instructions are less complicated.

■ EVALUATION

Favorable treatment outcome is judged by increased lengths of time in abstinence, decreased denial, acceptable occupational functioning, improved family relationships, and, ultimately, ability to relate normally and comfortably to other human beings.

The ability to use existing supports and skills learned in treatment is important for ongoing recovery. For example, recovery is actively viable if, in response to cues to use the substance, the client calls his or her sponsor or other recovering persons; increases attendance at 12-step meetings, aftercare, or other group meetings; or writes feelings in a log and considers alternative action. Continuous monitoring and evaluation increase the chances for prolonged recovery.

Mr. Young, aged 49 years, and his wife arrive in the emergency department one evening, fearful that he has had a stroke. His right hand is limp and he is unable to hyperextend his right wrist. Sensation to the fingertips in his right hand is impaired.

Mr. Young looks much older than his stated age; in fact, he looks about 65. His complexion is ruddy and flushed. History taking is difficult. Mr. Young answers only what is asked of him, volunteering no additional information. He states that he took a nap that afternoon and that when he awakened, he noticed the problems with his right arm.

Mr. Young reveals that he has been unemployed for 4 years because the company he worked for went bankrupt. He has been unable to find a new job but has a job interview in 10 days. His wife is now working full time, so the family finances are okay. They have two grown children who no longer live at home. As he relates this, momentarily his lips start to tremble and his eyes fill with tears.

He denies any significant medical illness except for high blood pressure, just diagnosed last year. His family history is positive for depression in his father, and his mother is a recovering alcoholic. Ms. Dee, the admitting nurse, asks Mr. Young questions about his mood and use of alcohol, including quantity, frequency, and withdrawal experiences. In general, he denies depression and any significant alcohol involvement. Ms. Dee shares with him the fact that depression and alcoholism run in families. She asks Mr. Young (1) whether he knows this and (2) whether it concerns him with regard to his own drinking. Mr. Young says that he knows and that he does not want to think about it.

Ms. Dee then speaks with Mrs. Young about the events of the day. Ms. Dee states that she spoke with Mr. Young and that she is concerned that he might have an alcohol problem. Ms. Dee shares the impressions that led her to that tentative conclusion and asks Mrs. Young to describe her husband's involvement with alcohol. Mrs. Young's shoulders slump; she sighs and says, "I have spent the entire day talking to a counselor at the local treatment center to see if I can get him in. He won't admit that he has a problem." Mrs. Young then recounts a 6-year history of steadily increasing alcohol use. She says that for a while she could not admit to herself that her husband was an excessive drinker. "He tried to hide it, but gradually I knew. I could tell from little changes that he was intoxicated. I couldn't believe it was happening because he had been through the same thing with his mother and we'd always had such a good relationship. I thought I knew him. Actually, I guess I did when he was a working man. Being unemployed and unable to find a job has really floored him. And now he's even going to job interviews intoxicated."

Mrs. Young recounts how her husband's drinking worsened dramatically with unemployment and how she tried ridding their home of liquor, only to find bottles hidden in their mobile home one day when she went to clean it. She describes her feelings, which are like an emotional roller coaster—elated and hopeful when he seems to be doing okay; dejected and desperate on other occasions, such as the time that she found the alcohol in their mobile home. She has threatened to leave him. Mrs. Young hates going to work for fear of what he might do while she is gone. She says she is terrified that one day her husband will crack up the car and kill himself, because he often drives when intoxicated. He tells her not to worry because the life insurance policy is paid up. Ms. Dee discusses with Mrs. Young her own involvement as part of the family system. Options for Mrs. Young and her husband are discussed.

Meanwhile, the physician in the emergency department has examined Mr. Young. The diagnosis is radial nerve palsy. Mr. Young most likely passed out while lying on his arm. Because Mr. Young was intoxicated, he did not feel the signals that his nerves sent out to warn him to move (numbness, tingling). Mr. Young continued to lie in this position for so long that the resultant cutoff of circulation was sufficient to cause some temporary nerve damage.

Mr. Young's BAL is 0.31 mg%. This is three times the legal limit for intoxication in many states (0.1 mg%). Even though he has a BAL of 0.31 mg%, Mr. Young is alert and oriented, not slurring his speech or giving any other outward signs of intoxication. The difference between Mr. Young's BAL and his behavior indicates the development of tolerance, a symptom of physical dependence.

■ ASSESSMENT

Ms. Dee organizes her data into objective and subjective components.

Objective Data
- Driving when intoxicated
- Covert references to death
- Nerve damage due to having passed out while lying on arm
- Increased alcohol use during stress of unemployment
- Capacity to obtain employment impaired by alcohol use
- Disruption in marital relationship caused by alcohol use
- Inability to see effects of his drinking
- Family history of alcoholism and depression
- BAL three times the legal limit of intoxication; has developed tolerance

Subjective Data
- Denies he has an alcohol problem
- Denies he has depression

Self-Assessment

The denial the alcoholic client exhibits often results in rejection by nurses, who feel that the alcoholic causes his or her own problems. Nurses generally feel sympathetic toward spouses and other family members but have a sense of helplessness about the ability to effect change.

Feelings of rejection, sympathy, and helplessness impair the nurse's ability to facilitate change. True, some alcoholic persons do maintain their denial and effectively resist intervention, but many others welcome the opportunity to begin to learn different ways of coping with life problems. Before dismissing alcoholic clients as "not wanting help" or being "the only ones who can change things," nurses need to ask themselves if they have done all that they can in an attempt to engage the client in the change process.

Ms. Dee has seen many clients with the disease of alcoholism make radical changes in their lives, and she has learned to view alcoholism as a treatable disease. She is aware also that it is the client who makes the changes, and she no longer feels responsible when a client is not ready to make that change.

■ NURSING DIAGNOSIS (NANDA)

From the data, the nurse formulates the following nursing diagnoses:

1. *Risk for suicide* related to depressed mood, as evidenced by
   - Dangerous behavior: driving when drinking
   - Full payment of life insurance policy

2. *Ineffective coping* related to alcohol use, as evidenced by
   - Increased alcohol use during stressful period of unemployment
   - Impairment in capacity to obtain employment caused by alcohol use
   - Disruption in marital relationship caused by alcohol use
   - Inability to see effect of his drinking on his life functioning

■ OUTCOME CRITERIA (NOC)

Long-term outcome: Client will consistently demonstrate effective coping.

■ PLANNING

The initial plan is to allow Mr. Young to sober up in the emergency department before discussing goals. After he is sober, the nurse establishes realistic outcomes with him.

■ INTERVENTION (NIC)

Mr. Young's plan of care is personalized as follows.

Nursing diagnosis: *Risk for suicide* related to depressed mood, as evidenced by dangerous behavior and full payment of life insurance policy
Outcome criteria: Client will consistently demonstrate suicide self-restraint.

Short-Term Goal	Intervention	Rationale	Evaluation
1. Client will seek treatment for depression.	**1a.** Determine presence and degree of suicidal risk. **1b.** Refer client to mental health care provider for evaluation and treatment.	**1a.** Risk of suicide is increased in substance-using clients. **1b.** Addressing both substance use and mental health treatment needs improves outcomes.	GOAL MET After 3 weeks, client attends appointment at local clinic and has started taking an antidepressant.

Nursing diagnosis: *Ineffective coping* related to alcohol use, as evidenced by increased alcohol use and impairment in life functioning
Outcome criteria: Client will demonstrate mild to no change in health status and social functioning due to substance addiction.

Continued

Short-Term Goal	Intervention	Rationale	Evaluation
1. Client will consistently acknowledge personal consequences associated with alcohol misuse.	**1a.** Identify with client those factors (genetics, stress) that contribute to chemical dependence. **1b.** Assist client to identify negative effects of chemical dependency.	**1a.** Emphasis on alcoholism as a disease can lower guilt and increase self-esteem. **1b.** Begins to decrease denial and increase problem-solving.	GOAL MET Client admits that he cannot find a new job when he is intoxicated.
2. Client will commit to alcohol use control strategies.	**2a.** Determine history of alcohol use. **2b.** Identify support groups in community for long-term substance use treatment (for wife also).	**2a.** Identifies high-risk situations. **2b.** Alcohol dependence requires long-term treatment; AA is effective.	GOAL MET After 3 weeks, client states that he attends AA every day. He is learning about his triggers and new coping skills. His wife attends Al-Anon.

■ EVALUATION

See individual outcomes and evaluation in the care plan.

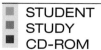 Visit the Evolve website at **http://evolve.elsevier.com/Varcarolis** for a full case study of this client and more case studies and nursing care plans.

■■■■ KEY POINTS to REMEMBER

- Substance use and dependence occur on a continuum, and addiction develops over a period of time.
- The cause of substance use disorders is a combination of genetic, biological, and environmental factors.
- Assessment of clients with substance use disorders needs to be comprehensive, aimed at identifying common medical and psychiatric comorbidities.
- Clients with a dual diagnosis have more severe symptoms, experience more crises, and require longer treatment for successful outcomes.
- Substance use disorders affect the family system of the client and may lead to codependent behavior in family members.
- Relapse is an expected complication of substance use disorders, and treatment includes a significant focus on teaching relapse prevention.
- Successful treatments include a dual-diagnosis approach, self-help groups, psychotherapy, therapeutic communities, and psychopharmacotherapy.
- Nurses need to be aware of their own feelings about substance use so that they can provide empathy and hope to clients.

- Nurses themselves are at higher risk for substance use disorders and should be vigilant for signs of impairment in colleagues to assure client safety and referral to treatment for the chemically dependent nurse.

■■■

Visit the Evolve website at **http://evolve.elsevier.com/Varcarolis** for a posttest on the content in this chapter.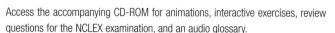

■ STUDENT
■ STUDY
■ CD-ROM

Access the accompanying CD-ROM for animations, interactive exercises, review questions for the NCLEX examination, and an audio glossary.

■ NURSE,
■ CLIENT, AND
■ FAMILY RESOURCES

For suggested readings, information on related associations, and Internet resources, go to **http://evolve.elsevier.com/Varcarolis**.

Critical Thinking and Chapter Review

Visit the Evolve website at **http://evolve.elsevier.com/Varcarolis** for additional self-study exercises.

evolve

■ ■ ■ CRITICAL THINKING

1. Write a paragraph describing your possible reactions to a drug-dependent client to whom you are assigned.

    A. Would your response be different depending on the substance, for example, alcohol versus heroin, or marijuana versus cocaine? Give reasons for your answers.

    B. Would your response be different if the substance-dependent person were a professional colleague? How?

2. Rosetta Seymour is a 15-year-old teenager who has started using heroin nasally.

    A. Briefly discuss the trend in heroin use among teenagers.

    B. When Ms. Seymour asks you why she needs to take more and more to get "high," how would you explain to her the concept of tolerance?

    C. If she had just taken heroin, what would you find on assessment of physical and behavioral-psychological signs and symptoms?

    D. If she came into the emergency department with an overdose of heroin, what would be the emergency care? What might be effective long-term care?

3. Tony Garmond is a 45-year-old mechanic. He has a 20-year history of heavy drinking and he says he wants to quit drinking but needs help.

    A. Role-play with a classmate an initial assessment. Identify the kinds of information you would need to have in order to plan holistic care.

    B. Mr. Garmond tried stopping by himself but is in the emergency department with delirium tremens. What are the dangers for Mr. Garmond? What are the appropriate medical interventions?

    C. What are some possible treatment alternatives for Mr. Garmond when he is safely detoxified? How would you explain to him the usefulness and function of AA? What are some additional treatment options that might be useful to Mr. Garmond? What are available as referrals for Mr. Garmond in your community?

■ ■ ■ CHAPTER REVIEW

Choose the most appropriate answer.

1. When intervening with a client who is intoxicated from alcohol, it is useful for the nurse to first

    1. let the client sober up.

    2. decide immediately on care goals.

    3. ask what drugs other than alcohol the client has recently used.

    4. gain compliance by sharing personal drinking habits with the client.

2. A principle of counseling intervention that should be observed by the nurse caring for a chemically dependent client is to

    1. look for therapeutic leverage.

    2. communicate that relapses are expected.

    3. recognize that recovery is considered complete and absolute.

    4. remove unhealthy defenses, then assist the client in building new ones.

3. As the nurse evaluates the client's progress, which treatment outcome would indicate a poor general prognosis for long-term recovery from substance abuse?

    1. Client demonstrates improved self-esteem.

    2. Client demonstrates enhanced coping abilities.

    3. Client demonstrates improved relationships with others.

    4. Client demonstrates positive expectations for ongoing drug use.

4. Which statement provides a basis for planning care for a client who has abused CNS stimulants?

    1. Symptoms of intoxication include dilation of the pupils, dryness of the oronasal cavity, and excessive motor activity.

    2. Medical management focuses on removing the drugs from the body.

    3. Withdrawal is simple and rarely complicated.

    4. Postwithdrawal symptoms include fatigue and depression.

5. The provision of optimal care for clients withdrawing from substances of abuse is facilitated when the nurse understands that severe morbidity and mortality are often associated with withdrawal from

    1. alcohol and CNS depressants.

    2. CNS stimulants and hallucinogens.

    3. narcotic antagonists and caffeine.

    4. opiates and inhalants.

REFERENCES

American Psychiatric Association. (2000a). *Diagnostic and statistical manual of mental disorders (DSM-IV-TR)* (4th ed., text rev.). Washington, DC: Author.

American Psychiatric Association. (2000b). *Practice guidelines for the treatment of psychiatric disorders: Compendium 2000.* Washington, DC: Author.

Bamford, Z., et al. (2003). Treatment outcome following day care for alcohol dependency: The effects of reducing programme length. *Health and Social Care in the Community, 11*(5), 440-445.

Becker, K. L., & Walton-Moss, B. (2001). Detecting and addressing alcohol abuse in women. *Nurse Practitioner, 26*(10), 13-16, 19-23; quiz, 24-25.

Brown, R. L., et al. (2001). A two-item conjoint screen for alcohol and other drug problems. *Journal of the American Board of Family Practice, 14*(2), 95-106.

Compton, W. M., et al. (2003). The role of psychiatric disorders in predicting drug dependence treatment outcomes. *American Journal of Psychiatry, 160*(5), 890-895.

Cornelius, J., et al. (2003). Alcohol and psychiatric comorbidity. *Recent Developments in Alcoholism, 16*, 361-374.

Dochterman, J. M., & Bulechek, G. M. (2004). *Nursing interventions classification (NIC)* (4th ed.). St. Louis, MO: Mosby.

Espeland, K. E. (2000). Inhalant abuse. *Lippincott's Primary Care Practice, 4*, 336.

Farris, C., et al. (2003). A comparison of schizophrenic patients with or without coexisting substance use disorder. *Psychiatric Quarterly, 74*(3), 205-222.

Frye, M. A., et al. (2003). Gender differences in prevalence, risk, and clinical correlates of alcoholism comorbidity in bipolar disorder. *American Journal of Psychiatry, 160*(5), 883-889.

HealthDayNews. (2004). *Helping alcoholics stay sober: Campral works to prevent relapses.* Retrieved March 12, 2005, from http://myhealth.medcenterone.com/healthnews/healthday/040802HD520435.htm?DisplayP.

Hopfer, C. J., et al. (2002). Adolescent heroin use: A review of the descriptive and treatment literature. *Journal of Substance Abuse Treatment, 23*(3), 231-237.

Judd, P., et al. (2003). A dual diagnosis demonstration project: Treatment outcomes and cost analysis. *Journal of Psychoactive Drugs, 35*(Suppl. 1), 181-192.

Leshner, A. I. (2000). A club drug alert. *NIDA Notes, 14*(6), 3-4.

Lingford-Hughes, A. R., et al. (2003). Addiction. *British Medical Bulletin, 65*(4), 209-222.

Martin, B., et al. (2003). Compliance to supervised disulfiram therapy: A comparison of voluntary and court-ordered patients. *American Journal of the Addictions, 12*(2), 137-143.

McComish, J. F., et al. (2000). Survival analysis of three treatment modalities in a residential substance abuse program for women and children. *Outcomes Management for Nursing Practice, 4*(2), 71.

Miller, T. R., Lestina, D. C., & Smith, G. S. (2001). Injury risk among medically identified alcohol and drug abusers. *Alcoholism: Clinical and Experimental Research, 25*(1), 54-59.

Minkoff, K. (2003). Dual diagnoses. In A. Tasman, J. Kay, & J. A. Lieberman (Eds.), *Psychiatry* (2nd ed., Vol. 2, pp. 2333-2341). West Sussex, England: Wiley.

Moorhead, S., Johnson, M., & Maas, M. (2004). *Nursing outcomes classification (NOC)* (3rd ed.). St. Louis, MO: Mosby.

Morgan, M. J. (2000). Ecstasy (MDMA): A review of possible persistent effects. *Psychopharmacology (Berlin), 152*(3), 230-241.

Mueser, K. T., et al. (2001). Community-based treatment of schizophrenia and other severe mental disorders: Treatment outcomes. *Medscape Mental Health, 6*(1), 1-31.

National Institute on Drug Abuse. (2001, April 23). *Study clarifies brain mechanisms of cocaine's high.* Retrieved February 22, 2005, from http://www.drugabuse.gov/MedAdv/01/NR4-23.html.

Negrete, J. (2003). Clinical aspects of substance abuse in persons with schizophrenia. *Canadian Journal of Psychiatry, 48*(1), 14-21.

O'Farrell, T. J., & Fals-Stewart, W. (2002). Behavioral couples and family therapy for substance abusers. *Current Psychiatry Reports, 4*(5), 371-376.

Resnick, B., et al. (2003). The impact of alcohol use in community-dwelling older adults. *Journal of Community Health Nursing, 20*(3), 135-145.

Sadock, B. J., & Sadock, V. A. (2003). *Synopsis of psychiatry: Behavioral science, clinical psychiatry* (9th ed.). Philadelphia: Lippincott Williams & Wilkins.

Schwartz, R. H., Milteer, R., & LeBeaur, M. A. (2000). Drug facilitated sexual assault ("date rape"). *Southern Medical Journal, 93*(6), 558-561.

Sees, K. L., et al. (2000). Methadone maintenance vs. 180-day psychosocially enriched detoxification for treatment of opioid dependence: A randomized controlled trial. *Journal of the American Medical Association, 283*(10), 1303.

Sinha, R., Drummond, D. C., & Orford, J. (2001). How does stress increase risk of drug abuse and relapse? *Psychopharmacology (Berlin), 158*(4), 343-359.

Sloan, A., & Vernarec, E. (2001). Impaired nurses: Reclaiming careers. *RN, 64*(2), 58-63, 64.

Sommers, M. S., et al. (2003). Assessing acute and critically ill patients for problem drinking. *Dimensions of Critical Care Nursing, 22*(2), 76-88.

Srisurapanont, M., & Jarusuraisin, N. (2005). Opioid antagonists for alcohol dependence (Cochrane Review). *The Cochrane Library*, Issue 4, 1-2.

Tuttle, J., et al. (2002). Adolescent drug and alcohol use. Strategies for assessment, intervention, and prevention. *Nursing Clinics of North America, 37*(3), 443-460, ix.

U.S. Department of Health and Human Services. (1999). *Mental Health: Culture, race and ethnicity. A supplement to Mental health: A report of the Surgeon General.* Retrieved February 6, 2004, from http://www.mentalhealth.org/cre/default.asp.

Webb, J. M., Carlton, E. F., & Geehan, D. M. (2000). Delirium in the intensive care unit: Are we helping the patient? *Critical Care Nursing Quarterly, 22*(4), 47-60.

Weir, E. (2000). Raves: A review of the culture, the drugs, and the prevention of harm. *Canadian Medical Association Journal, 162*(13), 1829-1830.

Severe Mental Illness: Crisis Stabilization and Rehabilitation

NANCY CHRISTINE SHOEMAKER ▪ ELIZABETH M. VARCAROLIS

KEY TERMS and CONCEPTS

The key terms and concepts listed here appear in color where they are defined or first discussed in this chapter.

OBJECTIVES

After studying this chapter, the reader will be able to

1. Discuss the behavior and symptoms of severe mental illness as they relate to the person's daily functioning and to family and other interpersonal relationships.
2. Describe three common problems associated with severe mental illness.
3. Explain six evidence-based practices for the care of the severely mentally ill person.
4. Explain the role of the nurse in the care of the severely mentally ill person.
5. Develop an outline for a psychoeducational teaching plan for a person with severe mental illness. (Choose one of your clients or a client in a facility you use in your clinical experience.)
6. Discuss the importance of medication and adherence to the medication regimen for the severely mentally ill client.

evolve Visit the Evolve website at **http://evolve.elsevier.com/Varcarolis** for a pretest on the content in this chapter.

SEVERE MENTAL ILLNESS

In this chapter, the focus is on the lifetime course of severe mental illness, such as schizophrenia, schizoaffective disorder, bipolar disorder, and even major depression. Characteristics of the population, particular problems, and important aspects of successful treatment are defined. Research has proven the effectiveness of six evidence-based practices for the treatment of the severely mentally ill. The perspective of the client is included through quotations from schizophrenic persons and vignettes describing the long-term treatment of a severely mentally ill client.

The term severe mental illness (SMI) refers to mental illness in individuals "that is characterized by pervasive impairments across different areas of function-ing, including social relationships, work, leisure, and self-care" (Mueser et al., 2001, p. 2). The illness is chronic, with remissions and exacerbations of varying lengths. Skill deficits range from an inability to prepare meals to an inability to cope with everyday stressors. Other terms that have been used in the literature for this population include *chronically mentally ill, seriously mentally ill,* and *severely and persistently mentally ill.*

The prevalence of serious mental illness in the United States was estimated in 2002 as 8.3% of adults, or 17.5 million Americans (Aquila & Emanuel, 2003). This population is at risk for multiple physical, emotional, and social problems as described later.

Chronicity can occur in persons of any gender, age, culture, or geographical location. However, this population includes two subgroups with unique characteristics: (1) those old enough to have experienced institutionalization (which was common before approximately 1975), and (2) those young enough to have been hospitalized only during acute exacerbations of their disorders.

Older Population

Before **deinstitutionalization** of the severely mentally ill beginning in 1975, psychiatric hospitals were the long-term residences for many people. Medical paternalism was a pervasive philosophical stance at that time. The health care approach to severely mentally ill persons was to make all their decisions for them. Clients became **institutionalized** (i.e., they could not think independently and lost the ability to problem solve). Much of an ill person's behavior came to reflect a combination of the disease process and the decreased sense of self that resulted from the lack of autonomy.

■ ■ ■ *VIGNETTE*

Marian was a resident at a facility for the severely and persistently impaired during her adolescence and young adulthood. On discharge, she moves to a community home, where she spends long periods sitting in front of the living room window. Marian does not ask to go out into the garden she watches for so many hours. Indeed, she rarely asks for anything, including snacks or recreational activities. The caregivers work with Marian for several months to help her to recognize her needs of the moment and then to articulate or act on them. There is a major celebration the day she walks into the kitchen and makes a peanut butter sandwich of her own volition. Some of the dependency caused by the institutionalization is being positively altered.

■ ■ ■

Younger Population

People young enough never to have been institutionalized do not have the problems of passivity and lack of autonomy. However, limited experience with formal treatment in short-term hospitalizations contributes to some clients' not truly believing that a problem exists. Denial, often coupled with the use of recreational drugs, puts severely ill young adults at particular risk for many additional problems, including legal difficulties and unemployment.

■ ■ ■ *VIGNETTE*

Robert is diagnosed with schizophrenia at the age of 26 years. For the next 15 years, he moves around the country, experiencing brief hospitalizations and receiving no outpatient treatment. Prior to his illness, he lived with his parents in a large eastern city and had graduated from high school. One day shortly after his twentieth birthday, he simply disappeared.

■ ■ ■

DEVELOPMENT OF A SEVERE MENTAL ILLNESS

Severe mental illness has much in common with persistent long-term physical illness. The original problem sets in motion an erosion of basic coping mechanisms and compensatory processes. As the disorder extends beyond the acute stage, more and more of the neighboring systems are involved. For example, with chronic congestive heart failure the lungs and kidneys begin to deteriorate. However, the disability of SMI may go much further in destroying a person's quality of life. In the case of an illness such as schizophrenia, a person's thought processes, ability to maintain contact with others, and ability to remain employed frequently deteriorate. For example, a person may have difficulty thinking clearly about even ordinary things such as grooming and conversation. This causes the person's interactions to be perceived as bizarre, unsatisfying, and anxiety provoking by both self and others. In turn, the person, friends, and even family members will hesitate to seek out interactions. Problematic communication escalates the tension in relationships and diminishes the person's self-esteem.

In the words of one schizophrenic client, "About this time my hallucinations began as voices. I remember walking to my room and hearing voices coming out of my closet. The voices of old friends and my sister were telling me that I was worthless and trash. These voices scared me" (Group for the Advancement of Psychiatry [GAP], 2000, p. 15).

People with SMI often miss out on making friends and sharing social activities that most people take for granted. In employment situations, the relationship between supervisor and employee is difficult to maintain. Social skills training and supportive interventions mentioned later in the chapter can make a positive difference in many of these people's lives.

Another similarity between physical illness and mental illness is the unpredictability of the disease course. Not knowing when the problem will exacerbate contributes additional stress. Those with SMI show a major deficit in mechanisms for coping with stress. The fear of relapse and avoidance of stress can cause a withdrawal from life that eventually heightens the person's social isolation and apathy, just as is the case with a physical dysfunction such as incontinence.

Exacerbations may decrease in frequency and intensity with careful attention to both the history of the disease itself and awareness of daily functioning. Assessment in these areas requires thorough and regular evaluation by an interdisciplinary psychiatric team (nurse, physician, social worker, occupational therapist). In this way, symptoms of relapse may be noted before the onset of more dramatic deterioration. As indicated by the aphorism "A stitch in time saves nine," assessing an early symptom and initiating treatment can decrease the severity of the exacerbation and the accompanying disruption of the person's life.

Rehabilitation is a critically important concept for people with an SMI. Rehabilitation addresses the disabilities and inabilities resulting from long-term mental illness and teaches alternative behaviors. Just as in medical-surgical nursing, the best mental health rehabilitation begins on the first day of acute care and continues after discharge from the facility. Achievement of success in discharge planning for community aftercare requires careful attention to the client's economic status. Lack of income and health insurance are barriers to effective treatment and rehabilitation (McAlpine & Mechanic, 2000). Appropriate referrals to enable the client to access public insurance programs are vital to assure adequate care.

Potential nursing diagnoses that apply to the severely mentally ill client are noted in Table 28-1.

COMMON PROBLEMS ASSOCIATED WITH SEVERE MENTAL ILLNESS

Access to Housing

Housing is the first priority of the seriously mentally ill once they are discharged from a hospital setting. Although 30% to 60% of clients with SMI return to their families, the remainder need safe housing (Mueser et al., 2001). People with SMI often cannot understand what others say, nor can they communicate their thoughts or needs to others. Some may retreat in confusion, others may have grandiose ideas of their abilities, and most cannot make sound judgments.

Without careful discharge planning and a strong social support system in place, many of the seriously mentally ill become homeless or missing. They often leave behind distraught families who are desperate for their return (National Alliance for the Mentally Ill [NAMI], 2000b). Studies consistently show that between 25% and 40% of homeless individuals have SMI,

TABLE 28-1

Potential Nursing Diagnoses for the Severely Mentally Ill Client

Signs and Symptoms	Nursing Diagnoses
Hallucinations	Disturbed sensory perception
Poor concentration	Disturbed thought processes
Inaccurate interpretation of environment	
Hypervigilance	
Non–reality-based thinking	
Inappropriate affect	
Mumbling or speaking too softly to be heard	Impaired verbal communication
Verbalization incongruent with the setting	Impaired social interaction
Absence of eye contact	Social isolation
Silence in groups or withdrawal when approached	
Failure to keep appointments	Noncompliance
Admitted missing of medication or observed return of symptoms	Ineffective coping
Repeated confusion about medication despite repeated teaching	
Self-negating verbalization	Chronic low self-esteem
Fear of trying new things or situations	Powerlessness
Nonassertiveness or passivity	
Inability to make decisions	
Unwashed face and body	Self-care deficit (bathing/hygiene, dressing/grooming)
Tangled, uncombed hair	
Inability to keep bathing supplies	
Mismatched clothing	
Indifference about appearance	
Distortion of client's health problem, often denial	Disabled family coping
Neglect of other members of family	Caregiver role strain
Excessive concern for and supervision of client	

not including people who have a primary diagnosis of substance abuse (NAMI, 2000b).

Some adults with SMI use temporary homeless shelters and local jails and prisons as permanent housing resources. What is even more disturbing is that many people with mental disabilities are using the public streets, sidewalks, parks, bus stations, and libraries as places to live (NAMI, 2000b).

There is a strong relationship between life without a home and the presence of a mental disorder. Life on the street or in a shelter, whether temporary or not, can have a very negative influence on a person's self-esteem. Homelessness on top of a fragile mental status may be all that is necessary to provoke a crisis leading to another hospitalization. Assistance in finding acceptable housing is critical if clients are to maintain themselves within the community and follow through on treatment and rehabilitation.

Nonadherence to Medication Regimen

The development of the atypical antipsychotic medications has renewed hope that more substantial improvement is possible for the chronically mentally ill client. Evidence-based pharmacological guidelines now recommend first-line treatment with atypical antipsychotics such as risperidone, olanzapine, or quetiapine (Risperdal Consta) (Mellman et al., 2001). In 2004, a long-acting injectable form of risperidone was released and may lead to decreased use of the older haloperidol decanoate and fluphenazine decanoate, which have more unpleasant side effects. The atypical antipsychotics do have possible side effects that require close medical monitoring: weight gain, hyperglycemia, type 2 diabetes mellitus, and cardiac problems (Nemeroff, 2004). The newer medications, when taken, do work. Treatment success rate is as follows (NAMI, 2000a):

- Bipolar disorder: 80%
- Major depression: 65%
- Schizophrenia: 60%

The severely mentally ill often fail to comply with the medication regimen, however. There are many reasons that people are nonadherent with their medication regimen. A review of the literature cites six common factors (Lacro & Glassman, 2004):

- Poor insight ("I don't have an illness")
- Negative attitude toward medication ("Taking medication is like taking dope")
- Previous history of nonadherence ("I get bad side effects every time they give me meds")
- Substance abuse ("I just smoke weed to help me relax")
- Inadequate discharge planning ("My medicine ran out and I didn't know where to go to get more")
- Poor therapeutic alliance with the treating clinician ("I don't trust my doctor")

In the words of one client who gave up on medication, "In the early years, I was consistently overmedicated and too doped up even to complain. . . . I failed at everything I tried" (GAP, 2000, p. 34).

There are other factors as well that decrease the effectiveness of medications (NAMI, 2000a). Not all clients with schizophrenia receive therapeutic dosages of medication, and long-term monitoring may be inadequate. Perhaps the most serious factor is the high cost of atypical antipsychotic medications. Lack of health insurance or limited medication choices in the public health care system pose barriers to access to this effective treatment.

Adequate monitoring of medication effects by the community-based health care provider is often difficult. Because the physical complications of pharmacotherapy are often subtle, they can be missed in the early stages. For example, constant smacking of the lips by a client may be mistaken for a manifestation of agitation and not recognized as an early sign of tardive dyskinesia. Baseline and periodic laboratory testing is needed to assess potential adverse effects of medications on liver and thyroid functions, blood cells, and lipid and blood glucose levels. Without early detection and treatment of medication complications, a person is at high risk for possible permanent impairment. For this reason, it is imperative for clients with SMI to see a physician regularly. In most clinical settings, the psychiatric nurse plays a significant role in medication teaching and monitoring.

Comorbid Medical Conditions

Ideally, there should be collaboration between the psychiatric team and the primary care provider. Multiple studies show that the severely mentally ill population is at higher risk for certain medical disorders. A large study of 26,000 Medicaid recipients showed increased prevalence of the following eight disorders in clients with a psychotic mental illness: diabetes, hypertension, heart disease, asthma, gastrointestinal disorders, skin infections, malignant neoplasms, and acute respiratory disorders (Dickey et al., 2002). When substance use was present, clients had even higher risks for some of these disorders. The mortality rate of individuals with schizophrenia is estimated to be twice that of the general population. Ten percent of deaths are due to suicide; other causes include accidents and medical illness (Patel et al., 2003).

Coexisting Substance Abuse

According to the 2002 National Survey on Drug Use and Health, 23.2% of adults with SMI had a substance use disorder, compared with 8.2% of adults without SMI (Aquila & Emanuel, 2003, p. 3). Persons with SMI suffer serious adverse consequences from substance use disorders. Research has demonstrated that integrated treatment programs that combine mental health and substance abuse interventions (dual-diagnosis treatment) offer more promise of success than traditional treatment through separate services (Drake & Mueser, 2000). Clinical consequences of substance abuse among the severely mentally ill include the following (Ryrie, 2000):

- Poor adherence to the medication regimen
- Increased rates of suicidal behavior
- Increased rates of violence
- Homelessness
- Worsening of psychotic symptoms
- Increase in human immunodeficiency virus (HIV) infection
- Increased use of institutional services

Stigma

Another problem experienced by the chronically mentally ill is the stigma of mental illness. Stigma is defined as "damage to reputation, the covert and sometimes overt shame and ridicule our society places on mental illness" (Vanderhorst, 2000, p. 41). It affects people through direct discrimination (e.g., refusal to hire), structural discrimination (e.g., fewer resources available for treatment or research), and social and psychological processes (e.g., negative beliefs based on family, peers, or media views) (Link et al., 2001). Studies have shown that clients with mental illness expect and fear rejection, which increases their tendency to avoid social contact. Clients feel that employment, friendships, and dating relationships are threatened by their illness. Surveys of the public reveal that many people believe that clients with mental illness are violent and unpredictable, despite research showing that violence occurs only in a minority of cases (Struening et al., 2001).

As one client explained, "We need to grieve the loss of normal lives, normal families, normal places in society. For me this is a continuous process that never ends. We are placed at the very lowest rung on the ladder of society. We are believed by many to be ax-murdering fiends—all of us, even though statistics do not bear this notion out" (GAP, 2000, p. 9).

■ ■ ■ *VIGNETTE*

After Robert leaves home, he enlists in the army and serves for 5 years. He settles on the West Coast and takes a job in the post office. In his first psychotic break, he becomes paranoid and threatening at work, and he is hospitalized briefly. Upon discharge, he refuses aftercare and will not take medication. He quits his job and moves to another city. For the next 15 years, he works intermittently, he is homeless off and on, and he drinks heavily whenever he has money. He is only hospitalized when his behavior is threatening to others. He consistently resists aftercare recommendations, showing no insight into his illness.

■ ■ ■

COMPREHENSIVE COMMUNITY RESOURCES

Ideally, the community-based mental health care system provides comprehensive, coordinated, and cost-effective care for the severely mentally ill client. However, in 2002, the President's New Freedom Commission on Mental Health evaluated the nation's mental health care system and concluded that services were fragmented and inefficient, particularly for the severely mentally ill. For example, services were very different from state to state, with blurring of responsibility among agencies, programs, and level of government. Many clients were noted to "fall through the cracks." Even those who received treatment had difficulty achieving financial independence because of limited job opportunities and the fear of losing health insurance in the workplace (President's New Freedom Commission on Mental Health, 2002).

The American Psychological Association released recommendations in 2003 for improving services to this population, including (1) passing federal legislation to provide full parity in insurance coverage for mental and physical health, (2) establishing mental health and suicide prevention as national priorities, (3) emphasizing consumer and family choices regarding care, and (4) identifying treatment modalities that have proven effective through research (American Psychological Association, 2003).

The overall goal of community psychiatric treatment is to improve the client's ability to function independently outside of the hospital setting (NAMI, 2000a). **Adult outpatient services** provide long-term mental health treatment, including depot intramuscular medication when necessary and response to crisis calls and walk-in requests for services, with evaluation for possible psychiatric hospitalization. **Psychosocial rehabilitation programs (PRPs)** are designed to provide daily structure for clients to promote socialization and vocational skills. **Case managers** serve as coordinators to ensure integration of and cooperation among the various elements of the system and to act as advocates for clients. Case management may be part of the role of the mental health therapist or may be a specific service offered by a comprehensive community mental health center.

A variety of services are focused on the mentally ill who have a dual diagnosis with alcohol or drug-related problems. Chemical dependency clinics provide therapeutic and rehabilitative services for alcoholics and drug abusers and their families. Services include medical and psychosocial assessment, detoxification, crisis intervention, and medication. Some clinics specialize in methadone treatment. Increasingly, treatment of mental illness and substance use is combined in the same facility, because of the abundant research that supports **dual-diagnosis treatment** as an evidence-based practice. Mental health staff are being trained in substance use treatment, and addiction staff are learning to address mental health issues (see Chapter 27).

Community mental health services are also designed to provide outreach and case management for seriously mentally ill persons who are homeless. Client participation in the program is voluntary. **Community outreach programs** send professional and nonprofessional workers into streets, parks, temporary shelters, bus stations, soup kitchens, and anywhere else the mentally ill may be found. A team approach is used to gain access to clients and to connect them with the various services available to meet their needs. The role of the outreach worker is to be an advocate in all areas of client need and to foster client self-care.

There are a variety of **housing options** for the seriously mentally ill client who is in treatment, ranging from facilities with 24-hour supervision to independent living. The highest level of structure is provided by a supervised residence associated with a PRP, which is a group home in which house staff are constantly available when the client is not attending the daytime program. Many clients who were institutionalized for years have been able to adjust to community life with intensive support. There are also group homes with intermittent staff supervision. Or clients may live with a caregiver in a board-and-care residence, where there is supervision with medication and a requirement for attendance at a day program. For clients who are more self-sufficient, apartments minimally supervised by a case manager are available. Eventually, some clients move to a totally independent apartment. Before appropriate housing is found, temporary shelters may provide a safe environment for individuals who have no other option.

Multiservice centers collaborate with the outreach unit in implementing individualized service plans for the persistently mentally ill. They supply hot meals, laundry and shower facilities, clothing, social activities, transportation to and from shelters, access to a telephone, and a mailing address for the person. Drop-in centers supported by mental health advocacy groups, which provide a safe environment for socialization and information on community resources, may also be available (see Chapter 6).

■ ■ ■ *VIGNETTE*

Finally, Robert returns home to his parents. Shortly thereafter, he is arrested for threatening a police officer with a steel pipe. He is found criminally not responsible and is released on the condition that he participate in mental health treatment. He attends a mental health clinic and receives intramuscular depot medication, due to his history of noncompliance. He is also enrolled in a PRP and is assigned a case manager. The case manager helps him to apply for Social Security income and also refers him to a group home when his elderly parents state that they can no longer live with him. Because he insists that he needs to work, he is referred to Goodwill Industries. He gets a job unloading delivery trucks and stays on that job for the next 5 years. When the requirements of his conditional release are completed, he continues in treatment and continues working nearly full time. Because he is stable, his medication is changed to an oral atypical antipsychotic, and he continues to receive supervision in his group home. He is discharged from the PRP.

■ ■ ■

OVERVIEW OF NURSING INTERVENTIONS

Nurses encounter the severely mentally ill in the acute psychiatric setting, community treatment setting, medical-surgical units, and clinics. All psychiatric nurses use the following basic interventions with these clients:

- Crisis intervention
- Psychobiological intervention
- Health teaching for clients and families
- Counseling
- Case management
- Milieu therapy
- Promotion of self-care activities
- Psychiatric rehabilitation

In addition, the advanced practice nurse may conduct group therapy or family therapy, or use cognitive-behavioral interventions. Refer to Box 28-1 for a sample of nursing interventions from the Nursing Interventions Classification (NIC) (Dochterman & Bulechek, 2004). The role of the nurse is illustrated in the following sections.

Case Management

Whether as a broker of services or as a therapist, the case manager can provide entrance into the system of care. Clients with SMI often have a variety of needs that span many different categories. Following through on multiple referrals to different agencies is beyond the coping capability of the chronically mentally ill. What is needed is "wraparound" services that care for the entire person. The role of the case manager is to coordinate access to psychiatric treatment, housing, rehabilitation or work setting, socialization assistance, and medical care (Aquila & Emanuel, 2003). One model of case management that has proven effective for severely mentally ill clients (another evidence-based practice) is known as **assertive community treatment (ACT)**, which provides all of the wraparound services noted (refer to Chapter 6 for an example). The case manager's role is completed when the client is able to independently access necessary services.

BOX 28-1

NIC Interventions for Severe Mental Illness

Reality Orientation

Definition: Promotion of patient's awareness of personal identity, time, and environment

Activities*:

- Approach patient slowly and from the front.
- Address patient by name when initiating interaction.
- Speak to patient in a slow, distinct manner with appropriate volume.
- Ask questions one at a time.
- Give one simple direction at a time.

Self-Care Assistance: Bathing/Hygiene

Definition: Assisting patient to perform personal hygiene

Activities*:

- Provide desired personal articles (e.g., deodorant, toothbrush, and bath soap).
- Monitor cleaning of nails, according to patient's self-care ability.
- Provide assistance until patient is fully able to assume self-care.

Self-Care Assistance: IADL

Definition: Assisting and instructing a person to perform instrumental activities of daily living (IADL) needed to function in the home or community

Activities*:

- Instruct individual on appropriate and safe storage of medications.
- Instruct individual on alternative methods of transportation (e.g., buses and bus schedules, taxis, city or county transportation for disabled people).
- Assist individual in establishing methods and routines for cooking, cleaning, and shopping.

Family Support

Definition: Promotion of family values, interests, and goals

Activities*:

- Determine the psychological burden of prognosis for family.
- Listen to family concerns, feelings, and questions.
- Accept the family's values in a nonjudgmental manner.
- Identify congruence between patient, family, and health professional expectations.

From Dochterman, J. M., & Bulechek, G. M. (2004). *Nursing interventions classification (NIC)* (4th ed.). St. Louis, MO: Mosby.
*Partial list.

OVERVIEW OF REHABILITATION

The long-term outcomes of rehabilitation for severely mentally ill clients include illness management and recovery (Mueser et al., 2002). *Illness management* refers to the focus in the early stage of treatment that assists the client in gaining control over symptoms. Clients are taught to

- Collaborate with professionals in mental health treatment.
- Reduce susceptibility to relapse.
- Cope more effectively with symptoms.

Recovery refers to outcomes following the relief of symptoms, with a focus on developing and accomplishing personal goals. Clients are assisted in developing

- Self-confidence.
- A self-concept beyond illness.
- A sense of well-being and hope.

As one client who succeeded in psychiatric rehabilitation stated, "Slowly I accepted my illness but wanted to live a full life in spite of it. I was desperate to succeed in the real world and I entered college. There I expanded my social ties so I wouldn't have to be forced into the identity of schizophrenia. My teachers gave me courage and respect" (GAP, 2000, p. 22).

Table 28-2 lists examples of specific nursing outcomes from the Nursing Outcomes Classification (NOC) (Moorhead, Johnson, & Maas, 2004).

The following sections discuss **crisis stabilization** as well as four evidence-based practices for clients with SMI:

1. Client and family psychoeducation
2. Social skills training and illness self-management
3. Vocational rehabilitation and supported employment
4. Cognitive interventions

Crisis Stabilization

People with SMI frequently experience crises. The incidence of crisis is increased in this population because of the nature of their vulnerability to stress, poor cognitive functioning, and lack of adequate problem-solving skills.

People usually have a number of coping responses they use when stressed in their everyday lives. For the severely mentally ill person with limited abilities, often the first response to a small stressor is to seek hospitalization. Seemingly small stressors might be changes in the routine at home, in treatment, or at work; physical or financial problems; or anniversaries of special events.

For example, a client with schizophrenia was hospitalized after making a scene in the lobby of her apartment building, falling to the floor and screaming incoherently. Upon admission, she told the nurse that she had run out of toilet paper and could not buy more because her check would not be in for another week. Another client went to the emergency department with paranoid delusions after receiving an eviction notice and fearing that he would be put out on the street immediately. Upon interview, it was discovered that he had forgotten to pay the rent for two months.

TABLE 28-2

NOC Outcomes for Severe Mental Illness

Nursing Outcome and Definition	Intermediate Indicators	Short-Term Indicators
Distorted Thought Self-Control: Self-restraint of disruptions in perception, thought processes, and thought content*	Interacts with others appropriately Exhibits reality-based thinking	Describes content of hallucinations or delusions Asks for validation of reality Refrains from responding to hallucinations or delusions
Self-Care: Hygiene: Ability to maintain own personal cleanliness and kempt appearance independently with or without assistive device†	Maintains neat appearance	Shampoos hair Washes hands Shaves Maintains oral hygiene
Self-Care: Instrumental Activities of Daily Living (IADL): Ability to perform activities needed to function in the home or community independently with or without assistive device†	Manages medications Manages money	Shops for groceries Prepares meals Uses phone Travels on public transportation
Family Coping: Family actions to manage stressors that tax family resources*	Uses available social support Cares for needs of all members	Involves family members in decision making Establishes family priorities Plans for emergencies

From Moorhead, S., Johnson, M., & Maas, M. (2004). *Nursing outcomes classification (NOC)* (3rd ed.). St. Louis, MO: Mosby.
*Evaluated on a five-point Likert scale from 1 (never demonstrated) to 5 (consistently demonstrated).
†Evaluated on a five-point Likert scale from 1 (severely compromised) to 5 (not compromised).

Crisis theory and intervention can be adapted successfully to treat people who have long-term mental illness. Traditionally, crisis intervention refers to treatment of a healthy individual who is temporarily suffering from disequilibrium in functioning. Crisis intervention helps people resume their previous level of functioning, and this is also the goal for people with severe and long-term mental health problems.

The nurse can adapt the crisis model for clients with SMI using the following principles: clarify the reality of the situation; focus on the client's strengths and support system; identify realistic goals and take a more active role in the problem-solving process. The nurse uses direct interventions such as calling on existing resources for additional support or finding new resources for the client. For example, in the two situations described earlier, the first client was discharged after 3 days with a referral to psychiatric home care; the second client was helped by a call to his case manager, who was able to resolve the issue with the landlord. In fact, much of the success of the case management approach with severely mentally ill clients is due to the availability of 24-hour support for crisis intervention, which averts hospitalization. See Chapter 22 for more discussion of crisis theory and interventions.

■ ■ ■ *VIGNETTE*

After 10 years of compliance with treatment, Robert announces one day that he wants to move out on his own and maybe get married. He has just celebrated his fiftieth birthday. Despite respectful disagreement from his nurse therapist and his caregiver, he finds himself a room to rent. Over the next 2 months, his mental status does not show any significant change: he is polite, quiet, and guarded as usual. But his psychiatrist, who routinely weighs him monthly, notices that he has lost 20 lb. Robert cannot explain any change in his eating habits, and he is referred to his primary care doctor for an evaluation. He gives various excuses for not going to the doctor for the next 4 weeks and loses another 10 lb. His nurse therapist then calls his job supervisor for additional observations. The supervisor reports that he is showing a change in behavior at work: he is talking out loud to himself and becoming more isolated, and one morning he smelled of alcohol. She is supportive about holding his job if he needs treatment. At his next clinic appointment, the psychiatrist and therapist discuss all of these changes and recommend that Robert go into the partial hospital program for medication reevaluation. He reluctantly agrees, denying that he has any problem.

■ ■ ■

Client and Family Psychoeducation

An important need of families caring for the severely and persistently mentally ill is psychoeducation to help them understand the disease process. Families need to be prepared to deal with the many issues related to safety, communication, medication compliance, and symptom management. Family interventions are now considered an evidence-based practice, with research showing improved outcomes in terms of decreased relapses and rehospitalizations for clients whose families participate in their care (Mueser et al., 2001). Effective teaching programs are implemented through outpatient centers and are relatively long term, lasting from 9 months to 2 years. Topics for education for both the family and the client include the following:

- Information about the illness
- Principles of management and treatment
- Information on medications and methods of improving adherence to the medication regimen
- Stress management for family members
- Improvement of functioning in all family members

The need to provide multiple types of support for families cannot be overemphasized. Dealing with a family member who has a mental illness is a major crisis for the family that pervades all aspects of family life. It is important that professionals not only recognize the problems facing the family but also identify the strengths from which the family can plan support. Often the family becomes the most accurate source of information for use in diagnosis and client management. Cooperative planning and respect for family members are essential in providing individualized client care as well as support for the caregivers. In this way, clients can develop coping skills to assist them throughout the lengthy and unpredictable course of the disease. Evidence from a study conducted by Cuijpers and Stam (2000) concluded that psychoeducation should concentrate on helping relatives to cope with the strain on the relationship with the severely mentally ill individual and with that individual's disruptive behavior.

Social Skills Training and Illness Self-Management

Social skills training is another evidence-based practice that involves using a variety of learning techniques to teach clients discrete skills. The two major goals of social skills training are improved functioning to reduce relapse and hospitalization, and improved quality of life with enjoyment of interpersonal relationships (Mueser et al., 2001). Research studies have shown that complex interpersonal skills can be taught by breaking them down into simpler behaviors, including verbal and nonverbal parts. A systematic approach using small steps is adopted, and clients observe and role-play new behaviors until they can perform the skill outside of the class. Teaching is often done in groups, although individual sessions can also be used. Social skills training can teach independent living skills, conversational skills, dating and job-seeking behavior, stress management, and symptom and medication management (Midence, 2000). Follow-up has shown that the learned skills persist over time

and may be transferred to new settings for some clients. Table 28-3 identifies specific interactions for which skills can be taught using a formal manual as a guide.

Vocational Rehabilitation and Supported Employment

Surveys of seriously mentally ill clients repeatedly show that they are interested in competitive employment (Drake et al., 2003). Vocational programs should be an integral part of the treatment of people with chronic

---

TABLE 28-3

Topics for Social Skills Training for Schizophrenia

Skill	Components
1. Conversation	Starting conversations Listening to others Maintaining conversations by expressing feelings Ending conversations
2. Conflict management	Compromising and negotiating Disagreeing without arguing Responding to untrue accusations Leaving stressful situations
3. Assertiveness	Making requests Refusing requests Making complaints Expressing angry feelings Making apologies
4. Community living	Handling a situation in which you think somebody has something of yours Handling a situation in which you do not understand what a person is saying Checking out your beliefs Eating and drinking politely
5. Friendship and dating	Expressing positive feelings Giving compliments Finding common interests Asking someone for a date Refusing unwanted sexual advances
6. Medication management	Making an appointment on the phone Asking questions about medication Asking questions about health-related concerns
7. Vocational activities, work	Interviewing for a job Asking for feedback about job performance Responding to criticism Solving problems

From Bellack, A. S., et al. (1997). *Social skills training for schizophrenia: A step-by-step guide.* New York: Guilford Press.

mental illnesses (Reker et al., 2000). A study conducted by Reker and colleagues of 471 chronically ill individuals with histories of repeated and long-term hospitalization provided support for giving clients opportunities to learn and improve vocational skills. After 3 years, 11% were in competitive employment, 67% were in sheltered employment, 7% were in outpatient work therapy programs, and only 15% were unemployed.

There have been a number of vocational rehabilitation models, but recent research has identified a more promising approach. In the past, clients were referred to state vocational rehabilitation agencies, which emphasized extensive prevocational training and employment in sheltered workshops before placement in competitive jobs. Success in maintaining employment was low. Recently, lessons have been learned from three successful community programs. Work with the developmentally disabled showed improved outcomes when the person was placed in the job first and then given individualized training. Psychosocial rehabilitation programs using a clubhouse model taught all members to perform a job in order to run the daily program. Assertive community case management proved the benefits of providing services in the field rather than in the clinic. These influences have led to the development of the supported employment model, which is now an evidence-based practice (refer to the Evidence-Based Practice box for research find-

ings). In this approach to vocational placement, there are four elements:

1. Rapid placement in a competitive job preferred by the client
2. Continuing support on the job (a coach) with training and communication with supervisors
3. Close integration between the job coach and the mental health team
4. Perspective that job endings are a learning experience instead of a failure

Cognitive Interventions

Studies have evaluated the use of cognitive interventions for clients with SMI who have persistent, residual psychotic symptoms. The same cognitive-behavioral approaches that are used with depressed and anxious clients are applied; that is, the challenging of beliefs about symptoms to alter feelings and reactions. Such strategies have been successfully applied to treat hallucinations, delusions, and negative symptoms, which makes cognitive interventions an evidence-based practice. For example, clients can be taught to use distraction techniques when auditory hallucinations occur, such as listening to music or humming. Refer to Chapter 20 for more discussion of the use of cognitive-behavioral techniques to address psychotic symptoms.

 EVIDENCE-BASED PRACTICE

Supported Employment

Background
Severely mentally ill clients often express the desire to work. In the past, vocational rehabilitation programs required extensive evaluation procedures and training before job placement was attempted. But these programs were unsuccessful at helping severely mentally ill clients to maintain jobs. Research efforts have identified a more productive model called supported employment.

Studies
Supported employment refers to specific principles for job placement for severely mentally ill clients. The most successful programs include five elements: (1) focus on competitive employment instead of sheltered work; (2) rapid job search instead of preemployment training; (3) selection of jobs related to the client's preferences and strengths; (4) provision of follow-up support indefinitely; (5) close integration of the supported employment with mental health treatment. Three quasi-experimental studies and eight randomized controlled trials have evaluated this model.

Results of Studies
In the three quasi-experimental studies, two-day treatment programs were compared: one converted to a supported employment model, and the other continued usual services. Clients in the converted program increased their employment rate, reported favorable reactions, and did not experience more adverse outcomes such as hospitalization.

Six randomized controlled studies compared supported employment with standard services. In all six, clients in the supported employment group showed significant gains in obtaining and keeping employment: a mean of 58% of such clients found and kept jobs compared to a mean of 21% in the control group. Two more randomized trials reported preliminary data in agreement with the first six studies.

Implications for Nursing Practice
Nurses need to be aware of clients' sincere desire to work. For a severely mentally ill client admitted to the acute care setting, the nursing assessment needs to identify any current work issues. Helping the client communicate with the job coach or supervisor may preserve the client's job. In the long-term care setting, the nurse can advocate for supported employment for the client, working closely with vocational staff to assure successful outcomes.

Bond, G. R., et al. (2001). Implementing supported employment as an evidence-based practice. *Psychiatric Services, 52*(3), 313-322.

In addition, studies are evaluating the use of cognitive rehabilitation; that is, attempts to improve general functioning in memory, attention, and abstract reasoning. Early results suggest that clients can enhance their social responses, working memory, and self-esteem even when there is no significant change in their symptoms (Mueser et al., 2001).

■ ■ ■ *VIGNETTE*

Robert attends the partial hospital program for 4 weeks. In the first week, the nurse calls the therapist to report that he is severely paranoid: he will not eat or drink out of any open containers and he is observed spitting out his pills. His medication is changed to a quickly disintegrating tablet form. He attends groups that focus on education about medication compliance, chronic illness, substance use, and healthy habits. He begins to eat normally, gaining 5 lb in 2 weeks. Finally, he admits that he has not taken any medication since he moved out of his group home. The discharge plan is developed in collaboration with the outpatient nurse therapist: referral to the psychosocial program again for daytime structure and case management to assist with finding a new home, medical care, and eventual return to work; and increased intensity of service at the clinic, with a biweekly medication injection and supportive group therapy. Over the next 3 months, Robert gradually returns to his baseline level of functioning. His case manager finds him another group home with his previous caregiver. He is able to return to work 2 days per week and still attends the day program for 3 days. Robert never is able to identify the trigger for his relapse, but his nurse therapist now observes his physical status more closely and inquires specifically about his work and social activities at each session.

■ ■ ■ KEY POINTS to REMEMBER

- Clients with SMI suffer from multiple impairments in their thinking, feelings, and interactions with others.
- The course of chronic mental illness involves exacerbations and remissions, as with chronic medical illness.
- Coordinated, comprehensive community services help the seriously mentally ill client to function at his or her optimal level.
- Severely mentally ill people often suffer complications due to insufficient housing, nonadherence to the medication regimen, comorbid medical or substance use problems, and the stigma of mental illness.
- Research has identified six evidence-based practices that produce positive outcomes for the seriously mentally ill.
- The family plays a major part in the care of many severely mentally ill persons and must be included as much as possible in education and treatment interventions.
- Through crisis stabilization and psychiatric rehabilitation, the nurse plays a significant role in helping the severely mentally ill client regain or attain the highest possible level of functioning in the community.

Visit the Evolve website at **http://evolve.elsevier.com/Varcarolis** for a posttest on the content in this chapter.   *evolve*

Critical Thinking and Chapter Review

Visit the Evolve website at **http://evolve.elsevier.com/Varcarolis** for additional self-study exercises.

■ ■ ■ CRITICAL THINKING

Lin Yang, age 42 years, just moved into town with his mother, who is now 70 years old. Lin has a severe mental illness and has a dual diagnosis (schizophrenia and alcohol plus marijuana abuse). Mrs. Yang brings Lin into the community mental health clinic, and you are doing an initial assessment. Mrs. Yang tells you that she has been caring for her son at home since Lin was 15 years of age; however, with the move to a new part of the country, she is at a complete loss regarding how best to handle her son and how to find out what is available in the community. Lin is currently taking haloperidol (Haldol), but Mrs. Yang says that Lin often does not take the drug because of the muscle rigidity and sexual side effects it causes. Mrs. Yang says they have tried many of the traditional antipsychotic drugs. Mrs. Yang tells you that they are currently living in an apartment, and her younger brother is coming to live with them in 6 months.

1. Given your understanding of the problems faced by a person with an SMI, what are some areas of Lin's life you might want to explore in your psychosocial assessment? Consider relationships, employment history, cognitive ability, behaviors, and such. How would knowledge in these areas help your long-term planning?

2. After you assess Lin's medication history, how can you be a client advocate in terms of Lin's nonadherence to a regimen of traditional antipsychotic medications? What are some of the problems in adherence for a client with severe mental illness and dual diagnosis? What approach seems to offer the best chance of success?

3. Of the resources mentioned in this chapter, what are some that might be potentially appropriate for Lin (assuming that a careful psychosocial and medical assessment has been performed and that all resources are available in your community)?

4. Identify three basic aims of psychoeducation for Mr. Yang and his mother.

Critical Thinking and Chapter Review—cont'd

Visit the Evolve website at **http://evolve.elsevier.com/Varcarolis** for additional self-study exercises.

■ ■ ■ CHAPTER REVIEW

Choose the most appropriate answer.

1. Care planning is facilitated when the nurse understands that a cornerstone of treatment for maintaining the individual with SMI within the community is
   1. intense psychotherapy.
   2. compliance with the medication regimen.
   3. respite care to ease family burden.
   4. referrals to numerous community resources.

2. For a client with chronic mental illness, exacerbations of mental illness may decrease in intensity with
   1. the client's willingness to meet with his or her social worker weekly for 1 year.
   2. the client's ability to work at a part-time rather than a full-time job.
   3. the nurse's attention to the history of the disease itself and an awareness of the client's daily functioning.
   4. the client's willingness to go to a respite facility 1 day per week.

3. When planning care for a client with a dual diagnosis, the nurse should consider that clients with dual diagnoses require
   1. less assistance in resolving situational crises.
   2. minimal training in skills for performing activities of daily living.
   3. treatment for both severe mental illness and substance abuse.
   4. intermittent therapy given at times when the client is least cognitively impaired.

4. Short hospitalization for crisis stabilization is more often recommended for a client with severe and persistent mental illness than for a client experiencing a crisis who is essentially mentally healthy because the client with severe mental illness
   1. often has inadequate situational supports.
   2. has a good sense of personal boundaries.
   3. has a realistic perception of the crisis event.
   4. can mobilize coping defenses to lower anxiety.

5. What topic would be *least* important to include in psychoeducation for severely mentally ill clients and their families?
   1. Understanding medications
   2. Monitoring levels of stress
   3. Improving communication skills
   4. Recognizing the impact of deinstitutionalization

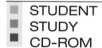 STUDENT
■ STUDY
■ CD-ROM

Access the accompanying CD-ROM for animations, interactive exercises, review questions for the NCLEX examination, and an audio glossary.

REFERENCES

American Psychological Association. (2003, July 22). *American Psychological Association applauds final report of President's New Freedom Commission on Mental Health* [Press release]. Washington, DC: Author.

Aquila, R., & Emanuel, M. (2003, September 25). *Managing the long-term outlook of schizophrenia.* Retrieved February 28, 2005, from http://www.medscape.com/viewprogram/2680_pnt.

Cuijpers, P., & Stam, H. (2000). Burnout among relatives of psychiatric patients attending psychoeducational support groups. *Psychiatric Services, 51*(3), 375-379.

Dickey, B., et al. (2002). Medical morbidity, mental illness, and substance use disorders. *Psychiatric Services, 53*(7), 861-867.

Dochterman, J. M., & Bulechek, G. M. (2004). *Nursing interventions classification (NIC)* (4th ed.). St. Louis, MO: Mosby.

Drake, R. E., et al. (2003). Recent research on vocational rehabilitation for persons with severe mental illness. *Current Opinions in Psychiatry, 16*(4), 451-455.

Drake, R. E., & Mueser, K. T. (2000). Psychosocial approaches to dual diagnosis. *Schizophrenia Bulletin, 26*(1), 105-118.

Group for the Advancement of Psychiatry. (2000). *Now that we are listening.* Dallas, TX: Committee on Psychiatry and the Community Group for the Advancement of Psychiatry.

Lacro, J., & Glassman, R. (2004). Medication adherence. *Medscape Psychiatry & Mental Health, 9*(1), 1-4.

Link, B. G., et al. (2001). The consequences of stigma for the self-esteem of people with mental illnesses. *Psychiatric Services, 52*(12), 1621-1626.

McAlpine, D. D., & Mechanic, D. (2000). Utilization of specialty mental health care among persons with severe mental illness: The roles of demographics, need, insurance, and risk. *Health Services Research, 35*(1 Pt 2), 277-292.

Mellman, T. A., et al. (2001). Evidence-based pharmacologic treatment for people with severe mental illness: A focus on guidelines and algorithms. *Psychiatric Services, 52*(5), 619-625.

Midence, K. (2000). An introduction to and rationale for psychosocial interventions. In C. Gamble & G. Brennan (Eds.), *Working with serious mental illness: A manual for clinical practice.* London: Baillière Tindall.

Moorhead, S., Johnson, M., & Maas, M. (2004). *Nursing outcomes classification (NOC)* (3rd ed.). St. Louis, MO: Mosby.

Mueser, K. T., et al. (2001). Community-based treatment of schizophrenia and other severe mental disorders: Treatment outcomes? *Medscape Mental Health, 6*(1), 1-31.

Mueser, K. T., et al. (2002). Illness management and recovery: A review of the research. *Psychiatric Services, 53*(10), 1272-1284.

National Alliance for the Mentally Ill. (2000a). *Access to effective medications: A critical link to mental illness recovery.* Retrieved February 28, 2005, from http://www.nami.org/update/000709b.html.

National Alliance for the Mentally Ill. (2000b). *NAMI offers testimony on homeless program consolidation legislation.* Retrieved February 28, 2005, from http://www.nami.org/update/000609.html.

Nemeroff, C. B. (2004, July). Atypical antipsychotics: Weighing the benefits. *Clinical Psychiatry News, 32*(Suppl., New findings in schizophrenia: An update on causes and treatment), 9-11.

Patel, J. K., et al. (2003). Schizophrenia and other psychosis. In A. Tasman, J. Kay, & J. A. Lieberman (Eds.), *Psychiatry* (2nd ed., Vol. 2, pp. 1131-1181). West Sussex, England: Wiley.

President's New Freedom Commission on Mental Health. *Interim Report of the President's New Freedom Commission on Mental Health.* (2002). Retrieved February 28, 2005, from http://www.mentalhealth.samhsa.gov/publications/allpubs/NMH02-0144/default.asp.

Reker, T., et al. (2000). Long term psychiatric patients in vocational rehabilitation programme: A naturalistic follow-up study over 3 years. *Acta Psychiatrica Scandinavica, 101*(6), 457-463.

Ryrie, L. (2000). Coexistent substance use and psychiatric disorders. In C. Gamble & G. Brennan (Eds.), *Working with serious mental illness: A manual for clinical practice.* London: Baillière Tindall.

Struening, E. L., et al. (2001). The extent to which caregivers believe most people devalue consumers and their families. *Psychiatric Services, 52*(12), 1633-1638.

Vanderhorst, K. J. (2000). Highways for the journey: The mental health system. In V. B. Carson, (Ed.), *Mental health nursing: The nurse-patient journey* (2nd ed.). Philadelphia: Saunders.

CHAPTER 29

Psychological Needs of the Medically Ill

ELIZABETH M. VARCAROLIS

KEY TERMS and CONCEPTS

The key terms and concepts listed here appear in color where they are defined or first discussed in this chapter.

coping strategies, 593

holistic approach, 588

holistic assessment, 594

human rights abuses, 597

psychiatric liaison nursing, 598

quality-of-life assessment, 595

stigmatized medically ill persons, 597

OBJECTIVES

After studying this chapter, the reader will be able to

1. Describe at least two common mental health sequelae and two psychological responses to a serious medical illness.
2. Construct a *DSM-IV-TR* diagnosis for an individual who has a substance abuse problem, has severe cardiac disease, and is soon to be evicted from his apartment.
3. Defend the teaching of relaxation and coping skills by nurses.
4. Perform a psychosocial (psychological-social-spiritual) nursing assessment.
5. Assess the client's coping skills: (a) identify areas for teaching, (b) identify areas of strength.
6. Identify two instances in which a consultation with a psychiatric liaison nurse might have been useful for one of your medical-surgical clients.

evolve Visit the Evolve website at **http://evolve.elsevier.com/Varcarolis** for a pretest on the content in this chapter.

The nurse's view of the individual as a complex blend of many parts is consistent with our holistic approach to nursing care. Nurses who care for people with physical illnesses ideally maintain a holistic view that involves an awareness of psychological, social, cultural, and spiritual issues.

A mentally healthy person who experiences psychological, social, cultural, and spiritual difficulties as a result of situational or maturational problems may be experiencing a crisis. Usually, some time-limited crisis intervention or brief supportive counseling is sufficient to bolster the person's already adequate coping skills until the crisis is past. However, when the situational crisis is a persistent life-threatening or disabling disease, or when a permanent change occurs in the person's situation, long-term interventions may be required. It helps us give more thorough and compassionate care when we are aware of the complex issues people confront when faced with a serious medical illness.

PSYCHOLOGICAL FACTORS AFFECTING MEDICAL CONDITIONS

Both the medical and the psychiatric communities recognize the interrelationships between psychiatric and medical comorbidity. Psychological factors may present a risk for medical disease, or they may magnify and/or adversely affect a medical condition (Levenson, 2003).

The expanded diagnostic category **psychological factor affecting medical condition (PFAMC)** in the *Diagnostic and Statistical Manual of Mental Disorders*, fourth edition, text revision *(DSM-IV-TR)* (American Psychiatric Association, 2000) includes the identification of psychological factors that interfere with medical treatment, pose health risks, or cause stress-related pathophysiological changes. This diagnosis includes both the psychological factor and the general medical condition. Axis I identifies the symptoms of the psychiatric disorder (e.g., depression, anxiety, substance abuse), whereas axis II codes the personality trait (e.g., type A personality trait). Axis III identifies the medical condition or maladaptive health behavior (diabetes, unsafe sex practices). For example, the diagnosis might read "a major depressive disorder aggravating coronary artery disease" (Levenson, 2003). Figure 29-1 lists the *DSM-IV-TR* criteria for PFAMC.

The subject of PFAMC is being intensively researched: first, because of the information gleaned on the basic disease mechanisms (e.g., psychoneuroimmunology; see Chapter 12); and, second, because of the deep interest in improving both the outcomes and the efficiency of health care delivery (Levenson, 2003). Collaboration between health care personnel in primary care and psychiatry can lead to more accurate diagnoses and an increased remission rate. Obtaining remission, improving care of the family, and decreasing suicide behavior are a major points of focus (Culpepper, 2003) (Box 29-1).

Stress is certainly a psychological factor. Axis IV (Psychosocial and Environmental Problems) identifies stressors in an individual's life that might become a primary focus of treatment. Hans Selye (1956) was the first to introduce the concept of stress into the fields of medicine and physiology. As you know from Chapter 12, stress can lead to changes in physical and mental health in many ways. Cannon's identification of the fight-or-flight response (1914) and Selye's description of the general adaptation syndrome provided insight into the biological and molecular reactions to stressors in the sympathetic nervous system, the pituitary-adrenocortical axis, and the immune system. Extensive studies have left little doubt that psychosocial stress can affect the course and severity of illness.

It has long been thought that an adverse psychosocial environment (e.g., stress, loneliness) can increase a person's risk of cardiovascular disease. Levenson

---

DSM-IV-TR Criteria for Psychological Factors Affecting Medical Condition

A. A general medical condition (coded on axis III) is present.

B. Psychological factors adversely affect the general medical condition in one of the following ways:
  (1) The factors have influenced the course of the general medical condition as shown by a close temporal association between the psychological factors and the development or exacerbation of, or delayed recovery from, the general medical condition.
  (2) The factors interfere with the treatment of the general medical condition.
  (3) The factors constitute additional health risks for the individual.
  (4) Stress-related physiological responses precipitate or exacerbate symptoms of the general medical condition.

Choose name based on the nature of the psychological factors (if more than one factor is present, indicate the most prominent):

  Mental disorder affecting... [indicate the general medical condition] (e.g., an axis I disorder such as major depressive disorder delaying recovery from a myocardial infarction)

  Psychological symptoms affecting... [indicate the general medical condition] (e.g., depressive symptoms delaying recovery from surgery, anxiety exacerbating asthma)

  Personality traits or coping style affecting... [indicate the general medical condition] (e.g., pathological denial of the need for surgery in a patient with cancer; hostile, pressured behavior contributing to cardiovascular disease)

  Maladaptive health behaviors affecting... [indicate the general medical condition] (e.g., overeating, lack of exercise, unsafe sex)

  Stress-related physiological response affecting... [indicate the general medical condition] (e.g., stress-related exacerbations of ulcer, hypertension, arrhythmia, or tension headache)

  Other unspecified psychological factors affecting... [indicate the general medical condition] (e.g., interpersonal, cultural, or religious factors)

FIGURE 29-1 Diagnostic criteria for psychological factors affecting medical conditions. (From American Psychiatric Association. [2000]. *Diagnostic and statistical manual of mental disorders* [4th ed., text rev.]. Washington, DC: Author.)

BOX 29-1

Patient-Specific Outcomes of Primary Care–Psychiatry Collaboration

Accuracy of diagnosis
Retention in care
Adherence with the treatment plan
Decreased medication problems
  ▪ Adverse/toxic effects
  ▪ Drug-drug interactions
Stabilization on long-term care plan
Attainment of remission
  ▪ Symptom control
  ▪ Functional improvement
Improved medical outcomes
  ▪ Preventive measures
  ▪ Chronic disease management
Improved care of family
Decreased suicidal behaviors

From Culpepper, L. (2003, May 18). The successful intervention: Management of the patient with medical comorbidities. In *Psychiatry and medicine: Common patients, different perspectives.* Symposium conducted at the 156th Annual Meeting of the American Psychiatric Association, San Francisco, CA.

(2003) cites studies finding evidence that psychological stressors can precipitate serious ventricular arrhythmias and sudden cardiac death. Psychological stress is also thought to adversely affect glucose control in individuals with diabetes (Levenson, 2003).

Numerous medical disorders have been studied extensively with regard to the effects of stress on the course of illness. Although personality traits and lifestyle may very well affect the course of disease, few of the earlier studies support the idea that a specific personality type causes or is an integral part of the cause of a medical disorder. Table 29-1 identifies some physical illnesses that benefit from stress reduction and support. In fact, anyone experiencing a serious medical condition needs a variety of supports and may benefit from learning new coping skills.

PSYCHOLOGICAL RESPONSES TO SERIOUS MEDICAL ILLNESS

People's responses can be many and varied when they find themselves faced with a serious medical problem:

- Will I be disfigured?
- Will I have a long-term disability?
- Will I be able to function as a wife or husband, parent, and person in society?
- Will I be able to continue to work?
- Will I suffer pain?

People who face the crisis of a serious medical diagnosis need the kind of emotional support that allows them to face their burdens without censure or fear of judgment (Zerbe, 1999). When strong emotional supports and social ties are not available, other questions may arise:

- How will I cope?
- How will this affect my life?
- Will I retain a reasonable quality of life?

Psychological sequelae of medical illness can be severe and can account for a higher rate of disruption in functional ability than just the medical illness alone would indicate. Among the most common psychological responses to physical illness are depression, anxiety, substance use, denial, and anger. A psychological condition, however, may supersede or be comorbid with a medical condition. Levenson (2003) states that, in general, individuals with medical disorders and psychological symptoms have poorer outcomes than those with the same medical disorders but without psychological problems.

Depression

The risk of a major depressive disorder is high among individuals with a serious medical illness and is thought to be as high as 20% to 25% (Valdivia & Rossy,

2004). Often depression is masked by the medical condition itself and goes unrecognized and thus untreated. Just a few of the medical illnesses that typically are associated with depression are coronary artery disease (depression rate of 23% in those with this illness), diabetes (depression rate of 9% to 27%), and stroke (depression rate of 22% to 50%) (Spollen & Gutman, 2003). It is known that depression can amplify the pathophysiology of endocrine and cardiac disease and diminish functional ability (Meyer, Klemme, & Herrmann, 2000). Depression is also prevalent in individuals with cancer, with rates as high as 40% to 50%.

Depression is a risk factor for nonadherence to medication and treatment regimen. Depressed clients are three times more likely to fail to adhere to the medical treatment recommendation than are nondepressed clients (Culpepper, 2003). Individuals who scored higher on the Hospital and Anxiety Depression Scale (HADS) were rated by physicians to have more severe illness and greater functional impairment (Meyer et al., 2000). Therefore, depression, if not recognized and treated, can affect the severity of the medical disorder, increase personal distress, impair functioning, and interfere with adherence to a prescribed medical regimen. However, people with medical conditions who do get treatment for co-occurring depression often experience an improvement in their overall medical condition, show better compliance with recommendations for general medical care, and experience a better quality of life.

Anxiety

Anxiety accompanies every illness, especially when pain, disability, hospitalization, economic loss, or fear of death is present. Anxiety disorders and medical illnesses are common comorbidities (Goddard & Shekhar, 2002). For example, adults with asthma, chronic bronchitis, or emphysema are more likely to experience panic attacks than are their healthy peers (Goodwin & Pine, 2002).

Verbalization is an effective outlet for anxiety, but the ability to verbalize may be compromised by cultural expectations, disability, or lack of a listener. A feeling of helplessness often accompanies anxiety in the person who feels a loss of control over events, such as when awaiting surgery or undergoing invasive treatments. In this case, defense mechanisms may be used with greater frequency, or compulsive behaviors may surface. Self-centeredness characterized by unreasonable requests of caregivers may also be a cover for feelings of inadequacy.

The following vignette shows how acute anxiety can affect a person's ability to take in information, can threaten his or her self-esteem ("I should be able to do this without help"), and can trigger expected and, at this point, adaptive denial.

TABLE 29-1

Common Medical Conditions Negatively Affected by Stress

Medical Condition	Incidence	Genetic and Biological Correlates	Common Precipitating Factors	Holistic Therapies in Addition to Medical Management
Cardiovascular disease (e.g., coronary heart disease)	Rates higher in males until age 60 years Rates higher in white population than in African American population	Family history of cardiac disease a risk factor Other risk factors include hypertension, increased serum lipid levels, obesity, sedentary lifestyle, and cigarette smoking Psychosocial risk factors (stress, depression, loneliness) High anxiety risk in client with prior cardiac events	Often, myocardial infarction occurs after sudden stress preceded by a period of losses, frustration, and disappointments	Relaxation training, stress management, group social support, and psychosocial intervention Support groups for type A personalities and type A modification helpful Anxiolytics (benzodiazepines) and antidepressants when indicated
Peptic ulcer (caused by *Helicobacter pylori* infection)	Occurs in 12% of men, 6% of women (more prevalent in industrialized societies)	Infection with *H. pylori* is associated with 95% to 99% of peptic ulcers Both peptic and duodenal ulcers cluster in families, but separately from each other	Periods of social tension and increased life stress After losses; often after menopause	Biofeedback can alter gastric acidity; cognitive-behavioral approaches are used to reduce stress (stress management)
Cancer	Men: most common in lung, prostate, colon, and rectum Women: most common in breast, uterus, colon, and rectum Death rate higher in men (especially African American men) than in women	Genetic evidence suggests dysfunction of cellular proliferation Familial patterns for breast cancer, colorectal cancer, stomach cancer, melanoma	Prolonged and intensive stress Stressful life events (e.g., separation from or loss of significant other 2 years before diagnosis) Feelings of hopelessness, helplessness, and despair (depression) may precede the diagnosis of cancer	Relaxation (e.g., meditation, autogenic training, self-hypnosis) Visualization Psychological counseling Support groups Massage therapy Stress management
Tension headache	Occurs in 80% of population when under stress Begins at end of workday or early evening		Associated with anxiety and depression	Psychotherapy usually prescribed for chronic tension headaches Learning to cope or avoiding tension-creating situations or people Relaxation techniques, stress management techniques, cognitive restructuring techniques
Essential hypertension	Rates higher in males until age 60 years	Family history of cardiac disease and hypertension a risk factor	Life changes and traumatic life events Stressful job (e.g., air traffic controller) Hypothesized to be found more in areas of social stress and conflict	Behavioral feedback, stress reduction techniques, meditation, yoga, hypnosis Note: pharmacological treatment is considered primary for the treatment of hypertension

■ ■ ■ *VIGNETTE*

At 27 years of age, Ted tests positive for human immunodeficiency virus (HIV) infection. During the posttest counseling session with the public health nurse at the health department, Ted is given referrals and information regarding the virus. The nurse notes that Ted is having difficulty focusing on details and needs to have information repeated several times. The nurse gives Ted the opportunity to explore his feelings, but Ted has difficulty in this area because he was raised to believe that it is a strength to deal with crisis alone. Ted is also experiencing a great deal of denial in this initial period of loss. For these reasons, the nurse anticipates the most common and immediate concerns that might be facing a person who has just discovered that he is HIV positive and gently leads Ted into discussion of these concerns over a period of several weeks, with the use of reflective statements and silence. This approach gives Ted the opportunity to verbalize his feelings and begin to unburden himself in a safe environment.

■ ■ ■

Long-term and pervasive anxiety or an anxiety disorder that precedes a medical disorder can actually be a risk factor for a medical disorder. A study by Bowen, Senthilselvan, and Barale (2000), which spanned a 10-year period, found that those with anxiety disorders had a significantly higher relative risk of developing a medical disease than did those without anxiety disorders. The highest relative risk was for cerebrovascular disease. Irritable bowel syndrome (IBS) is another example of a disease characterized by a high frequency of anxiety disorders in affected individuals (Levenson, 2003).

Substance Abuse

It is well documented that long-term abuse of various substances can lead to a variety of medical complications; for example, alcohol use is associated with hepatic conditions, marijuana use with lung disease, cocaine use with cardiac toxicity, and use of ecstasy (3,4-methylenedioxy-methamphetamine or MDMA) with neurotoxicity (problems with memory, reasoning, and impulse control). However, clients who are diagnosed with serious medical conditions often turn to alcohol and/or other substances of abuse to cope with overwhelming feelings of hopelessness, fear, anxiety, depression, or pain. Research is being funded by the National Institutes of Health to find ways to help link medical and mental health services with substance abuse services, because substance abuse is a concurrent diagnosis in large numbers of medical and mental health clients (Semet, Friedman, & Saitz, 2001). Untreated substance abuse can increase the number of hospitalizations and the severity of the disorder (medical and/or mental health) in clients with a dual diagnosis (Rosack, 2003). Thus, relevant research indicates that health care workers need to be diligent in their initial assessments, identifying any coexisting or resulting psychological response or disorder. In most cases of physical illness, the focus is on the complaints of physical symptoms, and minimal attention is given to the psychological responses of the client.

Grief and Loss

Very often, an individual with a serious medical illness experiences grief and loss. Any type of treatment or procedure intended to treat a physical illness that creates a major permanent change is accompanied by feelings of loss. The dynamics involved in coping with these feelings are similar to those in a person who is dealing with his or her own impending death or the death of a loved one. The person must grieve for this loss, just as the dying person must work through the confusion and darkness until a degree of acceptance and relative peace is achieved. Negotiating the loss of physical well-being involves movement through feelings of frustration, vulnerability, and sadness to become a whole person once again. This journey encompasses spiritual as well as emotional changes and, for this reason, requires spiritual assessment of the client as well as a focus on psychosocial issues.

Denial

As an unconscious defense mechanism, denial is a common response to physical illness. A person may believe that the pain is really nothing or will go away (even though it is severe and lasts for long periods) or may minimize dramatic bodily changes. Even after hearing a diagnosis with a poor prognosis, a person in denial may attend only to the more positive or hopeful message and may block out the negative. This is a protective measure, and it is necessary initially. However, there are times when denial does interfere with treatment. One danger of denial is that a person may minimize physical complaints; the nursing staff may unwittingly collude in the denial by not performing a complete assessment and accepting the person's subjective statements at face value.

■ ■ ■ *VIGNETTE*

After a car accident, Carol is being assessed by the triage nurse in the emergency department for possible injuries. She complains of a slight headache and dizziness but denies having any other pain or symptoms. Carol is preoccupied with seeing that her 2-year-old son, who was also in the car, is being examined, so she denies her own need for medical attention. Carol's blood pressure is 86/50 mm Hg and her body posture indicates that she is guarding her abdomen. These observations are reported to the examining physician immediately because they indicate possible internal bleeding and danger of shock. Carol is eventually taken to the operating room so the bleeding may be stopped.

■ ■ ■

Fear of Dependency

Responses to being dependent might be exhibited as the inability to accept warmth, nurturing, or tenderness from caregivers or as refusal to accept treatment or medical advice. This reaction is strongest in those who have unmet dependency needs and those who have had negative experiences when help was sought in the past. Anger with caregivers may mask acute embarrassment over being in a dependent position by one who needs to project an independent image.

Others find themselves becoming fearful of not having their dependency needs met and do not express any negative feelings to caregivers. These people feel the need to be "good" clients out of fear that they will be abandoned if they are perceived to be difficult. Any anxiety or anger they suppress may be exhibited through increased somatic complaints.

■ ■ ■ *VIGNETTE*

Lillian is a 47-year-old woman who is being treated with hemodialysis and has been complaining of frequent tension headaches and occasional stomach upsets before her treatment appointments. The hemodialysis nurse has always been impressed by Lillian's patience and compliant attitude in spite of her debilitating illness, which has robbed her of a normal family life. For this reason, the nurse suspects that Lillian's physical complaints could be a way of dealing with emotions, so the nurse makes a point of spending more time with Lillian to allow her to talk about her frustrations. Lillian expresses anger and some feelings of hopelessness. She resents others who are healthy, including the people who care for her. Frequent opportunities to verbalize these feelings gradually result in the lessening of her somatic complaints and a decrease in her sense of powerlessness and isolation.

■ ■ ■

Although medical procedures may extend or promote life, they often take their toll on the client's physical state because of the high degree of anxiety they evoke. The following have all been shown to affect a client's recovery positively:

- Educating the client regarding the specific medical treatment
- Identifying an anxious client and referring the client to community support groups (or systems)
- Evaluating the client's coping strategies (how the client has coped in past situations)
- Teaching more effective coping skills to clients

Focusing on a client's strengths and reinforcing and teaching coping skills (e.g., prayerfulness, participation in hobbies, and relaxation techniques) are important nursing interventions.

HOLISTIC ASSESSMENT OF A CLIENT'S NEEDS

Psychosocial factors are recognized as relevant to the course of disease, and the way a person thinks and feels can have a profound effect on how the disease progresses.

How can a health care worker know what a client thinks or feels unless the client's psychosocial situation is assessed? Although lip service is always paid to adopting a holistic approach to care, the health care environment often leaves little time for evaluating what could be pivotal information about what a client needs to best cope with illness. It is vital to understand how a client's illness affects his or her life and how the client copes with adversity. Because the best indicator of future behavior is past behavior, ineffective coping strategies used in the past can be identified and can be changed by teaching more adaptive skills. Nurse clinicians are in a primary position to effect change in the quality of life of a client with medical illness and to help that client find the best way to heal or to deal with the illness. An effective nurse-client or clinician-client relationship may depend on a shared understanding of the psychosocial stresses the client is undergoing (e.g., troubled family relationships, job pressures, problems with children) and any psychosocial impairment the client may be experiencing (e.g., substance abuse, lack of social supports).

Nurses and other health care workers are becoming increasingly aware of the role spirituality or religion plays in many clients' lives and its importance as a source of peace and nourishment. Support for the client from a priest, pastor, rabbi, or other religious leader may be indicated, especially in a case of *spiritual distress*. Many people derive a great deal of comfort and inner strength from their spiritual beliefs.

Stressors are events or circumstances in which demands of the internal and external environment challenge or exceed the adaptive resources of the individual. This definition allows for an understanding of the role of coping in moderating the effect of stressors and facilitating adaptation to environmental demands. There are many healthy ways people can cope with the stresses relating to their illnesses, and these should be encouraged. There are also unhealthy ways people cope with illness-related stresses. These less effective coping strategies can be assessed, and new and more effective coping skills (cognitive, behavioral, and psychosocial) can be taught.

An understanding of how a client has dealt with adversity in the past is important in caring effectively for that client. Assessing usual coping skills gives professional health care workers information about which coping skills they can support and encourage and an understanding of what kinds of coping skills may help a client to cope better with a serious medical or surgical situation. The effective coping skills that can be offered are many and varied (e.g., assertiveness training, cognitive reframing, problem-solving skills, social supports). A nurse is in a key position to assess, educate, or provide referrals to a client to enable healthier ways of looking at and dealing with illness.

For interventions to be most effective, the nurse must understand how a person's medical condition affects the person's quality of life. For example, how is the medical illness affecting the client's ability to function in the home, at work, or in school? How are the client's feelings about the illness (depression, anxiety, hopelessness) affecting his or her relationships and ability to function?

A holistic approach is by far the most effective. A holistic assessment of physical, social, psychosocial, and spiritual needs includes evaluation of the following:

- Psychosocial assessment
- Brief quality-of-life assessment
- Usual coping strategies
- Activities of daily living
- Spirituality and religiosity
- Social activities
- Social supports

- Perception of quality of life
- Feelings
- Pain

Psychosocial Assessment

The elements of a thorough psychosocial assessment are described in Chapter 9. The following are some highlights that can help the nurse plan needed interventions. When working with someone who is medically ill, it is important to know something about the person's life:

- Does the person have someone who can share his or her concerns and who cares for him or her?
- Does the person have friends and supports in the community?
- Does the person have any coexisting conditions that could negatively affect adjustment to the illness, the course of the illness, adaptation to the illness, or ability to heal (e.g., depression, personality disorder, substance abuse, compulsive behaviors such as gambling, eating, or cybersex)?
- Does the person practice risky health behaviors (e.g., has a sedentary lifestyle, smokes, engages in unsafe sex practices, and/or abuses alcohol or drugs)?

BRIEF QUALITY-OF-LIFE QUESTIONNAIRE

1. I worry about my medical condition.	4	3	2	1	0
2. My medical situation causes me to be apprehensive about resuming some of my previous activities.	4	3	2	1	0
3. My family is having a hard time dealing with my medical event.	4	3	2	1	0
4. I am having difficulty with sexual functioning.	4	3	2	1	0
5. I worry that I will not be able to return to my job and perform satisfactorily.	4	3	2	1	0
6. I am having difficulty with smoking cessation.	4	3	2	1	0
7. I feel depressed or discouraged about my medical problems.	4	3	2	1	0
8. I cry easily or am more irritable than before my medical event.	4	3	2	1	0
9. I have lost interest in activities that I used to enjoy.	4	3	2	1	0
10. I would rather be alone than with friends or family.	4	3	2	1	0
11. I am experiencing more memory or concentration problems since my medical problems.	4	3	2	1	0
12. I am having difficulty losing weight.	4	3	2	1	0
13. I feel as if I'm dealing with my health problems on my own with little support from others.	4	3	2	1	0

Rate your stress
On a scale of 1 (lowest) to 10 (highest) how would you rate your stress?

Circle the number that represents your overall stress level.
Low   1   2   3   4   5   6   7   8   9   10   High

FIGURE 29-2 Brief quality-of-life questionnaire. (Adapted from Scottsdale Health Care. [2004, September]. *Cardiopulmonary rehabilitation patient/history questionnaire*, Scottsdale, AZ: Author.)

- Does the person's cultural view of health and illness help or impede the process of seeking adequate care?

Table 29-2 provides an outline for a psychosocial assessment of a medically ill client. A psychosocial assessment is performed in tandem with a thorough physical workup and mental status examination (see Chapter 9).

Brief Quality-of-Life Assessment

How the individual's medical condition affects his or her daily living and quality of life can be gleaned through the use of a brief quality-of-life assessment. See Figure 29-2 for a brief quality-of-life questionnaire.

TABLE 29-2

Psychosocial Assessment for Medically Ill Clients

Social Supports and Cultural Issues	Areas to Assess
Family Friends	■ What were the effects of the client's illness, treatments, and recovery on the family in the past? ■ With whom can the client share painful feelings? ■ Does the client have friends to joke and laugh with? ■ Are there people the client believes would stand by him or her?
Religious or spiritual beliefs	■ Does the client find comfort and support in spiritual practices? ■ Is the client a member of a spiritual or religious group in the community (church, temple, other place of worship)? ■ Does the client find inner peace and strength in religious or spiritual practices? ■ The following statements may be used in performing a spiritual assessment of a client: 　—I believe that life has value, meaning, and direction. 　　Often　　Sometimes　　Seldom 　—I feel a connection with the universe. 　　Often　　Sometimes　　Seldom 　—I believe in a power greater than myself. 　　Often　　Sometimes　　Seldom 　—I believe that my actions make a difference. 　　Often　　Sometimes　　Seldom 　—I believe that my actions express my true self. 　　Often　　Sometimes　　Seldom
Cultural beliefs	■ Does the client use specific culture-oriented treatments or remedies for his or her condition? ■ Do the client's cultural beliefs allow for adequate treatment by Western medical standards?
Work	■ Are there colleagues at work on whom the client can count for support?
Concurrent Physical Conditions Affecting Psychosocial Well-Being	
Physical pain	■ Is the client in pain? 　—How does the client cope with it? 　—Is the pain disabling? 　—Are there pain-reducing techniques that might help?
Major illness	■ Does the client have a co-occurring major illness that will negatively affect his or her current condition? ■ Is the client undergoing treatments that are affecting daily life more than expected? ■ Are there interventions that would help the client to cope better with the sequelae of the illness and treatments? ■ Has the client been hospitalized in the past? 　—How many times? 　—For what? ■ How did the client cope?
Addictions and mental health	■ Does the client have a co-occurring mental health problem (depression, anxiety, compulsions)? ■ Has the client suffered a mental disease in the past? ■ Does the client participate in any compulsive behavior (e.g., smoking, overworking, excessive spending, gambling, cybersex)? ■ Does the client abuse substances (alcohol, drugs [illicit, over the counter, prescription])?

Assessment of Usual Coping Strategies

A person who has a life-threatening disease or chronic illness most often deals with distressing physical side effects and changes in body image. For example, a person who is given a colostomy to avoid death from cancer or ulcerative colitis is left with complex emotional as well as physical dilemmas. This is especially true for women. A client not only must learn techniques of dealing with the stoma but also must learn to deal with the lifelong consequences and their effects on the person's body image, appearance, and relationships. Concerns such as the following may arise (Zerbe, 1999):

- Will my partner still be attracted to me?
- Will I continue to be interested in sexual relationships?
- Will I be embarrassed by my friends' reactions to my situation?
- Will people still think of me and relate to me the way they did before this illness?

Breast cancer survivors have been helped by the camaraderie with other survivors who openly share their techniques for dealing with appliances or prostheses. Other survivors can also show clients how to respond to well-intended but probing or embarrassing questions. Women who have previously traveled the same path are the best resources for helping others establish appropriate boundaries regarding intrusive questions such as "Are you wearing a wig because you lost all your hair as a result of chemotherapy?" (Zerbe, 1999).

Table 29-3 is an assessment guide that highlights some of the characteristics that allow people to cope well and notes characteristics that may be changed or improved through psychosocial interventions or cognitive-behavioral approaches.

INTERVENTION STRATEGIES

In an ideal situation, a multidisciplinary team of caretakers, including a psychiatric liaison nurse, would be involved in the treatment of clients with serious medical illness. Using the data from the holistic assessment, nurse clinicians in tandem with a physician are in a position to provide useful and effective interventions.

People who are medically ill are vulnerable to a variety of psychosocial stresses. How they cope with these stresses may make the difference between living with an acceptable quality of life or giving in to despair, withdrawal, or helplessness and hopelessness. As has been stressed continuously in this chapter, people with serious medical illnesses, especially long-term illnesses, are at risk for psychological distress or even worse—depression, disabling anxiety, substance

TABLE 29-3

Assessment of Coping Skills

Effective Coping Behaviors	Ineffective Coping Behaviors
Has optimistic attitude	Sees glass as being half empty instead of half full
Confronts the issues; acts accordingly	Minimizes critical health status or signals
Seeks information; gets guidance	Shows tendency to find escape or withdraw
Shares concerns; finds consolation	Blames someone or something else
Has capacity for healthy denial	Denies as much as possible; shows prolonged denial
Redefines the situation, reviews alternatives, examines consequences	Feels things are hopeless, were meant to be; has attitude of "What's the use?"
Constructively uses distractions: keeping busy; maintaining positive emotional ties with family, friends, community	Withdraws; broods; is overwhelmed with self-pity, anger, envy, guilt about having caused the illness

abuse problems, and nonadherence to their medical regimen.

Nurses are in a position to assess and understand clients' psychosocial stressors, identify needed coping skills, and teach stress management techniques. Nurses can play a very important role not only in providing and managing clients' immediate medical care but also in helping clients to improve their ability to cope and increase the quality of life during the course of a chronic medical illness.

Does the client have sufficient social supports (family, friends, and religious or spiritual help) to enable him or her to share thoughts and feelings in safety? Would the client benefit from a medical support group? (Many people do.)

Is the pain management program used by the client working? Would complementary approaches (e.g., hypnosis, guided imagery, or biofeedback) be helpful in augmenting the client's pain control regimen? Does the client have a coexisting mental disorder? Anxiety, depression, substance abuse, and other disorders are treatable. If mental disorders are not treated, however, severe psychological responses or mental health phenomena can increase the severity of the disease and negatively affect functional ability and quality of life, as previously pointed out.

How does the client cope with stress? Chapter 12 provides tools for measuring levels of stress and suggestions for holistic approaches to stress management. Consider referring the client for instruction in a variety of relaxation techniques, such as meditation, guided imagery, breathing exercises, and others, or even teaching the client such techniques yourself. Behavioral techniques are useful, and nurses with special training can offer their clients progressive muscle relaxation or biofeedback.

Relaxation techniques, stress management, supportive education, and stress monitoring (e.g., SF-12 Health Survey) should be part of the care of the medically ill client regardless of the medical diagnosis.

There is growing evidence that psychotherapy can help people endure medical illness (Zerbe, 1999). Beneficial psychotherapy approaches include the following:

- Cognitive-behavioral psychotherapy
- Guided imagery, biofeedback, acupressure, and hypnosis
- Psychodynamic psychotherapy

Box 29-2 provides guidelines for helping clients and their families better adapt to a major medical illness.

HUMAN RIGHTS ABUSES OF THE STIGMATIZED MEDICALLY ILL

Some consumers of health care and some health care providers have voiced the need for examination of **human rights abuses** of persons stigmatized by the health care system. These **stigmatized medically ill persons** include those who have mental illnesses, those who are HIV positive, and those who have undergone transgender surgeries or treatments. These are abuses that can result in inadequate care and lead to undue stress, worsening of physical illness, and even death. By assuming that persons with certain illnesses are bad, disgusting, or even just unusual, health care workers fail to acknowledge and understand that the psychosocial issues of these people are similar to those of others and that the same nursing interventions for anger, anxiety, or grief are applicable. Examples of human rights abuse include the following:

- Failure to fully investigate somatic complaints made by emergency department clients with a history of psychiatric illness
- Avoidance of contact with, or refusal to care for, persons who are stigmatized, which results in worsening illness or death
- Hasty labeling with a psychiatric diagnosis and prescription of antipsychotic drugs for persons who are experiencing the normal emotional responses (e.g., sadness, anger) to chronic physical illness
- Inappropriate psychiatric admission of persons who are on medical units or in nursing homes based on the financial needs of the institution or on the staff's inability to manage emotional responses to physical illness or the aging process

---

BOX 29-2

Guidelines for Client and Family for Coping with a Major Medical Illness

Learn all you can about your illness—Knowledge reduces anxiety. Keeping your anxiety at manageable levels helps you understand your options and helps you make decisions you believe are right for you.

Practice healthy behaviors—Good sleep hygiene, diet, and exercise are always good policies. Even if you are physically limited, exercise promotes a positive state of well-being. Lack of sleep can increase pain, irritability, and fatigue. Proper nutrition in the face of a medical illness can preserve or promote a healthy immune system.

Take advantage of medical support groups—Support groups that focus on your medical issue can help give you information, help you learn how to handle difficult situations related to your illness, reduce isolation, and offer a safe place to share difficult thoughts and feelings.

Consider entering psychotherapy—There is growing evidence that psychotherapy helps people endure medical illness. Benefits include less pain, better coping skills, and even longer survival, in some situations.

Find a way to express your feelings—Studies have examined the profound healing power of putting upsetting experiences into words (e.g., writing them down, keeping a journal). Acknowledging thoughts and feelings can help your nervous system relax.

Seek additional help if you become depressed, demoralized, anxious, or panicky or have unremitting pain—Your clinician might not be aware of these changes, and there are approaches (e.g., acupuncture, acupressure, biofeedback) that can give people control over their physiological responses and reduce the need for high doses of medication.

Find a creative outlet—Writing poetry or prose, painting or making collages, playing an instrument or singing (anything creative) are powerful tools in working with the feelings of fear, anger, and loss that are stirred by illness.

If you are a caregiver, do not neglect your own self-care—Take time for rest and restoration, time to renew yourself in important life interests and activities. If you become depleted, you cannot give to another what is depleted and you no longer possess.

Data from Zerbe, K. J. (1999). *Women's mental health in primary care.* Philadelphia: Saunders.

These situations may occur more frequently for individuals who lack family support or the personal resources to advocate for themselves (e.g., those from the lower socioeconomic classes, newly arrived immigrants, those living socially "unacceptable" alternative lifestyles).

■ ■ ■ VIGNETTE

Cynthia Bruce was critically injured in a car accident on Monday, August 7, at 50th and C Streets, SE. The accident occurred at approximately 3:30 PM. Numerous witnesses report that when the fire department personnel working on Cynthia discovered she was biologically a male, they temporarily stopped treatment and made disparaging remarks and jokes about the victim. Cynthia was apparently semiconscious during this time. Cynthia died a short time later at D.C. General Hospital. (*Renaissance News & Views*, Vol. 9, No. 9, September 1995)

The key to increasing awareness of human rights issues in mental health care may be the integration of these concepts into nursing curricula. However, humanitarian values are often sown early in life, and nurses hesitate to confront employers regarding accepted practices that violate human rights. A committee composed of nurses who do not experience a conflict of interest while in the role of client advocate, as well as other hospital employees, could be formed to review such cases and make recommendations to the hospital administration. In this age of managed care and cuts in hospital budgets, human rights are one of nursing's greatest challenges.

ROLE OF THE PSYCHIATRIC LIAISON NURSE

Psychiatric liaison nursing is a subspecialty of psychiatric nursing that was initiated in the early 1960s. Usually, the psychiatric liaison nurse has a master's degree and a background in psychiatric and medical-surgical nursing. A psychiatric liaison nurse functions as a nursing consultant in managing psychosocial concerns and as a clinician in helping the client deal more effectively with physical and emotional problems. Throughout the steps of the nursing process, a psychiatric liaison nurse assists the nursing and medical staff in caring for hospitalized medically ill clients with mental health concerns. Often these individuals present management problems or have problems that impede their care. Therefore, the psychiatric liaison nurse is a resource for the members of a nursing staff who feel unable to intervene therapeutically with a client.

The psychiatric liaison nurse first meets with the nurse who initiated the consultation. The liaison nurse then reviews the medical records, talks with the physicians, and interviews the client. After interviewing the client, the liaison nurse discusses the assessment and suggestions with the referring nurse. If a psychiatric consultation is warranted, the psychiatric liaison nurse initiates the consultation by contacting the client's medical doctor. A case conference is sometimes needed to enhance communication and consistency in the care of a particular client.

▪ ▪ ▪ KEY POINTS to REMEMBER

- Just as physical illness is accompanied by emotional responses, so emotions often increase the severity of physical symptoms.
- The holistic philosophy of nursing dictates that all nurses, regardless of their roles or specialties, view clients as having a number of psychosocial needs as well as strengths that can be identified through a holistic assessment.
- The medical and psychiatric communities recognize the need to target both the psychological problems and medical problems of a client to increase adherence to the care regimen, maximize quality of life, and promote healing.
- Applying the theories and concepts of psychiatric mental health nursing to the care of all clients not only is a challenge to nurses but also is required by today's health care consumer. Illness disrupts the lives of clients and their families on many levels. By understanding a client's psychosocial needs and knowing when to intervene and where to refer the client, the nurse really practices holistic care and more effectively promotes health.
- Identifying the existence of depression, anxiety, and substance abuse and getting the client treatment can help promote a positive outcome of the medical disorder and improve the client's quality of life.
- A holistic approach to client care includes assessment of physical, psychosocial, social, and spiritual needs. Brief assessments are included in this chapter.
- A growing concern about clients is the state of their spiritual lives. Including this dimension in the holistic nursing assessment allows nurses to see inner strengths in their clients that might be overlooked by a more traditional approach. Interventions based on this holistic perspective may be more creative, as Eastern and Western approaches are united.
- Self-assessment allows nurses to explore what their own inner strengths are and how to use them in their professional lives in the service of clients who challenge nurses most—those who confront nurses with values, lifestyles, or beliefs that conflict with the nurses' own.
- It is incumbent upon nurses not only to care for clients but also to advocate for them in this ever-changing health care system, so that the psychological-social-spiritual needs of clients with medical disorders are not overlooked in their care.
- The psychiatric liaison nurse is a nurse clinician who is in the key position of being able to help other health care personnel look at their clients in a holistic manner and to help those who care for these clients understand nonmedical issues that are impeding medical progress.

Visit the Evolve website at **http://evolve.elsevier.com/Varcarolis** for a posttest on the content in this chapter.

■ **STUDENT**
■ **STUDY**
■ **CD-ROM**

Access the accompanying CD-ROM for animations, interactive exercises, review questions for the NCLEX examination, and an audio glossary.

Critical Thinking and Chapter Review

Visit the Evolve website at **http://evolve.elsevier.com/Varcarolis** for additional self-study exercises.

evolve

■■■ CRITICAL THINKING

Vincent Parello, 58 years old, is being discharged from the hospital after a serious myocardial infarction. His wife died a year earlier of cancer and he says he still feels down about it. He talks to his two children on a weekly basis, but he sees them only once a year for a few days around the holidays. He is a hard worker and complains, "I've got so much stress . . . but I am the only one who can do this job." He finds it hard to talk about his thoughts and feelings. "I'll be fine," he says, but the nurse notices that he appears anxious and admits to being lonely "with everyone out of the house." Although overly busy with work, he does go to church every week, and sometime he says he gets sad because it brings back memories of church social events he shared with his family and old friends in the past. When he is told of some limitations on his physical activities, he reacts in a belligerent manner: "I can do anything I used to do." But underneath, the nurse believes he is frightened and is feeling very alone.

1. How would you evaluate this man's social support system?
   A. What other information would you like to know about his situation that might help in your assessment?
   B. What do you need to know about his cultural beliefs and illness?
   C. What recommendations or referrals could you make for him?
   D. How would you approach these recommendations with this particular person?

2. From what you know of Mr. Parello, identify the strengths he has that you would support and encourage.
   A. What cognitive-behavioral coping skills have been proven useful for a client with cardiac problems (coronary heart disease)?
   B. What changes in Mr. Parello's approach to his work and life might help lessen his self-driven behaviors?
   C. Which cognitive-behavioral techniques would you choose to teach Mr. Parello?
   D. Would you include contact data for any medically related support groups in the information you would give him?

3. Discuss how you would approach the physician regarding Mr. Parello's need to be evaluated for depression. What are some of the compelling reasons depression (and any coexisting mental condition) should be treated in any and all seriously ill medically clients?

■■■ CHAPTER REVIEW

Choose the most appropriate answer.

1. Which psychological response to serious medical illness can the nurse expect to find in nearly all clients?
   1. Anger
   2. Anxiety
   3. Depression
   4. Substance abuse

2. Ms. Peters is a client who has been receiving hemodialysis for 3 months. During the psychosocial assessment with the psychiatric liaison nurse, Ms. Peters reports that she finds herself feeling angry whenever it is time for her dialysis treatment. The nurse can probably attribute this to
   1. organic changes in Ms. Peters's brain.
   2. a flaw in Ms. Peters's personality.
   3. a normal response to grief and loss.
   4. denial of the reality of a poor prognosis.

3. The psychiatric liaison nurse who assesses Ms. James realizes that depression is a complicating factor in the client's adjustment to newly diagnosed adult-onset diabetes. To what problem should the nurse advise clinic staff to be particularly alert?
   1. Development of agoraphobia
   2. Treatment noncompliance
   3. Frequent hypoglycemic reactions
   4. Silent urinary tract infections

4. Which client is least likely to be the victim of human rights abuse?
   1. Ms. Y., who is HIV positive and is being treated for a pulmonary infection
   2. Ms. H., who has received transgender surgery and has cholecystitis
   3. Mr. A., who is severely and persistently mentally ill and is being treated for cellulitis
   4. Mr. C., who has Duchenne's muscular dystrophy and is experiencing adult respiratory distress syndrome

5. Which client would the nurse assess as having ineffective coping skills?
   1. Ms. A., who has breast cancer and who confronts her health problem and devises an appropriate plan of action
   2. Ms. B., who has multiple sclerosis and keeps herself busy and maintains positive emotional ties with family and friends
   3. Mr. C., who is HIV positive and expresses guilt about his sexual behavior and broods about the hopelessness of his situation
   4. Mr. D., who has adult-onset diabetes mellitus and actively seeks information about management of his illness

REFERENCES

American Psychiatric Association. (2000). *Diagnostic and statistical manual of mental disorders (DSM-IV-TR)* (4th ed., text rev.). Washington, DC: Author.

Bowen, R. C., Senthilselvan, A., & Barale, A. (2000). Physical illness as an outcome of chronic anxiety disorders. *Canadian Journal of Psychiatry, 45*(5), 459-464.

Cannon, W. B. (1914). The emergency function of the adrenal medulla in pain and the major emotions. *American Journal of Physiology, 33,* 356-372.

Culpepper, L. (2003, May 18). The successful intervention: Management of the patient with medical comorbidities. In *Psychiatry and medicine: Common patients, different perspectives.* Symposium conducted at the 156th Annual Meeting of the American Psychiatric Association, San Francisco, CA.

Goddard, B. S., & Shekhar, A. (2002). Evaluating and treating anxiety disorders in medical settings. *Journal of Postgraduate Medicine, 48*(4), 317-321.

Goodwin, R. D., & Pine, D. S. (2002). Respiratory disease and panic attacks among adults in the United States. *Chest, 122*(2), 645-650.

Levenson, J. L. (2003). Psychological factors affecting medical conditions. In A. Tasman, J. Kay, & J. A. Lieberman (Eds.), *Psychiatry* (2nd ed.). West Sussex, England: Wiley.

Meyer, T., Klemme, H., & Herrmann, C. (2000). Depression but not anxiety is significant predictor of physicians' assessment of medical status in physically ill patients. *Psychotherapy and Psychosomatics, 69,* 147-154.

Rosack, J. (2003). Comorbidity common in addicts, but integrated treatment rare. *Psychiatric News, 38*(2), 30.

Selye, H. (1956). *The stress of life.* New York: McGraw-Hill.

Semet, J. H., Friedman, P., & Saitz, R. (2001). Benefits of linking primary medical care and substance abuse services: Patient provider and social services. *Archives of Internal Medicine, 161*(1), 85-91.

Spollen, J. J., & Gutman, B. S. (2003, May 18). The interaction of depression and medical disorders. In *Psychiatry and medicine: Common patients, different perspectives.* Symposium conducted at the 156th Annual Meeting of the American Psychiatric Association, San Francisco, CA.

Valdivia, I., & Rossy, N. (2004). Depressive disorder: Advice for the primary care physician. *Topics in Advance Practice eJournal* 4(1). Retrieved March 2, 2005, from http://www.medscape.com/viewarticle/467185.

Zerbe, K. J. (1999). *Women's mental health in primary care.* Philadelphia: Saunders.

CHAPTER 30

Care for the Dying and for Those Who Grieve

KATHY A. KRAMER-HOWE ▪ ELIZABETH M. VARCAROLIS

KEY TERMS and CONCEPTS

The key terms and concepts listed here appear in color where they are defined or first discussed in this chapter.

anticipatory grief, 607

bereavement, 612

caring presence, 604

disenfranchised grief, 613

Four Gifts of Resolving Relationships, 608

grief, 612

hospice, 602

mourning, 613

palliative care, 602

public tragedies, 613

OBJECTIVES

After studying this chapter, the reader will be able to

1. Contrast and compare the goals of end-of-life care inherent in the hospice model with those of the medical model and be specific about these differences.

2. Analyze the effects of specific tasks that health care workers (nurses and social workers) can perform when working with a dying person and his or her family and loved ones.

3. Analyze how the Four Gifts of Resolving Relationships could have affected the dying experience of someone you cared for in the past and consider how it could affect your response to a dying loved one in the future.

4. Using the seven motifs as a guide, describe how a loved one of yours might confront death in terms of how this person confronts life. Which motif might the person adopt and what guidelines might be best suited to the person at the time of dying?

5. Explain how the distinction between the words *bereavement* and *mourning,* as presented in this chapter, can help to enhance the effectiveness of a holistic approach.

6. Differentiate among some of the characteristics of normal bereavement and dysfunctional grieving.

7. Explain why frameworks (models) of understanding loss through stages (Kübler-Ross, Parkes, Engel, Lindemann, Bowlby, etc.) are helpful for people but are not the focus of care.

8. Apply some of the guidelines for helping people to cope with loss of a client, friend, family member, or classmate.

9. Discuss at least seven behavioral outcomes that indicate a successful bereavement.

10. Identify situations and circumstances that could affect a person's coming to terms with loss.

evolve Visit the Evolve website at **http://evolve.elsevier.com/Varcarolis** for a pretest on the content in this chapter.

Care for the Dying

KATHY A. KRAMER-HOWE

Caring for the terminally ill challenges and rewards nurses in deep and personal ways. In caring for the dying, nurses are called on both to find acceptance for their clients' deaths and to enter into a new relationship with their own mortality. They have the gratifica-tion of knowing that they helped another person die with minimal suffering and with the opportunity for life closure. In a culture that fears and denies aging and death, compassionate medical and social support at life's end is all the more appreciated for being unex-pected by most clients and families. Bringing dignity to dying and a sense of competency to caregivers and families helps shape an enduring positive memory. Thus, there are many lessons to be gained in caring for the terminally ill, and many gifts to be given and shared with the client and family.

In recent years, the burgeoning hospice and palliative care movement spurred research into the experience of dying in America. The realities can be grim. A recent study reported in the *Journal of the American Medical Association* asked family members of 1578 decedents about care in the setting in which death occurred. Questions centered on whether health care workers provided the desired physical and emotional comfort to the dying, supported shared decision making, treated the dying with respect, attended to the family's emotional needs, and provided coordinated care. Over 67% of deaths occurred in an institution, with the remainder occurring at home. Of these cases, just under half of individuals received home hospice services. Some key findings are that one in four people who died did not receive adequate pain medication; one in two received inadequate emotional supports; and between 20% and 33% of those surveyed expressed dissatisfaction with physician communication and treatment decisions, emotional support to families, and provision of consistently respectful treatment to the dying person. Families receiving home hospice care were the most satisfied on all these measures, with over 70% rating hospice care as excellent (Teno et al., 2004). The chances of dying in pain increase for people who do not speak English or who are poor, African American, Hispanic, elderly, or female (Byock, 1997). This study and others point to the need for across-the-board improvements in the care of the dying and their families.

Medical professionals in both institutional and home settings can become advocates for the terminally ill and their hardworking and often unsupported caregivers. The hospice and palliative care treatment model affirms that dying persons and their families have the right to honest answers to difficult questions; the right to have control over as much of their medical care and living situation as possible; the right to have advance directives completed and followed, including instructions to suspend or withhold curative efforts; the right to receive excellent palliative care and to be comfortable; and the right to be perceived as fully deserving of dignity and human worth. This chapter provides an overview of end-of-life care, with an emphasis on clinical strategies and interventions with clients and families.

HOSPICE AND PALLIATIVE CARE

Before the hospice movement began in England in the 1960s, dying people were routinely shunted into hospital rooms with phrases like "We're sorry, there's nothing more we can do for you," and with doctor's orders for "as needed" pain medication. Despite the ministrations of caring health professionals and visits from helpless relatives, dying people were often neglected, isolated, and in pain. In 1967, Dame Cicely Saunders established St. Christopher's Hospice in London to remedy this state of neglect (Stolberg, 1999). In her hospice house, clients' physical comfort was aggressively pursued with around-the-clock pain medication so that they could respond to other pressing issues and enjoy optimal quality of life. Effective management of physical symptoms restored meaningful quality of life to many. Some took care of legal and financial matters, some went shopping, some said their good-byes and restored damaged relationships, some aligned themselves with their God, and most were able to find peace in their lives.

During the late 1960s in the United States, Dr. Elisabeth Kübler-Ross began actively listening to the terminally ill, and out of her groundbreaking work came a construct of the human response to death and loss that has entered the mainstream. She identified distinctive phases, or cycles, in people's responses to terminal illness: denial, anger, bargaining, depression, and acceptance (Kübler-Ross, 1969). She also realized that personal growth did not necessarily cease in the last stages of life but, on the contrary, often accelerated. Encouraged by her findings, hospices staffed by volunteers began to appear in the 1970s. St. Christopher's comprehensive model was adapted, and the multidisciplinary care team evolved to include a physician, nurse, social worker, pastor or chaplain, bath aide, and volunteer. In 1983 Medicare instituted a hospice per diem reimbursement, and most commercial insurers have followed suit. Hospice organizations have proliferated, mostly nonprofit but also for-profit and governmental organizations. In 2003 the National Hospice and Palliative Care Organization (NHPCO) counted over 3300 operating or planned hospices in the 50 states. Approximately 950,000 Americans were served by hospices in the United States in 2002, the majority dying in their own homes (NHPCO, 2004b).

Palliative care is a medical specialty that has grown out of the hospice movement and an increasing international awareness of the need for better care for the dying. "Considered to be the model for quality, compassionate care for people facing a life-limiting illness or injury, hospice or palliative care involves a team-oriented approach to expert medical care, pain management, and emotional and spiritual support expressly tailored to the patient's needs and wishes. Support is provided to the patient's loved ones as well. At the center of hospice and palliative care is the belief that each of us has the right to die pain-free and with dignity" (NHPCO, 2004d). According to the NHPCO's Standards of Practice for Hospice Programs, "The test of palliative care lies in the agreement between the individual, physician(s), primary caregiver, and the hospice team that the expected outcome is relief from distressing symptoms, the easing of pain, and/or enhancing the quality of life. . . . The individual's choices and decisions regarding care are paramount and must be followed" (NHPCO, 2004a). In the United States, *palliative care* is usually regarded as the generic term, and *hospice* refers to a specific model for providing palliation to the terminally ill and the bereaved. "Palliative care is applicable from the beginning of an illness, in effect, whenever comfort, support and quality of life are significant concerns for a terminal illness" (Hutchings, 2002, p. 409). Teams of physicians, nurses, and social workers offer palliative care in many hospitals and other institutional settings to clients for whom hospice care is not an appropriate choice.

■ ■ ■ VIGNETTE

Mr. Spence contracted amyotrophic lateral sclerosis at the age of 52 years. He lived at home until his care overwhelmed his family and has now been in a care center for 9 months. He is almost totally paralyzed but can still use a letter board with a head-mounted laser pointer. He has a warm smile and a very pleasant gaze. He is experiencing shooting pains in his legs and has increasingly more difficulty swallowing and breathing. The staff worries about losing all communication with him and about his suffering at the end of life. He has rejected a feeding tube or any heroic measures. Will he starve to death? Will he be frightened once he can no longer communicate? Will he linger?

■ ■ ■

A palliative team consultation or hospice referral can offer practical help and guidance for staff, client, and family in treating Mr. Spence. The hospice nurse and social worker can talk with him about his future wishes as his condition declines, addressing his wishes to have control over eating and his fears of starvation. Breathing and any fears of choking or strangling toward the end of his life would also be discussed. Comfort-oriented medication and types of care can be talked about so that he can control as much as possible of the process of his illness and dying. Emotional, spiritual, and educational support can be offered to the family and staff about the course of the illness, anticipatory grieving, and ways of using the time remaining to meet goals and nurture their relationships. For example, a hospice volunteer might help Mr. Spence compose a memoir about the impact of his illness on his life and personal growth.

Hospice care is available to everyone, regardless of age, diagnosis, or the ability to pay. As a general rule, hospice care requires a physician's best clinical judgment that the client is terminally ill with a life expectancy of 6 months or less if the disease runs its normal course. In addition, the client chooses hospice care rather than curative treatments. The Medicare hospice benefit (provided under Part A) stipulates a certification period of several months, at the end of which time a physician recertifies the terminal illness and probable life expectancy. Clients with cancer and noncancer illnesses are eligible, and the client and family are con-

sidered the unit of care. Most clients receive care at home, but four levels of care are mandated: routine home care, continuous home care (with short-term around-the-clock nursing care at home), inpatient respite care, and general inpatient care. Ninety-six percent of hospice care is provided as routine home care (NHPCO, 2004c), which includes physician services, nursing and nurse's aide visits, medical equipment, medications related to the terminal illness, social work and counseling services, spiritual care, volunteer services, and bereavement services. Limited physical, dietary, speech, and occupational therapy are also covered. Medicare, and many commercial insurance plans, reimburse at a set per diem rate for all clients on service. The client's own physician usually continues to follow the client, although a hospice medical director is available.

Hospice programs accept dying as a natural and inevitable part of life. Care is delivered by a multidisciplinary team that integrates psychosocial, spiritual, and medical information to formulate and continually update a personalized plan of care. According to the NHPCO, the median length of stay in hospice care in 2003 was 22 days, and the mean was 55 days. This represents the first increase in these statistics in the past 2 years (NHPCO, 2004a). Hopefully, these numbers demonstrate more understanding and acceptance among physicians and the public of the significant benefits hospice care offers at life's end. Earlier access to hospice care can provide greater comfort, client control, and family satisfaction, and may reduce health care costs in the last year of life (Campbell et al., 2004). More than a physical place, hospice is a philosophy of care founded on the principles of

- Ensuring client dignity and respect.
- Treating the client and family as the unit of care.
- Supporting a peaceful, pain-free death.
- Providing client control and choice.
- Viewing the client holistically.
- Offering bereavement support for the family after the death.

NURSING GOALS IN END-OF-LIFE CARE

Nursing the terminally ill and supporting their families calls for a human and holistic approach. Client reports indicate that the caring presence of the nurse is valued as highly as is excellent symptom management. Paying attention to the client's religious and spiritual preferences can positively affect the plan of care. Hospice nurses draw on each other's and on physicians' knowledge to deliver expert palliative and comfort-oriented treatments. They have a heightened educational role with family caregivers and the client. Lastly, they must practice good self-care to manage and replenish their own emotional and professional reserves. These elements are explored in more depth in the sections that follow.

Practice the Art of Presence

Nursing the terminally ill, whether in home hospice or palliative care settings, requires many shifts in professional expectations. Because dying is a fundamentally personal and meaningful experience, the role of the nurse includes human presence and receptivity. Whole-person care involves seeing the client first and foremost as a human being and offering care for all aspects of suffering. Thus, the nurse's sense of competency and professionalism gained through taking action sometimes has to yield to a willingness to embrace the mystery and powerlessness of the dying process. As front-line caregivers in medical settings, nurses effectively bring symptom relief and comfort. They help clients get better, stronger, and more independent. The terminally ill are going to grow weaker and sicker and ultimately die. They experience levels of existential suffering that normal nursing interventions cannot resolve. Paradoxically, however, the caring presence of a health care professional in shared helplessness can bring solace and support to the dying person. The dying person has been compared to a composer of a unique melody. Hospice and palliative care nurses are the listeners of the music, and their role "is to be present with these person composers and invite them to guide their care" (Hutchings, 2002, p. 412).

In addition to excellent clinical skills and knowledge, what are the qualities of effective hospice nurses? In a recent study based on hospice family satisfaction surveys, field notes, and participant interviews with experienced hospice registered nurses, the first quality identified was the ability to be humanly present. This involved taking the time to be with the clients without distractions, attending to their needs and responding with flexibility. One client wrote, "There were times when I just needed someone to take time to talk to me—you did. Thanks. There were times when I just longed to be touched or hugged—you did. Thanks" (Wright, 2002, p. 212). Other qualities were the ability to think and act creatively, the ability to show compassion, appropriate technological knowledge, a spiritual dimension and sense of calling in their work, the ability to be interdisciplinary team players, and a sense of humor (Wright, 2002).

To cultivate the art of being humanly present, practice observing the client's nonverbal communications and pay attention to your own emotional response. Do you sense well-being? Sorrow? Suffering? Ask the client open-ended questions like, "Will you tell me what it is like to be at this point in your life?" "How do you see your illness right now?" "Where do you see things going?" "Are you suffering?" Practice staying silent and giving the client all the time he or she needs to respond. Offer a reassuring touch. Giving undiluted attention to the client may contribute to healing by communicating acceptance and shared humanity. Healing has been described as "being fully in the present, allowing a great spaciousness for life, for disease, for pain, and for death" (Gauthier, 2002, p. 221). The spaciousness created by a humanly present nurse can invite and permit the client to discover new dimensions to his or her own experiences. Nurses need the skills to assess and become sensitive to the spiritual themes embedded in a dying person's stories and conversation and silences.

Assess for Spiritual Issues

In addition to practicing human attentiveness, the hospice or palliative care nurse is asked to conduct a more formal **spiritual assessment.** Most professional nursing associations call for nurses to assess client spirituality in all health care delivery settings. Hospices have policies and sample assessments to address this issue, and spirituality in health care is increasingly a subject of research (Millison, 1995). Clients report that they feel cared about when medical personnel are interested in their spirituality. However, they seem to prefer that such discussions occur in the context of ordinary conversation and human sharing (Hart et al., 2003). Imbedded in the stories of a lifetime are spiritual themes such as how clients assign meaning and value, how they experience connections and becoming, and when they have sensed a transcendent realm or a dimension beyond the self (Stephenson, Draucker, & Martsolf, 2003, p. 52). Spirituality goes beyond religious affiliation and practices and can be an important component of how an individual defines hope and healing. Box 30-1 provides a spirituality assessment tool developed by a hospice nurse and social worker.

It is useful to distinguish between religion and spirituality, while acknowledging that they are aspects of the same human tendency to seek meaning and connection with something greater than self. Spirituality encompasses questions about how our lives relate to the rest of creation without requiring a specific religious affiliation, for example: What energizes our lives? What will survive our personal death, if anything? How do we explain to ourselves the things that happen in life? When do we feel most peaceful? How have we surmounted life's hardest challenges?

Religion refers to structured communities of support for people with shared spiritual beliefs, expressed as behaviors, roles, and expectations. Religiosity is most often indicated by membership, either current or past, in a church, synagogue, mosque, or other center of worship. Identifying a client's religious affiliation does not end the conversation. To understand how a client's spirituality may enhance end-of-life health

BOX 30-1

Spiritual Assessment Tool: S.H.A.R.E.

Spirituality
What does spirituality mean to you? How would you describe your belief or faith system?
Secular/Spiritual
What is the meaning of what is happening to you in your life?
How do you need to respond?
Religious/Spiritual
What is God's place in what is happening to you?
How do you need to respond?

How Important?
What role does your faith/spirituality have in your life?
Secular/Spiritual
What is most important in your life?
How would your life change if this were taken away?
Religious/Spiritual
What has been most meaningful to you in your faith community?
What is meaningful right now?

Activity
What actions connect you to your beliefs?
Secular/Spiritual
What calms your anxieties?
What puts you in touch with a sense of strength, peace, or hope?
Religious/Spiritual
What faith practices (prayer, music, movement, meditation, etc.) do you use to calm or center yourself?

Relationship
How do your beliefs and values relate to your present circumstances (diagnosis, prognosis, comfort, hope, etc.)?
Secular/Spiritual
Do you think there is a reason why this is happening to you?
Do you feel incomplete about aspects of your life?
Religious/Spiritual
Has this illness changed your relationship with God?
Do you feel incomplete in your relation to your church or faith?
Do you have any unmet needs?

Empower
How can we be most effective in supporting your faith/belief?
If we could do just one thing to help you with this part of your life, what would it be?
Do not seek to fix or answer everything that comes up.

Kramer-Howe, K., & Huls, P. T. (2004) *A spiritual assessment tool.* Phoenix, AZ: Hospice of the Valley.

care, it is important to assess his or her values, beliefs, and practices in an ongoing way. Of course, this requires the client's consent and is not applicable to every client. To assess spirituality in health care, the following guidelines may be helpful (Kramer-Howe & Huls, 2004):

Start the conversation. Allow yourself to be genuinely interested without feeling that you have to be an expert or have the answers. Just listen and ask again, in a spirit of seeking to understand the client, not to "fix" him or her.

This is the client's story. Avoid using the lens of your own belief system. This is the client and family's framework of values. You are there to learn and support, not to change their spirituality or faith, or lack thereof.

Refer to a counselor with spiritual expertise. There will be times when a client and/or family wishes to share with a counselor, or the palliative team thinks it would be helpful. A hospice chaplain can bring a perspective that complements that of the client and/or family's formal religious leader or community. The role of the hospice chaplain can be described as that of a nondenominational pastoral counselor with health care training and extensive experience in working with people in a similar situation.

Seek to hear unspoken questions. Sometimes a client's existential issues are not communicated in words. These may be unspoken questions such as: "Do you know what I am hoping for today?" "Can you tell if I am feeling despair?" "Do you know what brings me courage and peace?" "Can you help calm my fears?" Sometimes, by listening to a client's dreams, these unspoken emotional or spiritual states can also be explored and addressed.

Be empowered by the process. This ongoing assessment may help nurses explore their own spirituality. They can grow more comfortable hearing and expressing spiritual concepts in everyday language. The plan of care will become more individualized and meaningful when influenced by clients' spirituality.

Provide Palliative Symptom Management

Excellent **symptom management** is a hallmark of palliative nursing. The goals of care are defined by the client or by the client's advance directives and medical proxy. Restoring to clients control over medical decisions is part of a national trend toward greater client self-determination in health care, expressed in the Patient Self-Determination Act that became effective in 1991, the Project on Death in America, and the Missoula Demonstration Project, among other initiatives. Polls show that people fear being in pain, depleting family resources, having death prolonged artificially, and submitting to the suffering of death (Redford, 2000). Common to all of these is a sense of powerlessness. Palliative nursing returns a sense of control to dying individuals, as well as hope that uncomfortable symptoms can be alleviated through sophisticated use of medications (Redding, 2000). Hospice and palliative nurses continually update their medical knowledge and skills as they meet both routine and unusual challenges.

The palliative care philosophy is to accept clients' own reports of symptoms as accurate indicators for medical interventions. The most commonly reported symptoms are lack of energy, pain, lack of appetite, drowsiness, difficulty concentrating, sadness, shortness of breath, agitation, worrying, cough, nervousness, and constipation (Kutner, Kassner, & Nowels, 2001). Many of these symptoms are successfully managed with an array of medications and treatments. It is very gratifying to relieve a suffering person of unacceptable levels of pain or nausea, or to give them control over bowel medications and breathing treatments. As this list suggests, however, there are some symptoms that often are not adequately treated, such as lack of energy and appetite, drowsiness, sadness, worrying, and difficulty concentrating.

Palliative nurses assess for psychosocial sources of suffering, such as family discord, fears, lack of information, unacknowledged grief responses, poor coping skills, and so on. Counseling and behavioral interventions as well as complementary therapies such as massage, aroma therapy, art, and music are commonly offered to address these complex human issues. Although hospice and palliative care nurses usually succeed in greatly lessening clients' suffering, there is much yet to be learned about bringing holistic comfort to the dying and their families.

It is important to assess for dual diagnoses and past history. Although hospice nurses focus on the terminal condition, they must be aware of all comorbidities, such as diabetes or heart disease. A crucial question to ask is, "Who wanted this individual in hospice care and why now?" Sometimes an admitting diagnosis masks an underlying treatable condition. An example is admission of an elderly person for dementia or failure to thrive, with later discovery of a treatable underlying clinical depression. General debility can also result from a recent trauma, such as a serious fall or sudden loss. In those cases, behavioral therapy and/or psychotropic medications might resolve the symptoms. The abuse of drugs or alcohol in either the past or present will affect the types and amounts of analgesics needed to control pain. Mental illness can also affect the delivery and type of care. When a holistic approach is used, clients are seen and treated comprehensively in their environments.

BECOMING AN EFFECTIVE COMMUNICATOR

The palliative care nurse has a heightened **educational role** with the family, especially those at home who are usually providing direct care and administering med-

ications and treatments. In a national study to identify core competencies for nursing at the end of life, knowledge of how to talk to clients and families about dying was ranked first by the survey respondents across all age levels, educational levels, practice roles, and practice settings (the other core competency areas were pain control techniques, comfort care nursing interventions, palliative treatments, recognition of impending death, dealing with one's own feelings, dealing with angry clients and families, ethical issues, advance directives, bioethical legal issues, religion and cultural perspectives, and the meaning of hospice care) (White, Coyne, & Patel, 2001).

In a 2003 national poll conducted by the Hospice of the Florida Suncoast that underscored the need for heightened skills in communicating with families, 3000 caregivers with a dying or recently deceased family member were asked which kinds of support and information they considered most helpful. Over 900 responses indicated that caregivers value practical information such as information about the illness, how to give medications, what to expect at the time of death, and how to make end-of-life decisions (Florida Policy Exchange Center on Aging & The Hospice Institute of the Florida Suncoast, 2003). Nurses also play a key role in helping families identify and cope with their many grief reactions to loss. Anticipatory grieving (also called *premourning*) is grieving for the many losses caused by terminal illness, with the knowledge that death is inevitable (Shneidman, 1980). Its symptoms are very much like those of bereavement, but often they are unrecognized and unaddressed.

Whether in home hospice care or in an institutional setting, the palliative care nurse is called upon for information, education, and support. Confronting death is a stressful and often frightening experience. Even when death will end a long, debilitating condition such as dementia or failure to thrive, the loss of that individual heralds the occurrence of grief and change. Family systems usually make many adjustments to give care and to make the most of limited time with the client. If caregiving is prolonged, the family grows tired and may seek certainties and time lines from the hospice nurse. During stressful periods, two factors seem to make things more bearable: the ability to have, or believe one can have, some control over the situation, and the ability to predict changes. Information and education from the hospice nurse can improve a family's sense of control.

Convey Information to Enhance Competency

Both the client and the family often want to know how to interpret physical symptoms that are occurring. The nurse can share medical expertise about the normal progression of the disease, the effects of medications, reasons to change drug regimens, and ways to provide comfort care. Information can dispel myths and fears about symptoms and medications, and increase a sense of control. However, information should be conveyed slowly, given repeatedly, written down, and reviewed often. Communication experts estimate that people need *at least six reiterations of new information when they are under stress.*

In home hospice care, the family is usually administering treatments and medications. Nurses educate and train family members to organize and record medications given, even those unrelated to the hospice diagnosis. For example, a client with chronic obstructive pulmonary disease may have diabetes, or a cancer client may have congestive heart failure. Nurses commonly set up a medication tray every week, which includes the full array of client treatments. Families and clients often have misgivings and misconceptions about using opiates such as morphine. It is commonly thought that addiction will follow, that clients will get too sleepy or even stop breathing, or that morphine is administered "only at the very end." Hospice nurses enhance family competency and client comfort by repeatedly educating about drugs such as these and by explaining how palliative pain management differs from other approaches.

Another area of ongoing education is that of diminishing client energy and appetite. It is frightening to have a loved one refuse food and drink, or want to stay in bed much of the time. The hospice nurse can help the family deal with these symptoms by explaining that they are involuntary on the client's part and may actually serve an energy-conserving function. Another difficult symptom is the client's avoidance of discussion about dying or failure to complete end-of-life planning. The lack of advance care directives, powers of attorney, funeral plans, and final wishes causes added stress to family members who will have to confront the consequences later. Sometimes, the hospice nurse can counsel the client about the advantages of speaking more openly with the family, providing a safe channel for communication between them.

Make Limited but Realistic Predictions

Faced with the loss of a beloved person, families must live in extraordinary ways with the dual realities of impending death and continued life. At times, someone may confess that he or she wishes this were over. Either client or family may ask the nurse, "How long will this go on?" Once someone is receiving hospice care, the person has been told that the doctor estimates a life expectancy of 6 months or less, should the disease proceed at a normal pace. This is only a guess, however. The human inability to make accurate predictions until someone is actively dying can create a sense of interminable suffering for client or family. When the family seeks answers, a two-pronged approach can be helpful:

- Focus the family on the here and now, on opportunities to find respite and comfort, and on living one day at a time.
- Offer clinical data based on physical examination and paint a changing picture from which family and client can draw some conclusions.

The following case study illustrates the confusion and misery that can result from lack of information, the desire to take control of one's life situation, and the linguistic inadequacy of the word *dying.*

■ ■ ■ VIGNETTE

Susan, a 74-year-old divorced woman living alone, is told by her doctor that she is dying of liver cancer. Upon hearing that she cannot be cured, she assumes she will die in a few days or weeks. She goes home, settles all her affairs, calls everyone she cares about and says good-bye, accepts hospice care, and sits down to await death. As weeks and then months go by, Susan feels betrayed by her doctor, embarrassed to be alive, unsure how to behave, and uncomfortable with her friends and relatives. She has time to begin worrying about how her death will be, how much control she will lose, and how she can afford care at the end. She is confused and even disoriented by the unexpected improvement in her symptoms.

Susan is suffering from lack of knowledge and understanding. The hospice nurse works hard to educate Susan about her cancer and how to interpret her symptoms. It becomes important for Susan to return to her doctor several months later "to prove him wrong." The hospice team addresses this woman's emotions and needs in many ways, encouraging her to take a trip she had postponed and to begin seeing friends again. They educate her on the concept of "living with terminal illness" rather than dying from it. Susan needs to learn new approaches to living meaningfully with an uncertain future. When Susan finally enters the end stage of her disease, she is comfortable and cared for by her relatives at home.

■ ■ ■

Counsel About Anticipatory Grieving

As soon as a person receives a life-threatening diagnosis, anticipatory grief begins to affect him or her as well as family members and others who care. *Anticipatory grief* originally referred to grief reactions resulting from the expectation of death. However, "grief is a far broader concept. Grief results from a reaction to a loss—any loss, not just one related to death. . . . [Thus] anticipatory grief is a reaction not only to an expected loss, but to all the losses—past, present and future—that are encountered in an experience of illness or disability" (Doka, 2001, p. 217). In the course of a debilitating, lengthy, or fatal illness, there are innumerable losses—of health, ability to fulfill expected roles, financial status, plans for the future, body image and intimacy, and so on. Just as losses are inherent in these situations, so is grief. Doka writes that grief may be experienced physically as fatigue, tension, and aches and pains; emotionally as anxiety, anger, sorrow, guilt, jealousy, and many other emotions; cognitively as obsessive thinking about the ill person, forgetfulness, and other symptoms; and spiritually as loss or intensification of faith and a sense of meaning.

The symptoms of anticipatory grief are often unrecognized in the family system because attention is focused on other tasks. Sometimes, these grief reactions cause family and client to pull away from each other prematurely. It can be helpful if a hospice nurse educates the family on these grief reactions and explains that they are normal responses to losses and are not simply associated with anticipation of the client's death. The following are some helpful interventions (Doka, 2001, pp. 219-225):

Validate expressions of grief. Listening, understanding, accepting, and explaining the importance of the griever's reactions can be immensely freeing.

Inform clients and families about the disease and its symptoms. Common client behaviors such as social withdrawal, mood swings, fatigue, and vacillation between acceptance and denial can be taken personally by family members. It is essential to explain that these behaviors are part of the disease progression. The best approach is to follow the client's lead in knowing what information to share from one day to the next, and to know that the client, too, is following the lead of his or her body and its condition.

Invite clients and families to deal with affective issues. While the client is alive, families may feel disloyal or inhibited in sharing their feelings. Clients may be protecting family members by withholding their emotions. Inviting people to name and express their feelings can be done with comments such as "Other people in your situation have often told me they felt (depressed, guilty, angry, hopeless). Have you experienced that?"

Acknowledge the losses and changes in their lives. Many losses accumulate gradually and are secondary to the life-threatening condition central to the client and caregivers. Simply asking, "In what ways has your own life changed since _____?" can permit people to identify and begin to cope with these losses.

Explore ways of coping. Examining useful and unproductive ways of adjusting to change and loss can be helpful. Developing strategies for using informal and formal support systems can bring more support to the family and increase opportunities for respite and relief for both client and caregivers.

Anticipatory grieving is an extended process that "does not decrease or increase the amount of emotion generated by [the death], yet it can help work through feelings in advance and resolve unfinished business before the separation actually occurs" (Shearer & Davidhizar, 1994, p. 62). Box 30-2 lists some signs of anticipatory grief.

The Four Gifts of Resolving Relationships

An important role of hospice care in almost every family is to encourage people to accept and even consent to the dying of their loved one. Sometimes this is called "giving permission" for the client to die, but "consenting" to the inevitability of death is perhaps more accurate. Giving permission has connotations of approval or control of the process that do not really match the reality of dying. There are many barriers to openly acknowledging the coming death: the client and/or family's own style of facing or avoiding things; stress and exhaustion from sickness and/or caregiving; anticipatory grief processes that can threaten to overwhelm family members and/or clients with emotions; reticence about naming or expressing feelings. The Four Gifts of Resolving Relationships, or some version thereof, is used in many hospice settings as a relatively nonthreatening tool to open conversations about the coming loss. To invite people to share what they feel is important while there is still time and opportunity is to offer them an experience they can treasure later on.

The concept of the Four Gifts was interpreted from the writings of Elisabeth Kübler-Ross and used with her consent by Beverly Ryan, LCSW, of the Hospice of the Twin Cities in Minnesota. Dr. Kübler-Ross observed many couples and families in her workshops for the terminally ill and saw how often relationships shifted from being distant, cold, or angry to becoming warm,

---

BOX 30-2

Signs of Anticipatory Grief

- Feelings of emptiness or of being lost
- A sense of being numb and fatigued
- A feeling of unreality and disbelief
- Periods of weeping or raging
- A desire to run away from the situation
- A need to oversee every detail of the client's care to protect her or him from suffering and death
- Fear of the future and of the unknown
- Anger at the client or the medical professionals or both
- Pronounced clinging to or dependency on the client or other family members
- Fear of going crazy

loving, and close. The change followed a predictable sequence of emotional communications, and this sequence was eventually formulated into the Four Gifts. Family members often intuitively recognize the Four Gifts as processes they have already been experiencing. These processes seem to be innate within human relationships, but anxiety, sorrow, and denial can obstruct their expression. The hospice nurse can help by describing them in simple terms and encouraging families and clients to find their own ways toward using them. The gifts can work for both the giver and the receiver. When given with sincerity and simplicity, they invariably precipitate a healing shift in relationships.

1. **Forgiveness** ("I'm sorry"; "I forgive you"). The first step is to admit to the wrongs and hurts experienced at the hands of the other person. This can be frightening to do because it makes a person vulnerable to fresh injury. The other person may have no idea the speaker has been harboring a resentment or hurt and may respond with disbelief, defensiveness, or silence. The intention here is to forgive and release the hurt, and that must be the context in which this conversation takes place. Bear in mind two important caveats. One is that sometimes a face-to-face encounter is not possible (as when the client is sedated, comatose, or demented) and sometimes it is not advisable (as when there is a conviction that this would cause more distress than it would relieve). Forgiveness is a one-sided act. Reconciliation requires two people who wish to heal a broken relationship. The other caveat is that forgiveness does *not* mean that a truly injurious or abusive action has been condoned or accepted. It does not make a wrong right. What it does is signal a desire to let go of blame and anger, to release one's heart from the chains of resentment. As such, it is a gift to the one who offers forgiveness, whether reconciliation is possible or not.

   The willingness to say, "I forgive you," is accompanied by the question, "Is there anything I have done, or not done, for which I need to say I am sorry?" Being open to hearing about another person's injuries and asking him or her for forgiveness is the other side of the coin of this gift. The art of giving and receiving forgiveness is rarely practiced overtly in many families, so most people have had no experience with this remarkably healing practice. They may feel awkward and phony using the words. Doubtless this practice entails taking emotional risks. However, it is the gateway to the other three gifts. Time is running out, and families know it. With some practice and encouragement, many take the chance.

2. **Love** ("I love you"). The second gift is to express love to each other. Many adult children still yearn to hear their parents say, "I love you, and I am proud of you." In many long-term marriages, these words have faded away, to be replaced by daily togetherness and the practical caring of a shared life. The end of life is a wonderful time for people to fully express what they mean to each other. Especially meaningful are the many memories of things learned from another, such as values, attitudes, and beliefs. Ultimately, the message is that all people are loved for being just who they are, and they are loved just for being, rather than for what they have done or achieved.

3. **Gratitude** ("Thank you"). This is the moment for people to take the time to thank each other for what each has been in the other's life. People look back over life together and remember the good times and the tough times. They can take out photograph albums, show videotapes, reminisce, listen again to the client's' favorite stories. It is especially important to acknowledge the things that the client took for granted. Many fathers and husbands have never been thanked for going to work every day for 30 or 40 years. Many wives and mothers would never expect thanks for all the laundry, mending, and help with school projects. Many exhausted caregivers weep when they are told they really are doing a good job and are appreciated.

4. **Farewell** ("Good-bye, I'll be okay"). Many people say that they hate good-byes. Saying good-bye brings up feelings of grief at the finality of parting. Also, one hesitates to say good-bye before someone is actually leaving. It may appear to be rushing the person or even causing the departure. Yet when the final separation of death awaits us, the act of saying good-bye is deeply appropriate and meaningful. Survivors feel its absence when there was no chance to say good-bye and usually have to wrestle with this during bereavement.

   When one acknowledges the coming separation, one communicates acceptance that the death will occur. The person who is dying knows that the loved one is facing the death and will survive it. The person saying good-bye loosens his or her grasp and begins to surrender to the inevitability of the death. The phrases one uses can be softened. "I know the time will come when we'll have to part, and these are some of my feelings and thoughts. . . ." "I hate thinking about having to go on without you, yet I want you to know I am going to make it." "Thinking about saying good-bye makes me so terribly sad." However one finds the words, this final gift is a way of acknowledging and honoring the importance of the relationship in one's life, and it should be encouraged and even rehearsed if necessary.

Tom is a 28-year-old developmentally disabled man with bipolar disorder. He arrives at his dying father's home to see him for the last time, and the nurse tells him about the Four Gifts. The young man lives in a group home and has not seen his family for many months. The last time he visited, he had not taken his medication and his misbehavior had estranged his family. The young man sadly enters his father's bedroom and sits on the bed. He says, "Dad, I know you are going to die and I want you to know that I am so sorry for the ways I have acted before now, and the trouble I have caused. Please forgive me, Dad. You have always looked out for me, and I shouldn't have gone off my meds. I love you, Dad. You've never given up on me. Thank you for finding me the place where I live and people to love me and look after me. Thanks for being my Dad. I know I have to say good-bye. I promise I will keep on taking my meds so I will behave right. I promise I'll listen to my counselors and have a good life. I love you so much, Dad. Good-bye." He weeps with his father, who holds him for a little while. Then he comes out of the room with a tear-streaked face, knowing he will never see his father again alive. He feels complete, however. He has said the important things with courage and taken proper leave of his father.

■ ■ ■

In the preceding vignette, Tom did not rehearse, resist, or complicate the Four Gifts, but used the sequence to express a full range of his feelings. His story illustrates how simple and natural this process can be. Many families need no encouragement to forgive, cherish, thank, and release a loved one. The Four Gifts can be a helpful contribution, however, to those families whose members are overwhelmed, cling to false hope, or are emotionally reticent.

PRACTICING GOOD SELF-CARE

Finally, the greater call for human-to-human presence in end-of-life nursing leads to increased vulnerability to emotional attachments. This fact, along with the daily exposure to people who are suffering losses, calls nurses to practice **conscious self-care** in both their professional and private lives. Inevitably, health care personnel sometimes grow attached to clients and may experience both premourning and bereavement. To maintain emotional balance and health, it is essential to rely on the support of the multidisciplinary team and to practice good self-care. This is a journey that invites nurses and other health care personnel to greater self-understanding, wisdom, and compassion, and the team approach is integral to this process.

Nursing the dying and those who grieve challenges and enriches caregivers at a deep level. This is partly because each person has complex unconscious relationships to loss, grief, death, and dying. Reactions from "out of the blue" may be triggered by particular clients and situations; for example, when terminally ill clients are younger than the caregiver; when they resemble a significant person in the nurse's own life; when their diseases and symptoms are reminiscent of those of another difficult death; or when they offend the nurse's sense of fairness or acceptability. In addition, the nurse's own grief process may be stimulated so that she or he is not sure of the source of the sadness felt. Workplace conditions such as inappropriate caseloads, rapid turnover in office staff, too many losses in a short period of time, or too many demands for on-call time or overtime can intensify a nurse's vulnerability to feeling overwhelmed. Box 30-3 provides guidelines to

---

BOX 30-3

Guidelines for Self-Care by Health Care Professionals When Caring for the Dying

1. Remind yourself that what is happening to your clients and their families is not happening to you. This is their life drama right now, but not your own.
2. When you notice that you are having a particularly strong emotional reaction, either positive or negative (countertransference), take it as a signal to explore your deeper issues or needs by talking with a trusted friend, counselor, or colleague.
3. Protect your private life by practicing time management, avoiding overwork and working outside of normal hours, not giving out your pager or home telephone number, and taking regular days off and vacations.
4. Clearly state what you can and cannot do for your clients so that your human and professional limitations are known up front.
5. Expect the unexpected. This work can grab your heart at times and spin you around. It is vital and unpredictable work that exists on the very edge of human existential meaning.
6. Practice humility. The border at which life becomes death is beyond control and mastery. There is much you can do, but there is also much that is unknown and unknowable.
7. Do your own mourning when your heart is touched and you need to acknowledge the importance of others in your life. Even after a person has died, he or she continues a relationship with you in your memory. Attend funerals or create grieving rituals when this happens.
8. Create a healthy, balanced private life by releasing stress. This work creates stresses at many levels. As a human being, you are built for stress, but only when you can regularly discharge the stress and regain the homeostasis of the organism. Otherwise, your body can gradually go out of balance, and various symptoms and illnesses can result. Methods of discharging stress are well known and are endlessly paraded in the press and media. The challenge is to work them into your busy schedule and stay on course. Foremost among these methods are regular exercise, a balanced diet, adequate rest, vacations, fun and laughter, loving and accepting relationships, and a connection to spirituality.

help the health care professional maintain emotional health when working with death and the dying.

CONFRONTING THE PROSPECT OF DYING: SEVEN MOTIFS

At some point in the illness of an individual receiving hospice or palliative care, families usually are handed a description of the physical changes typical in dying individuals. A common reaction is, "I can't believe how closely she followed all the stages!" People are reassured to find that there is some order and predictability in the body's shutting down. Similarly, both families and hospice workers return to the Kübler-Ross stages of dying as a roadmap for a mysterious, complex, and very personal journey. Models, phases, and stages of the human response to dying help us understand what we have in common. Hopefully, they lead us to be more helpful and relevant in our interventions with particular individuals.

"Death belongs to the dying. The only person who can inform us, on an existential level, of what is needed at the end of life is the individual who is dying" (Redding, 2000, p. 204). Focusing on in-depth interviews with dying persons and using inductive, qualitative analysis can help us to find out about dying from the perspective of the clients themselves. How do they create meaning within their reality? How does the encounter with medical workers fit into the broader context of their lives? How can medical workers customize their approaches and interventions for each individual? One recent contribution to this field of research found seven distinct motifs emerging from extensive interviews with the research population—that is, "seven cohesive patterns characterizing the ways in which participants viewed the prospect of their own death" (Yedidia & MacGregor, 2001, p. 811).

These motifs are intriguing for several reasons. One is that they show that people's "responses to dying are seamlessly integrated with broader themes in their lives, and appreciation of their distinctive outlooks requires awareness of their life stories as well as other salient characteristics that distinguish them as people" (Yedidia & MacGregor, 2001, p. 817). In other words, to provide holistic care for the dying requires getting to know about them in a much broader context. They are so much more than an array of symptoms or tasks to be completed.

Second, the quality of their deaths should be evaluated in reference to their life motifs and not by anyone else's standards. They may confront death with struggle and chaos just as harmoniously as someone who meets death with inner strength and transcendent visions. Third, the study results suggest that dying is not necessarily or solely a crisis of meaning requiring reassessments of the past, new coping skills, or new visions of the future. Rather, it occurs in the context of a lifetime of experience, perception, and ways of assigning meaning. Health care workers may interpret a client's behavior in light of stages or phases, but they should also explore a behavior's unique meaning in that person's life. The seven motifs and how they might influence hospice interventions can be described briefly as follows (Yedidia & MacGregor, 2001):

1. **Struggle—living and dying are a struggle.** For these people, life has been hard and required tremendous effort. They may have dealt with abuse, mental illness, or addiction. Dying is a further manifestation of the struggle. In hospice care, psychotherapeutic efforts to reassess lifelong conflicts would not be successful, but basic safety, caring, and comfort can provide a haven of rest.

2. **Dissonance—dying is not living.** These people reflect positively on their past lives but do not think dying offers anything but the end of their story. They do not seek meaning in dying or wish to adapt to it. It represents an unacceptable quality of life that they hope will be over soon. Because physical symptoms are so unwelcome and burdensome to these people, aggressive pain and symptom management is advised. Life-prolonging care is unwelcome.

3. **Endurance—triumph of inner strength.** These people are determined to continue on with life on their terms as they are dying. They take control of their emotions, sustain an upbeat outlook, and wish to be strong in the face of adversity. Introspection or reflection does not interest them. Their strength is more an intrinsic character trait than linked to a belief system. Treatment plans capitalize on their inner strength, setting outcomes and rewarding challenges met. Their confidence should not be mistaken for denial but should be seen as an affirmation of their identity.

4. **Incorporation—belief system accommodates death.** These people have a belief system, whether religious or secular, that encompasses both life and death. Although they may regret the timing of their death, they accept it as in accordance with a larger purpose or higher power. It is important to acknowledge and respect the belief systems of these people and to harmonize it with the plan of care as much as possible.

5. **Coping—working to find a new balance.** These people work hard to adjust to change; they want to cope and find a new equilibrium in their lives. They do not use a core of inner strength or rely on an overarching belief system. Seeking meaning or resolving old issues does not attract them. They try hard to be realistic and practical. An appropriate intervention would be to help them marshal their own resources in confronting the challenges of dying.

6. **Quest—seeking meaning in dying.** The opportunity to grow and to learn has been paramount throughout these people's lives. Dying presents new perspectives from which to mine meaning in their lives. They are reflective and exploratory. They value the opportunity to speak about their experiences and to know that they are perceived as unique, whole individuals, apart from their age, symptoms, and disabilities.

7. **Volatile—unresolved and unresigned.** Throughout many life experiences, these people have confused, chaotic, and unresolved issues. They lack clarity of direction and express a lack of understanding or control over major forces in their lives. Psychosocial interventions may be welcomed in an effort to understand past conflicts, but these individuals may not be able to incorporate much purposeful change, and their deaths may engulf them as their lives have done. Acceptance and affirmation of their survival in life and their worthiness in dying can be helpful.

■ ■ ■ VIGNETTE

Arthur is a 62-year-old married man dying of liver failure brought on by an early life of heavy drug and alcohol use. He vehemently denies any belief in God or anything remotely "spiritual." When asked, during a spiritual assessment, what has brought him the most joy and sense of freedom in his life, he replies, "Oh, that's easy. Riding my Harley!" Conversely, his greatest loss during these days is not being able to ride his bike. Arthur has had a long illness during which he typically leaves the room when death or dying is discussed and will not talk about it with his teenaged children. Just before the onset of several days of acute delirium and agitation preceding his death, Arthur shares a dream with his wife that he has had on three consecutive nights. He has experienced himself riding his bike from city to city, visiting friends and family. His wife uses this powerful image of freedom, joy, and connection to comfort herself and the children as Arthur lies dying.

■ ■ ■

Based on the previous vignette, what would you identify as Arthur's dominant life motif? How might that information influence the plan of care, your own feelings as a nurse, and the response of the multidisciplinary team?

Obviously, these seven motifs for confronting the prospect of dying are just a starting place. To use them as a rubber stamp diagnosis would be to miss the human richness they describe. Any single person will combine motifs, will be a part of a larger social or familial system, and will contain surprising and unexpected potential. These findings, however, invite us to think about dying as the continuation of an already complex and individualized life. By seeking out distinctions amidst the experiences of those actually confronting death, this study contributes to a greater cul-

tural acceptance of death and dying. It moves us from the ideal to the real, and reminds us that dying is a deeply personal event, deserving of dignity, care, and respect.

Care for Those Who Grieve

ELIZABETH M. VARCAROLIS

Loss is part of the human experience, and grief and bereavement are the normal responses to loss. We grieve on a recurring basis as we face the commonplace losses in our lives, be they loss of a relationship (divorce, separation, death, abortion), health (a body function or part, mental or physical capacity), a friendship, status or prestige, security (occupational, financial, social, cultural), or a dream. Normal losses include changes in circumstances, such as retirement, promotion, marriage, and aging. Volkan and Zintl (1993) stated that the course of our lives depends on how we adapt to these losses and how we use change as a vehicle for growth. Changes that we do not adapt to—or fully mourn—may negatively affect our lives by sapping energy and impairing ability to connect (Volkan & Zintl, 1993).

Loss through death is a major life crisis. People grieve because they have become attached to the person dying and are deeply committed to that person. To sever that bond is to do without shared joy, security, satisfaction, growth, and comfort (Tschudin, 1997). On the whole, this is a physically painful process. Simone Weil (1998) described it as an "almost biological disorder caused by the brutal unloosing of an energy hitherto absorbed by an attachment and now left undirected" (p. 42). Losses of this kind can hurt and diminish the part of life that is shared with and related to others, but it can also hurt and diminish one's inner life, which is not so readily shared (Tschudin, 1997).

REACTIONS TO BEREAVEMENT

Grief is the reaction to loss. Normal grief reactions include depressed mood, insomnia, anxiety, poor appetite, loss of interest, guilt feelings, dreams about the deceased, and poor concentration. Psychological states include shock, denial, and yearning and searching for the deceased. The acute grief reaction typically lasts from 4 to 8 weeks, the active symptoms of grief usually last from 3 to 6 months, and the work of mourning may take from 1 to 2 years or more to complete.

Bereavement is the social experience of dealing with the death of a loved one. It refers to the event of losing an important person to death and is derived from the Old English word *berafian*, meaning "to rob." It is important for nurses to understand that cultural influences may dictate how people experience bereavement. Mourning refers to culturally patterned expressions of bereavement and grief (Bateman, 1999). Sensitivity to the ethnic, cultural, spiritual, and religious beliefs of a diverse cultural population can help nurses more effectively identify a person's needs (Bateman, 1999).

Denial and fear of death are strong in the American culture. This denial and fear affect the ways in which the bereaved, the family, and those who support the family experience and express grief. Advances in medicine have fed the cultural expectation that only the old will die, and little attention is paid to coping with grief throughout the life span. Geographic mobility has eroded communities that used to provide a context for grief support. Mourning and bereavement have been deritualized in economically developed countries, which further reduces cultural comfort with mourning (Cable, 1998).

Nurses are affected by cultural myths and conditions in the same way the rest of society is; when they are faced with a person who is dying, nurses may feel uncomfortable and unequipped to face the loss. They may remember their own losses that have not been fully grieved. Difficult memories and unresolved feelings are often awakened. When staff members have not been able to resolve their own conflicts with loss, their ability to help others is minimized. Psychological support and education should be available to help staff better understand the grieving process. When nurses examine their own feelings and their personal experiences of loss, verbal and nonverbal clues to the needs of grieving family members of a dying client become more apparent (Marks, 1976).

Sometimes, nurses grieve with family members at the death of a person they have cared for and become fond of. Sometimes, an entire staff may mourn the death of a client. After clients die, nurses may be faced with managing their own tasks of mourning, such as making sense of the death, dealing with mild to intense emotions, and realigning relationships. Albert (2001) states that "in the face of overwhelming, unending death, health care workers may come to question their deepest values, the meaning of their existence, and the value of the work they do." Losses such as these are often complicated and may come under the heading of disenfranchised grief. Disenfranchised grief and grief engendered by public tragedy are two specific types of grief worth examining here.

Disenfranchised Grief

There are circumstances under which an individual experiences an intense loss that is not congruent with a socially recognized and sanctioned role, for example, the role of lover, neighbor, foster parent, in-law, caregiver, roommate, co-worker, counselor, or health care worker (Albert, 2001). Often these mourners do not have the opportunity to publicly grieve the loss. Doka (1989) refers to these experiences as disenfranchised grief—"the grief a person experiences when they[sic] incur a loss that is not and cannot be openly acknowledged, publicly mourned, or socially supported." Thus, health care workers may experience real grief over the loss of a client, a grief that may not be recognized or acknowledged by others. This grief may be solitary and uncomforted (Albert, 2001) and may be difficult to resolve.

Grief Engendered by Public Tragedy

Another kind of loss can be caused by public tragedies. Public tragedies involve a loss whose impact is felt broadly across a community or the general public (Corr, 2003). Because of the scale of the loss, many are affected, and the events often involve strong elements of surprise and shock (Corr, 2003). Common public tragedies include, among others,

- Terrorist assaults (e.g., the terrorist attacks on September 11, 2001)
- Assassinations
- Tornados, earthquakes, or flooding
- Large-scale wildfires
- Well-publicized kidnappings of children who are later found to have been assaulted and killed
- School shootings (e.g., Columbine)

Responses to a public tragedy encompass two ongoing processes (Corr & Doka, 2001):

1. Coping with loss, grief, and trauma
2. Finding ways to adapt to a changing world

After a public tragedy, life will never be the same for many of those involved. As an example, since the September 11 terrorist attacks, life will never be the same for most of us in the United States. Certainly, life is forever altered for those who lost loved ones, for the first responders, and for all those living in the New York City environs during that time.

FRAMEWORKS FOR UNDERSTANDING LOSS

Grieving is a distinct psychological process that involves disengaging strong emotional ties from a significant relationship and reinvesting those ties in a new and productive direction. This reinvestment of emotional energy into new relationships or creative activities is necessary for a person's mental health and ability to function in society. When the mourning process is successfully completed, the griever is released from one interpersonal relationship and is able to form new relationships. The entire process of mourning may take a year or more to complete.

In a study of the grief responses of elderly widows, Hegge and Fischer (2000) found that the grief work followed an erratic cycle, with peaks and valleys, spurts and relapses, through the various phases of loss and bereavement mentioned in the literature. Studies of grief and loss by Parkes (1970, 1975), Caplan (1974), Engel (1964), Kübler-Ross (1969), and others postulated various phases of bereavement that proceed in orderly sequences within certain time frames. In reality, these phases overlap, and regression to previous phases is common and is usually marked by the erratic peaks and valleys mentioned. The distinct phases of human response to death and dying identified by Kübler-Ross (denial, anger, bargaining, depression, and acceptance) do not occur in a specific order; instead, an individual might go through all phases in the space of a few minutes, in varying order (Tschudin, 1997, p. 119).

The various frameworks for grieving and phases of grief are useful models for helping people to normalize the deeply felt and disturbing phenomena they experience when they confront profound loss. Denial and shock, anger and guilt, emotional turmoil, disorganization, panic, depression, loneliness, and, eventually, acceptance of the loss are all common during bereavement. Models and frameworks help organize the experience of loss, but models do not provide the focus of care when facilitating the process of mourning. The nurse's focus when facilitating bereavement holistically is on helping the bereaved deal with the most important issues emerging at a particular time. Often the nurse or other caregiver can best serve the grieving just by being present, listening with interest, and encouraging talking and the recounting of meaningful stories.

Many theorists have studied the grief process. Some of the most widely known are George Engel, Colin Parkes, Erich Lindemann, John Bowlby, and Edgar Jackson. Although each theorist uses different terminology, the process all of them outline is fundamentally the same. Each describes commonly experienced psychological and behavioral phenomena. These phenomena follow a pattern of response:

1. Shock and disbelief
2. Sensation of somatic distress
3. Preoccupation with the image of the deceased
4. Guilt
5. Anger
6. Change in behavior (e.g., depression, disorganization, or restlessness)
7. Reorganization of behavior directed toward a new object or activity

The process of mourning is often divided into stages (phases). The stages discussed here have been identified by Engel (1964) as (1) acute and (2) long term. All frameworks address the same phenomena.

Acute Stage

The acute stage (4 to 8 weeks after the death) involves shock and disbelief, development of awareness, and restitution.

Shock and Disbelief

The bereaved's first response is that of **denial.** The person is emotionally unable to accept his or her painful loss. Denial functions as a buffer against intolerable pain and allows the person slowly to acknowledge the reality of death. The mourner may appear to be functioning like a robot. Often, the bereaved person feels numb. A death may be accepted intellectually during this stage—"It's just as well, she was suffering"—although the emotional responses are still repressed. Denial is a needed defense that lasts for a few hours or a few days. Denial that persists longer than a few days may become dysfunctional, making it difficult to move through the process of mourning.

Development of Awareness

As denial fades, painful feelings begin to surface. The finality of the loved one's death becomes more of a reality. Waves of anguish and pain are experienced and may be localized in the chest or the epigastric area. **Anger** often surfaces at this time. Doctors and nurses are often the objects of blame. Awareness by staff that anger is often displaced onto people in the hospital environment may decrease defensive staff behaviors. **Guilt** is often experienced, and the bereaved blames himself or herself for taking or for failing to take specific actions. Impulsive and self-destructive acts by the mourner may occur, such as smashing a hand through a window or beating the head against a wall.

Crying is a common phenomenon during this stage. "It is during this time that the greatest degree of anguish or despair, within the limits imposed by cultural patterns, is experienced or expressed" (Engel, 1964). Crying can afford a welcome release from pent-up anguish and tension. Assessment of cultural patterns is important in making clinical judgments about the appropriateness of the bereaved's behavior. Failing to cry can be the result of cultural influences or environmental restraints. The person may cry in private. Inability to cry, however, may be the result of a high degree of ambivalence toward the deceased. A person who is unable to cry may have difficulty in successfully completing the work of mourning.

Restitution

Restitution is the formal, ritualistic phase of mourning during the acute stage. It is the institutionalization of mourning: it brings friends and family together in the rites of the funeral service and serves to emphasize the finality of death. The viewing of the body, the lowering of the casket or scattering of ashes, and the various religious and cultural rituals all help the bereaved shed any residual denial in an atmosphere of support. Every human society has its own moral and cultural standards according to which the rituals of mourning take place. The gathering in ritualistic farewell to the deceased provides support and sustenance for the family.

Long-Term Stage

After the acute stage has been completed, the main work of mourning goes on intrapsychically during the long-term stage, which lasts for 1 to 2 years or longer. The various phenomena experienced during bereavement are described in Table 30-1.

Most bereaved persons come to terms with their losses with support from family and friends. However, more than 30% may require professional support (Lloyd-Williams, 1995). Unresolved grief reactions over a lifetime have been called the hidden disease and may account for many of the physical symptoms seen in doctors' offices and hospital units. The existence of the broken-heart syndrome is supported by statistics that show that surviving spouses die within a year at a much higher rate than do members of control groups (Carr, 1985). Suicide is higher among people who have had a significant loss, especially if losses are multiple and grieving mechanisms are limited.

TABLE 30-1

Phenomena Experienced During Bereavement

Symptoms	Examples
Sensations of Somatic Distress	
The bereaved may experience tightness in the throat, shortness of breath, sighing, mental pain, or exhaustion; food tastes like sand; things feel unreal. Pain or discomfort may be identical to the symptoms experienced by the dead person. Normally, symptoms are brief.	A woman whose husband died of a stroke complains of weakness and numbness on her left side.
Preoccupation with the Image of the Deceased	
The bereaved brings up and thinks and talks about numerous memories of the deceased. The memories are positive. This process goes on with great sadness. The idealization of the deceased lets the bereaved relive the gratifications associated with the deceased and helps resolve any guilt the bereaved feels concerning the deceased. The bereaved may also take on many of the mannerisms of the deceased through identification. Identification serves the purpose of holding on to the deceased. Preoccupation with the dead person can continue for many months before it lessens.	A man whose wife has very recently died states, "I just can't stop thinking about my wife. Everything I see reminds me of her. We picked up this seashell on our honeymoon. I remember every wonderful moment we had together. The pain is so great, but the memories just keep coming." His friends notice that when he talks, his hand gestures and expressions are very like those of his recently deceased wife.
Guilt	
The bereaved reproaches himself or herself for real or fancied acts of negligence or omissions in the relationship with the deceased.	"I should have made him go to the doctor sooner." "I should have paid more attention to her, been more thoughtful."
Anger	
The anger the bereaved experiences may not be toward the object that gives rise to it. Often the anger is displaced onto the medical or nursing staff. Often it is directed toward the deceased. The anger is at its height during the first month but is often intermittent throughout the first year. The overflow of hostility disturbs the bereaved, resulting in the feeling that he or she is "going insane."	"The doctor didn't operate in time. If he had, Mary would be alive today." "How could he leave me like this . . . how could he?"
Change in Behavior: Depression, Disorganization, Restlessness	
A person may exhibit marked restlessness and an inability to organize his or her behavior. A depressive mood during routine activities is common, decreasing as the year passes and the intensity of the grief declines. Absence of depression is more abnormal than its presence. Loneliness and aimlessness are most pronounced 6 to 9 months after the death.	Six months after her husband died, Mrs. Faye states, "I just can't seem to function. I have a hard time doing the simplest tasks. I can't be bothered with socializing." "I feel so down . . . so, so empty."
Reorganization of Behavior Directed Toward a New Object or Activity	
Gradually, the person renews his or her interest in people and activities. The grieving thus releases the bereaved from one interpersonal relationship, and new ones are free to take its place.	Twenty months after her husband's death, Mrs. Faye tells a friend, "I'll be away this weekend. I am going fishing with my brother and his friend. This is the first time I've felt like doing anything since Harry died."

In some cases, bereaved persons become disorganized, neglect themselves, do not eat, use alcohol or drugs, and are susceptible to physical disease. Several studies have shown that the health of widows and close relatives of the deceased declines within 1 year of bereavement, and medical and psychiatric problems increase (Bowlby & Parkes, 1970; Carr, 1985). Health care workers are not immune to grief reactions. A study by Feldstein and Gemma (1995) found that oncology nurses scored higher than the norm in despair, social isolation, and somatization.

Table 30-2 identifies the common phenomena experienced during grief and describes the pathological intensification of these phenomena that indicates the need for counseling.

HELPING PEOPLE COPE WITH LOSS

Prolonged and serious alterations in social adjustment, as well as medical diseases, may develop if the phases of mourning are interrupted or if needed support is not available. Listening is the most important support for acute grief. The helping person should keep his or her own talking to a minimum. Telling the story over and over is therapeutic for the bereaved. Listening, **really listening,** not just to the words but to the whole person, can assist in healing. Tschudin (1997) states that "listening and not talking, not interrupting, being comfortable with silence when indicated, and using prompts like 'go on,' etc., to encourage the person to continue talking" (p. 105) are the most helpful behaviors.

Talking can release negative emotions. When a person is faced with loss, strong feelings of anger, guilt, and hate are normal reactions that have to be expressed to facilitate the process of mourning. It is important that someone listen and encourage the expression of feelings surrounding the person's loss or anticipated loss.

Banal advice and philosophical statements are useless. Unhelpful responses by others, such as "He's no longer suffering" or "You can always have another child" or "It's better this way," can lead the bereaved to believe that others do not understand the acute pain being suffered and that the personal impact of the loss is being minimized. Such statements can compound feelings of isolation.

More helpful responses are "His death will be a terrible loss" or "No one can replace her" or "He will be missed for a long time." Statements such as these validate the bereaved person's experience of loss and communicate the message that the bereaved is understood and supported. Table 30-3 provides guidelines for helping people grieve. Table 30-4 offers guidelines for what to say to a person suffering a profound loss.

TABLE 30-2

Common Experiences During Grief and Their Pathological Intensification

Phenomenon	Typical Response	Pathological Intensification
Dying	Emotional expression and immediate coping with the dying process	Avoidance; feeling of being overwhelmed, dazed, confused; self-punitive feelings; inappropriately hostile feelings
Death and outcry	Outcry of emotions with news of the death and turning for help to others or isolating self with self-soothing	Panic; dissociative reactions, reactive psychoses
Warding off (denial)	Avoidance of reminders and social withdrawal, focusing elsewhere, emotional numbing, not thinking of implications to self or of certain themes	Maladaptive avoidance of confronting the implications of death; drug or alcohol abuse, counterphobic frenzy, promiscuity, fugue states, phobic avoidance, feeling of being dead or unreal
Reexperience (intrusion)	Intrusive experiences, including recollections of negative experiences during relationship with the deceased, bad dreams, reduced concentration, compulsive reenactments	Flooding with negative images and emotions; uncontrolled ideation, self-impairing compulsive reenactments, night terrors, recurrent nightmares, distraught feelings resulting from the intrusion of anger, anxiety, despair, shame, or guilt; physiological exhaustion resulting from hyperarousal
Working through	Recollection of the deceased and a contemplation of self with reduced intrusiveness of memories and fantasies and with increased rational acceptance, reduced numbness and avoidance, more "dosing" of recollections, and a sense of working it through	Feeling of inability to integrate the death with a sense of self and continued life; persistent warding-off themes that may manifest as anxious, depressed, enraged, shame-filled, or guilty moods and psychophysiological syndromes
Completion	Reduction in emotional swings and a sense of self-coherence and readiness for new relationships; ability to experience positive states of mind	Failure to complete mourning, which may be associated with inability to work or create, or to feel emotion or positive states of mind

From Horowitz, M. J. (1990). A model of mourning: Change in schemas of self and others. *Journal of the American Psychoanalytic Association, 38*(2), 297-324.

TABLE 30-3

Guidelines for Helping People in Acute Grief

Intervention	Rationale
1. Employ methods that can facilitate the grieving process (Robinson, 1997). 1a. **Give your full presence:** use appropriate eye contact, attentive listening, and appropriate touch.	1a. Talking is one of the most important ways of dealing with acute grief. Listening patiently helps the bereaved express all feelings, even ones he or she feels are "negative." Appropriate eye contact helps to convey the awareness that you are there and are sharing the person's sadness. Suitable human touch can express warmth and nurture healing. Inappropriate touch can leave a person confused and uncomfortable.
1b. Be patient with the bereaved in times of silence. Do not fill silence with empty chatter.	1b. Sharing painful feelings during periods of silence is healing and conveys your concern.
2. Know about and share with the bereaved information about the phenomena that occur during the normal mourning process, because they may concern some people (intense anger at the deceased, guilt, symptoms the deceased had before death, unbidden floods of memories). Give the bereaved support during the occurrence of these phenomena and a written handout to refer to.	2. Although the knowledge won't eliminate the emotions, it can greatly relieve a person who is thinking there is something wrong with having these feelings.

3. **Encourage the support of family and friends.** If no supports are available, refer the client to a community bereavement group. (Bereavement groups are helpful even when a person has many friends or much family support.)	3. There are routine matters that friends can help with. For example:
	  ■ Getting food into the house
	  ■ Making phone calls
	  ■ Driving to the mortuary
	  ■ Taking care of the kids or other family members

4. **Offer spiritual support and referrals** when needed.	4. Dealing with an illness or catastrophic loss can cause the most profound spiritual anguish.
5. **When intense emotions are in evidence, show understanding and support** (see Table 30-4).	5. Empathetic words that reflect acceptance of a bereaved individual's feelings are healing (Robinson, 1997).

Some people find comfort and support in grief counseling or support groups. Six to ten sessions of psychotherapy have been found to be helpful during the crisis period. At a later stage, the use of 15 sessions or more has been found to have a good outcome. More complicated or pathological patterns of grief may require special techniques, such as re-grief work (Middleton & Raphael, 1992). One study demonstrated that highly religious clients with grief and bereavement issues tended to improve faster when religious psychotherapy was added to a cognitive-behavioral approach (Azhar & Varma, 1995).

Box 30-4 offers guidelines that can help people and their families cope with catastrophic grief.

UNRESOLVED AND DYSFUNCTIONAL GRIEF

Acute grief can be a time of exacerbation of any preexisting medical or psychiatric problems. A history of depression, substance abuse, or posttraumatic stress disorder can complicate grief, and such problems certainly deserve specific treatment (Prigerson et al., 1995).

TABLE 30-4

Guidelines for Communicating with a Bereaved Person

Situation	Sample Response
When you sense an overwhelming *sorrow*	"This must hurt terribly."
When you hear *anger* in the bereaved's voice	"I hear anger in your voice. Most people go through periods of anger when their loved one dies. Are you feeling angry now?"
If you discern *guilt*	"Are you feeling guilty? This is a common reaction many people have. What are some of your thoughts about this?"
If you sense a *fear* of the future	"It must be scary to go through this."
When the bereaved seems *confused*	"This can be a bewildering time."
In almost any *painful situation*	"This must be very difficult for you."

Adapted from Robinson, D. (1997). *Good intentions: The nine unconscious mistakes of nice people* (p. 249). New York: Warner Books.

Guidelines for Dealing with Catastrophic Loss

Take the time you need to grieve. The hard work of grief uses psychological energy. Resolution of the numb state that occurs after loss requires a few weeks at least. A minimum of 1 year, to cover all the birthdays, anniversaries, and other important dates without your loved one, is required before you can learn to live with your loss.

Express your feelings. Remember that anger, anxiety, loneliness, and even guilt are normal reactions and that everyone needs a safe place to express them. Tell your personal story of loss as many times as you need to—this repetition is a helpful and necessary part of the grieving process.

Establish a structure for each day and stick to it. Although it is hard to do, keeping to some semblance of structure makes the first few weeks after a loss easier. Getting through each day helps to restore the confidence you need to accept the reality of loss.

Don't feel that you have to answer all the questions asked you. Although most people try to be kind, they may be unaware of their insensitivity. Down the road, you may want to read books about how others have dealt with similar circumstances. They often have helpful suggestions for a person in your situation.

As hard as it is, try to take good care of yourself. Eat well, talk with friends, get plenty of rest. Be sure to let your primary care clinician know if you are having trouble eating or sleeping. Make use of exercise. It can help you let out pent-up frustrations. If you are losing weight, sleeping excessively or intermittently, or still experiencing deep depression after 3 months, be sure to seek professional assistance.

Expect the unexpected. You may begin to feel a bit better, only to have a brief emotional collapse. These are expectable reactions. Moreover, you may find that you dream about, visualize, think about, or search for your loved one. This, too, is a part of the grieving process.

Give yourself time. Don't feel that you have to resume all of life's duties right away.

Make use of rituals. Those who take the time to say good-bye at a funeral or a viewing tend to find that it helps the bereavement process.

If you do not begin to feel better within a few weeks, at least for a few hours every day, be sure to tell your doctor. If you have had an emotional problem in the past (e.g., depression, substance abuse), be sure to get the additional support you need. Losing a loved one puts you at higher risk for a relapse of these disorders.

From Zerbe, K. J. (1999). *Women's mental health in primary care* (pp. 207-208). Philadelphia: Saunders.

Indications that a person may have the potential for **dysfunctional grieving** may be gleaned by understanding some things about the bereaved. It is important to determine whether the bereaved person exhibits any of the following characteristics that can complicate bereavement:

- Was the bereaved heavily dependent on the deceased?
- Were there persistent unresolved conflicts between the bereaved and the deceased?
- Was the deceased a child (often the most profound loss)?
- Does the bereaved have a meaningful relationship or support system?
- Has the bereaved experienced a number of previous losses?
- Does the bereaved person have sound coping skills?
- Was the deceased's death associated with a cultural stigma (e.g., acquired immunodeficiency syndrome, suicide)?
- Was the death unexpected or associated with violence (murder, suicide)?
- Has the bereaved had difficulty resolving past significant losses?
- Does the bereaved have a history of depression, drug or alcohol abuse, or other psychiatric illness?
- If the bereaved is young, are there indications for special interventions?

Dysfunctional grieving essentially means that the grief work is unresolved. Prolonged depression is the most common response to unresolved grief. Disturbances in mood are associated with biological changes in the body during stress-related depressive illness. Some examples include electrolyte disturbance, nervous system alterations, and faulty regulation of the autonomic nervous system. Always assess the potential for suicide. Someone who is having difficulty negotiating the work of mourning and is suffering can benefit from counseling, as mentioned earlier.

SUCCESSFUL MOURNING

Worden (1991) developed a model that describes the tasks involved in the process of mourning:

1. Accept the reality of the loss.
2. Work through the pain of grief. (Sharing with others can facilitate this task.)
3. Adjust to an environment in which the deceased is missing.
4. Restructure the family's relationship with the deceased and reinvest in other relationships and life pursuits.

Have these tasks been accomplished? The work of mourning is over when the bereaved can remember realistically both the pleasures and the disappointments of the relationship with the lost loved one. Brief periods of intense emotions may still occur at significant times, such as holidays and anniversaries, but the person or family members have energy to reinvest in new relationships that bring shared joys, security, satisfaction, and comfort. If, after a normal period of time (12 to 24 months), a person has not completed the grieving process, reassessment and reevaluation are indicated.

■ ■ ■ KEY POINTS to REMEMBER

- Care for the terminally ill challenges health care providers in deep and personal ways. The hospice movement offers compassionate care for those who are dying. Hospice and palliative care focus on clients' physical and emotional comfort and offer holistic support for dying persons and their families.

- More hospitals are offering palliative expertise for end-of-life care, but in many hospitals, conflict continues to exist between the wishes of dying persons and their families and the medical model of treatment that focuses on the prolongation of life as opposed to client-defined quality of life.

- In work with the terminally ill, nursing goals include providing physical and emotional comfort, helping with adjustments in lifestyle and relationships, and offering spiritual support. Health care workers need to shift their thinking so as to see the value of providing a caring human presence even in the face of helplessness.

- It is important to assess regularly for spiritual themes embedded in ordinary conversations, develop expertise with palliative medicine and treatments, and assume a greater educational role with the client and family.

- Learning to follow the dying person's lead and understanding that relationships are usually the most important aspect of life for the dying person, once pain has been controlled, are important lessons.

- Assessing for multiple or hidden diagnoses can greatly improve a person's quality of life until the end, if the health care team takes appropriate steps.

- People who work with the dying need to maintain their own emotional health. End-of-life care is usually delivered by multidisciplinary teams so that no one discipline bears too much responsibility. Nurses need to learn to draw on team support, protect their private lives by setting clear personal boundaries, and recognize their human and professional limitations.

- Information about the disease and its effects and about physical and psychological signs of death, and education about effective caregiving can help the family deal with painful, confusing feelings.

- Health care workers involved in care of the dying can teach families communications skills, such as the Four Gifts of Resolving Relationships, that will help them to say good-bye, express love, and share memories. These abilities can help to give the dying person and the family a sense of closure and peace.

- Family members may experience anticipatory grief, and it is helpful for them to understand that it is normal, although painful. It can be helpful to understand that the way an individual confronts dying usually harmonizes with the ways he or she has faced other important aspects of life.

- Seven motifs have been proposed to sensitize health care workers to the different ways individuals deal with their impending death so that plans of treatment and approaches can be truly individualized.

- Hospice care seeks to treat every client and family with respect and dignity, viewing them holistically and supporting client choices and control. Ameliorating pain and other symptoms is paramount, so that persons can face the end of their lives in peace and comfort. Every person's dying process is unique and should be valued without comparisons to those of others.

- The process of bereavement is a distinct psychological process and is the normal reaction to a loss, real or perceived, including the loss of a person, loss of security, loss of self-confidence, and loss of a dream. Essentially, a loss results in a change in self-concept.

- The stage of acute grief may last from 4 to 8 weeks; the complete process of mourning (the long-term stage) may take a year or two or longer.

- Common phenomena are evident during the experience of grief, and people usually show similar patterns of grief and mourning within their cultural norms. Culture greatly affects the patterns of response to death and dying in both clients and nurses.

- Grief, when experienced by health care workers, can reactivate distressing feelings related to previous losses. If nurses have unresolved issues of grief and depression, their ability to help others is greatly minimized, so it is important to recognize that staff members need psychological support when they work with people who are grieving.

- Many people are experts on loss but not on coping with loss. There are a number of coping skills that health care workers can use to help comfort the bereaved and facilitate mourning. Really listening to a grieving person's story without offering banal or philosophical responses can assist in healing. Short-term grief counseling and groups are often helpful.

- Indicators of the potential for complicated or unresolved grief include social isolation, extensive dependency on the deceased person, unresolved interpersonal conflicts, loss of a child, violent and senseless death, and/or a catastrophic loss.

- Grief work is successful when the relationship to the deceased person has been restructured and energy is available for new relationships and life pursuits. The work of mourning is complete when the bereaved person or persons can remember realistically both the pleasures and the disappointments of the lost relationship. Outcomes for successful grief work have been identified.

■ ■ ■

Visit the Evolve website at **http://evolve.elsevier.com/Varcarolis** for a posttest on the content in this chapter. ***evolve***

Critical Thinking and Chapter Review

Visit the Evolve website at **http://evolve.elsevier.com/Varcarolis** for additional self-study exercises.

evolve

▪ ▪ ▪ CRITICAL THINKING

1. Using the examples supplied in this chapter, compare and contrast the hospice model of care with the medical model of care for dying persons. What would be done differently if the hospice model were used in caring for Mr. Spence (see the first vignette)?

2. How can you use the Four Gifts in working with the families of dying people in your practice of nursing? Do you think you would find this a useful tool for a personal family member in the future?

3. What are some concrete ways in which you can help another to cope with a loss? Identify specific components in the following areas:

   A. How can you let the person tell his or her story and what is the potential therapeutic value of doing so?

   B. Avoiding banal advice, what are some things you might say that could offer comfort? Use the guidelines in Table 30-4 to describe how you would help a person who is suffering a profound loss.

▪ ▪ ▪ CHAPTER REVIEW

Choose the most appropriate answer.

1. Grief is best described as
   1. a normal response to a significant loss.
   2. a mild to moderately severe mood disorder.
   3. the abnormal display of feelings associated with death.
   4. denial of the reality of the loss of a significant person, object, or state.

2. Which statement would be evaluated as indicating that successful mourning has taken place?
   1. "She was so strong after her husband died. She never cried the whole time. She kept a stiff upper lip."
   2. "She was a wreck when her sister died. She cried and cried. It took her about a year before she resumed her usual activities with any zest."
   3. "You know, he still talks about his mother as if she were alive today. . . . And she's been dead for 4 years."
   4. "He never talked about his wife after she died. He just picked up and went on life's way."

3. K., 34 years of age, is single and has very few close friends and relatives. He was very dependent on his mother before her death, although he often complained about her intrusiveness. What statement best describes his risk for problems in resolving his grief?
   1. He is at no particular risk because the death of parents is an expected event in one's life.
   2. He is at low risk because the task of young adulthood is to develop independence from the family of origin.
   3. He is at moderate risk.
   4. He is at high risk because he was dependent on his mother, demonstrated ambivalence toward her, and has a limited support system.

4. Which statement about palliative care could serve as a basis for the information a nurse gives to a client?
   1. Palliation focuses on aggressive comfort care when cure is no longer the goal.
   2. Clients receiving palliative care can realistically expect discomfort at life's end.
   3. Palliation addresses emotional and spiritual pain more than physical pain.
   4. Clients receiving palliative care are relieved of the responsibility of making care decisions.

5. Which nursing approach will be disruptive to the provision of nursing care for terminally ill clients?
   1. Seeing a dichotomy between the living and the dying
   2. Understanding that there is no "right" way to die
   3. Learning to follow the client's lead
   4. Maintaining one's emotional health

■ STUDENT
■ STUDY
■ CD-ROM

Access the accompanying CD-ROM for animations, interactive exercises, review questions for the NCLEX examination, and an audio glossary.

■ NURSE,
■ CLIENT, AND
■ FAMILY RESOURCES

For suggested readings, information on related associations, and Internet resources, go to **http://evolve.elsevier.com/Varcarolis.** *evolve*

REFERENCES

Albert, P. A. (2001). Grief and loss in the workplace. *Progress in Transplantation, 11*(3), 169-173.

Azhar, M. Z., & Varma, S. L. (1995). The religious psychotherapy as management of bereavement. *Acta Psychiatrica Scandinavica, 91*(4), 233-235.

Bateman, A. L. (1999). Understanding the process of grieving and loss: A critical social thinking perspective. *Journal of the American Psychiatric Nurses Association, 5*(5), 139-147.

Bowlby, J., & Parkes, C. (1970). Separation and loss within the family. In E. J. Anthony & C. Koupernik (Eds.), *Child in his family.* New York: Wiley.

Byock, I. (1997). *Dying well: Peace and possibilities at the end of life.* New York: Riverhead Books.

Cable, D. (1998). *Grief in the American culture.* In K. Doka & J. Davidson (Eds.), *Living with grief: Who we are, how we grieve.* Philadelphia: Brunner/Mazel.

Campbell, D., et al. (2004). Medicare program expenditures associated with hospice use. *Annals of Internal Medicine, 140*(4), 269-277.

Caplan, G. (1974). *Support systems and community mental health. Lectures on concept development.* New York: Behavioral Publications.

Carr, A. L. (1985). Grief, mourning, and bereavement. In H. I. Kaplan & B. J. Sadock (Eds.), *Comprehensive textbook of psychiatry* (4th ed.). Baltimore: Williams & Wilkins.

Corr, C. A. (2003). Loss, grief and trauma in public tragedy. In M. Lattanzi-Light & K. J. Doka (Eds.), *Living with grief: Coping with public tragedy.* Washington, DC: Hospice Foundation of America.

Corr, C. A., & Doka, K. J. (2001). Master concepts in the field of death, dying, and bereavement: Coping versus adaptive strategies. *Omega, 43,* 183-199.

Doka, K. (1989). *Disenfranchised grief—recognizing hidden sorrows.* New York: Lexington Books.

Doka, K. (2001). Grief, loss, and caregiving. In K. Doka & J. Davidson (Eds.), *Caregiving and loss.* Washington, DC: Hospice Foundation of America.

Engel, G. L. (1964). Grief and grieving. *American Journal of Nursing, 64*(9), 93-98.

Feldstein, M. A., & Gemma, P. B. (1995). Oncology nurses and chronic compounded grief. *Cancer Nursing, 18*(3), 228-236.

Florida Policy Exchange Center on Aging & The Hospice Institute of the Florida Suncoast. (2003, June). *Caregiving at life's end: The national needs assessment and implications for hospice practice.* Tampa and Largo, FL: Authors.

Gauthier, D. (2002). The meaning of healing near the end of life. *Journal of Hospice and Palliative Nursing, 4*(4), 220-227.

Hart, A., et al. (2003). Hospice clients' attitudes regarding spiritual discussions with their doctors. *American Journal of Hospice and Palliative Care, 20*(2), 135-139.

Hegge, M., & Fischer, C. (2000). Grief response of senior and elderly widows: Practice implications. *Journal of Gerontological Nursing, 26*(2), 35-43.

Hutchings, D. (2002). Parallels in practice: Palliative nursing practice and Parse's theory of human becoming. *American Journal of Hospice and Palliative Care, 19*(6), 408-414.

Kramer-Howe, K., & Huls, P. T. (2004) *A spiritual assessment tool.* Phoenix, AZ: Hospice of the Valley.

Kübler-Ross, E. (1969). *On death and dying.* New York: Macmillan.

Kutner, J., Kassner, D., & Nowels, D. (2001). Symptom burden at the end of life: Hospice providers' perceptions. *Journal of Pain and Symptom Management, 21*(6), 473-480.

Lloyd-Williams, M. (1995). Bereavement referrals to a psychiatric service: An audit. *European Journal of Cancer Care, 4*(1), 17-19.

Marks, M. J. (1976). The grieving client and family. *American Journal of Nursing, 76,* 1488-1491.

Middleton, W., & Raphael, B. (1992). Bereavement. In E. S. Paykel (Ed.), *Handbook of affective disorders* (2nd ed., pp. 619-634). New York: Guilford Press.

Millison, M. (1995). A review of the research on spiritual care and hospice. *Hospice Journal, 10* (4), 3-19.

National Hospice and Palliative Care Organization. (2004a). *An explanation of hospice and palliative care.* Alexandria, VA: Author. Retrieved April 14, 2005, from http://www.nhpco.org/i4a/pages/index.cfm?pageid=3657.

National Hospice and Palliative Care Organization. (2004b). *Hospice fact sheet.* Alexandria, VA: Author. Retrieved April 14, 2005, from http://www.nho.org.

National Hospice and Palliative Care Organization. (2004c). *Medicare hospice benefits.* Alexandria, VA: Author. Retrieved April 14, 2005, from http://www.nhpco.org/i4a/pages/index.cfm?pageid=3283.

National Hospice and Palliative Care Organization. (2004d). *What is hospice and palliative care?* Alexandria, VA: Author. Retrieved April 14, 2005, from http://www.nhpco.org/i4a/pages/index.cfm?pageid=3281.

Parkes, C. M. (1970). The first year of bereavement: A longitudinal study in the reaction of London widows to the death of their husbands. *Psychiatry, 33*(4), 444-467.

Parkes, C. M. (1975). *Bereavement: Studies of grief in adult life.* Harmondsworth, England: Penguin.

Prigerson, H. G., et al. (1995). Complicated grief and bereavement-related depressions as distinct disorders: Preliminary empirical validation in elderly bereaved spouses. *American Journal of Psychiatry, 152,* 22-30.

Redding, S. (2000). Control theory in dying: What do we know? *American Journal of Hospice and Palliative Care, 17*(3), 204-208.

Redford, G. (2000, September-October). Their final answers. *Modern Maturity,* pp. 66-68.

Robinson, D. (1997). *Good intentions: The nine unconscious mistakes of nice people.* New York: Warner Books.

Shearer, R., & Davidhizar, R. (1994). It can never be the way it was. *Home Health Care Nurse, 12*(4), 60-65.

Shneidman, E. (1980). *Voices of death: Letters, diaries and other personal documents from people facing death that provide comforting guidance for each of us.* New York: Harper & Row.

Stephenson, P., Draucker, C., & Martsolf, D. (2003). The experience of spirituality in the lives of hospice clients. *Journal of Hospice and Palliative Nursing, 5*(1), 51-58.

Stolberg, S. G. (1999, May 11). A conversation with Dame Cicely Saunders: Reflecting on a life of treating the dying. *New York Times,* Health and Fitness Section.

Teno, J., et al. (2004). Family perspectives on end-of-life care at the last place of care. *Journal of the American Medical Association, 291*(1), 88-93.

Tschudin, V. (1997). *Counseling for loss and bereavement.* London: Baillière Tindall.

Volkan, V. D., & Zintl, E. (1993). *Life after loss.* New York: Simon and Schuster.

Weil, Simone. (1998). *Simone Weil: Writings selected with an introduction by Eric Springsted.* New York: Orbis Books.

White, K., Coyne, P., & Patel, U. (2001). Are nurses adequately prepared for end-of-life care? *Journal of Nursing Scholarship, 33*(2), 147-151.

Worden, W. (1991). *Grief counseling and grief therapy* (2nd ed.). New York: Springer.

Wright, D. (2002). Researching the qualities of hospice nurses. *Journal of Hospice and Palliative Nursing, 4*(4), 210-218.

Yedidia, M., & MacGregor, B. (2001). Confronting the prospect of dying: Reports of terminally ill clients. *Journal of Pain and Symptom Management, 22*(4), 807-819.

CHAPTER 31

Psychiatric Forensic Nursing

JUDITH W. CORAM

KEY TERMS and CONCEPTS

The key terms and concepts listed here appear in color where they are defined or first discussed in the chapter.

competence to proceed, 627

correctional mental health nursing, 625

correctional nursing, 625

criminal profiler, 628

expert witness, 627

fact witness, 627

forensic nursing, 623

legal sanity, 626

psychiatric forensic nursing, 625

victimology, 624

OBJECTIVES

After studying this chapter, the reader will be able to

1. Define forensic nursing, psychiatric forensic nursing, correctional nursing, and correctional mental health nursing.
2. Describe the nature of the nurse-client relationship in each of these nursing specialties.
3. Discuss the difference between a fact witness and an expert witness.
4. Describe the role of a sexual assault nurse examiner.
5. Discuss the significance of the terms *legal sanity* and *competence to proceed.*

evolve Visit the Evolve website at **http://evolve.elsevier.com/Varcarolis** for a pretest on the content in this chapter.

In 2002, 15% of U.S. households experienced one or more violent or property crimes, according to the National Crime Victimization Survey (Rennison & Rand, 2004). These crimes included rape and sexual assault, robbery, aggravated and simple assault, household burglary, motor vehicle theft, and other theft. About 1 in every 26 households experienced violence in a household burglary or other violence by a stranger. Although these crimes are often cited as the most fear provoking, their total number has fallen steadily since 1994. This trend is encouraging; nevertheless, we know that significant violence is still occurring in homes, in schools, and in workplaces across the United States.

Traditionally, nurses have always dealt with the aftermath of violence—caring for rape victims in the emergency department, assisting in life-saving surgeries for victims of shootings and other violent crimes, providing care for injured alleged perpetrators, improving the lot of battered women and children, working with the criminally insane, and offering their nursing services within the correctional system. Only recently have many of these nurses formalized their interest in working with victims, perpetrators, and the legal system. This chapter introduces you to the relatively new specialty of psychiatric forensic nursing and gives you an overview of the critical roles and functions performed by these nursing pioneers.

DEFINITION OF FORENSIC NURSING

Forensic nursing is an emerging specialty area of practice that combines elements of nursing science, forensic science, and criminal justice. Some specialty areas of nursing practice are defined by the practice setting, such as critical care nursing, surgical nursing, home care nursing, and flight nursing. Some specialty areas are defined by the clients that are served, such as pediatric or geriatric nursing. Forensic nursing is determined by the nature of the nurse-client relationship and the nursing role functions performed.

623

The International Association of Forensic Nurses (IAFN) was formed in 1992 when 74 nurses, most of whom were sexual assault nurse examiners, came together to create an organization representative of nurses who practice in the arena of the law (IAFN, 2002a). This organization speaks for nurses who are death investigators, correctional nurse specialists, forensic psychiatric nurses, and nurse lawyers, as well as for those in other forensic nursing specialties that continue to evolve. A year after its creation, the organization had more than tripled in size, and by 1999 the IAFN's membership had grown to more than 1800 nurses. The goals of the IAFN include the following (IAFN, 2002b):

- To participate in active research projects and dissemination of research information
- To educate nurses to work in collaboration with law enforcement and the forensic sciences
- To develop the role of forensic specialist in nursing practice
- To introduce a new perspective in the holistic approach to victims of violent crime in clinical or community-based institutions
- To unite in a common concern for the plight of victims of criminal activity and traumatic accidents
- To develop formal education programs in forensic nursing at the undergraduate, graduate, and postgraduate levels, providing initial and continuing education and specific guidelines for the practice and policies that must be implemented in the investigation of trauma in both living and deceased victims
- To meet the challenges of sharing a mutual responsibility with the legal system to protect victims' legal, civil, and human rights, to protect the constitutional rights of perpetrators of criminal acts, and to protect the rights of the families of both

The American Nurses Association (ANA) officially recognized forensic nursing as a specialty practice area in 1995. The ANA combined efforts with the IAFN to develop the *Scope and Standards of Forensic Nursing* (1997).

Forensic nursing is still so new that nurses encounter professional resistance both in and out of nursing. They face challenges in education and training and barriers to employment, and most significantly, because currently there is no official credentialing process, they continue to struggle simply for the right to call themselves forensic nurses (Pyrek, 2004). Recognizing that every nursing discipline has had to go through this developmental phase, these pioneering nurses continue to forge ahead with passion in the belief that the role of the forensic nurse is a critical one with unlimited potential.

In forensic nursing, the nurse-client relationship is predicated on the possibility that a crime has been committed. One significant element of the forensic nurse's role is to contribute data toward answering questions such as whether the client is competent to stand trial, whether or not a crime has been committed, and whether a person judged incompetent to stand trial or adjudicated not guilty by reason of insanity poses a danger to society. There is an investigative quality to the nursing assessment that does not exist in other areas of nursing practice (Winfrey & Smith, 1999).

FORENSIC NURSING ROLE FUNCTIONS

Role functions are the nursing acts and skills related to a particular area of practice. For example, the role functions of a nurse in a cardiac care setting are very different from those of a nurse in a pediatric oncology setting. The role functions in forensic nursing center on the identification, collection, documentation, and preservation of potential evidence and complement client care roles with assessment and treatment roles related to competency, risk, and dangerousness.

■ ■ ■ *VIGNETTE*

Faye Battiste-Otto became interested in forensic nursing when she worked in an emergency department. She recalls that she was intrigued by forensic science and wanted to pursue it. This initial interest led her to the understanding that evidence handling was not only the responsibility of law enforcement officers but of nurses as well. She was also aware that nurses frequently compromised the very evidence they should be protecting. "If we encountered a chest injury caused by a bullet, for instance, the first thing we would do is clean the chest really well and throw away the bullet. I started to think, 'We really shouldn't do that.' I began to look for education and there was little or none" (quoted in Pyrek, 2004, p. 3).

■ ■ ■

Forensic nurses understand that there are two sides to any criminal act, which are brought together at a point in time and reflect the perpetrator's motivation, background, and values, and the characteristics of the victim (**victimology**). Forensic nurses working with either victim or perpetrator know that having an understanding of both enhances their evidence collection. For example, a forensic nurse completing a rape examination might use the Comprehensive Sexual Assault Assessment Tool (CSAAT) in the interview. The CSAAT provides law enforcement personnel with a detailed description of the perpetrator's sexual and postoffense behavior. Similarly, because of the possibility of victim selection, the criminal profiler includes victim-related factors in the data collection.

WORKING WITH VICTIM OR PERPETRATOR

There are several subspecialty areas of practice within forensic nursing (Saunders, 2000). All share the same medicolegal aspects, but the nurse-client relationship differs. Physiological forensic nurses focus on the alleged victim, whereas psychiatric forensic nurses work with the alleged perpetrator and focus the interaction on the needs of the court. The work done by physiological forensic nurses is described later in this chapter.

PSYCHIATRIC FORENSIC NURSING

Psychiatric forensic nursing is defined as the psychiatric nursing assessment, evaluation, and treatment of individuals pending or following a criminal hearing or trial (Coram, 1993). The defendant's thinking and behavior prior to and during the commission of the crime are the primary focus of the nurse-client relationship. Psychiatric forensic nurses work as forensic examiners, competency therapists, caregivers in forensic settings, and consultants to attorneys or law enforcement personnel.

The core of practice is psychiatric mental health nursing, but the relationship between client and nurse is markedly different from that in traditional psychiatric mental health nursing practice. For instance, in psychiatric forensic nursing the client is the attorney or the court. The roles fulfilled by the psychiatric forensic nurse are also quite unique. A listing of some of the role functions in psychiatric forensic nursing is presented in Box 31-1.

Evidence collection is central to the role of all forensic nurses. One way evidence collection is carried out within psychiatric forensic nursing is through evaluation to determine intent or diminished capacity in the perpetrator's thinking at the time of the crime. This evaluation aids in determining the degree of crime and may later influence the sentence. Psychiatric forensic nurses who work as competency therapists collect evidence by spending many hours with a defendant and carefully documenting the dialogue.

BOX 31-1

Psychiatric Forensic Nursing Role Functions

Assesses
- Perpetrator's ability to formulate intent
- Risk for violence and for committing additional crimes
- Factors such as race and culture that influenced crime
- Legal sanity
- Competence to proceed to trial
- Sexual predator behaviors

Investigates criminal history and reviews police reports

Provides competency therapy

Writes and submits formal reports to court

Serves as an expert witness

Participates in police training

Assists in jury selection

Consults with attorneys as well as law enforcement personnel at crime scene

Offers opinions regarding parole and probation

CORRECTIONAL AND CORRECTIONAL MENTAL HEALTH NURSES

Because both correctional nurses and psychiatric forensic nurses work with an incarcerated population, confusion exists between the practices of nurses in these two specialties. The difference between correctional nursing and psychiatric forensic nursing lies in the nature of the nurse-client relationship. Correctional nursing is defined by the location of the work or the legal status of the client, rather than by the role functions being performed. Correctional nurses work with inmates who are older and sicker and who remain imprisoned longer than the inmates of 20 years ago. Today's inmates suffer from a disproportionately greater number of chronic illnesses and infectious diseases than the nonincarcerated population. Correctional nurses provide care for inmates with tuberculosis, acquired immunodeficiency syndrome, and hepatitis C. These nurses also deal with the special medical needs of female prisoners, who have higher rates of diabetes, human immunodeficiency virus infection, and sexually transmitted diseases than do male inmates. Moreover, about 6% of female inmates are pregnant on admission to jail and prison, and the infants born to these inmates account for approximately 8820 of the 3.8 million births in the United States each year (Bickford, 2004). Correctional nurses do not contribute data regarding the alleged offense. In fact, they frequently care for inmates without knowing the nature of the inmates' crimes, because such knowledge would prejudice their level of care.

A psychiatric forensic nurse advocates for the process, whereas the correctional nurse advocates for the client. A correctional nurse may be directed to perform a forensic nursing function, such as a male rape examination or collection of a DNA specimen; however, many correctional nurses decline to perform these tasks because they believe doing them would interfere with their relationship with the inmate.

In correctional mental health nursing, nurses care for inmates housed in the psychiatric unit of a jail or prison, or on the long-term ward of a forensic hospital where persons adjudicated as not guilty by reason of insanity are being treated. However, the nature of the nurse-client relationship remains focused on the client's day-to-day needs, rather than the client's thinking and behavior in the past, at the time of the crime.

The correctional mental health nurse provides care for many of the seriously mentally ill who are caught in a cycle of homelessness, mental hospitals, and jail. Frequently these individuals become incarcerated as a result of psychiatric emergencies that generally include threats made to others. Because psychiatric facilities to manage these emergencies are sorely lacking, these clients end up in jail instead of in a hospital. Once they are in jail their psychiatric condition only worsens without adequate psychiatric intervention. The fortunate clients end up in a secure treatment unit within the jail, where they receive proper medication and psychiatric nursing care from correctional mental health nurses.

These nurses perform psychiatric nursing role functions, rather than forensic nursing role functions, including performing a comprehensive mental status examination. The following vignette illustrates a challenging situation facing the correctional mental health nurse who is responsible for completing a psychiatric evaluation of a client.

■ ■ ■ *VIGNETTE*

Jeffrey is a 29-year-old man charged with murder. Officers report that he allegedly murdered his girlfriend during an argument by stabbing her several times with a knife. During the booking process, officers observe Jeffrey's eyes darting around the room, and he appears to be in a heated conversation with "unseen others." He often cries out, "Leave me alone. I told you to leave me alone!" When his handcuffs are removed, he becomes combative. Jeffrey says the same voices that kept him awake for several days before his argument with his girlfriend are telling him to attack the officers. When asked about substance abuse or any medical problems, Jeffrey responds, "No way, I'm not sick, never have been, and I don't do dope!" (Coram, 2004b, p. 1).

■ ■ ■

The main differences between psychiatric forensic nursing, correctional nursing, and correctional mental health nursing can be summarized as follows:

Nurse-client relationship:
- For correctional nurses and correctional mental health nurses, the client is the jail or prison inmate.
- For the psychiatric forensic nurse, the client is the attorney or the court.

Approach of the nurse:
- Both correctional nurses and correctional mental health nurses use an empathetic, supportive, and accepting approach with the client.
- Psychiatric forensic nurses remain detached, objective, and neutral.

Purpose of the relationship:
- For correctional nurses, the purpose is to provide nursing care directed at the physical and mental health needs of inmates.
- For correctional mental health nurses, the purpose is to provide nursing care directed at the mental health needs of inmates.
- For psychiatric forensic nurses, the purpose is to evaluate the sanity and competency of the perpetrator prior to trial.

Practice setting:
- For correctional nurses, the practice setting is a cell, secured unit, or central clinic within a correctional facility.
- For correctional mental health nurses, the practice setting is a psychiatric unit within a jail or

prison or within a long-term unit of a forensic hospital.
- For psychiatric forensic nursing, the practice setting may be the community, an inpatient unit, or a jail or prison.

Examples of nursing functions:
- Correctional nurses might treat an injury or complete a suicide assessment.
- Correctional mental health nurses might provide medication teaching, offer one-to-one counseling, and run therapeutic groups.
- The functions of psychiatric forensic nurses are described in the following section.

ROLES WITHIN PSYCHIATRIC FORENSIC NURSING

The psychiatric forensic nurse may function as a forensic examiner, competency therapist, consultant to law enforcement agencies, or consultant to the criminal justice system. These roles involve providing expert witness testimony, services to a prosecutor or defense attorney, criminal profile reports, or hostage negotiation.

Forensic Examiner

A **forensic examiner** conducts court-ordered evaluations of legal sanity or competency to proceed, responds to specific medicolegal questions as requested by the court, and renders an expert opinion in a written report or courtroom testimony. An evaluation may be requested by the prosecution, the defense, or the judge. Evaluations are usually based on the defendant's history or behavior at the scene of the crime, in jail, or in the courtroom.

A complete report is based on clinical data, observations of the defendant's behavior, any forensic evidence contained in crime scene reports or laboratory reports, summary of any psychological testing, and a thorough psychosocial history. The forensic examiner interviews the defendant and notes behavior, past diagnoses, personality traits, emotions, cognitive abilities, any symptoms of mental disorder, and the psychodynamics of interpersonal relationships (Emiley, 2002).

Legal Sanity

Legal sanity is defined as the individual's ability to discriminate right from wrong with reference to the act charged, capacity to understand the nature and quality of the act charged, and capacity to form the intent to commit the crime. Legal sanity is determined for the specific time of the act. The forensic examiner must reconstruct the defendant's mental state by reviewing evidence left at the scene, any witness statements, the self-report of the defendant's symptoms, and the defendant's disclosed motivation. Some of the issues addressed in the forensic examiner's determination are (1) whether or not the defendant was using drugs, (2) whether the defendant's reasoning ability was affected by any medical condition, and (3) what the social context of the crime was.

A legal insanity defense is a choice. In most states, the presence of a major mental disorder is a prerequisite for a finding of legal insanity; however, a defendant who has a mental illness does not have to use this defense.

The forensic nurse specialist must have a clear knowledge of which legal standard is being used and must be able to articulate it to the court and jury. Such legal tests include the M'Naghten rules, irresistible impulse, and guilty but mentally ill (Coram, 2004a).

The *M'Naghten rules* derive from a trial in 1843 in which Daniel M'Naghten was tried for the murder of a public official. M'Naghten believed there was a conspiracy among the Tories of England to destroy him. In an attempt to assassinate the Prime Minister, who was the Tory leader, M'Naghten mistakenly shot and killed the Prime Minister's secretary. M'Naghten was judged to be criminally insane and acquitted of the murder. There was a public outcry over the leniency of this verdict. The House of Lords convened a special session of the judges to give an advisory opinion regarding the law of England governing the insanity defense. The judges advised that, to be considered criminally insane, the accused with a mental disorder either must not know the nature and quality of the act or must not know whether the act is right or wrong. Whether or not the individual is responsible for his or her action is the underlying issue in the M'Naghten rules.

Irresistible impulse was added to the M'Naghten rules in 1929. This addition stipulates that, even if the defendant knew the criminal act was wrong, if the defendant could not control his or her behavior because of a psychiatric illness or a mental defect, then the defendant is not guilty.

Guilty but mentally ill is another insanity defense. Those who plead guilty but mentally ill are remanded to the correctional system, where they receive treatment for their mental disorder. They are subject to the correctional system's parole decisions.

The ethical forensic examiner must be able to separate personal opinion from professional opinion. Personal opinion is based on one's background, upbringing, education, and value system. Professional opinion is based on scientific principle, advanced education in a specific field of endeavor, and the unbiased standards set by research in that area. Although members of the treatment staff on a forensic unit strive to be supportive, accepting, and empathetic, the forensic examiner strives to remain neutral, objective, and detached.

Competence to Proceed

Whereas legal insanity is determined by defendant's thinking in the past at the time of the offense, compulsion to proceed is determined by the defendant's thinking in the present at the time of the trial. It is defined as the capacity to assist one's attorney and to understand the legal proceedings. As many as 60,000 de-

fendants are evaluated annually in the United States (Poythress et al., 2001). Because competence to proceed is a determination of mental capacity in the present, the defendant's competency must be determined each time he or she goes to court. A prior finding of incompetence, even if due to a developmental disability or mental illness, does not preclude a subsequent finding of competency in a later, unrelated case.

Competency Therapist

Under American law, no person may be tried if he or she is deemed legally incompetent. A court will remand an incompetent defendant to a suitable facility (usually a locked unit in a mental hospital) for a specified time period for treatment to regain competency. Psychiatric forensic nurses working as competency therapists have greatly enhanced the treatment of legal incompetence, which in the past usually meant only the prescribing of antipsychotic medications. Psychiatric forensic nursing role functions for the **competency therapist** include using assessment tools, assessing competency and mental disorder, conducting a forensic interview, providing documentation, completing a formal report to the court, and testifying as an expert witness.

Competency therapists work with the defendant in one-to-one and group activities. It is important that the therapist maintain objectivity and not confuse this type of education and training with psychotherapy. Competency therapists realize that the client is the court, not the defendant, and that the work product is a competent defendant and a completed report. Becoming an advocate for the defendant, rather than for the process, is a breach of professional boundaries (Jacobson, 2002). The competency therapist who does so should seek supervision for countertransference issues.

Expert Witness

Most of the psychiatric forensic nursing role functions reflect the difference between a *fact witness* and an *expert witness* in the court system. By license, any nurse can be subpoenaed by the court to testify as a fact witness. A fact witness testifies regarding what was seen or heard, performed, or documented regarding a patient's care. A fact witness testifies regarding first-hand experience only.

An expert witness is recognized by the court as having a certain level of skill or expertise in a designated area. Usually, the expert witness testifies regarding his or her involvement with the client as well as any documentation completed by the expert witness. Following this testimony, the court allows the expert witness to give additional testimony in the form of a professional opinion. Forensic nurses with advanced degrees are more likely to be called upon as expert witnesses.

To establish credibility as an expert witness and to have one's opinion given equal weight in court to that of a psychiatrist, the forensic nurse specialist must have expertise, trustworthiness, and presentation style. These characteristics are described in Box 31-2.

BOX 31-2

Expert Witness: Credentials for Credibility

Establishment of Expertise
- Academic preparation
- Professional training
- Occupational and life experiences
- Involvement in professional organizations

Establishment of Trustworthiness and Objectivity
- Dress, manner, and performance that communicate professionalism
- Successful communication to jury

Expertise is established by professional credentials. Trustworthiness is the degree of honesty in demeanor and opinion evinced on the witness stand, as perceived by the judge or jury. The expert witness may be credible, trustworthy, and an authority in a specialty area, but unless he or she has the ability to communicate in a concise and convincing fashion, the testimony given is of limited value.

Consultant to Law Enforcement Agencies

Over the last decades, deinstitutionalization of the mentally ill has precipitated a need for interagency cooperation between mental health and law enforcement agencies. The mental health personnel summoned by law enforcement officers function as advocates for the perpetrator. The perpetrator's well-being is the focus of the interaction, which may result in civil detention and admission to a hospital. Community mental health nurses have traditionally served in this role.

Psychiatric forensic nurses are expanding their scope of practice by working as **consultants to law enforcement agencies** in hostage negotiation and criminal profiling. These roles differ from those described earlier in both purpose and philosophy.

Hostage Negotiator

In the late 1970s, the Federal Bureau of Investigation began expanding hostage negotiation team structure by recommending the use of consultants who could address the mental state of the perpetrator and recommend appropriate negotiation strategies. In the 1980s, local police agencies began to develop specialized teams and to use consultants. Police agencies that use a consultant in hostage situations report significantly more negotiated surrenders, significantly fewer incidents ending with tactical team assaults, and fewer incidents in which a hostage is killed or seriously injured by a perpetrator (Slatkin, 2000). The first use of a psychiatric forensic nurse as a consultant was reported in 1993.

When the psychiatric forensic nurse functions as a behavioral science expert, the role of the nurse differs markedly from that of the community mental health nurse. In this role the psychiatric forensic nurse is an advocate not for the perpetrator but rather for the process of hostage negotiation. Duties within this role include the following:
- Being on call around the clock to assist SWAT (special weapons and tactics) or tactical teams and patrol officers on the scene
- Providing suggestions regarding negotiation techniques
- Assessing the mental status of the perpetrator
- Providing a link to mental health agencies
- Participating in a critique of the hostage incident
- Assessing released hostages
- Assessing the stress level of the hostage negotiator
- Providing training in communication skills to law enforcement officers

The successful consultant thinks clearly under stress, is able to communicate with persons from all socioeconomic classes, demonstrates common sense and is "streetwise," is able to cope with uncertainty, can accept responsibility with no authority, and is able to express commitment to the negotiation process.

Criminal Profiler

Criminal profiling is an educated attempt to provide law enforcement officials with specific information regarding the type of individual who would have committed a certain crime. This is done after study of the behavioral and psychological indicators left at a violent crime scene (O'Toole, 1999). This service is usually requested when the crime scene indicates psychopathology or when serial crime is suspected.

Historically, before forensic nurses entered the area of behavioral science, profilers came from a variety of backgrounds, including law enforcement, psychology, psychiatry, and criminal justice. An understanding of psychopathology is necessary, but other specialized education is not as important as having investigative experience. The criminal profiler collects all the available data, attempts to reconstruct the crime, formulates a hypothesis, develops a profile, and tests it against the known data. This is familiar territory for the psychiatric forensic nurse, who is comfortable with the nursing processes of assessment, analysis, planning, implementation, and evaluation.

Skilled profilers are able to isolate their own emotions and attempt to reconstruct the crime using the criminal's reasoning process (Fintzy, 2000). Attempts to analyze the event based on the personal values of the profiler or on logic will lead to misinterpretation of the criminal's behavior.

Consultant to Attorneys

Psychiatric forensic nurses may be used as a resource for education and information about mental illness by either side in a court case. In this role the nurse may be asked to attend the hearing as a courtroom observer who listens to other witness testimony for the purpose of guiding further cross-examination or may be asked to assist in the preparation for trial by giving information about mental illness, personality disorders, or paraphilias. The nurse may be asked to testify regarding mental health treatment options, medications, and community resources.

OTHER SUBSPECIALTY AREAS OF FORENSIC NURSING

Physiological forensic nurses focus on the application of forensic aspects of health care in the scientific investigation and treatment of trauma and/or investigation of medicolegal issues (Goll-McGee, 1999). The client is the alleged victim, either living or dead. Role functions in **physiological forensic nursing** are listed in Box 31-3.

Physiological forensic nurses work as coroners or death investigators, sexual assault nurse examiners (Girardin, 2001), child abuse or elder abuse specialists (Fulton, 2000), spouse or partner abuse specialists, or legal nurse consultants (Lorenzo, 2000).

Death investigation and sexual assault investigation are two forensic subspecialties attractive to basic level registered nurses. These nurses usually testify as fact witnesses and provide their testimony via court-accepted documentation. Sometimes these nurses are called to testify regarding the identification and accuracy of their documentation. Certification in these areas can be obtained through the IAFN, various state boards, the forensic associations, or other educational groups.

■ ■ ■ VIGNETTE

The watershed moment in forensic nursing had its beginnings in late 2000 in a Virginia circuit court where a sexual assault case, *Commonwealth v. Johnson,* was underway. Suzanne Brown, RN, a SANE [sexual assault nurse examiner] considered to be an expert by the presiding judge, was allowed to testify about injuries she observed in a rape victim. Brown testified that physical injuries detectable by gross visualization are not found in individuals in whom the 'human sexual response' had been triggered. The prosecutor said that injuries visible without magnification indicated to Brown that the sexual activity occurred without consent, whereas the defense

said Brown's opinion was scientifically unreliable. The court consulted various studies and ruled that none of them supported Brown's opinion that genital injuries detectable by gross visualization do not result from consensual sexual intercourse. The court said that because the medical literature did not support Brown's opinion about the human sexual response relating to genital injury, there was not foundation to admit evidence and Brown's testimony about the human sexual response was excluded. Even though portions of Brown's testimony were thrown out of court, forensic nurses celebrated the significance that Brown, as a SANE, was an expert witness. (Pyrek, 2004, p. 4)

■ ■ ■

PROFESSIONALISM IN PSYCHIATRIC FORENSIC NURSING

Working within forensic psychiatry requires the nurse to be assertive and able to work with autonomy. The ability to cope with dangerous situations and hostile environments is necessary. It is a challenge to be viewed as an expert. For some female nurses, it is difficult to work in a predominantly male atmosphere or to find mentors in these arenas. Georgia Pasqualone shares one of her challenging moments as a nurse investigator in the following vignette.

■ ■ ■ VIGNETTE

Everything was going smoothly until the attorney applied for funding from the presiding judge on the case. The dialogue went a little like this:

Attorney: Your honor, I would like to present a motion for funding for my nurse investigator.

Judge: You want funds to pay a nurse? What do you need a nurse for? There aren't any hospital records to read. Nobody's sick. You don't need a nurse.

Attorney: But, Your Honor, she's my investigator, my crime scene photographer, my reconstructionist, my criminalist, my child abuse specialist, my DNA interpreter, my expert witness. . . .

Judge: She's just a nurse. There are no bedpans in this case. Funding denied.

The attorney eventually got the judge's attention and I was granted funding. However, this is one of the dilemmas that complicate the future of forensic nursing. Judges, police officers, detectives, attorneys, school superintendents, medical examiners, coroners, physicians, and psychiatrists, to name only a few, need to be educated and enlightened about our emerging specialty. (Pasqualone, 2004, pp. 10-11)

■ ■ ■

The psychiatric forensic nurse must be highly skilled in interpersonal communications and able to develop collegial relationships with those in other disciplines. Nurses should not practice in this area if they hold narrow views of the issues facing these clients or

---

BOX 31-3

Role Functions of Physiological Forensic Nursing

- Photographs crime scene
- Identifies bite marks, sharp injuries, and blunt trauma
- Assesses victim of sexual assault
- Identifies patterned injury
- Establishes chain of custody of evidence
- Assesses pattern of injury in abuse
- Documents gunshot wounds

if they are motivated by the desire to punish (Evans, 2000). A prerequisite is the ability to listen and accept others' values and motivations in a nonjudgmental fashion.

Psychiatric forensic nursing appeals to a particular type of nurse who thrives in a stimulating intellectual environment, who seeks out opportunities to apply clinical skills to complex legal problems, and who enjoys pushing the limits of traditional boundaries. Because of the value placed on tradition by the nursing profession, the psychiatric forensic nurse is sometimes viewed with skepticism within nursing and with a bit of caution within the legal system. These responses must be met with professionalism in practice, research, and education of future psychiatric forensic nurses. Individuals who meet these challenges are characteristically confident in their own knowledge and abilities.

■ ■ ■ **KEY POINTS to REMEMBER**

- Forensic nursing is an emerging specialty area of practice that combines elements of traditional nursing, forensic science, and criminal justice.
- The IAFN was established in 1992 as the professional association representing this specialty.
- Psychiatric forensic nurses fulfill a variety of roles, including that of forensic examiner; competency therapist; expert witness; consultant to law enforcement agencies, attorneys, and the court; hostage negotiator; and criminal profiler.
- Physiological forensic nurse focus on the investigation and treatment of trauma and investigation of medicolegal issues.
- Psychiatric forensic nurses must be assertive and autonomous.

■ ■ ■

Visit the Evolve website at **http://evolve.elsevier.com/Varcarolis** for a posttest on the content in this chapter. *evolve*

Critical Thinking and Chapter Review

Visit the Evolve website at **http://evolve.elsevier.com/Varcarolis** for additional self-study exercises.
evolve

■ ■ ■ **CRITICAL THINKING**

1. How would you describe the nurse-client relationship in forensic nursing? In what ways does this differ from the nurse-client relationship in correctional nursing?
2. Ralph, an angry and alienated 16-year-old high school student, rapes a young woman who is developmentally delayed. In Ralph's defense, he claims that he was criminally insane at the time of the rape. What are some issues that would face a forensic examiner in determining whether Ralph's behavior could be considered a result of insanity?
3. Explain the differences among the legal tests that are used in a criminal insanity defense.
4. Imagine you are working on a psychiatric inpatient unit as a new graduate. A patient on the unit commits suicide. You are called to testify as a fact witness. What would your role be as a fact witness? A nurse who is nationally recognized for her research on suicidal behavior is called as an expert witness. How would this nurse's role differ from yours?

■ ■ ■ **CHAPTER REVIEW**

Choose the most appropriate answer.

1. Mr. O. has the psychiatric diagnosis of paranoid schizophrenia. He stopped taking his medication, became more delusional, and started accosting people on the street and haranguing them. He was arrested and jailed. Once a medication regimen is reinstituted, a focus for intervention that the nurse in the jail should pursue is
   1. persuading Mr. O. to be screened for human immunodeficiency virus infection.
   2. identifying the reason Mr. O. stopped taking medication to prevent recurrence.
   3. advocating for Mr. O.'s charges to be dropped so he can return to the community.
   4. teaching Mr. O. the importance of maintenance of physical health via regular physical examinations.
2. Which responsibility would *not* be found in the job description of a psychiatric nurse working with mentally ill clients within a correctional facility?
   1. Providing direct care
   2. Planning health education
   3. Taking part in the punishment process
   4. Functioning as liaison between the correctional facility and the community mental health system
3. A specialty area of nursing practice that combines elements of nursing science, forensic science, and criminal justice is
   1. forensic nursing.
   2. psychiatric specialist nursing.
   3. criminal justice nursing.
   4. critical science nursing.
4. One main difference among the roles of a forensic nurse, a correctional mental health nurse, and a correctional nurse is
   1. the psychiatric forensic nurse may run therapeutic groups for psychiatric mental health patients in a noncorrectional setting.
   2. the psychiatric forensic nurse may function as a forensic examiner.
   3. for many correctional mental health nurses, the setting is a locked psychiatric unit in a community hospital.
   4. many correctional nurses are employed in a community hospital emergency room.

Critical Thinking and Chapter Review—cont'd

Visit the Evolve website at **http://evolve.elsevier.com/Varcarolis** for additional self-study exercises.

5. Ms T. is a forensic nurse and serves as a forensic examiner. She conducts court-ordered evaluations of clients to determine

1. the legal sanity of a client.
2. any history of abusive behavior.
3. an appropriate defense to bring to court.
4. the testimony that would predict the thought process of a psychiatric mental health client.

■ STUDENT
■ STUDY
■ CD-ROM

Access the accompanying CD-ROM for animations, interactive exercises, review questions for the NCLEX examination, and an audio glossary.

■ NURSE,
■ CLIENT, AND
■ FAMILY RESOURCES

For suggested readings, information on related associations, and Internet resources, go to **http://evolve.elsevier.com/Varcarolis.**

REFERENCES

American Nurses Association & International Association of Forensic Nurses. (1997). *Scope and standards of forensic nursing practice.* Washington, DC: American Nurses Publishing.

Bickford, C. (2004). Correctional nursing standards are undergoing revision; Comments are due. *Forensic Nurse,* July/August, 1-24. Retrieved November 23, 2004, from http://www.forensicnursemag.com/hotnews/48h181158 53.html?wts=20050405092217&hc=426&req= correctional+and+nursing+and+standards.

Coram, J. (1993). *Role development within a new subspecialty: Forensic nursing.* Unpublished master's thesis, Washington State University, Spokane.

Coram, J. (2004a). Forensic psychiatric nursing. In C. R. Kneisl, H. S. Wilson, & E. Trigoboff, *Contemporary psychiatric-mental health nursing* (pp. 819-834). Upper Saddle River, NJ: Pearson/Prentice Hall.

Coram, J. (2004b). *Psychiatric nursing in the correctional setting* (Nursing Spectrum Education/CE Self-Study Module). Retrieved October 13, 2004, from http://nsweb. nursingspectrum.com/ce/m30C-1.htm.

Emiley, S. F. (2002). Forensic psychological evaluations: Back to basics. *Forensic Examiner, 11*(1-2), 31-35.

Evans, M. (2000). Re-visioning the nurses' punitive attitudes within forensic psychiatric and correctional nursing: The significance of ethical sophistication. *Journal of Psychosocial Nursing, 38*(4), 8-13.

Fintzy, R. T. (2000). Criminal profiling: An introduction to behavioral evidence analysis. *American Journal of Psychiatry, 157,* 1532-1555.

Fulton, D. R. (2000). Recognition and documentation of domestic violence in the clinical setting. *Critical Care Nursing Quarterly, 23*(2), 26-34.

Girardin, B. (2001). Is this forensic specialty for you? *RN, 64*(12), 37-41.

Goll-McGee, B. (1999). The role of the clinical forensic nurse in the USA. In D. Robinson & A. Kettles (Eds.), *Forensic nursing and multidisciplinary care of the mentally disordered offender* (pp. 213-226). London: Jessica Kingsley Publishers.

International Association of Forensic Nurses. (2002a). *About IAFN.* Retrieved November 22, 2004, from http://www. iafn.org/about/default.html.

International Association of Forensic Nurses. (2002b). *About IAFN: Goals.* Retrieved November 22, 2004, from http:// www.iafn.org/about/goals.html.

Jacobson, G. (2002). Maintaining professional boundaries: Preparing nursing students for the challenge. *Journal of Nursing Education, 41,* 279-281.

Lorenzo, P. (2000). Distinguishing the legal nurse consultant, *Legal Assistant Today, 18*(1), 12-13.

O'Toole, M. E. (1999). Criminal profiling: The FBI uses criminal investigative analysis to solve crimes. *Corrections Today, 61*(1), 44-46.

Pasqualone, G. (2004). Perspectives on the future of forensic nursing. *Forensic Nurse,* November/December, 10-13. Retrieved November 23, 2004, from http://www.forensic-nursemag.com/articles/3b1cover.html?wts=200411230735 15hc=44.

Poythress, N., et al. (2001). The MacArthur adjudicative competence study: Executive summary. *Behavioral Sciences and the Law, 15,* 329-345.

Pyrek, K. M. (2004). Forensic nursing pioneers ponder the future. *Forensic Nurse,* November/December, 1-13. Retrieved November 23, 2004, from http://www.forensicnursemag. com/articles/3b1cover.html?wts=2004112373515&hc=44.

Rennison, C. M., & Rand, M. R. (2004). *Criminal victimization, 2002* (NCJ 201797). Washington, DC: Bureau of Justice Statistics.

Saunders, L. (2000). Forensic nursing. *Australian Nursing Journal, 8*(3), 49-50.

Slatkin, A. (2000). The role of the mental health consultant in hostage negotiations: Questions to ask during the incident phase. *Police Chief, 67*(7), 64.

Winfrey, M. E., & Smith, A. R. (1999). The suspiciousness factor: Critical care nursing and forensics. *Critical Care Nursing Quarterly, 22*(1), 1-7.

A FAMILY SPEAKS

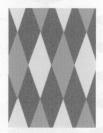

My mother is 78 years old and was living independently until May 6, 2004. I will never forget the day. She was found in her car in a ditch approximately 150 miles north of her home town. She had no memory of driving there and was very confused. She was taken to a local emergency department and then transferred to a large medical facility. The doctors thought she had suffered a small stroke and also had a serious urinary tract infection. After they began treating her, they decided she had Alzheimer's disease. When she was discharged back to her home, I took over making all her meals, cleaning her house, doing her errands, and making sure she got to all her medical appointments. I called many times during the day to check on her. Fortunately, she voluntarily gave me her car keys. After the incident in May she was afraid to drive.

My husband and I worked to prepare a room and small living area in our home for my mom; we moved her on June 19. Initially, Mom was being seen by a medical nurse from a local home care agency as well as a psychiatric nurse, who evaluated Mom's memory and her cognitive function. The psychiatric nurse helped us all as we made the adjustment to Mom's living with us, and she helped Mom adjust to the change as well. I was relieved to have Mom in our home—at least I didn't feel like I needed to be in two places at once.

Once Mom's medical condition stabilized, the psychiatric nurse took over my mother's care. Every week she visited our family; she always checked Mom for any physical problems or cognitive changes, but she spent most of her time with me, my husband, and our son. She taught us all about Alzheimer's disease and what we would need to do to take care of Mom. The nurse taught us about safety issues that are so important in caring for a loved one with Alzheimer's disease. For instance, during one of the nurse's visits, she and I walked through my house and she helped me to identify things that needed to be locked up, like medications and cleaning supplies; she pointed out the need for handrails in the hallways and bathroom; together we looked at future modifications such as a ramp to the front of the house. She helped me get Mom enrolled in the Safe Return program sponsored by the Alzheimer's Association.

Probably the most important thing that the nurse taught us was how to communicate with Mom. The best advice she gave us was "Thou shalt not reason." This alone has saved me, my husband, and son so much grief. I don't know if we will always be able to care for Mom, but right now we are managing. Sometimes things are tough. My mother has always been pretty focused on herself, and this has only gotten worse. But overall I think we are doing a good job.

LIFESPAN ISSUES AND INTERVENTIONS

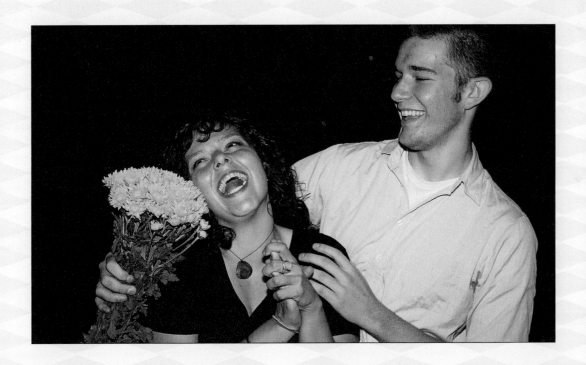

LAUGHTER IS THE SHORTEST DISTANCE BETWEEN TWO PEOPLE.

Victor Borge

CHAPTER 32

Disorders of Children and Adolescents

CHERRILL COLSON

KEY TERMS and CONCEPTS

The key terms and concepts listed here appear in color where they are defined or first discussed in this chapter.

adjustment disorder, 649

attention deficit hyperactivity disorder (ADHD), 635

bibliotherapy, 653

conduct disorder, 643

mental status assessment, 639

oppositional defiant disorder, 643

pervasive developmental disorder (PDD), 640

play therapy, 652

posttraumatic stress disorder (PTSD), 646

resilient child, 637

separation anxiety disorder, 646

temperament, 637

therapeutic drawing, 653

therapeutic games, 652

therapeutic holding, 651

time-out, 651

Tourette's disorder, 648

OBJECTIVES

After studying this chapter, the reader will be able to

1. Explore what factors and influences contribute to child and adolescent mental disorders and how they relate to multi-modal intervention strategies for these young clients.

2. Explain how the characteristics associated with resiliency can mitigate against etiological influences.

3. Identify characteristics of mental health in children and adolescents.

4. Discuss various components involved in constructing a holistic assessment of a child or adolescent.

5. Explore areas in the assessment of suicide that may be unique to children or adolescents.

6. Describe the clinical features and behaviors of at least three child and adolescent psychiatric disorders and identify useful intervention strategies for each.

7. Compare and contrast at least six treatment modalities for children and adolescents.

8. Formulate three nursing diagnoses, stating client outcomes with corresponding interventions, for at least three child and adolescent psychiatric disorders discussed in this chapter.

evolve Visit the Evolve website at **http://evolve.elsevier.com/Varcarolis** for a pretest on the content in this chapter.

PREVALENCE

One in five children and adolescents in the United States suffers from a major mental illness causing significant

Important psychiatric disorders in youth such as mood disorders, anxiety disorders, schizophrenia, and substance abuse are described elsewhere in this text. These are conditions that may be present during childhood or adolescence but are most often diagnosed when a child reaches maturity. Anxiety and depression are discussed here as they relate specifically to the child and adolescent.

impairments at home, at school, and with peers. An estimated two thirds of all young people with mental health problems are not getting the help they need. Mental illness can continue into adulthood, as evidenced by the fact that 74% of 21 year olds with mental disorders have had previous problems. Approximately 60% of all children in out-of-home care have moderate to severe mental health problems. Suicide is now the third leading cause of death among youth aged 15 to 24 years and the sixth leading cause of death for 5 to 15 year olds. For every older teen and young adult who takes his or her own life, 100 to 200 of their peers attempt suicide (National Mental Health Association, 2004).

The federal government's recognition of these mental health problems and efforts toward effective treatments were identified in *Mental Health: A Report of the Surgeon General* (U.S. Department of Health and Human Services, 1999). However, barriers to assessment and treatment remain. Identified barriers are (1) lack of clarity about why, when, and how children should be screened; (2) lack of coordination of multiple systems with different funding streams and eligibility requirements; (3) lack of resources; (4) lack of mental health providers; and (5) inadequate reimbursement (Children's Defense Fund, 2004). Table 32-1 gives the prevalence of common child and adolescent mental health disorders.

COMORBIDITY

Emotionally disturbed children often meet the criteria for more than one diagnostic category. Attention deficit hyperactivity disorder (ADHD), a prominent comorbid condition, occurs in 90% of individuals with juvenile-onset bipolar disorder, 90% of children with oppositional defiant disorder, and 50% of those with conduct disorder. Childhood depression is associated with a high incidence of comorbidity: 20% to 80% of children with depression have conduct or oppositional disorders, 30% to 75% have anxiety disorders, and 5% to 60% display symptoms of ADHD (Inder, 2000). Multiple services are needed by those with dual or co-existing diagnoses, such as individuals in whom depression and suicidal ideation coexist with substance abuse, conduct disorder, or ADHD.

Mental illness can become severe and persistent when effective early intervention is not provided. Between 20% and 50% of depressed children and adolescents have a family history of depression (Sadock & Sadock, 2004). A child raised by a depressed parent is at risk for developing anxiety disorder, conduct disorder, and alcohol dependence. The depressed parent's inability to model effective coping strategies leads to learned helplessness, which leaves the child anxious or apathetic and unable to learn how to master the environment. Another result may be the child's inability to make emotional attachments because the depressed parent is emotionally unavailable. A child with a conduct disorder may go on to develop an antisocial personality and end up in the criminal justice system. In fact, two thirds of youth in the juvenile justice system have one or more diagnosable mental disorders (Children's Defense Fund, 2004).

Abused and neglected children are at great risk for developing emotional, intellectual, and social handi-

---

TABLE 32-1

Prevalence Rates of Some Child and Adolescent Disorders

Disorder	Prevalence	Male/Female Ratio
Autism	3-5 per 10,000	3:1-4:1
Asperger's disorder	0.5-10 per 10,000	3:1-4:1
Rett's disorder	0.5-1.5 per 10,000	All female
Attention deficit hyperactivity disorder	School-aged children: 3%-7% Grade school children: 2%-20%	5:1
Conduct disorder	3%-5% lifetime prevalence 9% of males, 2% of females in children younger than 18 years of age	3:1-5:1

Depressive disorders	*Major depression:*
	  Children: 0.4%-2.5%
	  Adolescents: 0.4%-8.3%
	Dysthymic depression*:
	  Children: 0.6%-1.7%
	  Adolescents: 1.6%-8.0%
		Children 1:1
		Adolescents 2:1

Anxiety disorders	*Separation anxiety:*
	  School-aged children: 3%-4%
	  Adolescents: 1%
	Posttraumatic stress disorder:
	  General population: 0.1%-1.3%
	  Children who have suffered sexual abuse: 32%-53%
		1:1-2:1

Tourette's disorder	5-30 per 10,000	3:1 to 4:1

*Depression persists into adulthood with recurrence rates estimated to be 60% to 70%.

caps as a result of their traumatic experiences (U.S. Department of Health and Human Services, 1999). Abused children are also at risk for identifying with the aggressor and becoming the neighborhood bully, becoming an abuser in adulthood, or developing dysfunctional behavior patterns in close interpersonal relationships.

CHILD AND ADOLESCENT PSYCHIATRIC NURSE

The first roles assumed by the child psychiatric nurse generalist were those of parental surrogate, socializing agent, teacher, counselor, manager of a therapeutic milieu, and member of a multidisciplinary team. More recently, the American Nurses Association (ANA), together with the American Psychiatric Nurses Association and International Society of Psychiatric-Mental Health Nurses, has defined the basic level functions in the combined child and adult *Scope and Standards of Psychiatric-Mental Health Nursing Practice* (2000).

Although the number of acutely ill children is increasing, inpatient treatment time has steadily decreased. Treatment for children consists of brief hospitalization followed by interventions conducted in a wide spectrum of community support settings, including day treatment programs, partial hospitalization programs, clinics, and psychiatric home care. The nurse has less time to form a therapeutic alliance with the child, which makes it more difficult to facilitate lasting behavioral changes.

The majority of children who are hospitalized are diagnosed with a conduct disorder; they infrequently come from intact homes—and this is especially true in urban areas. These children are referred to as "functional orphans" because they have never received adequate parenting. This lack of a family support system in turn limits the nurse's ability to work with caregivers on parenting issues and to ensure that the gains made in treatment are sustained.

As psychiatric care has moved from inpatient to outpatient facilities and into the community, mental health nurses have become an integral part of home care and hospice teams, proving their ability to work with youth and their families in the home. Advanced practice nurses have established school-based primary prevention and treatment programs for children and adolescents (Costello-Wells et al., 2003; Eggert et al., 2002). Therapeutic work is also being carried out in nontraditional settings such as homeless shelters.

Meeting the mental health needs of youth and their families is a challenge for the nurse as needs steadily increase while funding resources and access to care steadily decrease. This chapter describes the assessment and interventions for selected mental disorders as well as broad treatment modalities that are implemented through the nursing process.

THEORY

The causes of mental illness in children and adolescents encompass multiple factors. The need to distinguish among the genetic, organic, and environmental causes of mental illness makes diagnosis difficult. Increasing numbers of children are born with, or develop, disordered brain function related to malnutrition, lead poisoning, human immunodeficiency virus (HIV) infection, fetal alcohol syndrome, drug addiction, and traumatic experiences such as child abuse.

Younger children are far more difficult to diagnose than older children because the boundaries between normal and abnormal behaviors are less distinct. Pediatricians and parents often must wait to see whether symptoms are the result of a developmental lag that will eventually correct itself or something more serious. Therefore, intervention may be delayed until the child reaches school age (Sadock & Sadock, 2004). Usually, a number of factors influence a child's or adolescent's mental health, so interventions need to be multimodal—that is, a variety of interventions are needed to improve the child's psychological, social, physical, and spiritual well-being and overall quality of life.

A child's vulnerability to emotional and mental disorders is the result of complex, multilayered interactions among the child's attributes (biological, psychological, and genetic), trauma, disease, interpersonal experiences, environment, and cultural factors, all of which shape the child's development (Popper et al., 2004). The degree of vulnerability changes over time. The resiliency of the growing child and the presence of positive environmental factors enable a child to continue learning and adapting, which in turn decreases the vulnerability to mental disorders.

Genetic Influences

Hereditary factors are implicated in a number of mental disorders, including autism, bipolar disorders, schizophrenia, attention deficit problems, and mental retardation (Sadock & Sadock, 2004). Genetic studies indicated an 80% heritability for ADHD (Inder, 2000). Vulnerability to these disorders exists even when a child is not being raised by the biological parents. Because not all vulnerable children develop mental disorders, it is assumed that constitutional resilience and a supportive environment play roles in keeping the disorders from developing. According to the *Diagnostic and Statistical Manual of Mental Disorders*, 4th edition, text revision *(DSM-IV-TR)* (American Psychiatric Association [APA], 2000), some disorders have a direct genetic link, such as the mental retardation seen in those with Tay-Sachs disease, phenylketonuria, and fragile X syndrome. These conditions may become manifest whenever the gene is passed to the child.

Biochemical Factors

Alterations in neurotransmitters play a role in causing child and adolescent disorders. Decreases in norepinephrine and serotonin levels are related to depression and suicide; elevated levels are related to mania. Abnormalities in dopamine receptors and dopamine transporters are implicated in ADHD (Sadock & Sadock, 2004).

Temperament

Temperament, according to Thomas and Chess (1977), is the style of behavior a child habitually uses to cope with the demands and expectations of the environment. Temperament is a constitutional factor and is thought to be genetically determined. It may be modified by the parent-infant relationship, with positive or negative results. In the case of an individual showing the difficult-child temperament, if the caregiver is unable to respond positively to the child, there is a risk of insecure attachment, developmental problems, and future mental disorders.

Social and Environmental Factors

External factors in the environment put stress on children and adolescents and shape their development. There are a number of familial risk factors that correlate with child psychiatric disorders (Popper et al., 2004; Sadock & Sadock, 2004): (1) severe marital discord, (2) low socioeconomic status, (3) large families and overcrowding, (4) parental criminality, (5) maternal psychiatric disorders, and (6) foster care placement. The greater the number of stressors, the greater the incidence of mental disorders.

The abuse of children and stressful life events are known to be associated with increased incidence of accidental injuries, anxiety, depression, and suicidal behaviors (Sadock & Sadock, 2004). Traumatic life events can lead to insecure attachments, posttraumatic stress disorder (PTSD), conduct disorders, delinquency, and impaired social and cognitive function (Popper et al., 2004). Physical and sexual abuse of young children puts them at risk for developing a dissociative identity disorder as a defense against the overwhelming anxiety associated with the abuse (Sadock & Sadock, 2004).

Cultural and Ethnic Factors

Culture shock and cultural conflicts related to assimilation issues put immigrant children at risk for a variety of problems. Yeh and colleagues (2004) noted that a disproportionate number of minority children are labeled as having mental and learning disorders and suffer from this stigma throughout life. These same researchers propose that the lack of cultural role models can put minority children at risk. The differences in cultural expectations, presence of stresses, and support or lack of support by the dominant culture have profound effects on a child's development and the risk of mental, emotional, and academic problems.

Resiliency

Most children who grow up at risk are able to develop normally, without mental problems. They have a resilience that enables them to handle the stresses of a difficult childhood. The term *resilience* has been used to denote the relationship between a child's constitutional endowment and environmental factors. Studies have shown that a resilient child has the following characteristics (Gallagher & Chase, 2002; Hall & Pearson, 2003): (1) a temperament that can adapt to changes in the environment, (2) the ability to form nurturing relationships with other adults when a parent is not available, (3) the ability to distance himself or herself from the emotional chaos of the parent or family, (4) good social intelligence, and (5) the ability to use problem-solving skills. Other studies have identified the cushioning effects of family stability in the face of poverty and adversity. The nurse's role is to foster these characteristics and environmental supports to keep the at-risk child from developing emotional and mental problems.

OVERALL ASSESSMENT

Mental Health Versus Mental Illness

A mentally disturbed child or adolescent is one whose progressive personality development is hindered or arrested by a variety of biopsychosocial and spiritual factors, which results in impairments in the capacities expected of a child of his or her age and physical and cognitive endowments. In comparison, the personality development of a mentally healthy child or adolescent progresses with only minor regressions as the individual masters developmental tasks and learns to love, work, and play with satisfaction (Box 32-1).

BOX 32-1

Characteristics of a Mentally Healthy Youth

- Trusts others and sees his or her world as being safe and supportive
- Can correctly interpret reality (reality test) and make accurate perceptions of the environment
- Has a positive, realistic self-concept and identity
- Copes with anxiety and stress using age-appropriate behavior
- Can learn and master developmental tasks
- Expresses self in spontaneous and creative ways
- Develops and maintains satisfying relationships

Assessment Data

The type of data collected to assess mental health depends on the setting, the severity of the presenting problem, and the availability of resources. The nurse is often the first health care professional to have contact with the child and should be aware of the types of data that can be collected. Box 32-2 identifies essential assessment data, including the history of the present illness; the medical, developmental, and family history; and developmental attributes, mental status, and neurological developmental characteristics. Agency policies determine which data are collected and documented, but a nurse in a primary care setting makes an independent judgment about what to assess and how to assess it. In all cases, a physical examination is part of a complete workup for serious mental problems.

Data Collection

Methods of collecting data include interviewing, screening, testing (neurological, psychological, intelligence), observing, and interacting with the child or adolescent. Histories are taken from parents, caregivers, the child (when appropriate) or adolescent, and other family members.

Structured questionnaires and behavior checklists can be completed by parents and teachers. A genogram can be used to document family composition, history, and relationships (see Chapter 36 for an example of a genogram). Numerous assessment tools are available, and with training, nurses learn to use them effectively.

The observation-interaction part of a mental health assessment begins with a semistructured interview in which the child or adolescent is asked about life at home with parents and siblings and life at school with teachers and peers. Because the interview is semistructured, the child is free to describe current problems, even giving information about his or her own developmental history. Play activities such as games, drawings, puppets, and free play are used for younger children who cannot respond to a direct approach. An important part of the first interview is observing the interactions among the child, the caregiver, and siblings (if available). Whenever possible,

---

BOX 32-2

Types of Assessment Data

History of Present Illness
- Chief complaint
- Development and duration of problems
- Help sought and tried
- Effect of problem on child's life at home and school
- Effect of problem on family and siblings' lives

Developmental History
- Pregnancy, birth, neonatal data
- Developmental milestones
- Description of eating, sleeping, and elimination habits and routines
- Attachment behaviors
- Types of play
- Social skills and friendships
- Sexual activity

Developmental Assessment
- Psychomotor skills
- Language skills
- Cognitive skills
- Interpersonal and social skills
- Academic achievement
- Behavior (response to stress, to changes in environment)
- Problem-solving and coping skills (impulse control, delay of gratification)
- Energy level and motivation

Neurological Assessment
- Cerebral functions
- Cerebellar functions
- Sensory functions

- Reflexes
- Cranial nerves

Functions can be observed during developmental assessment and while playing games involving a specific ability (e.g., "Simon says touch your nose")

Medical History
- Review of body systems
- Traumas, hospitalizations, operations, and child's response
- Illnesses or injuries affecting central nervous system
- Medications (past and current)
- Allergies

Family History
- Illnesses in related family members (e.g., seizures, mental disorders, mental retardation, hyperactivity, drug and alcohol abuse, diabetes, cancer)
- Background of family members (occupation, education, social activities, religion)
- Family relationship (separation, divorce, deaths, contact with extended family, support system)

Mental Status Assessment
- General appearance
- Activity level
- Coordination and motor function
- Affect
- Speech
- Manner of relating
- Intellectual functions
- Thought processes and content
- Characteristics of child's play

the child is observed in situations involving interactions with peers.

Mental Status Assessment

Mental status assessment in children is similar to that in adults except that the developmental level and characteristics of play are considered. The developmental and mental status assessments have many areas in common, and for this reason any observation or interaction will provide data for both assessments.

The mental status assessment provides information about the child's mental state at the time of the examination and identifies problems with thinking, feeling, and behaving. The broad categories that are assessed include general appearance, activity level, speech, coordination and motor function, affect, manner of relating, intellectual function, thought processes and content, and characteristics of play.

Developmental Assessment

The developmental assessment provides information about the child's current maturational level. These data are then reviewed in relation to the child's chronological age to identify developmental lags and deficits. The Denver II Developmental Screening Test for infants and children up to 6 years of age is a popular assessment tool that provides this comparison.

Abnormal findings in the developmental and mental status assessments are often related to stress and adjustment problems, rather than to more serious disorders. However, pediatricians no longer automatically say, "It's just a stage. The child will grow out of it." Although many children will outgrow a difficulty, nurses need to evaluate which behaviors indicate stress or minor regressions and which indicate more serious psychopathology. A child's stress behaviors or minor regressions can usually be handled by working with the parents. More serious psychopathology needs to be evaluated by the advanced practice nurse in collaboration with clinicians from other mental health disciplines.

Suicide Risk

Not only does the number of suicidal children and adolescents increase each year, but the number of suicides also rises with increasing age throughout the teenage years, so that suicide is the third leading cause of death in adolescence (Sadock & Sadock, 2004). Because the nurse is often the first health care professional to have contact with the child or adolescent, the nurse needs to know how to assess suicidal ideation and risk. Some children make idle threats about killing themselves. However, the nurse must listen carefully to any child or adolescent who expresses the wish to

die to determine the cause of the distress and the risk of suicide. The areas to explore when assessing suicidal risk include the following:

- Suicidal thoughts, threats, or attempts
- Circumstances and motivation at the time of suicidal thoughts or behaviors
- Concepts about suicide and death, and experiences with the same
- Depression and other moods or feelings (anger, guilt, rejection)

These areas are also applicable when assessing adolescents, but additional questions are asked about acting-out behaviors and about listening to music or reading books with morbid themes.

Assessing lethality in a child's or young adolescent's suicide plan is complicated by the distorted concept of death, immature ego functions, and lack of understanding of lethality. For instance, a child might be highly suicidal and believe that a few aspirin will cause death. The fact that the child is incorrect about the lethality of a few aspirin does not diminish the seriousness of the suicidal intent. Another child may threaten to jump off a bridge, believing that this would not be fatal. This child may be seeking attention and does not want to die. Early intervention is important, and parents need to understand that suicidal behavior must be evaluated by mental health professionals.

Cultural Influences

Psychiatric professionals recognize the importance of culture in evaluating psychiatric disorders, especially when working with families. The *DSM-IV-TR* identifies culture-bound syndromes of mental illness that are not diagnostic categories in Western medicine. Sensitivity to cultural influences in mental illness is a necessity to avoid behavior stereotyping and clouding of assessment.

The nurse considers the influence of culture on the child's behavior, thoughts, and emotions. A lack of eye contact when relating to adults is indicative of respect in African, Caribbean, and Vietnamese children. The Native American child is taught to withhold the expression of feelings, especially anger, both verbally and nonverbally. The Japanese child learns to play using polite, social manners in interactions, whereas other cultures encourage aggressive retaliation when one is bullied by another.

In assessing speech, both the characteristics and the content are considered. For example, the Navajo child's speech is slow and methodical, with pauses that could lead the nurse to believe the child has finished the sentence. The African American child is expected to be verbal, following the oral tradition in which there are multiparty conversations and children are encouraged to demonstrate their wit by outperforming peers. The Hawaiian child whose speech overlaps another's speech might be considered rude. The use of nonstandard English dialects makes speech difficult for the outsider to assess and can contribute to stereotyping. A child's bilingual ability always needs evaluation, because proficiency in interpersonal communication does not guarantee academic success. Whenever possible, a child should be interviewed in his or her native language to obtain a more accurate description of problems.

In evaluating a child's cognition, it is important to know whether expressed beliefs are in keeping with the child's cultural belief system or are bizarre and indicative of disturbed thought processes. For example, a belief in witchcraft or in communication with the spirits of the dead might not be pathological if the child is from a Caribbean culture. Folk medicine practices are also considered when evaluating the child. Cambodian refugees, who believe that illness is caused by a bad wind, will rub their child's skin with oil and a heated coin (*kos khyal*) to raise red welts through which the bad wind is thought to escape (Andrews & Boyle, 2003). In Western culture, these red welts might be mistaken for child abuse.

PERVASIVE DEVELOPMENTAL DISORDERS

A **pervasive developmental disorder (PDD)** is characterized by severe and pervasive impairment in reciprocal social interaction and communication skills, usually accompanied by stereotypical behavior, interests, and activities (APA, 2000). Mental retardation is often evident in these disorders. The latest diagnostic refinement in the *DSM-IV-TR* identifies the four subtypes as autism, Asperger's disorder, Rett's disorder, and childhood disintegrative disorder.

Autistic Disorder

Autism is viewed as a behavioral syndrome resulting from abnormal brain function of unknown etiology. Problems with left hemispheric functions (e.g., language, logic, reasoning) are evident, whereas music and visual-spatial activities may be enhanced, such as in savant syndrome (Popper et al., 2004). Autistic disorder is usually first observed before 3 years of age, and the prognosis is related to the child's overall intellectual level and the development of social and language skills (APA, 2000). Autism is first noticed by the mother or caretaker when the infant fails to be interested in others or to be socially responsive through eye contact and facial expressions. Some children show improvement as they develop, but puberty can be a turning point toward either improvement or further deterioration. Few individuals with autism are ever able to live and work independently, and only about one third can achieve partial independence.

Three presenting symptoms of autism, as adapted from the *DSM-IV-TR*, include the following:
1. Impairment in communication and imaginative activity
   - Language delay or total absence of language
   - Immature grammatical structure, pronoun reversal, inability to name objects
   - Stereotypical or repetitive use of language (echolalia, use of idiosyncratic words, inappropriate high-pitched squealing or giggling, repetition of phrases, unusual babbling or clicking, sing-song speech quality)
   - Lack of spontaneous make-believe play or imaginative play
   - Failure to imitate
2. Impairment in social interactions
   - Lack of responsiveness to and interest in others
   - Lack of eye-to-eye contact and facial responses
   - Indifference to or aversion to affection and physical contact
   - Failure to cuddle or be comforted
   - Lack of seeking to share enjoyment, interest, or achievement with others
   - Failure to develop cooperative play or imaginative play with peers
   - Lack of friendships
3. Markedly restricted, stereotypical patterns of behavior, interest, and activities
   - Rigid adherence to routines and rituals with catastrophic reactions to minor changes in them or to changes made in the environment (e.g., moving furniture)
   - Stereotypical and repetitive motor mannerisms (hand or finger flapping, clapping, rocking, dipping, swaying, spinning, dancing around and walking on toes, head banging or hand biting)
   - Preoccupation with certain repetitive activities (pouring water or sand, spinning wheels on toys, twirling string) that is abnormal in intensity or focus
   - Other abnormalities in behavior

Asperger's Disorder

Asperger's disorder differs from autistic disorder in that it appears to have a later onset and no significant delay in cognitive and language development is noted (APA, 2000). The etiology is also unknown, although there appears to be a familial pattern. As in autism, restricted and repetitive patterns of behavior and idiosyncratic interests (e.g., fascination with remembering train schedules or dates) may develop. Problems with empathizing and modulating social relationships become more noticeable when the child enters school and may continue into adulthood. In the movie *Rain Man*, Dustin Hoffman portrayed a man who fell into this diagnostic classification.

Rett's Disorder

Rett's disorder differs from autistic disorder and Asperger's disorder in that it has been observed only in females, with onset before 4 years of age (APA, 2000). The exact cause is unknown, but the disorder has been associated with electroencephalographic abnormalities, seizure disorder, and severe or profound mental retardation.

Childhood Disintegrative Disorder

Childhood disintegrative disorder is rare; it occurs in both sexes but is more common in males (APA, 2000). The age of onset is between 2 and 10 years, with most cases presenting between 3 and 4 years of age. The onset can be abrupt or insidious, and the cause is unknown, although it is thought to be related to an insult to the central nervous system. Refer to Table 32-2 for comparisons among this and the other PDDs.

Assessment Guidelines Pervasive
Developmental Disorders

1. Assess for developmental spurts or lags, uneven development, or loss of previously acquired abilities. Use baby books and diaries, photographs, films, or videotapes. (First-time mothers may not be aware of developmental lags, and family members may need to be consulted.)
2. Assess the quality of the relationship between the child and parents or caregivers for evidence

of bonding, anxiety, tension, and difficulty of fit between the parents' and child's temperaments.
3. Be aware that children with behavioral and developmental problems are at risk for abuse.

Nursing Diagnosis

The child with PDD has severe impairments in social interactions and communication skills, often accompanied by stereotypical behavior, interests, and activities. The severity of the impairment is demonstrated by the child's lack of responsiveness to or interest in others, lack of empathy or sharing with peers, and lack of cooperative or imaginative play with peers. Table 32-3 lists potential nursing diagnoses.

Other behaviors not specifically addressed by North American Nursing Diagnosis Association (NANDA) categories (NANDA, 2005) include the following:
- Anger
- Bizarre behaviors
- Low tolerance for frustration
- Abnormal, stereotypical body movements
- Clinging and dependent behaviors
- Poor impulse control
- Ritualistic behaviors

Outcome Criteria

The Nursing Outcomes Classification (NOC) (Moorhead, Johnson, & Maas, 2004) identifies a number of outcomes appropriate for the child with PDD. Table 32-4 includes a sampling of NOC outcomes and

TABLE 32-2

Characteristics and Differential Diagnosis of Pervasive Developmental Disorders

Characteristics	Autistic Disorder	Childhood Disintegrative Disorder	Rett's Disorder	Asperger's Disorder
Feature	Standard autism	Delayed onset but severe autism	Mid-childhood autism	High-functioning autism
Intelligence	Severe MR to normal	Severe MR	Severe MR	Mild MR to normal
Age at recognition	0-3 years	>2 years	0.5-2.5 years	Usually >2 years
Communication skills	Usually limited	Poor	Poor	Limited to fair
Social skills	Very limited	Very limited	Varies with age	Limited
Loss of skills	Usually none	Marked	Marked	Usually none
Restriction of interests	Variable	Not applicable	Not applicable	Marked
Seizure disorder	Uncommon	Frequent	Uncommon	Common
Family history of similar problems	Uncommon	No	No	Common
Gender predilection	M > F	M > F	F	M > F
Course in adulthood	Stable	Declining	Declining	Stable
Outcome	Poor	Very poor	Very poor	Fair to poor

Adapted from Volkmar, F. R., & Cohen, D. J. (1991). Nonautistic pervasive developmental disorders. In R. Michaels et al. (Eds.), *Psychiatry*. Philadelphia: Lippincott.
F, Female; *M*, male; *MR*, mental retardation.

TABLE 32-3

Potential Nursing Diagnoses for Disorders of Childhood and Adolescence

Signs and Symptoms	Nursing Diagnosis
Lack of responsiveness or interest in others	**Impaired social interaction**
Lack of empathy or sharing	
Lack of cooperation or imaginative play with peers	
Disruptive, hostile behavior leading to difficulty in making or keeping friends	
Language delay or absence, stereotyped or repetitive use of language	**Impaired verbal communication**
	Delayed growth and development
Head banging, face slapping, hand biting	**Risk for injury**
Catastrophic reactions (e.g., severe temper tantrums, rage reactions)	**Risk for other-directed violence**
Impulsiveness, anger, and aggression	**Risk for self-mutilation**
Thoughts or verbalizations regarding self-harm	**Risk for self-directed violence**
Frequent disregard for bodily needs	**Self-care deficit**
Inability to feed, bathe, dress, or toilet self at age-appropriate level	
Conflict with authority, refusal to comply with requests	**Impaired adjustment**
Failure to follow age-appropriate social norms	**Ineffective coping**
Blaming of others for problems or for causing his or her actions	**Defensive coping**
Fear of being separated from parent (e.g., going to school or a party)	**Anxiety**
	Fear
Refusal to attend school	**Ineffective coping**
Inability to concentrate, withdrawal, difficulty in functioning, feeling down, change in vegetative symptoms	**Risk for suicide**
Reexperiences of past trauma (dreams, illusions, flashbacks)	**Fear**
Fear of objects, people, or situations	**Anxiety (identify level)**

TABLE 32-4

NOC Outcomes for Pervasive Developmental Disorders

Nursing Outcome and Definition	Intermediate Indicators	Short-Term Indicators
Child Development: 3 Years: Milestones of physical, cognitive, and psychosocial progression by 3 years of age*	Speech understood by strangers	Gives own first name
Child Development: 4 Years: Milestones of physical, cognitive, and psychosocial progression by 4 years of age*	Engages in creative play	Draws person with three parts
Child Development: Preschool: Milestones of physical, cognitive, and psychosocial progression from 3 years through 5 years of age*	Follows simple rules of interactive games with peers	Recognizes most letters of the alphabet
Communication: Expressive: Expression of meaningful verbal and/or nonverbal messages†	Directs messages appropriately	Uses spoken language: vocal
Play Participation: Use of activities by a child from 1 year through 11 years of age to promote enjoyment, entertainment, and development*	Expresses emotions during play activities	Expresses satisfaction with play activities

From Moorhead, S., Johnson, M., & Maas, M. (2004). *Nursing outcomes classification (NOC)* (3rd ed.). St. Louis, MO: Mosby.
*Evaluated on a five-point Likert scale ranging from 1 (never demonstrated) to 5 (consistently demonstrated).
†Evaluated on a five-point Likert scale ranging from 1 (severely compromised) to 5 (not compromised).

supporting indicators that target developmental competencies and coping skills.

Intervention

Children with PDD are treated in therapeutic nursery schools, day treatment programs, and special education classes in public schools, because their education and treatment are mandated under the Children with Disabilities Act. Treatment plans include working with parents, who are taught how to modify the child's behavior and to foster the development of skills when the child is home. Pharmacological agents such as haloperidol and fenfluramine are used with some success.

Nursing interventions for *impaired verbal communication* and *risk for self-mutilation* are described in more detail on the Evolve website.

ATTENTION DEFICIT HYPERACTIVITY DISORDER AND DISRUPTIVE BEHAVIOR DISORDERS

Attention Deficit Hyperactivity Disorder

Children with ADHD show an inappropriate degree of inattention, impulsiveness, and hyperactivity. ADHD occurs in various cultures and is difficult to diagnose before 4 years of age. ADHD in the preschool child manifests itself as excessive gross motor activity that becomes less pronounced as the child matures. The disorder is most often detected when the child has difficulty making the adjustment to elementary school and exhibits excessive fidgeting, restlessness, talkativeness, impulsivity, and difficulty sticking to and completing tasks. The symptoms worsen in situations requiring sustained attention. The attention problems and the hyperactivity contribute to a low tolerance for frustration, temper outbursts, labile moods, poor school performance, rejection by peers, and low self-esteem (Sadock & Sadock, 2004). Children with ADHD are three times more likely to have nocturnal enuresis and five times more likely to have daytime enuresis than are children without ADHD (Popper et al., 2004).

Children with ADHD are often concurrently diagnosed as having oppositional defiant disorder or conduct disorder. ADHD is often associated with Tourette's disorder; at least 25% of males with Tourette's disorder have ADHD (Popper et al., 2004).

Presenting symptoms of ADHD, as adapted from the *DSM-IV-TR*, include the following:

1. Inattention
   - Has difficulty paying attention in tasks or play
   - Does not seem to listen, follow through, or finish tasks
   - Does not pay attention to details and makes careless mistakes
   - Is easily distracted, loses things, and is forgetful in daily activities (symptoms worsen in situations requiring sustained attention)
2. Hyperactivity
   - Fidgets, is unable to sit still or stay seated in school or at other times
   - Runs and climbs excessively in inappropriate situations
   - Has difficulty playing quietly in leisure activities
   - Acts as if "driven by a motor," constantly on the go
   - Talks excessively
3. Impulsivity
   - Blurts out answer before question has been completed
   - Has difficulty waiting for own turn
   - Interrupts, intrudes in others' conversations and games

Oppositional Defiant Disorder

Oppositional defiant disorder is a recurrent pattern of negativistic, disobedient, hostile, defiant behavior toward authority figures without serious violations of the basic rights of others (APA, 2000). Such children exhibit persistent stubbornness and argumentativeness, persistent testing of limits, an unwillingness to give in or negotiate, and a refusal to accept blame for misdeeds. This behavior is evident at home but may not be manifested elsewhere. These children and adolescents do not see themselves as defiant; instead, they feel they are responding to unreasonable demands or situations.

This disorder is usually evident before 8 years of age and is more common in males (until puberty, when male-female rates are equal).

Conduct Disorder

Conduct disorder is characterized by a persistent pattern of behavior in which the rights of others and age-appropriate societal norms or rules are violated (APA, 2000). It is the most frequently diagnosed disorder, with rates of 6% to 16% of all males and 2% to 9% of all females. Predisposing factors are ADHD, oppositional child behaviors, parental rejection, inconsistent parenting with harsh discipline, early institutional living, frequent shifting of parental figures, large family size, absence of father or alcoholic father, antisocial and drug-dependent family members, and association with a delinquent group.

Childhood-onset conduct disorder occurs prior to age 10 years and is found mainly in males, who are physically aggressive, have poor peer relationships and shows little concern for others, and lack feelings of guilt or remorse. These children frequently misperceive the intentions of others as being hostile and believe their aggressive responses are justified. Although they try to project a tough image, they have low self-esteem and low tolerance for frustration; they also show irritability and outbursts of temper. In individuals with childhood-onset conduct disorder, the disorder is more likely to persist through adolescence and develop into antisocial personality disorder.

In **adolescent-onset conduct disorder,** individuals demonstrate less aggressive behaviors and more normal peer relationships. These youths tend to act out their misconduct with their peer group (e.g., early onset of sexual behavior, smoking, drinking, substance abuse, risk-taking behaviors). Males are apt to fight, steal, vandalize, and have school discipline problems, whereas girls lie, are truant, run away, abuse substances, and engage in prostitution. The male/female ratio is not as high as for the childhood-onset type.

Complications associated with conduct disorder are academic failure related to below-average reading and verbal skills and learning disabilities, school suspensions and dropouts, juvenile delinquency, and the need for the juvenile court system to assume responsibility for youths who cannot be managed by their parents. Psychiatric disorders that frequently coexist with conduct disorder are anxiety, depression, ADHD, and learning disabilities. Studies indicate that the antisocial behaviors persist into adulthood and often result in the diagnosis of antisocial personality disorder.

Conduct disorder is identified by four types of behavior in the *DSM-IV-TR*: (1) aggression toward people and animals; (2) destruction of property; (3) deceitfulness or theft; and (4) serious violations of rules.

Assessment Guidelines Attention Deficit
Hyperactivity Disorder and Disruptive Behavior Disorders

1. Assess the quality of the relationship between the child and parents or caregivers for evidence of bonding, anxiety, tension, and difficulty of fit between the parents' and the child's temperaments, which can contribute to the development of disruptive behaviors.
2. Assess the parents' or caregivers' understanding of growth and development, parenting skills, and handling of problematic behaviors, because lack of knowledge contributes to the development of these problems.
3. Assess cognitive, psychosocial, and moral development for lags or deficits, because immaturity in developmental competencies results in disruptive behaviors.

Attention Deficit Hyperactivity Disorder

1. Observe the child for level of physical activity, attention span, talkativeness, and the ability to follow directions and control impulses. Medication is often needed to ameliorate problems in these areas.
2. Assess difficulty in making friends and performing in school. Academic failure and poor peer relationships lead to low self-esteem, depression, and further acting out.
3. Assess for problems with enuresis and encopresis.

Oppositional Defiant Disorder

1. Identify issues that result in power struggles—when they begin and how they are handled.
2. Assess the severity of the defiant behavior and its impact on the child's life at home, at school, and with peers.

Conduct Disorder

1. Assess the seriousness of the disruptive behavior, when it started, and what has been done to manage it. Hospitalization or residential placement may be necessary in addition to medication.
2. Assess the child's levels of anxiety, aggression, anger, and hostility toward others, and the ability to control destructive impulses.

3. Assess the child's moral development for the ability to understand the impact of hurtful behavior on others, to empathize with others, and to feel remorse.

Nursing Diagnosis

Children and adolescents with ADHD, oppositional defiant disorder, and conduct disorder display disruptive behaviors that are impulsive, angry-aggressive, and often dangerous. These children and adolescents are often in conflict with parents and authority figures, refuse to comply with requests, do not follow age-appropriate social norms, and have inappropriate ways of getting needs met. Refer to Table 32-3 for potential nursing diagnoses.

Other behaviors not specifically addressed by NANDA categories include the following:
- Attention seeking
- Intrusive behaviors
- Disregard for social norms or rules
- Lack of remorse
- Lying
- Promiscuity
- Poor school performance
- Dangerous risk taking
- Running away
- Stealing
- Truancy

Outcome Criteria

NOC identifies a number of outcomes appropriate for the child with ADHD, oppositional defiant disorder, or conduct disorder. Table 32-5 lists a sampling of NOC outcomes and supporting indicators that target hyperactivity, impulse self-control, the development of self-identity and self-esteem, positive coping skills, and family functioning.

Intervention

The interventions for ADHD are behavior modification and administration of pharmacological agents for the inattention and hyperactive-impulsive behaviors, special education programs for the academic difficulties, and psychotherapy and play therapy for the emotional problems that develop as a result of the disorder. Methylphenidate (Ritalin) is the most widely used psychostimulant because of its safety and simplicity of use. A mixed amphetamine preparation such as Adderall has proven effective, and Concerta, an extended-release formula, allows once-daily dosing, which helps keep the existence of the condition private. In 20% to 30% of children, however, the stimulant medications are ineffective or cause adverse effects such as tics, mood swings, insomnia, anorexia,

TABLE 32-5

NOC Outcomes for Attention Deficit Hyperactivity Disorder and Disruptive Behavior Disorders

Nursing Outcome and Definition	Intermediate Indicators	Short-Term Indicators
Hyperactivity Level: Severity of patterns of inattention of impulsivity in a child from 1 year through 17 years of age*	Inappropriate aggressive behavior	Lack of active listening
Impulse Self-Control: Self-restraint of compulsive or impulsive behaviors†	Maintains self-control without supervision	Identifies harmful impulsive behaviors
Self-Esteem: Personal judgment of self-worth‡	Feelings about self-worth	Acceptance of self-limitations
Coping: Personal actions to manage stressors that tax an individual's resources†	Reports increase in psychological comfort	Identifies effective coping patterns
Family Normalization: Capacity of the family system to maintain routines and develop strategies for optimal functioning when a member has a chronic illness or disability†	Maintains usual parenting expectations for affected child	Acknowledges existence of impairment and its potential to alter family routines

From Moorhead, S., Johnson, M., & Maas, M. (2004). *Nursing outcomes classification (NOC)* (3rd ed.). St. Louis, MO: Mosby.
*Evaluated on a five-point Likert scale ranging from 1 (severe) to 5 (none).
†Evaluated on a five-point Likert scale ranging from 1 (never demonstrated) to 5 (consistently demonstrated).
‡Evaluated on a five-point Likert scale ranging from 1 (never positive) to 5 (consistently positive).

and obsessive-compulsive symptoms (Popper et al., 2004).

Interventions for treating oppositional defiant and conduct disorders focus on correcting the child's or adolescent's faulty personality (ego and superego) development, which involves generating more mature and adaptive coping mechanisms. This process is gradual and cannot be accomplished during short-term hospitalization or brief treatment. With conduct disorder, inpatient hospitalization for crisis intervention, evaluation, and treatment planning, as well as transfer to therapeutic foster care or long-term residential treatment, is often needed. Youths with oppositional defiant disorder are generally treated on an outpatient basis using individual, group, and family therapy, with much of the focus on parenting issues.

To control the **aggressive behaviors** of these disorders, a wide variety of pharmacological agents have been tried, including antipsychotics, lithium, anticonvulsants, antidepressants, and β-adrenergic blockers. Cognitive-behavioral therapy is used to change the pattern of misconduct by fostering the development of internal controls, both cognitive and emotional. Development of problem-solving, conflict resolution, empathy, and social interaction skills is an important component of the treatment program.

Families are involved in therapy and are given support in parenting skills designed to help them provide nurturance and set consistent limits. They are the key players in carrying out the treatment plan, using behavior modification techniques at home, monitoring the medication and its effects, collaborating with teachers to foster academic success, and setting up a home environment that promotes the achievement of normal developmental milestones. When families are

abusive, drug dependent, or highly disorganized, the child may benefit from out-of-home placement. The following nursing interventions are helpful when working with parents and caregivers:

- Assess parents' or caregivers' knowledge of the disorder and the related behaviors and provide needed information.
- Explore the impact of the behaviors on family life.
- Assess the family's or caregivers' support system.
- Discuss how to make home a safe environment.
- Discuss realistic behavioral goals and how to set them.
- Teach behavior modification techniques.
- Give parents or caregivers support as they learn to apply techniques.
- Provide educational information about medications.
- Refer parents or caregivers to a local chapter of an appropriate self-help group.
- Be a child and parent advocate with the educational system.

Nursing interventions for *defensive coping* and *risk for other-directed violence* are described in more detail on the Evolve website. Techniques for managing disruptive behaviors are listed in Box 32-3.

ANXIETY DISORDERS

Not all anxiety is abnormal in childhood or adolescence; a number of fears and worries are part of normal development. Anxiety becomes a problem when the child or adolescent fails to move beyond the fears associated with a certain developmental stage or when the anxiety develops in response to physical or psychosocial stressors or trauma and interferes with nor-

Techniques for Managing Disruptive Behaviors

Planned ignoring: Evaluate surface behavior and intervene when the intensity is becoming too great.

Use of signals or gestures: Use a word, a gesture, or eye contact to remind the child to use self-control.

Physical distance and touch control: Move closer to the child for a calming effect, perhaps put an arm around the child.

Increased involvement in the activity: Redirect the child's attention to the activity and away from a distracting behavior by asking a question.

Additional affection: Ignore the provocative content of the behavior and give the child emotional support for the current problem.

Use of humor: Use well-timed kidding as a diversion to help the child save face and relieve feelings of guilt or fear.

Direct appeals: Appeal to the child's developing self-control: "Please, not now."

Extra assistance: Give early help to the child who "blows up" and is easily frustrated when trying to achieve a goal; do not overuse this technique.

Clarification as intervention: Help the child understand the situation and his or her own motivation for the behavior.

Restructuring: Change the activity in ways that will decrease the stimulation or the frustration (e.g., shorten a story or change to a physical activity).

Regrouping: Use total or partial changes in the group's composition to reduce conflict and contagious behaviors.

Strategic removal: Remove a child who is disrupting or acting dangerously, but consider whether this gives the child too much status or makes the child a scapegoat.

Physical restraint: Use therapeutic holding to control, to give comfort, and to assure the child that he or she is protected from own impulses to act out.

Limit setting and permission granting: Use sharp, clear statements about which behavior is not allowed and give permission for the behavior that is expected.

Promises and rewards: Use very carefully and very infrequently to avoid situations in which the child bargains for a reward.

Threats and punishment: Use very carefully; the child needs to internalize the frustration generated by the punishment and use it to control impulses rather than externalize the frustration in further acting out.

Data from Redl, F., & Wineman, D. (1957). *The aggressive child.* New York: Free Press.

mal functioning. There may be a genetic vulnerability to anxiety disorders, because they seem to run in families. Cognitive theorists propose that anxiety is the result of dysfunctional efforts to make sense of life's events. The physiological, behavioral, and cognitive

characteristics of anxiety in youth are basically no different from those in adults. Anxiety disorders affect as many as 10% of young people (National Mental Health Association, 2004). Separation anxiety disorder and PTSD are briefly discussed here as they relate to children and adolescents.

Separation Anxiety Disorder

Children and adolescents with separation anxiety disorder become excessively anxious when separated from or anticipating a separation from their home or parental figures (APA, 2000). Separation anxiety disorder may develop after a significant stress, such as the death of a relative or pet, an illness, a move or change in schools, or even a physical or sexual assault. The onset can be any time between preschool years and age 18. The prevalence of the disorder in children is estimated to be 4%, with a higher incidence of the disorder in females. The disorder is common in first-degree biological relatives of an affected individual, and the incidence may be higher in children whose mothers have a panic disorder. Although the remission rates are high, the disorder can persist and lead to panic disorder with agoraphobia. A **depressed mood** often accompanies the anxiety.

The *DSM-IV-TR* characteristics of separation anxiety disorder are the following:

- Excessive distress when separated from or anticipating separation from home or parental figures
- Excessive worries that one will be lost or kidnapped or that parental figures will be harmed
- Fear of being home alone or in situations without other significant adults
- Refusal to sleep unless near a parental figure and refusal to sleep away from home
- Refusal to attend school or other activities without a parental figure
- Physical symptoms as a response to anxiety

Posttraumatic Stress Disorder

Posttraumatic stress disorder (PTSD) can occur at any age and has now been recognized in children. Rather than reliving the traumatic event as an adult might, younger children with PTSD tend to react with behaviors indicative of internalized anxiety. In older children and adolescents the anxiety is more often externalized.

Posttraumatic Stress Behaviors

Preschool Children. Internalization of anxiety is common in the posttraumatic stress behaviors of preschool children, who exhibit the following responses (Popper et al., 2004; Sadock & Sadock, 2004):

- Agitated and disorganized behavior
- Separation anxiety

- Sleep difficulties (including problems in falling or staying asleep, or in sleeping alone)
- Nightmares or night terrors with unknown content or changing to dreams of monsters
- Reliving of the trauma in repetitive play of the event
- Increase in specific fears, especially those related to the trauma stimuli (storms, noise, a specific place)
- Irritability, whining, angry outbursts, temper tantrums
- Regression or loss of previously learned skills
- Somatic complaints
- Withdrawal from activities

School-Aged Children. Externalization of anxiety is common in the posttraumatic stress behaviors of school-aged children, who exhibit the following responses:

- Sleep difficulties, especially nightmares of monsters, rescuing others, or being threatened
- Irritability and increased fighting with friends and siblings
- Difficulty concentrating, with impaired academic performance
- Repetitive playing out of the traumatic event
- Jumpiness and hypervigilance, increased startle response
- Belief that his or her life will be short
- Belief that he or she can foresee untoward events in the future ("omen formation")
- Somatic complaints

Assessment Guidelines Anxiety Disorders

1. Assess the quality of the relationship between child and parents or caregivers for evidence of anxiety, conflicts, or difficulty of fit between child's and parents' temperaments.
2. Assess for recent stressors and their severity, duration, and proximity to the child.
3. Assess the parents' or caregivers' understanding of developmental norms, parenting skills, and handling of problematic behaviors (lack of knowledge contributes to increased anxiety).
4. Assess the developmental level and determine whether regression has occurred.
5. Assess for physical, behavioral, and cognitive symptoms of anxiety.

Separation Anxiety Disorder
Assess the child's previous and current ability to separate from parents or caregivers (the separation or individuation process may not be completed or the child may have regressed).

Posttraumatic Stress Disorder
Assess for personal exposure to an extreme traumatic stressor and evidence of internalized or externalized anxiety symptoms.

Nursing Diagnosis

As the name indicates, the anxiety disorders have as their chief characteristic disabling anxiety. Refer to Table 32-3 for potential nursing diagnoses.

Outcome Criteria

NOC identifies a number of outcomes appropriate for the child with an anxiety disorder. The two most relevant outcomes focus on decreasing the anxiety level of the child or adolescent and increasing the ability to control anxiety (Table 32-6).

Intervention

The nursing interventions for an anxious child or adolescent include the following:

- Protecting the child from panic levels of anxiety by acting as a parental surrogate and providing for biological and psychosocial needs
- Accepting regression but giving emotional support to help the child progress again
- Increasing the child's self-esteem and feelings of competence in the ability to perform, achieve, or influence the future

TABLE 32-6

NOC Outcomes for Anxiety Disorders

Nursing Outcome and Definition	Intermediate Indicator	Short-Term Indicator
Anxiety Level: Severity of manifested apprehension, tension, or uneasiness arising from an unidentifiable source*	Decreased school achievement	Problem behavior
Anxiety Self-Control: Personal actions to eliminate or reduce feelings of apprehension, tension, or uneasiness from an unidentifiable source†	Controls anxiety response	Monitors intensity of anxiety

From Moorhead, S., Johnson, M., & Maas, M. (2004). *Nursing outcomes classification (NOC)* (3rd ed.). St. Louis, MO: Mosby.
*Evaluated on a five-point Likert scale ranging from 1 (severe) to 5 (none).
†Evaluated on a five-point Likert scale ranging from 1 (never demonstrated) to 5 (consistently demonstrated).

▪ Helping the child accept and work through traumatic events or losses

Children and adolescents with anxiety disorders are most often treated on an outpatient basis using cognitive-behavioral techniques in individual, group, or family therapy. Medications such as antihistamines, anxiolytics, and antidepressants are also used. Cognitive therapy focuses on the underlying fears and concerns, and behavior modification is used to reinforce self-control behaviors. Children who refuse to start primary school are introduced gradually into the school environment with a parent or caregiver present for support for part of the day. When adolescents develop school phobia, the goal is to return them to the classroom at the earliest possible date and to give parents support in setting limits on truancy.

Specific nursing interventions for *anxiety* are described in more detail on the Evolve website.

MOOD DISORDERS

It was once believed that children do not suffer from the same type of depression that adults do and that a child's sadness in reaction to an event or situation will be short-lived. Now, with increasing suicide rates in childhood and with suicide the third leading cause of death in adolescence (National Mental Health Association, 2004), depression is being treated with psychotherapy and medication rather than being allowed to run its course. The most frequently diagnosed mood disorders in children and adolescents are **major depressive disorder, dysthymic disorder,** and **bipolar disorder.** Symptoms of depression in children and adolescents may be similar to the symptoms in adults, with feelings of sadness, pessimism, hopelessness, and anhedonia, as well as social withdrawal and thoughts of suicide. Children are more apt to have somatic complaints, be critical of themselves and others, and feel unloved. Adolescents are more likely to have psychomotor retardation and hypersomnia (APA, 2000). Both children and adolescents often manifest irritability leading to aggressiveness. They are less likely than adults to have psychotic symptoms, and auditory hallucinations are more common than delusions. The acting-out behaviors of children and adolescents, once considered symptoms of masked depression, can clearly be related to the presence of mood disorders. The signs of depression in both children and adolescents are listed in Box 32-4.

Factors associated with child and adolescent depression are physical and sexual abuse, neglect, homelessness, parental marital discord, death, divorce or separation of parents, separation from parents, learning disabilities, chronic illness, conflicts with family or peers, and rejection by family or peers. The complications of depression are school failure and dropout, drug and alcohol abuse, sexual promiscuity, preg-

---

BOX 32-4

Signs of Depression in Children and Adolescents

Mood or Affect
▪ Apathy
▪ Anhedonia
▪ Anger
▪ Sadness or crying
▪ Irritability
▪ Guilt
▪ Decreased self-esteem
▪ Decreased spontaneity
▪ Monotone speech

Cognition
▪ Apathy
▪ Boredom
▪ Decreased concentration
▪ Loss of interest in school
▪ Decreased school performance
▪ Decreased creativity
▪ Loss of interest in activities
▪ Preoccupation with illness
▪ Preoccupation with death
▪ Thoughts of dying
▪ Suicidal ideation
▪ Suicidal threats

Physical Activity
▪ Loss of energy
▪ Insomnia or hypersomnia
▪ Nightmares
▪ Appetite changes
▪ Weight loss or gain
▪ Physical complaints (aches in head, stomach, or legs)

Behavior and Social Function
▪ Isolation (self-imposed or rejection by peers)
▪ Change in friends
▪ Loss of girlfriend or boyfriend
▪ Risk taking
▪ Drug or alcohol use
▪ Running away or truancy
▪ Misuse of sex
▪ Decrease in after-school activity and playtime
▪ Interest in morbid music and literature
▪ Suicidal gestures or attempts

---

nancy, running away, illegal and antisocial behavior, and suicide.

TOURETTE'S DISORDER

Tourette's disorder is characterized by motor and verbal tics that cause marked distress and significant impairment in social and occupational functioning (APA, 2000). Tics may appear as early as 2 years of age, but the average age of onset for motor tics is 7 years. Motor tics usually involve the head but can also involve the torso or limbs, and they change in location, frequency, and severity over time. In one half of cases the first symptom is a single tic, most often eye blinking. Other motor tics are tongue protrusion, touching, squatting, hopping, skipping, retracing steps, and twirling when walking. Vocal tics include production of words and sounds (barks, grunts, yelps, clicks, snorts, sniffs, coughs). Coprolalia (uttering of obscenities) is present in fewer than 10% of cases. The disorder is usually permanent, but there can be periods of remission, and the symptoms often diminish during adolescence and sometimes disappear by early adulthood. There is a familial pattern in about 90% of cases. Vulnerability is transmitted in an autosomal dominant pattern, with 70% of females and 99% of males who have inherited the gene developing the disorder. Nongenetic Tourette's disorder often coexists with PDD, a seizure disorder, obsessive-compulsive disorder, or ADHD (Popper et al., 2004).

Symptoms associated with Tourette's disorder are obsessions, compulsions, hyperactivity, distractibility, and impulsivity. In addition, a child or adolescent with tics has low self-esteem as a result of feeling ashamed, self-conscious, and rejected by peers. The fear of having tic behavior in public situations causes the individual to limit activities severely. Central nervous system stimulants increase the severity of the tics, so medications must be carefully monitored in children with coexisting ADHD.

ADJUSTMENT DISORDER

Adjustment disorder is a residual category used for emotional responses to an identifiable stressor that do not meet the criteria for a *DSM-IV-TR* axis I psychiatric disorder (APA, 2000). It is a category commonly applied to children and adolescents whose problems are not severe enough to require hospitalization but who are showing decreased performance at school and temporary changes in social relationships. The disorder begins within 3 months of the stress and lasts no longer than 6 months after the stress has ceased. The subtypes are classified according to the presenting symptoms: adjustment disorder (1) with anxiety, (2) with mixed anxiety and depressed mood, (3) with disturbance of conduct, (4) with mixed disturbance of emotions and conduct, and (5) unspecified.

FEEDING AND EATING DISORDERS

Three feeding and eating disorders are pica, rumination disorder, and feeding and eating disorder of infancy or early childhood (APA, 2000). Pica is the persistent eating of nonnutritive substances, although there is no aversion to eating food. Infants and toddlers may eat paint, plaster, string, or cloth. Older children may eat sand, pebbles, insects, or even animal droppings. This behavior is frequently associated with mental retardation. Rumination disorder is the repeated regurgitation and rechewing of food without apparent nausea, retching, or gastrointestinal problems. This disorder may occur with developmental delays between 3 and 12 months of age. It occurs later in mentally retarded children. In a feeding and eating disorder, the infant or child fails to eat adequate amounts of food, despite availability, and there is no medical condition or mental retardation. The individual fails to gain weight or has a significant weight loss, which then contributes to developmental delays.

OVERALL INTERVENTIONS FOR CHILD AND ADOLESCENT DISORDERS

The forms of treatment described in this section can be used in a variety of settings: inpatient, residential, outpatient, day treatment, outreach programs in schools, and home visits. Many of the modalities involve the normal activities of a child's day, such as activities of daily living, learning activities, multiple forms of play and recreational activities, and interactions with adults and peers.

Family Therapy

In the past, children who were treated in long-term facilities had limited contact with parents. This approach changed as family dynamics came to be viewed as contributing factors in the child's disorder, and family therapy was developed as a treatment modality. Today parents are actively involved in treatment decisions and in designing a plan that considers potential parental competencies and family organization. The treatment team recognizes the importance of the family in the supportive and educative system for the child or adolescent.

In addition to therapy involving a single family, multiple-family therapy is frequently used. This modality engages families as cotherapists for other families in a process in which families learn to (1) like and respect others, (2) accept shortcomings and capitalize on strengths, (3) develop insight and improve judgment, (4) use new information, and (5) develop lasting and satisfying relationships.

Group Therapy

Group therapy for younger children takes the form of play; for grade school children, it combines play and talk about the activity. The child learns social skills by taking turns and sharing with peers. For adolescents, group therapy involves more talking and focuses largely on peer relationships and specific problems. The difficulty in using groups when working with children and adolescents lies in the contagious effect of disruptive behavior.

There is a wealth of information in the nursing literature about how to perform group therapy with children and adolescents. For example, adolescent group therapy might use a popular television show or soap opera as the basis for a group discussion. Groups have been used effectively to deal with specific issues in a child's life (e.g., bereavement and loss, physical and sexual abuse, substance abuse, sexuality and dating, teenage pregnancy, chronic illnesses, depression, suicidal ideation). The mental health promotion and prevention activities that nurses are now carrying out in school-based clinics involve working with multiple groups (e.g., students, teachers, parents, and community leaders).

Milieu Therapy

Milieu therapy remains the philosophical basis for structuring inpatient, residential, and day treatment programs. According to the *Scope and Standards of Psychiatric-Mental Health Nursing Practice*, the combined adult and child standards of practice developed by the ANA and other groups (ANA et al., 2000), the nurse collaborates with other health care providers in structuring and maintaining a therapeutic environment to

- Provide physical and psychological security.
- Promote growth and mastery of developmental tasks.
- Ameliorate psychiatric disorders.

The physical milieu is designed to provide a safe, comfortable place to live, play, and learn, with areas for private time as well as group activity. There may be a gym, outdoor playground, swimming pool, garden, cooking and other recreational facilities, and even pets. No matter what physical facilities exist, the essential parts of a therapeutic milieu are the multidisciplinary team and the therapeutic activities. The daily schedule structures the activities (e.g., school, therapy sessions, group activities and outings, family or home visits). The multidisciplinary team shares a philosophy regarding how to provide physical and psychological security, promote personal growth, and work with problematic behaviors. The child's or youth's behavior, emotions, and cognitive processes are the focus of the therapeutic interventions in the milieu. The therapeutic factors operating in the milieu's structure, activities, and interactions with staff are listed in Box 32-5.

Behavioral Therapy

Behavior modification is based on the principle that behavior which is rewarded is more likely to be repeated. Developmentally appropriate behaviors are normally

---

BOX 32-5

Therapeutic Factors in the Milieu

- Holding environment, with roles, boundaries, and limits
- Reduction in stressors
- Situations for expression of feelings without fear of rejection or retaliation
- Availability of emotional support and comfort
- Assistance with reality testing and support for weak or missing ego functions
- Interventions in impulsive or aggressive and inappropriate behaviors
- Opportunities for learning and testing new adaptive behaviors and mastering developmental tasks
- Consistent, constructive feedback
- Reinforcement of positive behaviors and development of self-esteem
- Corrective emotional experiences
- Role models for making healthy identifications and positive attachments
- Opportunities to develop better peer relationships and be influenced by positive peer pressure
- Opportunities to be spontaneous and creative
- Experiences leading to identity formation

---

rewarded with validation by a significant adult in the child's life, so modifying behavior in this manner is a standard parenting technique (**operant conditioning**). Behavior modification is easy to learn and does not require an understanding of the child's psychopathology. It is necessary only to identify the desired behavior and its reward and to apply the process systematically. To extinguish undesirable behavior, either the behavior is ignored or, if it is too disruptive, limits that have specified consequences are set.

Although there is an individualized treatment plan for each child or adolescent, most treatment settings use a behavior modification program to motivate and reward age-appropriate behaviors. One popular method is the **point and level system,** in which points are awarded for desired behaviors, and increasing levels of privileges can be earned. The point value for specific behaviors and the privileges for each level are spelled out on a large memo board. Each child's status and points acquired for the day are recorded. Older children and adolescents can be made responsible for keeping their own daily point sheet and for requesting points for their behaviors. Age-appropriate behaviors for which points are given can include dressing, attending school and activities on time and without disruptive behaviors, and demonstrating social skills. Children who work on individual behavioral goals (e.g., seeking out staff for help in problem solving) are also rewarded with points. Points are collected and used to obtain a specific reward, such as visiting the point store at the end of the week to pick out a toy or moving from one privilege level to the next.

The level system defines privileges, with the lowest level confining the child to the unit for all activities. Each level has increasing privileges (e.g., going off the unit with a staff member, enjoying a later bedtime on weekends). At the highest level, the privilege might be to go off the unit unescorted.

Modifying Disruptive Behavior

Managing and modifying disruptive behaviors in group activities and in the therapeutic milieu are real challenges for the nurse. If the disruptive behavior is not interrupted early, the contagion effect will derail the group activity and cause chaos. Intervention techniques for working with disruptive behaviors are rarely described in the nursing literature. A proactive approach to dealing with the contagion effect of disruptive behavior includes increasing the structure of a group activity, using all available resources (e.g., increasing staff presence), and anticipating the contagious effects by means of "antiseptic bouncing" of a disruptive child from the activity. Refer back to Box 32-3 for a description of classic intervention techniques developed by Redl and Wineman (1957) in their work with highly aggressive youth with conduct disorders. These techniques remain just as effective today in modifying disruptive behaviors and preventing the contagion effect.

Removal and Restraint

Seclusion

Controversy continues over the use of seclusion in dealing with children; there is no clear evidence that it is therapeutic. Child and adolescent units may have a seclusion room, but its use is limited because individuals who are out of control can become self-destructive. Seclusion is most frequently used to deal with noncompliant behaviors that might have been managed in other ways before the behavior escalated. The persistent use of seclusion reflects the staff's lack of confidence in their ability to handle behaviors and their adherence to traditional practices (Allen, 2000). Seclusion may bring about superficial compliance, but it has little to do with real behavioral change. Nursing staff must realize that the child or adolescent will always perceive seclusion as punishment, and the experience of being overpowered by adults is terrifying for one who has been abused.

Quiet Room

Instead of a seclusion room, a unit may have an unlocked **quiet room** for a child who needs to be removed from a situation for either self-control or control by the staff. Variations on the quiet room include the **feelings room,** which is carpeted and supplied with soft objects that can be punched and thrown, and the **freedom room,** which contains a large ball for throwing and kicking. The child is encouraged to express freely and work through feelings of anger, frustration, and sadness in private and with staff support. When a child has difficulty being in touch with or expressing feelings, staff can provide practice sessions and act as role models.

Time-Out

Imposing a time-out from the group or unit activity is another method for intervening to halt disruptive or inappropriate behaviors. Time-out procedures are designed so that staff can be consistent in their interventions. Taking a time-out may require going to a designated room or sitting on the periphery of an activity until the child gains self-control and reviews the episode with a staff member. The child's individual behavioral goals are considered in setting limits on behavior and using time-out periods. If they are overused or used as an automatic response to a behavioral infraction, time-outs lose their effectiveness.

Therapeutic Holding

At times a child's behavior is so destructive that physical restraint is needed. Although a mechanical restraint such as a helmet for head banging may be used, therapeutic holding is a long-established practice for the control of destructive behaviors. This intervention requires prompt, firm, nonretaliatory protective restraint that is gently and continuously personal to reduce the child's distress and to produce greater relaxation, a return of self-control, and trust in the staff. In one technique, the basket hold, the nurse holds the child from behind by the wrists, while the child's arms are crossed over the torso. The nurse can immobilize the child's legs if necessary by sitting and crossing one or both legs over the child's legs.

Throughout the episode, the nurse talks to the child in a reassuring manner, providing comfort and keeping the child's self-esteem intact. To make each restraint situation therapeutic, the nurse reviews the event with the child after restraint is released. This review of the event and a discussion of alternative ways of coping foster learning and self-control.

Cognitive-Behavioral Therapy

The goal of cognitive-behavioral therapy is to change cognitive and behavioral processes, and thereby reduce the frequency of maladaptive responses and replace them with new cognitive and behavioral competencies. This therapy is carried out in individual or group sessions. An example of its use in group work is Teaching Kids to Cope, a 10-session psychoeducational program for adolescents that teaches youth how to cope with problems and stress through a series of cognitive and behavioral activities (e.g., cognitive rehearsal, social skills and assertiveness training, relaxation techniques) (Puskar et al., 1997).

Play Therapy

Play is the work of childhood and the way a child learns to master impulses and adapt to the environment. Play is the language of childhood and the communication medium for assessing developmental and emotional status, determining diagnosis, and instituting therapeutic interventions. Melanie Klein (1955) and Anna Freud (1965) were the first to use play as a therapeutic tool in their psychoanalysis of children in the 1920s and 1930s. Axline (1969) identified the guiding principles of play therapy, and they are still used by mental health professionals:

- Accept the child as he or she is and follow the child's lead.
- Establish a warm, friendly relationship that helps the child express feelings completely.
- Recognize the child's feelings and reflect them back, so the child can gain insight into the behavior.
- Accept the child's ability to solve personal problems.
- Set limits only to provide reality and security.

There are many forms of play therapy that can be used individually or in groups. The term *play therapy* usually refers to a one-to-one session the therapist has with a child in a playroom. Most playrooms are equipped with art supplies, clay or play dough, dolls and dollhouses, hand puppets, toy telephones, building blocks, and trucks and cars. The dolls, puppets, and dollhouse provide the child with opportunities to act out conflicts and situations involving the family, to work through feelings, and to develop more adaptive ways of coping. The following vignette shows how play therapy can help a child cope with a significant loss.

■ ■ ■ *VIGNETTE*

Jennie, a 6 year old, begins having nightmares and refusing to go to school after her baby-sitter grandmother dies. Her parents do not let her attend the funeral, thinking it will upset her. Jennie becomes fearful and preoccupied with the events surrounding the death. In play sessions, she repeatedly uses dolls to act out her grandmother's hospitalization, death, and funeral. She then pretends to bury her grandmother in a small, coffinlike box. Her parents have told Jennie that Grandma has gone to heaven. Jennie demonstrates the concept by removing "Grandma" from the box and placing her high up on a bookshelf in the playroom, looking down on the rest of the doll family.

■ ■ ■

Dramatic Play

Psychodrama, now more commonly referred to as *theater,* is a treatment modality in which individuals use dramatic techniques to act out emotional problems, examine subjective experience, develop new perspectives, and try out new behaviors. This modality may be used with groups of verbal children and adolescents. If they are psychotic, reality-based role-plays are substituted for fantasies.

Dramatic play, less formal than psychodrama, is used in many settings and with one child or several children. Hand puppets and puppet shows are a favorite way to enable children to act out problems and solutions. Uninhibited children and adolescents enjoy acting roles in dramas that they have created spontaneously or scripted. The dramas can be videotaped so the nurse can review the experience and facilitate new learning with the group. A favorite type of dramatic play for children is dress up, and a box of clothes is all that is needed. It is normally unstructured, and the staff observes the activity and intervenes only if behavior becomes destructive.

Mutual storytelling is a psychodramatic technique developed by Gardner (1971) to help young children express themselves verbally. The child is asked to make up a story; it cannot be a known fairy tale, movie, or television show. The story must have a beginning, middle, and ending. At the end of the story, the child is asked to state the lesson or the moral of the story. The nurse determines the psychodynamic meaning of the story and selects one or two of its important themes. Using the same characters and a similar setting, the nurse retells the story, providing a healthier resolution. The lesson of the story is also reformulated to help the child become consciously aware of the better resolution. If the child has trouble starting a story, the nurse can assist by beginning the story with "Once upon a time in a faraway land there lived a . . ." and then pointing to the child to continue. After the child has identified the main characters, the nurse may need to keep prompting the child with comments such as "and then . . . " until the story is completed. The story can be audiotaped or videotaped, which increases the child's motivation to participate and allows for a review to reinforce the learning.

Therapeutic Games

Children enjoy games, so the therapeutic game treatment modality is ideal for children who have difficulty talking about their feelings and problems. Playing a game with the child facilitates the development of a therapeutic alliance and provides an opportunity for conversation. The game might be as simple as checkers, but therapeutic games are more effective in eliciting children's fears and fantasies. Gardner (1979) developed a series of therapeutic games for children, one of which, Board of Objects, can be used with children 4 to 8 years of age. The game pieces are small items (people, animals, various objects) that are placed on a checkerboard. The players roll dice. One side of each is colored red. If a red side lands face up, the player selects an object. To get a reward chip, the player must say something about the object; if the player tells a story about the object, he or she gets two reward chips. The child's statement or story can be used in a therapeutic interchange (e.g., to communicate empathy or make a statement suggesting a more adaptive way to cope with a difficult situation). In the end, the player with the most chips (usually the child) wins.

A board game appropriate for latency phase and preadolescent children is Gardner's Talking, Feeling, and Doing Game (1986). The player throws dice to advance his or her playing piece along a pathway of different-colored squares. Depending on the color landed upon, the player draws a talking, feeling, or doing card, which gives instructions or asks a question. A reward chip is given when the player responds appropriately. For example, a feeling card might read, "All the girls in the class were invited to a birthday party except one. How did she feel?" If this game is played with more than one child, the nurse can elicit additional responses and engage the whole group in the therapeutic interchange. The nurse may stack the deck to make sure that cards relating to the child's problems will be selected.

Bibliotherapy

Bibliotherapy involves using children's literature to help the child express feelings in a supportive environment, gain insight into feelings and behavior, and learn new ways to cope with difficult situations. When children listen to a story, they unconsciously identify with the characters and experience a catharsis of feelings. The books selected by the nurse should reflect the situations or feelings the child is experiencing. It is important to assess not only the needs of the child but also the child's readiness for the particular topic and the child's level of understanding. A children's librarian has access to a large collection of stories and knows which books are written specifically to help children deal with particular subjects. Whenever possible, the nurse consults with the family to make sure the books do not violate the family's belief systems. A choice of several books is offered, and a book is never forced on the child.

Therapeutic Drawing

Children love to draw and paint and will spontaneously express themselves in artwork. The drawings capture the thoughts, feelings, and tensions children may not be able to express verbally, are unaware of, or are denying. Children do not have to draw themselves. In drawing any human figure, children leave an imprint of the inner self, revealing personality traits, relationships with others, attitudes and values of the family and cultural group, behavioral characteristics, and perceived strengths or weaknesses. Drawings are most reliable as indicators after children are able to create objective representations of what is seen (usually between 5 and 7 years of age). Drawings are less reliable when children have cognitive impairments. To use this modality, the nurse needs to be familiar with the drawing capabilities expected of children at particular developmental levels.

Therapeutic drawing may be used in play therapy with individuals or groups. When this modality is used, the therapist observes children while they draw, asks questions about the pictures, and looks for messages in what has been drawn. Often children draw or are asked to draw human figures. The following characteristics of human figures in such drawings are general indicators of children's emotions, but the specific features described are not necessarily indicative of psychopathology:

- Size of figures: very large (aggression, poor impulse control); very small (shyness, insecurity)
- Emphasis on and exaggeration of body parts: large heads (desire to be smarter), large mouths (speech problems), large arms (desire for strength and power)
- Omissions of body parts: hands (trauma, insecurity), arms (inadequacy), legs (lack of support), feet (insecurity, helplessness), mouth (difficulty relating to others)
- Facial expressions: mood and affect
- Integration of body parts: scattered or disorganized parts indicate cognitive or psychological problems or both

Drawing can be used in working with children and families. In the following vignette, the art therapist and the nurse use a family art session to identify family dynamics and begin interventions.

■ ■ ■ VIGNETTE

Melvin, a highly intelligent 15 year old with obsessive-compulsive behaviors and severe insecurity, lives with his parents and younger sister. In the art session, all family members are given paper on an easel and asked to draw themselves and the other members of the family. Melvin draws his parents and sister as being the same size and standing together shoulder to shoulder. He draws himself as a tiny figure in a box that appears to be suspended in space. When questioned, he reports feeling as though he were trapped in a falling elevator and disconnected from the family.

The family is surprised that he feels isolated (he is a normal size in their drawings). After completing a series of drawings and discussing them, the family is asked to draw a joint picture that requires them to work together. The picture they draw shows a smiling family standing by a house near a tree and a fence. The picture clearly demonstrates that the family does view Melvin as separate and different, for although he is standing beside the family, he is placed behind the fence. This observation is discussed, and as an intervention, the family is given the task of finding ways to make Melvin feel included.

■ ■ ■

Psychopharmacology

Rarely, if ever, is medication alone the treatment of choice. However, there are many indications for the use of medications. Medications that target specific symptoms can make a decided difference in a family's ability to cope and quality of life, and they can enhance the child's or adolescent's potential for growth. Table 32-7 lists some child and adolescent disorders and identifies the medications used in the treatment of these disorders.

TABLE 32-7

Psychopharmacology for Child and Adolescent Disorders and Symptoms

Disorder or Symptom	Type of Drug	Examples and Comments
Pervasive developmental disorders	Antipsychotics	Risperidone (Risperdal) reduces hyperactivity, fidgetiness, and labile affect.
		Olanzapine (Zyprexa) reduces hyperactivity, social withdrawal, use of language, and depression.
Autistic disorder	Antipsychotics	Haloperidol (Haldol) can reduce irritability and labile affect.
	Propranolol (Inderal)	Propranolol reduces rage outbursts, aggression, and severe anxiety.
	Selective serotonin reuptake inhibitors (SSRI)	Clomipramine (Anafranil) may help treat anger and compulsive behavior.
Attention deficit hyperactivity disorder (ADHD)	Stimulants	Methylphenidate (Ritalin)
		Mixture of salts and L-amphetamine (Adderall)
		Dexmethylphenidate (Focalin)
		Pemoline (Cylert)
		All improve symptoms of ADHD.
	Antidepressants	Nortriptyline (Aventyl)
		Bupropion (Wellbutrin)
		Fluoxetine (Prozac)
		All produce improvements in hyperactivity, attention, and global functioning.
	α-adrenergic agonists	Clonidine (Catapres) can be used for aggressiveness, impulsivity, and hyperactivity in clients with ADHD.
Conduct disorders	Antipsychotics	Risperidone decreases aggression.
	Stimulants	Methylphenidate decreases antisocial behaviors.
	Antidepressants	Bupropion improves symptoms of conduct disorder.
	Mood stabilizers	Carbamazepine (Tegretol) and lithium both have demonstrated efficacy in decreasing aggression.
	α-adrenergic agonists	Clonidine may help with impulsive and disordered behaviors.
Anxiety disorders		
Panic and school phobia	Antidepressants	
	SSRIs	Citalopram (Celexa), fluoxetine, and paroxetine (Paxil)
	Tricyclic antidepressants (TCAs)	Imipramine (Tofranil) is commonly used.
Obsessive-compulsive disorder (OCD)	Antidepressants	
	SSRIs	Fluoxetine and paroxetine
	TCAs	Clomipramine
	Atypical anxiolytics	Buspirone (BuSpar) is used as adjunct treatment for refractory OCD.
Separation anxiety disorder	Antidepressants	
	TCAs	Imipramine
	SSRIs	Fluoxetine
Social phobia	Antidepressants	
	TCAs	Imipramine
	Anxiolytics	Buspirone
Posttraumatic stress disorder (PTSD)	Atypical antipsychotics	Risperidone is used to control the flashbacks and aggression in PTSD.
Anxiety symptoms		
Insomnia	Antihistamines	Diphenhydramine (Benadryl)

TABLE 32-7

Psychopharmacology for Child and Adolescent Disorders and Symptoms—cont'd

Disorder or Symptom	Type of Drug	Examples and Comments
Depressive symptoms		
Major depression and dysthymia	Antidepressants	
	SSRIs	Fluoxetine is effective in decreasing depressive symptoms.
	TCAs	No significant differences have been found between responses to TCAs and to placebo.
	Atypical antidepressants	Venlafaxine (Effexor): one small study reported no difference between venlafaxine and placebo.
		Nefazodone (Serzone) effective in treating depressive symptoms.
Psychotic symptoms	Antipsychotics	Quetiapine (Seroquel)
		Risperidone

Data from Wagner, K. D. (2004). Treatment of childhood and adolescent disorders. In Schatzberg, A. F., & Nemeroff, C. B. (2004). *Textbook of psychopharmacology* (3rd ed., pp. 949-1007). Washington, DC: American Psychiatric Publishing.

■ ■ ■ KEY POINTS to REMEMBER

- One in five children and adolescents in the United States suffers from a major mental illness causing significant impairments at home, at school, and with peers. An estimated two thirds of all young people with mental health problems are not getting the help they need.
- The mentally disturbed child or adolescent is one whose progressive personality development is hindered or arrested by a variety of factors, which results in impairments in the capacities expected given age and physical and cognitive endowment.
- Factors known to affect the development of mental and emotional problems in children and adolescents include genetic influences, biochemical (prenatal and postnatal) factors, temperament, psychosocial developmental factors, social and environmental factors, and cultural influences.
- The characteristics of a resilient child include an adaptable temperament, the ability to form nurturing relationships with surrogate parental figures, the ability to distance the self from emotional chaos in parents and family, and good social intelligence and problem-solving skills.
- The most commonly diagnosed child psychiatric disorders are ADHD, adjustment reactions, conduct and oppositional disorders, separation anxiety disorder, and mood disorder (depression). The PDDs are rare.
- Treatment of childhood and adolescent disorders requires a multimodal approach in almost all instances.
- Close work with schools, the provision of remediation services when needed, and behavior modification techniques should be part of the intervention.
- Cognitive-behavioral therapies, social skills groups, family therapy, parent training in behavioral techniques, and individual therapy focused on esteem issues are therapies that have been found useful.
- Skills training may focus on a variety of areas, depending on the child's or adolescent's presenting symptoms.
- Child and adolescent psychiatric nurses are increasingly becoming aware of the need to educate the family and involve its members in the treatment process. The family is an integral part of the supportive and educative system for the child and adolescent.

■ ■ ■

Visit the Evolve website at **http://evolve.elsevier.com/Varcarolis** for a posttest on the content in this chapter. *evolve*

Critical Thinking and Chapter Review

Visit the Evolve website at **http://evolve.elsevier.com/Varcarolis** for additional self-study exercises.

■ ■ ■ CRITICAL THINKING

1. T. S., a 4-year-old boy, has been diagnosed with a PPD—autism.

   A. Describe the specific behavioral data you would find on assessment in terms of (1) communication, (2) social interactions, (3) behaviors and activities.

   B. Name at least six realistic outcomes for a child with PPD.

   C. Which interventions do you think are the most important for a child with PPD? Identify at least six.

   D. What kinds of support should the family receive?

2. N. T. is a 7-year-old girl who has been diagnosed with ADHD.

   A. This child is in the second grade. What clinical behaviors might she be exhibiting at home and in the classroom? Give behavioral examples for her (1) inattention, (2) hyperactivity, and (3) impulsivity.

   B. Identify at least six intervention strategies one might use for her. What medications might help her?

   C. Describe the concept of time-out.

3. J. F. is an 8-year-old boy who has been diagnosed with conduct disorder.

   A. Explain to one of J. F.'s classmates his probable behaviors in terms of (1) aggression toward others, (2) destruction of property, (3) deceitfulness, and (4) violation of rules.

   B. What are the outcomes for this child? What is the overall prognosis for children with this disorder?

   C. What are at least seven ways you could support J. F.'s parents? Where could you refer this family within your own community?

■ ■ ■ CHAPTER REVIEW

Choose the most appropriate answer.

1. Which of the following should not be identified by the nurse as a risk factor associated with child psychiatric disorders?
   1. Resiliency
   2. Severe marital discord
   3. Low socioeconomic status
   4. Maternal psychiatric disorder

2. The nurse working in the emergency department usually assesses adult clients. To assess a child's suicide potential adequately, which additional topic must be explored in the assessment?
   1. Understanding about and experiences with suicide and death
   2. The presence of ideas about hurting self seriously or causing death
   3. Circumstances at the time suicidal thoughts are experienced
   4. Identification of feelings such as depression, anger, guilt, and rejection

3. G. L., age 5 years, has been diagnosed with a pervasive developmental disorder based on loss of previously acquired abilities, deficits in communication, lack of responsiveness to and interest in others, and rigid adherence to routines and rituals. An applicable nursing diagnosis would be
   1. impaired mobility.
   2. impaired social interaction.
   3. disturbed personal identity.
   4. risk for self-directed violence.

4. Which topic would be of the *least* relevance as a focus during the assessment of a 12 year old with suspected ADHD?
   1. Impact of defiant behavior on the child's life at home and school
   2. The child's level of physical activity and attention span
   3. The child's ability to make friends and perform in school
   4. Progress with toilet training and self-care habits

5. A method of modifying the disruptive behavior of a child that will be perceived by the child as punishment is
   1. therapeutic holding.
   2. planned ignoring.
   3. restructuring.
   4. seclusion.

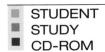

■ **STUDENT**
■ **STUDY**
■ **CD-ROM**

Access the accompanying CD-ROM for animations, interactive exercises, review questions for the NCLEX examination, and an audio glossary.

■ **NURSE,**
■ **CLIENT, AND**
■ **FAMILY RESOURCES**

For suggested readings, information on related associations, and Internet resources, go to **http://evolve.elsevier.com/Varcarolis**.

REFERENCES

Allen, J. (2000). Seclusion and restraint of children: A literature review. *Journal of Child and Adolescent Psychiatric Nursing, 13*(4), 159-167.

American Nurses Association, American Psychiatric Nurses Association, & International Society of Psychiatric-Mental Health Nurses. (2000). *Scope and standards of psychiatric-mental health nursing practice*. Washington, DC: American Nurses Publishing.

American Psychiatric Association. (2000). *Diagnostic and statistical manual of mental disorders (DSM-IV-TR)* (4th ed., text rev.). Washington, DC: Author.

Andrews, M., & Boyle, J. (2003). *Transcultural concepts in nursing care* (4th ed.). Philadelphia: Lippincott.

Axline, V. (1969). *Play therapy*. New York: Ballantine Books.

Children's Defense Fund. (2004). *The state of America's children 2004*. Washington, DC: Author.

Costello-Wells, B., et al. (2003). School-based mental health clinics. *Journal of Child and Adolescent Psychiatric Nursing, 16*(2), 60-70.

Eggert, L., et al. (2002). Preliminary effects of brief school-based prevention approaches for reducing youth suicide-risk behaviors, depression, and drug involvement. *Journal of Child and Adolescent Psychiatric Nursing, 15*(2), 48-64.

Freud, A. (1965). *Normality and pathology in childhood: Assessments of development*. New York: International Universities Press.

Gallagher, R., & Chase, A. (2002). *Building resilience in children in the face of fear and tragedy*. Retrieved September 16, 2004, from http://AboutOurKids.org./aboutour/articles/crisis_resilience.html.

Gardner, R. A. (1971). *Therapeutic communication with children: The mutual story-telling technique*. New York: Jason Aronson.

Gardner, R. A. (1979). Helping children cooperate in therapy. In J. D. Noshpitz & S. I. Harrison (Eds.), *Basic handbook of child psychiatry: Therapeutic interventions* (pp. 414-432). New York: Basic Books.

Gardner, R. A. (1986). The talking, feeling and doing game. In C. E. Schaefer & S. E. Reid (Eds.), *Game play: Therapeutic use of childhood games* (pp. 41-72). New York: Wiley.

Hall, D. K., & Pearson, J. (2003). *Resilience—giving the skills to bounce back*. Retrieved September 16, 2004, from http://www.voicesforchildren.ca/report-Nov2003-1.htm.

Inder, T. (2000). *Advances and application of psychopharmacology in pediatrics*. Paper presented at Advancing Children's Health 2000: Pediatric Academic Societies and American Academy of Pediatrics Year 2000 Joint Meeting. Retrieved April 2, 2005, from http://trainland.tripod.com/advancing.pdf.

Klein, M. (1955). The psychoanalytic play technique. *American Journal of Orthopsychiatry, 25*, 223-237.

Moorhead, S., Johnson, M., & Maas, M. (2004). *Nursing outcomes classification (NOC)* (3rd ed.). St. Louis, MO: Mosby.

National Mental Health Association. (2004). *Children's mental health statistics*. Retrieved September 15, 2004, from http://www.nmha.org/children/prevent/stats.cfm.

North American Nursing Diagnosis Association. (2005). *NANDA nursing diagnoses: Definitions and classification 2005-2006*. Philadelphia: Author.

Popper, C., et al. (2004). Disorders usually first diagnosed in infancy, childhood, or adolescence. In R. E. Hales & S. C. Yudofsky (Eds.), *Essentials of clinical psychiatry* (2nd ed.). Washington, DC: American Psychiatric Publishing.

Puskar, K., et al. (1997). Teaching kids to cope: A preventive mental health nursing strategy for adolescents. *Journal of Child and Adolescent Psychiatric Nursing, 10*(3), 18-28.

Redl, F., & Wineman, D. (1957). *The aggressive child*. New York: Free Press.

Sadock, B. J., & Sadock, V. A. (2004). *Kaplan & Sadock's concise textbook of clinical psychiatry* (2nd ed.). Philadelphia: Lippincott Williams & Wilkins.

Thomas, A., & Chess, S. (1977). *Temperament and development*. New York: Brunner/Mazel.

U.S. Department of Health and Human Services. (1999). *Mental health: A report of the Surgeon General*. Rockville, MD: U.S. Department of Health and Human Services, Center for Mental Health Services, National Institutes of Health. Retrieved March 9, 2004, from http://www.surgeongeneral.gov/library/mentalhealth/toc.html#chapter3.

Yeh, M., et al. (2004). Parental beliefs about causes of child problems: Exploring racial/ethnic patterns. *Journal of the American Academy of Child and Adolescent Psychiatry, 43*(5), 605-612.

CHAPTER 33

Adult Issues

VERNA BENNER CARSON

KEY TERMS and CONCEPTS

The key terms and concepts listed here appear in color where they are defined or first discussed in this chapter.

OBJECTIVES

After studying this chapter, the reader will be able to

1. Discuss the significance of sleep deprivation with regard to social problems, medical conditions, and psychiatric disorders.
2. Describe a normal sleep cycle.
3. Discuss the variation in normal sleep requirements, evaluate whether or not you are a short or a long sleeper, and analyze the impact of sleep deprivation on your daytime functioning.
4. Discuss the significance of primary insomnia.
5. Compare and contrast the use of polysomnography and the 2-week sleep diary in the assessment of sleep problems.
6. Discuss at least two interventions for primary insomnia.
7. Identify at least two sleep disorders that are life threatening.
8. Identify at least two factors that make diagnosis of adult attention deficit hyperactivity disorder (ADHD) difficult.
9. Discuss the importance of self-report questionnaires as well as family and spouse reports in the diagnosis of ADHD.
10. Describe the components of multimodal treatment for the adult with ADHD.
11. Discuss personal values and biases regarding sexuality and sexual behaviors.
12. Define at least three sexual disorders and describe their treatment.
13. Role-play with a classmate taking a sexual history and discuss how you feel and how your feelings influence your ability to perform this assessment.

evolve Visit the Evolve website at **http://evolve.elsevier.com/Varcarolis** for a pretest on the content in this chapter.

In this chapter we examine three issues that affect adults: sleep disorders, adult attention deficit hyperactivity disorder (ADHD), and gender identity and sexual disorders. Each of these disorders is receiving increased attention in health care. For instance, not so long ago sleep problems were considered either an insignificant nuisance not deserving of attention or a symptom of a psychiatric disorder, in which case the treatment focused on the psychiatric problem, not the sleep issue. As we will explore, sleep problems have a profound impact on the course of both medical and psychiatric disorders (Krahn, 2003; Roth et al., 2003).

ADHD was once thought to be a condition that affects children and some adolescents. Even though it was recognized that children with ADHD were more likely to have difficulties in adulthood, these difficulties were frequently misdiagnosed and treated as other conditions. Over the last 20 years, ADHD has been recognized as a disorder in older adolescents as well as adults that causes significant impairments in many aspects of life (Byrnes & Watkins, 2004).

Gender identity and sexual disorders historically have been shrouded in myth, misunderstanding, discomfort, and denial. Even in health care these issues are only beginning to be explored to the degree that is necessary for a holistic approach. It is important for both the basic level and advanced practice psychiatric mental health nurse to be aware of the role of nursing in relation to sexual functioning.

Let us begin this chapter with an exploration of sleep disorders.

Sleep Disorders

THE PROBLEM

Sleep is a basic human need, and unless we experience difficulty sleeping, we tend to take our sleep for granted. Sleep is receiving increasing attention in the media and medical research, however, because an estimated 47 million Americans suffer from sleep deprivation, which means that a person is not getting an optimal amount of sleep every night (Stickgold, Winkelman, & Wehrwein, 2004; Walsh, 2004; Weintraub, 2004a). Sleep deprivation leads to chronic fatigue, memory problems, energy deficit, mood difficulties, and a feeling of just generally being out of sorts (Sleep-deprivation.com, 2004).

We live in a fast-paced, high-tech world that operates 24 hours a day, and we expect around-the-clock access to supermarkets, airports, train and bus terminals, and a myriad of other services. Nurses, physicians, and fire and police personnel are part of the 20% of today's workforce who are required to work rotating shifts and because, of their work schedules, average only 5 hours

of sleep a night (Sleep-deprivation.com, 2004). Stimulation from television and radio that broadcasts day and night bombards us. Many of us are willing to trade hours of sleep to "catch up" on work or home projects. Estimates are that over the last century the average nightly sleeping time has been reduced by 2 hours from 9.0 hours a night in 1910 to 6.9 hours a night in 2002 (*Info on Sleep Deprivation*, 2002)!

In the following sections, we examine the significance of sleep deprivation as a problem co-occurring with other important social, medical, and psychiatric difficulties. We briefly review the components of normal sleep, sleep regulation, and the functions of sleep. An examination of the major sleep disorders follows. We apply the nursing process to a selected sleep disorder.

COMORBIDITY

Sleep deprivation is implicated in social problems, medical conditions, and psychiatric disorders.

Social Issues

According to the National Sleep Foundation, social problems such as road rage may be caused, in part, by a national epidemic of sleepiness (National Sleep Foundation, 2004). Sleep loss diminishes safety and results in loss of lives and property in occupations in which workers are expected to work shifts around the clock. Workers in such occupations includes those employed by the transportation industry, the armed forces, the space industry, health care, and law enforcement, as well as in other at-risk jobs in the construction, manufacturing, and service sectors of the American economy. The National Highway Traffic Safety Administration estimates that between 100,000 and 150,000 motor vehicle accidents per year are caused by drowsy drivers; 1550 of these crashes result in fatalities (National Center on Sleep Disorders Research, 2003). An individual who has been awake for 24 hours displays the same mental acuity as someone with a blood alcohol level of 0.1 mg%, who would be considered legally drunk in most states (Weintraub, 2004b).

Medical Conditions

Sleep problems are also associated with serious medical conditions. For instance, sleep apnea is closely related to hypertension, heart failure, and diabetes (Krakow et al., 2001; Walsh, 2004). Sleep deprivation leads to the production of fewer infection-fighting antibodies and thereby increases vulnerability to infection. Chronic sleep loss might lead to an earlier onset and an increase in severity of diabetes and obesity. A few age-related diseases such as arthritis and Alzheimer's disease also affect sleep. Arthritis causes pain that interferes with sleep; Alzheimer's disease leads to a reversal of sleep patterns, with increasingly more time spent in daytime sleeping and less time in nighttime sleeping. Alzheimer's disease also changes the normal sleep cycle, which results in a reduction in rapid eye movement (REM) sleep (Krahn, 2003; National Center on Sleep Disorders Research, 2003; Stickgold et al., 2004).

Psychiatric Disorders

Prolonged periods of sleep deprivation are linked to hallucinations and delusions (Sadock & Sadock, 2004). Sleep disturbance is part of the diagnostic criteria of many of the psychiatric disorders, including major depressive disorder, anxiety, and manic episodes (American Psychiatric Association, 2000). Current research indicates a relationship between sleep and dream disturbances and the development of posttraumatic stress disorder (National Center on Sleep Disorders Research, 2003). An increased risk for relapse of alcoholism and drug addiction is also linked to sleep deprivation.

NORMAL SLEEP CYCLE

Before sleep problems are discussed, it is helpful to review the normal sleep cycle, which consists of two distinct physiological states: non-REM (NREM) sleep and REM sleep. NREM sleep is characterized by a marked reduction in physiological function compared to the wakeful state and is composed of four stages (Figure 33-1).

REM sleep is quite different from NREM sleep. Whereas NREM sleep is a peaceful state compared to wakefulness, REM sleep is characterized by a high level of brain activity and physiological activity levels that are similar to those of the waking state. During REM sleep there is a generalized muscle atonia. Dreaming in REM sleep is frequently vivid with a strong emotional component and is associated with activation of the amygdala (Sanford et al., 2001). About 90 minutes after the beginning of sleep, the NREM sleep changes to the first REM cycle of the night. This 90-minute period is referred to as the REM latency period and is a consistent finding in most adults. The REM latency period is frequently shorter in depressed individuals.

The cycling between NREM and REM sleep is regular, with REM sleep occurring every 90 to 100 minutes. Except for the first REM cycle, which usually lasts less than 10 minutes, the REM periods last from 15 to 40 minutes each.

Sleep Patterns

Sleep patterns evolve over the lifetime. In the newborn, REM sleep comprises more than 50% of total sleep time, and NREM sleep does not progress through stages 1 through 4. This pattern gradually changes, with less time spent in REM sleep. The sleep of prepubertal children is characterized by a large proportion of REM and high-amplitude slow-wave sleep. During adolescence there is a sharp decrease in slow-wave sleep (Hales & Yudofsky, 2004). By young adulthood, about 75% of total sleep is NREM and 25% is REM. With advancing age, sleep becomes more fragmented and lighter. Older persons experience a reduction in both slow-wave sleep and REM sleep as well as a shift in the diurnal sleep-wake pattern, with more naps being taken. Box 33-1 shows the distribution of time spent in each of the sleep states.

Evaluation of Sleep

Sleep cycles are evaluated through polysomnography, a method of sleep study in which multiple processes are monitored during sleep, including electroencephalographic activity, electrooculographic activity (eye movement), and electromyographic activity (muscle movement). Additional measurements such as breathing effort, chest and abdominal wall movement, oral or nasal airflow, oxyhemoglobin saturation, or exhaled carbon dioxide concentration may be obtained to detect sleep apnea and evaluate its severity (American Psychiatric Association [APA], 2000; Neylan, Reynolds, & Kupfer, 2004).

Regulation of Sleep

The regulation of sleep is not totally understood. In fact, the 2003 National Sleep Disorders Research Plan emphasizes the need to better understand the role played in sleep by neurotransmitters and neuromodulators and other neurobiological factors, as well as by circadian rhythms under the control of the suprachiasmatic nucleus in the hypothalamus. Researchers have identified anatomic areas that promote sleep, such as the ventrolateral preoptic area of the hypothalamus (National Center on Sleep Disorders Research, 2003) and have recognized the impact of certain neurotransmitters such as serotonin in sleep regulation. Prevention of serotonin synthesis or destruction of the dorsal raphe nucleus of the brainstem where most of the brain's serotonergic cell bodies are located results in reduced sleep for a considerable amount of time. Norepinephrine-containing neurons with cell bodies located in the locus ceruleus also influence normal sleep patterns. Brain acetylcholine is involved in the production of REM sleep, so that any change in levels of this neurotransmitter affects the sleep cycle. Additional investigation is needed to understand the interconnections between hypothalamic and brainstem circuits that control REM sleep, NREM sleep, and wake states (Hales & Yudofsky, 2004).

HOW WE SLEEP

Every night, we drift through repeated sleep cycles lasting anywhere from 90 to 120 minutes. Each cycle ends in the famous, dreamy state known as rapid eye movement, or REM. The non-REM stages that cycle with REM bring progressively deeper states of unconsciousness. And as the night wears on, the REM stages and accompanying dream sequences grow longer.

STAGE 1 As we begin to nod off, we fall into the first—and lightest—phase of non-REM sleep. The senses switch off, so we no longer hear the light snoring of our spouse, nor do we feel the chill of the air coming through the window. But we can be easily aroused by the neighbor's screeching car alarm. Marker: Low-frequency **THETA WAVES.**

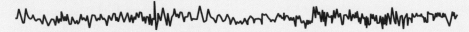

STAGE 2 Our breathing and heart rates even out, our body temperature drops, and we become increasingly disengaged from our waking senses. Marker: Brain waves alternate between short bursts called **SLEEP SPINDLES** and sudden, large waves called **K-COMPLEXES.**

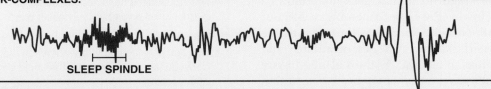

— K-COMPLEX

SLEEP SPINDLE

STAGE 3 and 4 In the deepest phases of sleep—also known as slow-wave sleep— blood pressure falls, breathing slows, and body temperature drops even lower. These phases are essential for restoring energy, strengthening the immune system, and prompting the body to release vital growth hormones. Marker: Wide, slow **DELTA WAVES.**

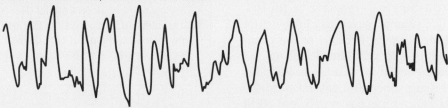

REM Eyes dart back and forth, breathing and heart rates flutter, and muscles are mostly paralyzed. While we dream vividly of performing gold-medal dives at the Olympics, portions of our brains may focus on real-world pursuits: Solving problems from the previous day and burning knowledge and experience into long-term memories. Marker: **BETA WAVES.**

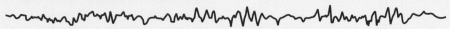

FIGURE 33-1 Stages of sleep. (From *BusinessWeek Online*. [2004, January 26]. Retrieved June 7, 2004, from http://www.businessweek.com/magazine/content/04_04/b3867005_ mz001.htm.)

Functions of Sleep

The functions of sleep are also a focus of research (National Center on Sleep Disorders Research, 2003), but most investigators believe that sleep serves to restore and maintain homeostasis. Sleep also appears to be essential to the body's thermoregulation and energy conservation (Sadock & Sadock, 2004).

Requirements of Sleep

Requirements for sleep vary from individual to individual. Some people are considered short sleepers and can function effectively on fewer than 6 hours of sleep per night. Others, considered long sleepers, require more than 9 hours of sleep each night. Long sleepers experience more REM periods than do short sleepers (Sadock & Sadock, 2004).

Distribution of Sleep in Adults

Non–rapid eye movement sleep: 75% of total sleep
- Stage 1: 5%
- Stage 2: 45%
- Stage 3: 12%
- Stage 4: 13%

Rapid eye movement sleep: 25%

Data from Sadock, B. J., & Sadock, V. A. (2004). *Kaplan and Sadock's concise textbook of clinical psychiatry* (2nd ed., p. 310). Philadelphia: Lippincott Williams & Wilkins.

The body has a natural internal clock that follows a 25-hour cycle. However, we are coaxed into a 24-hour clock by the influence of external factors such as the cycle of light and dark, daily routines, mealtimes, and other external clues. Biological rhythms also influence sleep. Most adults sleep once, sometimes twice, within a 24-hour period. During the phases of the menstrual cycle, some women experience changes in their sleep patterns (Sadock & Sadock, 2004).

It is a myth that a daytime nap compensates for lack of nighttime sleeping. Daytime naps differ in structure from normal nighttime sleeping because of the circadian cycle. For most people who sleep during the night, a nap taken in the morning or at noon includes a great deal of REM sleep, whereas a nap taken in the late afternoon or early evening has much less REM sleep. A change in the amount of REM sleep changes the physiology of sleep as well as the psychological and behavioral effects of sleep. This is especially important for those whose occupations require shift rotation (Sadock & Sadock, 2004).

SLEEP DISORDERS

The *Diagnostic and Statistical Manual of Mental Disorders,* fourth edition, text revision *(DSM-IV-TR)* (APA, 2000) classifies sleep disorders into three major categories, including primary sleep disorders, sleep disorders related to other mental disorders, and other sleep disorders.

There are five major symptoms associated with sleep disorders. These include insomnia, hypersomnia, somnolence, parasomnia, and sleep-wake schedule disturbance. Frequently these symptoms overlap. See Box 33-2 for descriptions of these symptoms.

Primary Sleep Disorders

The primary sleep disorders are further classified as dyssomnias and parasomnias.

Primary Symptoms of Sleep Disorders

Insomnia
- Difficulty initiating or maintaining sleep
- May be a temporary or a persistent condition and is associated with anxiety
- Most common sleep complaint

Hypersomnia
- Excessive amounts of sleep, excessive daytime sleepiness or somnolence, or both
- Not applied to those who are simply tired or weary
- Occurs less frequently than insomnia but is not rare

Somnolence
- Feeling of sleepiness accompanied by a tendency to suddenly fall asleep in the waking state

Parasomnia
- Unusual or undesirable phenomenon that occurs suddenly during sleep or at the threshold between waking and sleeping
- Includes nightmares, sleep terrors, sleepwalking, and bruxism or tooth grinding

Sleep-Wake Schedule Disturbance
- Displacement of sleep from its desired circadian period
- Characterized by complaints that one cannot sleep when one wishes to sleep but can sleep at other times, or cannot be fully awake when one wants to be but is awake at other times

Dyssomnias

Dyssomnias involve problems in initiating or maintaining sleep. The main symptoms of the dyssomnias are disturbances in the amount, quality, or timing of sleep (APA, 2000). Box 33-3 lists and defines the dyssomnias. The focus here is on primary insomnia.

Primary Insomnia. Individuals who experience primary insomnia complain that they have difficulty falling asleep and staying asleep and that their sleep is nonrestorative. According to the *DSM-IV-TR,* this condition must persist for 1 month and must not be related to any known physical or medical condition (Box 33-4).

To diagnose primary insomnia—in fact, to diagnose any sleep disorder—a thorough medical and psychiatric history must be taken. The entire 24-hour period must be explored with respect to sleep-wake behaviors. Clients should be asked what they believe constitutes healthy sleep. Frequently, clients who are naturally short sleepers become upset because they are unable to sleep for the popular standard of 8 hours, yet when questioned they do not report experiencing day-

BOX 33-3

Primary Sleep Disorders: Dyssomnias

Primary hypersomnia: Excessive sleepiness for at least 1 month evidenced by either prolonged sleep episodes or by daytime sleep episodes that occur almost daily and causes significant distress or impairment of functioning

Narcolepsy: Repeated irresistible attacks of refreshing sleep, recurrent intrusions of rapid eye movement sleep into the transition period between sleep and wakefulness, and cataplexy, which is a loss of muscle tone leading to a subtle sagging jaw or drooping eyelids, head, or arms, or to a dramatic buckling of the knees, falling, or dropping of objects

Breathing-related sleep disorder: Sleep disruption that leads to excessive sleepiness or sometimes insomnia caused by abnormalities of breathing during sleep— either sleep apnea or central alveolar hypoventilation

Circadian rhythm sleep disorder: Persistent or recurrent pattern of sleep disruption resulting from altered function of the circadian timing system or from a mismatch between the individual's natural circadian sleep-wake cycle and external demands regarding the timing and duration of sleep, such as in those who do shift work or who experience jet lag

Dyssomnia not otherwise specified: Insomnias, hypersomnias, or circadian rhythm disturbances that do not meet the criteria for any specific dyssomnia; includes

- *Restless legs syndrome,* in which people feel deep sensations of creeping inside the calves whenever sitting or lying down that result in an almost irresistible urge to move the legs and thus interfere with falling asleep and remaining asleep
- *Kleine-Levin syndrome,* a rare condition characterized by recurrent periods of prolonged sleep (lasting from one or several weeks) with intervening periods of normal sleep and alert waking
- *Menstrual-associated syndrome,* in which some women experience marked hypersomnia, a change in behaviors, and voracious eating at or before the onset of their menses
- *Sleep disturbance in pregnancy,* common in pregnant women due to hormonal factors, maternal respiratory physiology, body changes, and fetal movements
- *Insufficient sleep,* defined as an earnest complaint of daytime sleepiness and associated waking symptoms by a person who persistently fails to obtain adequate daily sleep to support alertness when awake
- *Sleep drunkenness,* a rare and abnormal form of awakening in which the individual experiences a confused state that often leads to individual or social inconvenience and sometimes to criminal acts

Adapted from American Psychiatric Association. (2000). *Diagnostic and statistical manual of mental disorders* (4th ed., text rev.). Washington, DC: Author; and Sadock, B. J., & Sadock, V. A. (2004). *Kaplan & Sadock's concise textbook of clinical psychiatry* (2nd ed.). Philadelphia: Lippincott Williams & Wilkins.

BOX 33-4

DSM-IV-TR Criteria for Primary Insomnia

A. The predominant complaint is difficulty initiating or maintaining sleep, or nonrestorative sleep, for at least 1 month.

B. The sleep disturbance (or associated daytime fatigue) causes clinically significant distress or impairment in social, occupational, or other important areas of functioning.

C. The sleep disturbance does not occur exclusively during the course of narcolepsy, breathing-related sleep disorder, circadian rhythm sleep disorder, or parasomnia.

D. The disturbance does not occur exclusively during the course of another mental disorder (e.g., major depressive disorder, generalized anxiety disorder, a delirium).

E. The disturbance is not due to the direct physiological effects of a substance (e.g., a drug of abuse, a medication) or a general medical condition.

From American Psychiatric Association. (2000). *Diagnostic and statistical manual of mental disorders* (4th ed., text rev.). Washington, DC: Author.

time functional deficits. The significance of insomnia can be fully appreciated only by examining its impact on the client's daytime functioning in terms of moods, fatigue, muscle aches, and ability to attend and concentrate. Eliciting information about the total number of hours spent sleeping typically has limited value. There are rating scales such as the Pittsburgh Sleep Quality Index (Buysse et al., 1989) that allow measurement of subjective sleep quality. A 2-week sleep diary or log is an invaluable tool for obtaining a history of irregular sleep-wake patterns; napping; use of stimulants, hypnotics, or alcohol; diet; activity during the day; number of arousals; and perceived length of sleep and its relationship to daytime mood and alertness (Neylan et al., 2004). Figure 33-2 provides a sample of a sleep diary developed by the National Sleep Foundation. However, the primary diagnostic tool is polysomnography. In the diagnosis of primary insomnia, polysomnography demonstrates sleep fragmentation (interruption of sleep), prolonged sleep latency (time required to fall asleep), decreased sleep efficiency (ratio of actual time asleep to time spent in bed, with higher numbers indicating better sleep), and a predominance of the lighter stages of NREM sleep (APA, 2000; Neylan et al., 2004).

Several effective approaches are available for the treatment of primary insomnia. The first is the use of medications such as the benzodiazepines (alprazolam [Xanax], chlordiazepoxide [Librium], chlordiazepoxide [Novapam], triazolam [Halcion], and diazepam [Valium]), zolpidem (Ambien), zaleplon (Sonata), and

NATIONAL SLEEP FOUNDATION SLEEP DIARY

	COMPLETE IN MORNING							COMPLETE AT END OF DAY				
Fill out days 1-4 below and days 5-7 on page 2	I went to bed last night at:	I got out of bed this morning at:	Last night, I fell asleep in: *(Record number of times)*	I woke up during the night: *(Record number of times)*	When I woke up for the day, I felt: *(Check one)*	Last night I slept a total of: *(Record number of hours)*	My sleep was disturbed by: *(List any mental, emotional, physical or environmental factors that affected your sleep; e.g., stress, snoring, physical discomfort, temperature)*	I consumed caffeinated drinks in the: *(e.g., coffee, tea, cola)*	I exercised at least 20 minutes in the:	Approximately 2-3 hours before going to bed, I consumed:	Medication(s) I took during the day: *[List name of medication/drug(s)]*	About 1 hour before going to sleep, I did the following activity: *(List activity; e.g., watch TV, work, read)*
DAY 1 DAY___ DATE___	___ PM/AM	___ PM/AM	___ Minutes	___ Times	□ Refreshed □ Somewhat refreshed □ Fatigued	___ Hours		□ Morning □ Afternoon □ Within several hours before going to bed □ Not applicable	□ Morning □ Afternoon □ Within several hours before going to bed □ Not applicable	□ Alcohol □ A heavy meal □ Not applicable		
DAY 2 DAY___ DATE___	___ PM/AM	___ PM/AM	___ Minutes	___ Times	□ Refreshed □ Somewhat refreshed □ Fatigued	___ Hours		□ Morning □ Afternoon □ Within several hours before going to bed □ Not applicable	□ Morning □ Afternoon □ Within several hours before going to bed □ Not applicable	□ Alcohol □ A heavy meal □ Not applicable		
DAY 3 DAY___ DATE___	___ PM/AM	___ PM/AM	___ Minutes	___ Times	□ Refreshed □ Somewhat refreshed □ Fatigued	___ Hours		□ Morning □ Afternoon □ Within several hours before going to bed □ Not applicable	□ Morning □ Afternoon □ Within several hours before going to bed □ Not applicable	□ Alcohol □ A heavy meal □ Not applicable		
DAY 4 DAY___ DATE___	___ PM/AM	___ PM/AM	___ Minutes	___ Times	□ Refreshed □ Somewhat refreshed □ Fatigued	___ Hours		□ Morning □ Afternoon □ Within several hours before going to bed □ Not applicable	□ Morning □ Afternoon □ Within several hours before going to bed □ Not applicable	□ Alcohol □ A heavy meal □ Not applicable		

FIGURE 33-2 Days 1 through 4 of a 7-day sleep diary. (From National Sleep Foundation. *National Sleep Foundation sleep diary.* Retrieved June 1, 2004, from http://www.sleepfoundation.org/publications/SleepDiaryChart.pdf.)

other hypnotics. Hypnotic drugs are always used with caution. Over-the-counter sleep aids have limited effectiveness. Long-acting sleep medications such as flurazepam (Dalmane) and quazepam (Doral) are most helpful for middle-of-the-night insomnia, whereas short-acting drugs such as zolpidem and triazolam are useful for individuals who have problems falling asleep. Generally speaking, sleep medications are not prescribed for more than 2 weeks' duration, because tolerance and withdrawal may occur (Sadock & Sadock, 2004). Table 33-1 provides information on medications commonly prescribed to treat insomnia.

Increasingly, melatonin is being used by the elderly to deal with insomnia. Melatonin appears to be helpful in treating sleep problems in older adults. However, this practice is not without risk. Melatonin is an over-the-counter hormone medication available in health food stores. Melatonin products are not approved by the U.S. Food and Drug Administration; therefore, the purity, safety, and effectiveness of the products may vary. There are two known risks in taking melatonin. First, the substance has been linked to orthostatic blood pressure changes, which can increase the risk of falls in the elderly. Second, there are two types of melatonin: one is natural and is made from the pineal glands of animals, and the other is synthetic. The **natural form** could be contaminated with a virus and **its use is not recommended;** the synthetic form does not carry this risk (American Academy of Family Physicians, 2003). Additional research is needed to determine the optimal dosage of melatonin, long-term effects, and possible drug interactions (Hoffman, 2003).

Another approach to treating insomnia involves the use of nonpharmacological interventions, including various relaxation therapies such as hypnosis, meditation, deep breathing, and progressive muscle relaxation, as well as education regarding establishment of habits for good sleep hygiene (Sadock & Sadock, 2004). These approaches, unlike medication, are not immediately helpful and may require several weeks of practice before improvement is experienced. The success of these techniques is dependent on a high degree of motivation in clients, who must devote time to practicing these methods and changing lifestyle habits. However, those clients who succeed in learning these techniques generally have longer lasting benefits than those who use pharmacological interventions (Neylan et al., 2004). Box 33-5 provides tips for good sleep hygiene.

Sleep restriction therapy is yet another intervention that is useful in dealing with insomnia and is directed at reducing the amount of time spent awake in bed. Clients are asked to record in a sleep diary the amount of time they estimate they are asleep. They are then instructed to restrict their time in bed so that it equals their total sleep time. Clients often experience their usual difficulties with sleep fragmentation during the first few nights, which results in sleep deprivation. Sleep deprivation leads to a consolidation of sleep on subsequent nights and thereby improves the quality of sleep. The length of time spent in bed then is then adjusted until daytime fatigue is eliminated (Krahn, 2003; Neylan et al., 2004).

TABLE 33-1

Medications Used to Treat Insomnia

Medication (Trade Name)	Usual Adult Therapeutic Dosage (mg/day)*	Time Until Onset of Action (minutes)
Clonazepam (Klonopin)†	0.5-2.0	20-60
Clorazepate (Tranxene)	15-60	30-60
Lorazepam (Ativan)†	2-4	30-60
Oxazepam (Serax)	10-30	30-60
Temazepam (Restoril)	15-30	45-60
Triazolam (Halcion)	0.125-0.5	15-30
Chloral hydrate (Noctec)	500-1000	30-60
Trazodone (Desyrel)†‡	50-150	30-60
Zaleplon (Sonata)‡	10	30
Zolpidem (Ambien)‡	5-10	30

Data from Skidmore-Roth, L. (2005). *Mosby's nursing drug reference.* St. Louis, MO: Elsevier.
*Consider lower dosages in the elderly.
†Sleep induction is not a use for which this drug is approved by the Food and Drug Administration.
‡These drugs are not benzodiazepines.

BOX 33-5

Tips for Promoting Good Sleep Hygiene

- Go to sleep at the same time each night and awaken at roughly the same hour each morning.
- Practice stress-reducing strategies; avoid taking worries to bed.
- Sleep in loose, comfortable clothes in a comfortable bed.
- Eliminate sources of noise or bright lights that may prevent or disrupt sleep.
- Maintain a comfortable temperature in the bedroom.
- Cut down on beverages containing caffeine during the day because the stimulating effects of caffeine can linger for as long as 12 hours.
- Avoid heavy meals before bedtime.
- Avoid alcohol before bedtime; initially it will cause drowsiness, but it disrupts normal sleep patterns and leaves the individual awake later in the night.
- Exercise daily.
- Take a warm bath before going to bed.

Adapted from Stickgold, R. A., Winkelman, J. W., & Wehrwein, P. (2004, January 19). *Newsweek Health: You will start to feel very sleepy. . . .* Retrieved June 7, 2004, from http://msnbc.msn.com/id/3928217/; and National Sleep Foundation. *Can't sleep? Healthy sleep tips.* Retrieved June 7, 2004, from http://www.sleepfoundation.org/hottopics/index.php?secid=9&id=31.

■ ■ ■ **VIGNETTE**

Josie Harris is a 52-year-old woman who complains that she experiences difficulty getting to sleep every night. Josie reports that this has been going on for at least a year and seems to be getting progressively worse with time. She states that once she falls asleep she sleeps soundly for about 6 hours, waking up to void. After going to the bathroom, she tosses and turns for the next 2 hours until her alarm clock goes off announcing the beginning of her day. She feels tired during her waking hours and has difficulty focusing on the task at hand in her accounting job. Family members complain that she is irritable and short-tempered with them. Josie completes a sleep diary for a 2-week period and undergoes a sleep study at a nearby sleep laboratory. Josie is diagnosed with primary insomnia.

■ ■ ■

Parasomnias

The parasomnias, which are also primary sleep disorders, are characterized by unusual or undesirable behaviors that intrude into sleep or occur at the threshold between waking and sleeping (APA, 2000). The parasomnias are listed and defined in Box 33-6.

Treatment for the parasomnias includes reduction of stress, measures to protect the client, provision of low-dose benzodiazepines, the use of a dental bite plate for sleep-related bruxism, and the administration of clonazepam (Klonopin) and/or carbamazepine (Tegretol) for REM sleep behavior disorder.

■ ■ ■ **VIGNETTE**

An 80-year-old man is referred to a sleep clinic by his primary care physician. The client's wife complains that her husband screams and strikes out at night. These behaviors seem to arise from sleep, and he does not awaken. He suddenly yells and punches at the air. On several occasions he has knocked over the bedside lamp and twice he has struck his wife. After the second incident, she decided to sleep in a nearby twin bed. She expresses concern for his safety as well as her own. A polysomnographic examination reveals that he does not experience the muscle atonia normally found in REM sleep. This lack of atonia leads to muscle twitching as well as more complex movements during REM sleep. He is literally acting out his dreams. He is diagnosed with REM sleep behavior disorder and is treated with clonazepam.

■ ■ ■

Sleep Disorders Related to Other Mental Disorders

There are two distinct classifications of sleep disorders associated with major mental disorders: *insomnia related to another mental (axis I or axis II) disorder* and *hypersomnia related to another mental (axis 1 or axis II) disorder*. Both of these disorders produce significant functional problems in the social and occupational domains and in other important areas. Although sleep

---

BOX 33-6

Primary Sleep Disorders: Parasomnias

Nightmare disorder: Nightmares are long, frightening dreams from which people awaken scared. They almost always occur during rapid eye movement (REM) sleep and usually after a long REM period late in the night. For some people this is a lifetime condition; for others nightmares occur at times of stress and illness.

Sleep terror disorder: Sleep terror represents an arousal in the first third of the night during deep non-REM (NREM) sleep (stages 3 and 4). It usually begins with a scream or cries and is accompanied by behaviors of intense anxiety bordering on panic. Night terrors occur frequently as isolated episodes in children and more often in boys than in girls.

Sleepwalking disorder: Sleepwalking is also referred to as somnambulism and consists of a sequence of complex behaviors that begin in the first third of the night during deep NREM sleep (stages 3 and 4) and usually progress without full consciousness or later memory to leaving bed and walking about (may include dressing, going to the bathroom, screaming, and even driving).

Parasomnia not otherwise specified: This diagnostic category includes the presence of abnormal behavior or physiological events during sleep or sleep-wake transitions that do not meet the criteria for a more specific parasomnia. Included in this category are the following:

- *Sleep-related bruxism,* which is tooth grinding that occurs throughout the night but most prominently in stage 2 sleep.
- *REM sleep behavior disorder,* a chronic, progressive condition found mostly in men and characterized by the loss of atonia during REM sleep followed by the emergence of violent and complex behaviors. The client is acting out his or her dreams. This disorder poses significant risk to the client as well as to the client's bed partner.
- *Sleeptalking,* which occurs in all stages of sleep and is common in children and adults.
- *Sleep-related head banging,* a sleep behavior consisting of rhythmic to-and-fro head rocking occurring just before or during sleep.
- *Sleep paralysis,* characterized by a sudden inability to perform voluntary movements either at the onset of sleep or on awakening from sleep.

Adapted from American Psychiatric Association. (2000). *Diagnostic and statistical manual of mental disorders* (4th ed., text rev.). Washington, DC: Author; and Sadock, B. J., & Sadock, V. A. (2004). *Kaplan & Sadock's concise textbook of clinical psychiatry* (2nd ed.). Philadelphia: Lippincott Williams & Wilkins.

---

disturbances accompany many mental disorders, an additional diagnosis of *insomnia or hypersomnia related to another mental disorder* is made when the client's chief complaint is the sleep disturbance. Clients with this type of insomnia or hypersomnia tend to focus on their sleep and ignore the symptoms of the related mental disorder, even to the point of denying that they have a mental disorder.

Clients with major depressive disorder frequently experience insomnia that involves relatively normal sleep onset followed by repeated awakenings during the second half of the night and very early awakening in the morning. This is usually followed by a difficult mood in the morning, which many clients identify as the worst time of the day for them. Results of polysomnography indicate reduced stage 3 and 4 sleep and frequently a short REM latency, with an extended first REM period. Total or partial sleep deprivation has been shown to speed up the client's response to antidepressant medication (APA, 2000; Sadock & Sadock, 2004).

■ ■ ■ *VIGNETTE*

Kathy has just been diagnosed with major depressive disorder. She tells her nurse Pat that the worst symptom is the wakening at 4 AM followed by the inability to fall back to sleep. Kathy says, "It is still dark; no one else is awake; I feel incredibly alone with my sadness. The night seems to stretch on forever. This is the time that I actually consider suicide. Thank God for the daybreak. Although I'm exhausted, the light of day gives me hope." Pat explains the doctor's order for sleep deprivation as a way of dealing with her sleep problems as well as speeding up her response to the antidepressant medication.

■ ■ ■

Anxiety disorders and insomnia are also closely related. Polysomnography indicates a different pattern than that seen in clients with major depressive disorder. Anxiety disorders are associated with normal REM latencies and a decreased percentage of REM sleep. Furthermore, sleep deprivation does not produce improvement in anxiety symptoms (Neylan et al., 2004).

Clients with schizophrenia frequently have prolonged sleep latencies, sleep fragmentation with many awakenings, decreased slow-wave sleep, variable REM latency, and decreased REM rebound after REM sleep deprivation. The decrease in slow-wave sleep is associated with poor performance on neuropsychological tests of attention and with negative symptoms (Neylan et al., 2004).

■ ■ ■ *VIGNETTE*

Sarah has been living with schizophrenia for many years. She has grown accustomed to what she describes as "less than satisfying" sleep. However, through her relationship with a psychiatric nurse at the clinic where her medications are monitored, Sarah has learned to pay attention to changes in her sleep pattern, because a change in Sarah's assessment from "less than satisfying" to "an awful night" frequently is one of the earliest signs of an exacerbation of her illness. When she responds to what she calls her "sleep alarm" and informs her nurse and physician about what is happening, they are able to help her ward off an exacerbation.

■ ■ ■

Hypersomnia related to another mental disorder is seen in many mental conditions, including mood disorders. Many clients report excessive daytime sleepiness in the beginning stages of a mild depressive disorder. A similar complaint is characteristic of the depressed phase of bipolar I disorder. Uncomplicated grief may temporarily be associated with hypersomnia. Personality disorders, dissociative disorders, somatoform disorders, and dissociative fugue are all associated with hypersomnia. Generally speaking, treatment is directed at the primary disorder (APA, 2000; Sadock & Sadock, 2004).

Other Sleep Disorders

The last category of sleep disorders includes *sleep disorder due to a general medical condition* and *substance-induced sleep disorder*. In both of these disorders, the sleep disturbance may be insomnia, hypersomnia, parasomnia, or a combination.

Many medical conditions are associated with insomnia. For instance, conditions accompanied by pain and discomfort such as arthritis and angina are frequently further complicated by the presence of insomnia. Insomnia is also associated with neoplasms, vascular lesions, infections, and degenerative and traumatic conditions. The treatment is directed at the underlying medical condition (APA, 2000; Sadock & Sadock, 2004).

■ ■ ■ *VIGNETTE*

Robbie Carson is a student nurse assigned to Mrs. Viatelli in a nursing home. Robbie is in his psychiatric nursing rotation, part of which is spent in a skilled nursing facility taking care of clients with dementia. When Robbie receives the report in the morning, he learns that Mrs. Viatelli has been experiencing significant sleep disturbance. She seems to have difficulty falling asleep and frequently wakes up groaning during the night. Robbie notes that Mrs. Viatelli is very confused as well as agitated. She grimaces whenever she moves. Robbie believes Mrs. Viatelli is in pain. He checks the client's history to find that she has had arthritis for many years. He then checks her medication profile and discovers that Mrs. Viatelli is not on any antiinflammatory medication for her arthritis. He speaks to the charge nurse, who calls the physician. Immediately, the physician orders an antiinflammatory agent for Mrs. Viatelli. Over the next few days, not only is there a dramatic improvement in Mrs. Viatelli's sleep but there is also an improvement in her confusion, and the agitation disappears.

■ ■ ■

A substance-induced sleep disorder can result from the use or recent discontinuance of a substance. The sleep disturbance can take the form of insomnia, hypersomnia, parasomnia, or a combination. Alcohol and hypnotic drugs are both associated with sleep disorders. These substances produce tolerance to the sleep-inducing effect of the substance as well as increased awakenings during periods of withdrawal. Stimulant drugs produce difficulty in falling asleep, and when these drugs are withdrawn a rebound hypersomnia is common. Other drugs such as antimetabolites and other cancer chemotherapeutic agents, thyroid preparations, anticonvulsant agents, antidepressant drugs, and oral contraceptives, to name a few, produce sleep problems. Cigarette smoking can have a paradoxical effect on sleep. The combination of a relaxing ritual and a low dose of nicotine may actually help sleep. However, high doses of nicotine can interfere with sleep. Typically, cigarette smokers sleep less than nonsmokers (Neylan et al., 2004; Sadock & Sadock, 2004).

Application of the Nursing Process

Discussion of the application of the nursing process is focused on primary insomnia because it is the most common of the sleep disorders and for this reason will be seen in all specialty areas of nursing.

ASSESSMENT

The nurse may assign the client the homework of completing a sleep diary for 2 weeks. This approach encourages the client not only to take ownership of the problem but also to begin to think that the solution is within his or her means. Even without the sleep diary, however, there are areas that the nurse assesses. The following questions and comments provide direction for that assessment:

- When did you begin having trouble with sleep?
- What time do you fall asleep?
- Do you awaken frequently? Are you able to return to sleep?
- Can you identify any stress or problem that may have initially contributed to your sleep difficulties?
- Does your sleep problem interfere with your ability to function when you are awake? If so, how?
- Can you identify any particular issue or problem that is currently troubling you?
- How have you dealt with that stress or problem?
- Describe your sleeping environment to me. Is it a peaceful and restful place that is conducive to sleep or is it an environment that interferes with relaxation? How would you describe the comfort level of your bed? The noise and light levels in your bedroom? The degree of privacy available to you?

- Tell me about your daily habits. I am interested in your diet, exercise, and medications that you take. I am interested in whether or not you smoke or drink caffeinated or alcoholic beverages.
- Describe your bedtime routine. What are the activities that you customarily engage in before sleep?
- Can you describe for me the thoughts that you experience when you are lying in bed unable to get to sleep?
- Is your sleeping area used for other activities besides sleep and sex?
- What changes if any have you made to improve your sleep? What were the results?

NURSING DIAGNOSIS

There are two appropriate North American Nursing Diagnosis Association (NANDA) nursing diagnoses for primary insomnia (NANDA, 2005):
1. *Sleep deprivation* related to insomnia with difficulty at sleep onset
2. *Disturbed sleep pattern* related to insomnia with difficulty maintaining sleep

OUTCOME CRITERIA

The Nursing Outcomes Classification (NOC) (Moorhead, Johnson, & Maas, 2004) identifies a number of appropriate outcomes for the client experiencing primary insomnia, including *Rest, Sleep, Mood Equilibrium,* and *Personal Well-Being.* Table 33-2 provides selected intermediate and short-term indicators for these categories.

PLANNING

The majority of clients with sleep disorders are managed in the community. The exceptions are cases in which the client has a primary psychiatric disorder or a medical condition that requires hospitalization. Because long-standing sleep problems are associated with a host of occupational, social, interpersonal, psychiatric, and medical conditions, the treatment is multifaceted and frequently requires a team approach under the leadership of a sleep disorder specialist. The role of the nurse is generally to conduct a full assessment, to provide support to the client and family while the appropriate interventions are determined, and to teach the client and family strategies that may improve sleep.

INTERVENTION

Basic Level Interventions

The interventions of the basic level psychiatric mental health nurse include counseling, health teaching, and psychobiological interventions.

TABLE 33-2

NOC Outcomes for Primary Insomnia

Nursing Outcome and Definition	Intermediate Indicators	Short-Term Indicators
Sleep: Natural periodic suspension of consciousness during which the body is restored*	Sleeps through the night consistently Not dependent on sleep aids Sleep quality Feels rejuvenated after sleep	Hours of sleep Sleep pattern Sleep routine Wakefulness at appropriate times
Rest: Quantity and pattern of diminished activity for mental and physical rejuvenation†	Physically rested Emotionally rested Mentally rested Feels rejuvenated after rest	Amount of rest Rest pattern Rest quality
Mood Equilibrium: Appropriate adjustment of prevailing emotional tone in response to circumstances‡	Exhibits appropriate energy level Accomplishes daily tasks	Reports adequate sleep (at least 5 hours of every 24 hours) Exhibits appropriate affect
Personal Well-Being: Extent of positive perception of one's health status and life circumstances§	Spiritual life Physical health Cognitive function	Performance of activities of daily living Performance of usual roles

From Moorhead, S., Johnson, M., & Maas, M. (2004). *Nursing outcomes classification (NOC)* (3rd ed.). St. Louis, MO: Mosby.
*Evaluated on a five-point Likert scale ranging from 1 (severely compromised) to 5 (not compromised).
†Evaluated on a five-point Likert scale ranging from 1 (extremely compromised) to 5 (not compromised).
‡Evaluated on a five-point Likert scale ranging from 1 (never demonstrated) to 5 (consistently demonstrated).
§Evaluated on a five-point Likert scale ranging from 1 (not at all satisfied) to 5 (completely satisfied).

Counseling

The nurse's counseling role begins with the assessment of the sleep disorder. The nurse's questions and responses provide support to the client and family as well as assurance that the sleep problems are amenable to treatment. For many clients the distress caused by chronic sleep difficulties sets up a conditioned barrier of hopelessness. Through the nurse's counseling approach this hopelessness is identified and countered with encouragement, positive suggestions, and the belief that the client will be able to manage his or her sleep difficulties.

Health Teaching

The nurse's role in health teaching cannot be overemphasized. As was mentioned at the beginning of the chapter, most individuals do not think about their sleep unless there is a problem. This means that they also do not recognize the importance of a sleep routine or consider factors that influence good sleep. In addition, there are many myths regarding what constitutes "good sleep" as well as what factors contribute to either a good night's sleep or a restless night's sleep. For instance, many people believe that 8 hours of sleep per night is normal and do not recognize that there are short sleepers and long sleepers who demonstrate quite a bit of variability in the hours of sleep obtained per night. Furthermore, many people are unaware of the normal sleep changes that occur with aging and cause themselves needless worry when these changes are noticed. The notion that a glass of wine or a couple of beers acts as a sedative is also an erroneous belief.

Although it is true that alcohol initially makes the individual feel relaxed and sleepy, it is also true that alcohol disrupts normal sleep patterns and leaves the individual awake later in the night. Refer back to Box 33-5 for educational points for teaching how to obtain a good night's sleep. The nurse may also be involved in teaching relaxation techniques such as meditation, the use of relaxation tapes, and practice of the relaxation response. Use of these techniques has been linked to sustained benefits for clients with primary insomnia (Neylan et al., 2004; Sadock & Sadock, 2004).

Psychobiological Interventions

Many clients use medication to address their sleep problems. Nurses frequently provide education about the benefits of a particular drug, the side effects, untoward effects, and the fact that medications are usually prescribed for no more than 2 weeks because tolerance and withdrawal may result (Sadock & Sadock, 2004). In many settings the nurse is also monitoring the effectiveness of the medication.

Box 33-7 lists interventions appropriate for sleep enhancement from the Nursing Interventions Classification (NIC) (Dochterman & Bulechek, 2004). These interventions are appropriate for primary insomnia as well as for all other sleep disorders.

Advanced Practice Interventions

Although psychotherapy offers little value in the treatment of primary insomnia, there is a component of primary insomnia that involves a conditioned response. The initial episode of insomnia is frequently associated

BOX 33-7

Sleep Enhancement (NIC)

Definition: Facilitation of regular sleep-wake cycles
Activities:

- Determine patient's sleep/activity pattern.
- Approximate patient's regular sleep-wake cycle in planning care.
- Explain the importance of adequate sleep during pregnancy, illness, psychosocial stresses, etc.
- Determine the effects of patient's medications on sleep pattern.
- Monitor/record patient's sleep pattern and number of sleep hours.
- Monitor patient's sleep pattern and note physical (e.g., sleep apnea, obstructed airway, pain/discomfort, and urinary frequency) and/or psychological (e.g., fear or anxiety) circumstances that interrupt sleep.
- Instruct patient to monitor sleep patterns.
- Monitor participation in fatigue-producing activities during wakefulness to prevent overtiredness.
- Adjust environment (e.g., light, noise, temperature, mattress, and bed) to promote sleep.
- Encourage patient to establish a bedtime routine to facilitate transition from wakefulness to sleep.
- Facilitate maintenance of patient's usual bedtime routines, presleep cues/props, and familiar objects (e.g., for children a favorite blanket or toy, rocking, pacifier, or story; for adults, a book to read, etc.), as appropriate.
- Assist to eliminate stressful situations before bedtime.
- Monitor bedtime food and beverage intake for items that facilitate or interfere with sleep.
- Instruct patient to avoid bedtime foods and beverages that interfere with sleep.

- Assist patient to limit daytime sleep by providing activity that promotes wakefulness, as appropriate.
- Instruct patient how to perform autogenic muscle relaxation or other nonpharmacological forms of sleep inducement.
- Initiate/implement comfort measures of massage, positioning, and affective touch.
- Promote an increase in numbers of hours of sleep, if needed.
- Provide for naps during the day, if indicated, to meet sleep requirements.
- Group care activities to minimize number of awakenings; allow for sleep cycles of at least 90 minutes.
- Adjust medication administration schedule to support patient's sleep-wake cycle.
- Instruct patient and significant other about factors (e.g., physiological, psychological, and lifestyle factors, frequent work shift changes, rapid time zone changes, excessively long work hours, and other environmental factors) that contribute to sleep pattern disturbances.
- Identify what sleep medications patient is taking.
- Encourage use of sleep medications that do not contain rapid eye movement sleep suppressor(s).
- Regulate environmental stimuli to maintain normal day-night cycles.
- Discuss with patient and family sleep-enhancing techniques.
- Provide pamphlet with information about sleep enhancement techniques.

From Dochterman, J. M., & Bulechek, G. M. (2004). *Nursing interventions classification (NIC)* (4th ed.). St. Louis, MO: Mosby.

with a stressful event or crisis that produces anxiety. This anxiety becomes associated with worry about not being able to get to sleep and leads to preoccupation with getting enough sleep. The more the client tries to sleep, the more elusive sleep becomes and the greater the client's experienced anxiety. The advanced practice nurse may be closely involved in the use of deconditioning techniques to improve sleep.

■ EVALUATION

Evaluation is based on whether or not the client experiences improved sleep quality as evidenced by decreased time to fall asleep initially, fewer nighttime awakenings, and a shorter time to get back to sleep after awakening. This evaluation is accomplished through client report and through maintenance of a sleep diary. Just as important as objective changes in the client's sleep pattern is the client's perception that there has been an improvement. The improvement may objectively be quite modest, but the client may perceive that he or she is no longer controlled by sleep

but is exerting control over sleep by changes in lifestyle and establishment of a sleep routine.

Adult Attention Deficit Hyperactivity Disorder

"When my young sons were diagnosed with ADHD by their pediatrician and a child psychologist, I had an 'Aha!' experience. A light came on in my head and within a few months, I was also diagnosed with ADHD and started multimodal treatment along with my sons. By multimodal I am speaking of a treatment approach that utilizes the resources of counseling, education, and medicine to address the client's needs. For our family, this was the first step toward more satisfying and productive lives" (Mary McDonald Richard, in Murphy & LeVert, 1995, p. x)

The experience described by Mary McDonald Richard is a common one for adults with ADHD. Many have had childhood experiences that convinced them that they were different. They may have struggled to fit in with what they saw as the "normal kids." Some may have fallen into serious trouble. The majority experienced pain from feelings of low self-esteem, anger, and frustration. Adults with ADHD, especially those who are undiagnosed and untreated, struggle with life. Some of their struggles stem directly from the disorder, and other struggles arise out of associated adjustment problems. These adults are not easily identified. Contrary to popular belief, there is no one ADHD personality profile. Adults with ADHD come in many shapes and sizes. Some are outgoing, whereas others are shy. Some are able to concentrate if they are particularly interested or excited; others find concentration difficult regardless of the circumstances. Some are extreme risk takers, whereas others pursue quiet activities. Some have poorly developed social skills, whereas others are people pleasers. Adults may have ADHD alone or in combination with other psychological conditions that often coexist with ADHD.

DIAGNOSIS

ADHD is characterized in the *DSM-IV-TR* as a disorder usually first diagnosed in infancy, childhood, or adolescence. The *DSM-IV-TR* criteria for *attention deficit hyperactivity disorder* and *attention deficit hyperactivity disorder not otherwise specified* are shown in Boxes 33-8 and 33-9. Many adults with ADHD were diagnosed with "hyperactivity" as children and received treatment until adolescence, when it was probably stopped because many professionals believed that the disorder resolved itself. This belief was supported by the fact that the hyperactive-impulsive qualities tend to diminish, whereas the inattentiveness and disorganized patterns of behavior remain constant (Goldstein, 2004a).

■ ■ ■ *VIGNETTE*

"What I had forgotten until recently was that my mother had taken me to a doctor when I was seven years old, and I'd been given medication—Ritalin, I think—for a number of

---

BOX 33-8

DSM-IV-TR Criteria for Attention Deficit Hyperactivity Disorder

A. Either (1) or (2):
  (1) Six (or more) of the following symptoms of **inattention** have persisted for at least 6 months to a degree that is maladaptive and inconsistent with developmental level:
    Inattention
    (a) Often fails to give close attention to details or makes careless mistakes in schoolwork, work, or other activities
    (b) Often has difficulty sustaining attention in tasks or play activities
    (c) Often does not seem to listen when spoken to directly
    (d) Often does not follow through on instructions and fails to finish schoolwork, chores, or duties in the workplace (not due to oppositional behavior or failure to understand instructions)
    (e) Often has difficulty organizing tasks and activities
    (f) Often avoids, dislikes, or is reluctant to engage in tasks that require sustained mental effort (such as schoolwork or homework)
    (g) Often loses things necessary for tasks or activities (e.g., toys, school assignments, pencils, books, or tools)
    (h) Is often easily distracted by extraneous stimuli
    (i) Is often forgetful in daily activities
  (2) Six (or more) of the following symptoms of **hyperactivity-impulsivity** have persisted for at least 6 months to a degree that is maladaptive and inconsistent with developmental level:

Hyperactivity
    (a) Often fidgets with hands or feet or squirms in seat
    (b) Often leaves seat in classroom or in other situations in which remaining seated is expected
    (c) Often runs about or climbs excessively in situations in which it is inappropriate (in adolescents or adults, may be limited to subjective feelings of restlessness)
    (d) Often has difficulty playing or engaging in leisure activities quietly
    (e) Is often "on the go" or often acts as if "driven by a motor"
    (f) Often talks excessively
    Impulsivity
    (a) Often blurts out answers before questions have been completed
    (b) Often has difficulty awaiting turn
    (c) Often interrupts or intrudes on others (e.g., butts into conversations or games)
B. Some hyperactive-impulsive or inattentive symptoms that caused impairment were present before age 7 years.
C. Some impairment from the symptoms is present in two or more settings (e.g., at school [or work] and at home).
D. There must be clear evidence of clinically significant impairment in social, academic, or occupational functioning.
E. The symptoms do not occur exclusively during the course of pervasive developmental disorder, schizophrenia, or other psychotic disorder and are not better accounted for by another mental disorder (e.g., mood disorder, anxiety disorder, dissociative disorder, or personality disorder).

From American Psychiatric Association. (2000). *Diagnostic and statistical manual of mental disorders* (4th ed., text rev.). Washington, DC: Author.

BOX 33-9

DSM-IV-TR Criteria for Attention Deficit Hyperactivity Disorder Not Otherwise Specified

This category is for disorders with prominent symptoms of inattention or hyperactivity-impulsivity that do not meet the criteria for attention deficit hyperactivity disorder. Examples of persons whose disorder is classified into this category include

- Individuals whose symptoms and impairment meet the criteria for *attention deficit hyperactivity disorder, predominantly inattentive type* but whose age at onset is 7 years or older.
- Individuals with clinically significant impairment who present with inattention and whose symptom pattern does not meet the full criteria for the disorder but who have a behavioral pattern marked by sluggishness, daydreaming, and hypoactivity.

Adapted from American Psychiatric Association. (2000). *Diagnostic and statistical manual of mental disorders* (4th ed., text rev.). Washington, DC: Author.

years," recalls Richard. "I don't remember anything specific about taking the drug, but I know I started going downhill in eighth grade, after they assumed I'd outgrown the hyperactivity and took away the medicine" (Murphy & LeVert, 1995, pp. 28-29).

Other adult ADHD sufferers may have experienced symptoms that went undetected; thus, they were able to compensate until the demands of adulthood overwhelmed their coping skills. The fact that coping was possible does not diminish the frustration and poor sense of self esteem experienced by the individual struggling with this disorder (Byrnes & Watkins, 2004). Still others were not diagnosed and were just considered "bad kids" with all the emotional baggage that such a label carries.

Current literature suggests that approximately 10% to 20% of adults with histories of ADHD experience few problems when moving into adult years. Approximately 60% continue to experience symptoms of ADHD that affect the social, academic, and emotional arenas of their lives. Finally, 10% to 30% exhibit serious problems, including antisocial behaviors coupled with their continued ADHD symptoms and other comorbid problems such as depression and anxiety (Goldstein, 2004b).

Diagnosis of adult ADHD is largely subjective. Many adults do not recall the specific details of their early lives. Obtaining information from relatives, spouses, or even old school records is sometimes helpful. There is no high-tech diagnostic procedure that identifies ADHD, no psychological or medical test, nor is there any confirmatory blood work. Sometimes, as

the opening quote indicates, the adult with ADHD is the parent of a child who has been diagnosed with the disorder. The parent sees himself or herself in the child and the stress of a lifetime begins to make sense—it has a name. The following vignette illustrates the freedom that comes to the adult as a result of the diagnosis.

■ ■ ■ VIGNETTE

"It surprised me how much getting the diagnosis changed the way I looked at my life," Richard confesses. "A lot of anger and frustration I'd turned in on myself dissipated. I redirected some of it at teachers who should have known better than to make a child feel so lousy about his shortcomings, whatever the cause. And some of it I redirected at the simple unfairness of the world. I realized that although I'd failed at some things in the past, I wasn't a failure. Instead of my enemy, my past became my friend" (Murphy & LeVert, 1995, pp. 30-31).

The use of self-report questionnaires, spouse reports, and parent reports are all useful in the diagnosis of adult ADHD. However, at this time no normative data are available for these questionnaires, so the evaluator must rely heavily on qualitative data derived from the client's self-report. Essential to making a diagnosis is a childhood history of ADHD symptoms or a childhood diagnosis of ADHD, as well as the client's report that inattention and disorganization are major life problems. Although restlessness and impulsivity may continue to some degree, they are not the hallmark symptoms of ADHD in the adult (Goldstein, 2004a).

Before settling on the diagnosis of adult ADHD, it is critical to rule out other possible causes. There is a high degree of co-occurrence of adult ADHD with other psychiatric disorders, including borderline personality disorder, substance abuse disorders, depression, and anxiety (Goldstein, 2004a). In fact, it is not uncommon for ADHD also to be diagnosed while a client is in treatment for another psychiatric problem. To tease out the ADHD symptoms from the symptoms of these other disorders requires great skill on the part of the psychiatric provider, because the symptoms of stress intolerance, inattention, disorganization, and impulsivity are not only extremely common but appear in quite a few psychiatric disorders (Byrnes & Watkins, 2003; Goldstein, 2004b; Murphy & LeVert, 1995).

TREATMENT

Adults with ADHD are treated with a combination of medication, cognitive therapy, and life coaching (Goldstein, 2004b). The stimulant and antidepressant medications used for children are equally effective in adults, producing a 60% to 80% response rate (Watkins, 2003).

Medication

Although the same medications used in children are also used in adults, there are some significant differences. Adults may require less of a particular medication per pound of body weight. Even though adults are generally larger than children, their kidney and liver function may not be as robust (Watkins, 2003). Furthermore, a given dose of a medication may linger in the adult's system. Adults are more likely to be taking medications to treat other medical conditions such as hypertension and diabetes. These medications may interact with the ADHD medication.

The psychostimulants, including methylphenidate (Ritalin-SR, Concerta, and Metadate CD), dexmethylphenidate (Focalin), and the amphetamines (Adderall, Adderall XR, Dexedrine, Dexedrine Spansules, and Desoxyn), constitute the cornerstone of treatment of both adult and childhood ADHD (Schatzberg & Nemeroff, 2004). Some tricyclic antidepressants, including desipramine (Norpramin), imipramine (Tofranil), amitriptyline (Elavil), and clomipramine (Anafranil), are comparable in efficacy to the psychostimulants. However, there are still individuals who respond either partially or not at all to these medications. Because of this, several second-line medications are used, including clonidine (Catapres), guanfacine (Tenex), bupropion (Wellbutrin), and pemoline (Cylert). Other medications often used for comorbid disorders or ADHD-related symptoms include the selective serotonin reuptake inhibitors (SSRIs) (e.g., fluoxetine [Prozac], sertraline [Zoloft], and others) and the mood stabilizers (lithium [Eskalith], divalproex [Depakote], and carbamazepine [Tegretol]).

Research continues on new drugs as well as new forms of older drugs. The year 2003 saw the release of two such drugs, Ritalin LA and atomoxetine (Strattera). Ritalin LA is a new formulation of methylphenidate that releases half the medication immediately and the other half slowly. Atomoxetine is an alternative for those who are unable to tolerate the psychostimulants due to irritability and weight loss (Watkins, 2003). New forms of long-acting stimulants, including a MethyPatch from Shire Pharmaceuticals, may soon be on the market. MethyPatch is a small patch worn on the skin under one's clothes. It delivers methylphenidate directly through the skin into the bloodstream. It is anticipated that, because the drug does not pass through the digestive system, smaller doses will be effective. Table 33-3 provides dosage information on the most commonly prescribed medications used to treat ADHD.

Therapy

For the adult with ADHD, therapy is essential and may take the form of cognitive-behavioral, group, and/or family therapy, as well as vocational counseling.

It is through the forum of therapy that questions long unanswered about potential, ability, and the barriers that have blocked success are resolved. For the adult with ADHD, the self, long shrouded in confusion and chaos, begins to come into focus. The understanding gained about ADHD allows the individual to reframe the past in a more positive and realistic light and to challenge internalized false beliefs such as "I am unlovable or unable to give love," "I am lazy and unmotivated," and "I am stupid." These beliefs are

TABLE 33-3

Medications Used to Treat Attention Deficit Hyperactivity Disorder

Medication (Trade Name)	How Supplied (mg)	Usual Daily Dosage Range (mg/day)	Usual Starting Dose (mg)	Maintenance Number of Doses per Day
Methylphenidate (Ritalin)	5, 10, 20 Sustained release 20	10-60	5-10 qd or bid	2-3
Methylphenidate (Concerta) (extended release)	18-36 Single dose system	18-54	18	1
Dextroamphetamine (Dexedrine)	5, 10 Elixir (5 mg/5 ml) Spansules 5, 10, 15	5-40	2.5 or 5.0 qd or bid	2-3
Amphetamine mixed salts (Adderall)	5, 10, 20, 30	5-40	2.5-5.0 qd	1-2
Atomoxetine (Strattera)	10, 18, 25, 40, 60	40-100	40	1-2
Pemoline (Cylert)	18.75, 37.5, 75.0	37.5-112.5	37.5 qd	1

Data from Wagner, K. D. (2004). Treatment of childhood and adolescent disorders. In A. F. Schatzberg & C. B. Nemeroff (Eds.), *The American Psychiatric Publishing textbook of psychopharmacology* (3rd ed., pp. 967-968). Washington, DC: American Psychiatric Publishing; Cozza, S. J., Crawford, G. C., & Dulcan, M. K. (2004). Treatment of children and adolescents. In R. E. Hales & S. C. Yudofsky (Eds.), *Essentials of clinical psychiatry* (2nd ed., p. 923). Washington, DC: American Psychiatric Publishing; and Skidmore-Roth, L. (2005). *2005 Mosby's nursing drug reference.* St. Louis, MO: Elsevier.

gradually replaced with positive beliefs and a sense of self-esteem. Once faulty thinking is corrected, new behaviors and skills, including improved time management, organizational abilities, and communication skills, are addressed.

Many adults with ADHD benefit from group therapy. The benefits go beyond the opportunity to commiserate with others who have the same diagnosis. The group setting is comparable to a laboratory in which skill-building methods can be tested and applied, coping strategies explored, and feedback provided. As valuable as group therapy is to the adult with ADHD, such groups are not widely available. However, support groups organized by associations such as Children and Adults with Attention-Deficit/Hyperactivity Disorder (CHADD) and Adults with Attention Deficit Disorder (AADD), although lacking the structure and organization of group therapy, still provide opportunities for emotional support and educational exchange, and can be an invaluable part of any treatment plan.

Family or Marriage Counseling

Living with an adult with ADHD can be extremely difficult, and in fact, sustaining healthy intimate relationships is the major challenge facing an adult with ADHD. Family or marriage counseling provides the opportunity for intimate partners and other family members to learn about the dynamics of ADHD and to begin to reframe their own feelings of hurt and frustration experienced because of behaviors that seemed to be willful, insensitive, and forgetful. In the course of therapy feelings such as blame, anger, and frustration can be gradually replaced with feelings of optimism and commitment to change.

Vocational Counseling

The employment records of many adults with ADHD tend to be erratic, characterized by short job tenures, frequent dismissals, mutual partings, and resignations. The adult with ADHD experiences more than the normal amount of personal angst in identifying an occupation that suits her or his personal abilities. However, with diagnosis and treatment, the individual notes a dramatic improvement in job skills and productivity. By enlisting the services of a vocational counselor to identify strengths and weaknesses and to help in matching occupations to skills and abilities, the individual is able to explore career options that are more sensible and satisfying.

■ ■ ■ **VIGNETTE**

Adam Hicks did his share of job jumping through his twenties. His wife was patient with him as he "found himself." When he is in his early thirties, after he forgets her birthday for the third year in a row, her patience runs out, and she gives him an ultimatum to find out why he can't keep a job and why he is disorganized, distracted, and so forgetful. Adam makes an appointment with the local mental health clinic, where he is initially interviewed by a psychiatric nurse. The nurse conducts a thorough assessment of Adam's history, his present difficulties, and his perception of his problems. Adam states, "I seem to fail at everything I do. I start out with a positive attitude and determination and almost immediately I get overwhelmed with the details. Once that happens, I sort of shut down." Although Adam seems depressed, the nurse notes that there is more than this going on. The nurse presents her findings to the psychiatric treatment team. The team recommends treatment for Adam's depression as well as additional assessment directed at the attentional issues he has identified. Adam, his wife, and his mother complete questionnaires that focus on behaviors consistent with a diagnosis of ADHD. Finally the diagnosis of adult ADHD is made. Adam is started on methylphenidate with excellent results. He also participates in a group co-led by a nurse and a clinical psychologist in which he learns organizational and time management skills. Eventually, he enlists the assistance of a vocational counselor, who administers vocational aptitude tests and recommends occupational choices that match his talents and skills. Adam has always enjoyed cooking, and pursuing the culinary arts is among the recommendations made by the vocational counselor. Adam and his wife decide that they will make the financial commitment for Adam to attend the local culinary institute. Two years later he graduates as a chef. Currently he is working as the executive chef of a large restaurant and doing well.

■ ■ ■

Application of the Nursing Process

■ ASSESSMENT

It is not uncommon for the client to come to a health care practitioner for treatment of a complaint that is unrelated to adult ADHD. For instance, a parent may bring a child into a mental health clinic or into the office of a private psychiatric provider because the parent is unable to cope with the child's behavior or the school system has recommended psychiatric evaluation of the child, or both. Another way the adult with ADHD may enter the health care system is for treatment of a co-occurring disorder such as depression, anxiety, or substance abuse. In the case of a parent initiating care for a child, the nurse's assessment includes not only the history of the child's present problem but also related family history. Frequently, it is during this initial assessment process that the parent begins to make connections between the child's present behaviors and the parent's lifelong difficulties. For many adults this begins not only their children's journey toward management of ADHD but their own healing journey as well.

In the case of a client coming for treatment of a co-occurring problem, symptoms of ADHD may not stand out in a significant manner from the symptoms of the presenting problem. Although the nurse's assessment always elicits information about difficulties the client is experiencing in interpersonal relationships and in social, educational, and occupational areas of life, such difficulties frequently accompany other disorders. There may be clues in the initial interview that there is more going on with the client than the presenting problem. The client may reveal a poor school history, early family difficulties, or patterns of failure and frustration; disorganization and distractibility are common. It is usually after the presenting problem is dealt with, however, that these issues begin to take on a life of their own and require additional assessment. This assessment usually involves the completion of self-report questionnaires as well as spouse and family questionnaires. If the client has access to early school records these can also shed light on ADHD.

Self-Assessment

In all clinical situations, it is imperative that the nurse examine personal experiences, feelings, and thoughts that might influence the care provided to a particular client. This is no less true in working with the adult with ADHD. Before diagnosis and treatment, this client may miss appointments and not follow through with treatment recommendations. Such behaviors can lead to irritation and judgment on the part of the nurse. The guiding philosophy that all behavior has meaning can help the nurse avoid negative responses and encourage further exploration regarding the reasons behind the client's behaviors.

Another issue that could influence the nurse's response is whether the nurse identifies with the client. Perhaps the nurse also has adult ADHD or has a child with ADHD. This shared experience has the potential for increasing understanding and compassion as well as for blurring the boundaries that are so necessary for the success of a therapeutic relationship.

■ NURSING DIAGNOSIS

Quite a few NANDA diagnoses are appropriate for clients with ADHD. Of course, the "related to" component of the diagnosis will differ depending on the individual client. Potential NANDA diagnoses include the following:

1. *Ineffective coping* related to inability to focus on important issues and establish priorities for action secondary to untreated symptoms of ADHD
2. *Readiness for enhanced coping* related to acceptance of diagnosis of adult ADHD and initiation of treatment
3. *Chronic low self-esteem* related to history of failure in school, in relationships, and in jobs secondary to untreated symptoms of ADHD

■ OUTCOME CRITERIA

NOC includes many outcomes appropriate for clients with adult ADHD. These include *Coping, Anxiety Self-Control, Role Performance, Decision Making,* and *Self-Concept.* However, NOC also includes *Hyperactivity Level* defined as "a severity of patterns of inattention or impulsivity in a child from 1 year through 17 years of age" (Moorhead, Johnson, & Maas, 2004, p. 315). Although this outcome is focused on the child and adolescent who may have ADHD, it includes indicators appropriate for the adult with ADHD. These indicators are evaluated on a scale from severe impairment to no impairment and include the following:

- Inattention
- Lack of active listening
- Difficulty organizing tasks
- Inability to stay "on task"
- Lack of follow-through or completion of activities
- Difficulty with tasks that require sustained mental effort
- Careless mistakes
- Frequency of losing things
- Excessive distractibility
- Excessive forgetfulness

■ PLANNING

Clients with adult ADHD are encountered in numerous settings. Nurses will provide care for these clients in medical-surgical units as well as outpatient settings, such as homes, clinics, and offices of private psychiatric providers. When these clients are encountered in the inpatient setting it is for treatment of a co-occurring diagnosis. Adult ADHD is not a primary diagnosis warranting hospitalization. Therefore, planning for care usually involves selecting interventions that can be implemented in a community setting. The client is an active participant in every aspect of the plan of care, from the decision to take medications to decisions regarding whether or not to participate in some type of therapy.

■ INTERVENTION

Basic Level Interventions

The primary interventions for the basic level psychiatric mental health nurse include counseling to enhance coping, decision making, and self-esteem; psychobiological interventions focused on medication management and teaching about the effects, side effects, and abuse potential of the various medications prescribed for ADHD; identification of appropriate community resources, including therapists and support groups that specialize in working with the adult with ADHD; and health teaching regarding strategies to deal with ADHD. Refer to Box 33-10 for useful strategies.

BOX 33-10

Tips for Managing Adult Attention Deficit Hyperactivity Disorder

Insight and Education

- Education is critical; it is important to understand attention deficit hyperactivity disorder (ADHD). Read books. Talk to professionals, Talk to other adults with ADHD.
- A coach is useful, someone who can "keep after you" with humor to assist you in organizing, staying on task, giving you encouragement. Your coach can be friend, colleague, or therapist, but preferably not your spouse.
- Encouragement is necessary to thriving.
- Realize what ADHD is *not* (i.e., conflicts with your mother, etc.).
- Realize that what you have is a neuropsychiatric condition that is genetically transmitted. It is caused by biology, by how your brain is wired. It is *not* a disease of the will or a moral failing or a weakness in character. *Always remember this.* Try as they might, many people with ADHD have trouble accepting the biological nature of ADHD.
- Listen to feedback from trusted others.
- Work on getting rid of negative feelings and thoughts.
- Try to help others with the condition.

Performance Management

- Get help establishing external structure. It is tedious to set up but it helps tremendously.
- Make frequent use of lists, color coding, reminders, notes to self, rituals, files.
- Acknowledge that inevitably there will be collapses of some projects, relationships entered into, and obligations incurred.
- Embrace challenges; many people with ADHD thrive with many challenges. Just avoid perfectionism; accept that not all challenges will pan out.
- Make deadlines.
- Break down large tasks into small tasks; attach deadlines to small parts.
- Prioritize and avoid procrastination.
- Accept fear of things going well; accept edginess when things are too easy—when there is no conflict. Avoid messing up just to make things more stimulating.
- Notice how and where you work best—in a noisy room, on the train, wrapped in three blankets, listening to music. You may find that you do your best under rather odd circumstances. Let yourself work under whatever conditions are best for you.
- Know that it is OK to do two things at once.
- Do what you are good at.
- Leave time between engagements to gather your thoughts. Transitions are difficult when you have ADHD. Mini-breaks help ease the transition.
- Keep a notepad in your car, by your bed, and in your pocketbook or jacket. You never know when a good idea will hit you or when you will want to remember something else.
- Read with a pen in hand, not only for making marginal notes or underlining, but also for writing notes on the inevitable cascade of "other" thoughts that will occur to you.

Mood Management

- Set aside time every week for just letting go.
- Recharge your batteries—take a nap, do something restful, something calm.

- Choose "good" helpful addictions such as exercise.
- Understand mood changes and ways to manage them. Know that your moods may change willy-nilly, independent of what is going on. Focus on learning to tolerate a bad mood, knowing it will pass, and learning strategies to make it pass sooner.
- Expect depression after success. People with ADHD commonly complain of feeling depressed, paradoxically, after a big success.
- Have strategies ready to deal with the inevitable blahs. Have a list of friends to call and a few videos on hand that you always enjoy. Have ready access to exercise. Have a punching bag or pillow handy if there's extra angry energy. Rehearse a few pep talks you can give yourself, such as, "You've been here before. These are the ADHD blues. They will soon pass. You are OK."
- Learn symbols, slogans, and sayings as shorthand ways of labeling and quickly putting into perspective your slip-ups, mistakes, or mood swings. When you turn left instead of turning right and take your family on a 20-minute detour, it is better to be able to say, "There goes my ADHD again" than to have a 6-hour fight over your unconscious desire to sabotage the whole trip. These are not excuses. You still have to take responsibility for your actions. It is just good to know where your actions are coming from and where they're not coming from.
- Learn how to advocate for yourself. Adults with ADHD are so used to being criticized that they are often unnecessarily defensive in putting their own case forward. Learn to get off the defensive.
- Avoid premature closure of a project, a conflict, a deal, or a conversation. Don't "cut to the chase" too often, even though you're itching to.
- Try to let the successful moment last and be remembered.
- Remember that ADHD usually includes a tendency to overfocus or hyperfocus at times. Be aware of the destructive potential of this, which is a tendency to obsess or ruminate over some imagined problem without being able to let go.
- Exercise vigorously and regularly.
- Make a good choice in a significant other. This is good advice for anyone. But it is striking how the adult with ADHD can thrive or flounder depending on the choice of mate.
- Learn to joke with yourself and others about your various symptoms, from forgetfulness, to getting lost all the time, to being tactless or impulsive. If you can be relaxed about it all and have a sense of humor, others will be much more willing to forgive you.
- Schedule activities with friends and stick to your schedule. It is crucial that you stay connected to other people.
- Find and join groups in which you are liked, appreciated, understood, and enjoyed. Conversely, don't stay long where you aren't appreciated or understood.
- Pay compliments. Notice other people. In general, get social training, as from your coach.
- Set social deadlines.

Adapted from Hallowell, E. M., & Ratey, J. J. (1992). *Adult ADHD: 50 tips on management.* Retrieved June 21, 2004, from http://www.addresources.org/article_50_tips_adult_ hallowell_ratey.php.

Advanced Practice Interventions

Many advanced practice psychiatric mental health nurses have developed a specialty in working with adults with ADHD. They may provide cognitive-behavioral therapy, lead therapy groups, provide family and/or marital counseling, and offer individual "life coaching" for clients interested in assistance in managing on a day-to-day basis.

■ EVALUATION

For the adult with ADHD, the success of treatment is measured qualitatively. The client reports improvement in areas such as self-esteem, time management and organizational skills, satisfaction with job performance, and family relationships.

Gender Identity and Sexual Disorders

The last section of this chapter deals with gender identity and sexual disorders, concepts that are increasingly viewed as essential components of a comprehensive health care approach. Traditionally, sexual concerns have not been a nursing focus. This is changing as well. It is within the purview of all nurses to assess a client's sexual practices and to be prepared to educate, dispel myths, assist with values clarification, refer to appropriate care providers when indicated, and share resources. Health promotion and disease prevention are key responsibilities for nurses. These actions alleviate or decrease client illness and suffering, and reduce health care costs. As a student of nursing, you are introduced to the complex issue of sexual behavior to facilitate thoughtful discussion of the topic and to develop personal belief systems that consider the broader perspective of sexual issues as they exist in contemporary society.

The following content provides enough knowledge about normal and abnormal human sexuality for you to conduct a sexual assessment, to explain what is meant by human sexuality and the sexual response cycle, and to enable recognition of sexual dysfunctions that can occur at different stages of the cycle. You will be able to identify deviations from normal sexual behaviors, recognize nursing implications, and formulate interventions. You will not be prepared to be a sex therapist.

All of us are aware of ourselves as sexual beings. This awareness is far broader than our awareness of lovemaking behaviors; it encompasses our views of ourselves as women and men, as mothers and fathers, as generative individuals who create and give to society in multiple ways. Multiple factors including societal attitudes and mores, parental views, cultural practices, spiritual and religious teaching, socioeconomic status, and education all greatly affect our sexual behaviors and our attitudes toward the sexual behaviors of others, including our clients. Box 33-11 provides questions to encourage sexual self-awareness.

DEFINITIONS

There is considerable confusion regarding terms such as *sex, gender identity, gender dysphoria, transsexualism,* and *sexual identity.* The term sex refers to a person's inherited biological sexual characteristics; that is, the

---

BOX 33-11

Questions to Encourage Sexual Self-Awareness

As you answer these questions, be aware of how you feel. Are you at ease? Uncomfortable? Embarrassed?

1. Am I comfortable being a woman (man)? When I consider my own sexuality, what do I mean? What behaviors and roles do I associate with my sexuality? Have I examined my own attitudes, feelings, and beliefs about sexual issues, such as
   - Gender roles.
   - Life-cycle changes, including menstruation, pregnancy, and menopause.
   - Sexually transmitted diseases, including acquired immunodeficiency syndrome.
   - All forms of sexual activity, including masturbation and self-pleasure, homosexual activity, bisexual activity, fellatio, cunnilingus, anal intercourse, sexual activity with multiple partners, nonmarital sexual activity.
   - Sexuality across the life cycle (i.e., in children, adolescents, elderly).
   - Sexuality in handicapped persons or in the mentally retarded.
   - Lubrication, orgasm, ejaculation.
   - Nudity (my own and others'), touching my own body or another's body.
   - Frequency of intercourse, positions for intercourse.
   - Abortion, contraception.
   - Talking about sexual issues, talking about sexual issues with clients.
2. As I look at my own attitudes, feelings, and beliefs, can I identify the sources of these? What part of my own attitudes, feelings, and beliefs can I attribute to my early upbringing? To my culture? To my religious beliefs? To my own sexual experiences?
3. Am I aware of what "turns me on" sexually? Conversely, what "turns me off" sexually?
4. Am I able to accept myself as a sexual human being? Am I able to accept my clients as such?
5. Am I willing to have my own beliefs challenged by learning accurate information regarding sexual issues?

From Carson, V. B. (2000). *Mental health nursing: The nurse-patient journey* (2nd ed., p. 822). Philadelphia: Saunders.

vagina, ovaries, uterus, and 46,XX karyotype or the penis, testicles, and 46,XY karyotype (Carson, 2000; Sadock & Sadock, 2004). Gender identity, the sense of maleness or femaleness, arises within the first 18 months of life. Gender identity develops along with the sense of being a self separate from mother and all others. Usually sex and gender identity are the same; that is, "I have a vagina and I am a woman," or "I have a penis and I am a man." When sex differs from gender identity, the individual suffers from gender dysphoria. Such an individual might have a physically normal female reproductive tract and yet have a sense that she is a male and might describe herself by saying, "I am a man trapped in a woman's body." This is an example of the most extreme case of gender dysphoria, called transsexualism, in which a person wishes to change his or her anatomical sexual characteristics to those of the opposite sex.

Another rare and poorly understood variant is hermaphroditism or intersexuality. In this condition, the individual is born with both ovarian and testicular reproductive tissue. Individuals with this condition have either ambiguous genitalia or genitalia that do not match the genetic makeup of the person (i.e., female genitalia in a genetically male individual). Treatment is based on the potential to correct the ambiguous genitalia rather than on the chromosomal determinants. It is easier to reconstruct female genitalia than male genitalia (*Medical encyclopedia: Hermaphroditism*, 2004).

Identification of oneself as being male or female, the appearance of traits of masculinity or femininity, and the emergence of appropriate eroticism result in the development of sexual identity. The majority of people develop a *heterosexual identity;* that is, they are attracted to members of the opposite sex. A percentage of individuals in all cultures develop a *homosexual identity,* in which a sexual preference is expressed for people of the same sex. Homosexuals can be either *ego-syntonic,* which means that the individual is emotionally comfortable with her or his sexuality, or *ego-dystonic,* which means that the individual is emotionally distressed by the same-sex attraction. Homosexual men are frequently referred to as *gay* and homosexual women as *lesbian.* Some people are not exclusively heterosexual or homosexual but are attracted to members of both sexes. These individuals are bisexual in their sexual identity (Carson, 2000).

SEXUAL RESPONSE CYCLE

To evaluate sexual dysfunction, one must have knowledge of normal sexual functioning as well as deviations from the norm. The *DSM-IV-TR* defines a four-phase response cycle: phase 1 is desire, phase 2 is excitement, phase 3 is orgasm, and phase 4 is resolution.

Desire Phase

Many factors in one's life may affect interest in sexual activity, including (but not limited to) age, physical and emotional health, availability of a sexual partner, and the context of the individual's life. In fact, for a number of individuals, the lack of sexual desire is not a source of distress either to the person or to his or her partner; in such a situation, decreased or absent sexual desire is not viewed as an illness. In general, however, hypoactive sexual desire is a challenging disorder, associated with other psychiatric or medical conditions. Conversely, excessive sexual desire becomes a problem when this creates difficulties for the individual's partner or when such excessive desire drives the person to demand sexual compliance from or force it upon unwilling partners.

Testosterone (which is normally present in the circulation of both males and females but in a much higher level in males) appears to be essential to sexual desire in both men and women. Men who, for one reason or another, have lost the ability to produce testosterone describe the change in their sexual feelings in terms such as "I still have the basic inclination for sex but do not seem to have the energy to put it into effect." In some of these men, testosterone replacement therapy appears to restore their sexual energy.

Testosterone increases interest in sexual activity in women. A serendipitous finding confirmed this when, many years ago, postmenopausal women with cancer of the breast were given testosterone to slow the rate of the cancerous growth. Many of these women reported strong and unusual interest in sexual activity, including fantasies, dreams, and urges to become sexually involved, none of which they had entertained for many prior years. Although testosterone has been used frequently to increase sexual desire in postmenopausal women, there have been no well-designed treatment outcome studies. There have, however, been many case reports such as that of Maria in the following vignette.

■ ■ ■ *VIGNETTE*

Maria is a 67-year-old woman, widowed many years, who has just been approached by a 75-year-old widower with a marriage proposal. Maria is concerned about the sexual implications of a marriage so late in life. She confides in her nurse practitioner, "I really haven't even thought about sex for so many years. I know Joe is just an old goat. He's always after me to take my clothes off." After discussing the possibility of a physiological cause for her lack of interest in sex, Maria's nurse practitioner gives her small doses of testosterone. Within a remarkably short time, Maria stops talking about Joe as "an old goat" and begins talking again about "how great life can be if you have the right partner."

■■■

Estrogen does not seem to have a direct effect on sexual desire in women. A secondary effect, however, may be present in the requirement of estrogen for the maintenance of normal vaginal distensibility and lubrication. If these functions are lost secondary to estrogen deficiency, as may occur in some postmenopausal women or in younger women who have had their ovaries removed, dyspareunia (painful coitus) and vaginismus (spasm of the vagina) may be the result. In addition to estrogen deficiency, other physical conditions, such as vaginal infections and lesions, can lead to dyspareunia and vaginismus. Once these occur, then the psychological anticipation of pain becomes a factor. At that point, the experience of painful coitus and the expectation of further coital discomfort may be hard to separate from the perceived lack of sexual desire (Carson, 2000).

In evaluating a client with a sexual desire disorder, the physical assessment, including laboratory studies, is performed before exploring psychological factors such as emotional issues, life situation, and experiences.

Excitement Phase

The excitement phase of the normal human sexual response cycle is that period of time during which sexual tension continues to increase from the preceding level of sexual desire. Traditionally, penile erection and vaginal lubrication have been used as indicators of the presence of sexual excitement. If erection or lubrication does not occur in what, for that individual, is a sexually stimulating and appropriate situation, then there has been an inhibition of sexual excitement, regardless of the causative factors.

Orgasm Phase

The orgasm phase of the human sexual response cycle is attained only at high levels of sexual tension in both women and men. Sexual tension (also described as sexual arousal) is produced by a combination of mental activity, including thought, fantasy, and dreams, and erotic stimulation of erogenous areas, which may be more or less specific for each individual. Most men require some penile stimulation and most women some clitoral stimulation, either directly or indirectly, to produce the high levels of sexual tension necessary for orgasm to occur. Orgasm may be described purely on the basis of its physical characteristics as a neurophysiological event with accompanying release of erotic tension. Orgasm is considered by most individuals who have experienced that event to be the acme of pleasure.

There is at least one major gender difference concerning orgasm: most women who have experienced one orgasm may have repeated orgasms during the continuation of the same sexual activity. The occurrence of multiple orgasms depends on the maintenance of high levels of sexual tension through continued stimulation. Men, on the other hand, once they ejaculate as a part of orgasm, go through a refractory period during which they cannot ejaculate again. The refractory period is the time required to produce another ejaculate and varies primarily with age; in a young man this refractory period is measured in minutes, whereas in an older man it may last several hours. Because women do not produce an ejaculate, they do not have a comparable refractory period. Premature ejaculation refers to the sudden release of semen with little or no penile stimulation. The inability to sustain high levels of sexual tension without ejaculating can seriously compromise the sexual act as a source of pleasure for both partners.

Resolution Phase

During the resolution phase, sexual tension developed in prior phases subsides to baseline levels provided sexual stimulation has ceased. The physiological changes that occurred during the earlier phases of the response cycle now tend to dissipate. This is a period of psychological vulnerability and either may be experienced as a period of pleasurable "afterglow" or may be described as being "uncomfortably emotionally exposed." With the restoration of normal physiological pulse, respiratory rate, and blood pressure, individuals frequently experience markedly increased perspiration.

Sexual dysfunctions are identified as occurring during three phases of the sexual response cycle: desire, excitement, and orgasm. The details of these dysfunctions are described in the following section.

SEXUAL DISORDERS

The *DSM-IV-TR* classifies sexual disorders into four categories: sexual dysfunction, gender identity disorder, paraphilias, and sexual disorder not otherwise specified.

Sexual Dysfunction

A sexual dysfunction is defined as a disturbance in the sexual response cycle or as pain on sexual intercourse (APA, 2000). Seven major classes of disorder are listed in the *DSM-IV-TR*: sexual desire disorders, sexual arousal disorders, orgasm disorders, sexual pain disorders, sexual dysfunction due to a general medical condition, substance-induced sexual dysfunction, and sexual dysfunction not otherwise specified (Box 33-12). Sexual dysfunctions can be the result of physiological problems or interpersonal conflicts or a combination of both. Stress of any kind can adversely affect sexual function (Sadock & Sadock, 2004).

BOX 33-12

Types of Sexual Dysfunction

Sexual desire disorders: These are subdivided into two classes: *hypoactive sexual desire disorder,* characterized by a deficiency or absence of sexual fantasies or desire for sexual activity, and *sexual aversion disorder,* characterized by an aversion to and avoidance of genital sexual contact with a sexual partner or by masturbation. An estimated 20% of the population has hypoactive sexual desire.

Sexual arousal disorders: These are subdivided into *female sexual arousal disorder,* characterized by persistent or recurrent partial or complete failure to attain or maintain the lubrication and swelling response of sexual excitement until the completion of the sexual act, and *male erectile disorder* (also called *erectile dysfunction* and *impotence*), characterized by the recurrent and persistent partial or complete failure to attain or maintain an erection to perform the sex act.

Orgasm disorders

Female orgasmic disorder: This is sometimes referred to as *inhibited female orgasm* or *anorgasmia* and is defined as the recurrent or persistent inhibition of female orgasm, as manifested by the recurrent delay in, or absence of, orgasm after a normal sexual excitement phase (achieved by masturbation or coitus).

Male orgasmic disorder: In male orgasmic disorder, sometimes called *inhibited orgasm* or *retarded ejaculation,* a man achieves ejaculation during coitus only with great difficulty. A man with a lifelong orgasmic disorder has never been able to ejaculate during coitus. Lifelong male orgasmic disorder indicates severe psychopathology. The disorder is diagnosed as acquired if it develops after previously normal functioning. Acquired male orgasmic disorder reflects interpersonal difficulties.

Premature ejaculation: A man persistently or recurrently achieves orgasm and ejaculation before he wishes to. Diagnosis is made when a man regularly ejaculates before or immediately after the penis enters the vagina.

Sexual pain disorders

Dyspareunia: Recurrent or persistent genital pain occurs in either men or women during or after intercourse. This condition is more common in women and is frequently associated with vaginismus.

Vaginismus: Involuntary muscle constriction of the muscles that close the vagina. This condition interferes with penile insertion and intercourse.

Sexual dysfunction due to a general medical condition: This category includes sexual desire disorders, orgasm disorders, and sexual pain disorders, but the cause of each is related to a medical condition such as cardiovascular, neurological, or endocrine disease.

Substance-induced sexual dysfunction: This diagnosis is used when evidence of substance intoxication or withdrawal is apparent from the history, physical examination, or laboratory findings. Distressing sexual dysfunction occurs within a month of significant substance intoxication or withdrawal. Specified substances include alcohol, amphetamines or related substances, cocaine, opioids, sedatives, hypnotics, anxiolytics, and other known and unknown substances. Abused recreational substances can have a variety of effects on sexual functioning. In small doses many substances enhance sexual performance. With continued use sexual difficulties become the norm.

Sexual dysfunction not otherwise specified: This category covers sexual dysfunctions that cannot be classified under one of the other categories. Examples include the experience of physiological sexual excitement and orgasm but with no erotic sensation or even with anesthesia. Women with a condition similar to premature ejaculation are classified as having this disorder. Disorders of excessive, rather than inhibited, sexual dysfunction, such as compulsive masturbation or coitus (sex addiction) or genital pain occurring during masturbation may be classified in this category.

Adapted from American Psychiatric Association. (2000). *Diagnostic and statistical manual of mental disorders* (4th ed., text rev.). Washington, DC: Author; and Sadock, B. J., & Sadock, V. A. (2004). *Kaplan & Sadock's concise textbook of clinical psychiatry* (2nd ed.). Philadelphia: Lippincott Williams & Wilkins.

Gender Identity Disorder

Gender identity disorder is defined as strong and persistent cross-gender identification (Sadock & Sadock, 2004). Little is known about the origins of gender identity disorder, but childhood patterns seem to be fairly consistent. As early as 2 to 4 years of age some children may have cross-gender interests and activities. However, only a small percentage of children who display gender identity disorder characteristics will continue to show these characteristics into adolescence or adulthood. Typically, children who become transsexual relate better to members of the sex opposite to their biological sex. Boys prefer female friends and activities and cross-dress whenever possible. Girls imitate what they consider masculine behavior and refuse to be involved in activities usually assigned to females.

At puberty, the individual is greatly concerned and often self-conscious about the physical changes taking place; this is not true for most homosexuals. About 75% of boys who had a childhood history of gender identity disorder report a homosexual or bisexual orientation. The remainder of these young men report a heterosexual orientation (APA, 2000). The corresponding percentages for women are not known. People with gender identity disorder continue to prefer the opposite-sex behavioral style into adulthood; often, they come to desire sexual reassignment as they find partners whom they wish to live with or marry. These individuals never consider themselves to be homosexual. The biological female who falls in love with a woman believes herself actually to be a man who loves that woman. Thus, a desire for congruity in gender identity and physiology becomes important for many individuals.

Adults with gender identity disorder seek various solutions when they suffer from gender dysphoria. Some people seek help in suppressing their cross-gender feelings, others want more information, and still others seek surgery to accomplish sex reassignment. When gender dysphoria is severe and intractable, sex reassignment may be the best solution. If the client is considered appropriate for sex reassignment, psychotherapy is usually initiated to prepare the client for the cross-gender role. The client is then instructed to go out into the world and live in the cross-gender role before surgery is performed. This includes going to work or attending school to help the client determine if he or she can interact successfully with members of society in the cross-gender mode. Legal and social arrangements are made: the name is changed on various documents, and new employment is obtained if it is necessary to leave a former job because of discrimination. Relationship issues, such as what to tell parents, children, and former spouses, must be resolved. Males are instructed to have electrolysis and practice female behaviors. Females are instructed to cut their hair, bind or conceal their breasts, and similarly take on the identity of a man.

After 1 or 2 years, if these measures have been successful and the client still wishes reassignment, hormone treatment is begun—males take estrogen and females take androgen. After another 1 to 2 years of hormone therapy, the client may be considered for surgical reassignment if this is still desired. In the male-to-female client, the procedure consists of bilateral orchiectomy, penile amputation, and creation of an artificial vagina. Female-to-male clients undergo bilateral mastectomy and optional hysterectomy with removal of the ovaries. Efforts to create an artificial penis have met with mixed results. Psychotherapy is indicated after surgery to help the client adjust to the surgical changes and discuss sexual functioning and satisfaction (Becker & Johnson, 2004).

Paraphilias

People do not decide voluntarily what arouses them sexually. Rather, in maturing, they discover the nature of their own sexual orientation and interests. Individuals differ from one another in terms of

- The types of partners whom they find to be erotically appealing.
- The types of behaviors that they find to be erotically stimulating.

They also differ in the intensity of the sexual drive, in the degree of difficulty that they experience in trying to resist sexual temptations, and in their attitudes about whether or not such temptations should be resisted. The sexual disorders include many forms of paraphilia, a term used to identify repetitive or preferred sexual fantasies or behaviors that involve preference for the use of a nonhuman object, repetitive sex-

ual activity with humans involving real or simulated suffering or humiliation, and repetitive sexual activity with nonconsenting partners. Most paraphiliacs are men, and in about 50% of these individuals the onset of the paraphiliac arousal is before age 18 years (APA, 2000). Currently, the following are considered unusual enough to be called paraphilias: fetishism, pedophilia, exhibitionism, voyeurism, transvestic fetishism, sexual sadism and masochism, and frotteurism. Paraphilia not otherwise specified is also a *DSM-IV-TR* category.

Fetishism is characterized by a sexual focus on objects such as shoes, gloves, pantyhose, and stockings that are intimately associated with the human body. The particular fetish is linked to someone involved with the client during childhood and thus is invested with a quality associated with this loved, needed, or even traumatizing person (APA, 2000; Sadock & Sadock, 2004).

Pedophilia involves sexual activity with a prepubescent child (generally 13 years or younger). Because pedophilia is illegal, its incidence is unknown. For the definition of pedophilia to be met, the perpetrator must be at least 16 years of age and at least 5 years older than the victim (Sadock & Sadock, 2004). The nature of the child molestation is generally genital fondling or oral sex. Vaginal or anal penetration is uncommon except in cases of incest. A significant number of pedophiles have previous or current involvement in exhibitionism, voyeurism, or rape (Sadock & Sadock, 2004).

Exhibitionism is the intentional display of the genitals in a public place. Sometimes the individual masturbates while exposing himself. Although exhibitionism is illegal, it seems to be done more for shock value than as a preamble to sexual assault or rape. Almost 100% of cases of exhibitionism involve a man exposing himself to a woman. Voyeurism is the viewing of other people in intimate situations (e.g., naked, in the process of disrobing, or engaging in sexual activity). Voyeurs are also called *peeping Toms.*

In **transvestic fetishism,** sexual satisfaction is achieved by dressing in the clothing of the opposite gender. This behavior is related to fetishism but often goes beyond the use of one particular object. Generally this behavior develops early in life. Unlike in gender identity disorders, there are no sexual orientation issues, and transvestites do not desire a sex change. Transvestites are usually heterosexual, many cross-dress only in specific sexual situations, and they often receive the cooperation and support of their partners. This paraphilia is more common in men than in women. Over time, some men as well as some women with transvestic fetishism desire to dress and live permanently as the opposite sex.

Sexual sadism involves the achievement of sexual satisfaction from the physical or psychological suffering (including humiliation) of the victim. The sadist inflicts pain and suffering on nonconsenting persons.

Sexual masochism involves the achievement of sexual satisfaction by being humiliated, beaten, bound, or otherwise made to suffer. Sexual masochistic practices are more common among men than among women (Sadock & Sadock, 2004).

Frotteurism is characterized by a man's rubbing his penis against the buttocks or other body parts of a fully clothed woman to achieve orgasm. This behavior usually occurs in busy public places, particularly in subways and buses, where the individual can escape after touching his victim (APA, 2000; Sadock & Sadock, 2004).

Paraphilia not otherwise specified includes various paraphilias that do not meet the criteria for the other categories. Included in this grouping are the following:

Telephone scatologia—obscene phone calling to an unsuspecting person

Internet sex—the use of interactive computer networks to sometimes compulsively send obscene messages by electronic mail or to transmit sexually explicit messages and video images

Necrophilia—obsession with having a sexual encounter with a cadaver

Partialism—a concentration of sexual activity on one part of the body to the exclusion of all other parts

Zoophilia—incorporation of animals into sexual activity

Urophilia—sexual activity that involves urinating on one's partner or being urinated on

Hypoxyphilia—desire to achieve an altered state of consciousness secondary to hypoxia while experiencing orgasm; a drug such as nitrous oxide may be used to produce hypoxia

Many of the people involved in nonstandard sexual practices find no need for therapy because their sexual activities are carried out with a consenting adult partner and they are neither illegal nor physically or emotionally harmful to either partner. If, however, the person is experiencing relationship difficulties, wishes to change the sexual behaviors, becomes involved in illegal activity, or is physically or emotionally harming others or being harmed, therapy is indicated.

The usual treatment design for working with clients with paraphilias is cognitive and behavioral therapy. An attempt is made to help the person learn a new sexual response pattern that will eliminate the need for the activity that is causing the problem. Techniques range from positive reinforcement for appropriate object choices to aversion techniques, in which mild electric shocks may be applied for inappropriate choices. Other treatment modalities include psychodynamic techniques designed to help the client understand the origin of the paraphilia. Psychotropic agents may also be used to treat clients whose practices are acutely or dangerously compulsive. Regardless of the treatment employed (pharmacological, cognitive, behavioral,

dynamic, or a combinations of these), it is unlikely to be effective unless extended over a very long period (Sadock & Sadock, 2004).

Other Sexual Problems

Sexual problems can also result from head trauma, chromosomal abnormalities, and psychosis.

Sexual Problems Resulting from Head Trauma

Clients who have experienced head trauma with damage to the frontal lobe of the brain may display symptoms of promiscuity, poor judgment, inability to recognize triggers that set off sexual desires, and poor impulse control.

Sexual Problems Resulting from Chromosomal Abnormalities

In Klinefelter's syndrome, a condition identified through genetic analysis, the client has an extra X chromosome in his genetic makeup instead of the normal XY genetic coding for the male. These clients frequently come for treatment with immature genitalia and show schizophrenic symptoms.

Sexual Problems Resulting from Psychosis

Sexual functioning may be adversely affected any time there is a disturbance in an individual's ability to develop and maintain stable relationships. This is especially true for clients with schizophrenia, who show difficulty coping with stress, a decrease in reality-based orientation to the world, and defense mechanisms that lead to withdrawn behavior.

■ ■ ■ ***VIGNETTE***

Josephine is admitted for inpatient psychiatric care after treatment on a medical unit for injuries sustained when she is struck by a car while wandering in the street. Josephine is well known to the staff and has had many previous hospital admissions to stabilize her schizophrenia. Referral to a community mental health center was not successful. Josephine did not return for treatment after the last discharge. However, she had been doing fairly well until 3 weeks before the automobile accident, when her purse containing her medication was stolen. Instead of going to the health center to get a new prescription, she went to a bar and drank heavily. This pattern continued for 3 weeks, during which time the auditory hallucinations that Josephine had experienced in the past returned.

Josephine heard a male voice telling her she was God's gift to men. These hallucinations, coupled with the effects of her heavy alcohol intake, led her into promiscuous behavior, soliciting sex with men in bars and proclaiming that she was doing "the Lord's work." Josephine's behavior put her into conflict with bar owners, and frequently she was asked to leave. On the night of the accident, after such an episode,

Josephine ran out of the bar and into the street and was hit by a passing car. She fell to the pavement complaining of leg pain. An ambulance brought her to the hospital, and x-ray examination showed that her leg was not broken. She was fully conscious and oriented but had no recall of the accident. The mental status examination revealed auditory hallucinations consisting of commands to share herself with men and become "the mother of the earth."

In the psychiatric unit, a review of Josephine's prior admissions shows that fluphenazine (Prolixin) has been effective in controlling her symptoms of schizophrenia. A treatment plan is formulated to start Josephine on oral fluphenazine and later change to fluphenazine decanoate (administered intramuscularly) to ensure better compliance. Hospital staff contact the mental health center that will follow up on Josephine's progress, and the center approves of the plan. Josephine accepts the plan because she is afraid that she will come to harm again and because she trusts the staff.

The challenge to the nursing staff is to prevent Josephine from engaging in inappropriate sexual behavior while the hallucinations are still present. To facilitate this goal, female nurses care for Josephine whenever possible. When male nurses are assigned to care for Josephine, they set limits with her when she becomes seductive. Another intervention to reduce the risk of inappropriate sexual behavior is to place Josephine in a room near the nurse's station, for closer monitoring. If these measures are not adequate, Josephine will be placed on close observation status (one nurse assigned to stay near Josephine at all times).

The policy on the unit is to monitor the hall during the night so that clients do not have access to the rooms of other clients. In addition, all clients are informed on admission that visiting in the rooms of other clients is not allowed. The unit rule also states that physical contact between clients is against policy and will result in discharge.

Because Josephine's sexually inappropriate behavior is driven by her command hallucinations, the staff expects that, as the hallucinations resolve, the behavior will stop. Because compliance with an oral medication regimen has been a problem for Josephine, the staff expects that the change in the form of Josephine's medication will result in improved compliance.

Other issues of concern to the nurses are the client's lack of "safer sex" practices, her failure to use birth control, her lack of information about sex, and her need for screening for sexually transmitted diseases. At a point when Josephine is able to hold a conversation free from the effects of her thought disorder, the staff initiate discussions with her about these issues. They provide Josephine with a referral to the gynecological clinic while she is still hospitalized.

The last issue of concern to the nurses is Josephine's self-esteem. As Josephine's symptoms abate, the behaviors that she had exhibited during her illness become a source of great embarrassment to her. The nurses respond to Josephine's embarrassment by being supportive, by being good listeners, and by encouraging her. The nurses frequently remind Josephine that her behaviors were symptoms of an illness—not manifestations of a character weakness.

The client with schizophrenia may experience an alteration in sexual drive only during the acute phase of illness or it may be ongoing. This could depend partly on the severity of the illness. In addition, clients with chronic schizophrenia have difficulty communicating their needs and concerns to others. For the client with schizophrenia, self-concept and ego strength deteriorate over time, further decreasing the client's ability to develop or maintain intimate relationships.

Schizophrenia is not necessarily associated with sexual dysfunction or deviant sexual behavior, but the symptoms of schizophrenia and even the treatment with neuroleptic medications may make the client vulnerable to disturbances in sexual functioning and often cause the client to be childlike and passive in relationships. The primary goal of the treatment team while the client is hospitalized is the control of acute symptoms. Sometimes the acute symptoms present as delusions. These delusions can be sexual, or they can be of a paranoid type that drives the client away from meaningful relationships and produces a sexual problem because of the resulting alienation. Delusions may also be of a grandiose nature, so that the client believes himself or herself to be a great lover or have a "special mission" of a sexual nature.

Sexually inappropriate or dangerous behaviors that have a delusional origin are noted during the initial psychiatric assessment. Even if the client does not initially share these thoughts, their presence could be recognized later in treatment as the nurse develops rapport with the client. Most clients respond to treatment with neuroleptic medications, and the inappropriate sexual behaviors resolve as the delusions subside. A client who does not have primarily sexual delusions may, in the course of the hospitalization, be willing to discuss issues of daily living that might include relationships and sexuality. A third type of client with schizophrenia may be admitted for control of acute symptoms but may also have a sexual problem that is not associated with the primary diagnosis. This problem may be detected through the client's self-report, the physician's physical examination, or the nursing assessment.

Some sexual problems require immediate interventions, such as alleviating the sexual symptoms caused by side effects of medications or controlling inappropriate sexual behavior. Other sexual problems are better managed through interventions identified in the long-term outcomes. These might include helping the client with schizophrenia to develop social skills that increase the probability of forming relationships. This may be accomplished by referring the client to a psychosocial rehabilitation program. Some sexual problems can be remedied by achieving short-term outcomes that use education as a nursing intervention. Frequently, sexual myths and misinformation can be corrected, which gives the client almost instant relief from perceived problems. For instance, some people continue to believe that there is a connection between masturbation and becoming "crazy." All clients can benefit from an assessment of their sexual knowledge. Sexual hygiene, methods of birth control, and sexual health are important issues, as is the client's understanding of sexual anatomy and physiology. Although these topics may not be the initial focus of nursing interventions, they become important at some point in the course of the hospitalization. The nurse assesses the client's sexual functioning and offers information when indicated. All clients on a psychiatric inpatient unit should be informed on admission about unit rules regarding personal contact between clients and between clients and staff. Limit setting is done consistently when indicated.

Application of the Nursing Process

■ ASSESSMENT

The sexual assessment includes both subjective and objective data. Many psychiatric hospitals use a nursing history tool that is biologically oriented but may have a few questions on sexual functioning. Health history questions pertaining to the reproductive system may be limited to menstrual history, parity, history of sexually transmitted diseases, method of contraception, and questions regarding "safer sex" practices. There may be some vague questions about sexual functioning or sexual concerns. Many nurses experience discomfort exploring sexual issues with clients, fearing that this discussion will be personally embarrassing as well as embarrassing to the client. Nurses may fear that they will not know what questions to ask or why the questions should be asked. Clients may sense the nurse's discomfort with the topic, or they may also be uncomfortable when discussing sexual issues.

Guidelines for Conducting a Sexual Assessment

The sexual history captures not only the client's physiological functioning, but also behavioral, emotional, and spiritual aspects of sexuality. It also includes cultural and religious beliefs with regard to sexual behavior and sexual knowledge base. During the assessment, both the nurse and the client are free to ask questions and to clarify information. It is reasonable to defer lengthy sexual health assessment when acute psychiatric symptoms preclude a calm, thoughtful discussion. As symptoms subside and rapport is developed, the assessment may be resumed. With experience, the nurse is able to identify those clients who are

at a greater risk for difficulties in sexual functioning. Key groups include clients with a history of medical problems such as diabetes, multiple sclerosis, myocardial infarction, Parkinson's disease, or epilepsy, or a history of surgical procedures (Sadock & Sadock, 2004); clients requiring maintenance medications (Sadock & Sadock, 2004); and clients who are experiencing relationship difficulties.

The initial sexual assessment may be a basic screening to detect areas of concern. It can be incorporated into the general physical assessment, which includes questions of a demographic nature, such as age, sex, marital status, religion, and educational level. The review of systems may reveal medical diagnoses that may affect sexual functioning. The reproductive history is a logical place in history taking to introduce nonthreatening questions of a sexual nature. In the psychiatric setting, many clients have illnesses that prevent them from developing relationships, yet they still have a need for sexual expression. A complete sexual assessment includes questions about the client's family, relationship between the parents, acquisition of sexual information (both formal and informal), gender roles, toilet training history, and attitudes about sexuality and sexual expression.

An important issue to explore is the relationship of spirituality or religious belief to sexuality. An individual may experience acute spiritual distress related to his or her choice of sexual expression. This distress may originate in religious dogma or tenets of moral behavior. Imagine the spiritual distress of a prominent religious leader accused of being a pedophile. The significance and meaning of sexuality to the individual is far reaching and is as important to understanding the individual's journey as are the physical and psychological aspects of the assessment.

Settings for a Sexual Assessment

Conducting a sexual interview requires a setting that allows privacy and eliminates distractions. Although note taking may be necessary for the beginner, it can be distracting to the client and can interrupt the flow of the interview. When note taking is necessary, it should be unobtrusive and kept to a minimum. The interview is conducted free from personal biases and judgmental attitudes that could block open discussion of sexual issues. Good eye contact, relaxed posture, and friendly facial expressions facilitate the client's comfort and communicate openness and receptivity on the part of the nurse.

Conducting the Interview

The interview begins with an introduction by the nurse, followed by an explanation of the purpose of the sexual assessment. The client is informed that confidentiality is strictly maintained. Questions proceed from least intrusive to more intrusive. The interview should be efficient but not hurried. The nurse uses a directive approach for gathering objective data that are less personal, whereas a less directive approach works well for more personal disclosure, allowing the client to freely express feelings and beliefs. Accepted medical terminology is used when discussing sexual issues, but the nurse must also have knowledge of commonly used slang expressions to understand what the client is saying. Through the use of medically correct terminology, the therapeutic relationship is maintained, and the client learns a way of communicating that is less embarrassing. Table 33-4 presents some common slang and colloquial expressions related to sexuality and the corresponding medical terms. It might be helpful to share this information with clients.

Throughout the interview, it is important to note the client's body language. Decreased eye contact, fidgeting, turning away from the interviewer, and hesitancy in answering questions may indicate an area of concern for the client. Box 33-13 lists client cues that may indicate concerns about sexuality.

At this point, the nurse may choose to ask the client if there is discomfort in the area of sexual functioning. Generally, it is more comfortable for the client if the nurse firsts asks questions in a general manner and then proceeds to the client's experience. For example: "Some people who are prescribed this medication find it difficult to achieve an erection. Have you had this problem?" This allows the client to feel that he or she is not alone in what he or she is experiencing. Table 33-5 provides facilitative statements for the interviewer conducting a sexual assessment. Table 33-6 provides some interviewing do's and don'ts to follow when obtaining sexual information.

Self-Assessment

When making judgments regarding sexual behavior, the nurse must appreciate the state of mind that contributed to the individual's behavior. Inappropriate sexual behaviors can occur for a variety of reasons. For example, a person with schizophrenia may behave in a particular way in response to hallucinations, whereas the alcoholic's behavior may be a reflection of diminished judgment secondary to intoxication. A mentally retarded client may become involved with a child (who may be of the same approximate mental age as the client) because of the lack of availability of adult partners and the lack of capacity to appreciate and understand fully the wrongful nature of his or her actions.

TABLE 33-4

Some Common Slang and Colloquial Expressions Related to Sexuality

Medical Term	Slang and Colloquial Expressions
Breasts	Tits, sacks, front, headlights, knockers, boobs, bosom, bonkers, bust, jugs, buds
Climax	Come, go off, shoot cream, blast off
Clitoris	Bedfellow, little gem, badge of shame, gaiety, madness, narrow strip
Cunnilingus	Eating it, going down, eating pussy
Erection	Hard-on, stiff, bone, boner, hot rocks, lover's nuts
Fellatio	Going down, sucking, blowing, getting a blow job, giving head, cocksucking
Homosexual	*Male:* Fairy, fag, faggot, gay, queen, nellie, homo, swish, pervert, pansy, back door artist *Female:* Lez, sister, lesbo, dyke, bull dyke
Hymen	Cherry, membrane, maidenhead
Impotence	Couldn't get it up, couldn't get a hard-on
Intercourse, coitus	Make love, screw, fuck, get down, ball, make it, get laid, mess around, score, bang, jive, frig, get a piece, sleep with, get some tail, hook up
Masturbation	Jacking off, jerking off, pocket pod, hand fuck, circle jerk, beat the meat, hand job
Menstruation	Curse, monthly period, devil's making ketchup, red-bearded cousin from the South, the flag's up, on the rag
Mutual oral-genital stimulation	Sixty-nine
Orgasm	Come, climax
Penis	Joystick, worm, dick, prick, stick, peter, rod, john, third leg, middle leg, joint, glans, cock, organ, thing
Pubic hair	Beaver, bush, pubes
Semen	Come, juice, egg white, gizzum
Sexual choice	Straight (heterosexual), gay (homosexual), AC-DC (bisexual)
Sexual desire	Horny, cold fish (decreased libido), nympho (increased libido)
Testes	Balls, nuts
Vagina	Pussy, hole, cunt, cat, pocketbook, treasure, twat, furburger, box, beaver, snatch, tunnel

Adapted from Green, R. (1975). *Human sexuality: A practitioner's text.* Baltimore: Williams & Wilkins.

BOX 33-13

Client Cues That May Indicate Concerns About Sexuality

Nonverbal Behaviors
- Showing discomfort by blushing, looking away, making tight fists, fidgeting, crying
- Openly engaging in overt sexual behaviors (e.g., touching own body parts, masturbating, exposing genitals, placing nurse's hand on genitals, making sexually suggestive sounds)

Verbal Behaviors
- Telling sexually explicit jokes
- Making sexual comments about the nurse
- Asking inappropriate questions about the nurse's sexual activity
- Discussing sexual exploits
- Asking the nurse to perform sexual acts
- Expressing concern about relationship with partner:
  "I don't feel the same about my partner."
  "My partner doesn't feel the same about me."
  "We're not as close."
  "Our relationship is changed."
  "My personal life has changed."
- Expressing concern that sexuality has been diminished (e.g., feeling less of a man, less of a woman):
  "I've lost my manhood."
  "I'm not as desirable as I once was."
- Expressing concern over lack of sexual desire:
  "I'm not horny anymore."
  "My desire has changed."
  "I'm not the man (woman) I used to be."
  "We don't click anymore."
- Expressing concern over sexual performance:
  "I don't get wet."
  "I've lost my power."
  "Will I still be able to get hard?"
  "What will happen to my ability to perform?"
  "I can't perform like I used to."
- Expressing concern about one's love life:
  "My love life has changed."
  "The spark has worn off."
- Expressing concern over the sexual impact of drugs, surgery, or some other medical treatment:
  "Will this drug interfere with my sex life?"
  "Will I still be able to perform sexually after surgery?"

TABLE 33-5

Facilitative Statements for the Interviewer Conducting a Sexual Assessment

Purpose	Facilitative Statement
To provide a rationale for a question	"As a nurse, I'm concerned about all aspects of your health. Many individuals have concern about sexual matters, especially when they are sick or when they are having other health problems."
To give statements of generality or normality	"Most people are hesitant to discuss . . ." "Many people worry about feeling . . ." "Many people have concerns about . . ."
To identify sexual dysfunction	"Most people have difficulties sometime during their sexual relationships. What have yours been?"
To obtain information	"The degree to which unmarried persons have sexual outlets varies considerably. Some have sexual partners. Others have none. Some relieve sexual tension through masturbation. Others need no outlet at all. What has been your pattern?"
To identify sexual myths	"While growing up, most of us have heard some sexual myths or half-truths that continue to puzzle us. Are there any that come to mind?"
To identify feelings about masturbation	"Many of us grown-ups have heard a variety of stories about masturbation and what problems it supposedly causes. This can cause worry even into adulthood. What have you heard?"
To determine whether homosexuality is a source of conflict	"Some say homosexuality is a mental disorder, others an emotional block, others a crime or sin, and still others view homosexuality as just an alternative lifestyle. What is your attitude toward your homosexual orientation?"
To identify an older person's concerns about sexual function	"Many people, as they get older, believe or worry that this signals the end of their sex life. Much misinformation continues this myth. What is your understanding about sexuality during the later years? How has the passage of time affected your sexuality (sex life)?"
To obtain and give information (miscellaneous areas)	"Frequently people have questions about . . ." "What questions do you have about . . ." "What would you like to know about . . ."
To close the history	"Is there anything further in the area of sexuality that you would like to bring up now? I hope that if questions or concerns do come to mind in the future we'll be able to discuss them."

Adapted from Green, R. (1975). *Human sexuality: A health practitioner's text.* Baltimore: Williams & Wilkins.

Do's and Don'ts When Obtaining Sexual Information

Do	Don't
Obtain information about all areas of need.	Focus only on sexuality.
	Obtain information when others are present or take copious notes.
Strive for an unhurried atmosphere.	Check your watch.
	Tap your foot.
Maintain an attitude that is frank, open, warm, objective, empathetic.	Project discomfort.
	Become defensive.
Use nondirective techniques when possible.	Ask many direct questions.
Have a prepared introduction to the stated purpose of interview.	Be vague about the purpose of interview.
Use appropriate vocabulary.	Use street terms.
"Check out" words to ensure that the client understands.	Assume the client understands what you're saying.
Adjust the order of questions according to the client's needs.	Follow a rigid form.
Give the client time to think and answer questions.	Answer questions for the client.
Recognize signs of anxiety.	Focus on getting information without recognizing the client's feelings.
Give permission not to do something.	Have preset expectations of the client's sexual activity.
Listen in an interested but matter-of-fact way.	Overreact or underreact.
Identify your attitudes, values, beliefs, and feelings.	Project your concerns or problems onto the client.
Identify significant others.	Assume that no one else is involved in the client's sexual concerns.
Identify philosophical, religious beliefs of the client.	Impose your moral judgments on the client.
Acknowledge when you don't have an answer to a question.	Pretend you know when you don't.

From Hogan, R. (1980). *Human sexuality: A nursing perspective* (p. 246). New York: Appleton-Century-Crofts.

It is also important when discussing sexual deviations to differentiate between an individual's sexual orientation and interest and the individual's temperament and traits of character, such as kindness versus cruelty, caring versus noncaring, sensitivity versus insensitivity, conscientiousness versus lack of conscience, and so on. Imagine the emotional and spiritual distress experienced by a pedophile who is unhappy with his sexual orientation. A person diagnosed with a sexual disorder may be a more concerned person dealing less than successfully with sexual temptations of a sort that are foreign to most individuals.

It is easy for a person who is not tempted by inappropriate sexual thoughts or behaviors to argue that any sex offender could have stopped the behavior if the person really wanted to and would simply make up his or her mind to do so. When it comes to appetites or drives such as hunger, thirst, pain, the need for sleep, or sex, however, biological regulatory systems may exist that can cause an individual to experience desires that cannot be successfully resisted by willpower alone.

One of the major issues in trying to understand human behavior relates to where to draw the line between considering a person to be the passive product of life experiences and biological makeup and considering him or her (by virtue of having subjective consciousness) to be an active agent capable of transcending previous determinants.

■ NURSING DIAGNOSIS

A comprehensive sexual assessment reveals areas of sexual concern and dysfunction for the client. These data are analyzed to determine the appropriate nursing diagnoses. Sample nursing diagnoses are as follows:

1. *Sexual dysfunction* related to marital problems evidenced in painful intercourse and inability to have orgasm
2. *Ineffective sexuality pattern* related to personal conflicts about sexual preferences evidenced by expressed desire to be the opposite gender

■ OUTCOME CRITERIA

NOC identifies a number of outcomes for clients with either sexual dysfunction or ineffective sexuality patterns. Included are *Abuse Recovery: Sexual; Risk Control: Sexually Transmitted Disease (STD); Sexual Functioning; Sexual Identity; Body Image; Role Performance;* and *Self-Esteem.* Table 33-7 provides selected intermediate and short-term indicators for *Sexual Identity* and *Sexual Functioning.*

■ PLANNING

Sometimes clients with sexual problems are seen as inpatients. They may be admitted for a primary diagnosis such as schizophrenia with sexual problems secondary to the psychotic process. In addition, there are

TABLE 33-7

NOC Outcomes for Sexual Dysfunction

Nursing Outcome and Definition	Intermediate Indicators	Short-Term Indicators
Sexual Functioning: Integration of physical, socioemotional, and intellectual aspects of sexual expression and performance*	Expresses ability to perform sexually despite physical imperfections Expresses comfort with sexual expression	Attains sexual arousal Adapts sexual technique as needed Sustains penile or clitoral erection through orgasm
Sexual Identity: Acknowledgment and acceptance of own sexual identity*	Sets resilient boundaries with respect to societal prejudice or discrimination Reports healthy sexual functioning	Affirms self as a sexual being Exhibits clear sense of sexual orientation Seeks support of peers

From Moorhead, S., Johnson, M., & Maas, M. (2004). *Nursing outcomes classification (NOC)* (3rd ed.). St. Louis, MO: Mosby.
*Evaluated on a five-point Likert scale from 1 (never demonstrated) to 5 (consistently demonstrated).

specialty units that focus solely on the treatment of clients with sexual disorders. However, most clients will be encountered in outpatient and community settings, and will come for treatment with a sexual disorder sometimes as a primary concern and other times as a secondary concern. The nurse must plan to respond to the client's sexual issues wherever they are seen.

▪ INTERVENTION

Basic Level Interventions

Although most nurses will never be sex therapists, all nurses need to be able to facilitate a discussion with the client about sexuality. To be a facilitator, the nurse must be nonjudgmental, have basic knowledge of sexual functioning, and have the ability to conduct a basic sexual assessment. Once the assessment is completed, the nurse needs to know when and to whom to refer the client with a sexual complaint. Depending on the nature of the problem, the client may need a referral to a professional such as a marital counselor, psychiatrist, gynecologist, urologist, clinical nurse specialist, or pastoral counselor.

Many nursing interventions were already discussed when specific deviations were considered. Appropriate strategies at the basic level include milieu therapy, counseling, education, behavioral therapy, and medication. Box 33-14 provides sample interventions from NIC for *Sexual Counseling.*

Generally, medication is not used independently as a treatment without other interventions. The drugs that are frequently used in treating sexual deviations are progestin derivatives, including medroxyprogesterone acetate (MPA) and cyproterone acetate (CPA). Both of these drugs act to decrease libido and break the individual's pattern of compulsive deviant sexual behavior. They work best in clients with paraphilias and a high sexual drive, such as pedophiles and exhibitionists, and less well in those with a low sexual drive or an antisocial personality (Becker & Johnson, 2004).

BOX 33-14

NIC Interventions for Sexual Counseling

Definition: Use of an interactive helping process focusing on the need to make adjustments in sexual practice or to enhance coping with a sexual event or disorder
Activities:
- ▪ Establish a therapeutic relationship, based on trust and respect.
- ▪ Provide privacy and ensure confidentiality.
- ▪ Discuss the effect of the illness or health situation on sexuality.
- ▪ Discuss the effect of medications on sexuality, as appropriate.
- ▪ Avoid displaying aversion to an altered body part.
- ▪ Provide factual information about sexual myths and misinformation that patient may verbalize.
- ▪ Provide reassurance that current and new sexual practices are healthy, as appropriate.
- ▪ Include the spouse/sexual partner in the counseling as much as possible, as appropriate.
- ▪ Refer patient to a sex therapist as appropriate.

From Dochterman, J. M., & Bulechek, G. M. (2004). *Nursing interventions classification (NIC)* (4th ed.). St. Louis, MO: Mosby.
*Partial list.

Current research is focusing on the use of SSRIs in the treatment of sexual disorders. Fluoxetine has been used successfully to treat clients with exhibitionism, voyeurism, and pedophilia and persons who have committed rape. In addition to fluoxetine, other drugs such as clomipramine and fluvoxamine (Luvox) have been used in the treatment of sexual obsessions, addictions, and paraphilias. The role of the nurse in pharmacotherapy is to educate regarding the specific drug prescribed and to monitor the drug's effectiveness as well as watch for untoward side effects (Becker & Johnson, 2004).

Advanced Practice Interventions

Advanced practice nurses require specialized training to work effectively with clients with sexual and gender identity disorders. This preparation allows the advanced practice nurse to practice sex therapy and conduct sex research. The Association of Sex Educators, Counselors and Therapists (AASECT) identifies the qualifications for practice in these roles.

■ EVALUATION

Evaluation of expected outcomes relates to the level of control and personal satisfaction that is achieved. Acceptance of sexual dysfunction such as impotence as being part of, but not necessarily the defining characteristic of, sexual behavior can result in greater satisfaction. The degree to which negative attitudes about sex are no longer problematic is also important.

■■■ KEY POINTS to REMEMBER

- Sleep disorders affect the individual's ability to function.
- Sleep deprivation is becoming a major problem in American society that affects medical, social, and psychological areas of functioning.
- Research into the physiology of normal sleep as well as of sleep disorders is expanding.
- The major symptoms seen in sleep disorders include insomnia, hypersomnia, and parasomnia.
- Primary insomnia is the most prevalent sleep disorder.
- Primary insomnia is treated with medications as well as non-pharmacological interventions such as relaxation techniques, hypnotherapy, meditation, sleep restriction, and behavioral therapy.
- Adult ADHD is difficult to diagnose; the practitioner must rely on self-report questionnaires as well as spouse and parent reports.

- The cardinal symptoms of adult ADHD include inattention and disorganization.
- There is a high degree of co-occurrence of adult ADHD with other psychiatric disorders, including borderline personality disorder, substance abuse disorders, depression, and anxiety.
- Clients with adult ADHD are treated with medication, cognitive therapy, and life coaching.
- Primary nursing interventions for the client with adult ADHD include counseling to enhance coping, decision making, and self-esteem; psychobiological interventions focused on medication management and teaching about the effect, side effects, and abuse potential of the various medications prescribed for ADHD; identification of appropriate community resources, including therapists and support groups that specialize in working with the adult with ADHD; and health teaching regarding strategies to deal with ADHD.
- A sexual dysfunction is defined as a disturbance in the sexual response cycle or as pain on sexual intercourse.
- There are seven different types of sexual dysfunction.
- Gender identity disorder is a strong and persistent cross-gender identification.
- *Paraphilia* is a term used to identify repetitive or preferred sexual fantasies or behaviors that involve preference for use of a nonhuman object, repetitive sexual activity with humans involving real or simulated suffering or humiliation, and repetitive sexual activity with nonconsenting partners.
- Paraphilias include fetishism, pedophilia, exhibitionism, voyeurism, transvestic fetishism, sexual sadism and masochism, frotteurism, and paraphilia not otherwise specified.
- In addition to conducting a sexual assessment, nurses are involved in milieu and behavioral therapy, counseling, education, and medication management.
- Interventions for paraphilias involve administration of medications such as medroxyprogesterone (Depo-Provera) and SSRIs, and therapy.

Visit the Evolve website at **http://evolve.elsevier.com/Varcarolis** for a posttest on the content in this chapter.

Critical Thinking and Chapter Review

Visit the Evolve website at **http://evolve.elsevier.com/Varcarolis** for additional self-study exercises.

■■■ CRITICAL THINKING

1. Your client has complained that he never sleeps. You have observed that he often takes frequent short naps during the day, and during this time he snores quite loudly. What questions would you ask to determine if this client has a sleep disorder?

2. You are working with a client who has recently been diagnosed with adult ADHD. He is very impulsive and frequently makes comments to you and others that are inappropriate and rude. You find yourself avoiding him and feeling angry toward him. Describe the approaches you could use to intervene in a therapeutic manner with this client.

Continued

Critical Thinking and Chapter Review—cont'd

Visit the Evolve website at **http://evolve.elsevier.com/Varcarolis** for additional self-study exercises.

3. As a nurse on an adolescent psychiatric nursing unit you often encounter teenagers who are misinformed about growth and development as well as about sexuality. Discuss information you might include in a series of teaching sessions that would help the adolescents acquire a greater understanding of the developmental changes they are going through.

4. Complete the questions asked in Box 33-11. What do your answers tell you about yourself? Are you comfortable with your own sexuality? With that of others? Are you judgmental? Could you be helpful to someone who has a sexual disorder? What factors have influenced your beliefs and values regarding sexuality? What do you think is the impact of sexually explicit television, music videos, and movies on your sexual attitudes, values, and beliefs?

■ ■ ■ CHAPTER REVIEW

Choose the most appropriate answer.

1. Mr. S., 76 years old, was told 4 days ago that his wife of 50 years has ovarian cancer. He is at the mental health clinic today because he is now complaining of not being able to sleep at night and wants to get help. He is afraid that, if he doesn't get enough sleep, he will be unable to care for his wife. As his nurse, you explain to Mr. S. that the primary goal to help him with his insomnia will be

   1. writing a prescription for short-term medication so that Mr. S. can get back into a regular sleep pattern.

   2. teaching Mr. S. relaxation techniques so that he will relax before bedtime and be able to sleep through the night.

   3. suggesting that Mr. S. have a glass of warm milk one half hour before bedtime to help him sleep.

   4. completing a medical and psychiatric history and assessment, including information on his sleep-wake behaviors.

2. Mrs. H., an elderly client, tells the nurse, "The only medication I take is trazodone (Desyrel), 50 mg." Based on this statement, the nurse should ask questions designed to assess for

   1. sleep disorder.

   2. schizophrenia.

   3. paraphilia.

   4. sexual dysfunction.

3. Which of the following sleep patterns observed in elderly clients would be assessed by the nurse as a sleep disorder?

   1. Reduction in REM sleep

   2. Decreased wakefulness at night

   3. Taking of several short naps daily

   4. Loud snoring followed by periods of not breathing

4. Which sexual disorder is illegal?

   1. Fetishism

   2. Transvestism

   3. Pedophilia

   4. Gender dysphoria

5. Which of the following nursing interventions would be considered essential when working with an adult with ADHD?

   1. Establishment of a regular exercise regimen

   2. Coaching of the client so he or she will not become discouraged about progress

   3. Education of the client about ADHD

   4. Daily encouragement to perform activities of daily living without help

STUDENT STUDY CD-ROM

Access the accompanying CD-ROM for animations, interactive exercises, review questions for the NCLEX examination, and an audio glossary

■ NURSE, ■ CLIENT, AND ■ FAMILY RESOURCES

For suggested readings, information on related associations, and Internet resources, go to **http://evolve.elsevier.com/Varcarolis.**

REFERENCES

American Academy of Family Physicians. (2003). *Melatonin.* Retrieved March 14, 2005, from Familydoctor.org website: http://familydoctor.org/x1903.xml?printxml.

American Psychiatric Association. (2000). *Diagnostic and statistical manual of mental disorders (DSM-IV-TR)* (4th ed., text rev.). Washington, DC: Author.

Becker, J. V., & Johnson, B. R. (2004). Sexual and gender identity disorders. In R. E. Hales & S. C. Yudofsky (Eds.), *Essentials of clinical psychiatry* (2nd ed.). Washington, DC: American Psychiatric Publishing.

Buysse, D. J., et al. (1989). The Pittsburgh Sleep Quality Index: A new instrument for psychiatric practice and research. *Psychiatry Research, 28,* 193-213.

Byrnes, G., & Watkins, C. (2004). *Adult attention deficit disorder: Diagnosis, coping and mastery.* Retrieved June 21, 2004, from http://www.ncpamd.com/adultadd.htm.

Carson, V. B. (2000). *Mental health nursing: The nurse-patient journey* (2nd ed.). Philadelphia: Saunders.

Dochterman, J. M., & Bulechek, G. M. (2004). *Nursing interventions classification (NIC)* (4th ed.). St. Louis, MO: Mosby.

Goldstein, S. (2004a). *Attention deficit hyperactivity disorder in adults.* Retrieved June 21, 2004, from http://www. addresources.org/article_adult_adhd_goldstein.php.

Goldstein, S. (2004b). *Update on adult ADHD.* Retrieved June 21, 2004, from http://www.addresources.org/article_ update_goldstein.php.

Hales, R. E., & Yudofsky, S. C. (2004). *Essential of clinical psychiatry* (2nd ed.). Washington, DC: American Psychiatric Publishing.

Hoffman, S. (2003). Sleep in the older adult: Implications for nurses. *Geriatric Nurse, 24(4),* 210-216.

Info on sleep deprivation. (2002). Retrieved June 2, 2004, from PageWise website: http://ky.essortment.com/ sleepdeprivatio_rloc.htm.

Krahn, L. E. (2003). Sleep disorders. *Seminars in Neurology, 23(3),* 307-314.

Krakow, B., et al. (2001). Prevalence of insomnia symptoms in patients with sleep-disordered breathing. *Chest, 120 (6),* 1923-1929.

Medical encyclopedia: Hermaphroditism. (2004, January 20). Retrieved from MedlinePlus website: http://www.nlm. nih.gov/medlineplus/ency/article/001669.htm.

Moorhead, S., Johnson, M., & Maas, M. (2004). *Nursing outcomes classification (NOC)* (3rd ed.). St. Louis, MO: Mosby.

Murphy, K. R., & LeVert, S. (1995). *Out of the fog: Treatment options and coping strategies for adult attention deficit disorders.* New York: Skylight Press.

National Center on Sleep Disorders Research. (2003). *National Sleep Disorders Research Plan.* Retrieved June 2, 2004, from http://www.nhlbi.nih.gov/health/prof/ sleep/res_plan/foreword.html.

National Sleep Foundation. (2004). *About NSF.* Retrieved June 7, 2004, from http://sleepfoundation.org/about. cfm.

Neylan, T. C., Reynolds, C. F., & Kupfer, D. J. (2004). Sleep disorders. In R. E. Hales & S. C. Yudofsky (Eds.), *Essentials of clinical psychiatry* (2nd ed., pp. 737-757). Washington, DC: American Psychiatric Publishing.

North American Nursing Diagnosis Association. (2005). *NANDA nursing diagnoses: Definitions and classification 2005-2006.* Philadelphia: Author.

Roth, T., et al. (2003, June 5). *Insomnia and beyond: The neurochemical basis for targeted sleep therapeutics.* Symposium conducted at the Hyatt Regency in Chicago, Illinois. Retrieved May 16, 2004, from http://www.medscape. com/viewprogram/2791_pnt.

Sadock, B. J., & Sadock, V. A. (2004). *Kaplan & Sadock's concise textbook of clinical psychiatry* (2nd ed.). Philadelphia: Lippincott Williams & Wilkins.

Sanford, L. D., et al. (2001). Influence of fear conditioning on elicited pon-to-geniculo-occipital waves and rapid eye movement sleep. *Archives Italiennes de Biologie, 139,* 169-203.

Schatzberg, A. F., & Nemeroff, C. B. (2004). *Textbook of psychopharmacology* (3rd ed.). Washington, DC: American Psychiatric Publishing.

Sleep-deprivation.com. (2004). *Sleep deprivation symptoms: Lack of energy, fatigue, and exhaustion.* Retrieved June 2, 2004, from http://www.sleep-deprivation.com.

Stickgold, R. A., Winkelman, J. W., & Wehrwein, P. (2004, January 19). *Newsweek Health: You will start to feel very sleepy. . . .* Retrieved June 7, 2004, from http://msnbc.msn. com/id/3928217/.

Walsh, J. K. (2004, March 30). *Testimony by James K. Walsh, Ph.D., Chairman, on behalf of the National Sleep Foundation: Fiscal year 2005 funding for the Department of Health and Human Services, House Labor, Health and Human Services, Education and Related Agencies Appropriations Subcommittee.* Retrieved June 7, 2004, from http://www. sleepfoundation.org/whatsnew/walsh_testimony.cfm.

Watkins, C. E. (2003). *New medications for adults with ADHD.* Retrieved June 21, 2004, from http://www.ncpamd. com/NewADD_Meds.htm.

Weintraub, A. (2004a, January 26). I can't sleep. *BusinessWeek Online.* Retrieved June 7, 2004, from http://www. businessweek.com/magazine/content/04_04/b3867001_ mz001.htm.

Weintraub, A. (2004b, January 26). Online extra: The deadly dangers of drowsy driving. *BusinessWeek Online.* Retrieved June 7, 2004, from http://www.businessweek. com/print/magazine/content/04_04/b3867010_mz001. htm?mz.

CHAPTER 34

Psychosocial Needs of the Older Adult

EVELYN L. YAP ■ SALLY K. HOLZAPFEL

■ KEY TERMS and CONCEPTS

The key terms and concepts listed here appear in color where they are defined or first discussed in this chapter.

adult day care, 700

advance directives, 706

ageism, 693

chemical restraints, 701

directive to physician, 706

durable power of attorney for health care, 707

living will, 706

Omnibus Budget Reconciliation Act (OBRA), 701

Patient Self-Determination Act (PSDA), 706

physical restraints, 701

■ OBJECTIVES

After studying this chapter, the reader will be able to

1. Discuss the facts and myths about aging.
2. Describe the impact of ageism in providing care to older adults.
3. Analyze how ageism affects your attitudes and willingness to care for the elderly.
4. Compare the different group interventions commonly used with elderly clients.
5. Explain the importance of a comprehensive geriatric assessment.
6. Describe the role of the nurse in different settings of care.
7. Identify the requirements for the use of physical and chemical restraints.
8. Discuss the importance of pain assessment and identify three tools used to assess pain in the elderly.
9. Identify the risk factors for elder suicide and the nurse's role in prevention of suicide.
10. Discuss institutional requirements related to the Patient Self-Determination Act (1990).
11. Discuss differences between a living will, a directive to physician, and durable power of attorney for health care.

evolve Visit the Evolve website at **http://evolve.elsevier.com/Varcarolis** for a pretest on the content in this chapter.

THE OLDER POPULATION AND THE HEALTH CARE SYSTEM

The aging of the population is a global phenomenon that is occurring at a record-breaking rate, especially in developing countries around the world (Kinsella & Velkoff, 2001). The economy as well as health and social services in the United States are affected by this marked increase in the proportion of the older adults in the population. By the year 2030, 23% of the population in the United States will consist of individuals older than 65 years of age. Among the elderly, the fastest-growing subgroups are the minorities, the poor, and those aged 85 years and older. By 2050, the population of seniors aged 65 years and older will double and the number of those aged 85 years and older will quadruple (Henderson, 2003).

As people live longer they are more likely to deal with chronic illness and disability (Miller, 2004). At least 80% of individuals older than age 65 years have one chronic condition; many elderly people have more than one. The likelihood of developing one or more chronic illnesses increases notably with age: individuals 75 years of age and older are the most prone to chronic illnesses and functional disabilities. After age

85 years, there is a one-in-three chance of developing dementia, immobility, incontinence, or another age-related disability.

According to the U.S. Census Bureau (Hetzel & Smith, 2001), today's life expectancy is 74.1 years for men and 79.5 years for women. Upon reaching 65 years of age, men can expect to live an average of 16.3 years longer and women can expect to live another 19.2 years (Miller, 2004). Elderly women outnumber elderly men in a ratio of 3:2. At age 85 years and older, this ratio increases to 5:2.

As the previous statistics indicate, women generally outlive men. Because husbands more often predecease their spouses, they benefit from the support of their wives to help with health-related issues. On the other hand, many older women lack this type of support. Women's greater longevity has significant ramifications for society at large and for the health care system in particular. Not only do women form the largest bloc among the elderly, they also use health care services more frequently than men and seek such services earlier, even for minor conditions.

Elderly individuals with mental health problems are less likely than young adults to be accurately diagnosed and to receive mental health treatment (Rabins et al., 2000). This is especially true for elderly individuals with depression and anxiety. Health providers frequently misinterpret clinical depression in older adults as a normal part of aging (Henderson, 2003). Anxiety is another important problem to assess because it interferes with normal functioning (Skoog, 2004).

Chronological age is considered an arbitrary indicator of function because there are significant variables that contribute to the capabilities of older adults. Surveys focusing on how the elderly see themselves reveal that nearly half of people 65 years and older consider themselves to be middle-aged or young. Only 15% of people aged 75 years and older consider themselves "very old" (Ebersole, Hess, & Luggen, 2004). However, current standards (Hogstel & Weeks, 2000) classify people into the following age categories:

Young old—those 65 to 74 years of age
Middle old—those 75 to 84 years of age
Old old—those 85 to 94 years of age
Elite old—those 95 years of age or older

There are noticeable differences between individuals in their sixties and people in their eighties. Whereas those in the younger group are relatively healthy, those in the older group are much more vulnerable, frail, and at risk for visual problems, cognitive impairment, and falls. They also have more limited economic resources and community supports, and are more affected by the chronic diseases and disorders of aging (Ebersole et al., 2004).

Health care expenses for the elderly are nearly four times higher than the expenses for the rest of the population, and with the predicted growth in the elderly population, health prevention and maintenance of functional ability must be a priority in nursing care. Issues pertaining to appropriate care of the elderly and health care delivery need to be addressed.

ROLE OF THE NURSE

Nurses make substantial contributions to care and health promotion for older adults. However, questions arise as to whether nurses in training are given enough information about and sufficient exposure to the elderly during their nursing education. It is important for all nurses to develop an interest in the elderly and to gain a better understanding of the older adult and the aging process. Adequate theory and principles are needed to provide safe and excellent care for the elderly. An outline of some major developmental theories of aging is provided in Box 34-1. Although these theories provide the framework for nurses to formulate appropriate nursing interventions in caring for the elderly, there is no specific theory that encompasses all the developmental stages. Research in these areas is ongoing (Miller, 2004). Overall, the goal of nursing is to deliver compassionate care while maintaining positive attitudes and realistic beliefs about the elderly when treating them.

The negative view of the elderly frequently held by nurses (as well as by the general population) is part of the phenomenon of ageism. Studies have found that recruits to nursing hold ageist views, which has significant implications for practice, education, and research (Lueckenotte, 2000).

Ageism Among Health Care Workers

Ageism has been defined as a bias against older people because of their age; it is a system of destructive, erroneous beliefs. In essence, ageism represents a dislike by the young of the old, reflecting the disparaging effects of society's attitudes toward the elderly. This age prejudice is based on the notion that aging makes people increasingly unattractive, unintelligent, asexual, unemployable, and senile.

Ageism is not limited to the way the young may look at the old. It is also seen in the views of older people, who tend to be critical about themselves and their peers. Indeed, the attitudes of the elderly toward their peers, particularly those with mental disabilities, are often more negative than the views held by the young (although this is not always the case). The threat of social contagion by association with the frail and infirm may simply be too strong to bear. Age proximity raises feelings of vulnerability. This may explain why older persons often do not like to be referred to as "old." By seeing themselves as "young" rather than "old," they adjust better to their advancing years.

BOX 34-1

Major Theories of Aging

Biological
Aging is influenced by molecular, cellular, or physiological systems and processes.
Gene theory: Harmful genes become active in later life.
Error theory: Error in protein synthesis results in impaired cellular function.
Free radical theory: Reactive molecules damage DNA.
Wear-and-tear theory: Internal and external stressors harm cells.
Programmed aging theory: Biological or genetic clock plays out on genes.
Neuroendocrine theory: There is neurohormonal regulation of life until death.
Immunological theory: Immune system diversifies with age.

Psychological
Kohlberg's theory: Crises and turning points in adult life are moral dilemmas.
Piaget's theory: Cognitive operations in youth influence aging.
Erikson's theory: Integrity is built on morality and ethics.
Bandura's theory: Self-efficacy is essential for longevity.
Sullivan's theory: Interpersonal responses influence behavior.
Freud's theory: Focuses on control of instinctual responses.
Psychobiological theory: Neurotransmitters modulate behaviors, emotions, and thoughts.
Dialectical theory: Crises and transitions release positive and negative forces that lead to developmental progress.
Behavioral theory: Learning determines the organization of behavior.

Psychosocial
Maslow's theory: Self-actualization and the evolution of developmental needs occur as the individual ages.
Disengagement theory: Mutual withdrawal occurs between the aging person and others.
Activity theory: Actions, roles, and social pursuits are important for satisfactory aging.
Continuity theory: Life satisfaction and activity are expressions of enduring personality traits.

Adapted from Hess, P. (2004). Theories of aging. In Ebersole, P., Hess, P., & Luggen, A. S. (Eds.), *Toward healthy aging: Human needs and nursing response* (6th ed.). St. Louis, MO: Mosby.

Ageism differs from other forms of discrimination in that it cuts across gender, race, religion, and national origin. In our culture, old age does not award a desirable status or membership in a sought-after club; rather, it is a social category with negative connotations. Today a new form of ageism puts the elderly in a no-win situation: well-to-do elderly are envied for their economic progress, the middle-class elderly are blamed for making Social Security too costly, and the poor elderly are resented for being tax burdens!

The results of ageism can be observed throughout every level of society. Even health care providers are not immune to its effects. Negative values can surface in a myriad of ways in the health care system. Financial and political support for programs for the elderly is difficult to obtain; their needs are addressed only after those of younger, albeit smaller, population groups. The Grey Panthers and the American Association of Retired Persons (AARP), however, are powerful lobbying groups that are fighting to change this trend.

Health care personnel do not always share medical information, recommendations, and opportunities with the elderly. Studies show that the elderly receive less information and sometimes less care than those who are younger. Ageism is also reflected in public policy, and this leads to discrimination against older adults (Hooyman, 2003; Nelson, 2002).

Health care workers who deal on a daily basis with the confused, ill, and frail older adult may tend to develop a somewhat negative and biased view of the elderly. Their attitudes often reflect society's views, which are characterized by negativism and stereotyping. The rendering of medical care to older adults has been burdened with pessimism, defeatism, and professional aversion. Such thinking can be found among professionals as well as among ancillary personnel working in nursing homes and other institutional settings.

Positive attitudes toward the elderly and their care need to be instilled during basic nursing education. If the goal of nursing programs is to prepare students to practice in the future, then preparing students to care for older adults in a wide variety of settings is mandatory, for that *is* the future (Lueckenotte, 2000). Education programs must include the following:

- Information about the aging process
- Discussion of attitudes relating to the care of the elderly
- Sensitization of participants to their clients' needs
- Exploration of the dynamics of nurse-client and staff-client interactions

Box 34-2 provides some facts and myths about aging, although this listing is not exhaustive. These issues influence how society perceives the older adult.

Unique Assessment Strategies

Nurses who work with the elderly benefit from specific knowledge about normal aging, drug interactions, and chronic disease. Those who work with elderly clients who have mental health problems also need to have special skills in interviewing and assessing, and special knowledge of effective treatment modalities. The National Institutes of Health recommend a comprehensive geriatric assessment to evaluate and manage the care and progress of the elderly

BOX 34-2

Facts and Myths About Aging

Facts

- The senses of vision, hearing, touch, taste, and smell decline with age.
- Muscular strength decreases with age. Muscle fibers atrophy and decrease in number.
- Regular sexual expressions are important to maintain sexual capacity and effective sexual performance.
- At least 50% of restorative sleep is lost as a result of the aging process.
- The elderly are major consumers of prescription drugs because of the high incidence of chronic diseases in this population.
- The elderly have a high incidence of depression.
- Many individuals experience difficulty when they retire.
- The elderly are prone to become victims of crime.
- Older widows appear to adjust better than younger ones.

Myths

- Most adults past the age of 65 years are demented.
- Sexual interest declines with age.
- Older adults are not able to learn new tasks.
- As individuals age, they become more rigid in their thinking and set in their ways.
- The aged are well off and no longer impoverished.
- Most elderly people are infirm and require help with daily activities.
- Most older adults are socially isolated and lonely.

client. A comprehensive geriatric assessment includes a focus on physical health; functional, economic, and social status; and environmental factors that might impinge on the elderly client's well-being (Dharmarajan & Norman, 2003). Figure 34-1 provides an example of a comprehensive geriatric assessment.

An examination and interview of an elderly person conducted in unfamiliar surroundings will most likely produce anxiety. Unlike younger clients, who may be comfortable discussing personal issues such as family conflicts, feelings of sadness, sexual practices, finances, and bodily functions, the elderly are part of a generation that viewed these topics as private, and as a result, they may be uncomfortable discussing these personal matters. It is important to respect these feelings while reviewing essential history by

- Conducting the interview in a private area.
- Introducing oneself and asking the client what he or she would like to be called.
- Establishing rapport and putting the client at ease by sitting or standing at the same level as the client.
- Ensuring that lighting is adequate and noise level is low in recognition of the fact that hearing and vision may be impaired in the elderly client.

- Using touch to convey warmth while at the same time respecting the elderly client's comfort level with personal touch.
- Summarizing the interaction and inviting feedback from the client.

Assessment of the cognitive, behavioral, and emotional status of the older adult is very important in managing the nursing care of the client. This is particularly vital for detecting dementia, delirium, and depression, because their prevalence increases with age (Dharmarajan & Norman, 2003). In addition, alcoholism and substance abuse among the elderly is a major health problem. To assess for depression, the Geriatric Depression Scale (Short Form) is a reliable tool (Sheikh & Yesavage, 1986) (Box 34-3). To screen for alcoholism, the Michigan Alcoholism Screening Test—Geriatric Version (MAST-G) is useful (Menninger, 2004) (Box 34-4). It is also essential to assess for suicidal thoughts and suicidal intent by asking specific questions such as the following:

- Have you ever thought about killing yourself?
- Have you ever tried to hurt yourself in the past?

In addition, harmful thoughts about other people need to be assessed and addressed. Suicide in the elderly is discussed in greater depth later in this chapter. In addition, Chapter 23 provides a comprehensive discussion of suicide assessment and intervention.

BOX 34-3

Geriatric Depression Scale (Short Form)

1. Are you basically satisfied with your life? Yes/No
2. Have you dropped many of your activities and interests? Yes/No
3. Do you feel that your life is empty? Yes/No
4. Do you often get bored? Yes/No
5. Are you in good spirits most of the time? Yes/No
6. Are you afraid that something bad is going to happen to you? Yes/No
7. Do you feel happy most of the time? Yes/No
8. Do you often feel helpless? Yes/No
9. Do you prefer to stay at home, rather than going out and doing new things? Yes/No
10. Do you feel you have more problems with memory than most? Yes/No
11. Do you think it is wonderful to be alive now? Yes/No
12. Do you feel pretty worthless the way you are now? Yes/No
13. Do you feel full of energy? Yes/No
14. Do you feel that your situation is hopeless? Yes/No
15. Do you think that most people are better off than you are? Yes/No

From Sheikh, J. I., & Yesavage, J. A. (1986). Geriatric Depression Scale (GDS): Recent evidence and development of a shorter version. In T. L. Brink (Ed.), *Clinical gerontology: A guide to assessment and intervention* (pp. 165-173). New York: Hawthorn Press.

COMPREHENSIVE GERIATRIC ASSESSMENT					
Name:		Date of birth:		Gender:	

Physical Health

Chronic disorder					
Vision	Adequate	Inadequate	Eyeglasses: Y N		Needs evaluation
Hearing	Adequate	Inadequate	Hearing aids: Y N		
Mobility	Ambulatory: Y N		Assistive device:		
	Falls: Y N				Needs evaluation
Nutrition	Albumin:	TLC:	HCT:		
	Weight:	Weight loss or gain: Y N			Needs evaluation
Incontinence	Y N	Treatment:	Y N		Needs evaluation
Medications	Total number:	Reviewed & revised:	Y N		
	Adverse effects/allergy:				
Screening	Cholesterol:	TSH:	B12:	Folate:	
	Colonoscopy: Date:		N/A		
	Mammogram: Date:		N/A		
	Osteoporosis: Date:		N/A		
	Pap smear: Date:		N/A		
	PSA: Date:		N/A		
Immunization	Influenza: Date:				
	Pneumonia: Date:				
	Tetanus: Date:		Booster:		
Counseling	Diet	Exercise	Calcium	Vitamin D	
	Smoking	Alcohol	Driving	Injury prevention	

Mental Health

Dementia	Y N	MMSE score:	Date:	Cause (if known):	
Depression	Y N	GDS score:	Date:	Treatment: Y N	

Functional Status

ADL	Bathing: I D	Dressing: I D	Toileting: I D
	Transferring: I D	Feeding: I D	Continence: Y N

FIGURE 34-1 Comprehensive geriatric assessment. *ADL,* Activities of daily living; *B12,* vitamin B_{12}; *D,* dependent; *GDS,* Geriatric Depression Scale; *HCT,* hematocrit; *I,* independent; *MMSE,* Mini-Mental State Examination; *N,* no; *PSA,* prostate-specific antigen; *TLC,* total lymphocyte count; *TSH,* thyroid-stimulating hormone; *Y,* yes.

Unique Intervention Strategies

The majority of older persons function quite well in their lives. For those who suffer from psychiatric problems, however, effective treatment is available. Certain psychotherapeutic methods are especially useful for the elderly client:

- Applying crisis intervention techniques (see Chapter 22)
- Providing empathetic understanding

BOX 34-4

Michigan Alcoholism Screening Test—Geriatric Version (MAST-G)

Please answer "yes" or "no" to each question by marking the line next to the question. When you finish answering the questions, please add up how many "yes" responses you checked and put that number in the space provided at the end.

1. After drinking have you ever noticed an increase in your heart rate or beating in your chest? ___ Yes ___ No
2. When talking to others, do you ever underestimate how much you actually drank? ___ Yes ___ No
3. Does alcohol make you sleepy so that you often fall asleep in your chair? ___ Yes ___ No
4. After a few drinks, have you sometimes not eaten or been able to skip a meal because you didn't feel hungry? ___ Yes ___ No
5. Does having a few drinks help you decrease your shakiness or tremors? ___ Yes ___ No
6. Does alcohol sometimes make it hard for you to remember parts of the day or night? ___ Yes ___ No
7. Do you have rules for yourself that you won't drink before a certain time of the day? ___ Yes ___ No
8. Have you lost interest in hobbies or activities you used to enjoy? ___ Yes ___ No
9. When you wake up in the morning, do you ever have trouble remembering part of the night before? ___ Yes ___ No
10. Does having a drink help you sleep? ___ Yes ___ No
11. Do you hide your alcohol bottles from family members? ___ Yes ___ No
12. After a social gathering, have you ever felt embarrassed because you drank too much? ___ Yes ___ No
13. Have you ever been concerned that drinking might be harmful to your health? ___ Yes ___ No
14. Do you like to end an evening with a nightcap? ___ Yes ___ No
15. Did you find your drinking increased after someone close to you died? ___ Yes ___ No
16. In general, would you prefer to have a few drinks at home rather than go out to social events? ___ Yes ___ No
17. Are you drinking more now than in the past? ___ Yes ___ No
18. Do you usually take a drink to relax or calm your nerves? ___ Yes ___ No
19. Do you drink to take your mind off your problems? ___ Yes ___ No
20. Have you ever increased your drinking after experiencing a loss in your life? ___ Yes ___ No
21. Do you sometimes drive when you have had too much to drink? ___ Yes ___ No
22. Has a doctor or nurse ever said they were worried or concerned about your drinking? ___ Yes ___ No
23. Have you ever made rules to manage your drinking? ___ Yes ___ No
24. When you feel lonely, does having a drink help? ___ Yes ___ No

TOTAL _____

From Menninger, J. (2004). Assessment and treatment of alcoholism and substance-related disorders in the elderly. *Bulletin of the Menninger Clinic, 66*(2), 166-183.
Scoring: A score of 3 points or less is considered to indicate no alcoholism; a score of 4 points is suggestive of alcoholism; a score of 5 points or more indicates alcoholism.

- Encouraging ventilation of feelings
- Normalizing emotions
- Reestablishing emotional equilibrium when anxiety is moderate to severe
- Providing health education—explaining alternative solutions
- Assisting in the use of problem-solving approaches

Box 34-5 provides helpful interview techniques to use with the elderly.

Nurses encounter the elderly in a variety of settings, and in each of these settings the nurse is responsible for application of the nursing process to the individual client's situation. The interventions provided by the basic level practitioner include counseling, milieu management, promotion of self-care activities, psychobiological interventions, health teaching, case management, and health promotion and health maintenance activities.

Inpatient Settings

An acutely ill older adult may require inpatient care in a hospital when he or she manifests signs and symptoms of severe acute psychiatric conditions, for example, major depression with suicidal thoughts and psychosis. Inpatient treatment is recommended when the client is at high risk of self-harm or poses a risk to harm other people. Depending on the needs and recovery potential of the elderly client, hospitalization may be either short term or long term. For those who are not able to be stabilized in short-term settings, the next option is a long-term stay in the hospital, usually for 3 to 6 months.

Nursing care of an acutely mentally ill older adult in a hospital, whether short term or long term, is a challenging opportunity. Nurses play a major role in providing around-the-clock care from admission to discharge.

Counseling. The basic level nurse uses counseling skills to assist the client in talking about present problems, examining his or her present situation, looking at alternatives, and planning for the future. Sometimes counseling is provided through group therapy because this helps to decrease the sense of disorientation and isolation. Remotivation therapy and reminiscence therapy are also appropriate interventions for the basic level nurse and are modalities that are useful for el-

---

BOX 34-5

Helpful Techniques for Interviewing the Older Adult

1. Gather preliminary data before the session and keep questionnaires relatively short.
2. Ask about often-overlooked problems, such as difficulty sleeping, incontinence, falling, depression, dizziness, or loss of energy.
3. Pace the interview to allow the client to formulate answers; resist the tendency to interrupt prematurely.
4. Use yes-or-no or simple choice questions if the older client has trouble coping with open-ended questions.
5. Begin with general questions such as "How can I help you most at this visit?" or "What's been happening?"
6. Be alert for information on the client's relationships with others, thoughts about families or co-workers, typical responses to stress, and attitudes toward aging, illness, occupation, and death.
7. Assess mental status for deficits in recent or remote memory and determine if confusion exists.
8. Be aware of all medications the client is taking and assess for side effects, efficacy, and possible drug interactions.
9. Determine how fast the condition of the client has been changing to assess the extent of the client's concerns.
10. Include the family or significant other in the interview process for added input, clarification, support, and reinforcement.

From National Institute on Aging. *Working with your older patient: A clinician's handbook.* Bethesda, MD: Author.

---

derly clients. Group psychotherapy, provided by advanced practice nurses, is another therapeutic intervention that may benefit the elderly client. Table 34-1 outlines the purpose, format, and desired outcomes for each type of therapy group. Box 34-6 gives an example of a remotivation therapy session.

Milieu Management. The major roles of the nurse are to assist the client in adjusting to the environment, to keep the client safe at all times, to minimize the adverse effects of hospitalization on functional capacity, to provide reality orientation, and to engage in therapeutic communication with the elderly client. In addition, the nurse orients the client to the environment, paying particular attention to the physical, sensory, and psychological needs of the elderly client.

Psychobiological Interventions. The nurse administers and monitors the effectiveness of the client's medication, and provides appropriate behavioral interventions (e.g., verbal deescalation and limit setting).

Health Teaching. The nurse provides health teaching to both client and caregiver on a variety of issues, including the nature of the client's illness, symptom

management, maintenance of safety, self-care strategies, management of medications, coping skills, steps necessary for recovery, and resources that will support recovery.

Promotion of Self-Care Activities. Hospitalized elderly adults often rapidly regress into a helpless state that ranges from needing assistance to requiring total care in accomplishing the activities of daily living. The goal is to encourage the client to regain independence in the realm of personal care. The nurse remains vigilant to changes in the client's mood, behaviors, and mental status. The treatment plan is developed and modified to reflect the unique needs of the individual.

Community-Based Programs

The hazards of institutionalization are numerous. Increased mortality may be caused by the increased risk for nosocomial infections. Injuries may occur due to initial disorientation to a new setting. Residents may develop learned helplessness, losing interest in self-care activities. There also may be a decrease in opportunities for socialization. In contrast, community-based programs are an alternative whose purpose is to promote the elder's independent functioning and reduce the stress on the family system. Community-based programs include partial hospitalization, behavioral health home care, and a variety of day treatment programs.

Partial Hospitalization. Partial hospitalization or acute psychiatric day hospital programs are sometimes recommended for clients who do not need 24 hours of nursing care but still require and would benefit from intensive and structured psychiatric treatment. The usual length of stay in such a program is between 1 and 2 weeks. A review of acute psychiatric day hospitals in the United Kingdom found that clients who received care in partial hospitalization programs showed a more rapid improvement in mental state than clients randomly assigned to inpatient care; this type of care also led to cost reductions ranging from 20.9% to 36.9% compared with inpatient care (Marshall, 2003).

As in an inpatient unit, the nurse must manage the milieu to provide safety for the client. Nursing care focuses on a continuation of the goals begun in the inpatient unit as well as preparation of the client and family and/or caregiver for discharge to home and community. In addition, the nurse continues to assess the client's physical and mental status, paying particular attention to functional status (e.g., ability to perform activities of daily living safely when at home, ambulation, and use of transportation). Health education includes symptom monitoring and management, medication management, relapse and stress preven-

TABLE 34-1

Useful Group Therapy Modalities for Elderly Clients

Remotivation Therapy	Reminiscence Therapy (Life Review)	Psychotherapy
Purpose of Group		
▪ Resocialize regressed and apathetic clients ▪ Reawaken interest in the environment	▪ Share memories of the past ▪ Increase self-esteem ▪ Increase socialization ▪ Increase awareness of the uniqueness of each participant	▪ Alleviate psychiatric symptoms ▪ Increase ability to interact with others in a group ▪ Increase self-esteem ▪ Increase ability to make decisions and function more independently
Format		

▪ Groups are made up of 10 to 15 people.
▪ Meetings are held once or twice a week.
▪ Meetings are highly structured in a classroomlike setting.
▪ Group uses props.
▪ Each session discusses a particular topic.
▪ See Box 34-6 for the five basic steps used in each session.
	▪ Groups are made up of 6 to 8 people.
	▪ Meetings are held once or twice weekly for 1 hour.
	▪ Topics include holidays, major life events, birthdays, travel, and food.
		▪ Group size is 6 to 12 members.
		▪ Group members should share similar
		  —Problems.
		  —Mental status.
		  —Needs.
		  —Sexual integration.
		▪ Group meets at regularly scheduled times (certain number of times a week, specific duration of session) and place.

Desired Outcomes		

▪ Increases participants' sense of reality
▪ Offers practice of health roles
▪ Realizes more objective self-image
	▪ Alleviates depression in institutionalized elderly
	▪ Through the process of reorganization and reintegration, provides avenue by which elderly can
	  —Achieve a new sense of identity.
	  —Achieve a positive self-concept.
		▪ Decreases sense of isolation
		▪ Facilitates development of new roles and reestablishes former roles
		▪ Provides information for other group members
		▪ Provides group support for effecting changes and increasing self-esteem

From Matteson, M. A., & McConnell, E. S. (Eds.). (1988). *Gerontological nursing: Concepts and practice* (p. 80). Philadelphia: Saunders.

tion, and problem solving of health maintenance issues to enable the client to adapt to active functioning in the community. The nurse also reviews with the team, in collaboration with the client and family or caregiver, additional referrals for needed services (e.g., Meals on Wheels, transportation services, church activities, and home care services).

Behavioral Health Home Care. Older individuals prefer the continuum of services to be delivered in the least-restrictive setting, and that is usually in their homes. Home-based behavioral health care is particularly recommended to assist the elderly person to adjust to and manage his or her illness and disability either before or after hospitalization. It is often the role of the behavioral health home care nurse to maintain a person affected by a cognitive brain disorder or a severe and persistent mental illness in the home or to facilitate a transfer to a temporary or permanent facility.

Behavioral health home care involves the provision of specialized and skilled nursing care on a visiting basis to clients in need of holistic care. Examples of ser-

vices provided are psychiatric and chemical dependency treatment, management of the psychosocial aspects of primary care, health and wellness teaching, and illness prevention. In addition to nursing, other medically necessary skilled services, including physical and occupational therapy, medical social work services, and home health aide assistance, are coordinated in keeping with the needs of the client and family and/or caregiver. The goals of behavioral health home care are (1) to restore and maintain the client's optimal state of health and independence, and (2) to minimize the effects of illness and provide rehabilitation.

The target population for behavioral health home care includes older adults with problems in daily living, behavioral issues related to their physical illness, and enduring mental illness. Nursing services are usually provided by a basic level practitioner or a certified generalist nurse in community health or home health care, or by a behavioral health clinical nurse specialist certified in adult psychiatric and mental health nursing. The nurse is guided by the American Nurses

BOX 34-6

Example of Remotivation Session (Bodies of Water)

Step 1: Climate of Acceptance

The leaders personally welcomed each participant as he or
she arrived at the group session. After the leaders introduced themselves, each group member made a self-
introduction. The leader used a calendar to orient the
members to the date and time of the current remotivation
session. The theme for session four was introduced by the
leader as "bodies of water—rivers, lakes, and oceans." All
group members had some familiarity with bodies of water
because of their residence in Seattle.

Step 2: Creating a Bridge to Reality

The world globe was used as a visual aid to stimulate discussion on bodies of water. The leader asked questions such
as "How are bodies of water formed from glaciers?"
Pictures of glaciers, rivers, and lakes were shown.
The leader read poems about tide pools, seashells, and fishing written by anonymous grade school children.
Discussion was stimulated by the leader's asking, "What
can we do at the ocean?" Visual aids and props were provided for direct sensory stimulation. Some examples of
these aids and props were (1) different types of seashells,
(2) fishing tackle and bait, (3) suntan lotion, (4) sun hat, and
(5) sunglasses.
A poem by an anonymous author about fishing was read to
the group. This was followed by recorded music with lyrics
about fishing experiences.

Step 3: Sharing the World We Live In

Group discussion focused on jobs related to bodies of water.
Topics the participants discussed in regard to self or others
included crabbing, clamming, shrimping, and fishing. Visual
aids were provided to stimulate further discussions of past-

related experiences involving bodies of water. Pictures of
river rafting, canoeing, scuba diving, and sailing were
shared.

Step 4: An Appreciation of the World of Work

This time was used for the members to think about work in
relation to others. More experiences in past-related work
roles as well as hobbies and pastimes were discussed.
The group then participated in singing a familiar old song,
"Love Letters in the Sand," written in 1931 by J. Fred
Coots and revived in 1957 when sung by Pat Boone.

Step 5: Climate of Appreciation

The group members were thanked individually by the leaders for coming to the group and sharing their experiences.
The next remotivation session theme and meeting date
were announced prior to terminating the session.

Group Response to Session Four

Most members of the group appeared to enjoy discussing
their experiences in relation to bodies of water. Many
members recalled fishing and boating experiences. Other
members expressed interest in this topic by their nonverbal participation in touching and smelling some physical
props and observation of visual aids. All but two participants touched the seashells and smelled the fish eggs.
One lady in the group stood up and modeled the sun hat
and glasses, while a man demonstrated how to reel in the
line on a fishing pole. Several participants remarked on
how beautiful the pictures of the glaciers were. All but a
couple of group members sang to the recorded lyrics on
fishing. One member stood up and danced to the music
while many others clapped to her movements.

From Janssen, J. A., & Giberson, D. L. (1988). Remotivation therapy. *Journal of Gerontological Nursing, 14*(6), 31-34.

Association (ANA) Standards of Care in support of
nursing processes of care (these standards are
reprinted at the back of the text).

The behavioral health home care nurse plays a
unique role in nursing the elderly client as well as the
family or caregiver. Strong physical assessment skills,
superb clinical judgment, effective communication and
organizational skills, knowledge of federally funded
and state-funded programs including third-party payers, flexibility, and ability to adjust to different settings
of care are among the most essential traits such a nurse
must possess. In addition, knowledge of cultural diversity is very critical, because nursing care is significantly
influenced by cultural differences related to the home
and community at large. Refer to Chapter 6 for more
information on home psychiatric mental health care
and to Chapter 7 for information on cultural influences.

Day Treatment Programs. Multipurpose senior
centers provide a broad range of services: (1) health
promotion and wellness programs; (2) health screening; (3) social, educational, and recreational activities;

(4) meals; and (5) information and referral services.
For those in need of nursing care and custodial care
services, adult day care is an appropriate choice
(Fultner & Raudonis, 2000).

As a result of economic factors and the negative
view of institutionalization, interest in day care programs has increased. Most individuals who use day
care centers are physically frail or cognitively impaired (Fultner & Raudonis, 2000). There are three
types of day care programs: (1) social day care, (2)
adult day health or medical treatment programs, and
(3) maintenance day care. In each, the elderly are cared
for during the day and stay in a home environment at
night. The boundaries of these programs blend and
overlap. See Chapter 6 for a complete discussion of
community-based care.

Social day care affords the participants the opportunity for recreation and social interaction. Nursing,
medical, or rehabilitative care is usually not provided.
This is the most common type of day care and is less
expensive to operate. Generally, the clients are older
adults who need socialization or continued physical

activities, or individuals with mild dementia or physical frailty.

The **adult day health** or medical treatment program goes beyond meeting recreational and social needs; it provides services such as medical interventions, psychiatric nursing, and rehabilitation for the high-risk elderly, and psychosocial interventions for the frail aged. Qualified personnel (nurses, pharmacists, physicians, physical therapists, occupational therapists, and social workers) are available, forming a broad base of support necessary for such care. This program, which requires physician referral, aims to prevent or slow down any mental, physical, or social deterioration and thus seeks to maximize the older adult's full potential regardless of disease or condition. If clients reach their full potential, they can be discharged from the program.

The **maintenance day care** program assists clients at high risk for institutionalization. Placement is usually on physician referral. An interdisciplinary team, including a psychiatrist, plans the care. The client mix includes frail persons with dementia and those with persistent and severe psychiatric disorders (e.g., schizophrenia, personality disorders). The program's emphasis is on maintaining clients' functional abilities. Although the inevitable cognitive decline cannot be prevented in clients with dementia, the clients' quality of life is enhanced and psychosocial dysfunction may be decreased. The restlessness, anxiety, and agitation that frequently occur in the demented client are kept to a minimum with the aid of individualized treatment plans. Discharge from this program is most often to an increased level of care such as an inpatient hospital or nursing home.

All three models are meant to provide a safe, supportive, and nonthreatening environment and fulfill a vital function for older adults and their families. The programs permit the elderly to continue their present living arrangements and maintain their social ties to the community. Day treatment programs relieve families of the burden of 24-hour daily care for their elderly dependents. If institutionalization becomes necessary, day care staff can work with elderly clients and their families to assess the present situation and make recommendations for placement.

ISSUES THAT AFFECT THE MENTAL HEALTH OF SOME ELDERLY

Six important problems affecting some older adults were chosen for discussion here:
1. Use of restraints
2. Pain management
3. Decision making about health care
4. Acquired immunodeficiency syndrome (AIDS)
5. Suicide
6. Alcoholism and substance abuse

Elder abuse, another serious problem for the elderly, is addressed in Chapter 25. Issues surrounding death, dying, and hospice care are additional concerns for the elderly and are discussed in Chapter 30.

Use of Restraints

The use of restraints in the elderly is an ethical, legal, and safety concern. Restraints can be both physical and chemical. Physical restraints are any manual methods or mechanical devices, materials, or equipment that inhibit free movement. Chemical restraints are drugs given for the very specific purpose of inhibiting a certain behavior or movement.

Physical Restraints

Surveys undertaken by the state and federal authorities in the United States between the 1970s and 1980s revealed levels of physical restraint use as high as 75% in some facilities and levels of psychotropic drug use as high as 90% (Marchello, 2003). Physical restraints are used with hospitalized confused clients primarily to prevent disruption of medical therapies and to prevent falls. Paradoxically, however, they are perceived as a form of physical and psychological abuse. Moreover, Arbesman and Wright (1999) concluded in their study that the risk of falling was highest soon after a person was placed in mechanical restraints.

Whether health care providers have the right to restrain another individual physically has always been a question. Being physically restrained can be a humiliating and demoralizing experience. The elderly have responded to such action with anger, fear, anxiety, depression, and stress-related syndromes (Meiner & Miceli, 2000).

In addition to the risk of falls, physical restraints pose a risk of death through strangulation or asphyxiation (Dharmarajan & Norman, 2003). Residents in restraint-free facilities have experienced fewer injuries from falls than those in facilities using restraints. A study by Neufield and colleagues (1999) found that serious injuries declined significantly when restraint orders were discontinued. The researchers concluded that restraint-free care is safe when a comprehensive assessment is performed and alternatives to restraints are used.

The Omnibus Budget Reconciliation Act (OBRA) of 1990 declares that each nursing home resident has the right to be free from unnecessary drugs and physical restraints. In addition, each resident must be provided with treatment to reduce dependency on chemical and physical intervention (Hogstel & Weeks, 2000). The Nursing Home Reform Amendment in OBRA details the regulatory framework governing the use of restraints in all states (Marchello, 2003). Since then, the prevalence of restraint use has decreased by 20%, and many facilities have created restraint-free environments or restraint-free policies and goals

(Guttman, Altman, & Karlan, 1999). The requirements governing the use of restraints include the following: (1) consultation with a physical and/or occupational therapist must be carried out, (2) the least restrictive measures must be considered and this must be documented, (3) a physician's order is required, (4) consent of the resident or family must be obtained, and (5) documentation must be provided that the restraint enables the resident to maintain maximum functional and psychological well-being.

The Joint Commission on Accreditation of Healthcare Organizations (JCAHO) developed recommendations on the use of physical restraints (JCAHO, 1999). Derived from OBRA regulations, the JCAHO guidelines for physical restraints are the following: (1) a physician's order must be obtained, (2) restraint application must be time limited, (3) attempts at alternative approaches must be documented, (4) ongoing observation and assessment of the client must be documented, and (5) care interventions (e.g., provision of food and fluids, toileting, help with activities of daily living, and response to attempted release) must be documented.

Nurses can avoid liability by knowing the law, adhering to the policies and procedures of the institution at which they work, and using good nursing judgment. All nursing homes and hospitals should have written restraint procedures and policies available to all health care providers. If restraints are used, the nurse is responsible for the safety of the client during the time of their use. The client should be restrained only for a minimal time and for a valid purpose. Use of restraints does not enhance client care. Creative nursing skills and interventions are frequently more beneficial.

Chemical Restraints

Drugs usually considered to be chemical restraints include antipsychotics, antianxiety drugs, minor tranquilizers, sedatives, hypnotics, and antidepressants (Ebersole et al., 2004). The National Citizens' Coalition for Nursing Home Reform (1991) wrote guidelines for the use of antipsychotic drugs in certain circumstances. For example, when a person with a cognitive disorder or dementia (with associated psychotic or agitated features) presents a danger to self or to others, and when psychotic symptoms cause the nursing home resident "frightful distress," the use of these drugs is considered medically appropriate and necessary. It is important for nurses to be aware that the use of chemical restraints increases the risk of falls.

Pain

Pain is very common in older adults and affects well-being and quality of life. Up to 85% of the older population is thought to have problems that predispose them to pain, such as arthritis, peripheral vascular disease, and diabetic neuropathy (Luggen, 2000). Pain can be chronic or acute. Although the prevalence of pain in older adults is not accurately known, pain is thought to occur in as many as 70% of community-dwelling adults, a level that may also be found in acute care settings. Pain management in the elderly frequently is not adequate and, in any event, is thought to be less effective than that provided for other age groups (Celia, 2000).

The elderly person's functioning and ability to perform activities of daily living such as walking, toileting, and bathing can be affected by pain, especially pain from musculoskeletal disease. Pain can also lead to increased stress, delayed healing, decreased mobility, interference with sleep, decreased appetite, and agitation with accompanying aggressive behaviors. Chronic pain can cause psychological and emotional distress, including depression, low self-esteem, social isolation, and feelings of hopelessness (Wynne et al., 2000).

Assessment and treatment of pain is one of the main tasks and responsibilities of the geriatric nurse. A full pain assessment is required that considers pain pattern, duration, location, and character; any exacerbating factors or relieving factors; and the most likely cause of the pain. Once an initial pain assessment has been completed, treatment is rendered, and the elderly client is monitored for changes in pain status.

Barriers to Accurate Pain Assessment

When assessing elderly clients, the health care provider takes into account the physical, sensory, psychological, and behavioral changes that affect the elderly. Older adults may give a low ranking to their pain in comparison to other health problems. They are often reluctant to talk about their pain because of a fear of what the pain really signifies, exposure to additional costs, fear of diagnostic tests or medications that may have side effects, and a belief that admitting to pain is a sign of weakness. They may be resigned to accepting serious disease or imminent death as a natural consequence of aging (Miakowski, 1999). Unlike younger adults, the elderly may refer to their pain using words such as *discomfort*, *hurting*, or *aching*. Changes in behavior may indicate pain and should be assessed, especially in clients who have difficulty communicating their needs (e.g., those with dementia).

In the aged, several chronic painful problems may occur together. Sorting out new pain from preexisting pain can be difficult. Sensory impairments, memory loss, dementia, and depression can exacerbate this. Any of these factors can add to the difficulty of obtaining an accurate pain assessment. An interview with close family members or friends is vital in such situations.

Assessment Tools

When pain is suspected, the nurse begins with a physical assessment for medical origins of the pain and assesses the pain itself. Many tools exist to assess pain.

All of them require some sort of communication (e.g., pictorial, verbal, or graphic) between the client and the health care provider. Because the elderly frequently suffer from sensory deficits or cognitive impairments, simply worded questions and simple drawings, which can be easily understood, are the most effective tools (Flaherty, 2000). **Visual analogue scales** (Jacox et al., 1994) (Figure 34-2) and the **Wong-Baker FACES Pain Rating Scale** (Wong et al., 2001) (Figure 34-3) are highly effective assessment instruments. Each visual analogue scale has a horizontal line between two pain extremes and divisions with numbers or words. Clients are asked to choose a position on the line that indicates their level of pain. The FACES scale shows facial expressions on a scale from 0 (a smile) to 5 (crying grimace). Respondents are asked to choose the face that depicts the pain they feel. Studies have shown that 86% of nursing home residents can successfully use either the visual analogue scale or the FACES scale (Flaherty, 2000).

The present pain intensity (PPI) rating from the **McGill Pain Questionnaire (MPQ)** (Davis & Srivastana, 2003) is another tool accepted for use with older clients. Clients are asked to respond by selecting the description (which goes from "no pain" [0] to "excruciating pain" [5]) that they believe identifies the pain they feel. Wynne et al. (2000) found that the PPI rating of the MPQ was the most useful instrument for pain assessment in nursing home residents, including both the cognitively intact and the impaired.

The **Pain Assessment in Advanced Dementia (PAINAD) scale** is used to evaluate the presence and severity of pain in clients with advanced dementia who no longer have the ability to communicate verbally (Figure 34-4). The scale evaluates five domains: breathing, negative vocalization, facial expression, body language, and consolability (Box 34-7). The score guides the caregiver in the appropriate pain intervention (Lane et al., 2003; Warden, Hurley, & Volicer, 2003).

Because pain assessment is an ongoing process, regular communication among staff along with the development of a comprehensive care plan is essential. Many health care workers refer to pain assessment as the fifth vital sign and make it a routine assessment in individuals who are likely to experience pain.

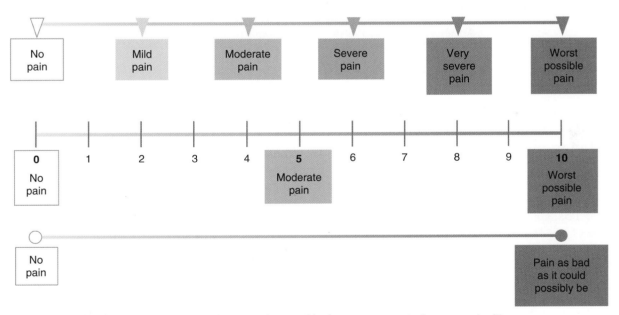

FIGURE 34-2 Visual analogue scales used in the management of cancer pain. (From Jacox A., et al. [1994, March]. *Management of cancer pain* [Clinical Practice Guideline No. 9, AHCPR Publication No. 94-0952]. Rockville, MD: U.S. Department of Health and Human Services, Public Health Service, Agency for Health Care Policy and Research.)

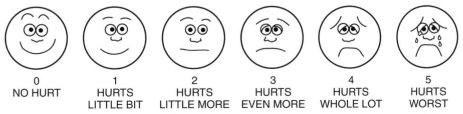

FIGURE 34-3 Wong-Baker FACES Pain Rating Scale. (From Wong D. L., et al. [2001]. *Wong's essentials of pediatric nursing* [6th ed., p. 1301]. St. Louis, MO: Mosby.)

	0	1	2	Score
Breathing Independent of vocalization	Normal	Occasional labored breathing; short period of hyperventilation	Noisy, labored breathing; long period of hyperventilation; Cheyne-Stokes respirations	
Negative Vocalization	None	Occasional moan or groan; low-level speech with a negative or disapproving quality	Repeated troubled calling out; loud moaning or groaning; crying	
Facial Expression	Smiling or inexpressive	Sad; frightened; frown	Facial grimacing	
Body Language	Relaxed	Tense; distressed pacing; fidgeting	Rigid; fists clenched; knees pulled up; pulling or pushing away; striking out	
Consolability	No need to console	Distracted or reassured by voice or touch	Unable to console, distract, or reassure	
			TOTAL	

FIGURE 34-4 Pain Assessment in Advanced Dementia (PAINAD) scale. (From Warden, V., Hurley, A. C., & Volicer, L. [2003]. Development and psychometric evaluation of the Pain Assessment in Advanced Dementia [PAINAD] Scale. *Journal of the American Medical Directors Association, 4*(1), 9-15.)

Pain Management

The cause of the pain should be addressed concomitantly with treatment of the pain itself. Pain should be managed with pharmacological and/or alternative measures. Pharmacological pain management relies on the use of prescriptive and nonprescriptive medications, frequently based on the recommendation of the health care provider. These include analgesics, opioid analgesics, and adjuvant medications. Some considerations in pharmacological pain management in the elderly are listed in Box 34-8.

Physical treatment may consist of exercise, positioning, acupuncture, heat and/or cold, massage, and transcutaneous electrical nerve stimulation (TENS). Cognitive strategies may emphasize relaxation, distraction techniques, biofeedback, and hypnosis. Clients may also seek out alternative medicine approaches such as the use of homeopathy, naturopathic preparations, and spiritual healing. Pain management education is very important for both the client and caregivers. The key to successful pain management lies in the application of a variety of techniques that the client must learn and practice.

Nursing Implications of Pharmacological Treatment of Pain. As the individual ages, the body's ability to eliminate drugs via the kidney decreases. Nurses must be aware of this change, which can result in overdosing. Fear of narcotic overmedication, which can cause respiratory depression, may lead the nurse to give less pain medication to elderly individuals than may actually be needed for effective treatment (Celia, 2000). Bergh and Sjostrom (1999) found that nurses tend to overestimate mild pain and underestimate severe pain. In the latter situation, the nurse may believe that appropriate pain relief medication was administered although the pain was not adequately alleviated. It is critical for nurses to evaluate the effectiveness of pain interventions at regular intervals and to be attentive to behavioral changes or verbal responses that indicate that the client is experiencing pain. It is a common misconception to assume that pain perception decreases with aging. No physiological changes in pain perception in the elderly have been demonstrated. In fact, older adults may feel pain even more keenly than do younger persons (Celia, 2000). Careful and continuing assessments and an understanding of pain physiology are necessary for effective

BOX 34-7

The Five Elements of the Pain Assessment in Advanced Dementia (PAINAD) Scale

1. Breathing
Normal breathing is effortless breathing characterized by quiet, rhythmic respirations.

Occasional labored breathing is characterized by episodic bursts of harsh, difficult, or wearing respirations.

Short period of hyperventilation is characterized by intervals of rapid, deep breaths lasting a short period of time.

Long period of hyperventilation is characterized by excessive rate and depth of respirations lasting a considerable time.

Cheyne-Stokes respirations are characterized by rhythmic waxing and waning of breathing from very deep to shallow respirations with periods of apnea.

2. Negative Vocalization
None is characterized by speech or vocalization that has a neutral or pleasant quality.

Occasional moan or groan: Occasional moaning is characterized by mournful or murmuring sounds, wails, or laments. *Occasional groaning* is characterized by louder than usual inarticulate involuntary sounds, often abruptly beginning and ending.

Low-level speech with negative or disapproving quality is characterized by muttering, mumbling, whining, grumbling, or swearing in a low volume with a complaining, sarcastic, or caustic tone.

Repeated troubled calling out is characterized by phrases or words being used over and over in a tone that suggests anxiety, uneasiness, or distress.

Loud moaning or groaning: Loud moaning is characterized by mournful or murmuring sounds, wails, or laments in a much louder than usual volume. *Loud groaning* is characterized by louder than usual inarticulate involuntary sounds, often abruptly beginning and ending.

Crying is characterized by an utterance of emotion accompanied by tears. There may be sobbing or quiet weeping.

3. Facial Expression
Smiling or inexpressiveness: Smiling is characterized by upturned corners of the mouth, brightening of the eyes, and a look of pleasure or contentment. *Inexpressive* refers to a neutral, at ease, relaxed, or blank look.

Sad is characterized by an unhappy, lonesome, sorrowful, or dejected look. Eyes may be teary.

Frightened is characterized by a look of fear, alarm, or heightened anxiety. Eyes may appear wide open.

Frown is characterized by a downward turn of the corners of the mouth. Increased facial wrinkling in the forehead and around the corners of the mouth may appear.

Facial grimacing is characterized by a distorted, distressed look. The brow is more wrinkled, as is the area around the mouth. Eyes may be squeezed shut.

4. Body Language
Relaxed is characterized by a calm, restful, mellow appearance. The person seems to be taking it easy.

Tense is characterized by a strained, apprehensive, or worried appearance. The jaw may be clenched.

Distressed pacing is characterized by activity that seems unsettled. There may be a fearful, worried, or disturbed element present. The rate may be faster or slower.

Fidgeting is characterized by restless movement. Squirming about or wiggling in the chair may occur. The person might be hitching a chair across the room. Repetitive touching, tugging, or rubbing body parts can also be observed.

Rigid is characterized by stiffening of the body. The arms and/or legs are tight and inflexible. The trunk may appear straight and unyielding (exclude contractures).

Fists clenched are characterized by tightly closed hands. They may be opened and closed repeatedly or held tightly shut.

Knees pulled up is characterized by flexing the legs and drawing the knees upward toward the chest (exclude contractures).

Pulling or pushing away is characterized by resistiveness upon approach or to care. The person is trying to escape by yanking or wrenching himself or herself free or by shoving you away.

Striking out is characterized by hitting, kicking, grabbing, punching, biting, or other forms of personal assault.

5. Consolability
No need to console is characterized by a sense of well-being. The person appears content.

Distracted or reassured by voice or touch is characterized by a disruption in the behavior when the person is spoken to or touched. The behavior stops during the period of interaction with no indication that the person is at all distressed.

Unable to console, distract, or reassure is characterized by the inability to soothe the person or stop a behavior with words or actions. No amount of verbal or physical comforting will alleviate the behavior.

Scoring
See Figure 34-4 for point allocation.
0-1 = No significant pain
2-3 = Mild to moderate pain
4-6 = Moderate to severe pain
7-10 = Severe to very severe pain

From Lane, P., et al. (2003). A pain assessment tool for people with advanced Alzheimer's and other progressive dementias. *Home Healthcare Nurse, 21*(1), 36.

BOX 34-8

Tips on Pharmacological Pain Management in the Elderly

- Remember that older adults often receive pain medication less often than younger adults, which results in inadequate pain relief. Compensate for this.
- Safe administration of analgesics is complicated because of possible interactions with drugs used to treat multiple chronic disorders, nutritional alterations, and altered pharmacokinetics in the elderly.
- Analgesics reach a higher peak and have a longer duration of action in the elderly than in younger individuals. Start with one fourth to one half the adult dose and titrate up carefully.
- Give oral analgesics around the clock at the beginning. Administer on an as-needed basis later on as indicated by the client's pain status.
- If acute confusion occurs, assess for other contributing factors before changing the medication or stopping analgesic use. Confusion in postoperative clients has been found to be associated with unrelieved pain rather than with opiate use.
- **Acetaminophen** is an effective analgesic in the elderly. Although there is an increased risk of end-stage renal disease with long-term use, it does not produce the gastrointestinal bleeding that is seen with the **nonsteroidal antiinflammatory drugs (NSAIDs).**
- Analgesics and adjuvants, such as **anticholinergics** and **pentazocine,** may produce increased confusion in the elderly. The **NSAIDs** can have the same effect during their initial period of administration.
- **Opiates** have a greater analgesic effect and longer duration of action than nonopioid analgesics. Avoid the use of **meperidine,** whose active metabolite may stimulate the central nervous system and lead to confusion, seizures, and mood alterations. If this drug is selected, do not use it for more than 48 hours. Avoid intramuscular administration because of tissue irritation and poor absorption. **Morphine** is a safer choice than meperidine because its duration of action is longer, so a smaller overall dose is required.
- Assess bowel function daily, because constipation can be a frequent side effect of opiates.

Data from Davis, M., & Srivastava, M. (2003). Demographics, assessment and management of pain in the elderly. *Drugs and Aging, 20*(1), 23-35.

pain management in the elderly (Luggen, 2000). Nurses must evaluate the effectiveness of pain interventions at regular intervals.

Decision Making

Patient Self-Determination Act

Since the 1960s, the public's desire to participate in decision making about health care has increased. This interest in client advocacy was recognized when Congress passed the Patient Self-Determination Act (PSDA) in 1990 requiring that health care facilities provide clear written information for every client regarding his or her legal rights to make health care decisions, including the right to accept or refuse treatment (Carson, 2000). It also establishes the right of a person to provide directions for clinicians to follow in the event of a serious illness. Increasing numbers of the elderly are creating written directives.

Advance directives is a term used to describe living wills, durable powers of attorney for health care, and health care surrogate appointments (Ebersole et al., 2004). Health care institutions that receive federal funds are now required to provide to each client at the time of admission written information regarding his or her right to execute advance health care directives and are required to inquire if such directives have been made by the client. The client's admission records should state whether such directives exist. The ANA (1992) recommends that specific questions be part of every nurse's admission assessment. Box 34-9 reproduces these questions and describes the responsibilities of health care workers under the PSDA.

Such a directive indicates preferences for the types of medical care or amount of treatment desired. The directive comes into effect should physical or mental incapacitation prevent the client from making health care decisions. These wishes can be communicated through one or more of the following instruments: (1) a living will, (2) a directive to physician, and (3) a durable power of attorney for health care. These documents must be in writing and the client's signature must be witnessed; depending on state and institutional provisions, notarization of the documents may be required.

Living Will. A living will is a personal statement of how and where one wishes to die (Ebersole et al., 2004). It is activated only when the person is terminally ill and incapacitated. A competent client may alter a living will at any time. The question of whether an incompetent person can change a living will is addressed on a state-by-state basis. Executing a living will does not always guarantee its application.

Directive to Physician. In a directive to physician, a physician is appointed by the individual to serve as proxy. Many of the features of a directive to physician parallel those of a living will, such as activation only when a terminal illness is present, need for verification of the terminal illness by the physician, and requirement for client competency at the time of signing. The directive to physician designating the physician as surrogate can be particularly useful in cases of terminal illness when an individual has no family. The physician must agree in writing to be the client's agent and must also be one of the two physicians who made the original determination that the

BOX 34-9

Nurses' Responsibilities and the Patient Self-Determination Act (1990)

Part of Nursing Admission Assessment

- Nurses should know the laws of the state in which [they] practice . . . and should be familiar with the strengths and limitations of the various forms of advance directive.
- The ANA recommends that the following questions be part of the nursing admission assessment:
  1. Do you have basic information about advance care directives, including living wills and durable power of attorney?
  2. Do you wish to initiate an advance care directive?
  3. If you have already prepared an advance care directive, can you provide it now?
  4. Have you discussed your end-of-life choices with your family or designated surrogate and health care workers?

Responsibilities of Health Care Workers Under the Patient Self-Determination Act of 1990

- Hospitals, skilled nursing facilities, home health agencies, hospice organizations, and health maintenance organizations serving Medicare and Medicaid clients must
  1. Maintain written policies and procedures for providing information to their clients for whom they provide care.
  2. Give written material to clients concerning their rights under state law to make decisions about medical care, including the right to accept or refuse surgical or medical care and to formulate advance directives and provide written policies and procedures for the realization of these rights.
  3. Document in clients' records whether they have advance directives.
  4. Not discriminate in care or in other ways against clients who have or have not prepared advance directives.
  5. Make sure that policies are in place to ensure compliance with state laws governing advance directives.

Data from Schlossberg, C., & Hart, M. A. (1992). Legal perspectives. In M. Burke & M. Walsh (Eds.), *Gerontologic nursing care of the frail elderly* (p. 469). St. Louis, MO: Mosby; and American Nurses Association. (1992). *Position statement on nursing and the patient self-determination act.* Washington, DC: Author.

client is terminally ill. Unlike the living will, the directive to physician can be revoked orally at any time without regard to client competency.

Durable Power of Attorney for Health Care.

The durable power of attorney for health care differs from the two instruments described earlier in that a person other than a physician is appointed to act as the client's agent. The client must be competent and of age when making the appointment and must also be competent in order to revoke the power. Individuals do not have to be terminally ill or incompetent to allow the empowered individual to act on their behalf. No physician's certification is required.

Nursing Role in the Decision-Making Process

The nurse explains the ethics and legal policies of the institution to both the client and family and helps them understand the concepts behind advance directives. The nurse explains that the family need not feel morally obligated to provide for all possible medical care when such care will only extend the suffering of a loved one. This is especially true when such extraordinary measures do not represent the person's values and beliefs. The nurse serves as an advocate and a knowledgeable resource person for the elderly client and family. The client is encouraged to verbalize his or her feelings and thoughts during this sensitive time of decision making. In addition, nurses are responsible for being knowledgeable about the state regulations on advance directives as well as the potential obstacles in completing the directives for the state in which they practice. Maintenance of an open and continuing dialogue among client, family, nurse, and physician is of principal importance. The nurse supports any surrogates appointed to act on the client's behalf and seeks consultation for ethical issues the nurse feels unprepared to handle.

Every health care facility receiving federal funds is required to have written policies, procedures, and protocols in compliance with the PSDA. Nurses must prepare themselves to deal with the legal, ethical, and moral issues involved when counseling about advance directives. The new law does not specify who should talk with clients about treatment decisions, but in many facilities nurses are being asked to discuss this issue with the client. If the advance directive of a client is not being followed, the nurse intervenes on the client's behalf. If the problem cannot be resolved with the physician, the facility's protocol providing for notification of the appropriate supervisor is followed.

Although nurses, especially in nursing homes, may discuss options with their clients, they may not assist clients in writing advance directives because this is considered a conflict of interest. The existence of an advance directive serves as a guide to health care providers in advocating for the elderly client's rightful wishes in this process.

Acquired Immunodeficiency Syndrome

Human immunodeficiency virus (HIV) infection and AIDS are rising faster among the older population than among those 24 years old and younger (Goodroad, 2003). Butler and Lewis (2002) indicate that 10% of people over age 50 years have active AIDS; one fourth of those are older than age 60 years and 4% are older than age 70 years. Blood transfusions are no longer the main cause for the spread of AIDS in the elderly. Research shows that elders are sexually active and thus at risk for HIV-AIDS due to failure to practice "safer sex." The aged and their spouses who received blood transfusions before 1985 are also at risk. In addition, the diagnosis and treatment of HIV-AIDS in the elderly are delayed because health care providers believe that elders are not sexually active. In general, lack of adequate knowledge about HIV-AIDS among the elderly, coupled with denial that this illness occurs in their generation, increases their risk for HIV infection and AIDS.

Older women who are sexually active are at higher risk for HIV-AIDS from an infected partner than are older men. Changes in vaginal tissue caused by the aging process can lead to tears in the vaginal mucosa during intercourse that allow HIV to penetrate. In addition, because pregnancy is no longer a threat, use of condoms in this age group is uncommon. This puts the older woman at greater risk of exposure (Hess, 2004).

Because dementia caused by AIDS and that caused by Alzheimer's disease can be easily confounded, a careful assessment and workup are required. The health care provider must be aware that AIDS can occur in the elderly. AIDS dementia has a rapid onset and may mimic symptoms of Alzheimer's disease such as confusion, forgetfulness, leg tremors, progressive weakness, apathy, fatigue, weight loss, and neurological abnormalities (Hess, 2004). Refer to Chapter 21 for a comprehensive discussion of Alzheimer's disease.

Generally, health care providers have directed their educational efforts in HIV prevention toward the younger age group. It is essential for the nursing and medical community to realize that age does not preclude sexual activity and that the potential for exposure to HIV exists among sexually active elderly clients. In recognition of the fact that the elderly may become victims of AIDS, educational programs need to address prevention strategies for both the elderly and health care providers as well as provide information on assessment and treatment of AIDS across the life span.

Suicide

Although suicide is often associated with the young, the suicide rates among the elderly in the United States are the highest of any age group. Suicide is now one of the top ten causes of death among the aged. Although older adults account for only 13% of the population, they are disproportionately affected by suicide: 20% of all suicides are committed by individuals 65 years of age or older (Luggen, 2004; McAndrews, 2001). Nationally, the highest rates of suicide are found in individuals over age 65 years (Ingram, 2001). Refer to Chapter 23 for a comprehensive discussion of suicide.

The highest prevalence of suicide occurs in elderly white males. One explanation for the high white male suicide rate may lie in changes of occupational status and measures of success in men at the time of retirement and thereafter (Ebersole et al., 2004). With retirement, a man may lose status, influence, and contact with fellow workers in the community. On the other hand, the older woman retains many of her earlier activities and roles. It remains to be seen whether women and other groups who have become more active in the workforce will experience the same effects as men on retirement. The Protestant white male older than 85 years of age living alone in his home is at highest risk. Although such a person appears neat and calm, he is often taking either antianxiety or antipsychotic medication (Hogstel & Weeks, 2000).

Other factors that can lead to suicide are feelings of hopelessness, uselessness, and despair. For older adults, suicide may be seen as a final gesture of control at a stage when independence is at risk or activities are limited. Severe medical illness, functional disability, alcohol abuse, history of suicide attempts, comorbid anxiety, and psychotic depression are added risk factors for suicide (Dharmarajan & Norman, 2003). For this reason, the suicide attempts of the elderly are more likely to succeed. Unlike younger persons, whose suicidal gestures may be intended to draw attention to their problems, those of older adults do not signify a call for help but rather a desire to die.

Financial need is another risk factor contributing to the high suicide rate. Federal reductions in programs such as Medicare, Medicaid, and food stamps, along with state-ordered cuts in medical care, cause many elderly Americans to worry about their future. An inverse relationship between economic conditions and suicide rate has been identified.

Even though suicide rates among the elderly are high, suicides in this group are probably underreported. Suicide is often not listed on the death certificate, even if it is suspected. The numbers also do not reflect those who passively or indirectly commit suicide by abusing alcohol, starving themselves, overdosing or mixing medications, stopping life-sustaining drugs, or simply losing the will to live. Many individuals who committed suicide visited their physicians within a week or month of their deaths (Andersen et al., 2000). Health care providers must promptly evaluate the potential for suicide of these high-risk individuals (Juurlink et al., 2004; Moscicki & Caine, 2004).

Assessment of Suicide Risk in the Elderly

The assessment of elderly clients must include attention to the high-risk factors that potentially contribute to suicide, such as widowhood, acute illnesses and intractable pain, status change, chronic illness, family history of suicide, chronic sleep problems, alcoholism, depression, and losses (Hogstel & Weeks, 2000). Losses may be personal (death of a family member or close friend), economic (loss of earnings or job), or social (loss of prestige or position). Multiple losses accompany the aging process, increasing stress at a time when the older adult may be the most vulnerable and least able to cope with stress and thus precipitating a depressive state. Nevertheless, many older adults are able to function despite their losses. Those who give in may do so because of hopelessness.

The nurse must remain vigilant for possible suicidal tendencies in clients later in life. In assessing suicide risk, the health care provider must examine previous suicidal behavior, seriousness of the intent, presence of active plans, availability of the means to commit the act, lethality of the method chosen, and the specific details of the plan. Compared to those in younger age groups, older adults are less likely to communicate their suicidal thoughts and plans (Hogstel &Weeks, 2000). Nurses play a vital role in the prevention of elderly suicide because of their presence in every care setting. Attention must be focused on building awareness and use of community resources in the high-risk population. Screening for depression and suicidal thinking in the elderly should be standard and would save lives.

The nurse is professionally obligated to respond and intervene with the elderly client in crisis, especially when the client believes that the willful destruction of life is the only option available. It is therefore very important to maintain a sensitive, compassionate, and therapeutic approach with the client. Communication with the elderly client must be skillful, clear, direct, and respectful of the individual's rights. For some people, these interventions may restore a sense of self and purpose so that life may be preserved (Ebersole et al., 2004). Questions such as the following may be asked in suicide assessment:

- What kinds of thoughts do you have about a person's right to take his or her life?
- What advantage does ending one's life offer?

In the elderly, suicide is most closely associated with untreated depression (National Center for Injury Prevention and Control, 2003). As the most frequent functional psychiatric disorder of later life, depression accounts for up to 70% of late-life suicides. Research has shown that most elderly who commit suicide suffer from the most treatable kind of depression and yet do not receive needed mental health services (National Institute of Mental Health, 2004). Early identification of and treatment for depression, therefore, are key measures for suicide prevention.

Right to Suicide

One concern of nursing is the question of whether an elderly individual has the right to commit suicide. Suicide always raises spiritual and moral issues. However, there are some in society who believe that elderly persons with terminal illnesses should be able to control their own deaths. If an alert elderly client is confronted with an intractable, lingering, and painful illness, with no hope of relief except by committing suicide, is the intervention of the health care provider to prevent suicide justifiable? The ANA advises nurses not to participate in assisted suicide. It is a violation of the ANA Code for Nurses to participate in assisted suicide; however, this does not mean that clients who want their life terminated should be abandoned (ANA, 1985).

Although suicide is discussed in Chapter 23, specific factors that concern the elderly are noted here, such as retirement-related difficulties, physical illness, economic problems, loneliness, social isolation, multiple losses, and ageism. Innovative methods to deal with these factors need to be developed for the elderly. Education of the public in general—and health care providers, in particular—is necessary to raise the level of awareness of this geriatric problem.

Depression Versus Dementia

Depression is often confused with dementia and is not always recognized. This is important for nurses to keep in mind. A careful, systematic assessment is therefore necessary to properly distinguish between the two. Unlike dementia, depression is treatable with medication and other interventions. In the elderly, symptoms of memory loss and other intellectual impairments or asocial or agitated behavior are generally associated with dementia but may actually be caused by depression. See Chapter 21 for comparisons between dementia and depression.

In making an assessment, the nurse needs to be familiar with the symptoms of later-life depression (National Institute of Mental Health, 2004), which include one or more of the following:

- Changes in sleep patterns (insomnia)
- Changes in eating patterns (loss of appetite)
- Loss of interest or pleasure in usual activities (anhedonia)
- Excessive fatigue (anergia)
- Increased concern with bodily functions
- Feelings of depression
- Apprehension and anxiety without any cause
- Low self-esteem (feelings of insignificance or pessimism)

A careful evaluation of the cause of the depression is also necessary. Depression can be caused by drugs (e.g., reserpine and other *Rauwolfia* derivatives, steroids, phenothiazines), by metabolic and endocrine disorders (e.g., hepatitis and adrenal and thyroid insufficiency), as well as by acute medical events such as cerebrovascular accident or myocardial infarction. Chronic health problems may also augment the depression and suicide potential. Thorough assessment for any medical or drug-induced side effects should be performed.

Antidepressant Therapy

In choosing a drug to treat depression in the elderly, primary emphasis is placed on avoidance of possible side effects rather than on efficacy. When antidepressant therapy is initiated, low dosages (usually half the routine recommended dosage) are suggested, and the dosage is then slowly and gradually increased if needed (Doddi, 2003). If the individual is at risk for suicide, then caregivers must be aware that, as the depression begins to lift, there is a greater chance that the individual will complete the suicide.

Selective serotonin reuptake inhibitors (SSRIs) are the first-line antidepressants for elderly individuals because of their more benign side effects profile and their lack of toxicity when taken in overdose (Ebersole et al., 2004; National Institute of Mental Health, 2004). The SSRIs are also helpful for those older adults with conduction defects, ischemic heart disease, glaucoma, and prostate disease (Rueben et al., 2003). However, SSRIs may also cause some problems, especially for elderly people who are more sensitive to medications and are therefore at greater risk for drug-drug interactions (Schatzberg & Nemeroff, 2004).

Fluoxetine and paroxetine can cause symptoms of central nervous system stimulation, including increased awakenings, reduced time in rapid eye movement sleep, and insomnia. Age does not appear to affect the pharmacokinetics of sertraline. However, the metabolism of fluoxetine and paroxetine is impaired in the elderly, which results in higher plasma levels. This makes sertraline a good choice among the SSRIs for antidepressant therapy for the older population. Reboxetine, a selective noradrenaline reuptake inhibitor, has also been found to be an effective and well-tolerated antidepressant for both long- and short-term treatment of the elderly (Aguglia, 2000).

The depressed elderly are at high risk for physical decline. Prevention and treatment of depression is a practical intervention to reduce physical decline in later years. Client and family education is an important component of successful management.

The advanced practice nurse may provide individual and/or group psychotherapy to the depressed elderly client. Groups are useful for the elderly because they can diminish social isolation and loneliness and help the members understand that they are not alone in their situation. Group members can learn creative ways to raise their mood and increase quality of life. Individual therapy, specifically cognitive-behavioral and psychodynamic therapy, is also useful. The best outcomes result from combining some kind of therapy with medication. Primary care providers therefore must acquire the skills to enable sensitive assessment for depression and suicide risk and must be knowledgeable about methods of intervention. See the Evidence-Based Practice box for study findings related to treatment of late-life depression.

Alcoholism and Substance Abuse

The American Medical Association has termed alcohol and substance abuse among the elderly a hidden epidemic. Identifying alcohol and substance abuse in the elderly is often difficult because personality and behavioral changes frequently go unrecognized and health care providers seldom assess the elderly for these problems (Riger, 2000). Let us first examine alcoholism.

Alcoholism

More than 10% of all older Americans in the community at large, and 20% of elders who are hospitalized, have serious problems with alcohol. Unfortunately, most (85%) receive no treatment. There are two major types of abusers: (1) the early-onset alcoholic or aging alcoholic, and (2) the late-onset alcoholic or geriatric problem drinker. The aging alcoholic has generally had alcohol problems intermittently throughout life, with a regular pattern of alcohol abuse starting to evolve in late middle age or later. The geriatric problem drinker, on the other hand, has no history of alcohol-related problems but develops an alcohol abuse pattern in response to the stresses of aging (Wagenaar, Mickus, & Wilson, 2001).

The stressful or reactive factors that precipitate late-onset alcohol abuse are often related to environmental conditions and may include retirement, widowhood, and loneliness. These stressors in the older adult, who may have retired, may not drive, and may be isolated from family and friends, are often greater than the problems faced by the middle-aged adult, who has to manage a job or career and care for a family and household. Work and family responsibilities may help keep a potential alcoholic from drinking too much. Once these demands are gone and the structure of daily life is disrupted, there is little impetus to remain sober. Older adults who lose a spouse through death, divorce, or legal separation are at the highest risk of becoming late-in-life alcoholics (Wagenaar et al., 2001).

Alcohol and Aging. Excessive consumption of alcohol can create particular problems for the elderly. The older adult has an increased biological sensitivity to (a decreased tolerance for) the effects of alcohol. This diminished resistance, combined with age-related changes such as weakened manual dexterity, balance, and postural flexibility, can increase the likelihood of falls, burns, or other accidents in elders who drink (Wagenaar, 2001).

Some drinkers, as they get older, note changes in their response to alcohol, such as the occurrence of headaches, reduction in mental abilities with memory losses or lapses, and feelings of malaise rather than well-being. These problems start to occur at lower levels of consumption than was the case in earlier years. Older persons are likely to drink more frequently but in lesser quantities than younger individuals, who tend to drink larger amounts less often. Thus, the possibility of alcohol abuse in cases of only moderate ingestion by the elderly often is not recognized by the alcoholic's friends or family.

With aging, the body becomes less resilient; healing from injury or infection is slower, and stress is more likely to cause a loss of physiological equilibrium. As the proportion of fatty tissues to lean body mass increases with age, the individual's metabolic rate usually slows down, which increases the amount of time it takes the body to eliminate drugs (Wagenaar et al., 2001).

Alcohol and Medication. The interaction of drugs and alcohol in the elderly can have serious consequences. There is a decreased functioning of the liver enzymes that break down the alcohol, which on a short-term basis has the effect of prolonging the action of many medications, potentiating their effect. On the other hand, chronic ingestion of alcohol speeds up the metabolism of many drugs (Wagenaar et al., 2001).

Older individuals can expect to reach higher blood alcohol levels than younger persons with an equivalent intake of alcohol. The effects of alcohol on the brain may be one reason that alcohol abuse sometimes mimics or exacerbates normal changes of aging, because even a moderate intake of alcohol can impair the cognition and coordination skills that are already decreased with age.

Extreme care is required when treating the older alcoholic with medication. Central nervous system toxicity from psychoactive drugs increases with aging. Ingestion of antidepressants or tranquilizers can be particularly harmful because their effect is further potentiated by alcohol. The toxicity of other drugs (e.g., acetaminophen) is enhanced by alcohol and by the age-related decrease in clearance (Luggen, 2004).

Alcohol consumption produces a change in sleep patterns, particularly in older adults. Unlike younger persons, the elderly take longer to fall asleep and do not sleep as restfully. Although alcohol may decrease the time it takes to fall asleep, this benefit is offset by frequent awakenings during the night caused by alcohol (Luggen, 2004).

 EVIDENCE-BASED PRACTICE

Collaborative Care Management of Late-Life Depression in the Primary Care Setting

Background
Depression occurs frequently in the elderly, who are sometimes unwilling to seek out psychotherapy. Efforts have been made to identify an effective model for treating the depressed elderly. The hypothesis of this study was that collaboration between psychiatrists and primary care providers could improve the mood of elderly clients experiencing late-life depression. The model is called IMPACT: Improving Mood-Promoting Access to Collaborative Treatment.

Study
A randomized controlled trial was conducted that recruited a total of 1801 clients aged 60 years or older between July 1999 and August 2001 from 18 primary care clinics and 8 health care organizations in five states. The clients were diagnosed with major depression, dysthymic disorder, or both. Clients were randomly assigned to the IMPACT intervention or to usual care. Clients receiving IMPACT intervention had access for up to 12 months to a depression care manager. The depression care manager was supervised by a psychiatrist and a primary care expert; was usually a nurse; and offered education, care management, and support of antidepressant management by the client's primary care physician or brief psychotherapy for depression, termed Problem-Solving Treatment in Primary Care. Assessments were performed at baseline and at 3, 6, and 12 months for depression, depression treatments, satisfaction with care, functional impairment, and quality of life.

Results of Study
At 12 months, 45% of the clients in the IMPACT intervention group had a 50% or greater reduction in depressive symptoms from baseline compared with a 19% reduction for participants receiving usual care; they also experienced greater rates of depression treatment, more satisfaction with depression care, lower depression severity, less functional impairment, and greater quality of life than participants assigned to the usual care group.

The IMPACT collaborative care model appears to be feasible and significantly more effective than usual care for treatment of depression in a wide range of primary care practices.

Implications for Nursing Practice
Nurses played a pivotal role in this study, which demonstrated that nurses working as primary care providers in collaboration with physicians are effective in improving the mood of elderly clients diagnosed with late-life depression. The results of this study suggest that nurses must play a critical role in coordinating care and working collaboratively with the physician. The nurse's ability to teach, counsel, case manage, and provide psychobiological interventions makes nursing a key to improving depression in the elderly.

Unutzer J., et al. (2002). Collaborative care management of late-life depression in the primary care setting: A randomized controlled trial. *Journal of the American Medical Association, 288*(22), 2836-2845.

Symptoms of Elder Dependence. Health practitioners working with the elderly need to be concerned with, and sensitive to, possible alcohol abuse among their older clients. Signs of alcohol abuse in younger individuals (e.g., alcohol-induced pancreatitis or liver disease, blackouts, major trauma) occur infrequently in older adults. Instead, the older alcoholic displays vague geriatric syndromes of contusions, malnutrition, self-neglect, depression, and falls (Wagenaar et al., 2001). Also present may be symptoms of diarrhea, urinary incontinence, a decrease in functional status, failure to thrive, and apparent dementia. Symptoms of poor coordination or visual changes may also mimic the normal aging process but actually be due to excessive drinking. Although confusion and disorientation in an older client are often associated with dementia or Alzheimer's disease, they could be caused by other factors, including alcohol abuse. Assessment of these conditions is necessary to differentiate the normal physiological changes of aging from those due to excessive drinking.

Treatment of the Elderly Alcoholic. Because many elderly people do not live in big families or have work-related contacts, they are less likely to be referred for treatment than are younger drinkers. Too often, by the time the elderly alcoholic comes to the notice of any treatment agencies, the client's support systems and resources are severely decreased or depleted. Declining social, physical, and psychological performance is frequently found in the elderly alcoholic, which exacerbates the difficulties of loneliness, depression, monotony, accidents, social conflict, loss, and the physiological changes of aging (Wagenaar et al., 2001).

Ageism has deterred the development of treatment programs designed specially for the elderly. Beliefs that the elderly are too isolated, too embedded in denial of their illness, and too old to function have been detrimental to encouraging health professionals to work with chemically dependent seniors. Another factor that may play a role is that older adults often try to hide alcohol dependence because they consider such abuse sinful or feel they can handle any problems themselves (Ebersole et al., 2004).

Whenever there is a suspicion or indication that an older adult is abusing alcohol, the health care provider should conduct a screening test. The CAGE-AID screening tool (Wagenaar et al., 2001) (Box 34-10) and the MAST-G (see Box 34-4) are instruments commonly used to assess the elderly (Menninger, 2004).

Treatment plans for the elderly problem drinker should emphasize social therapies. Elderly alcoholics tend to be more passive than younger alcoholics and may benefit from interpersonal involvement with professional health care personnel. Old people respond easily to emotional and social support. Family therapy should be encouraged. Group therapy with other mid-

---

BOX 34-10

CAGE-AID Screening Tool

C—Have you ever felt you ought to **C**ut down on your drinking (drug use)?

A—Have people **A**nnoyed you by criticizing your drinking (drug use)?

G—Have you ever felt bad or **G**uilty about your drinking (drug use)?

E—Have you ever had a drink (used drugs) first thing in the morning (**E**ye-opener) to steady your nerves or get rid of a hangover?

AID—adapted to include drugs. One positive answer indicates a possible problem; two positive answers indicate a probable problem.

From Ewing, J. A. (1984). Detecting alcoholism: The CAGE questionnaire. *Journal of the American Medical Association, 252,* 1905-1907.

---

dle-aged and older alcoholics as well as self-help groups like Alcoholics Anonymous can also be effective.

Although the aging alcoholic is difficult to treat, the prognosis for the geriatric problem drinker—a person who had lived to this point without recourse to alcohol and whose drinking is caused by losses and stress—is excellent. This individual often responds very positively to an alcoholic recovery program, especially if it is accompanied by environmental interventions (Salisbury, 1999). It is important that health care providers recognize this recovery potential. Proper education and awareness of a positive outcome for the geriatric problem drinker can increase the availability of resources; if the prognosis is good, providers and agencies should be more willing to spend resources on treatment.

Considering the magnitude of the problems and the likelihood that the number of older abusers will continue to increase, efforts need to be intensified to identify the causes of alcohol dependence among the elderly and to develop appropriate interventions for treating it. If not, such dependence can overwhelm those charged with meeting the health and social service needs of older adults.

Drug Abuse

Illegal Drug Use. Currently the prevalence of illicit drug use among the elderly is low (Patterson, Lacro, & Jeste, 1999). However, there is real concern that this will change dramatically as the baby boom generation moves into old age. Studies indicate that about 5% of baby boomers currently use illicit drugs, and projections are that this number will remain constant in the future. In 2011 the oldest members of the baby boom generation will turn 65 year of age, and during the following decade the number of individuals over the age of 65 years will increase by about 22 million. The sheer numbers of aging baby boomers threaten to overwhelm treatment resources. Today most substance abuse treatment is geared to the young abuser; major changes will need to occur to manage a large number of elderly abusers.

Prescription and Over-the-Counter Drug Use and Abuse. Because elderly clients use both prescription and over-the-counter drugs at a higher rate than the general population, it is difficult to accurately estimate the extent to which these drugs are abused and/or misused. The high exposure to medications coupled with age-related physiological changes, including decreased elimination, increased accumulation, and, in the case of the benzodiazepines, increased sensitivity, raises the likelihood of medication-related adverse events such as increased confusion, falls, and hip fractures (Patterson et al., 1999).

■ ■ ■ KEY POINTS to REMEMBER

- The elderly population continues to increase exponentially.
- The increase in the number of elderly poses a challenge not only to nurses but to the entire health care system to be prepared to respond to the special needs of this population.
- Attitudes toward the elderly are often negative, reflecting ageism—a bias against the elderly based solely on age.
- Ageism is found at all levels of society and even among health care providers, which affects the way we render care to our elderly clients.

- Nurses who care for the elderly in various settings may function at different levels. All should be knowledgeable about the process of aging and be cognizant of the differences between normal and abnormal aging changes.
- Older adults face increasing problems of alcoholism, abuse and misuse of prescription and over-the-counter drugs, and suicide.
- OBRA established guidelines and a philosophy of care that call for clients to be free from unnecessary use of drugs and physical restraints.
- Adequate pain assessment is important, and the nurse must bear in mind that the elderly tend to understate their pain. Sufficient pain medication should be administered and the drugs carefully titrated.
- Nurses working with the mentally ill client must know psychotherapeutic approaches relevant for the elderly, such as remotivation and reminiscence therapy. Advanced practice nurses may offer psychotherapy groups geared toward the special needs of this population.
- When it comes to dying and death, older adults' wishes and those of their families are frequently ignored. The implementation of the PSDA, passed in 1990, can afford some clients autonomy and dignity in death.

■ ■ ■

Visit the Evolve website at **http://evolve.elsevier.com/Varcarolis** for a posttest on the content in this chapter. *evolve*

Critical Thinking and Chapter Review

Visit the Evolve website at **http://evolve.elsevier.com/Varcarolis** for additional self-study exercises.
evolve

■ ■ ■ CRITICAL THINKING

1. Mr. Lopez is 70 years old and has been admitted to the intensive care unit with a diagnosis of alcohol withdrawal delirium. He is confused and combative, and threatens to strike the nurse who is trying to render care to him unless he is allowed to leave. The nurse applies wrist restraints to keep Mr. Lopez from striking her and leaving the room. What are the mandates of OBRA (1990) regarding the use of restraints?

2. Mr. Lopez has received treatment for alcohol withdrawal. He appears very quiet, refuses to eat, does not sleep at night, admits to thoughts of desperation, and wishes he could die. He also confides that he attempted suicide when his wife died 5 years earlier and at that time he started drinking heavily. Which is the appropriate depression assessment tool to use in assessing the severity of Mr. Lopez's condition? Explain your answer.

    A. Michigan Alcoholism Screening Test
    B. Geriatric Depression Scale
    C. Mini-Mental State Examination
    D. Patient Self-Determination Act

3. Mr. Simon, age 85 years, lives with his family. He has advanced Alzheimer's disease and often has short-lived angry outbursts. Mr. Simon's family wants to keep him at home for as long as possible, but family members are overwhelmed by his constant needs. Many well-meaning relatives have suggested that he be placed in a nursing home on a unit specifically designed for Alzheimer's clients. Which of the following community placements might be best for Mr. Simon? Explain your answer.

    A. Social day care
    B. Adult day health
    C. Maintenance day care
    D. Community mental health center

Continued

Critical Thinking and Chapter Review—cont'd

■ ■ ■ CHAPTER REVIEW

Choose the most appropriate answer.

1. Which of the following is most essential to the provision of high-quality nursing assessment of elderly clients? The nurse's knowledge of
    1. normal aging.
    2. drug interactions.
    3. chronic diseases.
    4. community supports.

2. Mrs. W. is an 82-year-old physically healthy widow who lives with her daughter and son-in-law, both of whom work during the day. Mrs. W. states that she is lonely at home, since all her friends are elderly and unable to visit her. Mrs. W.'s daughter reports that her mother "isn't as sharp as she once was" and mentions that she doesn't keep up with current news events and converses less during the evenings. The daughter asks if there are any programs that would be suitable for her mother. Assuming each is available, which should the nurse suggest?
    1. Social day care center
    2. Adult day health care center
    3. Maintenance day care center
    4. Skilled nursing facility

3. Which is knowledge the nurse needs when caring for an elderly client in restraint?
    1. Restraint use appreciably enhances the overall safety of the client.
    2. The nurse is responsible for client safety during the time the client is restrained.
    3. Chemical restraint presents less potential for client harm than physical restraint.
    4. Restraint may be used to prevent extubation if a nursing protocol exists.

4. Which view held by a nurse may prevent adequate intervention for an elderly client experiencing pain?
    1. Pain perception decreases with aging.
    2. Nonpharmacological interventions may provide control over pain.
    3. Research has demonstrated that nurses tend to underestimate severe pain.
    4. The nurse should assess verbal, facial, behavioral, and physical expressions of pain.

5. Which of the following is an action that is ethically unsuitable for a nurse?
    1. Ignoring a "Do not resuscitate" order for an elderly client in the intensive care unit
    2. Implementing a physician's orders to withhold artificial hydration from an elderly client in irreversible coma
    3. Adhering to the choices made for an elderly client by the individual with durable power of attorney for health care
    4. Advocating for an elderly client in the terminal stage of cancer who wishes to discontinue chemotherapy

---

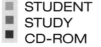
■ **STUDENT**
■ **STUDY**
■ **CD-ROM**

Access the accompanying CD-ROM for animations, interactive exercises, review questions for the NCLEX examination, and an audio glossary.

REFERENCES

Aguglia, E. (2000). Reboxetine in the maintenance therapy of depressive disorder in the elderly: A long-term open study. *International Journal of Geriatric Psychiatry, 15*(9), 784-793.

American Nurses Association. (1992). *Position statement on nursing and the patient self-determination act.* Washington, DC: Author.

Andersen, U., et al. (2000). Contacts to the health care system prior to suicide: A comprehensive analysis using registers for general and psychiatric hospital admissions, contacts to general practitioners and practicing specialists, and drug prescriptions. *Acta Psychiatrica Scandinavia, 102,* 126-134.

Arbesman, M. C., & Wright, C. (1999). Mechanical restraints, rehabilitation therapies, and staffing adequacy as risk factors for falls in an elderly hospitalized population. *Rehabilitation Nursing, 24*(3), 122-128.

Bergh, I., & Sjostrom, B. (1999). A comparative study of nurses' and elderly patients' ratings of pain and pain tolerance. *Journal of Gerontological Nursing, 25*(5), 30-36.

Butler, R., & Lewis, M. (2002). *The new love and sex after 60.* New York: Ballantine Books.

Carson, V. B. (2000). The older adult. In: *Mental health nursing: The nurse-patient journey* (pp. 561-580). Philadelphia: Saunders.

Celia, B. (2000). Age and gender differences in pain management following coronary artery bypass surgery. *Journal of Gerontological Nursing, 26*(5), 7-13.

Davis, M., & Srivastana, M. (2003). Demographics, assessment and management of pain in the elderly. *Drugs and Aging, 20*(1), 23-35.

Dharmarajan, T., & Norman, R. (Eds.). (2003). *Clinical geriatrics.* New York: Parthenon Publishing Group.

Doddi, S. R. (2003). Depression in the older adult. In T. Dharmarajan & R. Norman (Eds.), *Clinical geriatrics.* New York: Parthenon Publishing Group.

Ebersole, P., Hess, P., & Luggen A. (2004). *Toward healthy aging: Human needs and nursing response* (6th ed.). St. Louis, MO: Mosby.

Flaherty, E. (2000). Assessing pain in older adults. *Journal of Gerontological Nursing, 26*(3), 5-6.

Fultner, D., & Raudonis, B. (2000). Home care and hospice. In A. Lueckenotte (Ed.), *Gerontologic nursing* (p. 771). St. Louis, MO: Mosby.

Goodroad, B. K. (2003). HIV and AIDS in people older than 50. *Journal of Gerontological Nursing, 29*(4), 18-24.

Guttman, R., Altman, R., & Karlan, M. (1999). Report of the Council on Scientific Affairs: Use of restraints for patients in nursing homes. *Archives of Family Medicine, 8*(2), 101-105.

Henderson, J. (2003). Aging and public health. In T. Dharmarajan & R. Norman (Eds.), *Clinical geriatrics.* New York: Parthenon Publishing Group.

Hess, P. (2004). Intimacy, sexuality, and aging. In P. Ebersole, P. Hess, & A. S. Luggen (Eds.), *Toward healthy aging: Human needs and nursing response.* St. Louis, MO: Mosby.

Hetzel, L., & Smith, A. (2001, October). *The 65 years and over population: 2000.* Retrieved April 2, 2005, from the U.S. Census Bureau website: http://www.census.gov/prod/2001pubs/c2kbr01-10.pdf.

Hogstel, M., & Weeks, S. (2000). Mental health. In A. Lueckenotte (Ed.), *Gerontologic nursing* (p. 256). St. Louis, MO: Mosby.

Hooyman, N. (2003). Ageism. *Journal of Sociology and Social Welfare, 30*(2), 18.

Ingram, T. (2001). Risk for violence: Self-directed or directed to others. In M. Maas et al. (Eds.), *Nursing care of older adults: Diagnosis, outcomes, and intervention.* St. Louis, MO: Mosby.

Jacox A., et al. (1994, March). *Management of cancer pain* (Clinical Practice Guideline No. 9, AHCPR Publication No. 94-0952). Rockville, MD: U.S. Department of Health and Human Services, Public Health Service, Agency for Health Care Policy and Research.

Joint Commission on Accreditation of Healthcare Organizations. (1999). *Standards for behavioral health care.* Oakbrook, IL: Author.

Juurlink, D. N., et al. (2004). Medical illness and the risk of suicide in the elderly. *Archives of Internal Medicine, 164,* 1179-1184.

Kinsella, K., & Velkoff, V. (2001). *An aging world* (U.S. Census Bureau Series P95/01-1). Washington, DC: U.S. Government Printing Office.

Lane, P., et al. (2003). Assessment tool for patients with advanced Alzheimer's and other progressive dementias. *Home Healthcare Nurse, 21*(1), 30-37.

Lueckenotte, A. (2000). Gerontologic assessment. In A. Lueckenotte (Ed.), *Gerontologic nursing.* St. Louis, MO: Mosby.

Luggen, A. (2000). Pain. In A. Lueckenotte (Ed.), *Gerontologic nursing.* St. Louis, MO: Mosby.

Luggen, A. (2004). Mental wellness and disturbances. In P. Ebersole, P. Hess, & A. S. Luggen (Eds.), *Toward healthy aging: Human needs and nursing response.* St. Louis, MO: Mosby.

Marchello, V. (2003). Long-term care. In T. Dharmarajan & R. Norman (Eds.), *Clinical geriatrics.* New York: Parthenon Publishing Group.

Marshall, M. (2003). Adult psychiatric day hospital. *British Medical Journal, 327*(7407), 116-117.

McAndrews, M. M. (2001). Lighting the darkness. *Advance for Providers of Post-Acute Care, 73,* 40.

Meiner, S. E., & Miceli, D. G. (2000). Safety. In A. Lueckenotte (Ed.), *Gerontologic nursing.* St. Louis, MO: Mosby.

Menninger, J. (2004). Assessment and treatment of alcoholism and substance-related disorders in the elderly. *Bulletin of the Menninger Clinic 66*(2), 166-183.

Miakowski, C. (1999). Pain and discomfort. In J. Stone (Ed.), *Clinical gerontological nursing* (p. 647). Philadelphia: Saunders.

Miller, C. (2004). *Nursing for wellness in older adults: Theory and practice* (4th ed.). Philadelphia: Lippincott Williams & Wilkins.

Moscicki, E. K., & Caine, E. D. (2004). Opportunities of life: Preventing suicide in elderly patients. *Archives of Internal Medicine, 164,* 1171-1172.

National Center for Injury Prevention and Control. (2003). *Suicide: Fact sheet.* Retrieved April 6, 2005, from http://www.cdc.gov/ncipc/factsheets/suifacts.htm.

National Citizens' Coalition for Nursing Home Reform. (1991). *Nursing home reform law: The basics.* Washington, DC: Author

National Institute of Mental Health. (2004). *Older adults: Depression and suicide facts.* Washington, DC: Author. Retrieved March 21, 2005, from http://www.nimh.nih.gov/publicat/elderlydepsuicide.cfm.

Nelson, T. (2002). *Ageism: Stereotyping and prejudice against older persons.* Cambridge, MA: MIT Press.

Neufield, R. R., et al. (1999). Restraint reduction reduces serious injuries among nursing home residents. *Journal of the American Geriatrics Society, 47*(10), 1202-1207.

Patterson, T. L., Lacro, J. P., & Jeste, D. V. (1999). Abuse and misuse of medications in the elderly. *Psychiatric Times, 16*(4), 1-8. Retrieved March 21, 2005, from http://www.psychiatrictimes.com/p990454.html.

Rabins, P. V., et al. (2000). Effectiveness of a nurse-based outreach program for identifying and treating psychiatric illness in the elderly. *Journal of the American Medical Association, 283*(21), 2802-2809.

Reuben, D. B. (2003). *Geriatrics at your fingertips.* Malden, MA: Blackwell Science/American Geriatric Society.

Riger, S. K. (2000). Alcoholism in the elderly. *American Family Physician, 261,* 1710-1716.

Salisbury, S. (1999). Alcoholism. In J. Stone (Ed.), *Clinical gerontological nursing* (p. 537). Philadelphia: Saunders.

Schatzberg, A. F., & Nemeroff, C. B. (2004). *Textbook of Psychopharmacology* (pp. 1083-1106). Washington DC: American Psychiatric Publishing.

Sheikh, J. I, & Yesavage, J. A. (1986). Geriatric Depression Scale (GDS): recent evidence and development of a shorter version. In T. L. Brink (Ed.), *Clinical gerontology: A guide to assessment and intervention* (pp. 165-173). New York: Haworth Press.

Skoog, I. (2004). Psychiatric epidemiology of old age: The H70 study—the NAPE Lecture 2003. *Acta Psychiatrica Scandinavica, 109*(1), 46-54.

Wagenaar, D., Mickus, M., & Wilson, J. (2001). Alcoholism in late life: Challenges and complexities. *Psychiatric Annals, 31*(11), 665-672.

Warden, V., Hurley, A. C., & Volicer, L. (2003). Development and psychometric evaluation of the Pain Assessment in Advanced Dementia (PAINAD) scale. *Journal of the American Medical Directors Association, 4*(1), 9-15.

Wong D. L., et al. (2001). *Wong's essentials of pediatric nursing* (6th ed., p. 1301). St. Louis, MO: Mosby.

Wynne, C., et al. (2000). Comparison of pain assessment instruments. *Geriatric Nursing, 21*(1), 20-23.

A NURSE SPEAKS

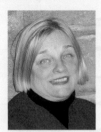

Working with clients who are actively hearing voices during group therapy is a rewarding, yet daunting, experience. Much of my current practice with one long-term group of six participants is counter to my early education over 40 years ago. Each member complied with the medication regimen, had extensive community support, and was diagnosed with some variant along the schizophrenic continuum. Of course, names and specifics have been altered. The frameworks used were a combination of Peplau's methods, Ericksonian hypnotherapy, and cognitive-behavioral therapy. These interventions were used with clients hearing nonthreatening, basically benign, yet critical voices, not with those hearing voices of lethal intent or command hallucinations.

The group members found the acceptance to talk about their voices and to talk with others who also experienced voices very helpful and healing. The participants informally started observing in themselves the intensity, duration, timing, numbers, and intent of the voices, and their relationship to them. They spontaneously started telling the group members ways they have coexisted and coped with the barrage of voices.

As leader, I normalized their experiences by reframing their negative voices as "inner critics" or "self-talk" that most people experience. We identified similarities to other people's self-talk in that the inner critic may continually comment on everything the person is doing, may play nonstop rap songs with sardonic overtones, or may yell lists of things not done well and all the mistakes the individual has made.

When Harold described his need to put all his CDs in the attic of his halfway house to try to decrease the incessant rap of negativity, I matched his metaphor by suggesting that in his head he slowly turn the volume control down on a make-believe CD player with each exhalation. Although he found this very helpful, he still kept his CDs in the attic. Kevin liked the suggestion that he develop a dialogue with his voices by saying things like: "Yep, that's a possibility. Thanks for the input." "I never thought of that. I'll give it a try." After reporting his ability to do this as his homework assignment, he then learned to pair his response with a physical activity, such as walking to the grocery store or around the block, to help divert his attention away from the voices. Other suggestions for dealing with negative and disturbing voices were the following: (1) Consider that the voice may be targeting an area of greatest insecurities and make a plan to improve that area. (2) Compare your list of all your positive traits, compiled by self-identification and group input, with the list of faults given by the voices and recognize that your voices are not always correct. (3) Put things in perspective. Will it matter tomorrow, next week, next year? Most of the time, the answer is no. (4) Compare yourself with your own yardstick of traits and accomplishments, not with your perceptions of someone else who appears to be perfect on the outside, when that may not necessarily be an accurate estimation of what is going on inside of that person.

Some of the voices were positive and offered alternatives. Jane described voices that sometimes encouraged her. We labeled these as her "guardians" or "angels." One member actually brought in a book about angels, and everyone actively participated in a discussion of his or her opinion and described how we can tap their resources.

Sharon Shisler

OTHER INTERVENTION MODALITIES

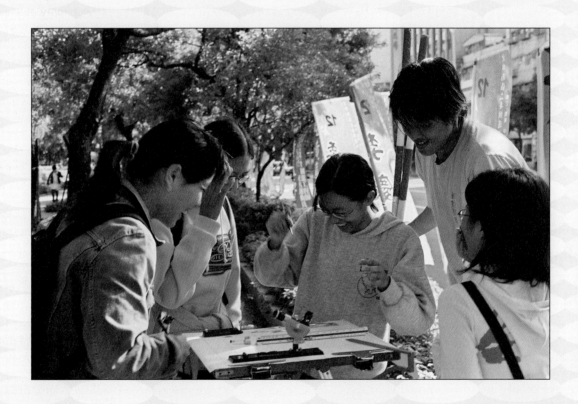

WISDOM BEGINS IN WONDER.

Socrates

CHAPTER 35

Therapeutic Groups

NANCY CHRISTINE SHOEMAKER ▪ CATHERINE M. LALA

KEY TERMS and CONCEPTS

The key terms and concepts listed here appear in color where they are defined or first discussed in this chapter.

group, 718

group content, 719

group norm, 719

group process, 719

group protocol, 722

group psychotherapy, 718

group themes, 719

psychoeducational groups, 724

self-help groups, 725

therapeutic factors, 721

OBJECTIVES

After studying this chapter, the reader will be able to

1. Identify basic concepts related to group work.
2. Describe the phases of group development.
3. Define task and maintenance roles group members may adopt within a group and give four examples.
4. Discuss the therapeutic factors that operate in all groups.
5. Name four facilitating techniques used by the group leader.
6. Describe a group intervention for a member who is silent or a member who is monopolizing the group.
7. Discuss four types of groups commonly led by basic level registered nurses.

evolve Visit the Evolve website at **http://evolve.elsevier.com/Varcarolis** for a pretest on the content in this chapter.

GROUP CONCEPTS

Definition of Group

All of us live and work in groups every day. We are born into a family group and grow up with various peer groups such as those at schools, spiritual centers, and neighborhoods. As adults, we establish a social network of friendships and work relationships, and our own family of significant others. Knowledge of groups and group process is beneficial to the nurse both personally and professionally.

A **group** is defined as "two or more people who develop an interactive relationship and share at least one common goal or issue" (Boyd, 2002, p. 277). Each group has specific characteristics, including the following:

- Size
- Defined purpose
- Degree of similarity among members
- Rules
- Boundaries

- Climate
- Apparent content (what is said in the group) and underlying process

Group psychotherapy is a specialized treatment intervention in which a trained leader (or co-leaders) establishes a group for the purpose of treating clients with psychiatric disorders. Nurses are involved in group psychotherapy as well as in many other types of therapeutic groups. These modalities are widely used in both hospital and community settings. Box 35-1 defines terms related to group work.

There are clear advantages and disadvantages of the group approach for psychiatric clients (Buffum & Madrid, 2003; Tunley Crenshaw, 2003). Advantages include the following:

- More clients can be treated in a cost-effective way.
- Members feel less isolated as they listen to peers discuss their problems.
- Members receive peer feedback about their styles of communication.

BOX 35-1

Terms Central to Group Work

Group content—all that is said in the group

Group norm—a pattern of behavior in the group that develops over time and provides structure for members (e.g., starting on time, not interrupting)

Group process—the verbal and nonverbal communication among the members (e.g., who talks to whom, facial expressions, and body language)

Group themes—ideas or feelings expressed by members in one meeting or in several meetings that have a common thread; the leader can clarify a theme to help members recognize it more fully

Feedback—letting group members know how they affect each other

Hidden agenda—individual, subgroup, or leader goals that are at cross purposes with the group's goals

Heterogeneous group—a group in which a range of differences exists among members

Homogeneous group—a group in which all members share certain traits (e.g., men's group, group of clients with bipolar disorder)

Conflict—open disagreement among members; may be positive, indicating involvement with the task, or negative, indicating frustration with an impossible task or intergroup conflict

Closed group—a group in which membership is restricted; no new members are added when others leave

Open group—a group in which new members are added as others leave

Subgroup—an individual or a small group that is isolated within a larger group and functions separately; members of a subgroup may have greater loyalty, more similar goals, or more perceived similarities to one another than they do to the larger group

- Groups teach different problem-solving approaches.
- Members learn about functional roles in groups.

Disadvantages include the following:

- A member's privacy may be violated if peers do not keep group content confidential.
- Some clients are unable to share intimate feelings or thoughts in a group.
- The individual may feel that he or she is not receiving enough attention because of other members' more active participation.

Not all clients can benefit from group treatment. Excluded would be persons who are acutely psychotic or manic and those who are cognitively impaired (e.g., those who have dementia or are intoxicated) (Buffum & Madrid, 2003).

Phases of Group Development

All groups go through developmental stages, which can be described in terms of the following four steps (Tunley Crenshaw, 2003).

In the **initial phase,** the leader's role is to set up an atmosphere of respect, confidentiality, and trust. The purpose of the group is stated, and members are helped to relax and feel comfortable. The group task is for members to get to know one another, to observe each other, and to begin to take steps toward the working phase. Members often give each other advice.

In the **working phase,** the leader's role is to encourage members to cooperate with each other and to handle conflict. Group tasks revolve around issues of power and control. Members may challenge the leader and begin to work together.

In the **mature phase,** the leader's role is to keep the group focused on therapeutic goals of individual members. The group develops functional norms and a sense of group identity. The members accept each other's differences and actively participate to help each individual to accomplish goals.

During **termination,** the group leader's task is to acknowledge the contributions of each member and the experience as a whole. Group members prepare for separation and help each other prepare for the future.

Roles of Group Members

There are only two formal group roles in each group: the leader and the members. But studies of group dynamics have identified informal roles of members that are necessary to develop a successful group. The most common descriptive categories for these roles are task, maintenance, and individual roles (Buffum & Madrid, 2003). Task roles serve to keep the group focused on its main purpose. Maintenance roles function to keep the group together, helping the members to compromise. There are also individual roles that can interfere with the group's functioning because they are not related to the group goals. Table 35-1 describes roles of group members.

Role of the Group Leader

The group leader has multiple responsibilities in starting, maintaining, and terminating a group. In the initial phase, the leader defines the structure, size, composition, purpose, and timing for the group. Task and maintenance functions may be discussed and demonstrated. To maintain the group, the leader facilitates communication and ensures that meetings start and end on time. In the termination phase, the leader ensures that each member summarizes individual accomplishments and gives positive and negative feedback regarding the group experience. Cultural characteristics of group members must also be taken into consideration when forming a functional group. Refer to the Culturally Speaking box for insight into this issue.

TABLE 35-1

Roles of Group Members

Role	Function
Task Roles	
Coordinator	Tries to connect various ideas and suggestions
Elaborator	Gives examples and follows up meaning of ideas
Energizer	Encourages the group to make decisions or take action
Evaluator	Measures the group's work against a standard
Information giver	Shares facts or own experience as an authority figure
Information seeker	Tries to clarify the group's values
Initiator-contributor	Offers new ideas or a new outlook on an issue
Opinion giver	Shares opinions, especially to influence group values
Orienter	Notes the progress of the group toward goals
Procedural technician	Supports group activity by distributing papers, arranging seating, etc.
Recorder	Keeps notes and acts as the group memory
Maintenance Roles	
Compromiser	In a conflict, yields to preserve group harmony
Encourager	Praises and seeks input from others
Follower	Agrees with the flow of the group
Gatekeeper	Monitors the participation of all members to keep communication open
Group observer	Keeps records of different aspects of group process and reports to the group
Harmonizer	Tries to mediate conflicts between members
Standard setter	Verbalizes standards for the group
Individual Roles	
Aggressor	Criticizes and attacks others' ideas and feelings
Blocker	Disagrees with group issues; oppositional
Dominator	Tries to control other members of the group with flattery or interruptions
Help seeker	Asks for sympathy of group excessively
Playboy	Acts disinterested in group process
Recognition seeker	Seeks attention by boasting and discussing achievements
Self-confessor	Verbalizes feelings or observations unrelated to group
Special interest pleader	Advocates for a special group, usually with own prejudice or bias

Data from Benne, K., & Sheats, P. (1948). Functional roles of group members. *Journal of Social Issues, 4*(2), 41.

▪▫▫ CULTURALLY SPEAKING

Cultural diversity among members of a group can have a profound effect on group process and presents a challenge for the group leader. Persons from different cultures may have a great deal to teach each other, but they may misunderstand communication or feel prejudiced. The risk for misunderstandings or negative feelings is increased by the intensity of a group experience, compared with one-to-one interaction.

Clients who belong to a minority group that feels oppressed may show anger and rejection toward others, or feelings of inferiority. Feelings related to oppression may be caused by other factors in addition to ethnic origin, such as sexual orientation. Sometimes clients, including minority members, deny feeling any prejudice at all.

It is important for the leader to address cultural differences early in the life of a group. A minority member may be asked to describe for the group pertinent cultural differences. Interactions among members are observed for signs of overreaction or misunderstanding. Clients are encouraged to express their here-and-now feelings and to explore how their beliefs developed. When a client denies any feelings of prejudice or is concealing a trait for fear of rejection, the leader allows time and encourages the person to communicate honestly.

At the same time, the leader does not overprotect a minority member, avoiding confrontation or allowing that person to repeatedly complain about prejudice. The group experience can be powerful for all members, and each member deserves a chance to clarify distortions about self and misunderstandings about others.

Data from Earley, J. (2002). *Interactive group therapy*. Philadelphia: Brunner/Mazel.

There are three main styles of group leadership. A leader selects the style that is best suited to the therapeutic needs of a particular group. The **autocratic leader** exerts control over the group and does not encourage much interaction among members. In contrast, the **democratic leader** supports extensive group interaction in the process of problem solving. A **laissez-faire leader** allows the group members to behave in any way that they choose and does not attempt to control the direction of the group. For example, staff leading a community meeting with a fixed, time-limited agenda may tend to be more autocratic. In a psychoeducational group, the leader may be more democratic to encourage members to share their experiences. In a creative group such as an art or horticulture group, the leader may choose a laissez-faire style, giving minimal direction to allow for a variety of responses. Table 35-2 describes communication techniques frequently used by group leaders.

THERAPEUTIC FACTORS COMMON TO ALL GROUPS

In a group, clients hear others share similar concerns, fantasies, and life experiences. The realization that one is not alone in one's situation may offer considerable relief and a "welcome to the human race" experience. The name of this concept is **universality.** Universality is one of the therapeutic factors of group therapy described by Yalom (1995), who has done extensive research into groups. Therapeutic factors are aspects of the group experience that clients and therapists have identified as facilitating therapeutic change. Different factors operate at different stages of a group, and the leader may role-model several behaviors during the initial phase, such as instilling hope and imparting information. Just as with other types of treatment, each person's response to a group is highly individualized, based on past experiences and level of participation.

TABLE 35-2

Group Leader Communication Techniques

Technique	Purpose	Example
Advice or information sharing—giving information that members may not know	Suggests useful information to a member or the group	"Here is the telephone number of the mental health drop-in center."
Clarification—making a statement or questioning to check the meaning of an interaction	Improves group communication by decreasing misunderstandings	"Are you saying that you are upset because two members were late today?"
Confrontation—questioning a member in a challenging but supportive way	Gives feedback to a member about behavior, especially disruptive interactions	"Mary, that is the third time that you interrupted Susan. Does her talking about her children upset you?"
Questioning—asking for more information	Encourages members to discuss the subject more extensively	"Could you describe the behaviors that led to your hospitalization?"
Reflection—identifying feelings or behavior more clearly	Supports members in talking more about their feelings or understanding how their behavior affects others	"You look sad, as if you are about to cry." "I noticed that you moved your chair away when John spoke about his anger."
Repetition or paraphrase—simply repeating a member's comment	Highlights information to emphasize it or to check for accuracy	*Member:* I forgot about group last week. *Leader:* You forgot about group last week.
Summarization—commenting at the end of the session to note issues discussed and incomplete topics	Helps to focus on themes and give continuity from one group to another	"Today we discussed sleep problems and different things you can do to help with sleep. I hope you try out one new tip before the next group meeting."
Support—giving feedback to encourage a member to continue communication	Develops a group climate to encourage members to express difficult feelings or relate painful stories	"Thank you for sharing that story with us. It seemed pretty painful."

Data from Sampson, E., & Marthas, M. (1990). *Group process for the health professions.* Albany, NY: Delmar; and Yalom, I. D. (1995). *The theory and practice of group psychotherapy* (4th ed.). New York: Basic Books.

Box 35-2 describes the eleven therapeutic factors that can benefit persons in groups.

There are significant differences between outpatient and inpatient groups, related to setting, length of stay, and the role of the leader. These differences are outlined in Table 35-3.

GROUP PROTOCOLS

A group protocol, or description of the specific characteristics of a therapeutic group, includes
- Name and objectives of the group.
- Types of clients or diagnoses for members.
- Group structure (frequency, times of meetings, etc.)
- Description of leader and member responsibilities.
- Methods or means to evaluate the outcomes of the group.

BOX 35-2

Therapeutic Factors in Groups

Instillation of hope—The leader shares optimism about group treatment, and members share their improvements.

Universality—Members realize that they are not alone with their problems, feelings, or thoughts.

Imparting of information—Participants receive formal teaching by the leader or advice from peers.

Altruism—Members feel a reward from giving support to others.

Corrective recapitulation of the primary family group—Members repeat patterns of behavior in the group that they learned in their families; with feedback from the leader and peers, they learn about their own behavior.

Development of socializing techniques—Members learn new social skills based on feedback from others.

Imitative behavior—Members may copy behavior from the leader or peers and can adopt healthier habits.

Interpersonal learning—Members gain insight into themselves based on the feedback from others. This is a complex process that occurs later in the group after trust is established.

Group cohesiveness—This powerful factor arises in a mature group when each member feels connected to the other members, the leader, and the group as a whole; members can accept positive feedback and constructive criticism.

Catharsis—Intense feelings, as judged by the member, are shared.

Existential resolution—Members learn to accept painful aspects of life (e.g., loneliness, death) that affect everyone.

Data from Yalom, I. D. (1995). *The theory and practice of group psychotherapy* (4th ed.). New York: Basic Books.

TABLE 35-3

Differences Between Outpatient and Inpatient Groups

Outpatient Groups	Inpatient Groups
The group has a stable composition.	The group is rarely the same for more than one or two meetings.
Clients are carefully selected and prepared.	Clients are admitted to the group with little prior selection or preparation.
The group is homogeneous with regard to ego function.	The group has a heterogeneous level of ego function.
Motivated, self-referred clients make up the group; therapy is growth oriented.	Clients are ambivalent, often therapy is compulsory; therapy is relief oriented.
Treatment proceeds as long as required: 1 to 2 years.	Treatment is limited to the hospital period: 1 to 3 weeks, with rapid client turnover.
The boundary of the group is well maintained, with few external influences.	Whatever happens on the unit affects the group.
Group cohesion develops normally, given sufficient time in treatment.	There is no time for cohesion to develop spontaneously; group development is limited to the initial phase.
The leader allows the process to unfold; there is ample time to set up group norms.	The group leader structures time and is not passive.
Members are encouraged to avoid extragroup contact.	Clients eat, sleep, and live together outside of the group; extragroup contact is endorsed.

Data from Mackenzie, K. R. (1997). *Time-managed group psychotherapy: Effective clinical applications.* Washington, DC: American Psychiatric Press.

An example of a group protocol for a medication education group is provided in Box 35-3.

If you were to start an inpatient medication group in accordance with this protocol, you would
1. Gather 8 to 10 clients in a meeting room for orientation to the group.
2. Define the boundaries of the group, including time, frequency, length of session (45 minutes), seating arrangement (circle), and the need to stay for the full session (but do not lock the door).
3. Structure the group interactions as you teach about major symptoms and medications, allowing for questions near the end of the meeting.
4. Maintain group safety by intervening immediately if a client becomes verbally or physically threatening.

Example of Medication Education Group Protocol

Description of Group

A group for all clients, regardless of level of concentration, that prepares clients for self-management of medication on discharge.

Criteria for Client Selection

Open to all clients except those who are displaying suicidal or homicidal behaviors or the potential for assault

Visual Aids

Overhead transparencies, films, patient medication education sheets

Purpose

1. To educate clients on the primary function of their medications
2. To provide information on side effects (that benefits can outweigh risks)
3. To describe a mechanism to negotiate relationships with health care workers
4. To enhance a sense of self-control over treatment

Procedure

1. Orientation and introduction to the group
2. Brief description of major symptoms in a diagnosis
3. Overview of antipsychotics or antidepressants
4. Use of Albany Medical Center patient medication education sheets
5. Specific open question period

Behavioral Objectives

At the end of the 45-minute session, clients will be able to

1. State one symptom they have that is treated by their medication.
2. Be able to ask at least one question about their medicine.
3. Identify one mechanism that helps in compliance with the medication regimen.

Theoretical Justification

Even people who think they are compliant only take 80% of doses. Counseling and therapy are always adjuncts to drug therapy.

Adapted from Ott, C. A. (2000). *Pediatric psychopharmacology.* South Easton, MD: American Healthcare Institute, a division of SC Publishing.

EXPECTED OUTCOMES

After a group experience, when members are presented with qualitative outcome criteria such as a questionnaire based on the therapeutic factors of groups (Yalom, 1995), they tend to respond in these ways:

- "I do not feel alone."
- "I need this."
- "Why don't they have more groups like this?"
- "Extend the group from 1 hour to 2 hours."
- "I'm more able to open up."
- "After being in this group, I am more capable of reaching out to others."
- "If I want to change a behavior or something about myself, I'll try it in group first."

It may be easier to achieve measurable outcomes with psychoeducation groups than with therapy groups. A nurse can define key quality indicators and can track those indicators over a period of time. For example, the key quality indicators for successful outcome (client education) in a medication education group could be any of the following: (1) the clients will verbalize names and purposes of medications; (2) the clients will maintain compliance with the medication regimen while hospitalized; and (3) the clients will report side effects. Refer to Figure 35-1 for an evaluation tool that can be used as a pretest and posttest to measure clients' learning.

Outcome criteria can also be used by an outside observer (e.g., another trained staff member) to help evaluate the effectiveness of group. The following are examples of such criteria (Paleg & Jongsma, 2000):

- Therapist gives feedback to group members about their behavior.
- Therapist facilitates interactions among group members.
- Therapist checks for understanding of what is being said.

ROLE OF THE NURSE IN THERAPEUTIC GROUPS

Psychiatric mental health nurses are involved in a variety of therapeutic groups in acute care and long-term treatment settings. Basic level registered nurses (RNs) lead psychoeducational groups and therapeutic milieu groups (Boyd, 2002; Buffum & Madrid, 2003). Advanced practice RNs (APRNs) also lead these groups and may independently perform group psychotherapy. For all group leaders, a clear theoretical framework is necessary to provide a structure to understand the group interaction. Clinical supervision is important for group leaders: it provides feedback about their performance and enhances their professional growth. Transference and countertransference issues occur in groups just as in individual treatment, and objective input from an outsider supports a focus on therapeutic goals. Co-leadership of groups is a common practice and has several benefits: it provides training for less experienced staff; it allows for immediate feedback between the leaders after each session; and it gives two role models for teaching communication skills to members.

Criteria	Strongly Agree	Somewhat Agree	Agree	Disagree	Strongly Disagree
1. I know the name(s) of the medication(s) I am taking.					
2. I know what symptoms the medication(s) can help me with.					
3. I know the common side effects of my medication(s).					
4. I feel comfortable talking to my prescriber if I am having problems with my medication(s).					
5. It is important to take my medication(s) at the same time every day.					

FIGURE 35-1 Medication group evaluation tool.

Basic Level Registered Nurse

Psychoeducational Groups

Psychiatric nurses, with their biopsychosocial and spiritual approach, are the ideal professionals to teach a variety of health subjects. Psychoeducational groups are groups set up to teach about a specific somatic or psychological subject; they also allow members to communicate about emotional concerns. These groups may be time limited or may be supportive for long-term treatment. Generally, written handouts or audio-visual aids are used to focus on specific teaching points. The following paragraphs describe psychoeducational groups commonly led by nurses.

The group for which the nurse most commonly assumes responsibility in all settings is the **medication education group.** The group setting facilitates discussion. Clients often listen to the experience of others who have taken medication and have an opportunity to ask questions without the fear that they will go against the prescriber's recommendations. Medication groups are designed to teach clients about their medications, answer their questions, and prepare them for self-management.

Nurses also frequently lead **sexuality groups.** Human immunodeficiency virus (HIV) infection/acquired immunodeficiency syndrome (AIDS) remains one of the most serious public health issues in the United States and throughout the world. Clients who have used poor judgment in sexual behavior because of mental illness are at high risk for HIV infection and other sexually transmitted diseases. Topics for discussion include the following:

- HIV/AIDS
- Modes of transmission and treatment of sexually transmitted diseases
- Education on condom use and other forms of safer sex practices
- The effect of medication on sexuality

Dual-diagnosis groups with a focus on psychiatric illness and substance use are becoming more widespread in acute and long-term settings. The RN may co-lead this group with a dual-diagnosis specialist (master's level clinician). The goal is to engage clients in treatment and to decrease their use of substances in a step-by-step process. Research has shown that combined treatment for the severely mentally ill population produces improved outcomes (Drake, 2001). Refer to the Evidence-Based Practice box for pertinent research findings.

Another evidence-based group therapy practice used with the severely mentally ill population is the **multifamily group** (Dyck et al., 2002). Usually found in the outpatient setting, the group is composed of family members and clients and continues for up to 2 years. The focus is on education about the mental illness and strategies for the family to cope with long-term disability. There is a strong emphasis on medication teaching, which makes the nurse a valuable co-leader for such a group.

Symptom management groups are designed for clients with a common problem such as anger or psychosis. The focus is on sharing positive and negative experiences so that members learn coping skills from each other. A primary goal is to increase self-control or prevent relapse by helping clients to develop a plan for action at the first sign of losing control. Even clients with chronic schizophrenia may benefit from a group approach if the sessions are kept highly structured and use a variety of short activities to accommodate the client's cognitive limitations (e.g., brief discussion, then paper-and-pencil exercises) (Ahmed & Boisvert, 2002).

Stress management groups are often time limited and teach members about various relaxation techniques, including deep breathing, exercise, music, and spirituality. One novel approach is the humor group. A nursing professor wrote about the positive outcomes

EVIDENCE-BASED PRACTICE

Dual-Diagnosis Services

Background
It is well known that up to 50% of clients with severe mental illness also have a substance use disorder. Clients with these dual diagnoses experience multiple negative outcomes: high relapse rates, increased hospitalization, violence, incarceration, and serious infections such as hepatitis or human immunodeficiency virus infection. Until the 1980s, treatment programs traditionally used one of two approaches: sequential treatment that focused on one disorder before starting to treat the second, or parallel treatment in which different clinicians or agencies treated the two disorders. Evaluation of these approaches showed high rates of dropout, poor coordination, and exclusion from services.

Studies
New models in integrated treatment were developed in the late 1980s for this dual-diagnosis population. Programs used various approaches, but all successful ones included outreach to engage clients; followed the concept of stages of treatment; used motivation-based interventions to assist clients in reaching personal goals; provided comprehensive services with counseling and social supports; and had a long-term focus. Dual-diagnosis groups are a key component of integrated treatment, in both the hospital and outpatient settings.

Results of Studies
Eight controlled studies showed improvement in engaging severely mentally ill clients and keeping them in treatment using the integrated approach. Three studies compared integrated and nonintegrated treatment. Two studies evaluated integrated treatment with a community outreach model and followed clients over 3 years. Three other studies compared substance abuse treatment integrated with case management, social skills training, or a 12-step program. All studies reported improvement in the substance use disorder. Other positive outcomes included decreased severity of symptoms and reduced hospitalizations.

Implications for Nursing Practice
In a variety of settings, the registered nurse has the opportunity to co-lead dual-diagnosis groups with a dual-diagnosis specialist. Starting the client in treatment during acute care and then referring the client to a community setting that provides integrated treatment can significantly improve outcomes for severely mentally ill clients with dual diagnoses.

Drake, R. E., et al. (2001). Implementing dual diagnosis services for clients with severe mental illness. *Psychiatric Services, 52*(4), 469-476.

---

achieved through the use of a humor group formed of state forensic hospital clients (Minden, 2003). Nursing students led a 16-week group that encouraged members to share jokes and to play a variety of humorous games. Members reported improvement in communication skills and enhanced coping with stress.

Therapeutic Milieu Groups

Therapeutic milieu groups aim to help increase clients' self-esteem, decrease social isolation, encourage appropriate social behaviors, and educate clients in basic living skills. These groups are often led by occupational or recreational therapists, although nurses frequently co-lead them. Examples of therapeutic milieu groups are recreational groups, physical activity groups, creative arts groups, and storytelling groups.

Other specific groups in the milieu led by nurses include community or goal-setting meetings and self-care groups. **Community meetings** usually include all clients and the treatment team, who meet frequently to discuss common goals. Functions include orienting new members to the unit, encouraging clients to engage in treatment, and evaluating the treatment program. Nursing staff are the largest group of providers and give valuable feedback to the team about group interactions. Goal-setting meetings may be held in a hospital or a partial hospital program to plan daily goals for each client to achieve.

Also in the acute care setting, nurses may lead **self-care groups.** These groups focus on basic hygiene issues such as bathing and grooming. Clients who are acutely overwhelmed with their symptoms can be gently encouraged to resume or increase independence in their activities of daily living.

Advanced Practice Registered Nurse

APRNs may lead any of the groups described earlier and may also lead psychotherapy groups. There are different theoretical frameworks for group therapy in which the APRN receives specialized training (Buffum & Madrid, 2003). As noted earlier, the APRN seeks ongoing clinical supervision related to group therapy to provide the most effective treatment for clients. Refer to Table 35-4 for an overview of theoretical foundations for group therapy. Note that the therapeutic factors described by Yalom (1995) (see Box 35-2) relate to several theories; a group therapist using Yalom's model would be considered eclectic.

SELF-HELP GROUPS

Self-help groups or support groups are based on the premise that people who have experienced a particular problem are able to help others who have the same problem. Nurses may serve as resource people for their clients and need to be aware of the wide array of self-help groups available. One of the most important functions of such groups is to demonstrate to individuals that they are not alone in having a particular

TABLE 35-4

Theoretical Foundations for Group Therapy

Theory	Concepts	Role of Therapist
Psychodynamic/ psychoanalytic	Applies Freud's concepts of psychoanalysis to individual members and to the group itself; focus is on unconscious conflicts and transference; goal is insight	Helps members to recognize unconscious conflicts and encourages peer feedback
Interpersonal	Applies Sullivan's theories about interpersonal learning; focus is on understanding how current relationships repeat early significant relationships; goal is to rebuild individual's personality	Helps to reduce anxiety and encourages members to validate feelings and thoughts with each other
Communication	Applies a systems model holding that the whole (group) is greater than the sum of its parts (members); focus is on subgroups and communication, both verbal and nonverbal; goal is to learn clear, congruent communication skills	Helps point out confusing or contradictory messages; acts as a role model for clear communication
Group process	Analyzes the group with a focus on individual roles and group patterns of behavior (stages, norms, etc.); goal is to resolve authority and intimacy issues	Helps develop a mature group in which members trust each other and give supportive feedback
Existential/Gestalt	Applies theories of Maslow and Rogers to encourage individuals to develop to full potential; focus is on the here and now to increase members' awareness of feelings; goal is self-actualization in which individual takes full responsibility for choices	Helps focus members on here-and-now experiences to promote self-learning; promotes emphasis on "what" of behaviors, not "why"
Cognitive-behavioral	Applies concepts of learning theory and Ellis's cognitive therapy; focus is on behavior and thinking patterns, with the group used to reinforce adaptive behavior and to extinguish maladaptive patterns; usually time limited; goal is to change behavior or thinking patterns	Helps develop a trusting group in which members give supportive feedback to reinforce healthier behavior; may provide formal teaching, along with homework assignments

Data from Dies, R. (1992). Models of group psychotherapy: Sifting through confusion. *International Journal of Group Psychotherapy, 42,* 1-16; and Scheidlinger, S. (1997). Group dynamics and group psychotherapy revisited: Four decades later. *International Journal of Group Psychotherapy, 47*(2), 141-159.

problem. Thus, these groups provide members with support, and their members help each other by telling their stories and providing alternative ways to view and to resolve problems. Box 35-4 describes characteristics of self-help groups.

CHALLENGING CLIENT BEHAVIORS

Finally, research into group dynamics has identified certain patterns of problematic behavior in individual members. Leading a group is anxiety provoking for most group leaders, and clients are equally anxious. Many defensive behaviors used by clients interfere with their attaining satisfaction in their lives. At the same time, these behaviors can be disruptive to group process and disturbing to the leader. The client who monopolizes the group, the client who complains but continues to reject help, the demoralizing client, and the silent client often challenge a group leader (Yalom, 1995).

Person Who Monopolizes the Group

The compulsive speech of a person who monopolizes the group is an attempt to deal with anxiety. As the client sees group tension grow, the client's level of anxiety rises and the client's tendency to speak increases

even more. Therefore, no one else gets a chance to be heard, and other group members eventually lose interest and begin to withdraw.

■ ■ ■ *VIGNETTE*

Holly is the most talkative member of the group until the nurse intervenes. Initially, Holly talks at length about her early experiences related to losing both of her parents and having to live with her grandparents. The other members of the group become bored with the same old story, and they drift off. They have heard these stories many times, not only in group therapy but also during other activities.

■ ■ ■

Intervention. The leader asks group members why they have permitted the monopolizer to go on and on. This serves to validate the other members' feelings of anger. After the group members become angry, they may see how they, too, are responsible for allowing themselves to be victimized. Some members may be angry with the therapist for pointing out their passivity, but they may subsequently realize that they are responsible adults with the right to say what they feel. They may then discuss their fears of being assertive or of hurting the feelings of the monopolizer. Placing responsibility on the group members also takes the therapist out of the authoritative position.

Supportive Self-Help Groups

Target Population
People who have experienced a common tragedy, crisis, illness, or self-destructive behavior, for example:

Support Groups

Bereavement: For those who have experienced the loss of a loved one

Rape: For those who have been raped

Cancer: For those families and clients coping with the ramifications of cancer and its treatment

RESOLVE: For couples experiencing infertility

Self-Help Groups

Alcoholics Anonymous (AA)—the prototype

Gamblers Anonymous (GA)

Overeaters Anonymous (OA)

Narcotics Anonymous (NA)

Co-Dependents Anonymous

Adult Children of Alcoholics (ACOA)

Goal
Overall goal: Provision of support and encouragement of positive coping behaviors:
- Decrease feelings of isolation
- Provide mutual support
- Provide psychoeducation and health education
- Reduce stress
- Help people cease self-destructive behaviors or come to terms with an overwhelming event or situation

Group Leader Activities
May or may not have a specific leader

Strengthens existing defenses

Is actively involved in the group process

Provides information to educate and give direction

Frequency and Duration
Meets: One or more times per week

For: Indefinite period of time, ongoing and open membership

Group members may need help disclosing their own feelings and responses. The therapist encourages the use of statements such as "When you speak this way, I feel . . . ." The therapist helps by noting that feelings are not right or wrong but simply exist. People feel less defensive when "I feel" statements are used than when "you are" statements are made. This approach helps members feel like part of the group, not alienated from it.

Person Who Complains but Continues to Reject Help (Yes . . . But)

The client who complains but continues to reject help continually brings environmental or somatic problems to the group and often describes them in a manner that makes the problems seem insurmountable; in fact, the client appears to take pride in the insolubility of his or her problems. The client seems entirely self-centered. The group's attempts to help the person are continually rejected. The person who uses these tactics generally has highly conflicting feelings about his or her own dependency. Any notice from the therapist temporarily increases the client's self-esteem; on the other hand, the client has a pervasive mistrust of all authority figures. Most clients who complain but continue to reject help have been subjected to severe deprivation early in their lives. For example, they may have been emotionally and physically abused.

■ ■ ■ VIGNETTE

Michelle is always complaining about how horrible her relationship with her boyfriend is, and she manages to get the entire group worked up over this. Members tell her to leave him, not to spend all her time with him, and not to spend all her money on him, but each week she reports a new escapade or crisis. In every session, the group members become concerned and offer encouragement, advice, and solutions. Each time, the group becomes angry at her lack of change, and she is frustrated by her own inability to change. She asserts that the group is not helpful.

■ ■ ■

Intervention. The therapist agrees with the content of the client's pessimism but maintains a detached affect. If the client stays in the group long enough and the group develops a sense of cohesion, this individual can be helped to recognize the pattern of his or her relationships. The therapist encourages the client to look at his or her "yes . . . but" behavior.

Person Who Demoralizes Others

Some people who are extremely self-centered or angry or depressed may lack empathy or concern for other members of the group. They refuse to take any personal responsibility and can challenge the group leader and negatively affect the group process.

■ ■ ■ VIGNETTE

Becky comes to the support group on the inpatient psychiatric unit. She is very angry, stating, "I don't know why I come to these groups anyway! They don't help." Becky is to be discharged the next day to a 28-day alcohol rehabilitation program. She has a previously scheduled dental appointment before the rehabilitation intake interview, and she is being strongly encouraged by her therapist to reschedule the appointment. The therapist fears she is at high risk for drinking again, because Becky states that she constantly has the urge to drink. When a group member who is an addictions therapist confronts Becky about not being flexible and prioritizing her need for alcohol treatment, she explodes. "I thought this group was for support. This is outrageous!" Group members are obviously uncomfortable with her anger.

■ ■ ■

Intervention. The group therapist needs to listen for the content that is being avoided by this client. Listening requires the leader to stay therapeutically objective. In being empathetic, however, the therapist must be aware that a narcissistic client may fear excessive warmth because it stimulates a great deal of anxiety or fear. Underneath, such a client may be extremely vulnerable, and devaluing or demoralizing others keeps them at a distance and maintains the client's own precarious sense of "safety." Therapists need to empathize with the client in a matter-of-fact manner (e.g., "You seem angry that the group wants to support you in putting sobriety over your dental needs.").

Silent Person

Clients who are silent in the group may be observing intently until they decide the group is safe for them or they may believe they are not as competent as other, more assertive group members. Often, these clients can offer valuable insights about others' behavior, but they may avoid speaking to avoid conflict. Note that silence does not mean that the member is uninvolved.

Intervention. The leader needs to exhibit patience but also to encourage active participation by each member, as a worthwhile contributor. This encouragement is offered in a supportive manner. The leader makes an observation without putting the client on the defensive. For example, the leader says, "What do you think, Jill?" instead of, "Do you want to say anything about Linda's problem, Jill?"

■ ■ ■ KEY POINTS to REMEMBER

- Nurses have many opportunities to lead or co-lead therapeutic groups, both in the hospital and in the community setting.
- Group psychotherapy offers the client significant interpersonal feedback from multiple persons, which is a different experience from individual therapy with one therapist.
- Groups develop through predictable stages over time.
- When a new group is formed, similarities and differences in many dimensions, including diagnosis, age, gender, and culture, must be considered.
- For a group to survive, members must fulfill specific functions known as task or maintenance roles.
- Research has identified 11 therapeutic factors that operate in groups and lead to therapeutic change for members.
- Psychoeducational groups and milieu groups are often led by nurses and provide significant treatment as part of the multi-disciplinary treatment plan.
- APRNs may lead psychotherapy groups based on various theoretical models.
- Clinical supervision is important so that group leaders can objectively analyze group interactions and leadership techniques.

Visit the Evolve website at **http://evolve.elsevier.com/Varcarolis** for a posttest on the content in this chapter.   *evolve*

Critical Thinking and Chapter Review

Visit the Evolve website at **http://evolve.elsevier.com/Varcarolis** for additional self-study exercises.
evolve

■ ■ ■ CRITICAL THINKING

1. Construct an outline for a medication teaching group that would cover information useful for your clients.
2. If possible, co-lead this group with a staff member or a fellow student with guidelines from your instructor. Use a pretest and posttest to evaluate learning.
3. Identify which milieu groups are offered in your clinical setting and ask either to co-lead or to participate in at least two, with your instructor's guidance.
4. Ms. Rodriguez is a 22-year-old Puerto Rico–born nursing student admitted to the psychiatric unit after a nearly lethal overdose of acetaminophen. She admits to drinking excessively for the past 6 months. She is at risk of failing school. She complains of depressed mood, a loss of interest in her studies, decreased concentration, and social isolation. In the dual-diagnosis group, she has been silent for the past two sessions and sits staring at the floor.

A. What is your evaluation of Ms. Rodriguez's situation?
B. What might Ms. Rodriguez's nonverbal behavior mean?
C. What approach would you use to involve her more in the group?
D. What criteria could you use to evaluate the effectiveness of your intervention?

Critical Thinking and Chapter Review—cont'd

Visit the Evolve website at **http://evolve.elsevier.com/Varcarolis** for additional self-study exercises.

evolve

■ ■ ■ CHAPTER REVIEW

Choose the most appropriate answer.

1. The nurse leader of the behavioral health inpatient unit wishes to assign a BSN-prepared staff nurse who has just completed orientation to co-lead a unit group. Which type of group should the nurse leader choose?
    1. Family therapy group
    2. Cognitive therapy group
    3. Dual-diagnosis group
    4. Medication education group

2. A nurse who plans to begin working with a new group of clients on the inpatient unit needs one additional client to complete the group. Of the clients listed below, the best choice would be
    1. Mr. F., who is diagnosed as having an antisocial personality.
    2. Ms. G., who is newly admitted for alcohol detoxification.
    3. Mrs. H., who has strong paranoid delusions and a high potential for violence.
    4. Ms. J., who was hospitalized following a suicide attempt.

3. In which self-help group would a nurse expect to observe the use of a 12-step method?
    1. Weight Watchers
    2. Alcoholics Anonymous
    3. Parents Without Partners
    4. National Alliance for the Mentally Ill

4. A student nurse tells the coassigned staff nurse, "I've been assigned to observe in a time-limited therapy group focusing on problems in interpersonal relationships. What can you tell me about the role of the group therapist?" The best explanation would be that the therapist focuses on
    1. creating harmony within the group.
    2. offering facts and personal experience.
    3. examining possible group solutions in light of group goals.
    4. stimulating group interaction and group analysis of the interaction.

5. Which factors can the nurse conducting a therapeutic group rely upon to promote client growth and behavioral change?
    1. Acting out and flooding
    2. Resistance and subgrouping
    3. Universality and imitative behavior
    4. Creation of defenses and alteration of the environment

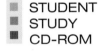

■ **STUDENT**
■ **STUDY**
■ **CD-ROM**

Access the accompanying CD-ROM for animations, interactive exercises, review questions for the NCLEX examination, and an audio glossary.

REFERENCES

Ahmed, M., & Boisvert, C. M. (2002). Cognitive skills group treatment for schizophrenia. *Psychiatric Services, 53*(11), 1476-1477.

Boyd, M. A. (2002). Group intervention. In M. A. Boyd (Ed.), *Psychiatric nursing: Contemporary practice* (2nd ed.). Philadelphia: Lippincott.

Buffum, M., & Madrid, E. (2003). Group therapy. In D. Antai-Otong (Ed.), *Psychiatric nursing: Biological & behavioral concepts.* New York: Thomson Delmar Learning.

Drake, R. E., et al. (2001). Implementing dual diagnosis services for clients with severe mental illness. *Psychiatric Services, 52*(4), 469-476.

Dyck, D. G., et al. (2002). Service use among patients with schizophrenia in psychoeducational multiple-family group treatment. *Psychiatric Services, 53*(6), 749-754.

Minden, P. (2003). The humor group: More than a joke. *Psychiatric Services, 54*(1), 106.

Paleg, K., & Jongsma, A. E., Jr. (2000). *The group therapy treatment planner.* New York: Wiley.

Tunley Crenshaw, B. G. (2003). Working with groups. In W. K. Mohr (Ed.), *Johnson's psychiatric-mental health nursing* (5th ed.). Philadelphia: Lippincott Williams & Wilkins.

Yalom, I. D. (1995). *The theory and practice of group psychotherapy* (4th ed.). New York: Basic Books.

CHAPTER 36

Family Therapy

VERNA BENNER CARSON ▪ ELIZABETH M. VARCAROLIS

■ KEY TERMS and CONCEPTS

The key terms and concepts listed here appear in color where they are defined or first discussed in this chapter.

behavioral family therapy, 736

boundaries, 731

clear boundaries, 731

diffuse or enmeshed boundaries, 731

double-bind theory, 735

family systems theory, 736

family triangle, 738

flexibility, 736

genogram, 740

insight-oriented family therapy, 736

multigenerational issues, 740

nuclear family, 739

psychoeducational family therapy, 745

rigid or disengaged boundaries, 731

sociocultural context, 739

■ OBJECTIVES

After studying this chapter, the reader will be able to

1. Discuss the characteristics of a healthy family using clinical examples.
2. Differentiate between functional and dysfunctional family patterns of behavior as they relate to the five family functions.
3. Compare and contrast insight-oriented family therapy and behavioral family therapy.
4. Identify five family theorists and their contributions to the family therapy movement.
5. Analyze the meaning and value of the family's sociocultural context when assessing and planning intervention strategies.
6. Construct a genogram using a three-generation approach.
7. Formulate seven outcome criteria that a counselor and family might develop together.
8. Identify some strategies for family intervention.
9. Distinguish between the nursing intervention strategies of a basic level nurse and those of an advanced practice nurse with regard to counseling and psychotherapy and psychobiological issues.
10. Explain the importance of the nurse's role in psychoeducational family therapy.

evolve Visit the Evolve website at **http://evolve.elsevier.com/Varcarolis** for a pretest on the content in this chapter.

In our culture the uniqueness of the individual is celebrated. We cheer the individual's search for an autonomous self (Nichols, 2004). We celebrate mythological champions like Spider-Man and Wonder Woman. We honor "heroes" whose accomplishments are larger than life and who seem to rise above the circumstances in which they find themselves. We wonder what our own potential would be if we were able to rise above our circumstances. At some point, though, most of us come to realize that the circumstances we wish to rise above are not only part of being human but also include our connection to our families.

We are defined and sustained by interlocking systems of human relationships, including the relationships we develop with our own family members. Yet many of us struggle with these personal family relationships and wish that these relationships were better. When families are discussed, the tone is frequently negative with a focus on differences and dissension. There is seldom acknowledgment of qualities such as loyalty, tolerance, mutual aide, and assistance that also characterize family life.

We hear a lot of talk about "dysfunctional" families. Sometimes such discussion serves as a thin veil for parent bashing, providing individuals with convenient scapegoats for all personal shortcomings. Most people struggle to fully understand the forces that influence family functioning, and when they are plagued with depression, anxiety, and or unhappy relationships, some will turn to family therapy.

Family therapy is essentially about changing this complex network of relationships by changing the interactions among the people who make up the family or marital unit. Therapy focuses on evaluating these relationships, as well as the communication patterns, structure, and rules that govern the nature of these relationships.

What is a family? Today there are many different types of families, each defined by reciprocal relationships in which people are committed to one another. A family is a married couple with children. A family is two people of the same sex committed to each other and living together. A family is a married couple without children. A family is a remarriage in which a parent, stepparent, and children and/or stepchildren all live together. A family is a single adult with an adopted child. A family can be a trigenerational group in which grandparent(s), parent(s), and child(ren) all live together as a cohesive unit. This is not an exhaustive list; pets are family members also.

The family is the primary system to which a person belongs, and in most cases, it is the most powerful system of which a person will ever be a member. Birth, puberty, marriage, and death are all considered to be family experiences. The family can be the source of love or hate, pride or shame, security or insecurity. Although individual family members have roles and functions, the overriding value in families lies in the relationships among family members. It is these family relationships that provide the primary context of human development. "Family" comprises the entire emotional system of at least three, and frequently four, generations. Many family theorists consider the intergenerational connectedness of the family to be one of our greatest human resources.

THEORETICAL PREMISES

Family Functions

Healthy families provide individuals with the tools that guide how they will function in intimate relationships, in the workplace, within their culture, and in society generally. These tools are acquired through the activities that are associated with family life. These activities can be divided into five functions: (1) management function, (2) boundary function, (3) communication function, (4) emotional-supportive function, and (5) socialization function (Nichols, 2004; Roberts, 1983). Although family counselors may use various assessment strategies, these five areas are always included. Figure 36-1 presents an assessment tool developed by Roberts that the family counselor can use to evaluate these five areas of function. The following sections explain these functions more fully.

Management Function

Every day in every family, decisions are made regarding issues of power, rule making, and provision of financial support. Other management issues include future planning and goods allocation (who gets what within the family). In healthy families, it is usually the adults in the family who agree as to how these functions are to be performed. In families with a single parent, these management functions may sometimes become overwhelming, and single parents can benefit from discussions with other adults. In more chaotic families, an inappropriate member, such as a teenager or a grandparent, may be the one who makes these decisions. Although children learn decision-making skills as they mature and increasingly make decisions and choices about their own lives, they should not have to take on this responsibility for the family of origin.

Boundary Function

Boundaries maintain a distinction between individuals in the family. Boundaries may be clear, diffuse, rigid, or inconsistent. Clear boundaries are well understood by all members of the family; they help to define the roles of members within the family and allow for differences among members. To a great extent, a person's emotional, social, and physical functioning is related to his or her level of role differentiation within the family and the amount of anxiety within the family system (Wetchler, 2003).

Diffuse or enmeshed boundaries refer to a blending together of the roles, thoughts, and feelings of the individuals so that clear distinctions among family members fail to emerge. The members of a family that operates with diffuse, or inconsistent boundaries are more prone to psychological or psychosomatic symptoms. A common phenomenon within families with diffuse boundaries is that individuals expect other members of the family to know what they are thinking ("Why did you take that? You know I wanted it!") and believe that they know what other family members are thinking ("I know exactly why you did that!").

Rigid or disengaged boundaries are those in which the rules and roles are adhered to no matter what; thus, rigid boundaries prevent family members from trying out new roles or, in some cases, from taking on more mature functions as time goes on. In families in which rigid boundaries predominate, isolation may be marked. Family members are often cut off from the community and outside influences, and even from each other.

FAMILY FUNCTION CHECKLIST

Client Family _____ Date of Assessment _____

Family Functions	Observed Behavior	Assessed Need Level (I-IV)	Suggested Nursing Responses

I. *Management function*
    A. Use of power for all family members
    B. Rule making clear, accepted
    C. Fiscal support adequate
    D. Successful negotiations with extrafamilial systems
    E. Future planning present			

II. *Boundary function*
    A. Clear individual boundaries
    B. Clear generational boundaries
    C. Clear family boundaries			

III. *Communication function*
    A. Straight messages
    B. No manipulation
    C. Safe expression of positive and negative feelings			

IV. *Emotional-supportive function*
    A. Mutual positive regard
    B. Deals with conflict
    C. Uses resources for all family members
    D. Allows growth for all family members			

V. *Socialization function*
    A. Children growing and developing in a healthy pattern
    B. Mutual negotiation of roles by age and ability
    C. Parents feeling good about parenting
    D. Spouses happy with each other's role behavior			

FIGURE 36-1 Family Function Checklist. (From Roberts, F. B. [1983]. An interaction model for family assessment. In I. W. Clements & F. B. Roberts [Eds.], *Family health: A theoretical approach to nursing care* [p. 202]. New York: Wiley. Copyright © 1983 John Wiley & Sons. Reprinted by permission of John Wiley & Sons, Inc.)

■ ■ ■ **VIGNETTE**

Lucy M. is a single parent with two preschool-aged children. The family is living on public assistance. Lucy is a teenaged mother who is working toward a general equivalency degree and who also works "under the table" part time as a seamstress. Her mother, Maria, watches the children for Lucy, and discipline is a hot issue between Lucy and Maria.

■ ■ ■

If the boundary functioning of this family were clear, Lucy and Maria would have worked out an arrangement in which Maria would be in charge of disciplining the children when Lucy is away, and Lucy would make the decisions without interference from Maria when both Lucy and Maria are present. The children would be made aware of these arrangements and would clearly understand who is in charge and when. They would know that Lucy and Maria have different operating styles, to which they would learn to adjust. If the boundary functioning of this family were blurred, Lucy and Maria would likely be interfering with each other's mode of discipline, which undoubtedly would lead to tension between them as their anxiety levels increased, and angry outbursts about many issues would eventually ensue. The children, in turn, would become confused as to where their loyalties lie and would probably engage in manipulative behaviors because of the unclear boundaries. If the boundary functioning of this family were rigid, Lucy and Maria would likely have great difficulty agreeing on issues of discipline if their perceptions of rules and roles differed. The children would probably be pulled into a no-win position between a warring mother and daughter in which no correct response exists. All family members would likely become stuck in this established, rigid pattern with no available alternatives.

Communication Function

Communication patterns are extremely important in family life. Healthy communication patterns are characterized by clear and comprehensible messages (e.g., "I would like to go now," or "I don't like it when you interrupt what I'm saying"). Healthy communication within the family encourages members to ask for what they want and to express their feelings appropriately. Feelings of affection and conflict are both openly expressed. Family members are able to ask for what they want and get the attention they need without resorting to manipulation to get their needs met. When communication among family members is not clear, it cannot be used as a means to solve problems or to resolve conflict; therefore, the cardinal rule for effective and functional communication in families is: "Be clear and direct in saying what you want and need."

As simple as this may seem, it is one of the hardest skills to activate in a family system. To be direct, individuals must first have a sense that the self is respected and loved; they then feel entitled to take a stand and to set boundaries with others. The consequences of being clear and direct may be unpleasant in a family system in which boundaries are enmeshed and confusion is the norm. To attempt to change a family pattern is to pit oneself against the status quo. Saying what one wants and needs is especially difficult when one believes that family members should already know—especially if the family member is a spouse, a parent, or a close sibling. In fact, most family members cannot read each other's minds, although emotionally undifferentiated members may think that this is possible. The following vignette describes a spousal situation that shows how easily communication can be misunderstood when clear and direct messages are not sent.

■ ■ ■ *VIGNETTE*

Mary would like to spend more time with her husband John on the weekends; however, John always seems to be busy doing projects around the house or talking with friends on the telephone. Mary feels that he does not notice her, or maybe is not interested in her, so she spends a lot of time working out or playing tennis. John figures that Mary is doing what she wants to do and that it makes her happy, so he contents himself with finding things to do alone. The net result is that Mary and John spend little time together.

Mary finally confronts John clearly and directly about his "disinterest" in her, saying what she wants and needs—that is, it is her desire to spend more time together on the weekends. John replies that he had no idea she felt that way. He had thought she enjoyed the way things were. Actually, he, too, would like to have more time together. What a learning experience for them both!

■ ■ ■

Box 36-1 identifies some unhealthy communication patterns.

Emotional-Supportive Function

All families encounter conflicts, and no family is 100% "functional." However, in a healthy family, feelings of affection are generally uppermost, and anger and conflict do not dominate the family's pattern of interaction. Healthy families are concerned with each other's

---

BOX 36-1

Examples of Dysfunctional Communication

Manipulating

Instead of asking directly for what is wanted, family members manipulate others in order to get what they want. For example, a child starts a fight with a sibling to get attention. Another example is a family member's making requests with strings attached, so that the other person has a difficult time refusing the request: "If you do this for me, then I won't tell Daddy that you are getting poor grades in school."

Distracting

To avoid functional problem solving and resolve conflicts within the family, family members introduce irrelevant details into problematic issues.

Generalizing

When dealing with problematic family issues, members use global statements like "always" and "never" instead of dealing with specific problems and areas of conflict. Family members may say "Harry is always angry" instead of "Harry, what is upsetting you?"

Blaming

Family members blame others for failures, errors, or negative consequences of an action to keep the focus away from themselves. This is a response to fear of being blamed by others.

Placating

Family members pretend to be inadequate but well meaning to keep peace in the family at any price: "Don't yell at the children, dear. I put the shoes on the stairs."

---

needs, and most of the family members' emotional and physical needs are met most of the time. When people's emotional needs are met, they feel support from those around them and are free to grow and explore new roles and facets of their personalities. A family that is dominated by conflict and anger alienates its members, leaving them isolated and fearful. This is not an atmosphere in which personality growth can take place, so this family would not be considered functional.

Socialization Function

It is within families that each member learns socialization skills. People learn how to interact, negotiate, and plan; they adopt coping skills. This is most evident in the socialization of children. Children learn how to function effectively within the family, and then they apply those skills in society. Parents are socialized into their family role by the demands of each child throughout the developmental stages of their children. The role of the parents changes again when the children mature and leave home, and the partners may renegotiate the pattern of their lives together. As time goes on, the parents may need their adult children's

TABLE 36-1

Family Life-Cycle Stages and Tasks for Three Types of Family Life Cycle

Stage	Task
I. Middle-Class North American Family Life Cycle	
1. Launching the single young adult	a. Differentiating self in relation to family of origin b. Developing intimate peer relationships c. Establishing self in relation to work and financial independence
2. Marrying: the joining of families	a. Establishing couple identity b. Realigning relationships with extended families to include spouse c. Making decisions about parenthood
3. Families with young children	a. Adjusting marital system to make space for child b. Joining in child-rearing, financial, and household tasks c. Realigning relationships with extended families to include parenting and grandparenting roles
4. Families with adolescents	a. Shifting parent-child relationships to permit adolescents to move into or out of system b. Refocusing on midlife marital and career issues c. Beginning to shift toward joint caring for older generation
5. Launching children and moving on	a. Renegotiating marital system as a dyad b. Developing adult-to-adult relationships between grown children and their parents c. Dealing with disabilities and death of grandparents
6. Families in later life	a. Maintaining own and/or couple functioning and interest in the face of physiological decline: exploration of new familial and social role options b. Making room in system for wisdom and experience of seniors c. Dealing with loss of spouse, siblings, and other peers and preparing for death
II. Divorce and Postdivorce Family Life Cycle	
1. Deciding to divorce	a. Accepting one's own part in the failure of the marriage
2. Planning the breakup of the system	a. Working cooperatively on problems of custody, visitation, and finances b. Dealing with extended family about the divorce
3. Separation	a. Mourning loss of nuclear family b. Restructuring marital and parent-child relationships and finances; adapting to living apart c. Realigning relationships with extended family; staying connected with spouse's extended family
4. Divorce	a. Retrieving hopes, dreams, and expectations from the marriage
Postdivorce: single parent (custodial)	a. Making flexible visitation arrangements with ex-spouse and his or her family b. Rebuilding own financial resources c. Rebuilding own social network
Postdivorce: single parent (noncustodial)	a. Finding ways to continue effective parenting relationships with children b. Maintaining financial responsibilities to ex-spouse and children c. Rebuilding own social network
III. Remarried Family Life Cycle	
1. Entering new relationship; conceptualizing and planning the new marriage and family	a. Recommitting to marriage and to forming a family b. Developing openness and avoiding pseudomutuality in new relationship c. Planning financial and coparental relationships with ex-spouse d. Planning to help children deal with fears, loyalty conflicts, and membership in two systems e. Realigning relationships with extended family to include new spouse and children f. Planning maintenance of connections for children with extended family of ex-spouse(s)
2. Remarriage and reconstruction of family	a. Restructuring family boundaries to allow for inclusion of new spouse-stepparent b. Realigning relationships and financial arrangements throughout subsystems to permit interweaving of several systems c. Making room for relationships of all children with custodial and noncustodial parents and grandparents d. Sharing memories and histories to enhance stepfamily integration

From Friedman, M. (1992). *Family nursing: Theory and practice* (3rd ed., pp. 82-105). Norwalk, CT: Appleton & Lange.

help if they become less able to care for their own needs. Each phase brings new demands and requires new approaches to deal with changes as people become socialized into new roles. Families have difficulty negotiating role change, and changes often increase the stress within families for a time. In response to the family's developmental life cycle, healthy families are flexible in adapting to new roles.

Family Life Cycle

The life cycle of the individual takes place within the family life cycle, which is the primary context of human development. The family is a system that moves through time, and family stress is often the greatest at transition points from one stage of the family developmental process to another. Symptoms are most likely to appear when an interruption or a dislocation occurs in the unfolding family life cycle. This interruption or dislocation could be a serious illness, a death, or a divorce. At these times, therapeutic efforts often need to be directed toward helping family members reorganize so that they can then proceed developmentally. Unlike all other organizations, families incorporate new members only by birth, adoption, or marriage, and members can leave only by divorce or death. If no way can be found to function within the system, the pressures of family membership with no available exit can, in the extreme, lead to mental illness or suicide. The development of symptoms should be viewed not only as a response to an interruption or a dislocation in the family life cycle but also as a solution to a stressful situation. This model assumes a traditional family organization and needs to be modified for less traditional family structures.

As identified in the middle-class North American family, six main stages exist in the changing family life cycle: (1) launching the single young adult, (2) joining families through couple formation, (3) becoming parents and caring for young children, (4) parenting adolescents, (5) launching children and moving on, and (6) experiencing later life. Four stages are identified in the life cycle of the divorcing and postdivorce family, and two phases in the remarried family life cycle (Table 36-1).

THEORIES, THEORISTS, AND APPROACHES TO FAMILY THERAPY

There are many different approaches to family therapy. Treatment possibilities have become too numerous to count (Hecker & Wetchler, 2003; Nichols, 2004). Many therapists today use an integrative approach.

The basic framework of family therapy took root in the 1960s and 1970s during societal upheaval. In clinical settings, therapists were beginning to notice the effects of the social milieu on their clients. The therapeu-

tic community was established as a treatment modality at this time, and group therapy and psychodrama were developed. All of these changes were based on observations of clients and a view of treatment as involving social systems. An **interactive** (interpersonal) rather than an **indwelling** (intrapsychic) model of mental illness was becoming more widely accepted. These influences paved the way for an interest in the family system as it related to psychiatric disorders.

One of the original shapers of family theory and therapy was Haley (1980), who was associated with the Mental Research Institute in Palo Alto, California, where the double-bind theory was developed. The double-bind theory describes a situation in which two conflicting messages are given simultaneously on two levels, verbal and nonverbal. Because the messages conflict, people find themselves in a double bind, in which no acceptable response exists. For example, a recently divorced and lonely mother says to her teenaged daughter, "Go on out, have fun with your friends. I'll be just fine." However, the nonverbal message is that the mother will be left alone and lonely. The nonverbal message is made clear by the mother's dejected face, slumped posture, and sad tone of voice. The daughter is now in a no-win situation: darned if she does and darned if she doesn't. Such a situation results in conflict and anxiety for the person caught in this double bind. If the daughter goes out with her friends, she will feel guilty for leaving her mother alone. If she stays home with her mother, she will miss out on the friendships and activities that are important for teenage development.

Virginia Satir (1972, 1983), a leading theorist of the same era, moved the focus from the client's symptoms to the client's position and relationships within the family. The Milan group, especially Palazzoli, Cecchin, and Prata (Wetchler, 2003), developed the use of paradox (i.e., "Don't change") as a way to work with families. Probably more than anyone, Minuchin (1974), a structural therapist, established the legitimacy of family therapy within psychiatry. Bowen (1985) was a leading proponent of the family systems model; he underplayed problem resolution, focusing instead on the long-term differentiation process of individual family members.

The terms *strategic* and *structural* are used to identify the frameworks adopted by specific therapists. A **strategic model of family therapy** assumes that changing any single element in the family system will bring about change in the entire system. Briefly, the aim of strategic therapy is to change the patterns, the rules, and the meaning of family interactions. For example, in the Gomez family, whom you will read about shortly, there is a pattern of communication, partly cultural, that excludes any discussion with the children. All decisions, whether or not they involve the children, are made without consulting them. Consequently, the children in this family often feel powerless, and the 8 year old has begun to engage in destructive behavior at school, which has precipitated a visit to a family therapist. A family therapist who uses the strategic model might work with the family to change their rigid pattern of communication to allow the children to be present when important decisions are being made. The children could comment and offer suggestions about how issues could be resolved. This could result in a resolution of the 8 year old's negative behavior by giving him a sense of control over aspects of his life and a more positive outlet for being heard and recognized. This intervention would result in a systemic change in the way the Gomez family communicates.

The **structural model of family therapy** is based on a normative concept of a healthy family and emphasizes the boundaries between family subsystems and the establishment and maintenance of a clear hierarchy based on parental competence. A therapist using the structural model with the Gomez family, rather than fo-

cusing on changing a specific pattern, would highlight the importance of boundaries between the parental and sibling (child) subsystems. At the same time, the therapist would emphasize the importance of flexibility in the family system that would allow for the changes inherent to normal growth and development.

The aims of family systems theory are to decrease emotional reactivity and to encourage differentiation among individual family members (i.e., increase each member's sense of self). In family therapy, no one model exists; all the shapers of family theory have made substantial contributions to the field of family therapy. In addition, all techniques are not applicable to all problems, and the experienced clinician must be discerning.

Most of the theoretical schools of or approaches to marital and family therapy fall into either insight-oriented family therapy or behavioral family therapy. Table 36-2 identifies some of the types of therapy in each group, describes their basic concepts and approaches, and lists the major theorists.

TABLE 36-2

Insight-Oriented and Behavioral Therapy

Type of Therapy	Concepts	Major Theorists
Insight-Oriented Family Therapy		
Psychodynamic therapy	Problems arise from ■ Developmental arrest ■ Current interactions ■ Projections ■ Current stresses Improvement through insight into problematic relationships originating in the past	Nathan Ackerman James Framo Ivan Boszormenyi-Nagy
Family-of-origin therapy	Family viewed as an emotional relationship system ■ Goal is to foster differentiation and decrease emotional reactivity ■ Concept of triangulation ■ Emphasis on the family of origin	Murray Bowen
Experimental-existential therapy	Goal of therapy is to encourage the growth of family ■ Symptoms express family pain ■ Family is responsible for its own solutions ■ Therapist uses nurturing and identifies dysfunctional communication patterns	Carl Whitaker Virginia Satir Leslie Greenberg Susan Johnson
Behavioral Family Therapy		
Structural therapy	Focus is on organizational patterns, boundaries, systems and subsystems, and use of scapegoating ■ Restructures dysfunctional triangles ■ Clarifies boundaries ■ Looks at enmeshment and disengagement (excessive distance) issues	Salvador Minuchin
Strategic therapy	Goal is to change repetitive and maladaptive interaction patterns ■ Identifies inequality of power, life-cycle perspectives, and use of double-bind messages ■ Uses paradox ■ Prescribes rituals	Jay Haley Chloe Madanes Milan group (Mara Palazzoli, Gianfranco Cecchin, Giuliana Prata)
Cognitive-behavioral therapy	Based on learning theory; focuses on changing cognition and behavior ■ Problem solving and solutions focus on present situations ■ Skills training is emphasized	Gerald Patterson Richard Stuart Robert Liberman

Basic Concepts in Family Therapy

Many concepts are widely used in working with families. The concepts of the identified client, the family triangle, and the nuclear family emotional system are discussed here. Box 36-2 describes other concepts relevant to family work.

The Family as a System

Every family can be viewed as a unique system. Each has its own structure, rules, and history of how it handles life problems and crises. Focusing on family patterns and interaction is basic to marital family therapy. The focus is *not* on an individual, as it is in traditional therapy, but rather on the interpersonal process of the family group (Nichols, 2004).

The Identified Client

The identified client is the individual in the family whom everyone regards as "the problem." This problem family member generally bears most of the family system's anxiety. When a family comes for treatment, the presenting problem, which is usually related to one member of the family, must be addressed before the underlying systemic problem is dealt with. The family member who is the identified client may or may *not* be the one who initially seeks help from inpatient or outpatient services.

Nurses generally tend to be more aware of the biophysical aspects of an individual than of the interpersonal aspects. Understandably, nurses also tend to subscribe to the medical model of cause-and-effect thinking. However, when a client is assessed in the context of the family, the nurse clinician must think less in a linear way (cause and effect) and more in terms of a circular causality. In considering circular causality, the presenting problem is viewed from many different perspectives. For example, the nurse considers a particular family's stressors and strengths in light of the family's current life-cycle stage, its sociocultural context and multigenerational issues, and the family's impact on the presenting problem. Thus, there is more than one perspective to be considered when looking at the identified client in terms of the family system. The focus is on the family system's anxiety.

▪ ▪ ▪ *VIGNETTE*

Eight-year-old Tommy Gomez, who is hyperactive and disruptive at school and at home, is brought to the community mental health clinic to be evaluated for attention deficit hyperactivity disorder. The nurse clinician performs an assessment and finds that a great deal of turmoil exists within the Gomez family. The family is composed of a heterosexual couple (married and the parents of the three children) and a grandmother. Tommy's father has just lost his job, and his grandmother was recently diagnosed with bladder cancer. Tommy's mother is planning to file for separation because of constant, unresolved arguments with her husband. The

BOX 36-2

Central Concepts of Family

Boundaries: Clear boundaries are those that maintain distinctions between individuals within the family and between the family and the outside world. Clear boundaries allow for balanced flow of energy between members. **Roles of children and parent or parents are clearly defined. Diffuse** or **enmeshed boundaries** are those in which there is a blending together of the roles, thoughts, and feelings of the individuals so that clear distinctions among family members fail to emerge. **Rigid** or **disengaged boundaries** are those in which the rules and roles are adhered to no matter what.

Triangulation: The tendency, when two-person relationships are stressful and unstable, to draw in a third person to stabilize the system through formation of a coalition in which the two join the third.

Scapegoating: A form of displacement in which a family member (usually the least powerful) is blamed for another's or another family member's distress. The purpose is to keep the focus off the painful issues and the problems of the blamers. **In a family, the blamers are often the parents and the scapegoat a child.**

Double bind: A situation in which a positive command (often verbal) is followed by a negative command (often nonverbal), which leaves the recipient confused, trapped, and immobilized because there is no appropriate way to act. A double bind is a "no-win" situation in which you are "darned if you do, darned if you don't."

Hierarchy: The function of power and its structures in families, differentiating parental and sibling roles and generational boundaries.

Family life cycle: The family's developmental process over time; refers to the family's past course, its present tasks, and its future course.

Differentiation: The ability to develop a strong identity and sense of self while at the same time maintaining an emotional connectedness with one's family of origin.

Sociocultural context: The framework for viewing the family in terms of the influence of gender, race, ethnicity, religion, economic class, and sexual orientation.

Multigenerational issues: The continuation and persistence from generation to generation of certain emotional interactive family patterns (e.g., reenactment of fairly predictable and almost ritual-like patterns; repetition of themes or toxic issues; and repetition of reciprocal patterns such as those of overfunctioner and underfunctioner).

---

nurse clinician who views this family from a perspective of circular causality would not focus solely on Tommy but would view Tommy's symptoms as a function of many difficult losses and transitions that are stressing the entire family's coping mechanisms.

The nurse identifies the multiple stressors in this family, believing that Tommy's symptoms of hyperactivity and acting out are related to the severe stresses in the family system. Once the issues within the family are addressed and plans are made to deal with these issues, perhaps Tommy's symp-

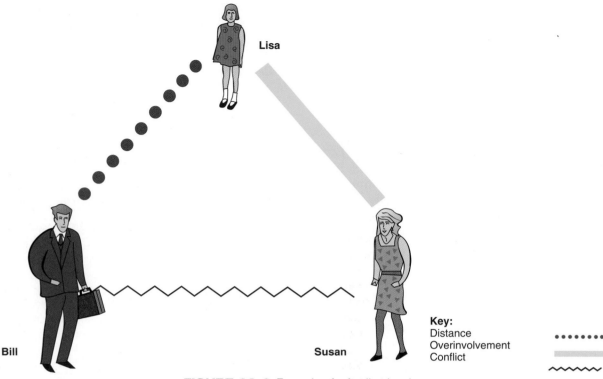

Key:
Distance
Overinvolvement
Conflict

FIGURE 36-2 Example of a family triangle.

toms will subside. She refers the couple to a family therapist. In the meantime, she encourages the couple to focus more on their own issues and less on Tommy's behavior. An appointment is made to go to the clinic in 1 month, where Tommy will be reevaluated.

Family Triangles

Bowen (1985) described a relationship process in families that can be seen as a system of interlocking triangles. In relationships between two people, the major tension lies in the struggle between closeness and independence. When the tension in a close twosome builds, a third person (child, friend, parent) may be brought in to help lower the tension. The family triangle (Figure 36-2) then becomes the basic building block of interpersonal relationships. All triangles contain a close side, a distant side, and a side in which conflict or tension exists between two people (Nelson, 2003). The intensity of the triangling process varies among families and within the same family over time. This is because triangles are related to lack of emotional stability. **Differentiation** refers to the ability of the individual to establish a unique identity and still remain emotionally connected to the family of origin. The lower the level of differentiation in a family, the higher the tension is, and the more important the role of triangling is to the lowering of tension and the preservation of emotional stability. As the family becomes stressed, for whatever reasons, the anxiety in

the system is triggered, and the triangles become more active.

A common problem that occurs in families is the setting up of a triangle among two parents and a child in which one parent is overinvolved with the child and the other plays a more peripheral role. In this situation, the child eventually becomes the means by which the parents communicate with each other about issues they cannot deal with directly. In other words, spousal conflicts may be brought into the parental arena, where they clearly do not belong.

■ ■ ■ *VIGNETTE*

Six-year-old Lisa is having trouble making friends. Her mother Susan has been feeling anxious and helpless as she tries to find ways to engage Lisa with other youngsters. Susan develops an overprotectiveness with Lisa that further inhibits Lisa from venturing out to make friends. Susan feels that her husband Bill is uncaring and disinterested because he thinks that she should be more relaxed about Lisa's social life and let things develop naturally. Bill's job requires that he travel most of the week, so he is not involved with Susan's daily experiences and struggles with Lisa.

In the spousal arena, Susan and Bill have been avoiding intimacy for almost a year. Susan is angry with Bill for spending so much time with his parents, which further casts him in a peripheral role in their nuclear family, and Bill is angry with Susan, sensing her rejection of him.

Both parents are feeling isolated and alienated and are consequently angry at each other. Neither Bill nor Susan addresses this issue directly. Instead, they play out their anger in the parental arena as they battle over how to handle Lisa's social isolation.

■ ■ ■

When working with families, advanced practice nurses must be aware that they carry their own family-of-origin issues, which may affect their responses to family work. When this happens, the nurse becomes triangled into the family's system. It is critical that the nurse's personal work on the nurse's own differentiation process continue even as she or he is involved in providing family therapy. The nurse's continuing work on self is an important way for the nurse to maintain emotional stability in the face of a chaotic family situation, in which the nurse's own issues may be playing out. Holding the family members accountable for themselves—making clear that the responsibility for change is theirs and not that of the nurse therapist—is a way of remaining clear of their triangles. For example, the nurse therapist could become triangled into a family system in any number of ways: perhaps the nurse recently experienced the loss of a family member; or maybe the nurse belongs to an enmeshed family system, in which the children are regularly drawn into spousal arguments; or perhaps stubbornness is an unresolved issue for the nurse. Any of these possibilities could allow the nurse to become triangled into a family system, which makes good therapeutic intervention difficult, if not impossible. The likelihood is great that nurse clinicians will become triangled into others' family systems to engage in their own family battles. Advanced practice nurses need to make regular concerted efforts to self-reflect and to understand their own personal family issues through therapy or supervision. Regular supervision is always recommended when nurse therapists work with individuals, couples, or families. Supervision can be conducted with peer professionals, in groups, or privately with a more experienced clinician. One indication that a nurse therapist is being triangled in is that his or her level of anxiety is greater than the situation warrants.

Although basic level nurses do not provide family therapy and do not generally seek out professional supervision, they also may bring their family issues into family teaching sessions and other interactions with family members. When the basic level nurse experiences either strong positive or negative reactions to a family, it is important to seek out a supervisor or peer to discuss what is happening.

The Nuclear Family Emotional System

The term nuclear family refers to a parent or parents and the children under the parents' care. Bowen (1985) developed the concept of a nuclear family emotional system, which is defined as the flow of emotional processes within the nuclear family. In this concept, symptoms are viewed as belonging to the nuclear family emotional system rather than to any one individual. Within the system, a distinction is made between conventional medical (psychiatric) diagnosis and family diagnosis; rather than viewing a symptom as reflecting a disease that is confined to a client, Bowen identified an emotional process that transcends the boundaries of a client and encompasses the family relationship system. The earlier example of 8-year-old Tommy, who was believed by his family and others to have attention deficit hyperactivity disorder, is one in which Tommy's symptoms could be viewed as reflecting the family's conflicts and changes.

Refer to Box 36-2 for a summary of concepts central to family life.

Application of the Nursing Process

■ ASSESSMENT

Assessment is typically intermixed with treatment, rather than constituting a distinct phase. Assessment should have multiple foci, including

- The family system.
- Its subsystems.
- The individuals in the family.

Essential information regarding sociocultural issues, past medical and mental illness, family interactions and communication styles, and areas of stress within the family needs to be obtained.

Nichols (2004) identifies a number of issues that should be assessed in family therapy:

- Stages of the family life cycle
- Sociocultural context
- Multigenerational issues

Sociocultural Context

The family must be viewed not as an isolated unit but in a sociocultural context, in which the issues of gender, race, ethnicity, class, sexual orientation, and religion are considered equally. Each of these contextual issues affects the family's specific values, norms, traditions, roles, and rules. For example, the way the family relates to a terminally ill family member may be decidedly different in a first-generation Italian American Catholic family than in an Asian family or in an African American Baptist family. Therefore, the nurse clinician needs to ask how this family's cultural and religious beliefs affect the client's presenting problem and what impact they have on the family's available options.

In regard to gender, for example, the position of women in U.S. society needs to be understood in terms of job opportunities, earning power, and status, which for most women are secondary to those of men. Gender and culture must be viewed together, because the relative status of males and females differs according to culture. In particular, people from Asian and Latin cultures living in the United States have difficulty understanding American gender roles. With regard to race and ethnicity, it is extremely important that nurses be aware of and understand the mores, practices, and beliefs of the many different cultures that currently make up America's fabric (refer to Chapter 7). This sensitivity prepares the nurse clinician to make effective interventions for families in times of crisis or psychiatric emergency. Because our American society does not outwardly make class distinctions (as do the British, for example), viewing the family in the context of class may not come easily and indeed may be downright uncomfortable; in fact, class is often considered by most therapists to be the "last taboo." Yet, although it is unspoken, most Americans do have a definite sense of the class to which they belong. It is most often defined in terms of money, education, and taste, and only with gentle questioning do these defining issues come to the fore.

Sexual orientation is another part of the context that often gets overlooked. When gathering family information, the nurse must ask questions regarding sexual orientation (e.g., in terms of long-term relationships). Finally, the context of religion figures prominently in a large percentage of the population, and this context includes many beliefs about why a person becomes ill and how that person should be treated. When the family is viewed in a sociocultural context, religion and spiritual values are important issues for consideration.

Multigenerational Issues

The influence of family is not restricted to the members of a household. Family is composed of the entire emotional system of at least three, and frequently four, generations. This means that the family is affected by multigenerational issues. Through this intergenerational system, various patterns (e.g., involving geographical distance between members, suicide, divorce, addiction, affairs, grief, triangles, and loss) are passed down through the generations. The messages and legacies of the multigenerational family relate in some way to the client's presenting problem. For example, in a family with adolescents in which the grandmother is terminally ill with cancer, if a pattern of addiction is already established in the family, the impending loss of an important family figure may exacerbate an incipient addiction in one of the family members. An astute nurse may express concern to the family regarding this possibility, perhaps preventing the development of a serious problem. This family may also have a preferred pattern of dealing with grief by using denial and by not allowing the outward expression of painful feelings. If

this is the case, the nurse guides the family into learning about other, more acceptable and healthier ways of dealing with grief, because unexpressed feelings of grief may lead to further symptomatic behaviors in other family members. One way to identify multigenerational issues is by constructing a genogram.

Constructing a Genogram

The genogram is a format for efficiently providing a clinical summary of information and relationships across at least three generations. It is an invaluable family assessment tool that provides a graphic display of complex patterns and serves as a source of hypotheses that indicate how the presenting problem connects to the family context and the evolution of the family over time (Nichols, 2004).

Bowen (1985) provided much of the conceptual framework for the analysis of genogram patterns. He proposed that the family is organized according to generation, age, sex, roles, functions, and interests, and suggested that where each individual fits into the family structure influences the family functioning, the relational patterns, and the type of family formed in the next generation. He further contended that sex and birth order shape sibling relationships and characteristics. Also, some issues tend to be played out from generation to generation through persisting interactive emotional patterns. A major concept is that of triangling, which was discussed earlier.

By creating a genogram, the nurse clinician is able to map the family structure and record family information. This information should include demographic data such as location, occupation, and educational level. Functional information regarding medical, emotional, and behavioral status is also recorded. Finally, critical events must be noted (e.g., important transitions, moves, job changes, separations, illnesses, and deaths). Figure 36-3 provides an example of a genogram derived from the data from the following vignette describing the Schneider family.

■ ■ ■ *VIGNETTE*

Hank and Catherine Schneider are both college educated, and each suffers from intermittent depression. Hank is an only child whose father died of a heart attack at age 55, Hank's present age. Hank's mother committed suicide at age 35. This is a toxic subject in Hank's family of origin. In Catherine's family of origin, she is the eldest, born after three miscarriages. Much pressure and many expectations were placed on Catherine. Catherine's brother Mike was born 4 years after Catherine. Their mother died during Mike's birth. Mike never finished high school, has a serious alcohol addiction, and has had three marriages that ended in divorce. One can speculate about the level of guilt Mike may feel regarding the loss of his mother.

Hank and Catherine have two children, Bill and Mary. Bill, the identified client, is 35 years old, has a college degree, and has not been able to hold down a job. He also has an

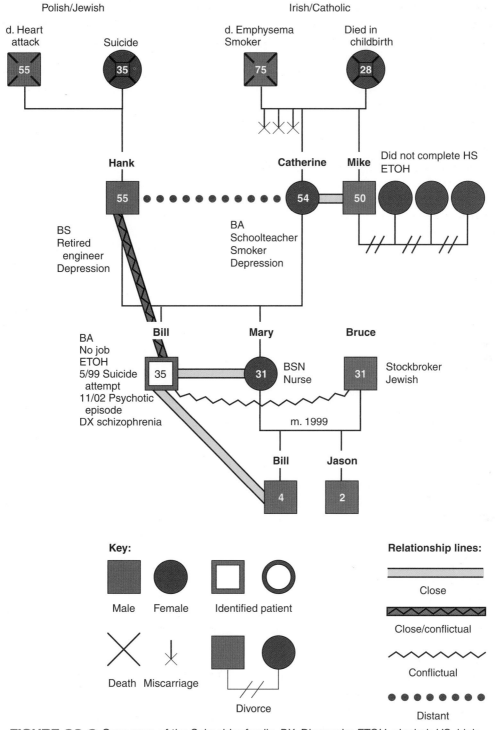

FIGURE 36-3 Genogram of the Schneider family. *DX,* Diagnosis; *ETOH,* alcohol; *HS,* high school; *m.,* married.

addiction to alcohol. In 1999, Bill made a suicide attempt. In November 2002, Bill experienced a psychotic episode for which he was hospitalized, and he was diagnosed as having schizophrenia. His younger sister Mary has a college degree and works as a nurse. She married Bruce in 1999, the year that Bill attempted suicide. Mary and Bruce have two young children, 4 and 2 years of age.

Self-Assessment

Nurses must be well trained when working with families in a counseling situation because the potential for multiple transferences and triangulations is high. Therefore, an advanced practice nurse educated at the master's level with special training in family work is usually best qualified to conduct family therapy. However, all nurses interact with families, whether in hospital acute care settings or in community-based settings. Most nurses come from a family, and because no family is perfect, all nurses are subject to forming triangles when anxious, to becoming defensive when personal family anxieties are aroused, or to experiencing role blurring or loosening of self-boundaries when sensitive personal issues and conflicts are triggered.

It is not uncommon for the nurse therapist to experience intense anxiety during the process of working with families. When this happens, it is important for the nurse to be able to draw back emotionally to examine the source of the anxiety; it may be that the nurse is responding to her or his personal family issues. When the nurse believes that he or she is getting drawn into the family dynamics rather than maintaining an objective stance, discussing these issues with a professional peer or supervisor is extremely important to maintain effectiveness. The nurse should identify a time when he or she reacted intensely (positively or negatively) to either a client or a client's situation. How was this issue dealt with later in conference? Common issues with which health care workers may intensely identify are alcohol or drug use, family abuse, codependency, rescue fantasies, and lifestyles. These and many other issues that evoke strong feelings need to be addressed before the nurse can see clearly the client and the client's situation and needs. Self-assessment is a crucial component of effective nursing care not only in psychiatric nursing but also in other nursing specialties.

Other Assessment Tools

Other tools are available to help the practitioner assess how the family functions as a unit and to identify individual members' perceptions of how the family communicates; how they deal with emotional issues such as anger, conflict, and affection; how they work together as a unit to plan and solve problems; how they make the important decisions for the family; and how they function generally. A focused interview, one in which the nurse can ask these questions directly, or an assessment device can be used to obtain this information.

A careful family assessment can be a vital part of the treatment if the family has as one of its members a person with a severe mental illness. Finkelman (2000) emphasizes the need to form a partnership with the family to reintegrate the ill person into the family and home.

■ NURSING DIAGNOSIS

Families have many needs at different times in their development. Family life often involves new members, deaths, mental and physical illnesses, economic challenges, developmental crises, and unanticipated

changes or decline. Severe dysfunctional patterns (e.g., marked relational conflict, sexual misconduct, abuse, violence, and suicide) exist within many families that cause physical or mental anguish to the members.

Numerous nursing diagnoses are useful in working with families. Box 36-3 identifies some useful family nursing diagnoses. The *Diagnostic and Statistical Manual of Mental Disorders*, fourth edition, text revision (*DSM-IV-TR*) (American Psychiatric Association, 2000) also identifies areas that can become the target of medical or psychiatric attention. These areas come under the heading of "other conditions that may be a focus of clinical attention." These *DSM-IV-TR* categories are as follows:

Relational problems	Relational problems related to a mental disorder or a generic medical condition, sibling relational problem or problems
Problems related to abuse or neglect	Includes physical and sexual abuse and neglect of a child, and physical or sexual abuse of an adult
Bereavement	Bereavement may cause considerable impairment and complications
Identity problems	
Religious or spiritual problems	
Age-related decline	
Acculturation problems	

■ OUTCOME CRITERIA

Although different therapists may adhere to different theories and use a wide variety of methods, the goals of family therapy are basically the same. These goals are the following (Nichols, 2004):

- To reduce dysfunctional behavior of individual family members
- To resolve or reduce intrafamily relationship conflicts

BOX 36-3

Possible Nursing Diagnoses for Family Interventions

- Impaired parenting
- Sexual dysfunction
- Interrupted family processes
- Dysfunctional family processes: alcoholism
- Caregiver role strain
- Risk for caregiver role strain
- Spiritual distress
- Impaired adjustment
- Ineffective denial
- Ineffective family therapeutic regimen management
- Deficient knowledge
- Impaired verbal communication
- Defensive coping

- To mobilize family resources and encourage adaptive family problem-solving behaviors
- To improve family communication skills
- To heighten awareness and sensitivity to other family members' emotional needs and help family members meet their needs
- To strengthen the family's ability to cope with major life stressors and traumatic events, including chronic physical or psychiatric illness
- To improve integration of the family system into the societal system (e.g., school, medical facilities, workplace, and especially the extended family)

Family psychoeducational treatment is often provided by nurses. Goals a nurse can use for psychoeducational teaching with a family include the following:

- Learning to accept the illness of a family member
- Learning to deal effectively with an ill member's symptoms, such as hallucinations, delusions, poor hygiene, physical limitations, paranoia, and aggression
- Understanding what medications can and cannot do and when the family should seek medical advice
- Learning what community resources are available and how to access them
- Feeling less anxiety and regaining or acquiring a sense of control and balance in family life

■ PLANNING

The immediate and long-term needs of the family should be determined. For example, is the family in crisis—that is, is one of the members homicidal, suicidal, abusive, or being abused? Do protective services need to be called? Is hospitalization necessary to protect a suicidal or self-mutilating member?

Is there a crisis at one of the family's developmental stages? What are the family's coping mechanisms at this time? What kinds of new skills can family members use at this time to help them facilitate resolution of normal life-cycle crises? Do family members need to be taught conflict management skills, problem-solving skills, parenting skills, limit-setting skills?

Is there a need for psychoeducational family interventions? Nurses are becoming adept at helping family members learn about the physical illness of an afflicted family member (e.g., severe mental illness, dementia), understand what medications can do (as well as side effects, etc.), and identify support groups and community resources to help the family cope with crisis and improve the quality of life for all of its members. How extensive is the family's knowledge deficit?

Where should a family be referred for optimal outcomes? Is there a problem with substance abuse, depression, unrealistic expectations of members, anger, or conduct disorder?

A careful analysis of the data from a sound assessment helps the nurse and other members of the health care team to identify the most appropriate family interventions for troubled families.

■ INTERVENTION

Family therapy has been applied to virtually every type of disorder among children, adolescents, and adults and has demonstrated efficacy for each population studied (Liddle & Rowe, 2004; Pinsof & Wynne, 2000). Family-based interventions enhance the involvement of clients and other family members, and impressive retention rates have been demonstrated for such therapy. Family therapy appears to be particularly effective in the treatment of substance abuse disorders, child behavioral problems, and marital relationship distress, and as an element of the treatment plan for schizophrenia (Liddle & Rowe, 2004).

Communication Guidelines

The roles of the basic level nurse and the advanced practice nurse vary in the ways in which these nurses work with families in both the hospital and the community settings. Differences exist in counseling and psychobiological interventions. The basic level nurse clinician may provide counseling through the use of a problem-solving approach to address an immediate family difficulty related to health or well-being. The advanced practice nurse, who has postgraduate training in family therapy, may conduct private family therapy sessions. With regard to psychobiological interventions, the advanced practice nurse may have prescriptive authority (depending on the state's nurse practice act and the nurse's qualifications).

The role of the basic level nurse, although different in scope from that of the advanced practice nurse, is equally important, especially in promoting and monitoring a family's mental health. Developing and practicing good listening skills and viewing family members in a positive, nonjudgmental way are critically important qualities for nurses at all levels, regardless of the practice setting.

An important function of basic level nurses is to assess cues from various family members that indicate the degree and amount of stress the family system is experiencing. These critical observations need to be readily reported so that appropriate interventions may be made in a timely manner. Some indicators of stress in a family system are the following:

- Inability of the family or a family member to understand and act on certain recommended treatment directives
- Various somatic complaints among family members
- High degree of anxiety
- Depression
- Problems in school
- Drug use

Promoting and monitoring a family's mental health can occur in virtually any setting and often requires making the most of an opportune moment. There does not have to be a formal meeting. Sometimes, an informal conversation **(therapeutic encounter)** can have the greatest effect. Following a few general guidelines can help the nurse remain nonjudgmental in the information presented as well as in the tone of voice and questions asked. For example, the question "Don't you think you should at least try to comply with your medical regimen?" would probably cause the client to tune the nurse out, whereas the invitation "Tell me what this medical regimen of yours is like" could open the door to understanding and problem solving in a collaborative rather than a hierarchical way.

- A nonblaming manner promotes open and flexible communication among all professionals and family members in the caregiving system. If other family members are involved in the conversation, be it on the hospital unit or in a family therapy session, the nurse should get each member's view, for example, by asking how the individual member's medical regimen affects the way the family functions and what the individual members consider a possible solution to the problem.
- Information should be imparted in a clear and understandable manner to all family members so they can decide what to do with the information. This is both a respectful and an empowering way to work with families, indicating to them that they are the ones who are accountable and responsible for how they choose to use the information.
- The perspective of each family member must be elicited and heard. Often, some family members hear another member's view for the first time in this democratic forum, and many times they are surprised ("I didn't know you felt that way"). The more family input there is, the more options usually exist for alternative ways of managing problematic situations. This approach defines the family as the central psychosocial unit of care. The following vignette provides an example of maintaining neutrality and hearing from all members.

■ ■ ■ *VIGNETTE*

Ms. Conway, the head nurse on the adolescent psychiatric unit, is concerned about all the negative comments the staff members are making regarding the fact that none of Chip's family has been in to visit him for over a week. In fact, she is concerned that Chip is picking up the staff's feelings as well. After many attempts, Ms. Conway finally reaches Chip's mother by telephone and begins to assess the situation. She discovers that Chip's mom is divorced and is working double shifts to meet the family's expenses. There is a 2 year old at home and a set of twins in the fourth grade.

Chip's mother had been planning to visit on the weekend, but the baby-sitter called to say she was sick. Once Ms. Conway

is able to see the situation from another perspective, that this is a family with young children that is struggling to make ends meet, she calls a staff meeting to address the situation.

■ ■ ■

Further interventions in this situation would be to problem-solve with Chip and his mother concerning what is realistic for each of them regarding visiting. Perhaps an extended family member or a friend can visit when the mother cannot. Longer-range planning for supervision for Chip when he is discharged should also be discussed as family supports are identified and assessed.

Unfortunately, negative comments about family members by staff occur all too often. This can present a difficult situation for the nursing student, who is entering the culture of the unit as an outsider and who realizes the negative effects that this behavior has on family members. It is appropriate for the student to first seek supervision from the instructor, so that the most effective approach can be planned out beforehand. One useful technique is for the student to ask questions of the supervising nurse and staff in such a manner that alternative ways of viewing the family in a broader perspective are embedded in the questions. An example of this is "Has anyone had a chance to contact Chip's mother to see if there are any problems?" or "I wonder what it's like for Chip's mother to have her son in a psychiatric unit."

Family Interventions

Family therapy is viewed by professionals as appropriate for most situations, although it may be contraindicated in some circumstances (Nichols, 2004):

- When the therapeutic environment is not safe and someone will be harmed by information, uncontrolled anxiety, or hostility
- When there is a lack of willingness to be honest
- When there is an unwillingness to maintain confidentiality

In most other situations, however, family therapy is useful, especially when it is combined with psychopharmacology in the treatment of families who have a member with a mental illness such as bipolar disorder, depression, or schizophrenia. Other families may choose psychoeducational family therapy and/or self-help groups, which are good options that may be less costly and time consuming. The following subsections introduce the student to (1) traditional family therapy intervention strategies, (2) psychoeducational groups, and (3) self-help groups that may benefit families and family members.

Traditional Family Therapy

Family therapists use a wide variety of theoretical philosophies and techniques to bring about change in dysfunctional patterns of behavior and interaction.

Some therapists may focus on the here and now, whereas others may rely more heavily on the family's history and reports of what happened between sessions. As stated earlier, most family therapists use an eclectic approach, drawing on a variety of techniques to fit the particular personality and strengths of the family.

Multiple-family group therapy is often used with families who have a hospitalized family member in an inpatient setting. These groups can help family members identify and gain insight into their own problems as they are reflected in the problems of other families. Several families meet in one group with one or more therapists, usually once a week until their ill family member is discharged; these groups often continue for a specific period of time after the client is discharged.

Psychoeducational Family Therapy

Psychoeducational family therapy has proven immensely effective, especially as a family treatment method combined with other modalities (e.g., psychopharmacology). One of the areas in which psychoeducational family training has been applied most successfully is in treatment of the client with schizophrenia. Some studies have shown that psychoeducational family therapy reduces the long-term need for rehospitalization by as much as 50% to 80% (Dixon et al., 2001; New York State Office of Mental Health, 2002; Steinglass, 1995). Families are extremely valuable and positive resources for clients. Family work promotes and supports families in coping with a family member with a severe mental illness.

The primary goal of psychoeducational family therapy is the sharing of mental health care information. Family education groups help family members better understand their member's illness, prodromal symptoms (symptoms that may appear before a full relapse), medications needed to help reduce the symptoms, and more. Psychoeducational family meetings or multiple family meetings allow feelings to be shared and strategies for dealing with these feelings to be developed. Painful issues of anger or loss, feelings of stigmatization or sadness, and feelings of helplessness can be shared and put in a perspective that the family and individual members can deal with more satisfactorily. Psychoeducational family groups are extremely useful for people with all kinds of mental as well as medical disorders.

Psychoeducational groups have also proven helpful in parent management training such as teaching a parent to work with a child with a conduct disorder.

Self-Help Groups

Self-help groups can be divided into two types. One type is for groups of people who have a personal problem or social deprivation. The second is for families with a member who has a specific problem or condition. Self-help groups acknowledge the needs of family members. Some groups may focus on families with healthy members, whereas others offer assistance to families whose members may be experiencing a health disorder or crisis. Most health professionals are aware that, for any developmental event, life crisis, or health disorder, a related mutual-aid group exists. These health professionals are in the best position to help clients and their families find additional support and information. For many people, self-help groups can be healing.

Case Management

Although the nursing profession has always interacted with families to some degree in the process of meeting a client's needs, our current knowledge of family systems dictates that the family be the primary focus when the management of the individual client is planned. The family's culture, ethnicity, socioeconomic status, and stage of family life cycle, as well as its unique patterns and beliefs about illness, all affect an individual's progress and response to case management. The family is the most powerful group to which an individual may ever belong, and it is vital that the nurse not discount or ignore the importance of the family's influence on its members when planning care.

To a great extent, case management entails teaching, giving appropriate referrals, and offering emotional support.

■ ■ ■ *VIGNETTE*

David Gardiner, age 21 years, is leaving the hospital after having experienced his first psychotic episode while taking his final examinations before graduation from college. David is being discharged back to his family, which consists of his mother and father; his maternal grandfather, who has been recently bedridden; and a younger brother Todd, who is 17 years of age. David's diagnosis is paranoid schizophrenia. The nurse takes a psychoeducational approach with the family.

Issues and needs are addressed by the nurse during family meetings while David is still hospitalized and later in follow-up family therapy after discharge. Initial interventions involve imparting information about David's mental illness through reading materials and discussion. The nurse also gives the family information on and telephone numbers of psychosocial support groups and a local chapter of the National Alliance for the Mentally Ill.

The nurse performs ongoing assessment of the family's strengths and weaknesses, including family supports as well as community support. She identifies some of the areas that may need to be addressed during the next few meetings.

Some of these issues include reorganizing family roles to accommodate a family member with a newly diagnosed severe and persistent mental illness; managing the bedridden grandfather; attending to Todd's probable fears that he, too, may have this illness; dealing with potential parental guilt feelings from a genetic point of view; planning how to mobilize should David experience another psychotic episode; managing medication and emphasizing the importance of compliance with the medication regimen; dealing with concerns about David's future and formulating realistic expectations; coping with feelings of loss for what was and what was hoped for; and, finally, maintaining the integrity and functioning of the spousal subsystem.

The nurse discusses these and other issues with the family and identifies where and how these issues can best be addressed. For example, a visiting nurse is called in to evaluate the grandfather's situation and need for support in the home, and a multiple-family psychoeducation group is formed to increase the family's understanding of David's illness, to help the family learn ways to cope with common problems that may arise, and to provide a place for family members to share their feelings of loss and grief.

■ ■ ■

Psychopharmacological Issues

The nurse is often the first to explain to the family the purpose of a prescribed medication as well as the desired effects and possible side effects and adverse reactions. The following vignette describes a situation that occurred at the time of discharge.

■ ■ ■ *VIGNETTE*

Susan Harris, a 45-year-old account executive and mother of three teenagers, has been referred by her physician to the mental health center for treatment of acute depression. The psychiatrist there has prescribed an antidepressant. Routinely, new clients are seen by the nurse clinician for a review of medications as a part of the health teaching. Unfortunately, the nurse clinician is engaged with another client in crisis at the time and misses meeting with Susan and her husband.

One week later, Susan makes an appointment with the clinical specialist complaining of symptoms of insomnia and lack of sexual desire, which is a concern for both Susan and her husband. Susan fears that she is getting worse and "going crazy." During the appointment, the nurse clinician reviews with Susan the side effects and adverse reactions associated with antidepressants. She informs Susan that the medication she is taking might not reach its full effects for 3 weeks or longer. She also explains that sleeplessness and lowered sexual drive are common side effects of the group of medications known as selective serotonin reuptake inhibitors, which includes the drug Susan is taking. They discuss ways to combat these side effects (see Chapter 18). The nurse urges Susan to continue taking the medication; however, if the side effects continue, the medication can be changed. Susan is due to visit the clinic 2 weeks later for follow-up. The nurse urges Susan to discuss the side effects of the medication with her husband and encourage him to come with her to the clinic at her next appointment.

■ ■ ■

Certainly, the more information family members have at their disposal, the less anxiety will distort their observations and decision making after discharge. Because of untoward circumstances in this case, the nurse clinician on the unit did not review Susan's medication with her before she was discharged. The clinical specialist needs to closely monitor Susan to determine whether her symptoms represent an exacerbation of her depression or a reaction to the antidepressant medication. If Susan is having a reaction to the medication, the nurse may consult with a physician so that another medication can be tried.

■ EVALUATION

The nursing process is not concluded until an evaluation is completed. In the treatment of families the evaluation focuses on whether family members are more functional, conflicts are reduced or resolved, communication skills are improved, coping is strengthened, and the family is more integrated into the societal system.

■ ■ ■ KEY POINTS to REMEMBER

- Family therapy is based on eclectic theoretical concepts.
- The aim of family therapy is to decrease emotional reactivity among family members and to encourage differentiation among individual family members.
- The primary characteristics that are essential to healthy family functioning are flexibility and clear boundaries.
- It is important to be aware of the stages in the changing family life cycle of a traditional family, a divorced family, and a remarried family.
- Family-oriented approaches that include helping a family gain insight and make behavioral changes are most successful.
- The genogram is an efficient clinical summary and format for providing information and defining relationships across at least three generations.
- The family's culture, ethnicity, socioeconomic status, and life-cycle stage, as well as its unique patterns and beliefs about illness, all affect the individual client's progress and response to case management.
- Assessment of the family includes a focus on the stage of the family life cycle, multigenerational issues, and the family's sociocultural status.
- Nurses with basic training are frequently called upon to conduct psychoeducation with families.
- Nurses who have specialized training and are certified provide family therapy using a variety of theoretical approaches.

■ ■ ■

Visit the Evolve website at **http://evolve.elsevier.com/Varcarolis** for a posttest on the content in this chapter.   *evolve*

Critical Thinking and Chapter Review

Visit the Evolve website at **http://evolve.elsevier.com/Varcarolis** for additional self-study exercises.

evolve

■ ■ ■ CRITICAL THINKING

1. Select a family from your clinical experience. Evaluate this family's status in terms of functionality-dysfunctionality with reference to the five family functions described in the text (i.e., management function, boundary function, communication function, emotional-supportive function, and socialization function).

2. Using the same family selected in the previous question, create a genogram that identifies the stage in the family life cycle and describe the sociocultural context of this family.

3. Create your own personal genogram, including at least three generations. Be sure to include the following:

    A. Location, occupation, and educational level

    B. Critical events, such as births, marriages, moves, job changes, separations, divorces, illnesses, deaths

    C. Relationship patterns, such as cutoffs, distancing, overinvolvement, and conflict

4. A family has just found out that their young son is going to die. The parents have been fighting and blaming each other for ignoring the child's ongoing symptom of leg pain, which was eventually diagnosed as advanced cancer. There are two other siblings in the family. How would you as the primary nurse apply family concepts to help this family? What would be your outcome criterion?

■ ■ ■ CHAPTER REVIEW

Choose the most appropriate answer.

1. When assessed within the context of the family system, the identified client is

    1. the family member who the others say is the problem.

    2. the individual member of the family who first seeks help.

    3. the person who is triangled in to help lower tension between spouses.

    4. the person who makes the rules about who participates in a particular family function.

2. When a nurse assesses a family system as being healthy, the two primary characteristics found to be present are

    1. generalizing and placating.

    2. flexibility and clear boundaries.

    3. diffusion and enmeshment.

    4. socialization and management.

3. A realistic goal for improved communication in a family engaged in family therapy can be stated as follows: Communication among family members will be

    1. clear and direct.

    2. altruistic and supportive.

    3. distant and guarded.

    4. emotional and conflictual.

4. A function of the entry-level staff nurse in promoting a family's mental health is to

    1. conduct family therapy sessions.

    2. identify each member's unmet needs and devise plans for meeting these needs.

    3. assess cues that indicate the amount of stress the family is experiencing.

    4. give assignments designed to change defensive coping styles and limit denial.

5. Jim, a 20-year-old college student, has been hospitalized for treatment of bipolar disorder. His discharge plan is to live with his parents and 17-year-old sister until his condition stabilizes. His return to college is planned for the following semester. The nurse believes rehospitalization can be avoided if Jim and his family understand his illness and his medication. The type of family therapy that will produce these outcomes is

    1. crisis intervention.

    2. traditional family therapy.

    3. psychoeducational family therapy.

    4. a self-help group for families with mentally ill members.

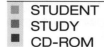

■ STUDENT
■ STUDY
■ CD-ROM

Access the accompanying CD-ROM for animations, interactive exercises, review questions for the NCLEX examination, and an audio glossary.

REFERENCES

American Psychiatric Association. (2000). *Diagnostic and statistical manual of mental disorders (DSM-IV-TR)* (4th ed., text rev.). Washington, DC: Author.

Bowen, M. (1985). *Family therapy in clinical practice.* New York: Jason Aronson.

Dixon, L., et al. (2001). Evidence-based practices for services to families of people with psychiatric disabilities. *Psychiatric Services, 52*(7), 903-910.

Finkelman, A. W. (2000). Psychiatric patients and families: Moving from catastrophic event to long-term coping. *Home Care Provider, 5*(4), 142-147.

Haley, J. (1980). *Leaving home.* New York: McGraw-Hill.

Hecker, L. L., & Wetchler, J. L. (2003). *An introduction to marriage and family therapy.* New York: Haworth Clinical Practice Press.

Liddle, H. A., & Rowe, C. L. (2004). Advances in family therapy research. In M. P. Nichols (Ed.), *Family therapy: Concepts and methods* (6th ed.). New York: Pearson Education.

Minuchin, S. (1974). *Families and family therapy.* Cambridge, MA: Harvard University Press.

Nelson, T. S. (2003). Transgenerational family therapies. In L. L. Hecker, & J. L. Wetchler (Eds.), *An introduction to marriage and family therapy.* New York: Haworth Clinical Practice Press.

New York State Office of Mental Health. (2002, February 6). *Evidence-based practice letter on family psychoeducation.* Retrieved August 7, 2004, from http://www.omh.state.ny.us/omhweb/ebp/letters/family.htm.

Nichols, M. P. (2004). *Family therapy: Concepts and methods* (6th ed.). New York: Pearson Education.

Pinsof, W. M., & Wynne, L. C. (2000). Toward progress research: Closing the gap between family therapy practice and research. *Journal of Marital and Family Therapy, 26*(1), 1-8.

Roberts, F. B. (1983). An interaction model for family assessment. In I. W. Clements & F. B. Roberts (Eds.), *Family health: A theoretical approach to nursing care* (pp. 189-204). New York: Wiley.

Satir, V. (1972). *Peoplemaking.* Palo Alto, CA: Science and Behavior Books.

Satir, V. (1983). *Conjoint family therapy.* Palo Alto: Science and Behavior Books.

Steinglass, P. L. (1995). Family therapy. In H. I. Kaplan & B. J. Sadock (Eds.), *Comprehensive textbook of psychiatry/VI* (6th ed., Vol. 1, pp. 1838-1846). Baltimore: Williams & Wilkins.

Wetchler, J. L. (2003). Structural family therapy. In L. L. Hecker & J. L. Wetchler (Eds.), *An introduction to marriage and family therapy.* New York: Haworth Clinical Practice Press.

CHAPTER 37

Integrative Care

CHARLOTTE ELIOPOULOS ▪ VERNA BENNER CARSON ▪ GLORIA KUHLMAN

KEY TERMS and CONCEPTS

The key terms and concepts listed here appear in color where they are defined or first discussed in this chapter.

acupuncture, 760

aromatherapy, 761

chiropractic, 754

complementary and alternative medicine (CAM), 749

conventional health care system, 750

herbal therapies, 761

homeopathy, 753

integrative care, 749

naturopathy, 753

prayer, 763

therapeutic touch, 760

OBJECTIVES

After studying this chapter, the reader will be able to

1. Describe integrative care.
2. Explore the philosophies behind various complementary and alternative therapies, including acupressure and acupuncture, aromatherapy, chiropractic medicine, herbal medicine, homeopathy, and massage.
3. Discuss the techniques used in major complementary therapies and the nurse's role.
4. Discuss how the public can be misled through quackery and fraud related to the use of alternative and complementary therapies.
5. Explore information resources available through literature and on-line sources.

evolve Visit the Evolve website at **http://evolve.elsevier.com/Varcarolis** for a pretest on the content in this chapter.

MOVEMENT TOWARD INTEGRATIVE CARE

This chapter explores issues and raises questions related to the trend toward integrative care, which refers to the blending of conventional or allopathic (mainstream) medical practices with those of complementary and alternative medicine (CAM). Integrative care represents a holistic approach, and for this reason it is of great importance to nurses who pride themselves on being holistic providers. Not only do nurses personally use CAM but they take care of clients who increasingly use CAM to meet health needs. To fully understand the needs of clients, it is essential that nurses ask questions about the use of CAM as part of a holistic assessment. It is equally important for nurses to be able to answer questions posed by clients regarding CAM (Stokowski, 2004).

OVERVIEW OF COMPLEMENTARY AND ALTERNATIVE MEDICINE

Complementary and Alternative Medicine Defined

CAM covers a broad range of healing philosophies. Most often it is defined as those treatments and health care practices that are not widely taught in medical schools, not generally used in hospitals, and not consistently reimbursed by insurance companies (National Center for Complementary and Alternative Medicine [NCCAM], 2004b). However, the insurance situation is gradually changing, and some major insurance companies now cover chiropractic care, acupuncture, and massage. CAM therapies are noninvasive and frequently described as "holistic"; that is, they incorporate the entire person—biological, psychological, social, and spiritual. CAM often espouses the promotion of health to prevent health problems rather than the treatment of symptoms once health problems arise. Therapies may be used as a substitute for conventional therapies (referred to as **alternative**) or in tandem with conventional treatments (referred to as **complementary**) (NCCAM, 2004b). In some cases, these therapeutic modalities incorporate treatments consistent with Western medicine, and in other cases, healing processes that have originated in other areas of the world are used. Some CAM practices are becoming incorporated into mainstream medical practice, but others are still considered outside the realm of accepted medical care.

Although in the United States the conventional health care system (also referred to as allopathic, mainstream, or orthodox medicine; regular medicine; and biomedicine) is based largely on scientific research, CAM therapies generally have not been scientifically tested. This does not necessarily mean that the therapies are ineffective; rather, insufficient valid, reliable research exists to establish their effectiveness and safety. To address this issue, Congress allocated $117 million toward alternative medicine research in 2004 (WNBC.com, 2004), and the World Health Organization (WHO) issued guidelines for ensuring the safety and efficacy of preparations in the multibillion-dollar herbal market (Hasselberger, 2004).

Most practitioners of conventional medicine treat the disease, whereas practitioners of CAM use a holistic approach; that is, they address the whole person: body, mind, and spirit. Integrative practitioners tend to perform thorough assessments with the client's active participation and then determine the best approach, which may be CAM, conventional medical care, or a combination of both (Eliopoulos, 1999; Kligler & Lee, 2004; Maizes, Koffler, & Fleishman, 2003). Assessments based on an integrative approach certainly include the traditional areas of inquiry such as history, present illness, family medical history, history of surgeries, as well as medications taken and response to these medications. However, the integrative assessment also includes areas such as the quality of social relationships, the meaning of work, the impact of major stressors in the person's life, strategies used to cope with stress (including relaxation, meditation, deep breathing, etc.), and the importance of spirituality and religion in the person's life. Clients also are asked what they really love, how this is manifested in their lives, what their strengths are, and what are the personal gifts that they bring to the world (Maizes et al., 2003). Even when the best treatment option is medication or surgery, practitioners following an integrative approach may use therapies from CAM to assist the client in relieving stress, promoting a sense of well-being, and establishing positive lifestyle habits. Drs.

Rakel and Weil (2003) contrast conventional and integrative health care as follows:

> In conventional medicine, healing occurs outside the body-mind and is viewed as something done to the client. In integrative medicine, healing occurs within the body-mind and requires active participation of the client. (p. 7)

Because of growing interest in and use of CAM, the National Institutes of Health (NIH) established the Office of Alternative Medicine (OAM) in 1992 and mandated the OAM to facilitate evaluation of alternative treatments, serve as an information clearinghouse, and support research training in therapies not usually incorporated into the educational programs for most health professions. In October 1998 the OAM was elevated to the status of a center and was renamed the National Center for Complementary and Alternative Medicine. The NCCAM does not advocate specific treatment modalities; instead, it supports fair and scientific evaluation of CAM therapies and dissemination of information that allows health care providers to make good choices regarding the safety and appropriateness of CAM.

In May 2004 the NCCAM and the National Center for Health Statistics (NCHS) released findings on Americans' use of CAM. These data came from the 2002 edition of the NCHS's National Health Interview Survey, which interviewed over 31,000 Americans regarding their health- and illness-related experiences. Included in this survey were questions that focused on a variety of CAM therapies that are commonly used in the United States. These included acupuncture and chiropractic, use of natural products, special dietary regimens, and megavitamin therapy. Box 37-1 lists the CAM therapies that were included in the 2002 National Health Interview Survey. The data focused on the use of CAM in the 12 months prior to the 2002 interview survey, and the data were analyzed including and excluding two therapies: (1) prayer used specifically for health reasons; and (2) megavitamin therapy. These two therapies were not consistently included in earlier national surveys (NCCAM, 2004b).

The findings of the survey indicated that 36% of American adults use some form of CAM. When prayer and megavitamin use were included in the definition of CAM, the proportion rose to 62%. The data were also analyzed to determine the frequency of CAM use in five specific categories, including mind-body medicine, biologically based practices, manipulative and body-based practices, whole medical systems, and energy medicine (these categories are defined and discussed later in the chapter). When prayer was included in the definition of CAM, mind-body medicine was the most commonly used form of CAM (53%). When prayer was excluded, biologically based practices (used by 22%) were found to be more popular than mind-body medicine (used by 17%).

BOX 37-1

Complementary and Alternative Medicine Therapies Included in the 2002 National Health Interview Survey

Acupuncture*
Ayurveda*
Biofeedback*
Chelation therapy*
Deep breathing exercises
Diet-based therapies
- Vegetarian diet
- Macrobiotic diet
- Atkins diet
- Pritikin diet
- Ornish diet
- Zone diet
Energy healing therapy*
Folk medicine*
Guided imagery
Homeopathic treatment
Hypnosis*
Massage*
Meditation
Megavitamin therapy
Use of natural products (nonvitamin and nonmineral, such as herbs and other products from plants, enzymes, etc.)
Prayer for health reasons
- Prayer for own health
- Prayer for own health by others
- Participation in prayer group
- Performance of healing ritual for self
Progressive relaxation
Qi gong
Reiki*
Tai chi
Yoga

From National Center for Complementary and Alternative Medicine. (2004b, September). *The use of complementary and alternative medicine in the United States.* Retrieved December 10, 2004, from http://nccam.nih.gov/news/camsurvey_fs1.htm.
*A practitioner-based therapy.

Many Americans who use CAM therapies do so without the knowledge of their conventional health care providers. This is not without risk. For instance, in the United States there are no standards or regulations that guarantee the safety or efficacy of herbal products. Some consumers operate under the impression that, if they can purchase a substance at a health food store without a prescription and it is a natural product, it also must be safe. This could not be further from the truth. "Natural" does not mean "harmless." Herbal products may contain powerful active ingredients that can cause damage if taken inappropriately. Furthermore, the consumer cannot be sure that the amount of the herb or other active ingredient listed on the label is actually the amount in the product. Another concern regarding CAM therapies is that clients may try many alternative interventions while delaying diagnosis and treatment of illnesses such as cancer. Of course, CAM practitioners can recount horror stories of clients who have been injured by a noncaring conventional medical system or who have suffered terrible consequences from the use of pharmaceutical drugs. An example of such a pharmaceutical nightmare was the administration of thalidomide to pregnant women to treat nausea, which resulted in the birth of babies with serious physical defects, including missing or shortened legs or arms.

The fact that increasing numbers of Americans use CAM has prompted conventional practitioners to establish bridges between conventional medicine and CAM so that clients not only can access the best therapies available from both arenas but also can use CAM safely and effectively.

Consumers and Health Care

Consumers are attracted to CAM for a variety of reasons:

- A desire to be an active participant in one's health care and engage in holistic practices that can promote health and healing
- A desire to find therapeutic approaches that carry lower risks than medications
- A desire to find less expensive alternatives to high-cost conventional care
- Positive experiences with CAM practitioners, who tend to spend more time with and learn about all facets of their clients
- Dissatisfaction with the practice style of conventional medicine (e.g., rushed office visits, short hospital stays)

The knowledgeable consumer, relying on medical information readily available through public libraries, popular bookstores, and the Internet, is questioning the traditional practice of conventional medicine. It is essential that nurses keep abreast of CAM, continue to evaluate the evidence supporting the effectiveness and safety of CAM, and be able to guide clients in the safe use of these treatments. For example, consumers are using some herbal remedies to treat a variety of psychiatric conditions because they believe these plants to be safe and effective; however, herbs can have serious side effects and interactions with other herbs and drugs.

Cost of Alternative Therapies

The growth in the use of CAM therapies is also linked to the rising cost of conventional medical care. There is mounting pressure to control health care spending in most countries, and efforts are focused on the development of less expensive means for the treatment of mental illnesses. Before we can adopt alternative methods of treatment, however, even those that are less expensive, it is essential that we have reliable information about the clinical effectiveness of these treatment methods. Herbs such as St. John's wort and ginkgo biloba may prove effective and less costly than prescription drugs that produce similar results; however, it is imperative that data be available to identify the desired and adverse effects of these treatments.

CATEGORIES OF COMPLEMENTARY AND ALTERNATIVE MEDICINE

Complementary alternative health care and medical practices may be grouped into five major domains according to the NCCAM. These domains include the following:

1. Alternative medical systems
2. Mind-body interventions
3. Biologically based therapies
4. Manipulative and body-based methods
5. Energy therapies

Alternative Medical Systems

Alternative medical systems are often traditional systems of medicine based on the religious beliefs and practices of cultures throughout the world. Two of these systems have a strong spiritual component that is grounded in an Eastern worldview. For instance, **ayurvedic medicine,** which originated in India around 5000 BC, is one of the world's oldest and most complete medical systems. The word *ayurveda* means "the science of life." Ayurveda stresses individual responsibility for health; it is holistic, promotes prevention, recognizes the uniqueness of the individual, and offers natural methods of treatment (Pai, Shanbhag, & Archarya, 2004).

Traditional Chinese medicine (TCM) also falls into the category of alternative medical systems. Because many other CAM therapies such as acupuncture, acupressure, transcendental meditation, and qi gong, to name a few, are derived from TCM, let us take an indepth look at this alternative medical system. TCM is derived from Taoism, which teaches the following (Chopra, 1991):

- Each person comprises the reality of existence.
- If one lives within the natural rhythms of the universe, he or she will be whole.
- Each person is one with all that surrounds him or her.
- Paying attention to nature and all its changes allows one to see that one is no different from what surrounds one.

- One must respect the life force of nature.
- Each person is essentially divine. Each person, therefore, possesses the creative energy or life force to change. This energy is called qi (or ch'i), or yin and yang.

According to Taoists, this life force is a two-part force, with each part complementary to the other and neither more important than the other. Good and evil, birth and death, action and inaction, flexibility and inflexibility, and love and hate are but a few facets of this two-part force. Health, according to Taoism, is the balance between these parts. Illness emanates from imbalances. The goal of life, according to Taoism, is transformation. This means returning to and being reabsorbed into the life force. Taoists also believe that individuals receive guidance from nature in the quest for balance.

TCM, based on Taoist natural philosophy, emphasizes the need to promote harmony (health) or bring order out of chaos (illness). TCM is a vast system of medicine based on a constellation of concepts, theories, laws, and principles of energy movement within the body. Specific modes of therapy in TCM include acupuncture, diet therapy, exercises, herbal therapy, and manipulation of the musculoskeletal system. These modes of therapy are aimed at addressing the client's illness in relation to the complex interaction of mind, body, and spirit. Adherents of TCM say that not only does it address symptoms but it also addresses what they call "cosmologic" events—events that relate to the dynamics of the universe.

According to TCM, the qi, or life force, circulates throughout the universe, as well as in our bodies, in precise channels called meridians. (These meridians become significant in the practice of acupuncture.)

TCM incorporates a five-element theory that is a concrete expression of the Taoist concept of qi, yin and yang, or life force. In this five-element theory, every substance, including substances of the body, is classified as one of five primordial elements: wood, fire, earth, metal, and water. For instance, a practitioner of TCM would say that the spleen and stomach "are of the realm of earth." The lungs and large intestines, on the other hand, "belong to metal."

These elements are said to act on one another as part of a dynamic system. For example, a practitioner of TCM would say that fire animates earth, that earth produces metal, that metal enriches water, that water produces wood, and that wood gives rise in turn to fire. In this system, the *transition* of the five elements reflects the human condition of transformation, and transformation, in this system, is the essence of healing (Carson, 2000).

According to TCM, the relationships among the elements can be both nurturing and destructive. Thus, they illustrate the delicate interaction between yin and yang and the need to maintain balance. In this view, not only does health depend on the web of relationships within the five-element energy system, it also depends on the relationships within the client's environment, including

- Relationships with individuals, families, and communities.
- Relationships with seasons, climates, and other physical phenomena.
- Relationships with emotional, mental, and spiritual influences.

Just as would any other health care practitioner, a practitioner of TCM assesses the client through a thorough history taking and physical examination. However, the practitioner of TCM uses the history and physical examination to gain an understanding of the imbalances of mind, body, and spirit that have caused the client's illness. Diagnosis, in TCM, involves not only questioning but also observing body structure, skin color, breath, body odors, nail condition, voice, gestures, mood, and pulse.

Practitioners of TCM say that *pulse diagnosis* is an art requiring years of practice. The practitioner palpates six pulses in each wrist, using both a light and a firm touch. She or he then describes the qualities of the pulses using terms such as *fast, slow, weak, slippery, astringent, stretched,* and *tardy.* This information is used to characterize not only the client's current health status but also past health history and the prognosis for future health (Carson, 2000).

To understand healing from an Eastern worldview, one must examine the goals, principles, and stages of healing. First, the goals of healing are

- To be in harmony with one's environment and with all of creation in mind, body, and spirit.
- To reawaken the spirit to its possibilities.
- To reconnect with life's meaning.

According to this worldview, the principles of healing are as follows:

- All nature (i.e., all living systems) tends toward order and harmony.
- All living systems are interdependent.
- Illness, or "dis-ease," is a pattern or patterns in the healing continuum of life.
- Healing is transformational and evolutional.
- All healing is manifested as a simultaneous yin and yang reflection of the whole being in a state of transition.
- All healing is engendered through love and compassion. Love is the "author" of all healing.
- All healing is spirit centered.

Finally, in an Eastern worldview, the stages of healing are the following:

- Awakening—represents a time, often triggered by crisis or illness, in which the person is said to sense a need for change, a feeling of diminution in the quality of life
- Intentionality and focus—occurs when the person desires to change his or her consciousness from

patterns of "disharmony" to patterns of healthy behaviors and seeks to ease the pain of spiritual discomfort and to obtain help

- Commitment—occurs when the person forges healing relationships and establishes goals for change
- Transformation—occurs when mutual, creative, active participation occurs between practitioner and client directed toward ongoing change in mind, body, and spirit
- Attainment—occurs when the client incorporates new, healthy behaviors, has a sense of well-being, and accepts new challenges for growth; he or she has a willingness to evaluate and change to move toward greater levels of wholeness
- Empowerment—occurs when the person feels a sense of stability and harmony

The following are some specific body-mind-spirit therapies based on an Eastern worldview:

- Acupuncture
- Imagery
- Therapeutic touch
- Therapeutic massage
- Relaxation
- Bioenergetics
- Biofeedback
- Qi gong
- Yoga

Several of these interventions are discussed later in the chapter.

Homeopathy and naturopathy are also examples of alternative medical systems. Although both of these systems emphasize holistic health, neither espouses a particular spiritual worldview. **Homeopathy** uses small doses of specially prepared plant extracts and minerals to stimulate the body's defense mechanisms and healing processes to treat illness. Immunizations and allergy treatments are examples of the use of homeopathic principles in medicine today. **Naturopathy** emphasizes health restoration rather than disease treatment and uses nutrition, homeopathy, herbal medicine, hydrotherapy, light therapy, therapeutic counseling, and other therapies. The underlying belief is that the individual assumes responsibility for his or her recovery.

Mind-Body Interventions

Mind-body interventions employ techniques designed to facilitate the mind's capacity to affect bodily function and symptoms. Conventional clinicians recognize the connection and interaction between mind and body, especially in the mental health field. This connection is understood in all areas of medicine, especially when symptoms are exaggerated by stress. Many of the mind-body interventions, such as cognitive-behavioral approaches, support groups, and education, are considered mainstream, but meditation, prayer, spiritual healing, and therapies using creative outlets such as dance, music, and art therapy are categorized as complementary and alternative.

Biologically Based Therapies

Biologically based therapies may overlap with conventional medicine's use of dietary supplements such as vitamins, minerals, herbs or other botanicals, amino acids, and substances such as enzymes, organ tissues, and metabolites.

Manipulative and Body-Based Methods

Manipulative and body-based methods employ manipulation or movement of the body. Chiropractic focuses on the relationship between structure and function, and the way in which that relationship affects the preservation and restoration of health by using manipulative therapy as a treatment tool. *Chiropractic* comes from the Greek words *praxix* and *cheir*, meaning practice or treatment by hand. This method of therapy originated with Daniel David Palmer, a grocery store owner, who had learned magnetic healing and mysticism. He distrusted much of the contemporary medicine of the late 1800s, and he was determined to heal others without using drugs. Palmer developed a series of manipulative procedures to bring health to muscles, nerves, and organs that had gotten out of alignment. His approaches are now called the Palmer method of chiropractic.

Palmer referred to misalignments as subluxations. He believed that subluxations were metaphysical and that they interfered with the flow through the body of "innate intelligence" (spirit or life energy). His theory had some commonalities with TCM. Palmer's son, Bartlett Joshua Palmer, was an attentive student of his father's approach. The son expanded his father's theory to assert that subluxations were the cause of all illnesses. Many chiropractic practitioners split away from the Palmer method because they could not accept this metaphysical explanation of illness, and they sought a scientific explanation for their interventions. Today there are chiropractors who embrace the Palmer method with its metaphysical roots as well as chiropractors who take a scientific approach to their profession and base their interventions on evidence-based guidelines (Erickson, Rosner, & Rainone, 2004; O'Mathuna & Larimore, 2001). Chiropractic manipulation is highly effective in relieving lower back pain; it is also used to treat neck pain, upper extremity disorders, headache, otitis media, sinusitis, asthma and chronic obstructive pulmonary disease, and digestive disorders.

Massage therapy includes a broad group of medically valid therapies that involve rubbing or moving the skin. Massage therapists employ four basic techniques: effleurage (long, gliding strokes over the skin), pétrissage (kneading of the muscles to increase circulation), vibration and percussion (a series of fine or brisk movements that stimulate circulation and relaxation), and friction (which is decreased with the use of massage oils). Probably the best-known massage technique in the United States is **Swedish massage,** which provides soothing relaxation and increases circulation. **Shiatsu massage** is of Japanese origin; it was strongly influenced by TCM and developed from acupressure. It originated as a way to detect and treat problems in the flow of life energy, which in Japanese is called *ki*. The shiatsu practitioner uses fingers, thumbs, elbows, knees, or feet to apply pressure by massaging various parts of the body, known as acupoints. **Rolfing** is another form of massage therapy that focuses on the treatment of connective tissue and fascia. The fascia and other connective tissue are believed to lose their elasticity under stress, which limits movement and breathing. A person generally receives 10 Rolfing sessions through which the connective tissue of the body is reset. **Reflexology** is yet another type of massage that focuses on the feet. This approach is based on the belief that there are zones and points on the feet that correspond to other parts of the body; thus, the foot is used as a map of the body. The purpose of treatments is to open blocked nerve pathways and improve circulation in the feet to treat problems that may exist elsewhere in the body (Riley, Ehling, & Saucier, 2004).

Energy Therapies

Energy therapy (also *energy medicine*) is a broad field that covers a variety of therapies originating in many parts of the world. Each of these therapies is based on the belief that there is a nonphysical energy force that pervades the universe. However, from culture to culture explanations vary regarding the nature of this energy, the form of the therapies, and the rationale for how healing is believed to occur. Energy therapies were traditionally part of Eastern medicine, and little attention was paid to them in the Unites States until the 1970s. When the United States opened up diplomatic relations with China, Americans along with others in the Western world were introduced to the use of acupuncture and other energy therapies common in TCM. The energy is referred to as *qi* in TCM, *prana* in Indian ayurvedic medicine, *ki* in Japanese medicine, and by a variety of other names. The NCCAM coined the term *biofield*.

The belief is that although this energy pervades the universe it takes a particular form in each person called the *human energy field* or *aura*. This energy field is said to contain a number of layers, each with energy of different frequencies. Energy is transferred between layers and eventually into the physical body through structures called *chakras*. Disturbances of the energy field are the cause of illness. Healing can occur only when the human energy field is balanced and energy is flowing freely. There have been many attempts to detect this human energy field. The most recent attempt involved the use of Kirlian photography as developed by two Russian researchers who claimed to be able to photograph human energy fields. The images captured by these scientists show auras and streams of light emanating from people's hands and even from the leaves of plants. The belief is that the health of the person or organism can be evaluated by noting the intensity, shape, and color of these emanations. These Kirlian photographs have been investigated by independent scientists, who have demonstrated that patterns seen on the images are explainable by variations in the techniques used in the photography. For instance, the intensity, color, shape, and size of the auras change according to the moisture level of the object photographed, the pressure exerted on the photographic film, the length of exposure, and the type of film used. Furthermore, when the same life energy field is repeatedly photographed using the same film, the results vary with each photograph; that is, the results are not consistently reproducible. Another issue is that Kirlian auras have been recorded for inanimate objects such as pennies, paperclips, and water droplets—none of which is believed to have a life energy field (O'Mathuna & Larimore, 2001). At this point there is no scientific proof that these energy fields exist (NCCAM, 2004b). In addition, it is important not to confuse the life force energy with electromagnetic radiation, which can be detected and does emanate from the human body. Electroencephalography, electrocardiography, and other conventional diagnostic techniques make use of these effects. This is not what energy medicine means by the human energy field.

Because the human energy field cannot be detected objectively, practitioners of energy medicine use meditation to increase their awareness of the human energy field. Through this heightened awareness, practitioners believe they can detect problems with someone's energy field. The practitioner may then suggest a healing approach that may relate to physical, emotional, mental, or spiritual issues. In the therapies based on energy medicine, the practitioner places his or her hands in or through these fields to direct the energy field through the application of pressure and/or manipulation of the body. Examples of energy therapies include acupressure, acupuncture, qi gong, reiki, and therapeutic touch.

The remainder of the chapter reviews some common complementary and alternative therapies that directly affect psychiatric treatment. The websites of both the NCCAM (http://nccam.nih.gov) and the NIH (http://www.nih.gov) provide information on and reviews of other complementary and alternative therapies. Table 37-1 summarizes integrative approaches to psychiatric disorders.

REVIEW OF SELECTED THERAPIES

Diet and Nutrition

Nutrition is an essential consideration when working with clients who have mental illnesses. Because psychiatric illnesses affect the whole person, it is not surprising that clients with mental illnesses frequently have inadequate diets. Often either their diets are deficient in the proper nutrients or they eat too much or too little. Research demonstrates an intimate connection between nutrition and behavioral disorders. For instance, anemia, which is the most common deficiency disease, often causes depression. It is essential that nurses assess the client's nutrition and address this area in health teaching.

Nurses must also be aware of the use of nutrients such as vitamins, protein supplements, herbal preparations, enzymes, and hormones that are considered dietary supplements. These dietary supplements are sold without the premarketing safety evaluations required of new food ingredients. Dietary supplements can be labeled with certain health claims if they meet published requirements of the Food and Drug Administration (FDA) and contain a disclaimer saying that the supplement has not been evaluated by the FDA and is not intended to diagnose, treat, cure, or prevent any disease.

Of additional concern to health care providers is the fact that many of the nutritional supplements may have problematic interactions with medications. There are known interactions with vitamins, but interactions with other supplements are not as easily recognized. Nurses should specifically ask about the use of supplements during the assessment and should not rely on clients to share this information without being questioned. When clients say that they are using supplements, nurses can review the use of the supplements and their related interactions with foods, drugs, and other supplements to help in reducing risks.

An example of a potential interaction between food and medication is the effect that can occur when a client who is taking a monoamine oxidase inhibitor (MAOI) for depression ingests a food that contains tyramine, such as aged cheese, pickled or smoked fish, or wine. Consumption of these foods along with MAOIs could cause a hypertensive crisis, in which the client's blood pressure soars to dangerous levels.

Megavitamin therapy, also called orthomolecular therapy, is a particular form of diet and nutrition therapy that involves taking large amounts of vitamins, minerals, and amino acids to treat a variety of physical and psychological illnesses. This therapy is based on

TABLE 37-1

Summary of Integrative Approaches to the Treatment of Psychiatric Disorders

Treatment	Depression	Anxiety	Schizophrenia	Bipolar Disorder
Acupuncture	±	+	±	
Antioxidants	+			
Behavioral therapies	+	+		
Biofeedback and neurofeedback	±	+		
Body therapies (touch)				
Chinese herbs	+		±	
Cognitive-behavioral therapy	+	+		
Comprehensive vitamin program			−	+
Cranial electrical stimulation	±			
Dehydroepiandrosterone	±			
Elimination diet		±		
Evening primrose oil		−		
Exercise	+	+		
Fish consumption	+		+	
Folic acid	+		+	
Gluten-free, casein-free diet			±	
Hypnosis	±	+		
Inositol	+	+		
Kava kava		+		
Light therapy	+			±
Magnesium	±			
Medication	+	+	+	+
Melatonin	+			
Negative ions	+			
Niacinamide		+		
ω-3 fatty acids	±		+	
Phenylalanine + pyridoxine			±	
Problem-solving psychotherapy	+			
Process psychotherapy	±			
Relaxation and meditation		+		
S-adenosyl methionine	+			
St. John's wort	+			
Supportive psychotherapy	+			
Therapeutic touch		+		
Thiamin		+	±	
Tryptophan and 5-hydroxytryptophan	+			
Valerian		+		
Vegetarian diet	+	+		
Vitamin A				
Vitamin B$_6$	+		±	
Vitamin B$_{12}$	+			
Vitamin C			±	
Zinc				

From Mehl-Madrona, L. (2004). Integrative approach to psychiatry. In B. Kligler & R. Lee (Eds.), *Integrative medicine: Principles for practice* (p. 625). New York: McGraw-Hill.
+, Effective; ±, inconclusive results.

the observation that, when a group of individuals is fed an identical diet containing everything needed for optimal health, some individuals in the group will absorb fewer nutrients than others. The theory is that the inability to absorb nutrients from a proper diet alone may lead to the development of different illnesses. The earliest use of megavitamin therapy was for the treatment of schizophrenia, for which niacin was recommended. Soon after this, in the 1960s, Dr. Linus Pauling, a biochemist and Nobel Prize winner, promoted his belief that megadoses of vitamin C could do everything from cure the common cold to treat some forms of cancer.

Although subsequent research demonstrated that vitamin C has many benefits, the claims made by Dr. Pauling were not validated, nor were his recommended daily megadoses of 10 g of vitamin C supported. In fact, the megadoses Dr. Pauling was taking are believed to cause an increased risk of kidney stones in some individuals (O'Mathuna & Larimore, 2001).

Megavitamin therapy became popular in the 1970s for treatment of children with attention deficit hyperactivity disorder as well as other developmentally challenged children. This therapy seems to move in and out of vogue and claims effectiveness in treating a variety of conditions, including acne, mild depression, arthritis, and Down syndrome (O'Mathuna & Larimore, 2001).

In 2000 the dietary reference intake recommendations included an upper limit (UL) to indicate the highest level likely to pose no risk of adverse health effects for most people. The UL for vitamin C was set at 2000 mg/day based on the risk of serious diarrhea and the possibility of pro-oxidant effects at higher dosages. The UL for vitamin E is 1000 mg/day based on the increased risk of hemorrhage due to vitamin E's anticoagulant properties. The maxim that if a little is good, then a lot must be better is certainly not true when it comes to vitamin intake. A single overdose of vitamin A can produce nausea, vomiting, headache, blurred vision, and lack of muscle coordination. The UL for vitamin A is 3 mg/day; it was set in January 2001 (O'Mathuna & Larimore, 2001).

Nutritional therapies are used to treat a variety of disorders, including depression, anxiety, attention deficit hyperactivity disorder, menopausal symptoms, and addictions. For instance, lower rates of anxiety and depression are reported among vegetarians than among nonvegetarians. An analysis of the vegetarian diet found a higher antioxidant level compared with the nonvegetarian diet, which suggests that antioxidants may play a role in the prevention of depression. Eating breakfast regularly improves mood, enhances memory, increases energy, and promotes feelings of calmness (Mehl-Madrona, 2004). Certain nutritional supplements, including S-adenosyl methionine (SAMe) and the B vitamins, especially vitamin B_6 and folic acid, also appear to improve depression (Mehl-Madrona, 2004). The following vignette contrasts conventional and integrative approaches in the treatment of depression.

▓ ▓ ▓ VIGNETTE*

Conventional Medicine Treatment of Depression. Megan was a 45-year-old woman suffering from chronic pancreatitis and biliary tract disease. She also had gluten sensitivity. Her family doctor suspected depression because she was

---

*From Mehl-Madrona, L. (2004). Integrative approach to psychiatry. In B. Klinger & R. Lee (Eds.), *Integrative medicine: Principles for practice*. New York: McGraw-Hill.

frequently irritable, had a disturbed sleep-wake cycle, had no source of pleasure in her life except for her children, and thought sometimes that death would be a desirable alternative to her life. Megan was started on venlafaxine 37.5 mg twice daily. This dose was gradually increased to 75 mg BID. Unfortunately, the higher dose worsened her pancreatic symptoms and the dose had to be decreased. She was tried on bupropion, but had side effects at the lowest dose. Then she was tried on sertraline, which gave her intense abdominal pain at the lowest dose. Next she was given low-dose lithium carbonate 300 mg/d to augment the lower dose of venlafaxine with some improvement in her symptoms. She was willing to tolerate a slight hand tremor from the lithium. Her symptoms of depression gradually improved.

Integrative Medicine Treatment of Depression. Teresa was a 48-year-old woman whose psychotherapist had referred her for a medication consult. Paradoxically, the last thing Teresa wanted was medication. Even though she had been in psychotherapy for 6 months and was becoming more depressed instead of less, she still believed that natural remedies could work better than drugs. Exploration of her life revealed major stress at her job. She worked for the public school system, and felt used, underpaid, and unhappy. As school budget cuts continued, the size of her classroom increased and the amount of aide time decreased. She felt unable to provide quality education under the circumstances, and felt trapped in her job by her need for benefits for her family, because her husband was self-employed, and not earning as much income as they had hoped. She was frustrated, angry, and hopeless.

First, supplements were recommended. She began taking a customized multiple vitamin, along with additional B-complex, omega-3 fatty acids, alpha-lipoic acid, vitamin C, S-adenosylmethionine, mineral complex (calcium, magnesium, zinc, copper, manganese, molybdenum, selenium, germanium), and inositol. She agreed to reduce her dietary intake of simple sugars and grains. We ordered a urine screening test for *Candida* breakdown products and other nutritionally correctable disorders. She agreed to increase her intake of root and green vegetables.

Next we discussed exercise. She was interested in taking yoga and planned to start. She increased her aerobic exercise by walking to and from work instead of taking the subway. She agreed to discuss with her therapist her options for stopping work. During one of these discussions, she decided that she could file for disability for work-related stress. She began this process, and her depression began to improve.

Yeast breakdown products indicative of excess *Candida* metabolism were found in her urine, so she was started on caprylic acid, garlic, green tea extract, berberis, and undecylenic acid. These substances are well-known in the naturopathic world as treatments for *Candida*. She felt quickly better. She modified her diet to decrease fermented foods, sugars, and grains. Some intestinal complaints that she had "learned to live with," disappeared.

Over the course of 6 months, her depression cleared and she became more organized, productive, and happier. She left her job, was exercising regularly, taking yoga class three times weekly, and was helping her husband in his business, which was becoming more successful. She knew that antidepressant medication was available if she wished it, but chose to treat herself nutritionally and with exercise and yoga. Changing adverse conditions in her life also contributed to her improvement.

■ ■ ■

There are no specific dietary guidelines for the treatment of anxiety except reducing or eliminating caffeine. However, several nutritional therapies and supplements are recommended for treatment of anxiety disorders. Thiamine has been used successfully at dosages of 250 mg/day to treat clients with anxiety disorders (Mehl-Madrona, 2004). Inositol (12 g/day) was used to treat 21 individuals with panic disorder with or without agoraphobia in a 4-week study with a double-blind, placebo-controlled, random-assignment, crossover design. The frequency and severity of panic attacks decreased significantly more after inositol administration than after placebo administration (Benjamin et al., 1995). Herbal preparations such as kava kava and valerian are both useful in ameliorating anxiety. Kava kava is an herb from the South Pacific used in traditional ceremonial rites in Micronesian culture. In the West, dosages of 300 mg/day (containing 210 mg of kavalactone) are used to treat anxiety. Kava kava was considered not only effective but safe until 2002, when at least 25 cases of liver toxicity, including hepatitis, cirrhosis, and liver failure, were linked to its use. The FDA issued a consumer advisory based on this potential risk (NCCAM, 2002c). Valerian not only is used as an antianxiety agent but also is reported to have antidepressant and sedative properties (Mehl-Madrona, 2004). The following vignette contrasts conventional and integrative approaches in the treatment of anxiety.

■ ■ ■ **VIGNETTE***

Conventional Medicine Treatment. Betty was a 38-year-old woman with chronic anxiety. She worried continually about family members having accidents. She would pace about the house, looking out the window frequently, whenever anyone drove into town, even for groceries. She had lost weight because she was too anxious to eat at meals. She would startle easily, and was described as "jumpy" by family members. Her anxiety made her irritable, and sometimes she would "snap" at her children, and then apologize profusely. The anxiety was becoming too severe for her to keep her job as a cashier at a restaurant.

Betty went to a local clinic and was started on clonazepam 0.5 mg BID. The dose was gradually increased to 1 mg PO TID, and she was also started on venlafaxine 37.5 mg to re-

duce her anxiety. The venlafaxine dose was gradually increased until she was taking 75 mg TID with the clonazepam constant at 1 mg TID. On this regimen, she was able to continue working at her job, and was more pleasant to be around, according to her family. She still worried incessantly, but it didn't bother her or her family as much.

Integrative Medicine Treatment. Andrea was a 24-year-old graduate student referred by her psychotherapist for medication for anxiety. Andrea came reluctantly because she did not really want to take medication. Her mother had developed kidney failure, possibly related to chronic and heavy ingestion of nonsteroidal anti-inflammatory drugs, so she worried about side effects. She didn't want to turn out like her mother. Nevertheless, her anxiety was disabling. She had trouble leaving her apartment unless her boyfriend accompanied her. She was missing classes. She feared being mugged in the subway. She worried about the future and about how she would support herself. She felt sure that her boyfriend would leave her imminently, even though he reassured her that he loved her and was happy with their relationship. She had many somatic symptoms of anxiety, including tremors, jitteriness, frequent sweating, cold hands and feet, headaches, shortness of breath, occasional tingling and numbness in her fingers, and feelings of disequilibrium and vertigo.

Because Andrea was opposed to medication, we discussed herbal approaches. She settled on taking kava kava 80 mg every 3 hours (with close monitoring of her liver enzymes) when she felt anxious. She would also make a strong tea of valerian root, hops, skullcap, and passion flower to take to class in a thermos and drink as needed throughout the day. We discussed decreasing her intake of caffeine and simple sugars, and increasing her intake of alkaline foods, particularly root and green vegetables. She also began drinking juices made from green and root vegetables when she felt particularly anxious. While no research has been conducted upon the use of alkaline foods and the raising of body pH to treat anxiety, it is common naturopathic practice, and appeared to work well with Andrea. Its effectiveness may relate to an inflammatory component to anxiety, as has been suggested in neurobiological research on depression.

We resolved that she would start learning meditation. Her boyfriend agreed to take her to the local Thich Nhat Hahn Buddhist sangha, where she could learn and practice mindfulness meditation. He was also interested in going with her to yoga class. She also began weekly acupuncture with the addition of Chinese herbs. She agreed to exercise in her apartment when she felt too scared to go out, and her boyfriend bought an exercise bicycle for both of them to use.

I met several times with them as a couple to explore the role that anxiety played in their relationship. I learned that they had separated for a time, and he had dated another woman. She had become quite anxious over the loss of his support, especially to someone else. In part, her anxiety showed him how much she loved him, and they reconciled. We developed other ways for her to express her love to him besides being anxious.

She continued to see her psychotherapist, who was invested in working on "childhood issues." Apparently this

---

*From Mehl-Madrona, L. (2004). Integrative approach to psychiatry. In B. Klinger & R. Lee (Eds.), *Integrative medicine: Principles for practice.* New York: McGraw-Hill.

also helped, because the combination of therapies led to a much improved anxiety rating 6 months later. She was able to go to class alone, to complete her assignments, and even gave a speech to a medium-sized colloquium.

■ ■ ■

Dietary therapies have also been used in the treatment of schizophrenia. In 1973 Dohan tested a gluten- and casein-free diet. Hospitalized schizophrenic clients were randomly assigned to consume either a grain-free, milk-free diet or a high-grain, unrestricted-milk diet. The mean discharge time for the group consuming the grain- and dairy-free diet was day 65, whereas that for the group consuming the high-grain, unrestricted-dairy diet was day 102 (Dohan & Grasberger, 1973; Mehl-Madrona, 2004). This study was replicated with similar results (Jansson, Kristjansson, & Nilsson, 1984; Mehl-Madrona, 2004; Vlissides, Venulet, & Jenner, 1986).

Folic acid, vitamin B_{12}, pyridoxine, and vitamin B_6 supplementation have been shown to be helpful for schizophrenic clients. A number of studies have looked at the impact of administering ω-3 fatty acids to clients with schizophrenia. Although the findings are only preliminary, the data suggest that such supplementation produces a significant improvement in both negative and positive symptoms (Bucci, 1973; Carney, 1992; Godfrey et al., 1990; Joy, Mumby-Croft, & Joy, 2003; Mehl-Madrona, 2004; Miodownik et al., 2002). The following vignette contrasts conventional and integrative approaches in the treatment of schizophrenia.

■ ■ ■ *VIGNETTE**

Conventional Medicine Treatment. Robert's parents brought him for consultation because he wouldn't leave the house. He spent hours on the Internet accomplishing nothing, appeared to have no interests in anything particular, and would doodle for hours. He had stopped producing art, which had been his passion during high school. He had stopped going to work, and sometimes sat alone for hours in a dark room talking to himself. They had to monitor his activities in the house, because he had almost set the kitchen on fire while cooking. Robert would start activities and then forget about them, wandering from room to room. He would leave food cooking on the stove until it burned. He would forget to turn off the shower, and would let the sink fill up with water and overflow.

On meeting, Robert was a pleasant, talkative 20-year-old male. He had long, rambling explanations for all of his parents concerns, which actually made no sense once they were completed, but fully occupied the listener. He insisted that he was perfectly normal and this was a phase he was going through. He insisted he could hold a job if he wanted to, but that he was trying to find his higher purpose, and

*From Mehl-Madrona, L. (2004). Integrative approach to psychiatry. In B. Klinger & R. Lee (Eds.), *Integrative medicine: Principles for practice.* New York: McGraw-Hill.

couldn't work until that was discovered. He occasionally heard voices giving him simple instructions to cook various foods, or to go to particular websites, or to try various keyboard combinations of letters and numbers. He was fascinated by the occult and was trying unsuccessfully to write a Tarot card computer program. He had been able to program during high school, but now felt befuddled by the simplest loop routine.

Robert was started on Risperdal (risperidone) 2 mg twice daily. The dose was gradually increased to a total of 10 mg daily. He began to have mild extrapyramidal symptoms, which were controlled with Cogentin (benztropine) 2 mg daily. He began to make more sense and to talk about more mundane concerns, but he was not able to get a job. He no longer searched for a higher purpose, was safer in the kitchen and the remainder of the house, did not overflow the bathroom, and spent most of his time playing various computer games.

Integrative Medicine Treatment. Tim was an 18-year-old male who was brought to a weekend workshop by his father and stepmother. They were concerned because Tim was disrupting all semblance of order in the house. The family lived in a rural area, but when they wanted to drive to town, it could take 2-3 hours to convince Tim to get in the car. He would walk back and forth in the driveway until finally he could be coaxed inside. Once in the car, he would moan repeatedly until the car had stopped. Then the same amount of time was required to get him back in the car to make the journey home. He could roll around in the parking lot or cry loudly, causing embarrassment to the family. At home, he would moan all night long, keeping the adults and their other three children awake. Tim had been a talented artist, but had stopped all art work. He spent his time drawing squares and circles and walking in squares and circles outside. He would repeat phrases said to him over and over. He interrupted conversation with bizarre and embarrassing questions. The family wondered what was wrong. Did he need Prozac?

Tim was clearly schizophrenic on mental status examination. During the weekend workshop he stood off by himself and was very anxious about being around people. He wandered into the desert and was briefly lost until his father went to find him. He was highly disorganized, and had lost all semblance of executive functioning ability.

The weekend workshop included two sweat lodge ceremonies. Tim participated in both of them—first with his father, then with his stepmother. Amazingly, during the ceremony, Tim was lucid and communicative, talking about painful areas in his life and his severe distress. Upon leaving the sweat lodge he became disorganized again.

The idea emerged of giving him a structure of ceremony and ritual. He was started on risperidone 1 mg at bedtime, and was taught a ceremony to conduct as an alternative to moaning. In this ceremony, he was to go outside to the tepee that his parents had raised behind the house. He was to go inside and to beat on a drum over and over, as hard as he could, until his discomfort had improved, or he broke the drum. He was taught a prayer song to sing, and was shown how to conduct a basic ceremony. Family therapy was conducted with all present (including his two younger and one older siblings). During these meetings, we discussed how anyone could recognize that Tim was improving and what the grades of improvement would be. We also wondered how long it would take Tim to reach each level of improvement. Family members unanimously agreed that the first grade of improvement would occur when Tim could go the entire night without moaning or waking anyone up. The second grade of improvement would occur when he could take himself out of the house and to the tepee when he needed to perform his ceremony. The third grade of improvement would occur when he could get into the car, at home or in town, within 20 minutes no matter how uncomfortable he felt.

Tim was started on a grain-, dairy-, and soy-free diet. He was also started on vitamin supplements, including a multivitamin; B-Complex 150; omega-3 fatty acids; omega-6 fatty acids; extra folic acid, B_6, B_{12}, and niacin; a comprehensive antioxidant supplement (Thorn Antioxidant); inositol; phosphatidylserine; taurine; SAMe; and a trace mineral complex.

Tim was referred to a homeopath in his own area, as well as a spiritually oriented psychotherapist, who would help him practice and refine his ceremony and practices.

I was in contact with Tim approximately every 6 months for the next 5 years. The psychotherapy continued. Tim improved one grade approximately every 4-6 months. After 2 years, he started drawing and painting again. After 4 years, he started attending junior college. After 5 years, he had a new girlfriend, felt very excited about his future, had paintings hanging in local galleries in the nearest big city, and was soon to graduate from junior college with a degree in art. He planned to transfer to the local 4-year college and earn a BFA in painting. He hoped that his girlfriend would fall in love with him. This was his first relationship, and his girlfriend, whom I met, was shy, but clearly not schizophrenic or seriously disabled in any way. Tim still showed some signs of obsessive-compulsive behavior but did not appear to be psychotic in any way. He continued on risperidone 1 mg at bedtime without side effects. He felt that it helped contain his fears and worries and allowed him to keep his compulsions in check. His vitamin program has been modified over the years, and continues to change as he does.

Acupressure and Acupuncture

Since the 1970s acupressure and acupuncture have become increasingly popular therapies in the United States. Acupuncture, a therapy used in TCM, involves the placement of needles into the skin at certain points to modulate the flow of energy, or qi, which moves through the body along specific nonvisible pathways called meridians. Research demonstrates that acupuncture stimulates physical responses such as changes in brain activity, blood chemistry, endocrine functions, blood pressure, heart rate, and immune system response. More specifically, medical research has shown that acupuncture can play a role in regulating blood cell counts, triggering endorphin production, and controlling blood pressure.

Sometimes acupuncture needles are inserted and removed immediately and at other times they are allowed to remain in place for a time. Sensations described as rushing, warmth, or tingling are experienced. As the immune system is stimulated, a sense of well-being is experienced. Acupuncture is used for maintaining health as well as for treating illness or pain.

Most people undergo acupuncture for pain relief (headache, back pain, osteoarthritis, neck pain, or organic pain), but this therapy also has been used to treat substance abuse and other emotional disorders (Freeman & Lawlis, 2001). There is interest in the use of acupuncture to treat alcoholism and other substance abuse because it is an intervention with few side effects and it seems to produce relaxation and minimize cravings (Bullock et al., 2002; Trumpler et al., 2003). In a randomized, controlled trial of auricular acupuncture for cocaine dependence, 82 clients were randomly assigned to receive appropriate acupuncture treatment, sham acupuncture, or relaxation therapy. Urine screenings for cocaine performed three times a week over an 8-week period showed that clients who were treated according to the appropriate acupuncture protocol were less likely to test positive for cocaine on urine screening than were clients in the sham acupuncture control group or the relaxation control group (Avants et al., 2000). More research is needed to support the use of acupuncture for treating addictions.

The NCCAM (2004a) fact sheet on acupuncture identifies anxiety, depression, insomnia, and other conditions appropriate for acupuncture therapy. These are among 40 conditions for which acupuncture can be used, as identified by the WHO. The researchers at the NCCAM are conducting randomized clinical trials for these and other conditions to identify the efficacy of the treatment. It is important to remember that acupuncture should be administered by a physician or a qualified practitioner.

Therapeutic Touch

Therapeutic touch is a technique developed in the 1970s by Dolores Krieger, a nursing professor at New York University, and Dora Kunz, a healer from Canada. Healing touch is an offshoot of therapeutic touch and includes a varied collection of energy techniques. Many nurses have been trained in these therapies, which are based on the belief that the healing force of the practitioner affects the client's recovery. Healing is promoted when the body's energies are in balance, and by passing their hands over the client, healers can identify energy imbalances. Practitioners *center* themselves in preparation for a treatment session so that they are totally consciously present for the client. Their focus is completely on the person receiving the treatment without any preoccupation or thoughts in any other direction. Practitioners assess the energy field, clear and balance it through hand movements, and/or direct energy in a specific region of the body. The therapist does not physically touch the client. After undergoing a session of therapeutic touch, many clients report a sense of deep relaxation.

Practitioners of therapeutic touch believe that the therapy is useful in relieving premenstrual syndrome, depression, complications in premature babies, and secondary infections associated with human immunodeficiency virus infection; in lowering blood pressure; in decreasing edema; in easing abdominal cramps and nausea; in resolving fevers; and in accelerating the healing of fractures, wounds, and infections. Therapeutic touch is unique among alternative therapies because it has been the subject of much research. However, the reviews of this research have generally found the results to be very weak. For example, there are at least five studies that examine the area of wound healing. Two of the studies show faster wound healing with therapeutic touch, two show slower wound healing, and one shows no difference. A review of other areas of research involving therapeutic touch reveals similar patterns (Aetna Intelihealth, 2003; CAMline, 2003; Eisenberg et al., 2001; Quinn, 1989; Rosa et al., 1998; Selby & Scheiber, 1996; Wheeler, 1997).

Given the lack of research support for therapeutic touch, perhaps the anecdotal reports of effectiveness reflect the benefit of what used to be called "good bedside manner," an approach that involves spending focused time with the client, talking, comforting, and reassuring. Sometimes these effects are derided as "just" a placebo response, when indeed they are beneficial to the client.

Aromatherapy

Aromatherapy, the use of essential oils for inhalation, works to activate the body's healing energy to balance mind, body, and spirit. Essential oils stimulate the release of neurotransmitters in the brain. The sense of smell connects with the part of the brain that controls the autonomic (involuntary) nervous system. Depending on the essential oil that is used, the resulting effects are calming, pain reducing, stimulating, sedating, or euphoria producing. These oils can also be applied to the skin in carrier oils or lotions.

An important nursing consideration is that some individuals, particularly those with pulmonary disease, may be sensitive or allergic to essential oils when these come into contact with the skin or are inhaled. To prevent an allergic reaction, it is essential to dilute oils before using them, to administer a small amount, and to perform a 24-hour skin patch test before massaging any essential oil into the skin. In the 24-hour skin patch

test, a small amount of diluted oil is applied to the forearm and the area is observed over 24 hours for erythema or rash. If either develops, the client is sensitive to the oil, and it should not be applied to the skin. Essential oils are also flammable and can be harmful if ingested. They should be stored in a safe place away from fire hazards where they cannot be accessed by confused clients who may inadvertently ingest them (AromaWeb, n.d.).

Aromatherapy is used in long-term care facilities during the bathing activity of clients with dementia. Lavender oil in particular is used for its calming effects (O'Mathuna & Larimore, 2001; Simpson, 2003). There are also anecdotal reports that aromatherapy is useful for pain relief, memory improvement, and wound healing.

Chiropractic Medicine

Chiropractic care is the most widely used complementary and alternative therapy. Contemporary chiropractic care most frequently involves relief of musculoskeletal pain. Chiropractic medicine is based on the theory that energy flows from the brain to all parts of the body through the spinal cord and spinal nerves. Manipulation of the spinal column, called adjustment, puts the vertebrae back into their normal positions. Back pain is the most common reason people seek chiropractic treatment, but chiropractic manipulation is used to treat a variety of other conditions, including pain, allergies, and asthma (NCCAM, 2003). Manipulation is also helpful in reducing migraine, tension, or cervicogenic headache pain. In randomized clinical trials investigating the treatment of tension headaches, one group of clients was treated with chiropractic manipulation and another group received pain medication. Both groups experienced relief of pain, but there were fewer side effects from the manipulation than from the use of medication (Freeman & Lawlis, 2001).

Herbal Medicine

A growing number of Americans are using herbal products for preventive and therapeutic purposes. At this time, manufacturers are not required to submit proof of safety or efficacy to the FDA. Providers must give close scrutiny to herbal therapies used by their clients. Food products now are being sold with herbs added. The druglike action of herbs is important to disease treatment, but the addition of herbs to foods may result in untoward reactions, especially when individuals do not realize that the supplement is in the food they are consuming. For example, a client may consume tea that contains ginseng, which has anticoagulant effects. If the client is taking a prescription anticoagulant, ingestion of this tea could have serious consequences. If the client does not know the contents of the tea, however, the client is less able to protect himself or herself.

With the widespread availability of lay literature on herbal remedies and the ready accessibility of the products in health food and other stores, growing numbers of consumers are using these products to manage symptoms. Information on the safe and effective use of these products is needed.

A number of herbs and supplements have recognizable effects on mood, memory, and insomnia. *Hypericum perforatum* (St. John's wort) is used to treat mild to moderate depression, and ginkgo biloba is used to treat dementia. Research is now being conducted on the use of vitamins, amino acids, and fatty acids to determine their effects on mood and other mental phenomena (Fugh-Berman & Cott, 1999; Kligler & Lee, 2004). People who seek conventional therapy commonly also use herbs and related products. All health care providers need to perform a careful assessment to determine if the client's symptoms are related to the ingestion of herbs and/or other supplements.

St. John's wort has been used for centuries to treat mental disorders and pain. In the past decade it has become the second most commonly used herbal remedy in Germany and the United States. It is estimated that 17% of Americans have taken products containing St. John's wort (Beaubrun & Gray, 2000). Herbalists in ancient times wrote about its efficacy as a sedative, antimalarial agent, and balm for burns and wounds (NCCAM, 2002d). People are turning to St. John's wort because the side effects of traditional antidepressants are unpleasant (dry mouth, nausea, headache, diarrhea, or impaired sexual function). St. John's wort is far less costly, has fewer side effects (dry mouth, dizziness, gastrointestinal symptoms, photosensitivity, and fatigue), and does not require a prescription (NCCAM, 2002d).

St. John's wort is thought to be useful in the treatment of mild to moderate depression. A study of the use of St. John's wort to treat major depression found no significant difference between placebo and St. John's wort ($N = 200$) (Shelton et al., 2001). Further studies comparing the effects of St. John's wort and the selective serotonin reuptake inhibitors (SSRIs) on mild to moderate depression will aid in clarifying its efficacy. It is important to understand that the different preparations available at natural food stores may vary in strength, quality, and potency of active ingredients, so individuals taking the compound may have varied responses (McEnany, 1999). Regulated preparations of St. John's wort are reasonably safe. The combining of St. John's wort with SSRIs is contraindicated because it can result in serotonin syndrome (tremors, hypertonicity, autonomic dysfunction, hyperthermia, and even death) (Beaubrun & Gray, 2000).

Ginkgo biloba has been used for the treatment of cerebral insufficiency, but this condition is broadly defined and ranges from memory loss to emotional instability. Ginkgo is well tolerated, with rare, nonspecific side effects of gastrointestinal distress, headache, and allergic skin reactions. Ginkgo has anticoagulant effects and can cause bleeding in individuals who are using anticoagulants and antiplatelet agents. Ginkgo should be used with caution by clients who consume alcohol or who have other risk factors for hemorrhagic stroke (Beaubrun & Gray, 2000; Kligler & Lee, 2004).

Black cohosh is an extract from a root that was used for centuries by Native Americans to ease the pain of rheumatism, sore throats, and menstrual problems. It continues to be popular as a way of decreasing hot flashes and as an alternative to hormone replacement therapy. Other uses are for treatment of premenstrual symptoms, menstrual cramping, and indigestion. Five clinical studies were done in Germany using a commercial black cohosh product called Remifemin, which is a standardized extract. These studies supported the effectiveness of black cohosh in relieving menopausal symptoms (O'Mathuna & Larimore, 2001).

Kava kava, previously discussed in the section on diet and nutrition therapies, has significant analgesic and anesthetic properties. It is considered a potential option in the treatment of anxiety but should not be combined with other tranquilizing agents, especially the benzodiazepines (Beaubrun & Gray, 2000; McEnany, 2000). Kava kava also may potentiate the effects of alcohol and other sedative-hypnotic agents (Beaubrun & Gray, 2000; Mehl-Madrona, 2004). As mentioned earlier in the chapter, kava kava has been implicated in cases of liver toxicity.

Valerian (also discussed under diet and nutrition therapies) is a root that when brewed as a tea has sedative, tranquilizing, and sleep-inducing effects (McEnany, 2000). Valerian can also be made into a variety of extracts and tinctures, which may also contain other ingredients (Beaubrun & Gray, 2000; Mehl-Madrona, 2004). It is generally recognized as safe for the treatment of insomnia when taken at the recommended dosages. Side effects at recommended dosages include headache and upset stomach. At higher than recommended dosages, side effects include blurred vision and severe headaches (NCCAM, 2004b). The major drug interactions are with other sedative-hypnotic agents, and the sedative effect of valerian may potentiate the effects of other central nervous system depressants (Beaubrun & Gray, 2000).

A variety of herbal teas have long been used for their sedative-hypnotic effects. Common ingredients in these teas, in addition to valerian, are hops, lemon balm, chamomile, and passion flower. The most studied of these is chamomile, a tea widely used as a folk remedy. Chamomile extract has been found to bind with γ-aminobutyric acid (GABA) receptors. Far less is known about the effectiveness of the other herbs (Beaubrun & Gray, 2000; O'Mathuna & Larimore, 2001).

Many other herbs are available as over-the-counter remedies at health food and other stores. Although these herbal remedies have been used for many years, most of them have not been extensively tested to determine their efficacy. Because these are dietary supplements (often found next to vitamins on store shelves), there is no FDA approval or standardization.

Homeopathy

Homeopathy is based on the concept that "like cures like"; this is referred to as the Law of Similars. Small doses of diluted preparations that produce symptoms mimicking those of an illness are used to heal the body or help the body heal itself. Basic principles of homeopathy are that healing occurs from the inside out and that symptoms disappear in the reverse order in which they appeared. Clients receiving homeopathic care frequently feel worse before they get better, because homeopathic medicines often stimulate, rather than suppress, symptoms. The treatments are designed to heal both physical and mental problems.

Homeopathic remedies are dilutions of natural substances from plants, minerals, and animals. Dilutions are prescribed that match the client's illness-symptom profile. Homeopathic treatments are individualized, and each individual, even one with the same diagnosis as another person, is given different medicines because the symptoms are different (Freeman & Lawlis, 2001). Homeopathy has been used in the treatment of short-term, acute illnesses, migraine pain, allergies, chronic fatigue, otitis media, immune dysfunction, digestive disorders, and colic. It is contraindicated as a treatment for advanced diseases, cancer, sexually transmitted diseases, conditions involving irreparable damage (e.g., defective heart valves), or brain damage due to stroke (Freeman & Lawlis, 2001).

Prayer

Prayer is an alternative therapy used by many Americans. Historically, there is a precedent for the inclusion of prayer and other spiritual practices as part of the care of the psychiatric client. In the mid-1840s, the very first form of psychiatric care took hold in the United States. It was called "moral treatment" and was based on a system developed in England by the devout Quaker William Tuke. Tuke had witnessed the common practices of bleeding, purging, and ice baths that were used in the treatment of the mentally ill and that were, of course, a total failure. He instituted a regimen of compassionate psychological and spiritual treatments based on the idea that insanity was a disruption of both mind and spirit. Tuke had remarkable

success, and this form of therapy spread across Europe and then to the United States. The first mental institutions in Philadelphia, Hartford, and Worcester were run by superintendents who were often quite religious. Spiritual care was very much part of the psychiatric care that clients received in those days. Chaplains lived on the grounds of the hospitals and held regular religious services for clients. This positive attitude toward the inclusion of prayer and other spiritual practices continued in the United States until the influence of Sigmund Freud changed thinking. From 1908 until his death in 1939, Freud spoke and wrote widely about the neurotic aspects of religion. Freud's views dramatically influenced psychiatry's attitude toward religion for many years to follow (Koenig, 2002).

Today, however, there is increasing interest in the use of spiritual interventions for some psychiatric clients. Many psychiatric clients have significant spiritual needs. Some may feel angry at God for allowing them to suffer with disorders that affect every aspect of their lives. Some clients have forgiveness issues to address. For example, the client's friends and family may have responded to the client with rejection and hurtful comments and attitudes just because the client has a psychiatric illness. Other clients may need to seek forgiveness because of hurt they have caused to others during a psychiatric episode. Many clients rely on God as their source of love and support and display a deep, abiding faith despite the circumstances of their illnesses (Carson & Koenig, 2004).

The challenge in meeting these spiritual needs in the psychiatric client is to remain aware of boundary issues. Boundary issues relate to defining the respective roles of caregiver and client and defining the limits of one's own identity. It is not uncommon in psychiatric illnesses for clients to have "loose boundaries," especially when a psychotic or personality disorder is present. Clients may experience difficulty in knowing where their own beliefs stop and those of the health care professional begin. This places the client in the vulnerable position of perhaps being unfairly influenced by someone with strong beliefs. In meeting the spiritual needs of psychiatric clients, it is imperative that nurses be continually aware and respectful of boundary issues and never impose beliefs on the client.

There is abundant research demonstrating the positive relationship between religion and measures of well-being, including marital status, health, participation in activities, social support, optimism, hope, purpose and meaning in life, and internal locus of control (Koenig, McCullough, & Larson, 2001). During the twentieth century, at least 724 quantitative studies examined these relationships. Nearly 500 (66%) found a significant relationship between religious involvement and better mental health. This is especially true for studies looking at positive emotions such as well-being, hope, and optimism; nearly 80% of these studies found significant associations between these emotions and religious faith and practices, including prayer (Koenig et al., 2001). These studies, however, do not reflect the experiences of the many persons with mental illnesses whose religious faith has deepened as a result of their suffering and yet who have continued to struggle (Carson & Koenig, 2004).

So how do we support the spiritual needs of psychiatric clients? First, we take a spiritual assessment to determine the beliefs and practices of the client. The assessment itself is a powerful intervention, because when we ask a client about the importance of spiritual issues in his or her life, we are not only providing an opening for this topic to be discussed, we are also communicating that we are interested in and comfortable talking about an area of the client's life that may be deeply important and meaningful to the client. Asking about issues such as prayer, sources of hope and strength, and the client's preferred spiritual practices allows us to know how we can provide spiritual support for the client.

QUACKERY AND FRAUD

Consumers waste billions of dollars on unproven, fraudulently marketed, and sometimes useless health care products and treatments. To make matters worse, some of the treatments can in fact cause harm. Plants and herbs are natural, but that does not mean they cannot be dangerous or abused. Herbs and other food supplements do not have to undergo the same safety review that over-the-counter and prescription medications must pass. Following are examples of claims that should serve as red flags in the advertising of CAM products and services (NCCAM, 2002b):

- The product is advertised as a quick and effective cure-all for a wide range of ailments.
- The promoters use words like *scientific breakthrough, miraculous cure, exclusive product, secret ingredient,* or *ancient remedy.*
- The text is written using impressive terminology to disguise lack of good science.
- The promoter claims the government, the medical profession, or research scientists have conspired to suppress the product.
- The advertisement includes undocumented case histories claiming amazing results.
- The product is advertised as available from only one source, and payment is required in advance.
- The promoter promises a "no-risk money-back guarantee."

Clients should be advised that claims such as these should be interpreted as warning signals that further investigation is necessary using sources such as the NCCAM.

CREDIBILITY OF CAM: RESEARCH, REIMBURSEMENT, AND CREDENTIALING

Although research on the efficacy of CAM is increasing, the field is still poorly studied compared with conventional medicine. There are several reasons for this, such as the relatively recent use of some of these therapies in the United States and the lack of financial incentive to support the research. (Consider that if a pharmaceutical company studies a drug, it can patent the drug and reap considerable financial return; however, an herb cannot be patented and exclusively marketed, so there is little incentive to invest in researching its uses and effects.) Governmental sources of funding such as the NIH, as well as nonprofit groups, are sponsoring research that should contribute to the understanding of CAM.

Payment for CAM services comes from a wide array of sources, although third-party coverage is still the exception rather than the rule. Research published in the early 1990s by David Eisenberg fueled a boom in CAM development. Dr. Eisenberg found that more money was being spent out of pocket on CAM than on primary care visits (Eisenberg, 1993). Out-of-pocket payments remain the principal source of spending on CAM. Some health insurance companies have begun to include coverage for certain modalities, particularly chiropractic medicine, nutritional care, massage, mind-body programs, and acupuncture (Dumoff, 2004). The covered benefits are quite narrowly defined, however; for instance, acupuncture can be used in some plans only as an alternative to anesthesia. These changes are finding their way into academia as well. In 2004 almost 75% of U.S. medical schools had some type of curriculum offering in the area of integrative medicine (Lee, Kligler, & Shiflett, 2004). Efforts are being made to legitimize integrative medicine through credentialing of integrative physicians and nonphysician practitioners, including nurses. Credentialing procedures are already in place for many of the specific modalities, such as acupuncture, chiropractic, naturopathy, and massage therapy.

INFORMATION RESOURCES

The NCCAM of the NIH conducts and supports basic and applied research and training. The center disseminates information on CAM to practitioners and the public through the NCCAM clearinghouse. The NCCAM provides fact sheets, information packages, and publications to increase the public's understanding of CAM and of research supported by the NIH. The NCCAM is not a referral agency; the agency conducts and facilitates biomedical research. Consumers and practitioners are able to access information from the clearinghouse through the center's website.

The NCCAM on-line database contains bibliographic records describing CAM research for which results have been published over the last several decades. Searches by various diseases or conditions, CAM products, and services, as well as bibliographic searches, are supported. The NCCAM and the National Library of Medicine (NLM) have partnered to create CAM on PubMed (NCCAM, 2002a). This is a subset of NLM's PubMed and provides access to a variety of citations, not only from MEDLINE but also from other life science journals.

The NCCAM website provides links to information that assists consumers in making wise choices regarding CAM. Medical regulatory and licensing agencies in each state also serve as clearinghouses for information.

■■■ KEY POINTS to REMEMBER

■ Complementary and alternative therapies are in growing demand as consumers seek a broader range of therapies than those offered by traditional medicine.

■ With the availability of information on the Internet, consumers are more likely to have researched their symptoms or condition and identified potential alternative or complementary treatments.

■ Nurses are in an ideal position to guide clients to reliable resources, such as the NCCAM, that provide up-to-date information for health care practitioners and consumers.

■ Nurses need to keep abreast of current research about major CAM therapies so that they can
  —Promote integrative care by informing clients and members of the health care team of CAM therapies that could be beneficial, affordable, and safe.
  —Prevent clients from wasting money on useless therapies.
  —Guide clients in discerning which therapies could be harmful for them.
  —Help clients to maximize the benefits of CAM therapies.

Visit the Evolve website at **http://evolve.elsevier.com/Varcarolis** for a posttest on the content in this chapter. *evolve*

Critical Thinking and Chapter Review

Visit the Evolve website at **http://evolve.elsevier.com/Varcarolis** for additional self-study exercises. *evolve*

■■■ CRITICAL THINKING

1. As a nurse you may have clients who use complementary and alternative therapies in conjunction with the therapies prescribed by the health care provider. Identify those communication techniques that would be most effective, during the assessment process, in determining the extent to which a client is following the therapeutic regimen. How would you determine whether a client was using complementary and alternative health care treatments in addition to prescribed treatments?

2. Discuss how herbal products sold in the United States can vary in quality. How does a client identify the efficacy of the herb? What can a client do to guarantee the quality and dosage of an herbal product?

3. Use the Internet to determine how the NCCAM provides information for the consumer and professionals.

■■■ CHAPTER REVIEW

Choose the most appropriate answer.

1. Kim, 24 years old, has been hospitalized several times for the treatment of schizophrenia. She presently takes psychotropic medication. She tells the nurse, "I'm going to stop taking the medication the psychiatrist prescribed. It makes me feel awful. I'm thinking of searching the Internet to find an alternative herbal remedy that will be a holistic treatment." The best response for the nurse would be

　　1. "Information on the Internet isn't always objective and reliable."
　　2. "You shouldn't do that! Herbals can be harmful to your general health."
　　3. "Tell me what you mean when you say the medicine makes you feel awful."
　　4. "Your medication treats your disease. Because nothing else is wrong with you, no other treatment is necessary."

Continued

Critical Thinking and Chapter Review—cont'd

Visit the Evolve website at **http://evolve.elsevier.com/Varcarolis** for additional self-study exercises.

2. A client tells the nurse, "I've been reading about Asian medicine. I think my alcoholism may be related to qi imbalance. I'm going to seek alternative treatment." The nurse can expect the client to turn to
   1. chiropractic care.
   2. acupuncture.
   3. aromatherapy.
   4. reiki.

3. A client tells the nurse, "I've been using St. John's wort to try to get back on track." The nurse should pursue assessment related to the client's experiencing symptoms of
   1. depression.
   2. diminished cognitive abilities.
   3. altered reality perception.
   4. sensory-perceptual disturbances.

4. The nurse who wishes to obtain accurate information on CAM should contact
   1. AMA.
   2. NLN.
   3. NAMI.
   4. NCCAM clearinghouse.

5. Mrs. Nash, 72 years of age, has had two small strokes. Her physician has prescribed warfarin (Coumadin) daily. Mrs. Nash tells the nurse that she is considering taking ginkgo biloba to help her with her failing memory. Which information should the nurse give Mrs. Nash?
   1. Ginkgo biloba seems to have a positive effect on memory.
   2. Warfarin and ginkgo biloba taken together may cause spontaneous bleeding.
   3. Ginkgo biloba may cause sedation and increased danger of falls.
   4. There is no medical reason not to try the herbal preparation.

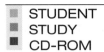

- **STUDENT**
- **STUDY**
- **CD-ROM**

Access the accompanying CD-ROM for animations, interactive exercises, review questions for the NCLEX examination, and an audio glossary.

- **NURSE,**
- **CLIENT, AND**
- **FAMILY RESOURCES**

For suggested readings, information on related associations, and Internet resources, go to **http://evolve.elsevier.com/Varcarolis**. *evolve*

REFERENCES

Aetna Intelihealth. (2003). *Therapeutic touch*. Retrieved April 17, 2005, from http://www.Intelihealth.com/IH/ihtIH/WSIHW000/8513/34968/358873.html?d=dmtContent.

AromaWeb. (n.d.). *Essential oil safety information*. Retrieved February 17, 2004, from http://www.aromaweb.com/articles/safety.asp.

Avants, S. K., et al. (2000). A randomized controlled trial of auricular acupuncture for cocaine dependence. *Archives of Internal Medicine, 160,* 2305-2312.

Beaubrun, G., & Gray, G. E. (2000). A review of herbal medicines for psychiatric disorders. *Psychiatric Services, 51*(9), 1130-1134.

Benjamin, J., et al. (1995). Double-blind, placebo-controlled, crossover trial of inositol treatment for panic disorder. *American Journal of Psychiatry, 152*(7), 1084-1087.

Bucci, L. (1973). Pyridoxine and schizophrenia [Letter]. *British Journal of Psychiatry, 122*(567), 240.

Bullock, M. L., et al. (2002). A large randomized placebo-controlled study of auricular acupuncture for alcohol dependence. *Journal of Substance Abuse Treatment, 22*(2), 71-77.

CAMline. (2003). *CAM therapies and practitioners: Therapeutic touch*. Retrieved December 17, 2004, from http://www.camline.org/therapiesPractitioners/therapeutic_touch/description.html.

Carney, M. W. (1992). Vitamins and mental health. *British Journal of Hospital Medicine, 48*(8), 451-452.

Carson, V. B. (2000). Alternative therapies. In V. B. Carson (Ed.), *Mental health nursing: The nurse-patient journey* (2nd ed., pp. 388-405). Philadelphia: Saunders.

Carson, V. B., & Koenig, H. G. (2004). *Spiritual caregiving: Healthcare as a ministry* (pp. 150-152). Philadelphia: Templeton Foundation Press.

Chopra, D. (1991). *Creating health*. Boston: Houghton Mifflin.

Dohan, F. C., & Grasberger, J. C. (1973). Relapsed schizophrenics: Earlier discharge from the hospital after cereal-free, milk-free diet. *American Journal of Psychiatry, 130*(6), 685-688.

Dumoff, A. (2004). Legal and ethical issues in integrative medicine. In B. Kligler & R. Lee (Eds.), *Integrative medicine: Principles for practice* (pp. 845-874). New York: McGraw-Hill.

Eisenberg, D. M. (1993). Unconventional medicine in the United States: Prevalence, costs, and patterns of use. *New England Journal of Medicine, 328*(4), 246-252.

Eisenberg, D. M., et al. (2001). Inability of an "energy transfer diagnostician" to distinguish between fertile and infertile women. *Medscape General Medicine 3*(1). Retrieved April 6, 2005, from http://www.medscape.com/viewarticle/408093.

Eliopoulos, C. (1999). Using complementary and alternative therapies wisely. *Geriatric Nursing, 20*(3), 139-143.

Erickson, K., Rosner, A., & Rainone, F. (2004). Chiropractic and osteopathic care. In B. Kligler & R. Lee (Eds.), *Integrative medicine: Principles for practice* (pp. 153-176). New York: McGraw-Hill.

Freeman, L. W., & Lawlis, G. F. (2001). *Mosby's complementary and alternative medicine: A research-based approach.* St. Louis, MO: Mosby.

Fugh-Berman, A., & Cott, J. M. (1999). Dietary supplements and natural products as psychotherapeutic agents. *Psychosomatic Medicine, 61*(5), 712-728.

Godfrey, P. S., et al. (1990). Enhancement of recovery from psychiatric illness by methylfolate. *Lancet, 336*(8712), 392-395.

Hasselberger, S. (2004). *WHO issues guidelines for herbal medicine:* Press exaggerates warnings. Retrieved May 22, 2005, from http://www.newmediaexplorer.org/Sepp/2004/06/30/who_issues_guidelines_for_herbal_medicine_press_exaggerates_warnings.htm#.

Jansson, B., Kristjansson, E., & Nilsson, L. (1984). Schizophrenic psychosis disappearing after patient is given gluten-free diet. *Lakartidningen, 81*(6), 448-449.

Joy, C. B., Mumby-Croft, R., & Joy, L. A. (2003). Polyunsaturated fatty acid supplementation for schizophrenia. *Cochrane Database of Systematic Reviews,* Issue 2, Art. No. CD001257.

Kligler, B., & Lee, R. (2004). *Integrative medicine: Principles for practice.* New York: McGraw-Hill.

Koenig, H. G. (2002). *Spirituality in patient care: Why, how, when and what* (pp. 17-18, 40-42). Philadelphia: Templeton Foundation Press.

Koenig, H. G., McCullough, M. E., & Larson, D. B. (2001). *Handbook of religion and health.* New York: Oxford University Press.

Lee, R., Kligler, B., & Shiflett, S. (2004). Integrative medicine: Basic principles. In B. Kligler & R. Lee (Eds.), *Integrative medicine: Principles for practice* (pp. 3-24). New York: McGraw-Hill.

Maizes, V., Koffler, K., & Fleishman, S. (2003). The integrative assessment. In D. Rakel (Ed.), *Integrative medicine* (pp. 11-16). Philadelphia: Saunders.

McEnany, G. (1999). Herbal psychotropics. Part 1: Focus on St. John's wort and SAMe. *Journal of the American Psychiatric Nurses Association, 5*(6), 192-196.

McEnany, G. (2000). Herbal psychotropics. Part 3: Focus on kava, valerian, and melatonin. *Journal of the American Psychiatric Nurses Association, 6*(4), 126-130.

Mehl-Madrona, L. (2004). Integrative approach to psychiatry. In B. Kligler & R. Lee (Eds.), *Integrative medicine: Principles for practice* (pp. 623-666). New York: McGraw-Hill.

Miodownik, C., et al. (2002). Vitamin B_6 as add-on treatment in chronic schizophrenic and schizoaffective patients: A double-blind, placebo-controlled study. *Journal of Clinical Psychiatry, 63*(1), 54-58.

National Center for Complementary and Alternative Medicine. (2002a, May 21). *CAM on PubMed.* Retrieved April 17, 2005, from http://www.nlm.nih.gov/nccam/camonpubmed.html.

National Center for Complementary and Alternative Medicine. (2002b, August). *Get the facts: Are you considering using complementary and alternative medicine (CAM)?* Retrieved December 1, 2004, from http://nccam.nih.gov/health/alerts.

National Center for Complementary and Alternative Medicine. (2002c, July 23). *Kava linked to liver damage.* Retrieved April 17, 2005, from http://nccam.nih.gov/health/alerts/kava/.

National Center for Complementary and Alternative Medicine. (2002d, April 9). *Questions and answers: A trial of St. John's Wort* (Hypericum perforatum) *for the treatment of major depression.* Retrieved April 17, 2005 at http://nccam.nih.gov/news/2002/stjohnswort/q-and-a.htm.

National Center for Complementary and Alternative Medicine. (2003, November). Research report: About chiropractic and its use in treating low-back pain. Retrieved April 17, 2005, from http://nccam.nih.gov/health/chiropractic/.

National Center for Complementary and Alternative Medicine. (2004a, December). *Get the facts: Acupuncture.* Retrieved April 17, 2005, from http://nccam.nih.gov/health/acupuncture/.

National Center for Complementary and Alternative Medicine. (2004b, September). *The use of complementary and alternative medicine in the United States.* Retrieved December 10, 2004, from http://nccam.nih.gov/news/camsurvey_fs1.htm.

O'Mathuna, D., & Larimore, W. (2001). *Alternative medicine: The Christian handbook* (pp. 404-407). Grand Rapids, MI: Zondervan.

Pai, S., Shanbhag, V., & Archarya, S. (2004). Ayurvedic medicine. In B. Kligler & R. Lee (Eds.), *Integrative medicine: Principles for practice* (pp. 219-240). New York: McGraw-Hill.

Quinn, J. (1989). Therapeutic touch as energy exchange: Replication and extension. *Nursing Science Quarterly, 2*(2), 79-87.

Rakel, D., & Weil, A. (2003). Philosophy of integrative medicine. In D. Rakel (Ed.), *Integrative medicine* (p. 7). Philadelphia: Saunders.

Riley, D., Ehling, D., & Saucier, K. (2004). Movement and body-centered therapies. In B. Kligler & R. Lee (Eds.), *Integrative medicine: Principles for practice* (pp. 241-254). New York: McGraw-Hill.

Rosa, L., et al. (1998). A close look at therapeutic touch. *Journal of the American Medical Association, 279,* 1005-1010.

Selby, C., & Scheiber, B. (1996, July). *Science or pseudoscience? Pentagon grant funds alternative health study.* Retrieved December 17, 2004, from http://www.csicop.org/si/9607/tt.html.

Shelton, R. C., et al. (2001). Effectiveness of St. John's wort in major depression: A randomized controlled trial. *Journal of the American Medical Association, 285*(15), 1978-1986.

Simpson, M. (2003). *The use of complementary therapies in long-term care facilities.* Medscape coverage of the National Conference of Gerontological Nurse Practitioners (NCGNP) 2003. Retrieved April 6, 2005, from http://www.medscape.com/viewarticle/464731.

Stokowski, L. (2004). Trends in nursing. *Topics in Advanced Practice Nursing eJournal, 4*(1). Retrieved April 6, 2005, from http://www.medscape.com/viewarticle/466711_1.

Trumpler, F., et al. (2003). Acupuncture for alcohol withdrawal: A randomized controlled trial. *Alcohol and Alcoholism, 38*(4), 369-375.

Vlissides, D. N., Venulet, A., & Jenner, F. A. (1986). A double-blind gluten-free/gluten-load controlled trial in a secure ward population. *British Journal of Psychiatry, 148,* 447-452.

Wheeler, T. (1997). *Review of TT cutaneous wound healing research.* Retrieved December 17, 2004, from http://www.phact.org/e/tt/wound.htm.

WNBC.com. (2004, February 10). *Complementary and alternative medicine undergoes new scrutiny: Americans spend $30 billion on alternative therapies.* Retrieved April 6, 2005, http://www.wnbc.com/print/2815485/detail.html.

APPENDIX A

DSM-IV-TR Classification*

NOS, Not Otherwise Specified.

An *x* appearing in a diagnostic code indicates that a specific code number is required.

An ellipsis (. . .) is used in the names of certain disorders to indicate that the name of a specific mental disorder or general medical condition should be inserted when recording the name (e.g., 293.0 Delirium Due to Hypothyroidism).

If criteria are currently met, one of the following severity specifiers may be noted after the diagnosis:
Mild
Moderate
Severe

If criteria are no longer met, one of the following specifiers may be noted:
In Partial Remission
In Full Remission
Prior History

*From American Psychiatric Association. (2000). *Diagnostic and statistical manual of mental disorders (DSM-IV-TR)* (4th ed., text rev.). Washington, DC: Author.

DISORDERS USUALLY FIRST DIAGNOSED IN INFANCY, CHILDHOOD, OR ADOLESCENCE

Mental Retardation

NOTE: These are coded on Axis II.
317   Mild Mental Retardation
318.0   Moderate Mental Retardation
318.1   Severe Mental Retardation
318.2   Profound Mental Retardation
319   Mental Retardation, Severity Unspecified

Learning Disorders

315.00 Reading Disorder
315.1   Mathematics Disorder
315.2   Disorder of Written Expression
315.9   Learning Disorder NOS

Motor Skills Disorder

315.4   Developmental Coordination Disorder

Communication Disorders

315.31 Expressive Language Disorder
315.32 Mixed Receptive-Expressive Language Disorder
315.39 Phonologic Disorder
307.0   Stuttering
307.9   Communication Disorder NOS

Pervasive Developmental Disorders

299.00 Autistic Disorder
299.80 Rett's Disorder
299.10 Childhood Disintegrative Disorder
299.80 Asperger's Disorder
299.80 Pervasive Developmental Disorder NOS

Attention-Deficit and Disruptive Behavior Disorders

314.xx Attention-Deficit/Hyperactivity Disorder
   .01 Combined Type
   .00 Predominantly Inattentive Type
   .01 Predominantly Hyperactive-Impulsive Type
314.9 Attention-Deficit/Hyperactivity Disorder NOS
312.xx Conduct Disorder
   .81 Childhood-Onset Type
   .82 Adolescent-Onset Type
   .89 Unspecified Onset
313.81 Oppositional Defiant Disorder
312.9 Disruptive Behavior Disorder NOS

Feeding and Eating Disorders of Infancy or Early Childhood

307.52 Pica
307.53 Rumination Disorder
307.59 Feeding Disorder of Infancy or Early Childhood

Tic Disorders

307.23 Tourette's Disorder
307.22 Chronic Motor or Vocal Tic Disorder
307.21 Transient Tic Disorder
       Specify if: Single Episode/Recurrent
307.20 Tic Disorder NOS

Elimination Disorders

___.__ Encopresis
787.6 With Constipation and Overflow Incontinence
307.7 Without Constipation and Overflow Incontinence
307.6 Enuresis (Not Due to a General Medical Condition)
       Specify type: Nocturnal Only/Diurnal Only/Nocturnal and Diurnal

Other Disorders of Infancy, Childhood, or Adolescence

309.21 Separation Anxiety Disorder
       Specify if: Early Onset
313.23 Selective Mutism
313.89 Reactive Attachment Disorder of Infancy or Early Childhood
       Specify type: Inhibited Type/Disinhibited Type
307.3 Stereotypic Movement Disorder
       Specify if: With Self-Injurious Behavior
313.9 Disorder of Infancy, Childhood, or Adolescence NOS

DELIRIUM, DEMENTIA, AND AMNESTIC AND OTHER COGNITIVE DISORDERS

Delirium

293.0 Delirium Due to . . . *[Indicate the General Medical Condition]*
___.__ Substance Intoxication Delirium *(refer to Substance-Related Disorders for substance-specific codes)*
___.__ Substance Withdrawal Delirium *(refer to Substance-Related Disorders for substance-specific codes)*
___.__ Delirium Due to Multiple Etiologies *(code each of the specific etiologies)*
780.09 Delirium NOS

Dementia

294.xx Dementia of the Alzheimer's Type, With Early Onset *(also code 331.0 Alzheimer's disease on Axis III)*
   .10 Without Behavioral Disturbance
   .11 With Behavioral Disturbance
294.xx Dementia of the Alzheimer's Type, With Late Onset *(also code 331.0 Alzheimer's disease on Axis III)*
   .10 Without Behavioral Disturbance
   .11 With Behavioral Disturbance
290.xx Vascular Dementia
   .40 Uncomplicated
   .41 With Delirium
   .42 With Delusions
   .43 With Depressed Mood
       Specify if: With Behavioral Disturbance
Code presence or absence of a behavioral disturbance in the fifth digit for Dementia Due to a General Medical Condition:
0 = Without Behavioral Disturbance
1 = With Behavioral Disturbance
294.1x Dementia Due to HIV Disease *(also code 042 HIV on Axis III)*
294.1x Dementia Due to Head Trauma *(also code 854.00 head injury on Axis III)*
294.1x Dementia Due to Parkinson's Disease *(also code 332.0 Parkinson's disease on Axis III)*
294.1x Dementia Due to Huntington's Disease *(also code 333.4 Huntington's disease on Axis III)*
294.1x Dementia Due to Pick's Disease *(also code 331.1 Pick's disease on Axis III)*
294.1x Dementia Due to Creutzfeldt-Jakob Disease *(also code 046.1 Creutzfeldt-Jakob disease on Axis III)*
294.1x Dementia Due to . . . *[Indicate the General Medical Condition not listed above] (also code the general medical condition on Axis III)*

___.__ Substance-Induced Persisting Dementia *(refer to Substance-Related Disorders for substance-specific codes)*

___.__ Dementia Due to Multiple Etiologies *(code each of the specific etiologies)*

294.8 Dementia NOS

Amnestic Disorders

294.0 Amnestic Disorder Due to . . . *[Indicate the General Medical Condition]*
Specify if: Transient/Chronic

___.__ Substance-Induced Persisting Amnestic Disorder *(refer to Substance-Related Disorders for substance-specific codes)*

294.8 Amnestic Disorder NOS

Other Cognitive Disorders

294.9 Cognitive Disorder NOS

MENTAL DISORDERS DUE TO A GENERAL MEDICAL CONDITION NOT ELSEWHERE CLASSIFIED

293.89 Catatonic Disorder Due to . . . *[Indicate the General Medical Condition]*

310.1 Personality Change Due to . . . *[Indicate the General Medical Condition]*
Specify type: Labile Type/Disinhibited Type/Aggressive Type/Apathetic Type/Paranoid Type/Other Type/Combined Type/Unspecified Type

293.9 Mental Disorder NOS Due to . . . *[Indicate the General Medical Condition]*

SUBSTANCE-RELATED DISORDERS

The following specifiers may be applied to Substance Dependence as noted:
[a]With Physiologic Dependence/Without Physiologic Dependence
[b]Early Full Remission/Early Partial Remission/Sustained Full Remission/Sustained Partial Remission
[c]In a Controlled Environment
[d]On Agonist Therapy

The following specifiers apply to Substance-Induced Disorders as noted:
[I]With Onset During Intoxication/[W]With Onset During Withdrawal

Alcohol-Related Disorders
Alcohol Use Disorders

303.90 Alcohol Dependence[a,b,c]
305.00 Alcohol Abuse

Alcohol-Induced Disorders

303.00 Alcohol Intoxication
291.81 Alcohol Withdrawal
Specify if: With Perceptual Disturbances
291.0 Alcohol Intoxication Delirium
291.0 Alcohol Withdrawal Delirium
291.2 Alcohol-Induced Persisting Dementia
291.1 Alcohol-Induced Persisting Amnestic Disorder
291.x Alcohol-Induced Psychotic Disorder
.5 With Delusions[I,W]
.3 With Hallucinations[I,W]
291.89 Alcohol-Induced Mood Disorder[I,W]
291.89 Alcohol-Induced Anxiety Disorder[I,W]
291.89 Alcohol-Induced Sexual Dysfunction[I]
291.89 Alcohol-Induced Sleep Disorder[I,W]
291.9 Alcohol-Related Disorder NOS

Amphetamine (or Amphetamine-Like)–Related Disorders
Amphetamine Use Disorders

304.40 Amphetamine Dependence[a,b,c]
305.70 Amphetamine Abuse

Amphetamine-Induced Disorders

292.89 Amphetamine Intoxication
Specify if: With Perceptual Disturbances
292.0 Amphetamine Withdrawal
292.81 Amphetamine Intoxication Delirium
292.xx Amphetamine-Induced Psychotic Disorder
.11 With Delusions[I]
.12 With Hallucinations[I]
292.84 Amphetamine-Induced Mood Disorder[I,W]
292.89 Amphetamine-Induced Anxiety Disorder[I]
292.89 Amphetamine-Induced Sexual Dysfunction[I]
292.89 Amphetamine-Induced Sleep Disorder[I,W]
292.9 Amphetamine-Related Disorder NOS

Caffeine-Related Disorders
Caffeine-Induced Disorders

305.90 Caffeine Intoxication
292.89 Caffeine-Induced Anxiety Disorder[I]
292.89 Caffeine-Induced Sleep Disorder[I]
292.9 Caffeine-Related Disorder NOS

Cannabis-Related Disorders
Cannabis Use Disorders

304.30 Cannabis Dependence[a,b,c]
305.20 Cannabis Abuse

Cannabis-Induced Disorders

292.89 Cannabis Intoxication
Specify if: With Perceptual Disturbances
292.81 Cannabis Intoxication Delirium
292.xx Cannabis-Induced Psychotic Disorder

.11   With Delusions[I]
.12   With Hallucinations[I]
292.89 Cannabis-Induced Anxiety Disorder[I]
292.9   Cannabis-Related Disorder NOS

Cocaine-Related Disorders

Cocaine Use Disorders

304.20 Cocaine Dependence[a,b,c]
305.60 Cocaine Abuse

Cocaine-Induced Disorders

292.89 Cocaine Intoxication
        Specify if: With Perceptual Disturbances
292.0   Cocaine Withdrawal
292.81 Cocaine Intoxication Delirium
292.xx Cocaine-Induced Psychotic Disorder
.11   With Delusions[I]
.12   With Hallucinations[I]
292.84 Cocaine-Induced Mood Disorder[I,W]
292.89 Cocaine-Induced Anxiety Disorder[I,W]
292.89 Cocaine-Induced Sexual Dysfunction[I]
292.89 Cocaine-Induced Sleep Disorder[I,W]
292.9   Cocaine-Related Disorder NOS

Hallucinogen-Related Disorders

Hallucinogen Use Disorders

304.50 Hallucinogen Dependence[b,c]
305.30 Hallucinogen Abuse

Hallucinogen-Induced Disorders

292.89 Hallucinogen Intoxication
292.89 Hallucinogen Persisting Perception Disorder
        (Flashbacks)
292.81 Hallucinogen Intoxication Delirium
292.xx Hallucinogen-Induced Psychotic Disorder
.11   With Delusions[I]
.12   With Hallucinations[I]
292.84 Hallucinogen-Induced Mood Disorder[I]
292.89 Hallucinogen-Induced Anxiety Disorder[I]
292.9   Hallucinogen-Related Disorder NOS

Inhalant-Related Disorders

Inhalant Use Disorders

304.60 Inhalant Dependence[b,c]
305.90 Inhalant Abuse

Inhalant-Induced Disorders

292.89 Inhalant Intoxication
292.81 Inhalant Intoxication Delirium
292.82 Inhalant-Induced Persisting Dementia
292.xx Inhalant-Induced Psychotic Disorder
.11   With Delusions[I]
.12   With Hallucinations[I]
292.84 Inhalant-Induced Mood Disorder[I]

292.89 Inhalant-Induced Anxiety Disorder[I]
292.9   Inhalant-Related Disorder NOS

Nicotine-Related Disorders

Nicotine Use Disorder

305.1   Nicotine Dependence[a,b]

Nicotine-Induced Disorder

292.0   Nicotine Withdrawal
292.9   Nicotine-Related Disorder NOS

Opioid-Related Disorders

Opioid Use Disorders

304.00 Opioid Dependence[a,b,c,d]
305.50 Opioid Abuse

Opioid-Induced Disorders

292.89 Opioid Intoxication
        Specify if: With Perceptual Disturbances
292.0   Opioid Withdrawal
292.81 Opioid Intoxication Delirium
292.xx Opioid-Induced Psychotic Disorder
.11   With Delusions[I]
.12   With Hallucinations[I]
292.84 Opioid-Induced Mood Disorder[I]
292.89 Opioid-Induced Sexual Dysfunction[I]
292.89 Opioid-Induced Sleep Disorder[I,W]
292.9   Opioid-Related Disorder NOS

Phencyclidine (or Phencyclidine-Like)–Related Disorders

Phencyclidine Use Disorders

304.60 Phencyclidine Dependence[b,c]
305.90 Phencyclidine Abuse

Phencyclidine-Induced Disorders

292.89 Phencyclidine Intoxication
        Specify if: With Perceptual Disturbances
292.81 Phencyclidine Intoxication Delirium
292.xx Phencyclidine-Induced Psychotic Disorder
.11   With Delusions[I]
.12   With Hallucinations[I]
292.84 Phencyclidine-Induced Mood Disorder[I]
292.89 Phencyclidine-Induced Anxiety Disorder[I]
292.9   Phencyclidine-Related Disorder NOS

Sedative-, Hypnotic-, or Anxiolytic-Related Disorders

Sedative, Hypnotic, or Anxiolytic Use Disorders

304.10 Sedative, Hypnotic, or Anxiolytic Dependence[a,b,c]
305.40 Sedative, Hypnotic, or Anxiolytic Abuse

Sedative-, Hypnotic-, or Anxiolytic-Induced Disorders

292.89   Sedative, Hypnotic, or Anxiolytic Intoxication

292.0   Sedative, Hypnotic, or Anxiolytic Withdrawal
Specify if: With Perceptual Disturbances

292.81   Sedative, Hypnotic, or Anxiolytic Intoxication Delirium

292.81   Sedative, Hypnotic, or Anxiolytic Withdrawal Delirium

292.82   Sedative-, Hypnotic-, or Anxiolytic-Induced Persisting Dementia

292.83   Sedative-, Hypnotic-, or Anxiolytic-Induced Persisting Amnestic Disorder

292.xx   Sedative-, Hypnotic-, or Anxiolytic-Induced Psychotic Disorder
.11   With Delusions[I,W]
.12   With Hallucinations[I,W]

292.84   Sedative-, Hypnotic-, or Anxiolytic-Induced Mood Disorder[I,W]

292.89   Sedative-, Hypnotic-, or Anxiolytic-Induced Anxiety Disorder[W]

292.89   Sedative-, Hypnotic-, or Anxiolytic-Induced Sexual Dysfunction[I]

292.89   Sedative-, Hypnotic-, or Anxiolytic-Induced Sleep Disorder[I,W]

292.9   Sedative-, Hypnotic-, or Anxiolytic-Related Disorder NOS

Polysubstance-Related Disorder

304.80   Polysubstance Dependence[a,b,c,d]

Other (or Unknown) Substance–Related Disorders

Other (or Unknown) Substance Use Disorders

304.90   Other (or Unknown) Substance Dependence[a,b,c,d]

305.90   Other (or Unknown) Substance Abuse

Other (or Unknown) Substance–Induced Disorders

292.89   Other (or Unknown) Substance Intoxication
Specify if: With Perceptual Disturbances

292.0   Other (or Unknown) Substance Withdrawal
Specify if: With Perceptual Disturbances

292.81   Other (or Unknown) Substance–Induced Delirium

292.82   Other (or Unknown) Substance–Induced Persisting Dementia

292.83   Other (or Unknown) Substance–Induced Persisting Amnestic Disorder

292.xx   Other (or Unknown) Substance–Induced Psychotic Disorder
.11   With Delusions[I,W]
.12   With Hallucinations[I,W]

292.84   Other (or Unknown) Substance–Induced Mood Disorder[I,W]

292.89   Other (or Unknown) Substance–Induced Anxiety Disorder[I,W]

292.89   Other (or Unknown) Substance–Induced Sexual Dysfunction[I]

292.89   Other (or Unknown) Substance–Induced Sleep Disorder[I,W]

292.9   Other (or Unknown) Substance–Related Disorder NOS

SCHIZOPHRENIA AND OTHER PSYCHOTIC DISORDERS

295.xx   Schizophrenia
The following Classification of Longitudinal Course applies to all subtypes of Schizophrenia:
Episodic With Interepisode Residual Symptoms (*specify if:* With Prominent Negative Symptoms)/ Episodic With No Interepisode Residual Symptoms
Continuous (*specify if:* With Prominent Negative Symptoms)
Single Episode in Partial Remission (*specify if:* With Prominent Negative Symptoms)/Single Episode In Full Remission
Other or Unspecified Pattern
.30   Paranoid Type
.10   Disorganized Type
.20   Catatonic Type
.90   Undifferentiated Type
.60   Residual Type

295.40   Schizophreniform Disorder
Specify if: Without Good Prognostic Features/With Good Prognostic Features

295.70   Schizoaffective Disorder
Specify type: Bipolar Type/Depressive Type

297.1   Delusional Disorder
Specify type: Erotomanic Type/Grandiose Type/Jealous Type/Persecutory Type/Somatic Type/Mixed Type/Unspecified Type

298.8   Brief Psychotic Disorder
Specify if: With Marked Stressor(s)/Without Marked Stressor(s)/With Postpartum Onset

297.3   Shared Psychotic Disorder

293.xx   Psychotic Disorder Due to . . . *[Indicate the General Medical Condition]*
.81   With Delusions
.82   With Hallucinations

___.___   Substance-Induced Psychotic Disorder (*refer to Substance-Related Disorders for substance-specific codes*)
Specify if: With Onset During Intoxication/With Onset During Withdrawal

298.9   Psychotic Disorder NOS

MOOD DISORDERS

Code current state of Major Depressive Disorder or Bipolar I Disorder in fifth digit:

1 = Mild
2 = Moderate
3 = Severe Without Psychotic Features
4 = Severe With Psychotic Features
Specify: Mood-Congruent Psychotic Features/ Mood-Incongruent Psychotic Features
5 = In Partial Remission
6 = In Full Remission
0 = Unspecified

The following specifiers apply (for current or most recent episode) to Mood Disorders as noted:
aSeverity/Psychotic/Remission Specifiers
bChronic
cWith Catatonic Features
dWith Melancholic Features
eWith Atypical Features
fWith Postpartum Onset

The following specifiers apply to Mood Disorders as noted:
gWith or Without Full Interepisode Recovery
hWith Seasonal Pattern
iWith Rapid Cycling

Depressive Disorders

296.xx	Major Depressive Disorder
.2x	Single Episode[a,b,c,d,e,f]
.3x	Recurrent[a,b,c,d,e,f,g,h]
300.4	Dysthymic Disorder
	Specify if: Early Onset/Late Onset
	Specify: With Atypical Features
311	Depressive Disorder NOS

Bipolar Disorders

296.xx	Bipolar I Disorder
.0x	Single Manic Episode[a,c,f]
	Specify if: Mixed
.40	Most Recent Episode Hypomanic[g,h,i]
.4x	Most Recent Episode Manic[a,c,f,g,h,i]
.6x	Most Recent Episode Mixed[a,c,f,g,h,i]
.5x	Most Recent Episode Depressed[a,b,c,d,e,f,g,h,i]
.7	Most Recent Episode Unspecified[g,h,i]
296.89	Bipolar II Disorder[a,b,c,d,e,f,g,h,i]
	Specify (current or most recent episode): Hypomanic/Depressed
301.13	Cyclothymic Disorder
296.80	Bipolar Disorder NOS
293.83	Mood Disorder Due to . . . *[Indicate the General Medical Condition]*
	Specify type: With Depressive Features/With Major Depressive-Like Episode/With Manic Features/With Mixed Features

___.__	Substance-Induced Mood Disorder *(refer to Substance-Related Disorders for substance-specific codes)*
	Specify type: With Depressive Features/With Manic Features/With Mixed Features
	Specify if: With Onset During Intoxication/ With Onset During Withdrawal
296.90	Mood Disorder NOS

ANXIETY DISORDERS

300.01	Panic Disorder Without Agoraphobia
300.21	Panic Disorder With Agoraphobia
300.22	Agoraphobia Without History of Panic Disorder
300.29	Specific Phobia
	Specify type: Animal Type/Natural Environment Type/Blood-Injection-Injury Type/Situational Type/Other Type
300.23	Social Phobia
	Specify if: Generalized
300.3	Obsessive-Compulsive Disorder
	Specify if: With Poor Insight
309.81	Posttraumatic Stress Disorder
	Specify if: Acute/Chronic
	Specify if: With Delayed Onset
308.3	Acute Stress Disorder
300.02	Generalized Anxiety Disorder
293.84	Anxiety Disorder Due to . . . *[Indicate the General Medical Condition]*
	Specify if: With Generalized Anxiety/With Panic Attacks/With Obsessive-Compulsive Symptoms
___.__	Substance-Induced Anxiety Disorder *(refer to Substance-Related Disorders for substance-specific codes)*
	Specify if: With Generalized Anxiety/With Panic Attacks/With Obsessive-Compulsive Symptoms/With Phobic Symptoms
	Specify if: With Onset During Intoxication/ With Onset During Withdrawal
300.00	Anxiety Disorder NOS

SOMATOFORM DISORDERS

300.81	Somatization Disorder
300.82	Undifferentiated Somatoform Disorder
300.11	Conversion Disorder
	Specify type: With Motor Symptom or Deficit/With Sensory Symptom or Deficit/With Seizures or Convulsions/With Mixed Presentation
307.xx	Pain Disorder
.80	Associated With Psychologic Factors
.89	Associated With Both Psychologic Factors and a General Medical Condition
	Specify if: Acute/Chronic

300.7	Hypochondriasis
	Specify if: With Poor Insight
300.7	Body Dysmorphic Disorder
300.82	Somatoform Disorder NOS

FACTITIOUS DISORDERS

300.xx	Factitious Disorder
.16	With Predominantly Psychologic Signs and Symptoms
.19	With Predominantly Physical Signs and Symptoms
.19	With Combined Psychologic and Physical Signs and Symptoms
300.19	Factitious Disorder NOS

DISSOCIATIVE DISORDERS

300.12	Dissociative Amnesia
300.13	Dissociative Fugue
300.14	Dissociative Identity Disorder
300.6	Depersonalization Disorder
300.15	Dissociative Disorder NOS

SEXUAL AND GENDER IDENTITY DISORDERS

Sexual Dysfunctions

The following specifiers apply to all primary Sexual Dysfunctions:
  Lifelong Type/Acquired Type
  Generalized Type/Situational Type
  Due to Psychologic Factors/Due to Combined Factors

Sexual Desire Disorders

302.71	Hypoactive Sexual Desire Disorder
302.79	Sexual Aversion Disorder

Sexual Arousal Disorders

302.72	Female Sexual Arousal Disorder
302.72	Male Erectile Disorder

Orgasmic Disorders

302.73	Female Orgasmic Disorder
302.74	Male Orgasmic Disorder
302.75	Premature Ejaculation

Sexual Pain Disorders

302.76	Dyspareunia (Not Due to a General Medical Condition)
306.51	Vaginismus (Not Due to a General Medical Condition)

Sexual Dysfunction Due to a General Medical Condition

625.8	Female Hypoactive Sexual Desire Disorder Due to . . . *[Indicate the General Medical Condition]*
608.89	Male Hypoactive Sexual Desire Disorder Due to . . . *[Indicate the General Medical Condition]*
607.84	Male Erectile Disorder Due to . . . *[Indicate the General Medical Condition]*
625.0	Female Dyspareunia Due to . . . *[Indicate the General Medical Condition]*
608.89	Male Dyspareunia Due to . . . *[Indicate the General Medical Condition]*
625.8	Other Female Sexual Dysfunction Due to . . . *[Indicate the General Medical Condition]*
608.89	Other Male Sexual Dysfunction Due to . . . *[Indicate the General Medical Condition]*
___.__	Substance-Induced Sexual Dysfunction *(refer to Substance-Related Disorders for substance-specific codes)*
	Specify if: With Impaired Desire/With Impaired Arousal/With Impaired Orgasm/With Sexual Pain
	Specify if: With Onset During Intoxication
302.70	Sexual Dysfunction NOS

Paraphilias

302.4	Exhibitionism
302.81	Fetishism
302.89	Frotteurism
302.2	Pedophilia
	Specify if: Sexually Attracted to Males/Sexually Attracted to Females/Sexually Attracted to Both
	Specify if: Limited to Incest
	Specify type: Exclusive Type/Nonexclusive Type
302.83	Sexual Masochism
302.84	Sexual Sadism
302.3	Transvestic Fetishism
	Specify if: With Gender Dysphoria
302.82	Voyeurism
302.9	Paraphilia NOS

Gender Identity Disorders

302.xx	Gender Identity Disorder
.6	In Children
.85	In Adolescents or Adults
	Specify if: Sexually Attracted to Males/Sexually Attracted to Females/Sexually Attracted to Both/Sexually Attracted to Neither
302.6	Gender Identity Disorder NOS

302.9   Sexual Disorder NOS

EATING DISORDERS

307.1   Anorexia Nervosa
         Specify type: Restricting Type; Binge-Eating/
         Purging Type
307.51   Bulimia Nervosa
         Specify type: Purging Type/Nonpurging Type
307.50   Eating Disorder NOS

SLEEP DISORDERS

Primary Sleep Disorders

Dyssomnias

307.42   Primary Insomnia
307.44   Primary Hypersomnia
         Specify if: Recurrent
347   Narcolepsy
780.59   Breathing-Related Sleep Disorder
307.45   Circadian Rhythm Sleep Disorder
         Specify type: Delayed Sleep Phase Type/Jet
         Lag Type/Shift Work Type/Unspecified
         Type
307.47   Dyssomnia NOS

Parasomnias

307.47   Nightmare Disorder
307.46   Sleep Terror Disorder
307.46   Sleepwalking Disorder
307.47   Parasomnia NOS

Sleep Disorders Related to Another Mental Disorder

307.42   Insomnia Related to . . . *[Indicate the Axis I or
         Axis II Disorder]*
307.44   Hypersomnia Related to . . . *[Indicate the Axis
         I or Axis II Disorder]*

Other Sleep Disorders

780.xx   Sleep Disorder Due to . . . *[Indicate the
         General Medical Condition]*
  .52   Insomnia Type
  .54   Hypersomnia Type
  .59   Parasomnia Type
  .59   Mixed Type
___.__   Substance-Induced Sleep Disorder *(refer to
          Substance-Related Disorders for substance-spe-
          cific codes)*
          Specify type: Insomnia Type/Hypersomnia
          Type/Parasomnia Type/Mixed Type

Specify if: With Onset During Intoxication/
With Onset During Withdrawal

IMPULSE-CONTROL DISORDERS NOT ELSEWHERE CLASSIFIED

312.34   Intermittent Explosive Disorder
312.32   Kleptomania
312.33   Pyromania
312.31   Pathologic Gambling
312.39   Trichotillomania
312.30   Impulse-Control Disorder NOS

ADJUSTMENT DISORDERS

309.xx   Adjustment Disorder
  .0   With Depressed Mood
  .24   With Anxiety
  .28   With Mixed Anxiety and Depressed Mood
  .3   With Disturbance of Conduct
  .4   With Mixed Disturbance of Emotions and
            Conduct
  .9   Unspecified
            Specify if: Acute/Chronic

PERSONALITY DISORDERS

NOTE: These are coded on Axis II.
301.0   Paranoid Personality Disorder
301.20   Schizoid Personality Disorder
301.22   Schizotypal Personality Disorder
301.7   Antisocial Personality Disorder
301.83   Borderline Personality Disorder
301.50   Histrionic Personality Disorder
301.81   Narcissistic Personality Disorder
301.82   Avoidant Personality Disorder
301.6   Dependent Personality Disorder
301.4   Obsessive-Compulsive Personality Disorder
301.9   Personality Disorder NOS

OTHER CONDITIONS THAT MAY BE A FOCUS OF CLINICAL ATTENTION

Psychologic Factors Affecting Medical Condition

316   . . . *[Specified Psychologic Factor] Affecting . . .
         [Indicate the General Medical Condition]*
Choose name based on nature of factors:
   Mental Disorder Affecting Medical Condition
   Psychological Symptoms Affecting Medical
      Condition
   Personality Traits or Coping Style Affecting Medical
      Condition
   Maladaptive Health Behaviors Affecting Medical
      Condition

Stress-Related Physiological Response Affecting Medical Condition

Other or Unspecified Psychological Factors Affecting Medical Condition

Medication-Induced Movement Disorders

332.1	Neuroleptic-Induced Parkinsonism
333.92	Neuroleptic Malignant Syndrome
333.7	Neuroleptic-Induced Acute Dystonia
333.99	Neuroleptic-Induced Acute Akathisia
333.82	Neuroleptic-Induced Tardive Dyskinesia
333.1	Medication-Induced Postural Tremor
333.90	Medication-Induced Movement Disorder NOS

Other Medication-Induced Disorder

995.2	Adverse Effects of Medication NOS

Relational Problems

V61.9	Relational Problem Related to a Mental Disorder or General Medical Condition
V61.20	Parent-Child Relational Problem
V61.10	Partner Relational Problem
V61.8	Sibling Relational Problem
V62.81	Relational Problem NOS

Problems Related to Abuse or Neglect

V61.21	Physical Abuse of Child (*code 995.5 if focus of attention is on victim*)
V61.21	Sexual Abuse of Child (*code 995.5 if focus of attention is on victim*)
V61.21	Neglect of Child (*code 995.5 if focus of attention is on victim*)
___.__	Physical Abuse of Adult
V61.12	(if by partner)
V62.83	(if by person other than partner) (*code 995.81 if focus of attention is on victim*)
___.__	Sexual Abuse of Adult
V61.12	(if by partner)
V62.83	(if by person other than partner) (*code 995.83 if focus of attention is on victim*)

Additional Conditions That May Be a Focus of Clinical Attention

V15.81	Noncompliance With Treatment
V65.2	Malingering
V71.01	Adult Antisocial Behavior
V71.02	Child or Adolescent Antisocial Behavior
V62.89	Borderline Intellectual Functioning **NOTE:** *This is coded on Axis II.*
780.9	Age-Related Cognitive Decline
V62.82	Bereavement
V62.3	Academic Problem
V62.2	Occupational Problem
313.82	Identity Problem
V62.89	Religious or Spiritual Problem
V62.4	Acculturation Problem
V62.89	Phase of Life Problem

ADDITIONAL CODES

300.9	Unspecified Mental Disorder (nonpsychotic)
V71.09	No Diagnosis or Condition on Axis I
799.9	Diagnosis or Condition Deferred on Axis I
V71.09	No Diagnosis on Axis II
799.9	Diagnosis Deferred on Axis II

Historic Synopsis of Psychiatric Mental Health Nursing

Pre-1860

Nursing care for the young, ill, and helpless historically has existed as long as the human race. Care was given by family members, other relatives, servants, neighbors, or members of religious orders or humanitarian societies, or by convalescing patients or prisoners.

1860

Florence Nightingale. Established Nightingale School at St. Thomas's Hospital in London after the Crimean War and worked with untrained women caring for soldiers. *Founder of modern-day nursing.*

1860-1880

Emphasized maintenance of healthful environment, personal hygiene, cleanliness, and healthful living habits, such as adequate nutrition, exercise, and sleep, so that nature could heal. Emphasized kindness toward clients along with custodial care.

Linda Richards. *First graduate nurse and first psychiatric nurse in the United States.* After study under Florence Nightingale, organized nursing services and educational programs in Boston City Hospital and in several state mental hospitals in Illinois.

Dorothea Dix. *Worked to reform psychiatric care in mental hospitals* and to correct overcrowding and the insufficient number of physicians and attendants.

1882

First school to prepare nurses to care for acutely and chronically mentally ill opened at McLean Hospital, Waverly, Massachusetts, through collaboration of Linda Richards and Dr. Edward Cowles.

1890-1930

Nurses with special preparation recognized by some administrative psychiatrists in state and private hospitals for their preparation. Nurses relieved of menial housekeeping chores to engage in physical custodial care of clients. Role primarily to assist physician or carry out procedures for physical care. Few psychological nursing skills. Psychologically concerned with maintaining kind, tolerant attitude and humane treatment.

1920

Harriet Bailey. *First nurse educator to write a psychiatric nursing text,* Nursing Mental Disease, 1920. She wrote of the importance of a nurse's knowing mental illness and of teaching mental health nursing, and she worked for provision of student experiences in psychiatry. She argued for more holistic care of clients.

1926

Euphemia "Effie" Jane Taylor. Became the first psychiatric nurse to be appointed Professor of Nursing at Yale University School of Nursing.

1937

National League for Nursing recommended that psychiatric nursing be included in the basic nursing curriculum.

1940

Publication of *Psychiatry for Nurses* by Louis Karnosh and Edith Gage, RN.

1946

National Mental Health Act passed, authorizing establishment of the National Institute of Mental Health, with funds and programs to train professional psychiatric personnel, conduct psychiatric research, and aid in the development of mental health programs at the state level. Provided impetus for psychiatric nursing as a specialty.

1950-1960

Nurse's role included physical care and administration of medications, and maintenance of therapeutic milieu. Less emphasis on physical restraints.

Ruth Matheney and Mary Topalis. Emphasized importance of milieu therapy and the nurse's use of this intervention.

1952

Hildegard E. Peplau. *Formulated first systematic theoretical framework in psychiatric nursing, presented in* Interpersonal Relations in Nursing, *1952.* Emphasized that nursing is an interpersonal process and that psychological techniques and theoretical concepts are essential to nursing practice. Defined steps in nurse-client relationship:

1. Nurse helps client examine situational factors through observation of behavior.
2. Nurse helps client describe and analyze behavior.
3. Nurse formulates with client connections between feelings and behavior.
4. Nurse encourages client to improve interpersonal competence through testing new behavior.
5. Nurse validates with client when new behavior is integrated into personality structure.

1953

The Therapeutic Community by Maxwell Jones, in Great Britain, laid basis for movement in United States toward milieu therapy and for nurse's role in this therapy.

1954

Advent of the use of the antipsychotic medication chlorpromazine (Thorazine) in the United States; synthesized in France in 1950.

1956

National Conference on Graduate Education in Psychiatric Nursing introduced concept of psychiatric clinical nurse specialist. Theoreticians begin to differentiate functions based on master's level of preparation in nursing.

1957

June Mellow. *Introduced second theoretical approach to psychiatric nursing, called "nursing therapy," which applied psychoanalytical theory in one-to-one interactions with schizophrenic clients. Emphasized providing corrective emotional experience rather than investigating pathological processes or interpersonal developmental processes to facilitate integration of overwhelmed ego.*

1958

American Nurses Association established Conference Group on Psychiatric Nursing.

1959

Accredited schools of nursing had to have own psychiatric nursing curriculum and instructor, per National League for Nursing. Could no longer buy services of hospitals to supply education.

1960-1970

Hildegard E. Peplau, Gertrude Ujhely, Joyce Travelbee, Shirley Burd, Loretta Bermosk, Joyce Hays, Catherine Norris, Gertrude Stokes, Anne Hargreaves, Dorothy Gregg, and Sheila Rouslin. Nursing leaders emphasized importance of self-awareness and use of self, nurse-client relationship therapy, therapeutic communication, and psychosocial aspects of general nursing. Peplau identified the manifestations of anxiety and formulated steps in anxiety intervention, now used by all health care professions. All of these nursing leaders converted various psychological concepts into operational definitions for use in nursing.

1960-1965

Sheila Rouslin and Suzanne Lego. Opened private practices in psychotherapy.

1961

Anne Burgess and Donna Aguilera. Engaged in crisis work and short-term therapy as well as long-term therapy. Applied crisis theory to psychiatric nursing.

Ida Orlando. *Initiated term* nursing process *and began to delineate its components.* Presented general theoretical framework for all nurse-client relationships, with focus on client's ascertaining meaning of behavior and explaining help needed. Wrote the classic book *The Dynamic Nurse-Patient Relationship.*

Hildegard E. Peplau. Promoted primary role of nurse as psychotherapist or counselor rather than as mother surrogate, socializer, or manager.

1963

Comprehensive Community Mental Health Act passed; provided impetus for nurses to move from hospital to community setting.

1967

American Nurses Association presented "Position Paper on Psychiatric Nursing," endorsing role of clinical specialist as therapist in individual, group, family, and milieu therapies.

American Nurses Association, Division on Psychiatric and Mental Health Nursing Practice, published first *Statement on Psychiatric and Mental Health Nursing Practice.*

1970-1980

Sheila Rouslin. *Because of her leadership, certification of clinical specialists in psychiatric nursing begun by Division of Psychiatric Mental Health Nursing, New*

Jersey State Nurses Association. Later, certification developed by American Nurses Association.

Shirley Smoyak. *Defined client as individual, group, family, or community; defined nurse as family therapist; defined expanded role of nurse.*

Gwen Marram and Irene Burnside. *Emphasized that nurses with graduate-level preparation could conduct group and family psychotherapy.*

Carolyn Clark. *Emphasized the usefulness of a systems framework for psychiatric nurses.* Also emphasized the importance of nurses acting as change agents and researchers.

Bonnie Bullough. *Emphasized legal and ethical aspects of psychiatric care.*

Madeleine Leininger. *Reemphasized care of whole person.* Introduced implications of cultural diversity for mental health services and psychiatric treatment.

1973

Standards of Psychiatric-Mental Health Nursing published. Certification of Psychiatric-Mental Health Nurse Generalists established by the ANA.

1976

American Nurses Association Division on Psychiatric and Mental Health Nursing Practice published revised *Statement on Psychiatric and Mental Health Nursing Practice.*

1978

Report of presidential commission concluded that deinstitutionalization and discharge of clients to community facilities had not worked as expected because of lack of financial, social, medical, and nursing resources and lack of coordination of services.

1979

ANA established certification of Psychiatric-Mental Health Nurse Specialists.

1980-1990

Anne Burgess. *Formulated theory of victimology,* based on extensive studies of adult and child victims of rape and abuse, child victims of neglect, and family violence of incest and battering. Described rape-trauma syndrome, silent rape trauma, and compound reactions to rape.

Lee Ann Hoff. *Expanded crisis theory to be used in nursing practice. Contributed to theory of suicidology.* Described battering syndrome after performing research on battered women and battered elderly.

1982

American Nurses Association Executive Committee and Standards Committee, Division on Psychiatric and Mental Health Nursing Practice, published

Standards of Psychiatric and Mental Health Nursing Practice.

Century Celebration of Psychiatric Nursing, Washington, DC.

1987

Maxine E. Loomis, Anita O'Toole, Marie Scott Brown, Patricia Pothier, Patricia West, and Holly S. Wilson. Began the development of a classification system for psychiatric and mental health nursing, first published in the new journal *Archives of Psychiatric Nursing, 1(1),* 16-24, 1987.

1988

NIMH Epidemiological Catchment Area Study published.

1990

Suzanne Lego. Opened the first psychoanalytic training program for nurses at Columbia University School of Nursing.

Americans with Disabilities Act passed by U.S. Congress. Presidential proclamation by George Bush declared the 1990s the "Decade of the Brain."

1994

Carolyn V. Billings, Jean Blackburn, Mickie Ceimone, Carol Dashiff, Kathleen Scharer, Anita O'Toole, and Carole A. Shea. Composed a task force to
- Revise *Statement on Psychiatric and Mental Health Nursing Practice,* updating the scope and functions for nurses certified at the basic level and those certified at the advanced practice level.
- Revise *Standards of Psychiatric and Mental Health Nursing Practice,* describing professional nursing activities that are demonstrated by the nurse throughout the nursing process for both the basic level certified psychiatric nurse and the advanced practice psychiatric nurse, and standards of professional performance.

Publication of *Essentials of Psychiatric Nursing,* 14th Edition, by Cecelia Taylor; originally published as *Psychiatry for Nurses* in 1940.

1995

Publication of *Journal of the American Psychiatric Nurses Association* began.

2000

Grayce Sills, Karen A. Ballard, Carolyn V. Billings, and others. Composed a task force to revise *Scope and Standards of Psychiatric Mental Health Nursing.*

Adapted from Murray RB (1991). The nursing process and emotional care. In Murray RB, Huelskoetter MMW (Eds.), *Psychiatric mental health nursing—giving emotional care* (3rd ed., pp. 94-97). Norwalk, CT: Appleton & Lange.

NANDA-Approved Nursing Diagnoses

Activity intolerance
Activity intolerance, Risk for
Adjustment, Impaired
Airway clearance, Ineffective
Allergy response, Latex
Allergy response, Risk for latex
Anxiety
Anxiety, Death
Aspiration, Risk for
Attachment, Risk for impaired parent/infant/child
Autonomic dysreflexia
Autonomic dysreflexia, Risk for

Body image, Disturbed
Body temperature, Risk for imbalanced
Bowel incontinence
Breastfeeding, Effective
Breastfeeding, Ineffective
Breastfeeding, Interrupted
Breathing pattern, Ineffective

Cardiac output, Decreased
Caregiver role strain
Caregiver role strain, Risk for
Communication, Impaired verbal
Communication, Readiness for enhanced
Conflict, Decisional
Conflict, Parental role
Confusion, Acute
Confusion, Chronic
Constipation
Constipation, Perceived
Constipation, Risk for
Coping, Ineffective
Coping, Defensive
Coping, Readiness for enhanced
Coping, Ineffective community
Coping, Readiness for enhanced community
Coping, Compromised family
Coping, Disabled family
Coping, Readiness for enhanced family

Death syndrome, Risk for sudden infant
Denial, Ineffective
Dentition, Impaired
Development, Risk for delayed
Diarrhea
Disuse syndrome, Risk for
Diversional activity, Deficient

Energy field, Disturbed
Environmental interpretation syndrome, Impaired

Failure to thrive, Adult
Falls, Risk for
Family processes: alcoholism, Dysfunctional
Family processes, Interrupted
Family processes, Readiness for enhanced
Fatigue
Fear
Fluid balance, Readiness for enhanced
Fluid volume, Deficient
Fluid volume, Excess
Fluid volume, Risk for deficient
Fluid volume, Risk for imbalanced

Gas exchange, Impaired
Grieving, Anticipatory
Grieving, Dysfunctional
Grieving, Risk for dysfunctional
Growth and development, Delayed
Growth, Risk for disproportionate

Health maintenance, Ineffective
Health-seeking behaviors
Home maintenance, Impaired
Hopelessness
Hyperthermia
Hypothermia

Identity, Disturbed personal
Incontinence, Functional urinary
Incontinence, Reflex urinary

Incontinence, Stress urinary
Incontinence, Total urinary
Incontinence, Urge urinary
Incontinence, Risk for urge urinary
Infant behavior, Disorganized
Infant behavior, Risk for disorganized
Infant behavior, Readiness for enhanced organized
Infant feeding pattern, Ineffective
Infection, Risk for
Injury, Risk for
Injury, Risk for perioperative-positioning
Intracranial adaptive capacity, Decreased

Knowledge, Deficient
Knowledge, Readiness for enhanced

Lifestyle, Sedentary
Loneliness, Risk for

Memory, Impaired
Mobility, Impaired bed
Mobility, Impaired physical
Mobility, Impaired wheelchair

Nausea
Neglect, Unilateral
Noncompliance
Nutrition: less than body requirements, Imbalanced
Nutrition: more than body requirements, Imbalanced
Nutrition, Readiness for enhanced
Nutrition: more than body requirements, Risk for imbalanced

Oral mucous membrane, Impaired

Pain, Acute
Pain, Chronic
Parenting, Readiness for enhanced
Parenting, Impaired
Parenting, Risk for impaired
Peripheral neurovascular dysfunction, Risk for
Poisoning, Risk for
Post-trauma syndrome
Post-trauma syndrome, Risk for
Powerlessness
Powerlessness, Risk for
Protection, Ineffective

Rape-trauma syndrome
Rape-trauma syndrome: compound reaction
Rape-trauma syndrome: silent reaction
Religiosity, Impaired
Religiosity, Readiness for enhanced
Religiosity, Risk for impaired
Relocation stress syndrome
Relocation stress syndrome, Risk for
Role performance, Ineffective

Self-care deficit, Bathing/hygiene
Self-care deficit, Dressing/grooming
Self-care deficit, Feeding
Self-care deficit, Toileting
Self-concept, Readiness for enhanced
Self-esteem, Chronic low
Self-esteem, Situational low
Self-esteem, Risk for situational low
Self-mutilation
Self-mutilation, Risk for
Sensory perception, Disturbed
Sexual dysfunction
Sexuality pattern, Ineffective
Skin integrity, Impaired
Skin integrity, Risk for impaired
Sleep deprivation
Sleep pattern, Disturbed
Sleep, Readiness for enhanced
Social interaction, Impaired
Social isolation
Sorrow, Chronic
Spiritual distress
Spiritual distress, Risk for
Spiritual well-being, Readiness for enhanced
Suffocation, Risk for
Suicide, Risk for
Surgical recovery, Delayed
Swallowing, Impaired

Therapeutic regimen management, Effective
Therapeutic regimen management, Ineffective
Therapeutic regimen management, Readiness for enhanced
Therapeutic regimen management, Ineffective community
Therapeutic regimen management, Ineffective family
Thermoregulation, Ineffective
Thought processes, Disturbed
Tissue integrity, Impaired
Tissue perfusion, Ineffective
Transfer ability, Impaired
Trauma, Risk for

Urinary elimination, Impaired
Urinary elimination, Readiness for enhanced
Urinary retention

Ventilation, Impaired spontaneous
Ventilatory weaning response, Dysfunctional
Violence, Risk for other-directed
Violence, Risk for self-directed

Walking, Impaired
Wandering

From North American Nursing Diagnosis Association. (2005). *NANDA nursing diagnoses: Definitions and classification 2005-2006.* Philadelphia: Author.

Answers to Chapter Review Questions

evolve Visit the Evolve website at **http://evolve.elsevier.com/Varcarolis** for rationales and text page references.

Chapter 1
1. 3
2. 4
3. 3
4. 2
5. 4

Chapter 2
1. 1
2. 3
3. 1
4. 3
5. 1

Chapter 3
1. 1
2. 3
3. 1
4. 2
5. 2

Chapter 4
1. 3
2. 2
3. 4
4. 4
5. 2

Chapter 5
1. 1
2. 4
3. 3
4. 3
5. 4

Chapter 6
1. 2
2. 1
3. 2
4. 2
5. 1

Chapter 7
1. 3
2. 3
3. 4
4. 2
5. 3

Chapter 8
1. 4
2. 1
3. 1
4. 1
5. 3

Chapter 9
1. 2
2. 1
3. 2
4. 1
5. 3

Chapter 10
1. 1
2. 3
3. 4
4. 3
5. 4

Chapter 11
1. 1
2. 3
3. 1
4. 2
5. 1

Chapter 12
1. 1
2. 2
3. 4
4. 3
5. 2

Chapter 13
1. 3
2. 3
3. 3
4. 1
5. 2

Chapter 14
1. 1
2. 3
3. 4
4. 4
5. 2

Chapter 15
1. 2
2. 3
3. 4
4. 2
5. 2

Chapter 16
1. 4
2. 2
3. 4
4. 2
5. 1

Chapter 17
1. 1
2. 3
3. 2
4. 1
5. 1

Chapter 18
1. 2
2. 4
3. 1
4. 3
5. 2

Chapter 19
1. 1
2. 2
3. 1
4. 2
5. 2

Chapter 20
1. 4
2. 4
3. 1
4. 1
5. 3

Chapter 21
1. 1
2. 4
3. 1
4. 1
5. 1

Chapter 22
1. 1
2. 3
3. 1
4. 1
5. 1

Chapter 23
1. 4
2. 2
3. 4
4. 4
5. 3

Chapter 24
1. 3
2. 1
3. 1
4. 4
5. 3

Chapter 25
1. 1
2. 4
3. 2
4. 1
5. 4

Chapter 26
1. 1
2. 4
3. 4
4. 2
5. 4

Chapter 27
1. 3
2. 1
3. 4
4. 1
5. 1

Chapter 28
1. 2
2. 3
3. 3
4. 1
5. 4

Chapter 29
1. 2
2. 3
3. 2
4. 4
5. 3

Chapter 30
1. 1
2. 2
3. 4
4. 1
5. 1

Chapter 31
1. 2
2. 3
3. 1
4. 2
5. 1

Chapter 32
1. 1
2. 1
3. 2
4. 4
5. 4

Chapter 33
1. 4
2. 1
3. 4
4. 3
5. 3

Chapter 34
1. 1
2. 1
3. 2
4. 1
5. 1

Chapter 35
1. 4
2. 4
3. 2
4. 4
5. 3

Chapter 36
1. 1
2. 2
3. 1
4. 3
5. 3

Chapter 37
1. 3
2. 2
3. 1
4. 4
5. 2

Glossary

abstract thinking The ability to conceptualize ideas (e.g., finding meaning in proverbs).

abuse An act of misuse, deceit, or exploitation; wrong or improper use of or action toward another, resulting in injury, damage, maltreatment, or corruption.

accommodation The ability to change one's way of thinking to introduce new ideas, objects, or experiences.

acrophobia Fear of high places.

acting-out behaviors Behaviors that originate on an unconscious level to reduce anxiety and tension. Anxiety is displaced from one situation to another in the form of observable responses (e.g., anger, crying, or violence).

activities of daily living For a person with a chronic mental illness, the activities necessary to live independently as an adult.

acute anxiety Anxiety that is precipitated by an imminent loss or a change that threatens an individual's sense of security.

addiction Loss of control with respect to use of a drug (e.g., alcohol), use of the drug despite the presence of related problems, and a tendency to relapse after stopping use. Addiction is an older term that has been replaced by the term *drug dependence*.

Adult Children of Alcoholics (ACOA) A support group for adult children of alcoholics, who often experience similar difficulties and problems in their adult lives as a result of having an alcoholic parent or parents.

adventitious crisis A crisis that is not part of everyday life but involves an event that is unplanned and accidental. Adventitious crises include natural disasters and crimes of violence such as rapes or muggings.

affect The external manifestation of feeling or emotion, which can be assessed by the nurse by observing facial expression, tone of voice, and body language. For example, a client may be said to have a flat affect, meaning that there is an absence or a near absence of facial expression. Some people, however, use the term loosely to mean a feeling, emotion, or mood.

ageism A system of destructive, erroneous beliefs about the elderly; a bias against older people based solely on their age.

aggression Any verbal or nonverbal (actual or attempted, conscious or unconscious) forceful means of harm or abuse of another person or object.

agnosia Loss of the ability to recognize familiar objects. For example, a person may be unable to identify familiar sounds, such as the ringing of a doorbell (auditory agnosia), or familiar objects, such as a toothbrush or keys (visual agnosia).

agoraphobia Anxiety/panicky feelings about being in places or situations in which escape might be difficult or embarrassing or in which help may not be available should an anxiety attack occur. For some individuals, these feelings occur at home, in crowded supermarkets, in places of worship—places that clearly are not open. Persons with agoraphobia actively avoid places or situations associated with anxiety. For some, life becomes increasingly constricted until, in the most severe cases, they may not be able to leave the home.

agraphia Loss of a previous ability to write resulting from brain injury or brain disease.

akathisia Regular rhythmic movements, usually of the lower limbs; constant pacing may also be seen; often noticed in people taking antipsychotic medication.

akinesia Absence or diminution of voluntary motion. Akinesia is usually accompanied by a parallel reduction in mental activity.

Al-Anon A support group for spouses and friends of alcoholics.

Alateen A nationwide network for children over 10 years of age who have alcoholic parents.

alcohol withdrawal delirium An organic mental disorder that occurs 40 to 48 hours after cessation or reduction of long-term heavy alcohol intake and that is considered a medical emergency; often referred to by the older term *delirium tremens* (DTs).

alcoholic hallucinations Visual and tactile hallucinations reported to occur in alcohol-dependent clients suffering from alcohol withdrawal delirium.

Alcoholics Anonymous (AA) A self-help group for recovering alcoholics that provides support and encouragement to those involved in continuing recovery.

alcoholism The end stage of the continuum that includes addiction to and dependence on the drug alcohol.

Alzheimer's disease A primary cognitive impairment disorder characterized by progressive deterioration of cognitive functioning, with the end result that the person may not recognize once-familiar people, places, and things. The ability to walk and talk is absent in the final stages.

ambivalence The holding, at the same time, of two opposing emotions, attitudes, ideas, or wishes toward the same person, situation, or object.

amnesia Loss of memory for events within a specific period of time; may be temporary or permanent.

anergia Lack of energy; passivity.

anger An emotional response to the perception of frustration of desires or threat to one's needs.

anhedonia The inability to experience pleasure.

anorexia A medical term that signifies a loss of appetite. A person with anorexia nervosa, however, may not have any loss of appetite and often is preoccupied with food and eating. A person with this disorder may suppress the desire for food in order to control his or her eating.

Antabuse (disulfiram) A drug given to alcoholics that produces nausea, vomiting, dizziness, flushing, and tachycardia if alcohol is consumed.

anticholinergic side effects Side effects caused by the use of some medications (e.g., neuroleptics and tricyclic antidepressants). Symptoms include dry mouth, constipation, urinary retention, blurred vision, and dry mucous membranes.

anticipatory grief Grief that occurs before an actual loss. During this time, painful feelings may be partially resolved.

antidepressants Drugs predominantly used to elevate mood in people who are depressed.

antimanic drugs Drugs used in the treatment of a manic state to lower an elevated and unstable mood and to reduce irritability and aggressiveness.

antipsychotic drugs (neuroleptics, major tranquilizers) Drugs that have the ability to decrease psychotic, paranoid, and disorganized thinking and positively alter bizarre behaviors; they are thought to reduce the effects of the neurotransmitter dopamine by blocking the dopamine receptors.

antisocial (sociopathic, psychopathic) Terms often used interchangeably to refer to a syndrome in which a person lacks the capacity to relate to others.

These people do not experience discomfort in inflicting pain on or observing pain in others, and they constantly manipulate others for personal gain. Common characteristics and behaviors seen in people with this disorder include crimes against society, aggressiveness, inability to feel remorse, untruthfulness and insincerity, unreliability, and failure to follow any life plan.

anxiety A state of feeling apprehension, uneasiness, uncertainty, or dread resulting from a real or perceived threat whose actual source is unknown or unrecognized.

anxiolytics (antianxiety drugs, minor tranquilizers) Drugs prescribed, usually on a short-term basis, to reduce anxiety.

apathy A state of indifference.

aphasia Difficulty in the formulation of words; loss of language ability. In extreme cases, a person may be limited to a few words, may babble, or may become mute.

apraxia Loss of ability to perform purposeful movements. For example, a person may be unable to shave, to dress, or to perform other once-familiar and purposeful tasks.

assault An intentional act that is designed to make the victim fearful and that produces reasonable apprehension of harm.

assertiveness Asking for what one wants or acting to get what one wants in a way that respects the rights and feelings of other people.

assertiveness training Instruction in communication skills that help people ask directly in appropriate (nondemanding, nonthreatening, and nondemeaning) ways for what they want.

assimilation The incorporation of new ideas, objects, and experiences into the framework of one's thoughts.

associative looseness A disturbance of thinking in which ideas shift from one subject to another in an oblique or unrelated manner. When this condition is severe, speech may be incoherent.

attention deficit hyperactivity disorder A behavioral disorder usually manifested before the age of 7 years that includes overactivity, chronic inattention, and difficulty dealing with multiple stimuli.

autistic thinking Thoughts, ideas, or desires derived from internal, private stimuli or perceptions that often are incongruent with reality.

automatic obedience The performance of all simple commands in a robotlike fashion; may be present in catatonia.

aversion therapy A behavioral technique that uses negative reinforcement or conditioning to alter or eliminate an unwanted or negative behavior.

avolition Lack of motivation.

axon The part of the neuron that conveys electrical impulses away from the cell body.

B

basal ganglia Pockets of integrating gray matter deep within the cerebrum that are involved in the regulation of movement, emotions, and basic drives.

battering Physical attack, such as hitting, kicking, biting, throwing, and burning.

battery The harmful or offensive touching of another person.

behavior modification A treatment modality that focuses on modifying and changing specific observable dysfunctional patterns of behavior by means of stimulus-and-response conditioning. Examples of behavioral therapy techniques include operant conditioning, token economy, systematic desensitization, aversion therapy, and flooding.

binge-purge cycle An episodic, uncontrolled, rapid ingestion of large quantities of food over a short period of time, followed by purging (vomiting; overexercising; misusing laxatives, diuretics, or other medications); seen in people with bulimia nervosa.

biofeedback A technique for gaining conscious control over unconscious body functions, such as blood pressure and heartbeat, to achieve relaxation or the relief of stress-related physical symptoms; involves the use of self-monitoring equipment.

bipolar disorders Mood disorders that include one or more manic episodes and usually one or more depressive episodes.

bisexuality Sexual attraction toward both males and females, which may be acted on by engaging in both heterosexual and homosexual activities.

blocking A sudden obstruction or interruption in the spontaneous flow of thinking or speaking that is perceived as an absence or deprivation of thought.

blurred or diffuse boundaries A blending together of roles, thoughts, and feelings of individuals so that clear distinctions among family members (or others) fail to emerge.

body image One's internalized sense of the physical self.

borderline personality disorder A disorder characterized by disordered images of self, impulsive and unpredictable behavior, marked shifts in mood, and instability in relationships with others.

boundaries Those functions that maintain a clear distinction among individuals within a family or group and between family members and the outside world. Boundaries may be clear, diffuse, rigid, or inconsistent.

bulimia Episodes of excessive and uncontrollable intake of large amounts of food (binges), usually alternating with compensatory activities such as self-induced vomiting, use of cathartics and/or diuretics, and self-starvation. These alternating behaviors characterize the eating disorder bulimia nervosa.

C

case management Duties of a health care worker (e.g., a nurse) that involve assuming responsibility for a client or group of clients—arranging assessments of need, formulating a comprehensive plan of care, arranging for delivery of services to address individual client needs, and assessing and monitoring the services delivered.

catatonia A state of psychologically induced immobilization at times interrupted by episodes of extreme agitation.

catecholamines A group of biogenic amines that are derived from phenylalanine and contain catechol as the aromatic portion. Certain of these amines, such as epinephrine, norepinephrine, and dopamine, are neurotransmitters and exert an important influence on peripheral and central nervous system activity.

cathexis A psychoanalytical term used to describe the emotional attachment or bond to an idea, an object, or, most commonly, a person.

character The sum of a person's relatively fixed personality traits and habitual modes of response.

chemical restraint A drug given for the specific purpose of inhibiting a certain behavior or movement.

child abuse—battering Physical assault of a child such as hitting, kicking, biting, throwing, and burning.

child abuse—neglect A type of child abuse that can be physical (e.g., failure to provide medical care), developmental (e.g., failure to provide emotional nurturing and cognitive stimulation), educational (failure to provide educational opportunities to the child in accordance with the state's education laws), or a combination of these.

child abuse—physical endangerment Reckless behaviors toward a child that could lead to the child's serious physical injury, such as leaving a young child alone or placing the child in a hazardous environment.

child abuse—sexual Sexual maltreatment of a child, which can take many forms. Essentially it is those acts designed to stimulate the child sexually or to use a child for sexual stimulation, either of the perpetrator or of another person.

chronic anxiety Anxiety that a person has lived with for a long time. Chronic anxiety may take the form of chronic fatigue, insomnia, discomfort in daily activities, or discomfort in personal relationships.

chronic illness An illness that has persisted over a long period of time and that generally involves progressive deterioration, with a resulting increase in functional impairment, symptoms, and disability.

chronic pain Pain that a client has had for longer than 6 months.

circadian rhythm A 24-hour biological rhythm that influences specific regulatory functions such as the sleep-wake cycle, body temperature, and hormonal and neurotransmitter secretions. The 24-hour biological rhythm is controlled by a "pacemaker" in the brain that sends messages to various systems in the body such as those mentioned.

circumstantial speech   A pattern of speech characterized by indirectness and delay before the person gets to the point or answers a question; the person gets caught up in countless details and explanations.

clang association   The meaningless rhyming of words, often in a forceful manner.

clinical (or critical) pathway   A written plan or "map" identifying predetermined times that specific nursing and medical interventions (e.g., diagnostic studies, treatments, activities, medications, teaching, discharge teaching) will be implemented (e.g., day 1 or day 2 for hospital settings, or week 1 or month 2 for community-based settings).

codependent   A term used to describe coping behaviors that prevent individuals from taking care of their own needs and have as their core a preoccupation with the thoughts and feelings of another or others. It usually refers to the dependence of one person on another person who is addicted in one form or another.

cognition   The act, process, or result of knowing, learning, or understanding.

cognitive impairment syndrome/disorder   A disturbance in orientation, memory, intellect, judgment, and affect due to physiological changes in the brain. Delirium and dementia are two examples of cognitive impairment syndromes. An older term is *chronic mental disorder.*

cognitive rehearsal   A technique in which a client imagines each successive step in the sequence leading to the completion of a task, identifying potential "roadblocks" (cognitive, behavioral, or environmental) and planning strategies to deal with them before they produce an unwanted failure experience.

cognitive therapy   A treatment method (particularly useful for depressive disorders) that emphasizes the revision of a person's maladaptive thought processes, perceptions, and attitudes.

community nursing center (CNC)   A nurse-managed center that provides direct access to professional nurses who offer holistic, client-centered health services for reimbursement.

compensation   Making up for deficits in one area by excelling in another area in order to raise or maintain self-esteem.

compulsion   Repetitive, seemingly purposeless behaviors performed according to certain rules known to the client to temporarily reduce escalating anxiety.

concrete thinking   Thinking grounded in immediate experience rather than abstraction. There is an overemphasis on specific detail as opposed to general and abstract concepts.

confabulation   The filling in of a memory gap with a detailed fantasy believed by the teller. The purpose is to maintain self-esteem. It is seen in organic conditions such as Korsakoff's psychosis.

confidentiality   The ethical responsibility of a health care professional that prohibits the disclosure of privileged information without the patient's informed consent.

conscious   Denoting experiences that are within a person's awareness.

consensual validation   The reality checking of thoughts, feelings, and actions with others. If a child grows up in an environment in which the chance to validate thoughts, feelings, and behaviors is decreased, the child's ability to perceive reality is greatly impaired.

conversion   An unconscious defense mechanism in which anxiety is expressed as a physical symptom that has no organic cause.

coping mechanism   A way of adjusting to environmental stress without altering one's goals or purposes. A coping mechanism may be either conscious or unconscious.

cotherapist   A therapist who shares responsibility for therapeutic work, usually work done with groups or with families.

countertransference   The tendency of the nurse (therapist, social worker) to displace onto the client feelings that are a response to people in the nurse's past. Strong positive or strong negative reactions to a client may indicate countertransference.

crisis   A temporary state of disequilibrium (high anxiety) in which a person's usual coping mechanisms or problem-solving methods fail. Crisis can result in personality growth or disorganization.

crisis intervention   A brief, active, and collaborative therapy that draws on an individual's personal coping abilities and resources within the family, health care setting, or community.

culture   The total lifestyle of a given people, the social legacy the individual acquires from his or her group, or the environment that is the creation of humankind.

cunnilingus   Oral sexual contact with the female sex organs.

cyclothymia   A chronic mood disturbance (of a least 2 years' duration) involving both hypomanic and dysthymic mood swings. Delusions are never present, and these mood swings usually do not warrant hospitalization or grossly impair a person's social, occupational, or interpersonal functioning.

D

decode   Interpret the meaning of autistic communications, such as those characterized by looseness of associations.

defense mechanism An unconscious intrapsychic process used to ward off anxiety by preventing conscious awareness of threatening feelings. Defense mechanisms can be used in a healthy or a not-so-healthy manner. Examples are repression, projection, sublimation, denial, and regression.

delayed grief A dysfunctional reaction to grief in which a person may not experience the pain of loss; however, the pain is manifested as chronic depression, intense preoccupation with body functioning (hypochondriasis), phobic reactions, or acute insomnia.

delirium An acute, usually reversible alteration in consciousness typically accompanied by disturbances in thinking, memory, attention, and perception; the syndrome has multiple causes.

delirium tremens (DTs) See *alcohol withdrawal delirium*.

delusion A false belief held to be true even with evidence to the contrary (e.g., the false belief that one is being singled out for harm by others).

dementia A progressive and usually irreversible deterioration of cognitive and intellectual functions and memory without impairment in consciousness.

dendrite The part of the neuron that conveys electrical impulses toward the cell body.

denial Escaping of unpleasant realities by ignoring their existence.

depersonalization A phenomenon whereby a person experiences a sense of unreality of or estrangement from the self. For example, one may feel that one's extremities have changed, that one is seeing oneself from a distance, or that one is in a dream.

depressive mood syndrome Defined by the American Psychiatric Association as a depressed mood or loss of interest that lasts at least 2 weeks and is accompanied by symptoms such as weight loss and difficulty concentrating.

derealization The false perception by a person that his or her environment has changed. For example, everything seems bigger or smaller, or familiar objects appear strange and unfamiliar.

desensitization The reduction of intense reactions to a stimulus (as in a phobia) by repeated exposure to the stimulus in a weaker or milder form.

detachment An interpersonal and intrapersonal dissociation from affective expression. Therefore, the individual appears cold, aloof, and distant. This behavior is thought to be learned and is viewed as defensive.

Diagnostic and Statistical Manual of Mental Disorders, Fourth Edition Text Revision (DSM-IV-TR) A classification of mental disorders that includes descriptions of diagnostic categories. The *DSM-IV-TR* is the most widely accepted system of classifying abnormal behaviors used in the United States today.

diffuse boundaries See *blurred or diffuse boundaries*.

disorientation Confusion and impaired ability to identify time, place, and person.

displacement Transfer of emotions associated with a particular person, object, or situation to another person, object, or situation that is nonthreatening.

dissociation An unconscious defense mechanism that allows blocking of overwhelming anxiety stemming from disintegration of functions of consciousness, memory, identity, or perception of environment.

dissociative disorders Disorders reflecting a disturbance in the normally well-integrated continuum of consciousness, memory, identity, and perception (see Chapter 15).

distractibility Inability to maintain attention; tendency to shift from one area or topic to another with minimal provocation.

double-bind message A communication that contains two contradictory messages given by the same person at the same time, to which the receiver is expected to respond. Constant double-bind situations result in feelings of helplessness, fear, and anxiety in the recipient of such messages.

drug abuse Defined by the American Psychiatric Association as the maladaptive and consistent use of a drug despite the presence of social, occupational, psychological, or physical problems exacerbated by such drug use; or recurrent use in situations that are physically hazardous, such as driving while intoxicated.

drug dependence Impaired control of drug use despite adverse consequences, the development of tolerance to the drug, and the occurrence of withdrawal symptoms when drug intake is reduced or stopped.

drug interaction The reciprocal action between two or more drugs taken simultaneously, which produces an effect different from the usual effects of either drug taken alone. The interacting drugs may be potentiating or inhibitory, and serious side effects may result.

drug tolerance A need for higher and higher dosages of a drug to achieve intoxication or the desired effect.

dual diagnosis The coexistence of a psychiatric disease with substance abuse. A person with a dual diagnosis is chronically dependent on a drug or alcohol and also has another psychiatric disorder such as a depressive or personality disorder.

dyskinesia Involuntary muscular activity, such as tic, spasm, or myoclonus.

dyspareunia Persistent genital pain in either a male or a female before, during, or after sex.

dysthymia A mild to moderate mood disturbance characterized by a chronic depressive syndrome that is usually present for many years. The depressive mood disturbance is hard to distinguish from the person's usual pattern of functioning, and the person has minimal social or occupational impairment.

dystonia Abnormal muscle tonicity resulting in impaired voluntary movement. May occur as an acute side effect of neuroleptic (antipsychotic) medication, in which it manifests as muscle spasms of the face, head, neck, and back.

E

echolalia Mimicry or imitation of the speech of another person.

echopraxia Mimicry or imitation of the movements of another person.

ego One of three psychological processes that make up the Freudian system of personality (id, ego, superego). The ego is one's sense of self and provides such functions as problem solving, mobilization of defense mechanisms, reality testing, and the capability of functioning independently. The ego is said to be the mediator between one's primitive drives (the id) and internalized parental and social prohibitions (the superego).

ego boundaries The individual's perception of the boundaries between himself or herself and the external environment.

ego-alien/ego-dystonic Synonymous terms used to describe symptoms that are unacceptable to the person who has them and are not compatible with the person's view of himself or herself (e.g., fear of cats).

ego-syntonic A term used to describe symptomatic behaviors or beliefs that do not seem to bother the person or that seem right to the person. For example, a very paranoid person who wrongly believes that the government is out to get him or her truly believes this thought, and it is consistent with the way this person experiences life.

egocentric Self-centered.

electroconvulsive therapy (ECT) An effective treatment for depression in which a grand mal seizure is induced by passing an electrical current through electrodes that are applied to the temples. The administration of a muscle relaxant minimizes seizure activity and prevents damage to long bones and cervical vertebrae.

elopement Escape.

emotional abuse Essentially, depriving an individual of a nurturing atmosphere in which he or she can thrive, learn, and develop. Emotional abuse takes many forms (e.g., terrorizing, demeaning, consistently belittling, withholding warmth).

empathy The ability of one person to get inside another's world and see things from the other person's perspective and to communicate this understanding to the other person.

enabling Helping a chemically dependent individual avoid experiencing the consequences of his or her drinking or drug use. It is one behavioral component of a codependency role.

endorphins Naturally produced chemicals (peptides) with morphinelike action. They are usually found in the brain and are associated with reduction of pain and feelings of well-being.

enmeshed boundaries See *blurred or diffuse boundaries*.

enuresis Nocturnal and/or daytime involuntary discharge of urine.

epinephrine (adrenaline) A catecholamine secreted by the adrenal gland and by fibers of the sympathetic nervous system. It is responsible for many of the physical manifestations of fear and anxiety.

ethics The discipline concerned with standards of values, behaviors, or beliefs adhered to by individuals or groups.

eustress A positive type of stress that reflects a person's confidence in the ability to successfully master given demands or tasks.

euthymia A normal mood state.

extrapyramidal side effects A variety of signs and symptoms that are often side effects of the use of certain psychotropic drugs, particularly the phenothiazines. Three reversible extrapyramidal side effects are acute dystonia, akathisia, and pseudoparkinsonism. A fourth, tardive dyskinesia, is the most serious and is not reversible.

F

family system Those individuals who make up the family unit and contribute to the functional state of the family as a unit.

family therapy A treatment modality that focuses on the relationships within the family system.

family triangle A dysfunctional phenomenon in which a third person is brought into a two-person relationship to help relieve anxiety or stress between two family members. Triangles are dysfunctional because the lowering of anxiety comes from diversion from the conflict rather than from resolution of the conflict between the two members.

fantasy Mental imagery that is unrestrained by reality and represents an attempt to solve problems in a private world. One difference between a healthy person and a schizophrenic, for example, is that a schizophrenic may not know where fantasy ends and reality begins.

fear A reaction to a specific danger.

feedback Communication of one person's impressions of and reactions to another person's actions or verbalizations.

fellatio Oral sexual contact with the penis.

fetish An object or part of the body to which sexual significance or meaning is attached.

fight-or-flight response (sympathetic response) The body's physiological response to fear or rage that triggers the sympathetic branch of the autonomic nervous system as well as the endocrine system. This response is useful in emergencies; however, a sustained response can result in pathophysiological changes such as high blood pressure, ulcers, and cardiac problems.

flight of ideas   A continuous flow of speech in which the person jumps rapidly from one topic to another. Sometimes the listener can keep up with the changes; at other times, it is necessary to listen for themes in the incessant talking. Themes often include grandiose and fantasized evaluation of personal sexual prowess, business ability, artistic talents, and so forth.

formication   A tactile hallucination or illusion involving the sensation of insects crawling on the body or under the skin.

frustration   The curtailment of personal goals, satisfaction, or security by conditions of external reality or by internal controls.

fugue   An altered state of consciousness involving both memory loss (as in psychogenic amnesia) and travel away from home or from one's usual work locale; that is, fugue involves flight as well as forgetfulness. Often called *psychogenic* or *dissociative fugue*.

G

general adaptation syndrome (GAS)   The body's organized response to stress, as elucidated by Hans Selye. It progresses through three stages: (1) the stage of alarm, (2) the stage of resistance, and (3) the stage of exhaustion.

genogram   A systematic diagram of the three-generational relationships within a family system.

grandiosity   Exaggerated belief in or claims about one's importance or identity.

grief   The subjective feelings and affect that are precipitated by a loss.

group   Two or more individuals who have a relationship with one another, are interdependent, and may share some norms.

group dynamics   The interactions and interrelations among members of a therapy group and between members and the therapist. The effective use of group dynamics is essential in group treatment.

group process   The interaction continually taking place among members of a group.

group therapy   Psychotherapy based on the examination of group interaction with a view toward understanding and eventually changing the ways in which clients interact with others.

H

hallucination   A sense perception (seeing, hearing, tasting, smelling, or touching) for which no external stimulus exists (e.g., hearing voices when none are present).

health maintenance organization (HMO)   An organization that contracts with a group or individuals to offer designated health care services to plan members for a fixed, prepaid premium (an example of a managed care program).

histrionics   A dramatic presentation of oneself with pervasive and excessive emotionality in order to seek attention, love, and admiration.

homelessness—chronic   Long-term lack of a home or permanent residence. It represents the final stage in a lifelong series of crises and missed opportunities and is the culmination of a gradual disengagement from supportive relationships and institutions.

homosexuality   Sexual attraction to or preference for persons of the same sex.

hopelessness   The belief of a person that no one can help him or her; extreme pessimism about the future.

hospice philosophy   A philosophy characterized by the acceptance of death as a natural conclusion to life and the belief that clients rather than health care providers should make the end-of-life decisions regarding how they want to live and die.

hostility   Anger that is destructive in nature and purpose.

hotline   A telephone crisis counseling service often used in crisis intervention centers to provide immediate contact between a person in crisis and a counselor.

hypermetamorphosis   The desire to touch everything in sight.

hyperorality   The desire to taste everything, chew everything, and put everything into one's mouth.

hypersomnia   The spending of increased time in sleep, possibly to escape from painful feelings; however, the increased sleep is not experienced as restful or refreshing.

hypochondriasis   Excessive preoccupation with one's physical health in the absence of any organic pathology.

hypomania   An elevated mood with symptoms less severe than those of mania. A person in hypomania does not experience impairment in reality testing, nor do the symptoms markedly impair the person's social, occupational, or interpersonal functions.

hysterical personality disorder   A disorder characterized by dramatic, emotionally intense, unstable behavior.

I

id   One of three psychological processes that make up the Freudian system of personality (id, ego, and superego). The id is the source of all primitive drives and instincts and is considered to be the reservoir of all psychic energy.

idea of reference   The false impression that outside events have special meaning for oneself.

identification Unconscious assumption of the thoughts, mannerisms, or behaviors of a person or group in order to decrease anxiety.

identity The sense of one's self based on experience, memories, perceptions, and emotions.

illusion An error in the perception of a sensory stimulus. For example, a person may mistake polka dots on a pillow for hairy spiders.

impotence The inability to achieve or maintain a penile erection of sufficient quality to engage in successful sexual intercourse.

impulsiveness The tendency to engage in actions that are abrupt, unplanned, and directed toward immediate gratification.

incest A sexual relationship between persons who are close biological relatives.

insight Understanding and awareness of the reasons for and meaning behind one's motives and behavior.

insomnia Inability to fall asleep or to stay asleep, early morning awakening, or both.

intellectualization The excessive use of reasoning, logic, or words to avoid confronting undesirable impulses, emotions, and interpersonal situations.

intimacy Emotional closeness.

intoxication Maladaptive behavioral or psychological changes caused by excessive use of a drug or alcohol.

intrapsychic Within the self.

introjection The process by which a person incorporates or takes into his or her own personality qualities or values of another person or group with whom intense emotional ties exist.

intuition Knowledge or insight gained without conscious rational thinking.

isolation The separation of thought, ideas, or actions from their emotional aspects.

J

judgment The ability to make logical, rational decisions.

L

la belle indifférence An affect or attitude of unconcern about a symptom that is seen when the symptom is unconsciously used to lower anxiety. The lack of concern is thought to be a sign that the primary goal has been achieved.

labile Characterized by rapid shifts; unstable.

lesbian A female homosexual.

libido Sexual drive.

limbic system The part of the brain that is related to emotions and is referred to by some as the "emotional brain." It is involved in the mediation of fear and anxiety; anger and aggression; love, joy, and hope; and sexuality and social behavior.

limit setting The reasonable and rational setting of parameters for client behavior that provide control and safety.

lithium carbonate Known as an antimanic drug because it can stabilize the manic phase of a bipolar disorder. When effective, it can modify future manic episodes and protect against future depressive episodes.

living will An expression by a person, while competent, of his or her preference that life-sustaining treatment be continued, withheld, or withdrawn if he or she becomes terminally ill and is no longer able to make health care decisions.

looseness of association A pattern of thinking that is haphazard, illogical, and confused, and in which connections in thought are interrupted; it is seen primarily in schizophrenic disorders.

M

magical thinking The belief that thinking something can make it happen; it is seen in children and psychotic clients.

malingering A conscious effort to deceive others, often for financial gain, by pretending to have physical symptoms.

managed care A term referring to an organized system that integrates cost management and provision of health care. Health maintenance organizations (HMOs), preferred provider organizations (PPOs), and managed care options offered by government and private indemnity health insurance plans are the basic types of managed care organization.

mania An unstable elevated mood in which delusion, poor judgment, and other signs of impaired reality testing are evident. During a manic episode, clients have marked impairment of social, occupational, and interpersonal functioning.

manipulation Purposeful behavior directed at getting one's needs met, sometimes without regard for the needs, goals, and feelings of others.

masochism The deriving of unconscious or conscious gratification from the experience of mental or physical pain; often used to refer to deviant sexual behaviors.

maturational crisis A normal state in growth and development in which a specific maturational task must be learned but old coping mechanisms are no longer adequate or acceptable.

mental status examination A formal assessment of cognitive functions such as intelligence, thought processes, and capacity for insight.

milieu The physical and social environment of an individual.

milieu therapy Therapy that focuses on manipulation of the environment (both physical and social) to effect positive change.

mnemonic disturbance Loss of memory.

modeling A technique in which desired behaviors are demonstrated. The client learns to imitate these behaviors in appropriate situations.

mood   Defined by the American Psychiatric Association as a pervasive and sustained emotion that, when extreme, can markedly color the way the individual perceives the world.

mood syndrome   An alteration in mood with associated symptoms that occurs for a minimal period.

mourning   The process by which grief is resolved.

multiple personality disorder   A severe dissociative disorder in which one or more distinct subpersonalities exist within an individual, each of which may be dominant at different times. Each subpersonality is a complex unit with its own memories, behavioral patterns, and social relationships, which may be very different from those of the primary personality.

N

narcissism (narcism)   Self-involvement with lack of empathy for others; the narcissistic person is very self-centered and self-important; narcissism is normal in children but pathological when it occurs in adults to the same degree.

narcissistic personality disorder   A disorder characterized by a pervasive pattern of grandiosity, need for admiration, and lack of empathy for others.

National Alliance for the Mentally Ill   A national support group for families of the mental ill with many local and state affiliates; provides educational programs and political action.

negativism   Opposition or resistance, either covert or overt, to outside suggestions or advice.

negligence   An act, or failure to act, that breaches the duty of due care and results in or is responsible for another person's injuries.

neologism   A word a person makes up that has meaning only for that person; often part of a delusional system.

neuroleptic malignant syndrome   A rare and sometimes fatal reaction to high-potency neuroleptic drugs. Symptoms include muscle rigidity, fever, and elevated white blood cell count. It is thought to result from dopamine blockage at the basal ganglia and hypothalamus.

neuron   A specialized cell in the central nervous system. Each neuron has a cell body, an axon, and dendrites.

neurotransmitter   A chemical substance that functions as a neural messenger. Neurotransmitters are released from the axon terminal of the presynaptic neuron when stimulated by an electrical impulse.

nihilism   A delusion that the self or part of the self does not exist.

no-suicide contract   A contract made between a nurse or counselor and a client, outlined in clear and simple language, in which the client states that her or she will not attempt self-harm and in which specific alternatives are given for the person instead.

nonverbal communication   Communication without words, such as body language, facial expressions, or gestures.

nursing   The diagnosis and treatment of human responses to actual or potential health problems.

O

obesity   A condition characterized by a body weight that is at least 20% higher than the acceptable standard or ideal weight.

obsession   An idea, impulse, or emotion that a person cannot put out of his or her consciousness; the condition can be mild or severe.

organic mental disorder   As defined by the American Psychiatric Association, a specific brain syndrome for which a cause is known; for example, alcohol withdrawal delirium or Alzheimer's disease.

orientation   The ability to relate the self correctly to time, place, and person.

overt anxiety   Anxiety in which the attendant physical, physiological, and cognitive symptoms are evident and may be assessed.

P

panic   Sudden, overwhelming anxiety of such intensity that it produces disorganization of the personality, loss of rational thought, and inability to communicate, along with specific physiological changes.

paranoia   A state characterized by the presence of intense and strongly defended irrational suspicions. These ideas cannot be corrected by experience and cannot be modified by facts or reality.

passive-aggressive behavior   Behavior that represents an indirect expression of anger or aggressive feelings. Behavior may seem passive but is motivated by unconscious anger and often triggers anger and frustration in others. Examples of passive-aggressive behavior are being late, forgetting, making "mistakes," and acting obtuse.

peer review   Review of clinical practice with peers, supervisors, or consultants.

perception   The mental process by which intellectual, sensory, and emotional data are organized logically or meaningfully.

perseveration   The involuntary repetition of the same thought, phrase, or motor response (e.g., brushing teeth, walking); it is associated with brain damage.

personality   Deeply ingrained personal patterns of behavior, traits, and thoughts that evolve, both consciously and unconsciously, as a person's style and way of adapting to the environment.

phobia   An intense irrational fear of an object, situation, or place. The fear persists even though the object of the fear is harmless and the person is aware of the irrationality.

physical restraint Any manual method or mechanical device, material, or equipment that inhibits free movement.

play therapy An intervention that allows a child to symbolically express feelings such as aggression, self-doubt, anxiety, and sadness through the medium of play.

pleasure principle A tendency to seek immediate gratification of impulses and tension reduction; the id operates according to the pleasure principle.

polydrug abuse The pathological use of more than one drug.

polypharmacy The taking of more than one drug at any given time.

postvention Therapeutic interventions with the significant others of an individual who has committed suicide.

poverty of speech A speech pattern characterized by brevity and uncommunicativeness.

pressure of speech A speech pattern characterized by forceful energy manifested in frantic, jumbled speech as when a manic individual struggles to keep pace with racing thoughts.

primary anxiety Anxiety that is due to intrapersonal or intrapsychic causes, such as a phobia.

primary depression Defined by the American Psychiatric Association as a depressive mood episode that is not due to known organic factors and is not part of another psychotic disorder, such as schizophrenia.

primary gain The anxiety relief resulting from the use of defense mechanisms or symptom formation such as somatization (e.g., getting a headache instead of feeling angry).

primary process In psychoanalytic theory, a primitive and unconscious psychological activity in which the id attempts to reduce tension by forming an image of or hallucinating the object that would satisfy its need.

projection The unconscious attributing of one's own intolerable wishes, emotions, or motivations to another person.

projective identification A primitive form of projection used to externalize aggressive feelings. Once projection has occurred, fear of the person who is the object of the projection is coupled with a desire to control the person.

prolonged grief A dysfunctional grief reaction in which the bereaved remains intensely preoccupied with memories of the deceased many years after the person has died.

psychiatric liaison nurse A nurse with a master's degree and a background in psychiatric and medical-surgical nursing. The liaison nurse functions as a nursing consultant in addressing psychosocial concerns and as a clinician in helping the client deal more effectively with physical and emotional problems.

psychiatry The science of treating disorders of the psyche. It is the medical specialty involved in the study, diagnosis, treatment, and prevention of mental disorders.

psychoeducational therapy A strategy of teaching clients and their families about disorders, treatments, coping techniques, and resources. It helps empower clients and families by having them become more involved and prepares them to participate in their own care once they have the requisite knowledge.

psychogenic Denoting a physical condition caused by psychological factors.

psychogenic amnesia The loss of memory for an event or period of time that is associated with overwhelming anxiety and pain. The loss of memory is related to psychological stress.

psychomotor agitation Constant involvement in some tension-relieving activity, such as constantly pacing, biting one's nails, smoking, or tapping one's fingers on a tabletop.

psychomotor retardation Extreme slowness of and difficulty in movements that in the extreme can entail complete inactivity and incontinence.

psychosexual development Emotional and sexual growth from birth to adulthood.

psychosis An extreme response to psychological or physical stressors that leads to pronounced distortion or disorganization of affective response, psychomotor function, and behavior. Reality testing is impaired, as evidenced by hallucinations or delusions.

psychosocial rehabilitation The development of the skills necessary for a person with chronic mental illness to live independently.

psychosomatic An older term describing the interaction of the mind (psyche) and the body (soma). The term was used in reference to certain disease thought to be caused by psychological factors. Referred to in the first edition of the *Diagnostic and Statistical Manual of Mental Disorders*.

psychotherapy A treatment modality based on the development of a trusting relationship between the client and therapist for the purpose of exploring and modifying the client's behavior in a positive direction.

psychotropic Affecting the mind.

psychotropic drugs Drugs that have an effect on psychic function, behavior, or experience.

R

racism A belief that inherent differences between races determine people's achievement and that one's own race is superior.

rape   See *sexual assault/rape.*

rape-trauma syndrome   A syndrome characterized by an acute phase and a long-term reorganization process that occurs after an actual or attempted sexual assault. Each phase has separate symptoms.

rationalization   Justification of illogical or unreasonable ideas, actions, or feelings by the development of acceptable explanations that satisfy the teller as well as the listener.

reaction-formation (overcompensation)   The process of keeping unacceptable feelings or behaviors out of awareness by developing the opposite emotion or behavior.

reality principle   The ability to delay immediate gratification and modify desires in accordance with the demands of society and external reality. The ego operates according to the reality principle.

receptor   A protein molecule located within or on the outer membrane of cells of various tissues, such as neurons, muscle, and blood vessels. A receptor receives chemical stimulation that causes a chemical reaction resulting in either stimulation or inhibition of the activity of the cell.

reframing   A technique of changing the viewpoint of a situation and replacing it with another viewpoint that fits the facts equally well but alters the entire meaning.

regression   In the face of overwhelming anxiety, the return to an earlier, more comforting (although less mature) way of behaving.

relapse   A recurrence of the manifestations of a disease after a period of improvement; in a substance use disorder, the process of becoming dysfunctional in sobriety that ends in a return to chemical use.

relaxation response   A set of physiological changes that result in decreased activity of the sympathetic part of the autonomic nervous system and a shift to the parasympathetic mode, which induces a state of relaxation. It is the opposite of the fight-or-flight response and has a stabilizing effect on the nervous system.

repression   The exclusion of unpleasant or unwanted experiences, emotions, or ideas from conscious awareness; considered the first line of psychological defense.

respite care   Temporary supervision and care of a client who lives with his or her family. The purpose of respite care is to provide the family with some relief from the demands of the client's need for continuous care.

restraint   See *physical restraint* and *chemical restraint.*

reuptake   The return of neurotransmitters to the presynaptic cell after communication with receptors on the postsynaptic cell.

rigid or disengaged boundaries   Adherence to the "rules and roles" within a family no matter what the situation. Rigid boundaries prevent family members from trying out new roles or taking on more mature functions.

ritual   A repetitive action that a person must execute over and over until he or she is exhausted or anxiety is decreased; it is often performed to lessen the anxiety triggered by an obsession.

role playing   A technique used in individual, group, or family therapy in which the therapist or a group member acts out the behavior of another member to increase that individual's ability to see a situation from another point of view. It is also a useful tool that therapists, teachers, and others employ to help people practice skills in a safe environment before they try them in real-life situations, such as practicing asking for a raise, discussing a crucial topic with a person in authority, or saying no to someone without becoming defensive or angry.

S

sadism   The deriving of sexual pleasure and erotic gratification from the infliction of pain, abuse, or humiliation on another.

scapegoat   A member of a group or family who becomes the target of others' aggression but who may not be the actual cause of their hostility or frustration.

schizoaffective disorder   A disorder that includes a mixture of schizophrenic and affective symptoms (i.e., alterations in mood as well as disturbances in thought); it is considered by some to be a severe form of bipolar disorder.

schizoid personality disorder   A personality disorder in which there is a serious defect in interpersonal relationships. Characteristics include lack of warmth, aloofness, and indifference to the feelings of others.

schizophrenia   A group of mental disorders characterized by severe disturbance of thought and associative looseness, impaired reality testing (hallucinations, delusions), and limited socialization.

seasonal affective disorder (SAD)   A recently studied syndrome that appears to affect mostly women and is characterized by hypersomnia, fatigue, weight gain, irritability, and interpersonal difficulties during the winter months. It has been successfully managed with daily treatments of 2 to 3 hours of bright light.

seclusion   The last step in a process to maximize the safety of a client and others in which the client is placed alone in a specially design room for protection and close observation.

secondary anxiety   Anxiety that is due to physiological abnormalities such as certain medical disorders (e.g., neurological, endocrine, or circulatory) or is secondary to a pervasive psychiatric disorder such as depression.

secondary dementia   Dementia that is due to an underlying disease process, such as a metabolic, nutritional, or neurological disorder. Dementia related to acquired immunodeficiency syndrome is an example.

secondary depression A depressive mood syndrome that is caused by a physical illness or another psychiatric disorder or is part of an organic mental disorder; essentially, it is depression secondary to other causes.

secondary gain Those advantages a person realizes from whatever symptoms or relief behaviors he or she employs. These advantages include increased attention from others, avoidance of expected responsibilities, financial gain, and the ability to manipulate others in the environment.

secondary process In psychoanalytic theory, a process consistent with the reality principle; that is, realistic thinking.

selective inattention The failure to notice or attend to an almost infinite number of more-or-less meaningful details of one's own living that might cause anxiety. A concept articulated by H. S. Sullivan.

selective serotonin reuptake inhibitors (SSRIs) First-line antidepressants that block the reuptake of serotonin, permitting serotonin to act for an extended period at the synaptic binding sites in the brain.

self-concept A person's image of the self.

self-esteem The individual's feeling that he or she has worth or value.

self-help group A group of people with similar problems or concerns who meet to receive peer support and encouragement and work together using their strengths to gain control over their lives.

self-mutilation The act of self-induced pain or injury without the intent to kill oneself.

sexual assault/rape Forced and violent vaginal, anal, or oral penetration against the victim's will and without the victim's consent. Legal definitions vary from state to state.

situational crisis A crisis arising from an external as opposed to an internal source. Most people experience situational crises to some extent during the course of their lives (e.g., the death of a loved one, marriage, divorce, or a change in health status).

social phobia A phobia of an interpersonal nature, such as fear of public speaking, fear of eating in front of others, or fear of writing or performing in public.

social skills training Training that uses the principles of guidance, demonstration, practice, and feedback to enhance a client's skills in community living. Training focuses on skills such as introducing oneself, starting and ending a conversation, asking for assistance, and other simple yet essential social interactions; it is often helpful in combating the negative symptoms of schizophrenia.

somatic therapy Treatment that involves the body, such as the use of medications or electroconvulsive therapy.

somatization The expression of psychological stress through physical symptoms.

specific phobia Fear and avoidance of a single object, situation, or activity. Specific phobias are very common in the general population.

spirituality The devotion or receptiveness to religious or moral values. Spirituality includes a search for meaning and purpose; a relationship with a higher being; and adherence to transcendent values such as hope, love, forgiveness. It is frequently experienced through a formal faith tradition.

splitting A primitive defense mechanism in which the person sees self or others as all good or all bad, failing to integrate the positive and negative qualities of the self and others into a cohesive whole.

spouse abuse The intentional physical or emotional injury of one's spouse.

stereotype The assumption that all people in a similar cultural, racial, or ethnic group think and act alike.

stereotyped behavior A motor pattern that originally had meaning to the person (e.g., sweeping the floor or washing windows) but has become mechanical and lacks purpose.

stress The body's arousal response to any demand, change, or perceived threat.

stupor A state in which a person is dazed and awareness of his or her environment appears deadened. For example, a person may sit motionless for long periods of time and in extreme cases may appear to be in a coma.

subconscious Experiences, thoughts, feelings, and desires that are not in immediate awareness but can be recalled to consciousness; often called the preconscious. The subconscious mind helps repress unpleasant thoughts or feelings.

sublimation The unconscious process of substituting constructive and socially acceptable activities for strong impulses that are not acceptable in their original form, such as strong aggressive or sexual drives.

suicidal ideation Thoughts a person has regarding killing himself or herself.

suicide The ultimate act of self-destruction in which a person purposefully ends his or her own life.

suicide attempt Any willful, self-inflicted, life-threatening attempt at suicide that did not lead to death.

suicide gesture A suicide attempt that is planned to be discovered and is made for the purpose of influencing or manipulating others.

sundown syndrome Increasing destabilization of cognitive abilities (e.g., confusion) and lability of mood during the late afternoon, early evening, or night. Seen in people with cognitive disorders.

superego One of three psychological processes that make up the Freudian system of personality (id, ego, and superego). The superego is the internal representative of the values, ideals, and moral standards of society. The superego is said to be the moral arm of the personality.

support group   A group that uses a variety of modalities to help people cope with overwhelming situations or alter unwanted behaviors during stressful periods.

suppression   The conscious removal from awareness of disturbing situations or feelings; the only defense mechanism that operates on a conscious level.

symbolization   The process by which one object or idea comes to represent another. For example, the nurse's keys on a locked unit may represent power and autonomy, or a fancy house may represent prestige and power.

synapse   The gap between the membrane of one neuron and the membrane of another neuron. The synapse is the point at which the transmission of the nerve impulse occurs.

synesthesia   A condition in which the stimulation of one sense also gives rise to a subjective sensation in another sense, such as hearing colors or seeing sounds; the phenomenon may be experienced by people taking hallucinogenic drugs.

T

tangentiality   A disturbance in associative thinking in which the speaker goes off the topic. When it happens frequently and the speaker does not return to the topic, interpersonal communication is destroyed.

Tarasoff **decision**   A California court decision that imposes a duty on the therapist to warn the appropriate person or persons when the therapist becomes aware that a client presents a risk of harm to a specific person or persons.

tardive dyskinesia   A serious and irreversible side effect of the phenothiazines and related drugs that consists of involuntary tonic muscle spasms typically involving the tongue, fingers, toes, neck, trunk, or pelvis.

therapeutic encounter   A brief, informal meeting between nurse and client in which the relationship is useful and important for the client.

therapeutic nurse-client relationship   A therapeutic relationship requiring that the nurse maximize his or her communication skills, understanding of human behaviors, and personal strengths in order to enhance personal growth in the client. This relationship occurs in all clinical settings, not just those on a psychiatric unit.

time-out   The removal or disengagement of an individual (especially a child) from a situation so that the person can regain self-control.

token economy   A behavioral approach to eliciting desired behaviors that involves application of the principles and procedures of operant conditioning;

it is generally used in the management of a social setting such as a ward, classroom, or halfway house. Targeted behaviors are awarded tokens that can be exchanged for desired goods or privileges.

tort   A civil wrong for which money damages (or other relief) may be obtained by the injured party (plaintiff) from the wrongdoer (defendant).

transference   The experiencing of thoughts and feelings toward a person (often the therapist) that were originally held toward a significant person in one's past. Transference is a valuable tool used by therapists in psychoanalytical psychotherapy.

transsexual   A person who has an early and persistent feeling that he or she is trapped in a body with the wrong genitals. The individual believes that he or she is, and was always meant to be, of the opposite sex.

triangle   See *family triangle.*

U

unconscious   The repressed memories, feelings, thoughts, or wishes that are not available to the conscious mind. Usually, these unconscious memories, feelings, thoughts, or wishes are associated with intense anxiety and can greatly affect an individual's behavior.

undoing   An act or behavior unconsciously designed to make up for or negate a previous act or behavior (e.g., bringing the boss a present after talking about the boss unfavorably to co-workers).

V

validate   See *consensual validation.*

values clarification   A process of self-discovery in which a person explores and determines his or her personal values and identifies what priority these values hold in personal decision making. This process can lead to increased awareness of why the person behaves in certain ways.

vegetative signs of depression   Significant changes from normal functioning in those activities necessary to support physical life and growth, such as eating, sleeping, elimination, and sex, during a depressive episode.

W

waxy flexibility   Excessive maintenance of posture; for example, after the arms or legs are placed in a certain position, the individual holds that same position for hours.

withdrawal symptoms   The negative physiological and psychological reactions that occur when a drug taken for a long period of time is reduced in dosage or no longer taken.

word salad   A mixture of words meaningless to the listener and to the speaker as well.

Index

Page numbers followed by *f* indicate figures; *t*, tables; *b*, boxes.

"Standards of Care" pertain to professional nursing activities that are demonstrated by the nurse through the nursing process. These involve assessment, diagnosis, outcome identification, planning, implementation, and evaluation. The nursing process is the foundation of clinical decision making and encompasses all significant action taken by nurses in providing developmentally and culturally relevant psychiatric–mental health care to all patients.

Standard I. Assessment

The psychiatric–mental health nurse collects patient health data.

RATIONALE

The assessment interview, which requires linguistically and culturally effective communication skills, interviewing, behavioral observation, record review, and comprehensive assessment of the patient and relevant systems, enables the psychiatric–mental health nurse to make sound clinical judgments and plan appropriate interventions with the patient.

Standard II. Diagnosis

The psychiatric–mental health nurse analyses the assessment data in determining diagnoses.

RATIONALE

The basis for providing psychiatric–mental health nursing care is the recognition and identification of patterns of response to actual or potential psychiatric illnesses, mental health problems, and potential comorbid physical illnesses.

Standard III. Outcome Identification

The psychiatric–mental health nurse identifies expected outcomes individualized to the patient.

RATIONALE

Within the context of providing nursing care, the ultimate goal is to influence mental health outcomes and improve the patient's health status.

Standard IV. Planning

The psychiatric–mental health nurse develops a plan of care that is negotiated among the patient, nurse, family, and health care team and prescribes evidence-based interventions to attain expected outcomes.

RATIONALE

A plan of care is used to guide therapeutic interventions systematically, document progress, and achieve the expected patient outcomes.

Standard V. Implementation

The psychiatric–mental health nurse implements the interventions identified in the plan of care.

RATIONALE

In implementing the plan of care, psychiatric–mental health nurse use a wide range of interventions designed to prevent mental and physical illness, and promote, maintain, and restore mental and physical health. Psychiatric–mental health nurses select interventions according to their level of practice. At the basic level, nurses may select counseling milieu therapy, promotion of self-care activities, intake screening and evaluation, psychobiological interventions, health teaching, case management, health promotion and health maintenance, crisis intervention, community-based care, psychiatric home health care, telehealth, and a variety of other approaches to meet the mental health needs of patients. In addition to the intervention options available to the basic-level psychiatric–mental health nursing, at the advanced level the APRN-PMH may provide consultation, engage in psychotherapy, and prescribe pharmacological agents in accordance with state statutes or regulations.

Standard Va. Counseling
Standard Vb. Milieu Therapy
Standard Vc. Promotion of Self-Care Activities
Standard Vd. Psychobiological Interventions
Standard Ve. Health Teaching
Standard Vf. Case Management
Standard Vg. Health Promotion and Health Maintenance

The following interventions (Vh-Vj) may be performed only by the APRN-PMH.

Standard Vh. Psychotherapy
Standard Vi. Prescriptive Authority and Treatment
Standard Vj. Consultation

Standard VI. Evaluation

The psychiatric–mental health nurse evaluates the patient's progress in attaining expected outcomes.

RATIONALE

Nursing care is a dynamic process involving change in the patient's health status over time, giving rise to the need for data, different diagnoses, and modifications in the plan of care. Therefore, evaluation is a continuous process of appraising the effect of nursing and the treatment regimen on the patient's health status and expected outcomes.

Key to Special Features